HYPERTENSIVE CARDIOVASCULAR DISEASE: PATHOPHYSIOLOGY AND TREATMENT

DEVELOPMENTS IN CARDIOVASCULAR MEDICINE

VOLUME 16

Series ISBN 90-247-2336-1

HYPERTENSIVE CARDIOVASCULAR DISEASE: PATHOPHYSIOLOGY AND TREATMENT

edited by

A. AMERY, R. FAGARD, P. LIJNEN
and J. STAESSEN

Hypertension and Cardiovascular Rehabilitation Unit
Department of Pathophysiology
University of Leuven
Leuven, Belgium

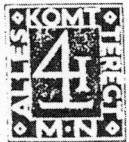

1982

MARTINUS NIJHOFF PUBLISHERS
THE HAGUE / BOSTON / LONDON

Distributors:

for the United States and Canada

Kluwer Boston, Inc.
190 Old Derby Street
Hingham, MA 02043
USA

for all other countries

Kluwer Academic Publishers Group
Distribution Center
P.O. Box 322
3300 AH Dordrecht
The Netherlands

Library of Congress Cataloging in Publication Data   CIP

Main entry under title:

Hypertensive cardiovascular disease.

  (Developments in cardiovascular medicine; v. 16)
  Includes index.
  1. Hypertension. 2. Hypertension—Chemotherapy.
I. Amery, Antoon K.P.C. II. Series. [DNLM: 1. Hypertension. W1 DE997VME
v. 16/WG 340 H99685] RC685.H8H9447   616.1'32   81-18955
                AACR2

ISBN-13: 978-94-009-7478-4   e-ISBN-13: 978-94-009-7476-0
DOI: 10.1007/978-94-009-7476-0

CONTENTS

VII. ANTIHYPERTENSIVE THERAPY

FOREWORD

Hypertension is a major world-wide health problem. With high blood pressure there is a greater risk of stroke, heart attack, heart failure, kidney disease and renal failure. Far too few people realize what the risks are and what can be done to prevent these risks even in the countries where programs in hypertension research are active and the full significance of hypertension is best understood. Some studies of the known hypertensive population indicate that one-half or less are receiving adequate treatment, and, of those on therapy, only half have their high blood pressure satisfactorily controlled. These realizations emphasize the need to inform all segments of society throughout the world on the importance of detection and control of high blood pressure. The great incidence of hypertension makes it of paramount importance that all practicing physicians have available the latest information on diagnosis and treatment of hypertensive cardiovascular disease.

This treatise on hypertension arrives at a time when there is an increasing recognition the world over of the importance of detecting and treating high blood pressure. The book has been edited by Dr. A. Amery and his associates in the University of Leuven. Professor Amery is one of the leaders in the field of hypertension and serves on the Council of the International Society of Hypertension. The many chapters and contributions of this volume were written by more than a hundred of the most outstanding physicians and investigators in the field of hypertension research from nineteen countries scattered around the globe.

The scope of this book is broad and its objectives are to provide a comprehensive coverage including the latest advances on the pathogenesis, diagnosis and treatment of the various types of hypertensive disease. It begins with a description of the mechanisms involved in the control of arterial pressure under normal conditions and includes such factors as the central nervous system, the kidneys, the arterial baroreflexes, and the hormonal mechanisms. A brief section describes experimental models and their contribution to the pathogenesis of hypertension. Fifteen chapters are devoted to the pathogenesis of primary hypertension which comprises about 90 percent of patients with hypertensive cardiovascular disease. In these chapters the material presented ranges from such basic concepts as ion transport in vascular smooth muscle, cell receptors and genes to organ physiology in the kidney and heart and to cardiovascular hemodynamics. Nine types of secondary hypertension are described in terms of the pathogenic mechanisms involved.

The serious complications of high blood pressure and its impact on the major target organs (heart, kidney, brain and ocular fundus) are considered in part IV under 'Repercussions of high blood pressure'. This section very appropriately includes an excellent discussion on malignant hypertension.

The last chapters are addressed more directly to the practicing physician and this part of the book is concerned with the clinical, laboratory and radiological examination of the patient. Antihypertensive therapy is covered extensively by considering the many specific types of treatment now available and the general strategy in antihypertensive therapy. Emphasis is placed on the importance of early and continuous treatment which is imperative to prevent the complications (discussed in part IV) which can be fatal. The benefits from treatment, the quality of life in the hypertensive patient, and the problem of compliance are other important topics covered.

James O. Davis, M.D.
Professor and Chairman of Physiology
University of Missouri School of Medicine
Columbia, Mo., U.S.A.

Former President of the
International Society of Hypertension

PREFACE

Hypertension is one of the major risk indicators for coronary heart disease, cerebrovascular disease, renal disease, and for death from all causes. However, this relationship has only been demonstrated in recent decades, and shown to be present not only in middle-aged people but also in elderly subjects. At the same time, potent new antihypertensive agents have become available with fewer subjective side effects. These drugs not only lower blood pressure over long periods, but also reduce morbidity, cerebrovascular accidents, and cardiovascular mortality, at least in certain well-defined groups. Thus, among the chronic diseases most frequent in industrialized societies, such as cancer and cardiovascular diseases, hypertension has become one of the diseases in which the natural history can be profoundly influenced, to the extent that better treatment may influence total mortality in the community at large.

The frequency of this disease, its importance as a major risk factor for other diseases, and the availability of drugs which influence its course, probably explain the extensive growth of research work on hypertension. It should be realized, however, that neither the course of hypertension, nor its many pathophysiological mechanisms have been satisfactorily explained and that more research is needed.

Many excellent books on hypertension are available. Most of them either are directed toward research topics or are introductions to the subject. This volume does not concentrate on research and the section on animal research is very short; nor is it intended as an introduction to the field. It is mainly aimed at doctors with more than a casual interest in hypertension such as practising physicians, residents in training, cardiologists, nephrologists and internists, who want to have a book available showing the recent advances in the field and their practical applications.

Since this field is rapidly expanding, it was felt that such a book could neither be written by one person, nor by one research team, but needed the collaboration of many authorities in the field. We would like to express our gratitude to all of them. The editors would also welcome any suggestion for topics that should be reviewed in future editions.

A. AMERY
R. FAGARD
P. LIJNEN
J. STAESSEN

LIST OF CONTRIBUTORS

A. Amery, Hypertension and Cardiovascular Rehabilitation Unit, Department of Pathophysiology, University of Leuven, K.U. Leuven, 3000 Leuven, BELGIUM.

Gunnar H. Anderson, Jr., Departments of Surgery and Medicine, State University of New York, Upstate Medical Center, 750 E. Adams Street, Syracuse, New York 13210, U.S.A.

Frederic C. Bartter, Audie L. Murphy Memorial Veterans Hospital, 7400 Merton Minter Boulevard, San Antonio, Texas 78284, U.S.A.

William H. Beierwaltes, Instructor in Physiology and Biophysics, Mayo School of Medicine, Rochester, Minnesota 55901, U.S.A.

Giuseppe Bianchi, Istituto Clinica Medica I, Padiglione Granelli, Via F. Sforza 35, 20122 Milano, ITALY.

W. H. Birkenhäger, Department of Medicine, Zuiderziekenhuis, Groene Hilledijk 315, 3075 EA Rotterdam, THE NETHERLANDS.

Henry R. Black, Associate Professor of Internal Medicine, Section of General Medicine, Yale University School of Medicine, 333 Cedar Street, Post Office Box 3333, New Haven, Connecticut 06510, U.S.A.

Fritz R. Bühler, Division of Cardiology, University Hospital, CH-4031 Basel, SWITZERLAND.

C. J. Bulpitt, London School of Hygiene and Tropical Medicine, Department of Medical Statistics and Epidemiology, Keppel Street (Gower Street), London WC1E 7HT, ENGLAND.

J. P. Cecile, Service de Radiologie Vasculaire, CHR, Lens, FRANCE.

Jolanta Chodakowska, Department of Angiology, Academy of Medicine, Nowogrodzka 59, 02-006 Warsaw, POLAND.

David G. Cogan, National Eye Institute, National Institutes of Health, Bethesda, Maryland 20205, U.S.A.

Thomas G. Coleman, Department of Physiology and Biophysics, University of Mississippi Medical Center, 2500 North State Street, Jackson, Mississippi 39216, U.S.A.

Pierre Corvol, Hôpital Saint-Joseph, 7, Rue Pierre-Larousse, 75674 Paris Cédex 14, FRANCE.

J. F. de Fremont, Service de Néphrologie, CHU, Hôpital Nord, 80000 Amiens, FRANCE.

Patrice Degoulet, Hôpital Saint-Joseph, 7, Rue Pierre-Larousse, 75674 Paris Cédex 14, FRANCE.

P. W. de Leeuw, Department of Medicine, Zuiderziekenhuis Groene Hilledijk 315, 3075 EA Rotterdam, THE NETHERLANDS.

Michael de Swiet, Senior Lecturer in Paediatrics, Cardiothoracic Institute, Fulham Road, London SW3 6HP, ENGLAND.

A. Distler, Department of General Internal Medicine and Nephrology, Free University of Berlin, Klinikum Steglitz, D-1000 Berlin, FEDERAL REPUBLIC OF GERMANY.

Geoffrey A. Donnan, University of Melbourne, Department of Medicine, Austin Hospital, Heidelberg, Victoria 3084, AUSTRALIA.

Austin E. Doyle, University of Melbourne, Department of Medicine, Austin Hospital, Heidelberg, Victoria 3084, AUSTRALIA.

Rainer Dusing, Department of Medicine, Erie County Medical Center, 462 Grider Street, Buffalo, New York 14215, U.S.A.

H. E. Eliahou, Department of Nephrology, Chaim Sheba Medical Center, Tel-Hashomer 52621, ISRAEL.

R. Fagard, Hypertension and Cardiovascular Rehabilitation Unit, Department of Pathophysiology, University of Leuven, K.U. Leuven, 3000 Leuven, BELGIUM.

Peter Fayers, Medical Research Council, Tuberculosis & Chest Diseases Unit, Cardiothoracic Institute, Fulham Road, London SW3 6HP, ENGLAND.

Desmond Fitzgerald, Department of Clinical Pharmacology, Royal College of Surgeons in Ireland, St. Stephen's Green, Dublin 2, IRELAND.

John S. Floras, Department of Medicine, Toronto General Hospital, Toronto, Ontario, CANADA.

Björn Folkow, Department of Physiology, University of Göteborg, Medicinaregatan 11, 400 33 Göteborg, SWEDEN.

F. Forette, Service de Gériatrie, Hôpital Charles Foix, 7, Avenue de la République, 94 206 Ivry-sur-Seine, FRANCE.

A. Fournier, Service de Néphrologie, CHU, Hôpital Nord, 80000 Amiens, FRANCE.

Edward D. Frohlich, Vice-President, Education and Research, Alton Ochsner Medical Foundation, 1516 Jefferson Highway, New Orleans, Louisiana 70121, U.S.A.

J. C. Gaignault, Centre de Recherches Roussel-UCLAF, 102 Route de Noisy, BP N° 9, 93230 Romainville, FRANCE.

Detlev Ganten, Department of Pharmacology, University of Heidelberg, Im Neuenheimer Feld 366, D-6900 Heidelberg, FEDERAL REPUBLIC OF GERMANY.

Ray W. Gifford, Jr., Department of Hypertension and Nephrology, Cleveland Clinic, 9500 Euclid Avenue, Cleveland, Ohio 44106, U.S.A.

Lee Goldman, Department of Medicine, Peter Bent Brigham Division, Brigham and Women's Hospital, 75 Francis Street, Boston, Massachusetts 02115, U.S.A.

J. Grumbach, Service de Radiologie, CHU, Hôpital Nord, 80000 Amiens, FRANCE.

Edgar Haber, Cardiac Unit, Massachusetts General Hospital, Boston, Massachusetts 02114, U.S.A.

Margareta Hallbäck-Nordlander, Department of Physiology, University of Göteborg, Medicinaregatan 11, 400 33 Göteborg, SWEDEN.

Lennart Hansson, Associate Professor, Department of Medicine, University of Göteborg, Ostra Hospital, 416 85 Göteborg, SWEDEN.

J. F. Henry, Service de Gériatrie, Hôpital Charles Foix, 7, Avenue de la République, 94 206 Ivry-sur-Seine, FRANCE.

M. P. Hervy, Service de Gériatrie, Hôpital Charles Foix, 7, Avenue de la République, 94 206 Ivry-sur-Seine, FRANCE.

Peter C. Houck, Cardiovascular Training Program, Mayo School of Medicine, Rochester, Minnesota 55901, U.S.A.

James C. Hunt, University of Tennessee, Center for the Health Sciences, College of Medicine, 800 Madison Avenue, Memphis, Tennessee 38163, U.S.A.

Wodzimierz Januszewicz, Department of Angiology, Academy of Medicine, Nowogrodzka 59, 02-006 Warsaw, POLAND.

James Gibb Johnson, University of Tennessee, Center for the Health Sciences, College of Medicine, 800 Madison Avenue, Memphis, Tennessee 38163, U.S.A.

Stevo Julius, Division of Hypertension, Department of Internal Medicine, University of Michigan Medical School, Ann Arbor, Michigan 48109, U.S.A.

William B. Kannel, Boston University Medical Center, School of Medicine, 80 East Concord Street, Boston, Massachusetts 02118, U.S.A.

Norman M. Kaplan, Professor of Internal Medicine, University of Texas Health Science Center, 5323 Harry Hines Boulevard, Dallas, Texas 75235, U.S.A.

Priscilla Kincaid-Smith, University of Melbourne, Department of Medicine, Royal Melbourne Hospital, Victoria 3050, AUSTRALIA.

Bernard E. Kreger, Boston University Medical Center, School of Medicine, 80 East Concord Street, Boston, Massachusetts 02118, U.S.A.

Rudolf E. Lang, Department of Pharmacology, University of Heidelberg, Im Neuenheimer Feld 366, D-6900 Heidelberg, FEDERAL REPUBLIC OF GERMANY.

Herbert G. Langford, Departments of Medicine and Physiology, University of Mississippi Medical Center, 2500 North State Street, Jackson, Mississippi 39216, U.S.A.

John M. Ledingham, Medical Unit, The London Hospital Medical College, Whitechapel, London E1 1BB, ENGLAND.

James B. Lee, Department of Medicine, Erie County Medical Center, 462 Grider Street, Buffalo, New York 14215, U.S.A.

Ellin Lieberman, Children's Hospital of Los Angeles, Post Office Box 54700, Los Angeles, California 90054, U.S.A.

P. Lijnen, Hypertension and Cardiovascular Rehabilitation Unit, Department of Pathophysiology, University of Leuven, K.U. Leuven, 3000 Leuven, BELGIUM.

Per Lund-Johansen, Professor in Medicine, Medical Department A, University of Bergen, School of Medicine, 5016 Haukeland Sykehus, 5000 Bergen, NORWAY.

R. Makdassi, Service de Néphrologie, CHU, Hôpital Nord, 80000 Amiens, FRANCE.

William M. Manger, Associate Professor of Clinical Medicine, New York University Medical Center, National Hypertension Association, Inc., 400 East 34th Street, New York, New York 10016, U.S.A.

Giuseppe Mancia, Istituto di Clinica Medica IV, Università di Milano, CNR, Milano, ITALY.

Morton H. Maxwell, Hypertension Division, Cedars-Sinai and UCLA Medical Centers, Box 48750, Los Angeles, California 900048, U.S.A.

Joël Menard, Hôpital Saint-Joseph, 7, Rue Pierre-Larousse, 75674 Paris Cédex 14, FRANCE.

Franz H. Messerli, Education and Research, Alton Ochsner Medical Foundation, 1516 Jefferson Highway, New Orleans, Louisiana 70121, U.S.A.

Philippe Meyer, Inserm U7, CNRS LA 318, Hôpital Necker, Department of Néphrology, 161 Rue de Sèvres, 75015 Paris, FRANCE.

William R. Murphy, Department of Physiology and Biophysics, University of Mississippi Medical Center, 2500 North State Street, Jackson, Mississippi 39216, U.S.A.

J. C. Nainby-Luxmoore, St. Bartholomew's Hospital, Medical College, West Smithfield, London EC1A 7BE, ENGLAND.

Helen F. Oates, Cardio-Renal Unit, Medical Research Department, Kanematsu Memorial Institute, Sydney Hospital, Sydney, N.S.W. 2000, AUSTRALIA.

Eoin O'Brien, Department of Clinical Pharmacology, Royal College of Surgeons in Ireland, St. Stephen's Green, Dublin 2, IRELAND.

Kevin O'Malley, Department of Clinical Pharmacology, Royal College of Surgeons in Ireland, St. Stephen's Green, Dublin 2, IRELAND.

Axel Overlack, Medizinische Universitäts-Poliklinik Bonn, Wilhelmstrasse 35-37, 5300 Bonn 1, FEDERAL REPUBLIC OF GERMANY.

Frederick B. Parker, Jr., Departments of Surgery and Medicine, State University of New York, Upstate Medical Center, 750 E. Adams Street, Syracuse, New York 13210, U.S.A.

Pierre-François Plouin, Hôpital Saint-Joseph, 7, Rue Pierre-Larousse, 75674 Paris Cédex 14, FRANCE.

B. N. C. Prichard, Department of Clinical Pharmacology, School of Medicine, University College London, 5 University Street, London WC1E 6JJ, ENGLAND.

Wolfgang Rascher, Department of Pharmacology, University of Heidelberg, Im Neuenheimer

Feld 366, D-6900 Heidelberg, FEDERAL REPUBLIC OF GERMANY.

A. Remond, Service de Radiologie, CHU, Hôpital Nord, 80000 Amiens, FRANCE.

John L. Reid, Department of Materia Medica, Stobhill General Hospital, Glasgow G21 3UW, SCOTLAND.

J. Carlos Romero, Associate Professor of Physiology and Biophysics, and Internal Medicine, Mayo School of Medicine, Rochester, Minnesota 55901, U.S.A.

Michel E. Safar, Hôpital Broussais, 96, Rue Didot, 75674 Paris Cédex 14, FRANCE.

Mohinder P. Sambhi, San Fernando Valley Medical Program, Sepulveda V.A. Medical Center, 16111 Plummer Street, Sepulveda, California 91343, U.S.A.

Rune Sannerstedt, Carlanderska Hospital, S-412, 55 Göteborg, SWEDEN.

Elliot Anthony Shinebourne, Senior Lecturer in Paediatrics, Cardiothoracic Institute, Brompton Hospital, Fulham Road, London SW3 6HP, ENGLAND.

F. Olaf Simpson, Wellcome Medical Research Institute, Department of Medicine, University of Otago Medical School, Post Office Box 913, Dunedin, NEW ZEALAND.

Peter Sleight, Department of Cardiovascular Medicine, University of Oxford, John Radcliffe Hospital, Headington, Oxford OX3 9DU, U.K.

Thomas L. Smith, Department of Physiology and Biophysics, University of Mississippi Medical Center, 2500 North State Street, Jackson, Mississippi 39216, U.S.A.

J. Staessen, Hypertension and Cardiovascular Rehabilitation Unit, Department of Pathophysiology, University of Leuven, K.U. Leuven, 3000 Leuven, BELGIUM.

Karen A. Stanek, Department of Physiology and Biophysics, University of Mississippi Medical Center, 2500 North State Street, Jackson, Mississippi 39216, U.S.A.

Gordon S. Stokes, Cardio-Renal Unit, Medical Research Department, Kanematsu Memorial Institute, Sydney Hospital, Sydney, N.S.W. 2000, AUSTRALIA.

Toma Strasser, Cardiovascular Diseases, World Health Organization, 1211 Geneva 27, SWITZERLAND.

David H.P. Streeten, Departments of Surgery and Medicine, State University of New York, Upstate Medical Center, 750 E. Adams Street, Syracuse, New York 13210, U.S.A.

Klaus O. Stumpe, Medizinische Universitäts-Poliklinik Bonn, Wilhelmstrasse 35-37, 5300 Bonn 1, FEDERAL REPUBLIC OF GERMANY.

E. Malcolm Symonds, Department of Obstetrics and Gynaecology, University of Nottingham, City Hospital, Hucknall Road, Nottingham NG5 1PB, ENGLAND.

R.C. Tarazi, Professor of Medicine, Cleveland Clinic, 9500 Euclid Avenue, Cleveland, Ohio 44106, U.S.A.

S.H. Taylor, University Department of Cardiovascular Studies and Department of Medical Cardiology, The General Infirmary, Leeds LS1 3EX, ENGLAND.

M. Tonnelier, Service de Radiologie, l'Hôtel Dieu, Paris, FRANCE.

Thomas Unger, Department of Pharmacology, University of Heidelberg, Im Neuenheimer Feld 366, D-6900 Heidelberg, FEDERAL REPUBLIC OF GERMANY.

Herman Villarreal, Instituto Nacional de Cardiologia, "Ignacio Chavez", Juan Badiano No. 1, Mexico 22, D.F., MEXICO.

R.J. Weir, Consultant Physician, Gartnavel General Hospital, Western Infirmary, 1053 Great Western Road, Glasgow G12 0YN, SCOTLAND.

Yves A. Weiss, Hôpital Broussais, 96, Rue Didot, 75674 Paris Cédex 14, FRANCE.

M. Worcel, Centre de Recherches Roussel-UCLAF, 102 Route de Noisy, BP N° 9, 93230 Romainville, FRANCE.

Yukio Yamori, Japan Stroke Prevention Center, Department of Pathology, Shimane Medical University, Izumo 693, JAPAN.

Alberto Zanchetti, Istituto di Clinica Medica IV, Università di Milano, CNR, Milano, ITALY.

HYPERTENSIVE CARDIOVASCULAR DISEASE: PATHOPHYSIOLOGY AND TREATMENT

I. BLOOD PRESSURE CONTROL IN NORMOTENSIVE SUBJECTS

1. ROLE OF THE KIDNEY IN BLOOD PRESSURE REGULATION

THOMAS G. COLEMAN, WILLIAM R. MURPHY, THOMAS L. SMITH and KAREN A. STANEK

An important part of normal physiological function is that arterial pressure remains within relatively narrow limits. A lower than normal pressure produces disorientation and acute intolerance to upright posture. A higher than normal pressure is much more insidious. Hypertension over the long term causes little acute discomfort while increasing mortality and morbidity in a statistical fashion. Typical sequelae include obstruction or rupture of major blood vessels with frequent involvement of the brain, heart, and kidneys.

Most would agree that genetic influences and physiological mechanisms combine to minimize fluctuations in arterial pressure. The importance of genetic influences is underscored by the observation that hypertension is likely to occur in the children of hypertensive parents. And, strains of animals have been developed by repetitive inbreeding that become predictably hypertensive, while other strains have been inbred to remain, just as predictably, normotensive [1]. Such demonstrations of the heritability of blood pressure have added much to our understanding of blood pressure control in general, but they have not helped much in settling the question of exactly which physiological mechanisms are involved.

All of the organs of the body must have adequate perfusion and, teleologically, all might be suspected of having some direct or indirect involvement in the control of blood pressure. The brain is most conspicuous, since normal cerebral function is lost when arterial pressure in the brain is insufficient for only a few moments. Further, hydrostatic forces reduce pressure as blood travels toward the head during upright posture and this puts the brain in special jeopardy. In response to these needs, it appears that the autonomic nervous system has evolved in such a way that a rapid and forceful neural response will occur if cerebral perfusion is threatened.

The baroreceptor reflexes tend to preserve pressure and flow in the brain and heart at the expense of other tissues. This is not likely to be a suitable method of blood pressure control over prolonged periods. Consider the case of upright posture. In the absence of the baroreceptor reflexes, arterial pressure decrease is secondary to a fall in cardiac output. The fall in cardiac output, in turn, results from gravitational translocation of blood to the lower

Amery, A. (ed.) Hypertensive Cardiovascular Disease: Pathophysiology and Treatment
© *1982, Martinus Nijhoff Publishers. The Hague / Boston / London*
ISBN-13: 978-94-009-7478-4

torso with concomitant impairment of venous return. The baroreceptor reflexes do not provide full hemodynamic compensation. Reflex vasoconstriction in organs other than the heart and brain tends to maintain the systemic arterial pressure and cerebral perfusion; but, vasoconstriction per se will further depress, rather than enhance, many regional flows and cardiac output in general. The short-term merits of such a response would undoubtedly become liabilities over prolonged periods of time.

In considering the special metabolic requirements of *all* of the tissues of the body, the regulation of arterial pressure is tightly linked to the overall maintenance of adequate blood flow. Adequate flow, in turn, depends on some fundamental aspects of cardiovascular function: the pumping ability of the heart, vascular (and especially venous) tone, and the adequacy of body fluid volumes. With respect to the last factor, the volume and composition of body fluids involve salt and water balance and the kidney. Therefore, as the kidney participates in the control of arterial pressure, its most important role may be in stabilizing cardiovascular performance over the long term rather than in responding to acute disturbances.

1. THE KIDNEY AND BLOOD PRESSURE: CLINICAL AND EXPERIMENTAL EVIDENCE

The occurrence of hypertension is usually cited as a primary example of dysfunction within the systems that control blood pressure. It is that and more. A persistent change in blood pressure involves the whole body: there are neural, humoral, and biochemical components; the structure and composition of the blood vessels are altered; the heart's work load increases; the volume and distribution of body fluids are altered; and so forth. It is very difficult to clearly separate cause from effect in such a complex response. Accordingly, many different concepts of blood pressure control have found supporting (but often indirect) evidence in studies investigating the genesis of hypertension. Several observations are cited below that seem specifically to support the kidney's importance in blood pressure control.

1.1. Blood pressure control after nephrectomy

One way to assess the kidney's role in blood pressure control is to see what happens when the kidneys are removed. The answer is that blood pressure becomes poorly controlled and hypertension often results. Early experimental studies used bilaterally nephrectomized animals; arterial pressure usually increased after nephrectomy but the accompanying uremia complicated such protocols. One of the prevailing explanations for postnephrectomy (renoprival) hypertension was that the kidneys secreted an antihypertensive substance that normally maintained normotension. Secretion theoretically stopped, of course, when the kidneys were removed. Another explanation might be that the body's salt and water stores were inadequately controlled and became expanded after nephrectomy.

Many additional observations have been made since maintenance hemodialysis of anephric patients became a common practice. It has been shown that hypertension does *not necessarily* develop after nephrectomy. However, the body's fluids must be properly controlled if normotension is to be maintained, as is illustrated in Figure 1. Increases in weight and the body's salt and water stores are associated with rising pressure; conversely, reduction of volume through ultrafiltration will lower pressure.

The activity of the renin–angiotensin system is negligible after nephrectomy. While overactivity of this system has been implicated in several forms of hypertension, it is improbable in the case of postnephrectomy hypertension. But, there is a further consideration. Changes in the activity of the renin-angiotensin system are usually in the direction that is opposite to changes in body fluids. This reciprocity undoubtedly helps to stabilize blood pressure. Reciprocity is lost with nephrectomy and this may be part of the explanation as to why some hemodialysis patients develop an intolerable hypotension during only small volume decreases with ultrafiltration (see also section 2.3).

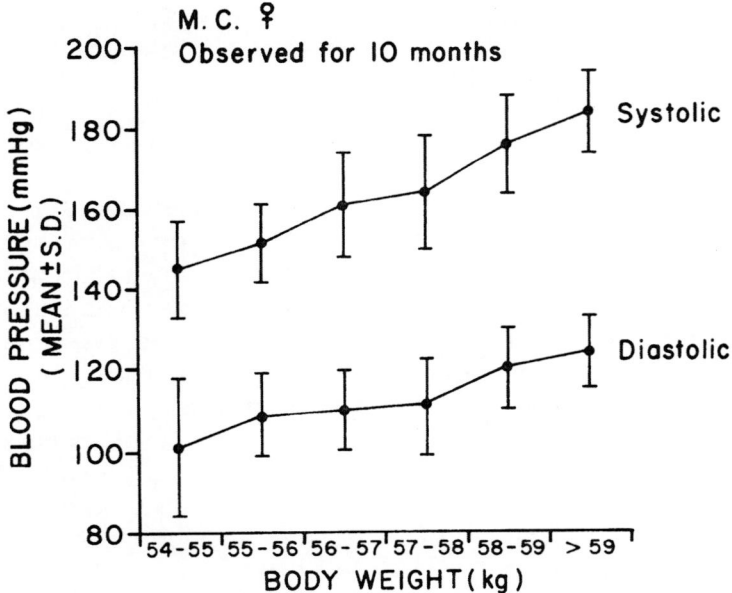

Figure 1. Long-term correlation between body weight and blood pressure in an anephric hemodialysis patient. Changes in weight are usually associated with changes in exchangeable sodium.

In total, arterial pressure is normally controlled with precision, but a significant part of this control disappears when the kidneys are removed. Both excretory function (related to salt and water balance) and secretory function (related to the effects of renin) are lost.

1.2. Renal transplantation

Arterial pressure can change when a kidney is surgically removed and a replacement kidney is implanted. This has been demonstrated in patients undergoing renal transplantation subsequent to deterioration of kidney function. Although the results are rather variable and the number of subjects reported on are often meager, some general ideas are emerging. Firstly, hypertension is most likely to develop or to continue if the remnant kidney is not removed during transplantation [2]. Remnant nephrectomy is usually beneficial in these instances [3]. Secondly, when only a transplanted kidney is present, the posttransplant arterial pressure correlates poorly with the pretransplant pressure. Normotensive recipients can become hypertensive while hypertensive recipients can become normotensive [4]. When hypertension does occur after transplantation, it often occurs in conjunction with overt renal artery stenosis. Thirdly, while there are instances of elevated plasma renin activity, the plasma renin activity in single-kidney transplant hypertension can be normal [5, 6]. Sodium retention with developing hypertension has been observed and positive correlations between blood pressure and the body's sodium stores have been reported [5-7]. Therefore, it appears that a transplanted kidney can have a significant effect on the blood pressure of the recipient, and both sodium and renin have been implicated in this influence.

Renal transplantation in experimental animals, particularly in special strains of rats, has also been informative. Selective inbreeding has been used to develop strains of rats that become hypertensive without added provocation; companion strains have been developed that remain normotensive in comparable circumstances. Cross-transplantation of kidneys, a difficult technical feat, has been employed in several instances to assess the role of the kidneys in this genetic or spontaneous hypertension. In the cases of the Okamoto strain [8] and the Bianchi or Milan strain [9] of spontaneously hypertensive rats, implantation of a kidney from a normotensive rat into a hypertensive recipient lowers blood pressure and results in lasting normotension. Likewise, implantation of a kidney from a hypertensive rat into a normotensive recipient results in persistent hypertension. Similar results have been obtained using cross-transplantation in Dahl (or Brookhaven) rats. One substrain of Dahl rats becomes hypertensive when given a salt-rich diet while the other substrain does not. Cross-transplantation has demonstrated that the hypertension follows the kidney [10]. It has been suggested that a kidney from a hypertensive donor may produce hypertension in a normotensive recipient because the transplanted kidney has sustained previous pressure-induced damage (see also section 1.4). If true, this would represent more of a pathological than a physiological role for the kidney in blood pressure control. However, the ability of a donor kidney from a normotensive rat to persistently lower the blood pressure in a previously hypertensive recipient should probably be considered to be a dramatic demonstration of the physiological importance of the kidney in long-term blood pressure regulation.

1.3. Lessons from experimental hypertension

Hypertension was a clearly identified clinical problem in the early twentieth century, but no comparable animal models were available to allow experimental study of this disease. A variety of attempts to produce experimental hypertension ended in failure. Then, in 1934, Goldblatt and colleagues showed that hypertension could be reliably produced in dogs by partial constriction of the renal artery [11]. Later, Wilson and Byrom introduced a variation of this procedure by producing hypertension in the rat while leaving the contralateral kidney intact [12]. Therefore, the first (and still foremost) methods of producing hypertension involve the kidneys.

Other renal insults will also produce hypertension. In 1939, Page showed that compression and/or irritation of the renal capsule by foreign substances such as silk or cellophane reliably produce hypertension [13]. In 1944, Grollman showed that compression of the renal capsule with an external ligature would also produce hypertension [14]. Partial nephrectomy will sometimes produce hypertension but will also produce serious uremia with excessive loss of renal tissue. Partial nephrectomy combined with increased sodium intake, however, is a reliable way of producing hypertension [15, 16].

Hypertension can also be produced by altering the extrinsic influences on the kidney that normally modulate sodium excretion. Most notably, mineralocorticoid excess has been used. Continuous administration of deoxycorticosterone or aldosterone, frequently in combination with increased sodium intake, is a popular laboratory procedure. Infusion of angiotensin or norepinephrine directly into the renal artery will elevate blood pressure for as long as the infusion continues.

Hence, in the past four and a half decades a variety of experimental procedures have been developed to produce hypertension in laboratory animals. Most of these procedures, like those cited above, involve a direct manipulation of the kidneys or alteration of the extrinsic influences on renal function. The procedures are characterized by their reliability and popularity.

1.4. Renal damage and self-sustaining hypertension

High blood pressure damages kidneys. Lesions develop in the large and small arteries of the kidney and these lesions are likely to affect the performance of the kidneys by increasing renal vascular resistance. The similarity between these lesions and the Goldblatt clamp, and the effectiveness of the Goldblatt clamp in raising arterial pressure, should be kept in mind.

An early demonstration of the influence of renal damage on blood pressure can be found in the work of Wilson and Byrom [17]. They produced hypertension in rats by clamping one renal artery and leaving the contralateral kidney intact. The contralateral kidney was exposed to the full force of the elevated blood pressure. After hypertension was well established, the clamped kidney was removed. Some elevation in arterial pressure persisted. Therefore, hypertension could be maintained in these animals after the original hypertension-producing stimulus was (surgically) removed.

It is likely that clinical and experimental hypertensions of all etiologies undergo a similar transition, i.e., pressure-induced renal damage becomes increasingly more important as time passes in maintaining some part or all of the blood pressure increase. The time course of such a transition and the physiological mechanisms underlying such a transition remain for the most part unknown. However, the data available to date suggest that a damaged kidney can, at times, dominate other pressure control mechanisms.

2. EXCRETORY AND SECRETARY FUNCTIONS OF THE KIDNEY

The kidney excretes, under precise control, many different substances in contributing to homeostasis. Among these are potassium, chloride, acids, and many metabolic end products which are unwanted and potentially toxic. However, with respect to blood pressure control, excretion of the sodium ion keeps coming to the forefront. Similarly, the endocrine or secretory function of the kidney includes release of prostaglandins and kinins, but it is the renin–angiotension system which has been most directly implicated in blood pressure control to date.

A very stable arterial pressure could theoretically be achieved by physiological mechanisms that incorporate the principle of negative feedback. Negative feedback means that information about the consequences of some disturbance are fed back to a controller and corrective action is instituted, which reduces (hence the term negative) the impact of the disturbance. The baroreceptor reflex is often used as an example. Arterial pressure is monitored by receptors in the major arteries of the upper body. Perceived disturbances in arterial pressure are interpreted in the brain stem and changes in autonomic outflow provide the vasoconstriction or vasodilation needed to minimize the impact of the original disturbance. A similar, but longer-acting, negative feedback scheme might involve the kidneys and be involved in the long-term control of arterial pressure. Many different possibilities exist, but two of these seem to be the most fully advanced and documented at the present time: (a) arterial pressure may affect sodium excretion and sodium excretion, in turn, may affect (negatively) arterial pressure, contributing to blood pressure stability; (b) arterial pressure may (negatively) affect renin secretion and, in turn, renin secretion may affect arterial pressure, again contributing to blood pressure stability. While these are attractive explanations on theoretical grounds, they must be accepted cautiously. For instance, blood pressure often increases without overt changes in either sodium balance or renin activity. And, the way in which changes in sodium excretion might influence blood pressure is not entirely clear (see section 3). A further complication is that the excretory and secretory aspects of the kidney are continually interacting. Nevertheless, many of the individual components of these two (potential) blood pressure control mechanisms have been experimentally documented.

2.1. Sodium excretion

Sodium excretion depends on the relative difference between the amount of sodium filtered and reabsorbed. These two processes, in turn, depend on arterial pressure, neural activity, blood levels of aldosterone and angiotensin, the composition of the blood, and other factors.

With such an extensive list of influences on sodium excretion, it is not clear why the arterial pressure–sodium excretion relationship should be singled out for emphasis. One reason is that this relationship is maintained even in the isolated kidney without the need for additional, extrinsic influences; this indicates that pressure-induced natriuresis is an intrinsic and fundamental property of the kidney. Many of the other influences on renal function change in conjunction with arterial pressure, thereby amplifying the pressure–excretion relationship. From a different point of view, it might be argued that the pressure–excretion relationship should be highlighted because it appears to be the *dominant* relationship. For instance, sodium excretion is negligible at an arterial pressure of 50 mm Hg whether humoral influences are present or absent. Conversely, sodium balance can be maintained even in the presence of maximal amounts of mineralocorticoids when arterial pressure reaches about 150 mm Hg.

The premise then is that sodium excretion and arterial pressure are pro-

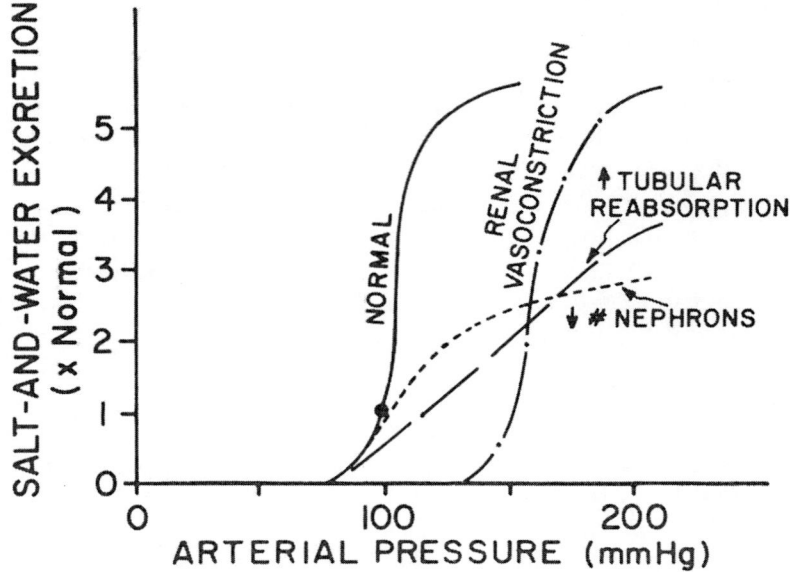

Figure 2. Hypothetical arterial pressure–sodium excretion relationships for normal and abnormal situations.

portional, that this relationship is important, and that this relationship can be modified by neural and humoral factors, pathology, and experimental intervention. Several possibilities are shown schematically in Figure 2. For instance, renal vasoconstriction by a Goldblatt clamp decreases renal perfusion pressure; arterial pressure must increase an amount equal to the pressure drop across the clamp in order to bring renal perfusion pressure and sodium excretion back to normal. The arterial pressure-excretion relationship for renal vasoconstriction is accordingly displaced to the right by an amount approximately equal to the pressure drop across the clamp. The influence of changes in tubular reabsorption and the total number of nephrons are also illustrated. This graph can be interpreted in two ways: if read from top to bottom, it suggests that those interventions that produce hypertension will decrease sodium excretion at any given arterial pressure; if read from left to right, it suggests that sodium balance can be maintained only at elevated arterial pressures when antinatriuretic influences are at work.

2.2. Renin secretion and angiotensin formation

Renin secretion can be altered by changes in sympathetic nerve activity, changes in renal blood flow and filtration, and changes in renal arterial pressure. This last relationship is illustrated in Figure 3. Decreasing renal perfusion pressure provokes renin release that may be related to a decrease

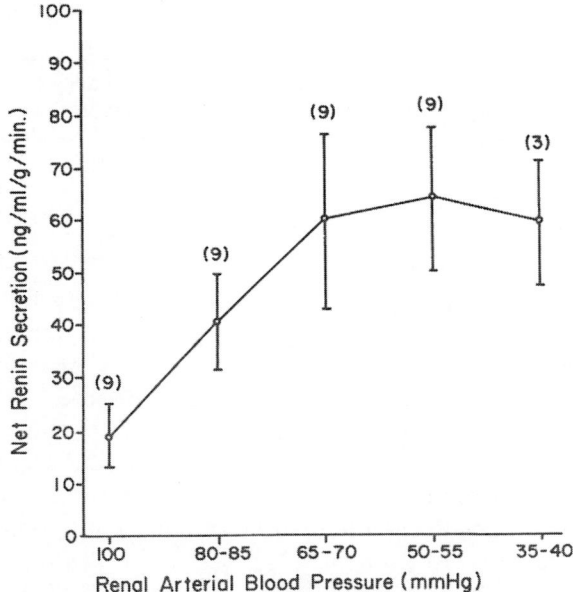

Figure 3. Renin secretion in response to changes in renal arterial pressure (from [18] with permission of the American Heart Association).

in tubular flow, a decrease in blood pressure within the small arteries of the kidney, or both. The net result is that falling arterial pressure stimulates renin secretion and the resultant increase in angiotensin formation tends to oppose or minimize the initial pressure decrease.

2.3. Renin–sodium interactions

Renin and sodium interact both within the kidney and within the systemic circulation. Therefore, an analysis of the kidneys' role in blood pressure control becomes considerably more complicated than if the sodium and renin mechanisms were completely independent.

An early demonstration of renin–sodium interaction can be found in the work of Gavras and colleagues [19]. They showed that blood pressure was decreased neither by sodium depletion nor by a blockade of angiotensin receptors with an angiotensin analog. But, sodium depletion *and* blockade of angiotensin receptors produced a dramatic decrease in arterial pressure.

This acute interrelationship has also been shown to occur over the long term [20], as summarized in Table 1, and it is therefore relevant to the long-term control of arterial pressure. One month of dietary sodium restric-

Table 1. Mean arterial pressure (BP, mmHg) and plasma renin activity (PRA, ngA$_1$/ml/h) with sodium restriction and/or converting enzyme inhibition

Diet	No treatment		Converting enzyme inhibition
	BP	PRA	BP
Normal sodium	99	1.1	88
Low sodium	99	8.5	77

tion in the rat did not change mean arterial pressure but did raise plasma renin activity. One week of blockade of angiotensin formation, using orally administered converting enzyme inhibitor, lowered mean arterial pressure in salt-replete animals but caused an even larger pressure decrease in sodium-restricted rats. Hence, arterial pressure is sensitive to changes in sodium intake in the absence of a functioning renin–angiotensin system. But, compensatory changes in renin activity in the intact animal provide a strong compensation for changes in sodium balance and thereby maintain a normal arterial pressure.

A more detailed view of the renin–sodium interaction is shown in Figure 4. Four different levels of sodium intake were used as a perturbation and enough time was allowed to elapse at each level to achieve sodium balance [21]. The blood pressure–renal sodium excretion relationship was derived for three sets of circumstances: endogenous angiotensin II had a fixed,

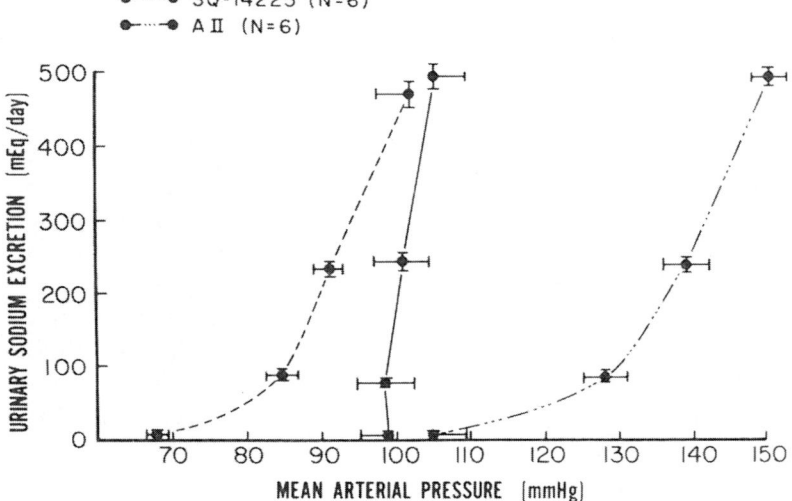

Figure 4. Steady-state arterial pressure–sodium excretion relationship in intact animals (CONTROL), during chronic converting enzyme inhibition (SQ-14225) and during continuous angiotensin infusion at 5 ng/kg/min (AII). From [21].

negligible level; endogenous plus added angiotensin II had a higher, but still fixed level; and, endogenous angiotensin II was allowed to change in response to varying dietary sodium intakes. Comparing the two rightmost curves, the effects of excessive angiotensin are most noticeable at high sodium intakes; comparing the two leftmost curves, the effects of an absence of angiotensin are most noticeable at low sodium intakes. Reading the graph from top to bottom it can be said that at a given arterial pressure, sodium excretion is much lower in the presence of angiotensin. Reading the graph from left to right it can be said that at any given level of sodium intake, arterial pressure is much higher in the presence of angiotensin than in the absence of it.

These various observations can be categorized with regard to sodium–pressure interactions, renin–pressure interactions, and sodium–renin interactions. With regard to sodium and pressure, the data in total suggest the following: (1) arterial pressure is proportional to sodium balance – as it appears from Figure 1; (2) net sodium retention is inversely proportional to arterial pressure. In other words, sodium *excretion* is proportional to blood pressure, as illustrated in Figures 2 and 4. With regard to renin–pressure interactions, the data in total suggest: (1) arterial pressure is proportional to angiotensin levels – from many studies showing that chronic angiotensin infusion produces hypertension; (2) renin secretion is inversely proportional to arterial pressure (see Figure 3). With regard to sodium and renin, the data in total suggest: (1) at a given arterial pressure, sodium excretion is decreased by increasing levels of angiotensin – from a comparison of the left hand and right hand curves in Figure 4; (2) at a given arterial pressure, renin secretion is increased by negative sodium balance – from data in Table 1.

Hence, both the excretory and secretory functions of the kidneys appear to have the necessary characteristics to contribute to blood pressure stability. Further, these two systems interact in a complementary way. Comparing the middle curve in Figure 4 with the other two, it can be seen that blood pressure changes little in the transition from a low salt diet or high salt diet if exogenous angiotensin changes freely. But, hypotension follows sodium restriction if angiotensin is not allowed to increase and hypertension follows sodium excess if angiotensin cannot be suppressed.

3. CONTROL OF VASCULAR RESISTANCE

According to the concepts of modern control theory, if the kidney is to have a dominant role in the long-term control of arterial pressure, there must be interactions between the arterial pressure and the kidney *and* between the kidney and arterial pressure. A complete circle or connected chain of interactions would thereby stabilize arterial pressure. Further, disease or dys-

14

function within the loop might impair blood pressure control and allow hypertension to develop. Two relationships between arterial pressure and the kidney have been described above. Possible relationships between the kidney and arterial pressure are less well understood.

Blood flow is relatively normal in hypertension. Hence, an increase in vascular resistance or, more directly, an increase in vascular smooth muscle tension, is one of the most significant events in the development of hypertension. Among many potential vasoconstrictors, angiotensin comes readily to mind. Angiotensin is known to be a potent vasoconstrictor and this observation completes the blood pressure-to-renin and renin-to-blood pressure loop. But, plasma renin activity and blood angiotensin concentrations are often normal or low in hypertension and this leaves many cases – possibly the majority of them – in need of a more complete explanation.

In many instances in which increased renin activity seems to be ruled out,

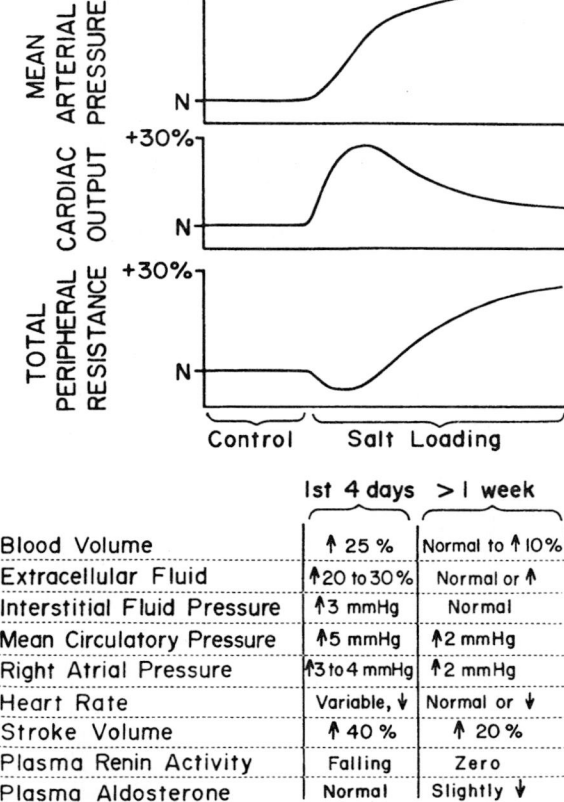

	1st 4 days	> 1 week
Blood Volume	↑ 25 %	Normal to ↑ 10%
Extracellular Fluid	↑20 to 30%	Normal or ↑
Interstitial Fluid Pressure	↑3 mmHg	Normal
Mean Circulatory Pressure	↑5 mmHg	↑2 mmHg
Right Atrial Pressure	↑3 to 4 mmHg	↑2 mmHg
Heart Rate	Variable, ↓	Normal or ↓
Stroke Volume	↑ 40 %	↑ 20 %
Plasma Renin Activity	Falling	Zero
Plasma Aldosterone	Normal	Slightly ↓

Figure 5. Hemodynamic and endocrine changes during the development of hypertension due to subtotal nephrectomy and saline loading. Data have been compiled from [22–24].

there are often signs of (albeit mild) sodium retention. Many strong statistical correlations have been developed between the body's exchangeable sodium and blood pressure. However, a physiological connection between the sodium ion and arteriolar vasoconstriction is not obvious.

One popular idea is that sodium has a direct effect on the vascular smooth muscle; there may be attractiveness in simplicity, but this idea has little persuasive evidence to support it. Another idea is that sodium retention increases both interstitial and plasma volumes. The expanded plasma volume, in turn, enhances venous return and cardiac output. A consequence of elevated flow is an autoregulatory vasoconstriction that normalizes blood flow while maintaining the elevated arterial pressure. This concept is supported by a series of experiments [22–24] in which hypertension was produced by combining subtotal nephrectomy and increased sodium intake. The total response is summarized in Figure 5. An initial increase in cardiac output is followed in time by a secondary increase in total peripheral resistance and this temporal relationship might be interpreted as autoregulatory vasoconstriction. There are other instances, however, in which sodium retention and autoregulatory vasoconstriction might be a perfectly acceptable explanation except that the expected hemodynamic transients have not been observed. Experimental evidence both for and against the sodium retention–autoregulation hypothesis must be interpreted with caution, since highly complex interactions may produce quite different observations from protocol to protocol [25]. In the absence of a totally acceptable explanation connecting changes in sodium balance and systemic vasoconstriction, it has been postulated that the connection is made by humoral intermediates [26, 27] which, as of today, have not been shown to exist. This matter remians unresolved because of a lack of evidence that is both direct and confirmatory.

4. SUMMARY

The renal influence on arterial blood pressure interacts with contributions from other systems, such as the autonomic nervous system, in providing overall blood pressure control. Several experimental observations indicate that the importance of the kidney is in the long-term control of arterial pressure: chronic blood pressure control is often defective after the kidneys are removed. Renal transplantation shows that blood pressure is often more strongly influenced by the donor kidney than by the recipient. Most forms of experimental hypertension involve manipulation of the kidneys or alterations in extrinsic influences on the kidneys. Persistent hypertension injures the kidneys in such a way that kidney damage per se appears to be capable of controlling blood pressure and sustaining hypertension.

16

The kidneys have both excretory and secretory functions. Excretion refers primarily to sodium excretion and the maintenance of sodium balance. In the absence of the renin–angiotensin system, changes in sodium balance can have a profound influence on blood pressure. Secretion refers primarily to secretion of renin by the kidney and the effects of the angiotensin that results. Angiotensin influences blood pressure both directly (via changes in vascular resistance) and indirectly (via changes in sodium excretion). Renin activity and sodium balance usually change in opposite directions, thereby stabilizing blood pressure. But, if exchangeable sodium and renin activity both become either low or high, hypotension or hypertension, respectively, will result.

A change in the caliber of the arterioles is the ultimate step in any long-term change in arterial pressure (specifically, in the development of hypertension). The connection between this vasoconstriction and the kidneys is not clear. Increased renin secretion can be responsible. In the many instances in which renin activity is normal or low, however, other connections must be sought. Sodium retention, local overperfusion and autoregulatory vasoconstriction in combination is one possible explanation. Action of intermediary vasoactive hormones under renal control has also been postulated.

REFERENCES

1. Schlager G: Spontaneous hypertension in laboratory animals. J Hered 63:35–38, 1972.
2. Cohen SL: Hypertension in renal transplant recipients: role of bilateral nephrectomy. Br Med J 3:78–81, 1973.
3. Grünfeld JP, Kleinknecht D, Moreau JF, Kamoun P, Sabto J, Garcia-Torres R, Osorio M, Kreis H: Permanent hypertension after renal homotransplantation in man. Clin Sci Mol Med 48:391–403, 1975.
4. Klarskov P, Brendstrup L, Knarup T, Jorgensen HE, Egeblad M, Palbol J: Renovascular hypertension after kidney transplantation. Scand J Urol Nephrol 13:291–298, 1979.
5. Horvath JS, Baxter C, Furby F, Hood V, Johnson J, McGrath B, Tiller DJ: Plasma renin activity, plasma angiotensin II and extracellular fluid volume in patients after renal transplantation. Clin Sci Mol Med 51 (Suppl 3):227–230, 1976.
6. Kornerup HJ: The significance of body sodium content in hypertension following renal transplantation: exchangeable sodium and plasma renin concentration before and after renal transplantation. Scand J Clin Lab Invest 37:295–301, 1977.
7. Kornerup HJ, Pedersen EB: Plasma renin, plasma aldosterone and exchangeable sodium in normotensive and hypertensive kidney transplant recipients with and without transplant renal artery stenosis. Acta Med Scand 202:509–516, 1977.
8. Kawabe K, Watanabe TX, Shiono K, Sokabe H: Influence on blood pressure of renal isografts between spontaneously hypertensive and normotensive rats, utilizing the F hybrids. Jap Heart J 19:886–899, 1978.
9. Bianchi G, Fox U, DiFrancesco GF, Giovanetti AM, Pagetti D: Blood pressure changes produced by kidney cross-transplantation between spontaneously hypertensive rats and normotensive rats. Clin Sci Mol Med 47:435–448, 1974.

10. Dahl LK, Heine M, Thompson K: Genetic influence of the kidneys on blood pressure. Circ Res 34:94–101, 1974.
11. Goldblatt H, Lynch J, Hanzal RF, Summerville WW: Studies on experimental hypertension-I. The production of persistent elevation of systolic blood pressure by means of renal ischemia. J Exp Med 59:347–379, 1934.
12. Wilson C, Byrom FB: Renal changes in malignant hypertension. Lancet 1:136–139, 1939.
13. Page IH: The production of persistent arterial hypertension by cellophane perinephritis. J Am Med Assn 113:2046–2048, 1939.
14. Grollman A: A simplified procedure for inducing chronic renal hypertension in the mammal. Proc Soc Exp Biol Med 57:102–104, 1944.
15. Koletsky S: Role of salt and renal mass in experimental hypertension. Arch Pathol 68:11–22, 1959.
16. Langston JB, Guyton AC, Douglas BH, Dorsett PE: Effect of changes in salt intake on arterial pressure and renal function in partially nephrectomized dogs. Circ Res 12:508–513, 1963.
17. Wilson C, Bryom FB: Vicious cycle in chronic Bright's disease: experimental evidence from the hypertensive rat. Quart J Med 10:65–93, 1941.
18. Cowley AW Jr, Guyton AC: Quantification of intermediate steps in the renin–angiotensin–vasoconstrictor feedback loop in the dog. Circ Res 30:557–566, 1972.
19. Gavras H, Brunner HR, Vaughan ED Jr, Laragh JH: Angiotensin–sodium interaction in blood pressure maintenance of renal hypertensive and normotensive rats. Science 180:1369–1372, 1973.
20. Bengis RG, Coleman TG, Young DB, McCaa RE: Long-term blockade of angiotensin formation in various normotensive and hypertensive rat models using converting enzyme inhibitor (SQ 14,225). Circ Res 43 (Suppl 1):45–53, 1978.
21. Hall JE, Guyton AC, Smith MJ Jr, Coleman TG: Blood pressure and renal function during chronic changes in sodium intake: role of angiotensin. Am J Physiol 239:F271–F280, 1980.
22. Douglas BH, Guyton AC, Langston JB, Bishop VB: Hypertension caused by salt loading – II. fluid volume and tissue pressure changes. Am J Physiol 207:669–671, 1964.
23. Coleman TG, Guyton AC: Hypertension caused by salt-loading – III. Onset transients of cardiac output and other circulatory parameters. Circ Res 25:153–160, 1969.
24. Manning RD Jr, Coleman TG, Guyton AC, Norman RA Jr, McCaa RE: Essential role of mean circulatory filling pressure in salt-induced hypertension. Am J Physiol 236:R40–R47, 1979.
25. Coleman TG, Samar RE, Murphy WR. Autoregulation versus other vasoconstrictors in hypertension. A critical review. Hypertension 1:324–330, 1979.
26. Haddy F, Pamnani M, Clough D: Review. The sodium–potassium pump in volume expanded hypertension. Clin Exp Hyper 1:295–336, 1978.
27. deWardener H, MacGregor GA: Dahl's hypothesis that a saluretic substance may be responsible for a sustained rise in arterial pressure. Its possible role in essential hypertension. Kid Inter 18:1–9, 1980.

2. ROLE OF CENTRAL MECHANISMS IN THE BLOOD PRESSURE REGULATION

THOMAS UNGER, WOLFGANG RASCHER, RUDOLF E. LANG and DETLEV GANTEN

This chapter is not meant to provide the reader with a comprehensive review on central blood pressure control mechanisms. We will instead discuss some selected topics on central blood pressure regulation that have recently gained interest due to the discovery of new substances in the brain and due to the introduction of new techniques allowing for more specific investigation of brain structures involved in the transmission of nerve signals within blood pressure controlling pathways.

The following four questions are posed: 1) What is the neuroanatomical basis of central cardiovascular control and what has recently been added to our knowledge in morphology?, 2) What is the functional significance of the different brain areas involved in cardiovascular regulation?, 3) What are the biochemical correlates, i.e., neurotransmitters or neuromodulator systems?, and 4) What is currently known about mutual interactions between these systems within the central blood pressure controlling pathways?

Baroreceptor mechanisms and other reflex circuits are omitted from this chapter; they are dealt with in a separate part of this book. For the same reason, pathophysiological data on the role of the central nervous system in different types of hypertension are limited to a miminum. For more extensive reviews on the topic, the reader is referred to the references given in the reading list.

1. NEUROANATOMICAL BASIS OF CENTRAL CARDIOVASCULAR CONTROL [1–3]

In spite of the accumulation of a wealth of data indicating marked cardiovascular effects following electrical stimulation of various brain areas, a precise definition of the role of the central nervous system in the control of arterial blood pressure and hemodynamics has been lacking. A major reason for this lack of functional concepts resides in the difficulties in studying the neuroanatomical organization of central autonomic pathways. The lesioning of suspected cardiovascular control centers in the brain has not always provided useful information because of many experimental problems. The introduction of two new techniques some years ago advanced our neuroa-

Amery, A. (ed.) Hypertensive Cardiovascular Disease: Pathophysiology and Treatment
© *1982, Martinus Nijhoff Publishers. The Hague / Boston / London*
ISBN-13: 978-94-009-7478-4

natomical knowledge considerably; these were the anterograde autoradiography and the retrograde horseradish peroxidase technique. By employing these two methods, it is now possible to trace neuronal pathways and to study their involvement in cardiovascular control. Biochemical correlates for these anatomical substrates can be investigated by the techniques of histofluorescence and immunohistochemistry which have also recently been added to the armament of neuroanatomists.

It has become clear from such studies that the previous idea of a single vasomotor center in the medulla oblongata, fostered for many generations since the studies by Dittmar [4] more than a hundred years ago, cannot be maintained. Rather, there exists a system of multiple neuronal pathways converging on cells in the brain stem and giving rise to the sympathetic and parasympathetic outflow.

Many areas of the brain are directly or indirectly involved in hemodynamic adaptation mechanisms. A limited number of distinct brain nuclei, however, play a direct role in cardiovascular regulation. Neuroanatomical studies have revealed a dense network of interconnections between these nuclei. This is described briefly in the following.

Nucleus of the solitary tract (NTS)

The NTS receives afferents from, among others, arterial baroreceptors and from chemoreceptors in the glomus caroticum, heart and lung via the ninth

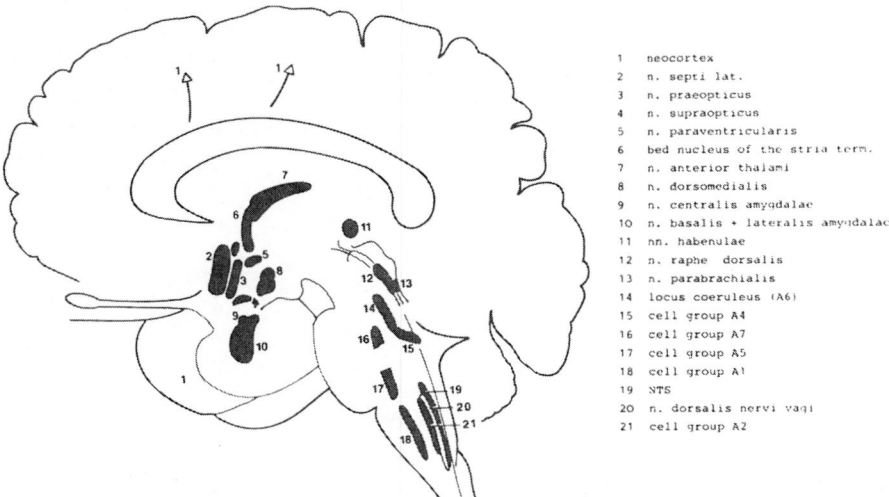

1	neocortex
2	n. septi lat.
3	n. praeopticus
4	n. supraopticus
5	n. paraventricularis
6	bed nucleus of the stria term.
7	n. anterior thalami
8	n. dorsomedialis
9	n. centralis amygdalae
10	n. basalis + lateralis amygdalae
11	nn. habenulae
12	n. raphe dorsalis
13	n. parabrachialis
14	locus coeruleus (A6)
15	cell group A4
16	cell group A7
17	cell group A5
18	cell group A1
19	NTS
20	n. dorsalis nervi vagi
21	cell group A2

Figure 1. Schematic drawing summarizing a number of sagittal cross-sections of the brain at various levels showing the brain areas known to be involved in cardiovascular control. Neuronal pathways interconnecting these areas as well as ascending and descending projections are described in the text.

and tenth nerve. Central afferents come from other parts of the medulla oblongata such as the A_5 cell group, from the paraventricular nucleus of the hypothalamus, the central amygdaloid nucleus and even the cerebral cortex. Efferent fibers project from the NTS to the vagal nuclei, to the cerebellum, the paraventricular and other hypothalamic nuclei, to the periventricular thalamic nucleus, the central amygdaloid nucleus and the medial preoptic area.

The key role for blood pressure control of the NTS as the first synapse within the baroreceptor reflex arch will be described in a separate chapter on baroreceptor reflex function in this volume.

Parabrachial nucleus

This area lies in the dorsolateral pons adjacent to the brachium conjunctivum. It is involved in cardiovascular regulation, control of respiration, and seems to play a role in the release of adrenocorticotrophic hormone (ACTH). Afferent and efferent fibers connect the parabrachial nucleus with the NTS and other brain stem regions, the hypothalamus and the central nucleus of the amygdala.

Paraventricular nucleus of the hypothalamus

The paraventricular hypothalamic nucleus receives afferents from the above nuclei, the commissural nucleus, the locus coeruleus and others and projects to the spinal cord, the periaqueductal gray, the parabrachial nucleus, the locus coeruleus, the dorsal vagal motor nucleus, the NTS of the brain stem, etc. It participates in the synthesis and release of the peptide hormones oxytocin and vasopressin (ADH) into the hypothalamic-hypophyseal tract, thus being also part of the neurohumoral control system of body fluid and volume homeostasis.

Central nucleus of the amygdala

This nucleus is connected with various regions of the hypothalamus and the medulla oblongata. It is known to participate not only in cardiovascular control, but also in several visceral and behavioral functions. It has been shown for instance, that electrical stimulation of the central amygdala in conscious cats produced a complex behavioral and cardiovascular response pattern which included components of attack; the cardiovascular portion consisted of a rise in blood pressure, tachycardia and increased peripheral resistance, all sensitive to peripheral alpha-adrenergic blockade. In contrast, stimulation of the magnocellular part of the basal amygdala resulted in a typical defense reaction with tachycardia, biphasic blood pressure responses, increased aortic blood flow and lowered peripheral vascular resistance, the latter effects being sensitive to atropine blockade [5].

Other brain areas

Apart from the closely interconnected nuclei described above several others have to be mentioned that are implicated in cardiovascular control, such as the bed of the stria terminalis, the anterior third ventricle (AV3V) region, the periaqueductal gray or the dorsomedial nucleus of the hypothalamus. These and others will have to be included into what has become of the 'vasomotor center', namely an 'anatomically widely dispersed, reciprocally interconnected system, pervaded by continuous activity' (Manning).

2. FUNCTIONAL SIGNIFICANCE OF DIFFERENT BRAIN AREAS IN CARDIOVASCULAR REGULATION [1–3, 6, 7]

Although the idea of one or several distinct vasomotor centers in the brain had to be abandoned for reasons described above, there is experimental evidence suggesting that some cardiovascular regulatory functions can be ascribed to certain brain areas. Many of these studies have been performed by employing lesioning or ablation procedures as well as electrical stimulation in anesthetized animals, and the results have to be interpreted with caution since they may not always be representative for intact conscious individuals. The following description gives a brief and somewhat simplified overview of these findings.

Areas within the medulla oblongata

The medullary cardiovascular centers comprising parts of the reticular formation, bulbar parts of the pons, and including areas such as the NTS, area postrema and others have been extensively investigated. Decerebration studies have demonstrated that this part of the brain is, by itself, able to maintain complete homeostasis of the cardiovascular system. The basal sympathetic vasoconstrictor tone as well as the sympathetic and vagal drive to the heart originate here, constantly modified by afferent impulses from peripheral cardiovascular receptors, e.g., the high pressure baroreceptors and cardiac or lung low pressure receptors, and modified by descending impulses from higher parts of the brain such as hypothalamic, limbic and cortical brain areas.

Electrical stimulation of these structures produces different responses: stimulation of lateral sites of the medulla oblongata entails mostly pressor responses, while mediocaudal stimulation rather has blood pressure lowering effects. The pressor responses are associated with sympathoadrenergic activation as evidenced by a rise in heart rate, increased cardiac contractility, increased vascular tone of resistance vessels and adrenal catecholamine release, while the sympathetic tone is reduced following stimulation of the depressor areas. Ablation of the brain stem at the level of the nucleus cuneatus separates the pressor from the depressor areas (the latter being partly preserved) and leads to a dramatic blood pressure fall and to a suppression of lower 'spinal centers'. Spinal centers come into play after dissection of the medulla oblongata caudally from the obex and are able to maintain blood pressure at a normal level and even a certain reflex activity to compensate for, e.g., blood loss.

Hypothalamic areas

Electrical stimulation of hypothalamic structures can produce a wide range of cardiovascular effects depending on the site of stimulation and other experimental conditions. Careful localization studies have demonstrated that selective vasoconstriction can be induced in distinct vascular beds, such as the renal or muscular vessels or those of the splanchnic territory from specific hypothalamic areas. Under basal conditions, the hypothalamus exerts a tonic influence on basal and reflex-induced activity of the medullary centers.

In addition, some hypothalamic areas are closely connected with emotional behavior such as the arousal or defense reactions, while others take part in the control of body temperature.

For instance, stimulation of sites within the posterior hypothalamus leads to an activation of the sympathetic cholinergic dilatatory system innervating the skeletal muscle, but can also lead to an adrenergic sympathetic activation with increases in blood pressure, heart rate and cardiac output. This may be accompanied by a generalized 'alarm' reaction with the well-known cardiovascular and emotional adaptation for fight and defense.

On the other hand, ventral parts of the hypothalamus have been shown to lower blood pressure by exerting an inhibitory influence on cardiovascular determinants which are involved in the control of body fluid homeostasis such as thirst and antidiuretic hormone release. The hypothalamus also contains target sites for the action of peptide hormones such as angiotensin and enkephalins that play a role in cardiovascular and volume regulation.

Cortical areas

Pressor and depressor reactions have been observed following electrical stimulation of various cortical brain areas. Clusters of 'cardiovascular spots' are found within the motor and premotor areas of the neocortex and within some paleocortical areas, such as the basal surface of the parietal or frontal lobe.

Stimulation of neocortical areas often produces a complex cardiovascular and emotional pattern, an 'apprehension' or 'start' reaction leading to a harmonization of vegetative and somatomotoric body functions in order to meet different kinds of challenges. Part of this cortical efferent output seems to converge in the hypothalamus since selective hypothalamic lesions can abolish the adaptive cardiovascular responses, while other vasoconstrictor efferents, and also fibers of the sympathetic cholinergic vasodilatory system originating in the cortex, directly descend to the lateral horn of the spinal cord.

3. NEUROTRANSMITTERS AND NEUROMODULATOR SYSTEMS INVOLVED IN CENTRAL CARDIOVASCULAR CONTROL [1, 8–11, 14]

A number of classical and putative neurotransmitters have been implicated in central cardiovascular control. The transmitters known for some time to be involved in blood pressure regulation are the catecholamines adrenaline and noradrenaline, while the role of dopamine is still less defined. Others include serotonin, acetylcholine, GABA, the amino acids glycine and glutamate and some peptides such as leucine-enkephalin, methionine-enkephalin, the endorphins, substance P and angiotensin, which have been found partly to fulfill the criteria for acceptance as transmitters within the central nervous system. However, it is also possible that these substances do not only act as neurotransmitters in the classical sense, but also as neuromodulators or neurohormones, i.e., control transmitter synthesis, release or uptake at more or less distant target neurons within the central nervous system (Figure 2).

Catecholamines

Noradrenaline has been demonstrated to be a transmitter in excitatory neurons descending in the spinal cord and ending in the sympathetic lateral columns which form part of a central pressor system. On the other hand, catecholaminergic nerves within the medulla oblongata also participate in central cardiovascular depressor function, especially within the baroreceptor reflex. These may be adrenergic or noradrenergic.

The following catecholaminergic pathways have been described: the intermediolateral cell column of the spinal cord, from which fibers to the peri-

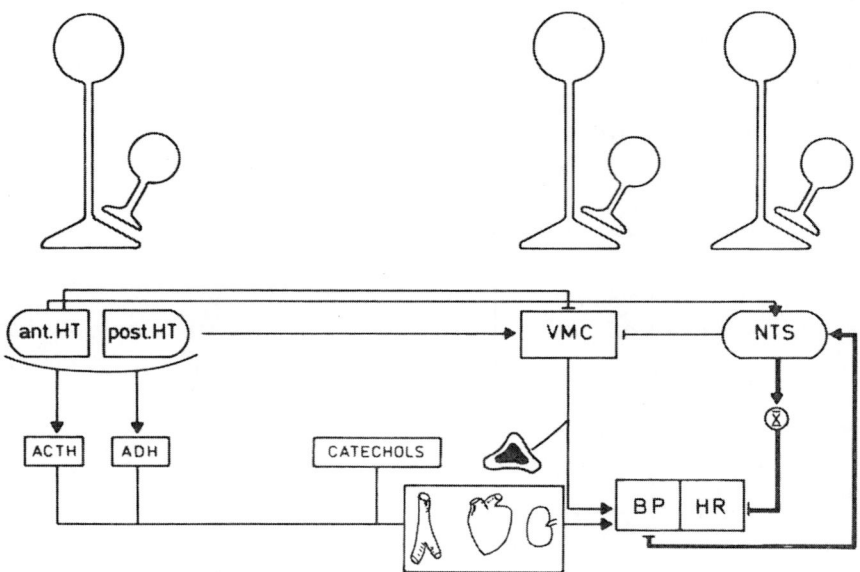

Figure 2. Schematic illustration of the sites and mechanisms of central blood pressure and volume regulation. Ant. HT: anterior hypothalamus; post. HT: posterior hypothalamus; VMC: 'vasomotor center'; NTS: nucleus tractus solitarii, both areas of the medulla oblongata; ACTH: adrenocorticotrophic hormone; ADH: antidiuretic hormone: blood pressure; HR: heart rate. Lines connecting brain areas with each other and with peripheral organs indicate stimulating (→) or inhibitory (–) effects. The lower part on the right depicts the baroreceptor reflex arch with afferent input to the NTS and reflex-induced bradycardia via the vagal nerve (X) and inhibition of sympathetic outflow from other areas of the medulla oblongata ('vasomotor center'). The close morphological and functional association of the baroreceptor reflex pathways with hypothalamic nuclei is also shown. Apart from the baroreceptor reflex, the central cardiovascular control can be mediated through hormones released from the hypothalamic-hypophyseal system (ACTH, ADH) and through the catecholamines released from peripheral nerve endings and the adrenal medulla which act on peripheral target organs (Blood vessel wall, heart, kidney). The schematic neurons of the upper part indicate that modulation of cardiovascular control through brain peptides or other transmitters (E.G., GABA, serotonin, glutamate) may occur at the level of the hypothalamus or the medulla oblongata. The action of the neuromodulator itself may be modified presynaptically by another controlling system. Such a mechanism has, for instance, been described for enkephalins, which can inhibit the release of substance P. Within the hypothalamus, neuromodulators could influence the synthesis and release of hormones or hormone precursors such as ACTH, ADH, oxytocin, neurophysin and others. They may also have a direct excitatory or inhibitory influence on nervous traffic from the hypothalamic to higher or lower brain areas. The blood pressure lowering effects of GABA and GABA agonists as well as their inhibitory action on central peptidergic pressor responses could be explained by such a mechanism. In the medulla oblongata, the neuromodulatory peptides such as the enkephalins or ADH are probably involved in the control of the baroreceptor reflexes, the enkephalins being inhibitory, while ADH possibly augments reflex sensitivity. Both substance P and glutamate can mimic the action of the baroreceptor reflex when applied locally into NTS structures, suggesting a possible role as transmitters in the mediation of the reflex. Neuromodulatory agents may also stimulate or inhibit adrenergic activity at hypothalamic or below hypothalamic sites, thereby modifying the sympathetic outflow to the peripheral organs.

pheral sympathetic ganglia arise, receives a dense input from catecholam-
ine-containing cell groups of the brain stem. A descending spinal noradrenergic projection originates from the so-called A_1 cell group which lies in the
area of the nucleus reticularis lateralis of the medulla oblongata and from
the A_2 cell group located in the nucleus commissuralis and the caudal part
of the NTS. Adrenaline-containing cell groups C_1 and C_2 are located in the
vicinity of the A_1 and A_2 loci. They have been claimed to have descending
projections to the NTS and to the spinal cord as well as ascending projections to several hypothalamic nuclei, the preoptic area and subcortical limbic structures such as amygdala and septum. The noradrenaline-containing
A_5 cell group, close to the olivary nuclei, projects caudally to the sympathetic intermediolateral cell column, to the medial and paramedian reticular
formation, the dorsal motor nucleus of the vagus and the NTS, and cranially
probably to various hypothalamic nuclei as well as to the piriform cortex.
The A_6 cell group, identical with the locus coeruleus, is rich in noradrenaline cells, some of which project caudally and innervate the NTS and other

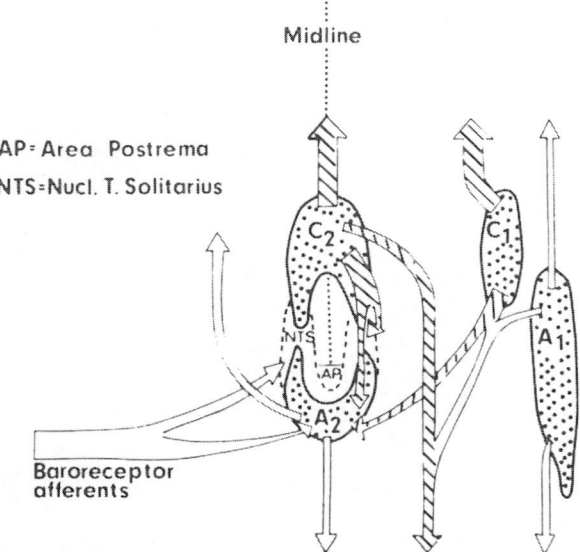

Figure 3. Schematic drawing of a frontal cross-section of the
medulla oblongata showing the noradrenergic areas A_1 and
A_2, the adrenergic areas C_1 and C_2 and their relationship to
the NTS and the area postrema. Interconnections and possible
projections are indicated by the arrows. For localization compare also with Figure 1 (areas 18, 19, 21). Note that the A_2 and
the C_2 cell groups are situated centrally, A_2 forming the caudal
part of the NTS, while the A_1 and C_1 cell groups are localized
more laterally, projecting into the hypothalamus, subcortical
limbic areas and the sympathetic lateral column of the spinal
cord. (Reproduced from Fuxe et al., with kind permission.)

parts of the dorsal caudal medulla oblongata, but the majority of the fibers ascend into higher brain centers. Other catecholaminergic cell groups have been defined in addition; their exact projections and role in blood pressure regulation remain to be investigated.

It has been postulated that a vasodepressor adrenaline system exists within the medulla oblongata, functionally opposed to the noradrenergic pressor system [11]. Evidence supporting this concept stems, for the most part, from pharmacological studies involving the use of alpha- and beta-adrenoceptor-agonists and -antagonists, but the pathophysiological significance of this concept has to be further clarified. Studies with antihypertensive agents such as clonidine, on the other hand, suggest that alpha-adrenoceptor-mediated inhibition of the noradrenergic pressor system, by stimulation of alpha-adrenoceptors in the brain stem and possibly in the posterior hypothalamus, exerts an inhibitory effect on excitatory cardiovascular neurons and thereby causes a decrease of blood pressure [12].

The precise definition of these facilitatory and inhibitory systems remains a major challenge to neuroanatomical and neuropharmacological research. It has been established, however, that neurons involved in central cardiovascular control and catecholaminergic nerves have similar pathways, and it is generally accepted that catecholaminergic neurotransmission plays an important role within central cardiovascular regulation.

The release of noradrenaline from nerve terminals into the synaptic cleft does not only depend on the action potentials that travel down to the nerve endings, but can also be modulated by a number of substances acting on presynaptic structures including the transmitter, noradrenaline, itself. This mechanism is called presynaptic regulation [13].

Apart from noradrenaline acting on alpha-receptors, acetylcholine acting on muscarinic receptors, histamine, enkephalins, some prostaglandins, dopamine, adenosine, and serotonin can, via presynaptic inhibition, decrease the amount of noradrenaline released by a nerve impulse. On the other hand, noradrenaline and adrenaline through beta-adrenoceptors, acetylcholine through nicotine receptors and angiotensin II can all enhance noradrenaline release via presynaptic facilitation.

Since presynaptic regulation can occur at any presynaptic structure within the central nervous system or at peripheral nerve endings, an enormous regulatory potential lies in a mechanism susceptible to such a variety of local influences.

Serotonin (5-hydroxytryptamine)

Evidence suggesting that serotonin may act as a neurotransmitter within cardiovascular control stems from anatomical and neurophysiological studies. It has been shown that the intermediolateral cell column of the spinal cord receives its high content of serotonin from the raphe nuclei of the pons. An inhibitory input to sympathetic paraganglionic neurons by a serotonergic pathway originating from one of the raphe nuclei has been reported. On the other hand, excitatory transmitter actions have been ascribed to serotonin as well, and electrical stimulation of the raphe nuclei has yielded pressor and depressor effects depending on the site of stimulation. Thus, the potential function of serotonin in cardiovascular control awaits further exploration.

Gamma amino butyric acid (GABA)

GABA has been recognized as the major inhibitory neurotransmitter in the brain. Its distribution appears to be discrete within the central nervous system, a characteristic shared by the monoamine transmitters. Concentrations were found to be highest in basal ganglia (substantia nigra, globus pallidus) and in the hypothalamus, the superior and inferior collicular region and in the periaqueductal gray; lower GABA concentrations were found in the pons and in the medulla oblongata. It is noteworthy that brain GABA concentrations in general are high, i.e., in the order of μmoles/g tissue as compared to nmoles/g tissue for many other brain neurotransmitters. The anatomy of the GABA-containing neurons in the mammalian central nervous system has not yet been clearly defined, although recently specific GABAergic input has been described for the nucleus ambiguus and possibly the hypothalamus [14].

Evidence suggesting an inhibitory influence of GABA on cardiovascular functions stems from pharmacological studies. It has been shown that intracerebroventricularly or topically applied GABA or the GABA agonist muscimol produce a hypotensive response which appears to be mediated by reduction of sympathetic outflow. On the other hand, GABA antagonists such as picrotoxin or bicuculline increase blood pressure when applied to the brain. The hypotensive effects of GABA were not affected by interference with central noradrenergic or dopaminergic transmission but attenuated by central acetylcholinergic or serotonergic activation. One could therefore conclude that the GABA effects may rather involve acetylcholinergic or serotonergic transmitter systems than catecholamines, but it has also been reported that GABA can enhance the pressor responses to hypothalamic stimulation through a release of central noradrenaline. Interference with peptidergic blood pressure controlling systems has recently been found in our laboratory: accumulation of endogenous GABA in the brain or application of the GABA agonist muscimol drastically reduced the pressor effects of central angiotensin and inhibited the release of vasopressin.

2. ROLE OF CENTRAL MECHANISMS IN THE BLOOD PRESSURE REGULATION

THOMAS UNGER, WOLFGANG RASCHER, RUDOLF E. LANG and DETLEV GANTEN

This chapter is not meant to provide the reader with a comprehensive review on central blood pressure control mechanisms. We will instead discuss some selected topics on central blood pressure regulation that have recently gained interest due to the discovery of new substances in the brain and due to the introduction of new techniques allowing for more specific investigation of brain structures involved in the transmission of nerve signals within blood pressure controlling pathways.

The following four questions are posed: 1) What is the neuroanatomical basis of central cardiovascular control and what has recently been added to our knowledge in morphology?, 2) What is the functional significance of the different brain areas involved in cardiovascular regulation?, 3) What are the biochemical correlates, i.e., neurotransmitters or neuromodulator systems?, and 4) What is currently known about mutual interactions between these systems within the central blood pressure controlling pathways?

Baroreceptor mechanisms and other reflex circuits are omitted from this chapter; they are dealt with in a separate part of this book. For the same reason, pathophysiological data on the role of the central nervous system in different types of hypertension are limited to a miminum. For more extensive reviews on the topic, the reader is referred to the references given in the reading list.

1. NEUROANATOMICAL BASIS OF CENTRAL CARDIOVASCULAR CONTROL [1–3]

In spite of the accumulation of a wealth of data indicating marked cardiovascular effects following electrical stimulation of various brain areas, a precise definition of the role of the central nervous system in the control of arterial blood pressure and hemodynamics has been lacking. A major reason for this lack of functional concepts resides in the difficulties in studying the neuroanatomical organization of central autonomic pathways. The lesioning of suspected cardiovascular control centers in the brain has not always provided useful information because of many experimental problems. The introduction of two new techniques some years ago advanced our neuroa-

Amery, A. (ed.) Hypertensive Cardiovascular Disease: Pathophysiology and Treatment
© 1982, *Martinus Nijhoff Publishers. The Hague / Boston / London*
ISBN-13: 978-94-009-7478-4

then stimulate specific receptors in the brain. This leads to characteristic cardiovascular, behavioral and neurohumoral effects, namely to an increase in blood pressure, stimulation of salt and water intake, and to a release of the hypothalamic hormones vasopressin (ADH), oxytocin and of ACTH from the pituitary gland. In addition, increases in plasma noradrenaline and adrenaline and a marked natriuretic effect have been observed. The central pressor effect of angiotensin II is partly due to ADH release, and partly due to central sympathetic activation; the latter has been demonstrated not only by experiments with sympathetic blocking agents, but also by the fact that brain angiotensin II can stimulate noradrenaline turnover in the hypothalamus and in the dorsal caudal medulla oblongata (DCMO).

The above mentioned central effects of angiotensin II can (with the exception of natriuresis) also be produced by circulating angiotensin II acting directly on central sites outside the blood brain barrier, which the peptide cannot freely cross. Brain sites sensitive to circulating angiotensin II are the subfornical organ, the organum vasculosum laminae terminalis (OVLT) and the area postrema.

Evidence for a pathophysiological role of brain angiotensin in the maintenance of high blood pressure has mainly been gathered in the spontaneously hypertensive rat. In these animals, increased renin levels have been observed in blood pressure controlling brain areas during the development of hypertension and, at a later stage, the intraventricular administration of specific inhibitors of the renin–angiotensin system has been found to lower the elevated blood pressure.

Opioid peptides

Opioid peptides (endorphins, dynorphins, enkephalins) are widely distributed within the central nervous system. The occurrence of short-chain enkephalins in the hypothalamus and the NTS points towards a participation in central blood pressure control. However, pharmacological studies with centrally applied endorphins and enkephalins have yielded contradictory results with respect to their cardiovascular action depending on the type of peptide, site of application, species or state of consciousness of the animal.

According to the present state of knowledge, the pentapeptide enkephalins seem to be pressor when applied to the brain ventricular system of conscious dogs, cats and rats, but can also induce depressor effects in anesthetized animals. The long-chain opioid peptides such as beta-endorphin, in contrast, appear to be mainly depressor. An interesting finding is that the vagal component of the baroreceptor reflex can be markedly attenuated by central enkephalin treatment. In spontaneously hypertensive rats, a supersensitivity to central enkephalins is observed, and blood pressure can be lowered by central opioid receptor blockade with diprenorphine, suggesting that opioid peptides may, in addition to angiotensin, be involved in the maintenance of high blood pressure in these animals.

Kinins

Bradykinin, a nonapeptide known for its potent vasodilating peripheral action, has been found to exert pressor effects when applied to the brain. These appear to be mediated by cholinergic pathways, but alpha-adrenergic and even histaminergic receptors have been implicated as well. Bradykinin-like immunoreactivity has recently been found in the hypothalamus. The identity of converting enzyme which generates angiotensin II with the kinin-degrading enzyme kininase II closely links the kinin system to the renin-angiotensin system in the periphery and in the brain, but central interactions of both peptide systems remain to be further explored.

Substance P

Substance P is an undecapeptide with a wide distribution within the central and peripheral nervous system. In the central nervous system, particularly high concentrations have been found in the hypothalamus. Substance P has a broad spectrum of biological activities and is traditionally associated with neurotransmission in the perception of pain.

Like bradykinin, this peptide produces potent depressor effects when applied peripherally but has marked pressor activity when applied to the brain ventricular system in conscious and anesthetized animals. The GABA derivative baclofen, β-(4-chlorophenyl)GABA, was shown to inhibit the central pressor responses to substance P almost completely, suggesting a central interaction of GABAergic neurons with those mediating the effects of the peptide. When applied directly to the hypothalamus, substance P augments hypothalamic blood flow. This effect was abolished by a variety of procedures including chemical sympathectomy with 6-hydroxydopamine, adrenoceptor or cholinoreceptor blockade or destruction of a so-called intracerebral noradrenergic pathway [18].

It is conceivable that some peptides like substance P or kinins could exert their central cardiovascular actions by changing blood flow in discrete cardiovascular control centers of the brain, thereby changing the function of, e.g., hypothalamic circuits, whereas such a mechanism seems less likely for angiotensin.

From pharmacological studies, it can be concluded that the central blood pressure responses to substance P are mediated by the sympathetic nervous system. In contrast to angiotensin II, this peptide has not been found to release ADH when applied centrally, although increases of vasopressinergic neuron activity in the nucleus supraopticus after intraventricular injection of substance P have been reported. Based on neuroanatomical and pharmacological findings, it has been claimed that substance P is a transmitter in the first synapse of the baroreceptor reflex arch within the NTS. However, this is still a matter of controversy, particularly since such a role has also been attributed to glutamate [19].

4. SIGNIFICANCE OF CENTRAL BLOOD PRESSURE CONTROL

Anatomical structures and biochemical correlates, which take part in the brain-mediated control of the cardiovascular system, have been presented in the foregoing parts of this chapter. The functional significance of these central pathways is undisputed, but it is not generally agreed upon whether the central cardiovascular control mechanisms are necessary under all circumstances for the homeostasis of cardiovascular function. This has, indeed, been questioned for several reasons [20]. It has, for example, been pointed out that, in animals with the nervous system either totally or partially destroyed, parameters such as local blood flow, cardiac output, blood volume and even arterial blood pressure over long periods of time can be precisely controlled in the total absence of the nervous system. According to this view, only four important control functions have been conceded to the nervous system that cannot be performed by other intrinsic control systems, namely 1) the control of fluid and electrolyte intake, 2) acute control of arterial pressure, 3) acute control of blood volume and 4) acute control of the heart's pumping capacity. Thus, with the exception of the nervous drive for water and electrolyte intake, which is a continuous necessity, the role of the nervous system in circulatory control would not appear to be that of the regular government but rather that of an emergency police squad which helps the organism to overcome acute threats to circulatory homeostasis or regain law and order, i.e., normal blood pressure and blood volume whenever they have been put out of order by stress, injury, blood loss or other intruding factors.

Although this is an attractive view based on impressive experimental data, it does not take into account the great number of observations that point towards an eminent integrating and control function of the nervous system not only in short-term but also in long-term cardiovascular regulation. Only a few can be mentioned here. It is known that emotional and behavioral factors can influence blood pressure to a large extent. Sustained hypertension has been produced in experimental animals by stressing procedures such as avoidance conditioning, long-term aversive conflict situa-

32

tions or psychosocial stress. Studies in man have linked certain personality patterns to hypertension and have demonstrated that emotional response patterns such as anger or frustration often produce the cardiovascular changes seen in hypertension. Moreover, the elevated blood pressure can return to lower values if an opportunity is provided to express and release the anger. In addition, the distinct cardiovascular changes associated with emotional behavior that have been shown to be generated in hypothalamic and limbic brain areas, underline the important pacemaker role of the central nervous system in cardiovascular adaptation. Other examples include the antihypertensive potency of drugs interfering almost exclusively with the central nervous system such as clonidine, reserpine or alpha-methyldopa. The fact that certain types of experimental hypertension even of renal origin can be prevented by central chemical sympathectomy with 6-hydroxydopamine also points to the sympathetic nervous system as an important regultor of arterial blood pressure.

In conclusion, there is no doubt that blood pressure is closely controlled by the relationship of effective blood volume and diameter of the vascular bed, i.e., peripheral resistance, the main direct regulators of which are the kidney, the resistance blood vessels and the heart. It is also evident, however, that the function of these primary and other secondary blood pressure-regulating peripheral organs is controlled and integrated by the brain. This is achieved by the projections of the brain into the periphery which are the sympathetic and parasympathetic nervous system and the hypothalamic and pituitary hormones. The brain structures, neurotransmitters and possible mechanisms involved in the control of the activity of these peripheral mediators of brain function in relationship to blood pressure regulation, were the subjects of this chapter.

REFERENCES

1. Loewy AD, McKellar S: The neuroanatomical basis of central cardiovascular control. Fed proc 39:2495–2503, 1980.
2. U.S. Department of Health, Education and Welfare: Report of the Hypertension Task Force. Vol. 4: Current Research and Recommendations from the Task Force Subgroup on 'Neural Control of the Circulation', 'Vascular Smooth Muscle, Nerve Terminals'. NIH Publication No. 79-1626, 1979.
3. Smith OA: Reflex and central mechanisms involved in the control of the heart and circulation. Ann Rev Physiol 36:93–123, 1974.
4. Dittmar C: Über die Lage des sogenannten Gefäßzentrums in der Medulla oblongata. Ber. Verh. Sächs. Ges. Wiss. Leipzig, Math. Phys. Kl. 25:449–469, 1873.
5. Stock G, Schlör KH, Heidt H, Buss J: Psychomotor behavior and cardiovascular patterns during stimulation of the amygdala. Pflüger's Arch 376:177–184, 1978.
6. Korner PI: Integrative neural cardiovascular control. Physiol Rev 51:312, 1971.
7. Smith OA, Astley CA, DeVito JL, Stein JM, Walsh KE: Functional analysis of hypothal-

amic control of the cardiovascular responses accompanying emotional behavior. Fed Proc 39:2487–1494, 1980.

8. Cooper JR, Bloom FE, Roth RH (eds): The Biochemical Basis of Neuropharmacology. New York: Oxford University Press, 1978.
9. Chalmers JP: Nervous system and Hypertension. Clin Sci Mol Med 55:45s–56s, 1978.
10. Ganten D, Stock G: Humoral and neurohormonal aspects of blood pressure regulation. Klin Wochenschr 56 (Suppl I):31–41, 1978.
11. Fuxe K, Bolme P, Agnati LF, Jonsson G, Andersson K, Köhler C, Hökfelt T: On the role of central adrenaline neurons in central cardiovascular regulation. In: Central Adrenaline Neurons. Wenner-Gren Center International Symposium Series, Vol. 33, pp. 161–182. Fuxe K et al., eds; Oxford: Pergamon 1980.
12. Isaac L: Clonidine and the central nervous system: site and mechanism of action. J Cardiovasc Pharmacol 2 (Suppl I):S5–S19, 1980.
13. Langer SZ: Presynaptic receptors and their role in the regulation of transmitter release. Br J Pharmacol 60:481–497, 1977.
14. Persson B: GABAergic mechanisms in blood pressure control, a pharmacological analysis in the rat. Acta Physiol Scand (Suppl) 491, 1980.
15. Hökfelt T, Elde R, Johansson O, Ljungdahl A, Schultzberg M, Fuxe K, Goldstein M, Nilsson G, Pernow P, Terenius L, Ganten D, Jeffcoate SL, Rehfeld J, Said S: Distribution of peptide containing neurons. In: Psychopharmacology, a Generation of Progress, pp. 39–66. Lipton MA, DiMascio A, Killam KF, eds. New York: Raven Press, 1978.
16. Schelling P, Speck G, Unger Th, Ganten D: The brain renin-angiotensin system: biochemistry, localization and functional aspects. In: Advances in experimental Medicine: A Centenary Tribute to Claude Bernard, pp. 243–288. Parvez H, Parvez S, eds. Amsterdam: Elsevier/North-Holland Biomedical Press, 1980.
17. Unger Th, Rockhold RW, Yukimura T, Rettig R, Rascher W, Ganten D: Role of kinins and substance P in blood pressure regulation of normotensive and spontaneously hypertensive rats. In: Central Nervous system Mechanisms in Hypertension, pp. 115–129. Buckley JP, Ferrario CM, eds. New York: Raven Press, 1981.
18. Klugman KP, Lembeck F, Markowitz S, Mitchell G, Rosendorff C: Substance P increases hypothalamic blood flow via an indirect adrenergic–cholinergic interaction. Br J Pharmacol 71:623–629, 1980.
19. Reis DJ, Tallman WF, Peroni M: Role of glutamate in the regulation of arterial pressure mediated through the nucleus tractus solitarii (NTS). In: Central Nervous System Mechanisms in Hypertension, pp. 37–48. Buckley JP, Ferrario CM eds. New York: Raven Press, 1981.
20. Guyton AC, Cowley JR, Young DB, Coleman TG, Hall JE, De Clue JW: Integration and control of circulatory function. In: Intern REV Physiol: Cardiovascular Physiology II, Vol. 9, pp. 341–385. Guyton AC, Cowley AW, eds. Baltimore: University Press, 1976.

3. ARTERIAL BAROREFLEXES IN NORMOTENSIVE AND HYPERTENSIVE MAN

GIUSEPPE MANCIA and ALBERTO ZANCHETTI

In the past thirty years a large body of experimental evidence has been collected on the cardiovascular control reflexly exerted by the arterial baroreceptors. Studies in both conscious and anaesthetized animals of several species have shown that: (1) this control is of paramount importance for insuring blood pressure stability and homeostasis under a variety of normal circumstances; (2) it is exerted to an important degree both by baroreceptors in the carotid sinuses and in the aorta; (3) it is not similar for these two reflexogenic areas and does not involve all cardiovascular target organs to a quantitatively similar extent; and (4) it is modified, often to a marked degree, in a number of pathological conditions [1].

However, little of this information has been directly verified in man, the reason being primarily the lack of suitable methods of study. Few satisfactory techniques are available in this field. The one most extensively used consists of altering the activity of the arterial baroreceptors by injecting vasopressor and vasodepressor drugs [2, 3]. This allows exploration of the baroreceptor control of heart rate (and also of other cardiac functions), but obviously it does not offer any information on the reflex control of blood pressure and more generally of peripheral circulation. Another technique makes use of the Valsalva manoeuvre. Although in this instance measurements have been made of both the cardiac and vasomotor reflex responses [4] there is no doubt that a major drawback is the complexity of the stimulus that is being applied to the various reflexogenic areas, which prevents the contribution of the arterial baroreflexes to be selectively sorted out. Another technique consists of reducing central blood volume and arterial blood pressure by application of negative pressure to the lower half of the body [5, 6]. This allows measurement of reflex changes in some vascular beds (those of the upper side of the body) as well as in the heart, and also exploration of possible differences between reflex control exerted by receptors in the high and low pressure areas. However, only one side of the reflexes (i.e. reduction in receptor activity) can be investigated. Moreover, in these circumstances no reflex blood pressure responses can be assessed.

A fourth technique for studying reflex control of circulation in human subjects is the variable pressure neck chamber [7]. This technique consists

Amery, A. (ed.) Hypertensive Cardiovascular Disease: Pathophysiology and Treatment
© *1982, Martinus Nijhoff Publishers. The Hague / Boston / London*
ISBN-13: 978-94-009-7478-4

of the use of a plastic collar with double rubber valves which adhere below to the shoulders and above, to the chin, the ear lobes and the occiput of the subjects. Pneumatic pressure inside the chamber can be altered in a positive and in a negative direction with corresponding reduction and increase in transmural pressure across the carotid arteries, and therefore with corresponding reduction and increase in the activity of the carotid sinus baroreceptors. This technique allows the study of reflex control from a baroreceptor area of paramount importance, and the estimation of a large number of reflex effects, which include arterial blood pressure. In addition, the reflex function can be evaluated over a range of baroreceptor activities from below to above the existing level.

In the past few years we have applied the variable pressure neck chamber technique in normotensive subjects and in subjects with arterial hypertension, while measuring blood pressure and other reflex responses. As a result a number of data have been collected on the characteristics of the carotid baroreceptor reflex in normal conditions and in conditions in which blood pressure is chronically elevated. A description of these data is provided in the following pages, along with other data in which other techniques were used, in combination with the neck chamber or alone, to enlarge our information on reflex circulatory control in human beings.

THE VARIABLE PRESSURE NECK CHAMBER TECHNIQUE

Before applying the variable pressure neck chamber in systematic studies a number of theoretical uncertainties about the technique were investigated [9]. For example, we observed that application of positive chamber pressure up to 60 mm Hg did not cause a reduction in cerebral blood flow, thus ruling out the possibility that cerebral ischemia was involved in the genesis of the cardiovascular response to be measured. We also gained evidence against a participation of the carotid chemoreceptors in the reflex changes that could be observed. Most importantly, however, we were able to determine the amount of positive and negative neck chamber pressures that are transmitted through the neck tissues to the region of the carotid sinuses. This point was investigated by applying a series of different positive and negative pressures within the neck chamber, while simultaneously measuring pressure from a tissue catheter placed close to the walls of a carotid sinus. The results of 10 subjects (6 normotensives and 4 hypertensives) studied in this way are shown in Figure 1 [9]. There was a very strict linear relationship between changes in positive or negative neck chamber pressure and changes in neck tissue pressure ($r > 0.989$, $p < 0.001$, in each subject). However, transmission, though prompt, was incomplete since 86% of the positive neck chamber pressure, and only 64% of the negative one were on average transmitted to the tissue catheter. It can be noticed from the confi-

36

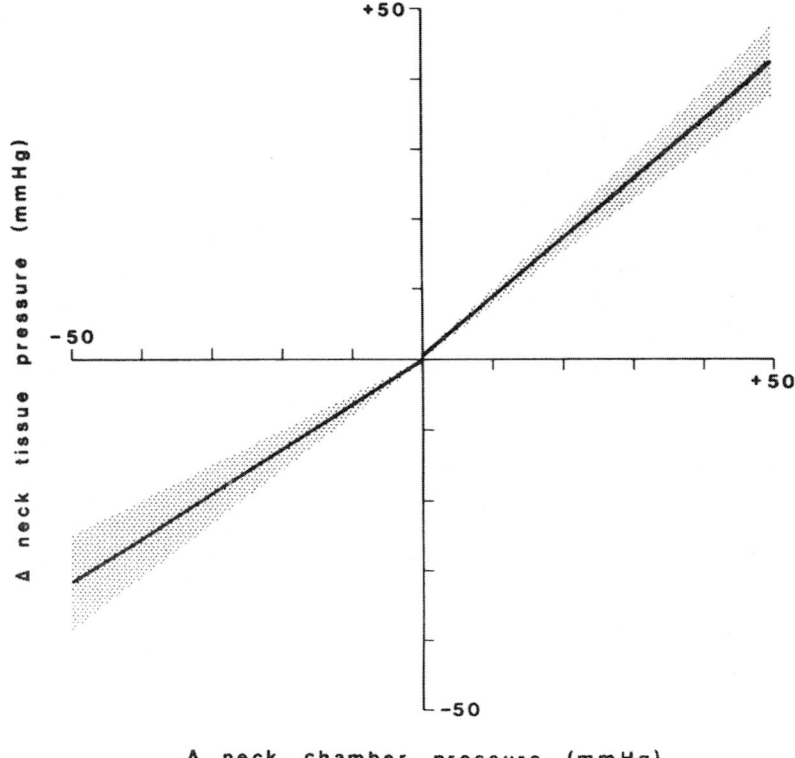

Figure 1. The relation of change in neck chamber pressure to change in tissue pressure adjacent to a carotid sinus. Separate mean regression lines and 90% confidence limits are shown for positive and negative applied pressures. Each of the lines and its limits was constructed from the individual calculated regressions of 10 subjects (5 to 10 observations for each regression in each subject). (from [9], with permission.)

dence limits shown in Figure 1 that individual regression coefficients were close to the means. These can therefore be meaningfully used as correction factors for the applied pneumatic pressures in order to achieve a more correct estimation of the stimuli applied to the carotid baroreceptors under the various circumstances of the study.

CAROTID BARORECEPTOR REFLEX IN NORMOTENSIVE SUBJECTS

Reflex effects of carotid baroreceptors on blood pressure and heart rate were investigated in 11 normotensive subjects whose mean age was 36 ± 4 years [10]. In each subject a series of 4–6 negative and 4–6 positive neck chamber pressures were applied within the range of ± 50 mm Hg. Each stimulus was maintained for 2 min, its reflex effects being evaluated both

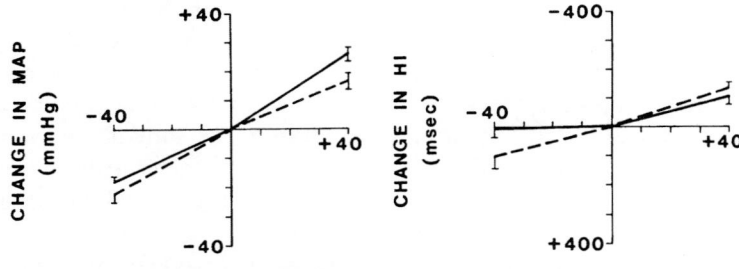

Figure 2. Changes in mean arterial pressure (MAP) and R–R interval (HI) induced by changes in tissue pressure outside the carotid sinuses (neck tissue pressure). Data are shown as means ±SE of individual regression coefficients in 11 subjects. The dashed line represents the early response (average of the values between the 5th and the 15th s following the change in neck tissue pressure) and the continuous line the steady-state response (the average value that occurred in the last 30 sec of the change in neck tissue pressure). Changes in neck tissue pressure were calculated from changes in neck chamber pressure, using correction figures for pressure transmission through neck tissue (see text). (From [10], with permission.)

shortly after stimulus application and in the last phase of it (for their characteristics, these responses were called 'early or transient' and 'late or steady-state', respectively). In almost each circumstance the magnitude of the applied stimulus and the resulting response displayed a linear relationship, which allowed us to take the regression coefficient as the measure of the reflex function.

The results of our study on normotensive subjects are summarized in Figure 2, which shows the relationship between changes in tissue pressure outside the carotid sinuses and resulting changes in mean arterial pressure and heart rate (expressed as R–R interval). The data are represented as means ± standard errors of the regression coefficients obtained in the individual subjects, the dashed lines representing the early responses and the continuous lines the steady-state responses.

Three findings are worth mentioning. Firstly, heart rate responses were not invariably sustained throughout the duration of the stimulus; in particular the bradycardia accompanying the negative neck chamber pressure, though evident in the early phase, almost disappeared in the late phase. Secondly, blood pressure changes were invariably sustained throughout the duration of the stimulus, as indicated by the fact that the steady-state responses were either greater than or similar to the early responses. Thirdly, the responses obtained with positive neck pressures were greater than those with negatives neck pressures, a finding which was particularly significant during the steady-state. The latter result in in line with that obtained by other investigators [11] and we have discussed elsewhere two hypotheses that can explain it [12]. One is that carotid baroreceptors discharge at basal blood pressure near their maximal level, thus making the decrease in baroreceptor firing induced by a decrease in carotid transmural pressure greater than the increase in baroreceptor firing induced by an increase in carotid transmural pressure. This must not be regarded as unlikely because the carotid sinuses have thin and well-compliant walls that can be easily distended by the pulse pressure wave to provide a strong stimulus for the local stretch receptors. A second hypothesis is that what has been speculated for the carotid baroreceptors (near-maximal stimulus provided by the existing blood pressure value) does in fact occur for the aortic (or cardio-aortic) baroreceptors. In this case the depressor response induced by an increase in carotid baroreceptor activity would be more effectively buffered than the pressor response induced by the decrease in carotid baroreceptor activity, thus accounting for the asymmetry that we observed. However, this is less likely for a number of reasons, viz. the fact that the aortic walls are much less compliant than the carotid sinuses, that no asymmetry of this sort has ever been shown in animals (if anything, the aortic baroreceptors have been shown to be close to threshold at normal blood pressure values), and that no pressor response ensues in normotensive humans if the ongoing cardioaortic baroreceptor influence is suddenly eliminated by vagal anaesthesia [13].

It seems likely therefore that the asymmetry we and Thron et al. [11] have observed refers to a peculiar role of the carotid baroreflex, which in human being with normal blood pressure levels may well have a greater ability to counteract a decrease rather than an increase in carotid transmural pressure, thus acting as a more effective anti-hypotensive than anti-hypertensive mechanisms.

CAROTID BARORECEPTOR REFLEX IN SUBJECTS WITH ARTERIAL HYPERTENSION

The carotid baroreceptor reflex was studied in a population of 35 subjects with essential hypertension (mean age 45 ± 5 years). The study was conducted in the same way as for the normotensives and the results are represented in Figure 3. As for the normotensives means $\pm$ standard errors of individual regression coefficients are shown, the dashed and continuous lines representing the early and steady-state responses respectively.

In this case three major conclusions were reached. Firstly, the carotid baroreceptor reflex continues to have a homeostatic role in essential hypertension, as reduction and increase in carotid baroreceptor activity both cause reflex responses linearly related to the stimuli. Secondly, also in hypertensive subjects there is a significant asymmetry of the reflex, but the asymmetry is opposite to that observed in normotensives and consists of

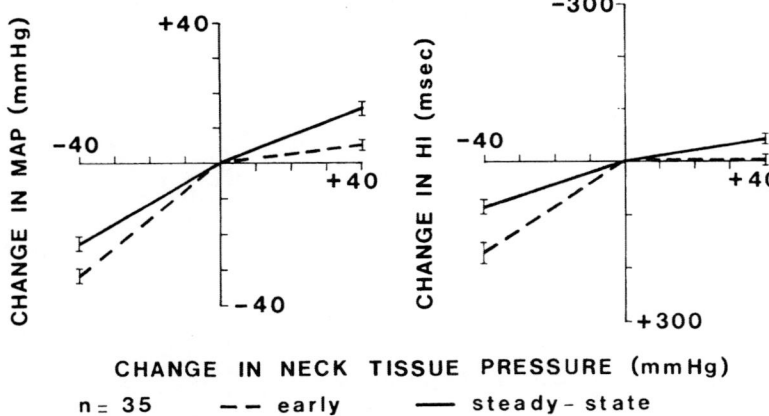

Figure 3. Changes in mean arterial pressure (MAP) and R–R interval (HI) induced by changes in tissue pressure outside the carotid sinuses (neck tissue pressure). Data are shown as means ±SE of individual regression coefficients in 35 subjects with essential hypertension. All Symbols and details as in Figure 2. For further explanation see text. (From [18], with permission.)

greater responses to increase rather than to decrease in carotid sinus transmural pressure. This means that in essential hypertension there is a reset of the baroreceptor reflex which favours its anti-hypertensive function.

Thirdly, not only differences in shape but also differences in magnitude of the reflex functions exist between normotensives and patients with essential hypertension. By comparison of the two sets of data with the unpaired T test, the responses to reduction in carotid transmural pressure appear to be less in hypertensives than in normotensives, while the responses to increase in carotid transmural pressure appear to be greater. This point is further developed in Figures 4 and 5 which show individual regression coefficients (expressing the magnitude of the reflex responses) as a function of the individual basal mean arterial pressure for three separate groups of subjects defined as normotensive, moderate and severe hypertensive (Figure 4) and for the whole group of normotensive and hypertensive subjects taken together (Figure 5). It is clear that these two variables were linearly related. That is, the depressor response to increase in carotid transmural pressure became progressively greater as mean arterial pressure moved from the lowest to the highest values, while the pressor response to reduction in carotid transmural pressure showed an opposite pattern.

Again, the hypotheses that can be made to explain these findings have been discussed in detail elsewhere [12]. One of them is clarified by expressing the data as in Figure 6 and by applying to them the scheme of Figure 7. In brief, it can be suggested that the progressively reversing asymmetry that the carotid baroreflex shows in going from normotensive to mild and more

40

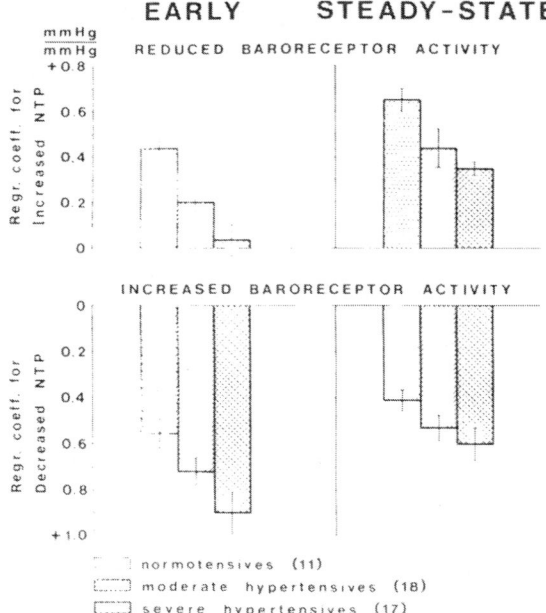

Figure 4. Carotid baroreceptor influence on blood pressure in 11 normotensive, 18 moderately hypertensive and 17 more severely hypertensive subjects. The data are shown as the averages (± standard error) of individual regression coefficients (regr. Coeff.) relating changes in mean arterial pressure (mmHg) to changes in tissue pressure outside the carotid sinuses (NTP, mmHg). Data for increased NTP, i.e. reduced baroreceptor activity, are shown at the top, data for decreased NTP, i.e. increased baroreceptor activity at the bottom; both early (left panels) and late or steady-state responses (right panels) are shown. (From [18], with permission.)

severe hypertensive subjects is due to the fact that under these circumstances the basal blood pressure level becomes a progressively less effective stimulus for the carotid baroreceptors. In normotensive subjects the basal blood pressure level may be capable of inducing a near-maximal carotid baroreceptor activation (see above) thereby allowing large decreases but only small further increases in the receptor activity to occur with the use of the neck chamber. In hypertensive subjects, however, the stimulus provided by the basal blood pressure may become progressively less effective and finally it may just move above the baroreceptor threshold, creating conditions in which smaller decreases but now larger increases in the receptor activity can be produced by the neck chamber. This is tantamount to suggesting that the carotid baroreflex undergoes a resetting in essential hyper-

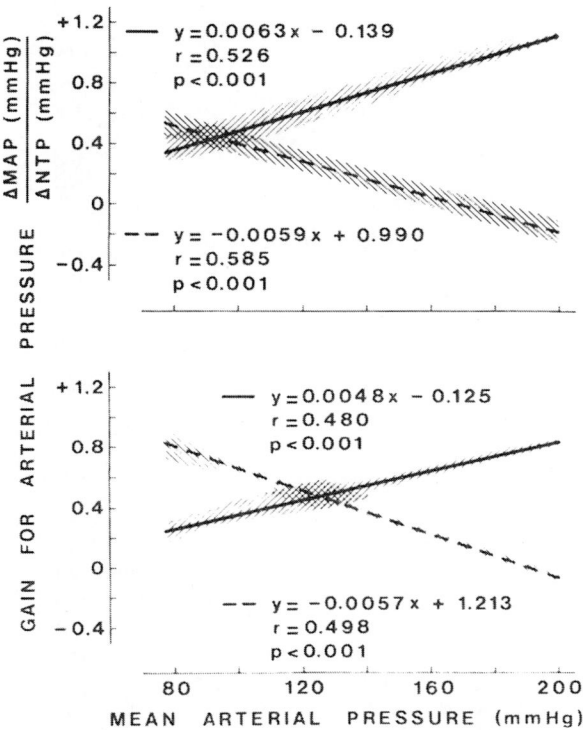

Figure 5. Relation between regression coefficients for mean arterial pressure (gain) and basal mean arterial pressure in 11 normotensive and 35 hypertensive subjects. The gain is expressed as changes in mean arterial pressure (MAP) induced by changes in tissue pressure outside the carotid sinuses (NTP); the early response is shown in the upper panel, and the late or steady-state response in the lower panel. Gains for reflex responses to increased baroreceptor activity are indicated by the continuous lines, gains for reflex responses to reduced baroreceptor activity by the dashed lines. The hatched areas represent the standard errors of the regressions. The equations of the regressions are also shown (p: probability; r: correlation coefficient). (From [12], with permission.)

tension and that such resetting is so marked that it does not limit itself to maintain the set-point of the reflex along the stimulus–response curve but actually moves it in a direction opposite to that which is predictable on the basis of the increasing pressure stimulus. A resetting of the baroreceptors in hypertension has been repeatedly shown in animal hypertensive models [14–16] and it may well be that the larger duration of human hyperten-

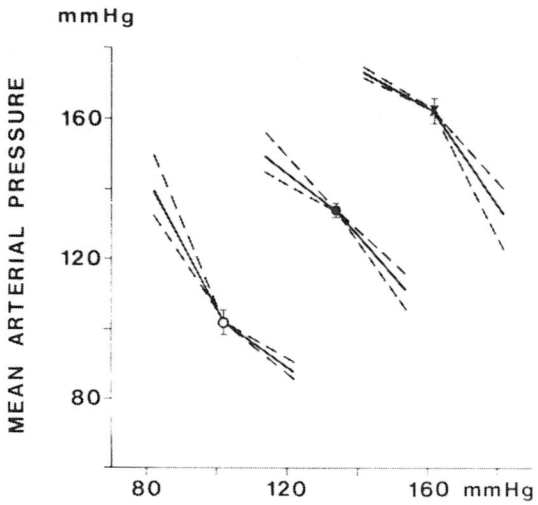

Figure 6. Carotid baroreceptor influence on blood pressure in the same three groups of subjects of Figure 4. The open circle, the closed circle and the cross represent the average (± standard error) mean arterial pressure during the control period in each group, respectively. The continuous lines represent the average of individual regression coefficients relating mean arterial pressure to increased or decreased carotid transmural pressure with respect to control values, the dashed lines indicating the standard errors of the regressions. The data are shown for the late or steady-state effects of the neck chamber, the carotid transmural pressure being calculated as the difference between the mean arterial pressure and the tissue pressure outside the carotid sinuses. (From [18], with permission.)

sion makes it an even more prominent event that it was originally supposed.

To date a controversial issue has been the change in the baroreflex sensitivity induced by essential hypertension. While there is no doubt that the sensitivity of the baroreceptor control of heart rate is reduced in this disease [2, 17] (and our data would suggest that this is so because of an impairment of aortic baroreflexes, see below), there are data which suggest that carotid sinus reflex control of blood pressure may be better preserved [18–21]. This may be due to the fact that in hypertension an increased wall to lumen ratio enhances the responses of the arterioles to sympathetic stimuli [22]. However, recent findings suggest that more complex reasons may be involved in this phenomenon. For example, in spontaneously hypertensive rats not only blood vessels [23], but also efferent sympathetic activity was

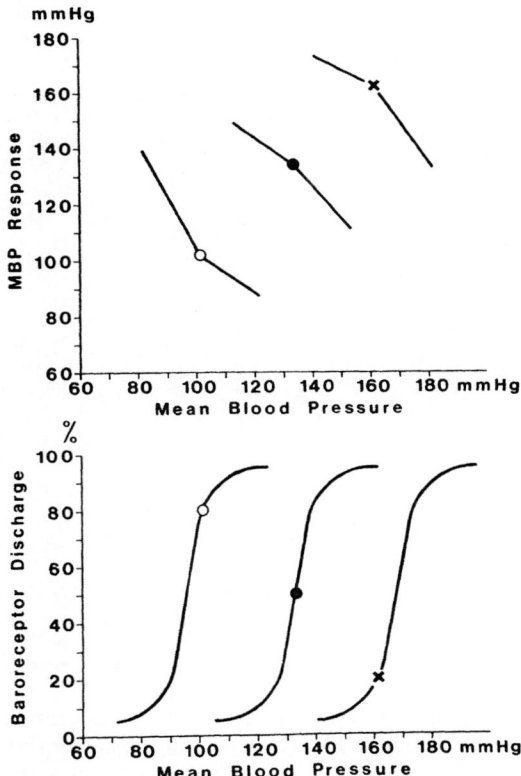

Figure 7. Schematic drawing of the stimulus–response curves relating arterial blood pressure with carotid baroreceptor firing. The set-point of the reflex (i.e. the point corresponding to the stimulus provided by the existing blood pressure) may be located nearby baroreceptor saturation in normotensive subjects (line to the left) and migrate progressively towards the baroreceptor threshold in moderate and severe hypertension.

found to be normally modulated by arterial baroreceptors [24]. Furthermore, the blood pressure response to carotid baroreceptor stimulation was unchanged, and the heart rate response largely impaired, even after an acute rise in blood pressure was produced by isometric exercise (Figure 8) [25, 26]. This suggests that the differential effect of hypertension on the heart rate and the blood pressure components of the baroreflex may be produced at least in part at a central level [27].

At any rate our data have a number of clinical implications. For example the greater response to increase in carotid transmural pressure that we found in hypertensives suggests a better protection of these subjects against further

44

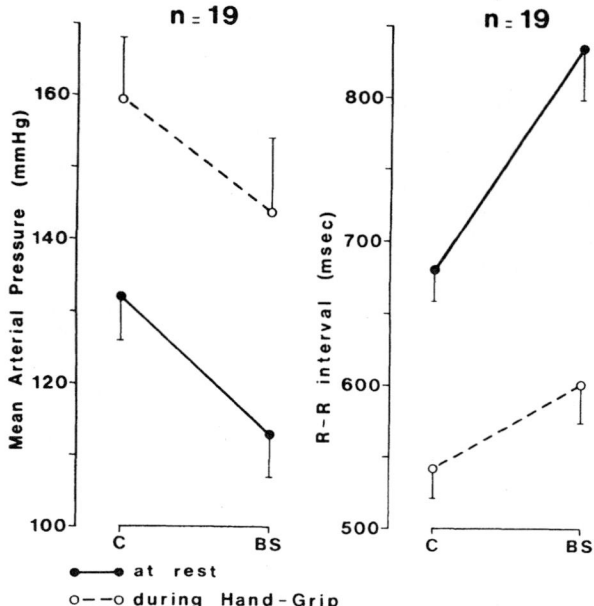

Figure 8. Reduction in mean arterial pressure and increase in R-R interval induced by stimulating the carotid baroreceptors at rest and during and isometric exercise (hand-grip). Data are shown as means $\pm$ SE from 19 subjects with essential hypertension. The stimulus to the carotid baroreceptors was provided by a neck-chamber-induced reduction in neck tissue pressure outside the carotid sinuses of 28.5 ± 1.6 mmHg at rest and of 29.4 ± 1.9 mmHg during hand-grip. C: control; BS: during baroreceptor stimulation. Note that during hand-grip the R-R interval responses to baroreceptor stimulation were markedly reduced, while the blood pressure responses were largely preserved. (From [26], with permission.)

sudden rises in pressure above the already high existing levels. On the other hand, the blunted response to reduction in carotid transmural pressure should leave hypertensive subjects less resistant to the effects of haemorrhage and perhaps explains why they are more prone to orthostatic hypotension [28]. This decrease in the reflex function favours antihypertensive therapy, in that attempts at pharmacological reductions of blood pressure should in theory be facilitated by attenuation of a negative feed-back system controlling this variable. A further facilitation of the effects of antihypertensive drugs may come from the baroreflex resetting that seems to be produced by several antihypertensive agents (see below).

Three other topics we have investigated in subjects with arterial hypertension will be briefly mentioned. One refers to reflex changes in cardiac output and total peripheral resistance induced by increase and decrease in

Table 1. Haemodynamic responses to changes in neck chamber pressure in 27 subjects with essential hypertension *

	Control	Decrease in NTP	Control	Increase in NTP
Mean arterial pressure (mmHg)	139.3±3.8	121.9 ±4.2	137.1 ±3.9	153.1 ±4.0
Cardiac output (L/min)	6.20±0.23	5.77±0.24	6.12±0.25	6.11±0.29
Total peripheral resistance (Units)	23.3±1.0	22.1 ±1.0	22.8 ±1.1	26.6±1.3

* Data are shown as means ±SE. Cardiac Output was measured during the steady-state phase of the blood pressure responses to the decrease and increase in neck tissue pressure (NTP) which amounted to $-35.8±0.8$ and $32.6±1.0$ mmHg.

the activity of the carotid baroreceptors. This point was examined in 27 subjects with essential hypertension in whom cardiac output (thermodilution technic) was measured before and during the steady-state phase of the blood pressure response to changes in neck chamber pressure over ±40 mm Hg [12]. The results (Table 1) indicate that the depressor responses to increases in carotid transmural pressure can be accounted for both by reduction in cardiac output and by decrease in total peripheral resistance. On the other hand, the pressor responses to reductions in carotid transmural pressure are not associated with any increase in cardiac output, and therefore appear to be caused entirely by an increase in total peripheral resistance. These findings reveal a major difference with the patterns of response observed by other investigators in normotensives, as in the latter subjects an increase in cardiac output was found to be the major cause for the reflex pressor response. It may be that subjects with established hypertension have less ability to increase cardiac output in face of an increasing afterload above the already elevated existing level.

A second topic is related to the possibility that carotid baroreceptors reflexly influence secretion of renin from the kidney. It has long been established that renin secretion can be powerfully modified by neural factors [29] and recent evidence has involved various reflexes in renin control [30–33]. However, in this case, too, information refers to animal experiments with hardly any direct evidence in man.

In our study [34] 11 supine patients with essential hypertension were fitted with the neck chamber while they were having catheterisation of the aorta and a renal vein for clinical reasons. Positive and negative neck chamber pressures (all above ±40 mm Hg) were applied for 5 min, and plasma renin activity was measured by radioimmunoassay from blood samples withdrawn via the catheters before and during the 5th minute of pressure application. Basal values of plasma renin activity from the aorta and a renal vein were 0.30 ± 0.06 and 0.40 ± 0.10 ng/ml/h. These values became 0.34 ± 0.10 and 0.44 ± 0.15 ng/ml/h during application of negative, and 0.32 ± 0.08 and 0.47 ± 0.10 during application of positive neck chamber pressure. Only the last difference (plasma renin activity in the renal vein before and during positive neck pressure) was statistically sigificant at $p<0.05$, though this difference was indeed very small. In 5 of the 11 subjects the results obtained with application of positive neck pressures, were compared to those obtained with 5 min of head-up tilting (Figure 9). This was done because tilting reduces central blood volume as well as arterial blood pressure at the carotid sinus level, and thus deactivates a much larger pop-

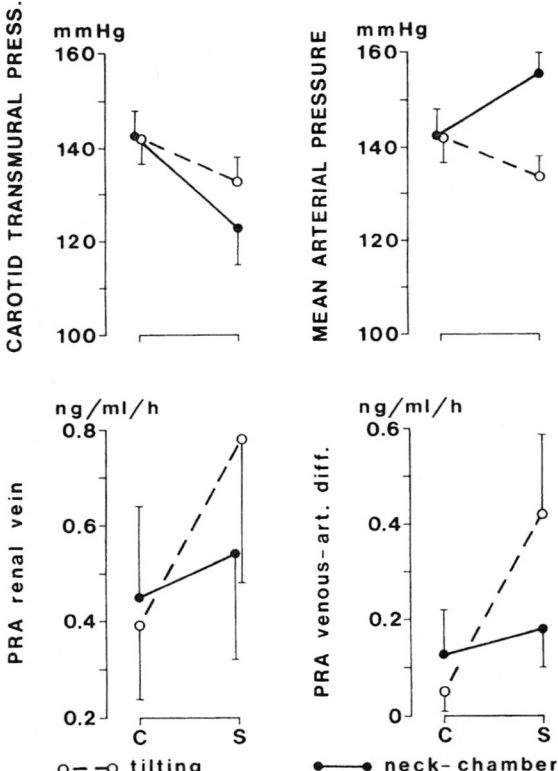

Figure 9. Effects of head-up tilting (broken lines) and application of positive pressures in the neck chamber (continuous lines) on plasma renin in 5 patients with essential hypertension. Results are shown as means $\pm$ SE. C: values during control; S: values during 5 minutes of tilting or positive neck pressure; PRA: plasma renin activity; venous-art. diff.: difference in PRA between a renal vein and the aorta.

ulation of receptors than the positive neck chamber application. With tilting, plasma renin activity from the renal vein increased significantly and markedly, though the calculated reduction in carotid transmural pressure was not greater than that induced by the neck chamber. Similar findings were obtained in hypertensive subjects with a high renin secretion (Figure 10) [35, 36]. From these data we concluded that the carotid baroreceptors do not exert a relevant control of renin release in essential hypertension. A reflex control of renin is present in this condition, but is likely to be due to receptors in the low pressure area.

The third topic refers to possible differences of the carotid baroreceptor reflex function in the different forms of hypertension. This was investigated by comparing the carotid baroreceptor control of blood pressure in renovascular vs. essential hypertension [25]. The results indicated that whenever age and basal blood pressure values of the subjects match there is no major

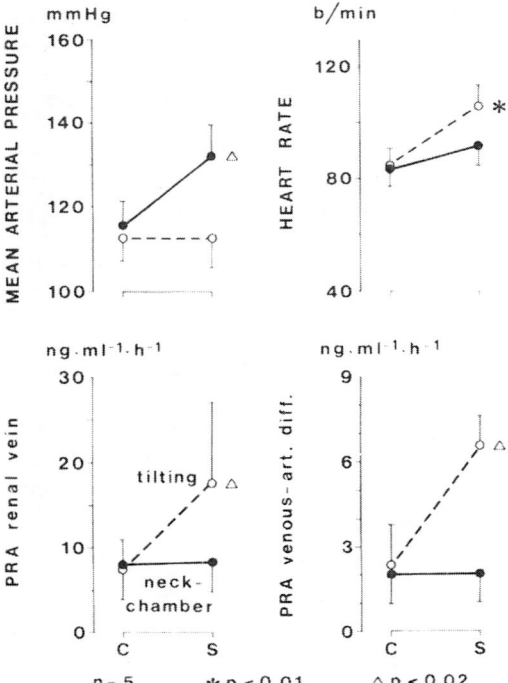

Figure 10. Effects of head-up tilting (broken lines) and applications of positive pressures in the neck chamber (continuous lines) on plasma renin in 5 patients with essential hypertension and high renin secretion rates induced by a short-lasting administration of diuretic (Chlorthalidone 50 mg for 3 days). Results are shown as means ± SE. Symbols as in Figure 9.

48

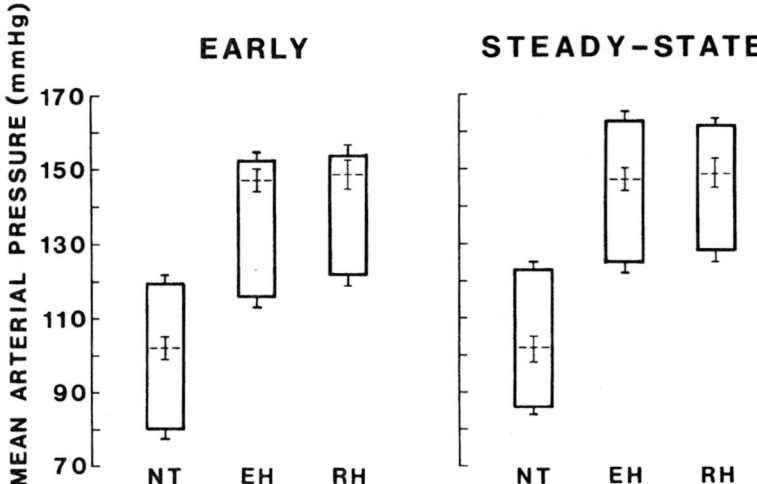

Figure 11. The histograms represent the reflex changes in mean arterial pressure induced by altering carotid transmural pressure approximately from −20 to +20 mmHg with respect to the baseline level. Data are shown as means (±SE) of a group of 11 normotensive subjects (NT), 35 subjects with essential hypertension (EH) and 18 subjects with renovascular hypertension (RH). The broken line within each histogram represents the baseline blood pressure value before the increase or the reduction caused respectively the reduction and the increase in carotid transmural pressure. The blood pressure changes observed during the early and the late or steady-state response to the alterations in baroreceptor activity are separately shown. Note that both in EH and RH subjects the pressor responses were reduced and the depressor responses increased with respect to the NT subjects. The magnitude of the reflex blood pressure excursion was not significantly different in the EH and RH subjects as compared to NT subjects.

difference in the baroreflexes of these two pathological conditions (Figure 11). This suggests that a secondary rather than primary phenomenon may be largely responsible for the baroreflex modifications that can be observed at elevated blood pressure values in human beings.

CAROTID BARORECEPTOR REFLEX DURING ANTIHYPERTENSIVE THERAPY

The problem of whether baroreceptor control of blood pressure is altered during treatment with antihypertensive drugs is of both practical and theoretical interest. Practical interest derives from the well-known fact that in animals interference with the baroreflex function induces a pronounced lability of arterial blood pressure [37–39]. Theoretical interest is related to the hypothesis (also derived mainly from animal experiments) that currently used drugs such as clonidine and alpha-methyldopa exert their hypotensive effect by reducing the activity of the sympathetic vasoconstrictor nerves [40, 41] and that in the case of clonidine this is in part due to potentiation of the baroreflexes [40, 42].

We have tested the carotid baroreceptor reflex function in 16 patients with essential hypertension before and after intravenous administration of clonidine at doses of 150 µg (8 patients) and 300 µg (8 patients) [43]. As mentioned above, the magnitude of the reflex response was established by the regression coefficient of the changes in mean arterial pressure or heart rate (expressed as R–R interval) and the changes in neck tissue pressure. The difference in the reflex responses induced by the drug was assessed in individual subjects by covariant analysis and in the group by paired T test. The results of the study are shown in Figure 12. In brief, no significant difference was found in the reflex responses to both increase and decrease in carotid transmural pressure before and after administration of clonidine.

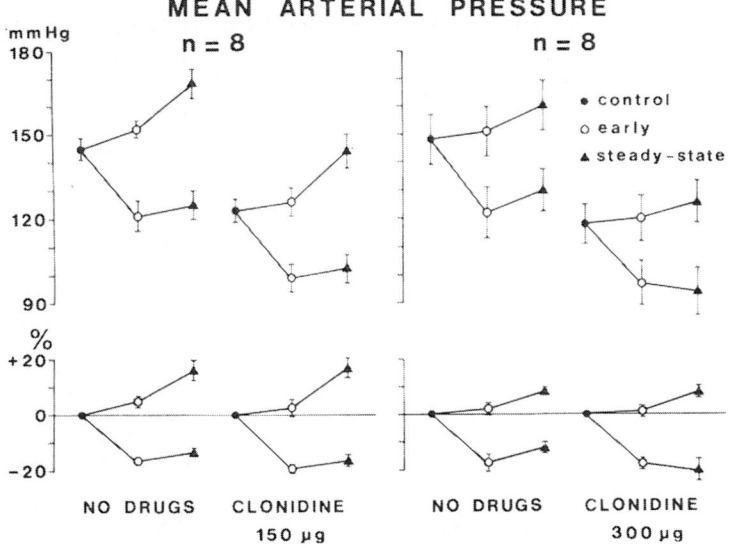

Figure 12. Carotid baroreceptor control of arterial blood pressure before and after i.v. administration of 150 µg of clonidine (left panel, 8 subjects) and of 300 µg of clonidine (right panel, 8 subjects). Data are shown as absolute mean (±SE) values in the upper panels, and as percent changes from control in the lower panel. Control refers to values before carotid manipulation, early and steady-state to values respectively between the 5th and the 15th s and inthe last 30 s of a two.minute manipulation. With respect to control the pressor responses were obtained by deactivating baroreceptors through positive pressure application within a neck chamber, and the depressor responses by stimulating baroreceptors through negative pressure application within a neck chamber. The baroreceptor manipulations were identical before and after clonidine.

50

Thus, it seems unlikely that potentiation of the baroreflexes is a mechanism for the hypotension clinically induced by clonidine. As far as other drugs are concerned we found a profound reduction of the carotid baroreceptor reflex response during administration of the ganglion blocking agent trimetaphan, but little change in the reflex during chronic therapy with alpha-methyldopa and prazosin [44, 45]. Thus several drugs which are reputed to lower blood pressure by interfering with the autonomic nervous system, do not affect baroreceptor reflex, at least as far as its gain is concerned. It should be mentioned, however, that preservation of similar baroreflex responses at lower blood pressure levels may indicate a resetting of the baroreflex and that this may represent an effect of these drugs which contribute to the persistence of their antihypertensive action.

There are, however, antihypertensive drugs whose action is accompanied by baroreflex potentiation, such as those that inhibit the activity of angiotensin converting enzyme [46]. Figure 13 shows the pressor responses to carotid baroreceptor deactivation, and the depressor responses to carotid baroreceptor stimulation in 8 subjects studied before and after an oral dose of 50 mg captopril. The depressor responses were similar before and after

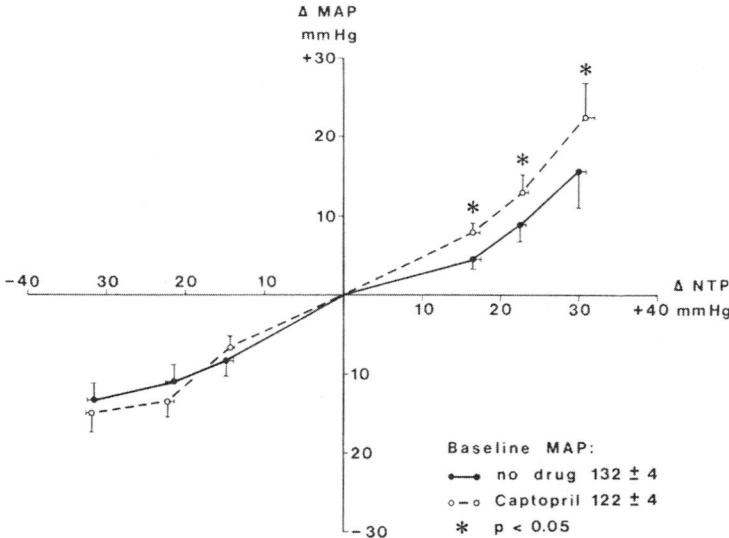

Figure 13. Effects of reducing and increasing neck tissue pressure on mean arterial pressure before and after administration of captopril. Data are shown as means (±SE) from 8 subjects with essential hypertension. Reduction and increase in neck tissue pressure were obtained through negative and positive pressure applications within a neck chamber, and were accompanied by carotid baroreceptor stimulation and deactivation respectively. (From [46], with permission.)

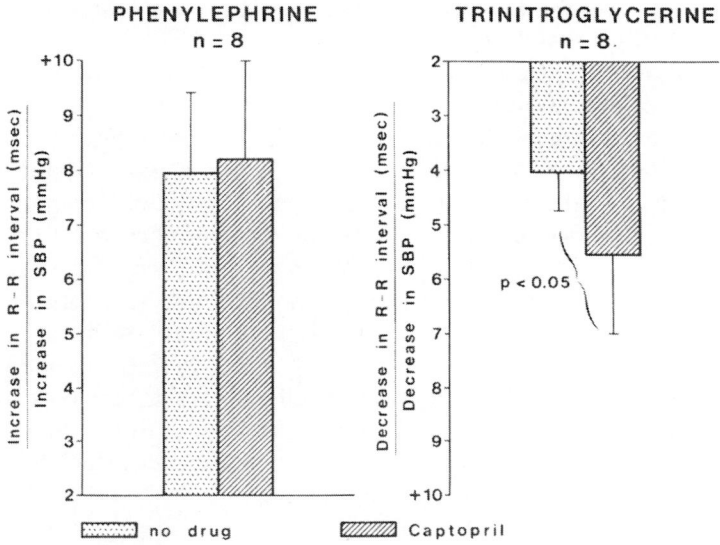

Figure 14. The histograms represent the slopes of the linear relationships between: (1) the increase in systolic blood pressure (SBP) induced by phenylephrine and the resulting lengthening in R–R interval, and (2) the reduction in SBP induced by trinitroglycerine and the resulting shortening in R–R interval. Data are shown as means ($\pm$SE) from the 8 subjects mentioned in Figure 12 which were showed before and after captopril.

captopril, but the pressor responses were clearly greater after than before administration of the drug. This was the case also when the heart rate responses to arterial baroreceptor stimulation and deactivation (obtained via injection of vasoactive drugs) were examined in the same patients (Figure 14). Thus both the heart rate and the blood pressure component of the baroreflex are potentiated by captopril, although the phenomenon only involves the lower portion of the stimulus-response curve of the reflex, i.e. the portion which goes from its threshold to its tonic level of activity. This may contribute to the hypotensive effect of this drug, it may account for the concomitant absence of tachycardia, and it may also suggest that in hypertension angiotensin II exerts a depressor influence on the baroreflex.

REFLEXES FROM AREAS OTHER THAN THE CAROTID SINUSES

Despite the unequivocal demonstration in animals of a powerful reflex control from the aortic arch [47] and from the heart and lungs [48] in man data on baroreflexes from areas other than the carotid sinuses are somewhat conflicting. Several investigators have reported vascular responses attribut-

52

able to receptors in the low pressure area [5]. However, other investigators have denied this possibility [13].

We had thought that information on the topic of the extracarotid baroreceptor reflexes in man might derive from comparing, in the same subjects, the reflex changes in heart rate induced by the two techniques; the variable pressure neck chamber which alters primarily the activity of the carotid baroreceptors, and the technique of intravenous injections of pressor and depressor drugs which induce a change in the stimulus to baroreceptors located at any possible arterial site. We have performed this study in 8 normotensive subjects and in 8 subjects with essential hypertension (mean ages 40 ± 3 and 38 ± 5 years). For comparison the stimuli were calculated as changes in transmural pressure; for the drugs these were represented by the changes in mean arterial pressure, while for the neck chamber they were the changes in tissue pressure outside the carotid sinuses minus the resulting reflex alterations in mean arterial pressure. The response induced by the drugs were calculated 10–15 s after the injection when the reflex changes in

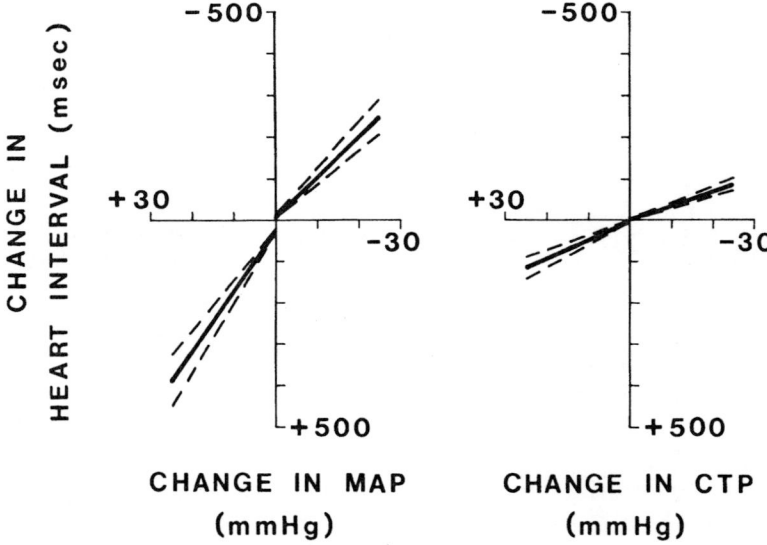

Figure 15. Changes in R–R interval (heart interval) with drug-induced changes in mean arterial pressure (MAP) (left) and with neck chamber-induced changes in carotid sinus transmural pressure (CPT) (richt); means (continuous lines) $\pm$SE (dashed lines) of individual regression coefficients taken from 8 normotensive subjects in whom both techniques were used. For the neck chamber the early heart interval responses were considered, the changes in carotid sinus transmural pressure being those at the time at which the responses were developed. Control mean arterial pressure and heart interval were 101 ± 5 mmHg and 864 ± 61 msec for the drug studies and 791 ± 59 msec for the neck chamber studies. (From [10], with permission.)

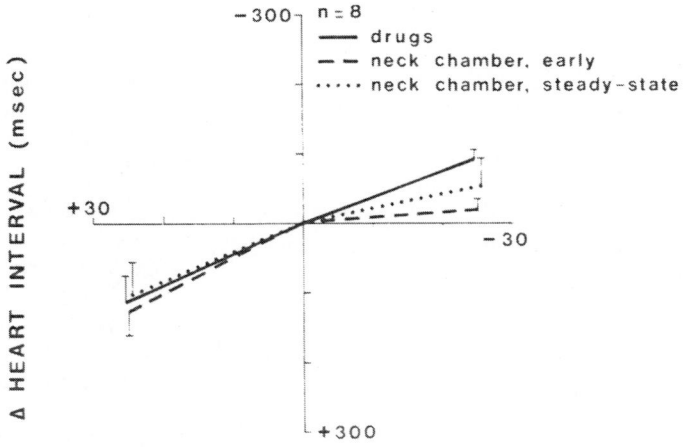

Figure 16. Changes in R–R interval (heart interval) with changes in arterial transmural pressure induced by drugs or by the neck chamber. Means ±Se of individual regression coefficient taken from 8 subjects with essential hypertension in whom techniques were used. For the neck chamber both the early and the steady-state heart interval responses were considered, the changes in arterial transmural pressure being those at the actual time at which the response was measured. Control mean arterial pressure and heart interval were 138±4.5 mmHg and 707±28 msec for the drug studies and 138±5 and 706±32 msec for the neck chamber studies. For further details see text. (from [13], with permission.)

heart rate were maximal and relatively stable. These responses were compared with the early or the steady-state responses induced by the neck chamber.

The results are shown in Figures 15 and 16 which represent means ± standard errors of individual regression coefficients of the relationship between stimuli and reflex responses. As in previous examples, changes in heart rate are shown as changes in R–R interval.

Two major points are evident. One, in normotensive subjects the reflex changes in heart-rate induced by the drugs were about three times as great as those induced by the neck chamber. In hypertensives the reflex changes in heart rate induced by the drugs were about three times less than in normotensives, thus becoming similar to those induced by the neck chamber which did not show appreciable modifications. This suggests that reflexes originating from extracarotid baroreceptor areas are important in heart rate control in normotensive man, and that this function is markedly diminished in hypertensives [18].

54

REFERENCES

1. Kirchheim HP: Systemic arterial baroreceptor reflexes. Physiol Rev 56:100, 1976.
2. Korner PI, West MJ, Shaw J, Uther JB: 'Steadystate' properties of the baroreceptor-heart rate reflex in essential hypertension in man. Clin Exp Pharmacol Physiol 1:65, 1974.
3. Pickering TG, Gribbin B, Sleight P: Comparison of reflex heart rate responses to rising and falling arterial pressure in man. Cardiovasc Res 6:277, 1972.
4. Korner PI, Tonkin AM, Uther JB: Reflex and mechanical circulatory effects of graded Valsalva maneuvers in normal man. J Appl Physiol 40:434, 1976.
5. Roddie IC, Shepherd JT: Receotors in the High-pressure and low-pressure vascular system. Their role in the reflex control of human circulation. Lancet 1:493, 1958.
6. Zoller RP, Mark AI, Abboud EM, Schmid PG, Heistad DD: The role of low-pressure baroreceptors in reflex vasoconstrictor responses in man. J Clin Invest 51:2967, 1972.
7. Ernsting J, Parry DJ: Some observations on the effect of stimulating the carotid arterial stretch receptors in the carotid artery of man. J Physiol (Lond) 137:45P, 1957.
8. Ludbrook J, Mancia G, Ferrari A, Zanchetti A: The variable pressure neck chamber method for studying the carotid baroreflex in man. Clin Sci Mol Med 53:165, 1977.
9. Mancia G, Ferrari A, Gregorini L, Ludbrook J, Zanchetti A: Baroreceptor control of heart rate in man. In: Nervous Control of Cardiac Arrhythmias, p. 323. Brown A, Malliani A, Schwartz PJ, Zanchetti A, eds. New York: Raveb Oress, 1978.
10. Mancia G, Ferrari A, Gregorini L, Valentini R, Ludbrook J, Zanchetti A: Circulatory reflexes from carotid and extracarotid baroreceptor areas in man. Circ Res 41:309, 1977.
11. Thron HI, Brechmann W, Wagner J, Keller K: Quantitative Untersuchungen über die Bedeutung der Gefassdehnungsrezeptoren im Rahmen der Kreislaufhomeostase beim wachen Menschen. Pflueg Arch 293:68, 1967.
12. Mancia G, Ferrari A, Gregorini L, Parati G, Ferrari MC, Pomidossi G, Zanchetti A: Control of blood pressure by carotid sinus baroreceptors in human beings. Am J Cardiol 44:895, 1979.
13. Guz A, Noble MIM, Trenchard D, Cochrane HJ, Makey AR: Studies on the vagus nerve in man: Their role in respiratory and circulatory control. Clin Sci 27:293, 1964.
14. McCubbin JW, Green JH, Page IH: Baroreceptor function in chronic renal hypertension. Circ Res 4:205, 1956.
15. Angell-James JE: Characteristics of single aortic and right subclavian baroreceptor fibre activity in rabbits with chronic renal hypertension. Circ Res 32:149, 1973.
16. Salgado HC, Krieger EM: Resetting of the baroreceptor in hypotension in rats. Clin Sci Mol Med 51:351s, 1976.
17. Bristow SD, Honour AS, Pickering GW, Sleight P, Smyth HS: Diminished baroreceptor sensitivity in high blood pressure. Circulation 39:48, 1969.
18. Mancia G, Ludbrook J, Ferrari A, Gregorini L, Zanchetti A: Baroreceptor reflexes in essential hypertension. Circ Res 43:170, 1978.
19. Wagner S, Wackerbauer S, Hilger HH: Arterieller Blutdruck und Herzfrequenz erhalten bei Hypertonikern unter Änderung des transmuralen Druckes im Karotissinusbereich. Z Kreislauf 57:703, 1968.
20. Kezdi P: Sino-aortic regulatory system. Arch Intern Med 91:26, 1953.
21. Bevegard S, Castenfors J, Danielson M: Carotid baroreceptor function in hypertensive patients. Scand J Lab Invest 37:495, 1977.
22. Folkow B, Hallback M, Lundgreen Y, Siertsson R, Weiss L: Importance of adaptive changes in vascular design for establishment of primary hypertension, studied in man and in spontaneously hypertensive rats. Circ Res 32 (Suppl 1):1–2, 1973.
23. Nosaka S, Wang SC: Carotid sinus baroreceptor functions in the spontaneously hypertensive cat. Am J Physiol 222:1079, 1972.

24. Ricksten SE, Thorèn P: Reflex control of sympathetic nerve activity and heart rate from arterial baroreceptors in conscious normotensive and spontaneously hypertensive rats. Proc VIII Meeting Int Soc Hypert, Milan, p. 375, 1981.
25. Mancia G, Ferrari A, Leonetti G, Pomidossi G, Zanchetti A: Carotid sinus baroreceptor control of blood pressure in renovascular hypertensive subjects. Hypertension (In Press).
26. Mancia G, Ferrari A, Gregorini L, Parati G, Pomidossi G: Effects of isometric exercise on the carotid baroreflex in hypertensive subjects. Hypertension (In press.)
27. Korner PI, West MJ, Shaw J: Central nervous resetting of baroreceptor reflexes. Austr J Med SCi 51:53, 1973.
28. Cuche JL, Kuchel O, Barbeau A, Boucher R, LangloisY, Genest J: Autonomic nervous system and benign essential hypertension. Circ Res 35:290, 1974.
29. Davis JO, Freeman RH: Mechanisms regulating renin release. Physiol Rev 56:1, 1976.
30. Bunag D, Page IH, McCubbin JW: Neural stimulation of renin release. Circ Res 19:851, 1966.
31. Stella A, Zanchetti A: Effects of renal denervation on renin release in response to tilting and furosemide. Am J Physiol 232:H500, 1977.
32. Mancia G, Romero JC, Shepherd JT: Continuous inhibition of renin release by vagally innervated receptors in cardiopulmonary region in dogs. Circ Res 36:529, 1975.
33. Zehr JE, Hasbargen JA, Kurtz KD: Reflex suppressing of renin secretion during distension of cardiopulmonary receptors in dogs. Circ Res 38:232, 1976.
34. Mancia G, Leonetti G, Terzoli L, Zanchetti A: Reflex control of renin release in essential hypertension. Clin Sci Mol Med 54:217, 1977.
35. Mancia G: Reflex control of renin release. Int Cong Series 470, Proc. VIII World Congr Cardiol, Tokio, p. 450. Hayase S, Murao S, eds. Amsterdam: Excerpta Medica, 1978.
36. Mancia G, Ferrari A, Leonetti G, Gregorini L, Terzoli L, Parati G, Bianchini C, Zanchetti A: Carotid sinus reflex control of renin release in hypertensive subjects with high renal secretion. Clin sci 61:505, 1981.
37. Heymans C, Neil E: Reflexogenic areas of the cardiovascular system. London, J and A Churchill Ltd, 1958.
38. Cowley AW, Liard JF, Guyton AG: Role of baroreceptor reflex in daily control of arterial pressure and other variables in dogs. Circ. Res 32:564, 1973.
39. Kumazawa T, Baccelli G, Guazzi M, Mancia G, Zanchetti A: Hemodynamic patterns during desynchronized sleep in intact cats and in cats with sino-aortic deafferentation. Circ Res 24:923, 1969.
40. Kobinger W: Catapres as a tool for evaluation of cardiovascular regulating system in CNS. In: The Nervous System in Arterial Hypertension, p. 430. Julius S, Esler M, eds. Springfield: Thomas CC, 1976.
41. Van Zwieten PA: Centrally mediated action of alphamethyldopa. In: Regulation of Blood Pressure by the Central Nervous System. p. 293, Onesti G, Fernandes M, Kim KE, eds. New York: Grune-Stratton, 1976.
42. Korner PI, Oliver JR, Sleight P, Chalmers JP, Robinson JS: Effects of clonidine on the baroreceptor-heart rate reflex and on single baroreceptor fibre discharge. Eur J Pharmacol 28:189, 1974.
43. Mancia G, Ferrari A, Gregorini L, Zanchetti A: Clonidine and Carotid baroreflex in essential hypertension. Hypertension 1:362, 1979.
44. Mancia G, Ferrari A, Gregorini L, Terzoli L, Leonetti G, Zanchetti A: Methyldopa and neural control of circulation in essential hypertension. Am J Cardiol 45:1237, 1980.
45. Mancia G, Ferrari A, Gregorini L, Ferrari MC, Bianchini C, Terzoli L, Leonetti G, Zanchetti A: Effects of prazosin on autonomic control of circulation in essential hypertension. Hypertension 2:700, 1980.

56

46. Mancia G, Parati G, Pomidossi G, Grassi G, Bertinieri G, Buccino N, Ferrari A, Zanchetti A: Modification of arterial baroreflexes by captopril in essential hypertension. Am J Cardiol (In press.)
47. Pelletier CL, Shepherd JT: Circulatory reflexes from mechanoreceptors in the cardio-aortic area. Circ Res 33:131, 1973.
48. Mancia G, Lorenz RL, Shepherd JT: Reflex control of circulation by heart and lungs. Int Rev Science, Cardiovasc Physiol II, 9:111, 1976.

4. ROLE OF CATECHOLAMINES IN BLOOD PRESSURE REGULATION

A. DISTLER

Catecholamines are compounds composed of a catechol nucleus (a benzene ring with two adjacent hydroxyl groups) and an amine-containing side-chain. The catecholamines occurring in man are dopamine, noradrenaline, and adrenaline. *Dopamine* serves as a neurotransmitter in the central nervous system. Furthermore, this amine functions as a precursor for noradrenaline and adrenaline. *Noradrenaline* is synthesized in the chromaffin tissue, in parts of the brain, and in the postganglionic sympathetic nerves, where it serves as the neurotransmitter substance. *Adrenaline* is synthesized in the brain and in the chromaffin cells. Most of the adrenaline is formed in the chromaffin cells of the adrenal medulla, from where it is secreted into the blood.

STRUCTURE AND ORGANIZATION OF THE SYMPATHETIC NERVOUS SYSTEM

Preganglionic sympathetic neurons originating from the medullary segments C 8 to L 2 synapse with a second neuron at the sympathetic ganglia located along the thoracolumbar part of the spinal column and in the peritoneal cavity. The postganglionic neurons are stimulated at the ganglionic level by the release of acetylcholine from the preganglionic nerve endings. The adrenal medulla can also be viewed as a sympathetic ganglion which is innervated by preganglionic fibers and stimulated by the release of acetylcholine.

All vascular beds (with the exception of the intracerebral vessels) and the heart are covered by a dense network of postganglionic sympathetic fibers, the most densely innervated areas being the arterioles, which are of crucial importance for regulation of peripheral resistance. In the vascular tissue, the adrenergic nerve terminals are distributed in the adventitia and the underlying portion of the media. Postganglionic sympathetic nerve fibers also extend to the juxtaglomerular apparatus of the kidney thereby mediating the secretion of renin.

The sympathetic impulses that lead to vasoconstriction and/or to an increase in heart rate and stroke volume arise from the vasomotor center in

Amery, A. (ed.) Hypertensive Cardiovascular Disease: Pathophysiology and Treatment
© *1982, Martinus Nijhoff Publishers. The Hague / Boston / London*
ISBN-13: 978-94-009-7478-4

the medulla. The vasomotor center is the major site for integrating the excitatory and inhibitory inputs that determine the final level of traffic in peripheral sympathetic neurons. The vasomotor center receives *excitatory impulses* from higher centers, in particular from the hypothalamus, the limbic system and the cortex. Furthermore, it is activated by physical exercise, wakefulness, pain or mental stress. A major source of *inhibitory impulses* travelling to the vasomotor center is the nucleus tractus solitarii, an area of the medulla, where afferent baroreceptor fibers synapse with inhibitory neurons.

The integration of excitatory and inhibitory impulses by the central and autonomic nervous system results in a continuous readjustment of the tone of the cardiovascular system which is mediated by sympathetic and parasympathetic efferents.

The role of the central nervous system in blood pressure regulation is described in more detail in chapter 2.

BIOSYNTHESIS, STORAGE AND RELEASE OF CATECHOLAMINES

All enzymatic reactions involved in the biosynthesis of catecholamines take place within the adrenergic neurons and the adrenal medulla. In the dopaminergic neurons of the central nervous systems the synthesis is terminated at the level of dopamine and in the adrenergic neurons at the level of noradrenaline. In the chromaffin tissues, which contain the enzyme phenylethanolamine N-methyltransferase, the synthesis progresses to adrenaline (Figure 1).

Postganglionic sympathetic nerves

In the postganglionic sympathetic nerves noradrenaline synthesizing and storing vesicles are located in varicosities, which represent thickenings along the course of the fibers and at the nerve endings. Most of the varicosities lie in close proximity to the effector cells.

L-tyrosine from the blood is transported across the membrane of the sympathetic nerves and the medulla by a special transport mechanism. L-tyrosine is then converted by the enzyme tyrosine hydroxylase to L-dihydroxy-phenylalanine (dopa). Tyrosine hydroxylase is inhibited by catecholamines and this inhibition is supposed to control the rate of biosynthesis of noradrenaline. Dopa is rapidly decarboxylated to L-dihydroxyphenylethylamine by aromatic L-amino acid decarboxylase. Dopamine then enters granulated vesicles of 400–600 Å in diameter, where it is hydroxylated to noradrenaline by dopamine β-hydroxylase (DBH). The contents of these

59

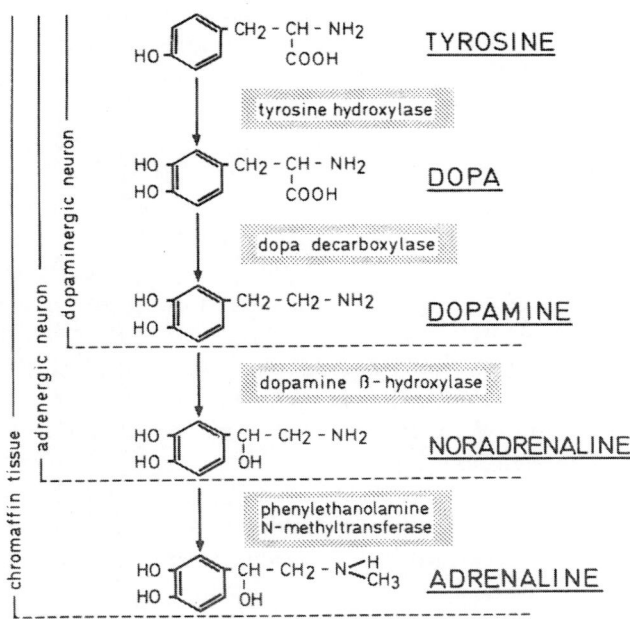

Figure 1. Biosynthesis of catecholamines. In the dopaminergic neurons of the central nervous system the synthesis is terminated at the
level of dopamine and in the adrenergic neurons at the level of
noradrenaline. In the chromaffin tissues the synthesis progresses to
adrenaline.

vesicles consist of noradrenaline and adenosine triphosphate, plus soluble
DHB, and a small amount of a protein substance which is called chromogranin. Excitation of the sympathetic nerves results in a process of exocytosis whereby storage granules move to the surface of the nerve membrane,
where they expel their contents into the synaptic cleft. The exocytosis
appears to be triggered by the following sequence of events: depolarization
of the terminal causes an increase in membrane calcium conductance, thereby leading to a net calcium entry and an increase in intracellular $[Ca^{2+}]$
which in turn induces the transmitter release [1].

Recent studies on adrenergic transmission have uncovered a number of
mechanisms by which the release of noradrenaline can be modulated [2].
Noradrenaline itself acts upon neuronal a-receptors, triggering a negative
feedback mechanism which inhibits subsequent transmitter release. In addition to a-receptors there is also evidence for presynaptic β-receptors. Stimulation of presynaptic β-receptors enhances the noradrenaline release during
adrenergic stimulation and thus constitutes a positive feedback control of
noradrenaline secretion (Figure 3). It has also been postulated that prostaglandins of the E series can exert a negative feedback inhibition of trans-

60

mitter release [3]. Moreover, a negative feedback control of neurotransmitter release can also be exerted by an action of acetylcholine on presynaptic muscarine receptors [4].

Adrenal medulla

In the adrenal medulla the biosynthesis and storage of noradrenaline is esentially the same as in the sympathetic nerves. However, most of the noradrenaline synthesized is converted to adrenaline by the enzyme phenylethanolamine N-methyltransferase (PNMT).

Since PNMT is located in the cytoplasm of chromaffin cells, noradrenaline must migrate from the storage granules to the cytoplasm for methylation, and then return to the granules for storage. The formation of PNMT is induced by glucocorticoids.

The release of catecholamines follows the liberation of acetylcholine from splanchnic nerve endings within the medulla. Acetylcholine increases the permeability of the chromaffin cells to calcium and the granular contents are extruded by exocytosis.

Bilateral adrenalectomy markedly reduces the concentration of adrenaline in the plasma and urine in man, whereas the noradrenaline concentration is not altered significantly [5]. Any remaining adrenaline is presumed to come from chromaffin cells present elsewhere in the body (e.g. in the heart or in prevertebral sympathetic ganglia).

INACTIVATION OF CATECHOLAMINES

Only minute amounts of the noradrenaline released from sympathetic nerve endings (some 15–20% according to a study by Reid et al. [6]) reach the systemic circulation, the rest being rapidly inactivated. Radioactive noradrenaline and adrenaline, when injected into animals in physiologic concentrations, have an initial half-life of 10–30 s [7, 8].

The most important mechanism for removing and inactivating released or circulating catecholamines is the neuronal re-uptake by an active transport mechanism localized in the axonal membrane, followed by renewed storage in the vesicles. The noradrenaline which is free in the cytoplasm of sympathetic nerves may be deaminated by mitochondrial monoamine oxidase (MAO) to form an unstable aldehyde, which can then be oxidized to 3,4-dihydroxymandelic acid (DHMA) by aldehyde dehydrogenase. MAO is widely distributed and is particularly abundant in the brain, liver, and kidney. This enzyme is probably primarily concerned with disposing of excess stores of catecholamines [9].

61

The noradrenaline and adrenaline which is released into the circulation (and which is not inactivated by re-uptake) is largely converted by O-methylation to normetanephrine and metanephrine by the action of catechol-O-methyltransferase (COMT). This enzyme is present in almost all tissues and particularly concentrated in liver and kidney. Further degradation of normetanephrine and metanephrine by MAO and of DHMA by COMT results in the formation of 3-methoxy-4-hydroxymandelic acid (vanillyl-mandelic acid, VMA), which is the main metabolite of the catecholamines. Another major metabolite of catecholamines is 3-methoxy-4-hydroxyphenylglycol (MHPG), which is generated by the enzymatic reaction of MAO plus aldehyde reductase with normetanephrine and metanephrine and by the reaction of COMT with a reduction product of noradrenaline and adrenaline, 3,4-dihydroxyphenylglycol (DHPG) (Figure 2).

Under resting conditions the amount of unchanged noradrenaline and adrenaline excreted with the urine is very low (Table 1). The ratio of VMA

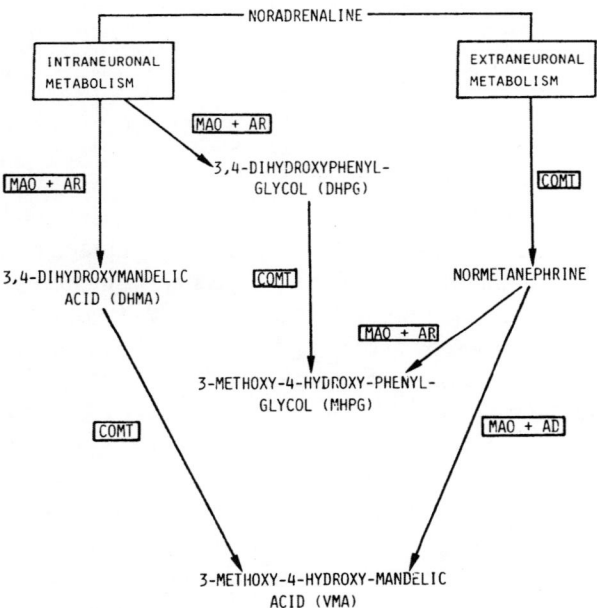

MAO = MONOAMINE OXIDASE
COMT= CATECHOL-O-METHYLTRANSFERASE
AD = ALDEHYDE DEHYDROGENASE
AR = ALDEHYDE REDUCTASE

Figure 2. Metabolic inactivation of noradrenaline (the inactivation of adrenaline is similar to that of noradrenaline, see text).

Table 1. Urinary excretion of endogenous catecholamines (data from [10])

	μ moles/day	% total
Noradrenaline	0.15	0.5
Adrenaline	0.04	0.1
Normetanephrine	1.4	3.5
Metanephrine	1.1	4.5
MHPG	8.7	27.9
VMA	19.0	60.9
Other	0.8	2.6
Total	31.2	100

to normetanephrine and metanephrine excretion is normally less than 10:1, reflecting that intraneuronal oxidation by MAO is the predominant pathway of degradation.

Urinary excretion of catecholamines may be considered to provide a useful index of the level of sympatho-adrenal medullary activity over intervals sufficiently long (i.e. greater than one hour) to collect adequate urine specimens [10].

ACTION OF NORADRENALINE AND ADRENALINE ON EFFECTOR CELLS

Most of the noradrenaline released from sympathetic nerve endings is taken up again into the storage granules by an efficient re-uptake mechanism and only a relatively small fraction of the active neurotransmitter reaches the effector cell receptors (e.g. vascular smooth muscle, myocardium, bronchoconstrictor muscles), thereby activating these cells. The circulatory effects of noradrenaline are mediated by `a`-receptors, which are located on the vascular smooth muscle cells, and by β-receptors, which are present in the myocardium and which represent so-called β_1-receptors.

Stimulation by noradrenaline of vascular a-receptors induces vasoconstriction. Recently, two types of postsynaptic a-receptors have been differentiated [11]: a_1-type receptors (which can be blocked competitively by prazosine) appear to have a synaptic location and are stimulated by neuronally released noradrenaline, whereas a_2-receptors (which can selectively be blocked by rauwolscine) are located extrasynaptically and are stimulated by circulating (or injected) noradrenaline (Figure 3).

Adrenaline secreted from the adrenal medulla stimulates a- as well as β-receptors. Small amounts of adrenaline released from the adrenal medulla stimulate vascular β-receptors (so-called β_2-receptors) thereby inducing vasodilation. Larger amounts activate vascular a-receptors thereby leading to vasoconstriction.

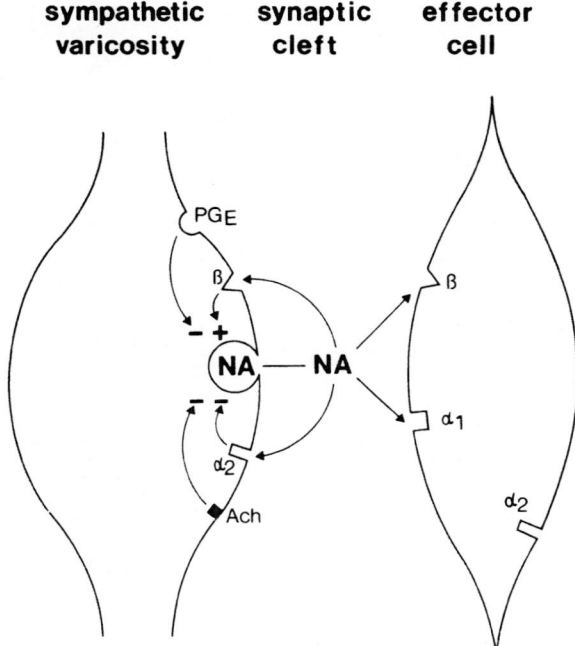

Figure 3. Action of noradrenaline released from a storing vesicle of a sympathetic varicosity on pre- and postsynaptic receptors. The transmitter release can be modulated by an inhibitory effect (−) of noradrenaline which is mediated by presynaptic α_2-receptors as well as by an enhancing effect (+) mediated
by presynaptic β-receptors. Inhibitory effects on transmitter
release can also be exerted by prostaglandins of the E series
(PG_E) and by acetylcholine (Ach). The effects of noradrenaline
on the effector cell are mediated by postsynaptic α- and β-
receptors. The postsynaptic α_2-receptors are supposed to be
located extrasynaptically (see text).

Stimulation by noradrenaline and adrenaline of myocardial β-receptors
leads to an increase in heart rate, in contractility and in conductivity.

ROLE OF THE SYMPATHO-ADRENAL SYSTEM IN CIRCULATORY
CONTROL

The most important role of the sympatho-adrenal system in the circulatory
control in man is to maintain the blood pressure against the gravitational
force which becomes effective in the upright posture and to adapt the blood
flow to the various organs to their needs during physical activity. Activation
of the sympathetic nervous system can influence the blood pressure and the
distribution of regional blood flow by several mechanisms (Figure 4):

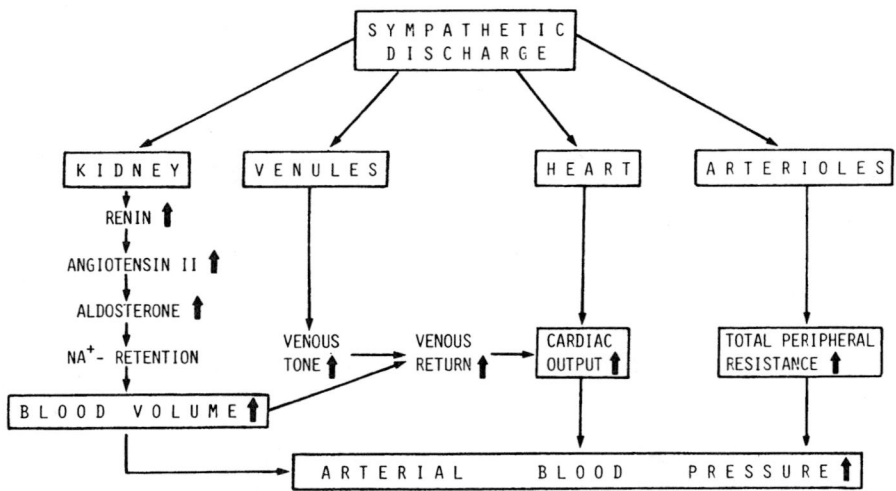

Figure 4. Action of the sympathetic nervous system on arterial blood pressure.

i) It may lead to an increased cardiac output by an effect on venous tone, thereby augmenting venous return, and/or by increasing heart rate and stroke volume.

ii) By an effect on the arterioles it may increase total peripheral resistance.

iii) Sympathetic nervous activity has been shown to be one of the most important factors in regulating renin release [12]. The autonomic control of renin release thus contributes to the volume regulation via angiotensin II, aldosterone and sodium retention as well as to the direct regulation of arteriolar resistance via angiotensin II. At the same time an augmented neurotransmitter release in autonomic ganglia, sympathetic nerve endings and adrenal medulla appears to be an important mediator of the vasoconstrictive action of angiotensin [13].

There are still many other interactions between the sympathetic nervous system, reactivity to noradrenaline, endocrine function, and blood pressure. For instance, plasma noradrenaline concentration (probably reflecting sympathetic tone) is high and reactivity to noradrenaline is low in hypothyroid state, whereas the reverse is true in hyperthyroid state [14]. Other substances which may interfere with catecholamine release and action are prostaglandins of the E series, the kallikrein–kinin system, vasopressin, 5-hydroxytryptamine, estrogens, and progesterone.

Activation of the sympathetic nervous system need not extend to all parts of the system. Although a more generalized response of the sympathetic nervous system may occur in severe stress, more often sympathetic outflow is regulated more selectively, with the pattern of response depending upon the specific input signal [15]. An increase in sympathetic neurotransmitter release may occur without significant adrenal discharge [16]. The selectivity of autonomic effects is illustrated by the ability of the rat to learn to vaso-dilate in one ear without changing flow to the other [17].

ASSAY METHODS FOR PLASMA CATECHOLAMINE DETERMINATION

The introduction by Engelman et al. in 1968 [18] of a sensitive and specific radioenzymatic method which, on subsequent modification, would permit the accurate determination of minute quantities of noradrenaline and adren-aline [19, 20], has allowed the reliable determination of plasma catechol-amine levels in physiological concentrations. Also the fluorimetric methods which were previously in use have been improved so as to produce results comparable to those obtained by the radioenzymatic procedures [21]. How-ever, despite the methodologic progress made, it must not be overlooked that the normal values for plasma noradrenaline given by different authors vary considerably (Table 2). Certainly, this difference is partly due to the methods used. Assays using phenylethanolamine N-methyltransferase as the methylating enzyme usually give values some 50–100% higher than those using catechol-O-methyltransferase [22]. Another reason for the differences in normal values reported seems to be the influence of age and emotional status. It has been shown repeatedly [23–25] (although not consistent-ly [26, 27]) that the plasma noradrenaline concentration tends to increase with age (and so does sympathetic activity recorded from muscle nerves [28]). As has been demonstrated by Reid and co-workers [6], medi-

Table 2. Resting plasma noradrenaline (NA) and adrenaline (A) levels (ng/l) in normotensive subjects (mean values ±SD)

Bertel et al. [43]	NA 250±121	R-COMT
	A 35± 19	
Brecht and Schoeppe [42]	NA 128± ?	F
Engelman et al. [47]	NA 200± 80	R-COMT
	A 50± 30	
Lake et al. [23]	NA 304±183	R-PNMT
Pedersen and Christensen [24]	NA 254± ?	R-COMT
	A 47± ?	
Philipp et al. [44]	NA 173± 45	F
Sever et al. [25]	NA 403±184	R-PNMT
Weidmann et al. [46]	NA 169± 91	R-COMT
	A 62± 62	

F = Fluorimetric method
R-COMT = Radioenzymatic method using COMT
R-PNMT = Radioenzymatic method using PNMT

66

cal and paramedical personnel tend to have considerably lower noradrenaline levels than normotensive patients who are not familiar with blood collecting procedures. Anxiety therefore appears to be a factor contributing to higher plasma noradrenaline levels.

Despite large interindividual variations the values for a given individual are fairly well reproducible when obtained under identical conditions on different occasions [29, 30]. There are no consistent differences in plasma noradrenaline concentration when samples are taken from multiple arterial and venous sites [31, 32] except for lower noradrenaline levels in the hepatic vein [32], presumably a consequence of catecholamine uptake and metabolism by the liver.

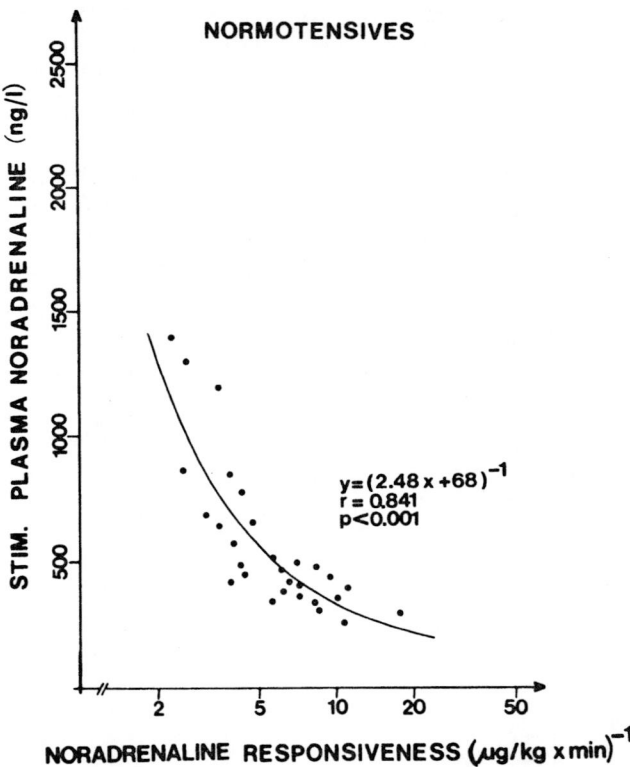

Figure 5. Relationship between plasma noradrenaline concentration following dynamic exercise (200 W for 2 min) and responsiveness to exogenous noradrenaline in 28 normotensive subjects. Noradrenaline responsiveness is expressed by the amount of noradrenaline (per kg and min) required to produce an increase in mean arterial blood pressure by 20 mmHg above control level. The data demonstrate that there is an inverse relationship between plasma noradrenaline and responsiveness to noradrenaline (data from [44]).

SOURCE OF PLASMA NORADRENALINE

Although it is now clear that the major source of plasma noradrenaline is the sympathetic nerve endings, it remains uncertain which sympathetic region is most important in detemining the plasma concentration. Resting plasma noradrenaline concentration (although not determined simultaneously) has been shown to be positively correlated to sympathetic activity recorded in muscle branches of the peroneal nerve in normotensive healthy subjects [28]. From this observation and since muscles (which may be assumed to contain large numbers of sympathetic nerve terminals) comprise about 40% of total body weight it has been suggested that overflow of transmitter from sympathetic terminals in muscles contributes significantly to the plasma concentration of noradrenaline at rest [28].

PLASMA NORADRENALINE AS AN INDEX OF SYMPATHETIC ACTIVITY

Plasma levels of noradrenaline have often been used as an index of sympathetic activity [10, 30, 33]. This was based on the fact that noradrenaline is the sympathetic neurotransmitter substance and that plasma levels of noradrenaline increase in the venous effluent when the sympathetic nerves to specific organs such as the cat spleen [34] or the dog heart [35] are stimulated electrically. Moreover, in the dog heart it has been shown that endogenous catecholamine levels increase in the coronary sinus blood with stimulation frequency and that a correlation exists between the amplitude of the response of the heart to sympathetic stimulation and the release of catecholamines into the coronary sinus blood [35]. Also in man a rise in plasma noradrenaline concentration could be demonstrated in response to maneuvers known to activate the sympathetic nervous system. This has been shown for dynamic [6, 36. 37] and isometric [30, 38] exercise, upright posture [6, 25, 30], sodium restriction [39] and mental stress [38]. In patients with essential hypertension a highly significant positive correlation has been found between the increase in plasma noradrenaline and the rise in systolic blood pressure following bicycle work load [6, 37].

Further evidence for the usefulness of plasma noradrenaline determination as an index of sympathetic activity comes from studies of patients with autonomic insufficiency. In these subjects, defective cardiovascular reflexes are associated with orthostatic hypotension. Resting levels of plasma noradrenaline are low in most patients with progressive autonomic failure and no rise can be demonstrated with orthostasis [40].

In conclusion, plasma levels of catecholamines in the venous blood seem to reflect adequately the state of sympathetic neuron and adrenal medullary activity and appear to be particularly useful in measurement of short-term changes in activity.

RELATIONSHIP BETWEEN PLASMA NORADRENALINE AND BLOOD PRESSURE

Although some authors [41-43] have reported on a direct relationship between plasma noradrenaline concentration and height of blood pressure in patients with essential hypertension, no such correlation – or only a weak one – appears to exist in normotensive subjects [43-45]. The lack of a positive association between plasma noradrenaline and blood pressure is not surprising since an inverse relationship exists between plasma noradrenaline and reactivity of the blood pressure to exogenous noradrenaline (Figure 5). This means that normally a high sympathetic tone (as reflected by high plasma noradrenaline levels) is compensated for by a low reactivity to the sympathetic neurotransmitter and vice versa. A likely explanation is that the availability of noradrenaline receptors falls with increasing sympathetic activity and vice versa [44]. Therefore, when considering the role of the sympathetic nervous system for blood pressure regulation, sympathetic activity has to be considered in conjunction with its effectiveness, i.e. reactivity to noradrenaline. Both factors together appear to form an important determinant of the arterial blood pressure level both in normotensives and in patients with essential hypertension [44].

REFERENCES

1. Blaustein MP: The role of calcium in catecholamine release from adrenergic nerve terminals. In: The Release of Catecholamines from Adrenergic Neurons, pp. 39–58. Paton DM, ed. Oxford: Pergamon, 1979.
2. Starke K, Taube HD, Borowski E: Presynaptic receptor systems in catecholaminergic transmission. Biochem Pharmacol 26:259–268, 1977.
3. Stjärne L: Role of prostaglandins and cyclic adenosine monophate in release. In: The Release of Catecholamines from Adrenergic Neurons, pp. 111–142. Paton DM ed. Oxford: Pergamon, 1979.
4. Muscholl E: Peripheral muscarinic control of norepinephrine release in the cardiovascular system. Am J Physiol 239:H713–H720, 1980.
5. von Euler US, Franksson C, Hellström J: Adrenaline and noradrenaline output in urine after unilateral and bilateral adrenalectomy in man. Acta Physiol Scand 31:1–5, 1954.
6. Reid JL: Plasma noradrenaline as an index of sympathetic activity. In: Hypertension. Mechanisms and Management, pp. 65–71. Philipp T, Distler A, eds. Berlin: Springer-Verlag, 1980.
7. Whitby LG, Axelrod J, Weil-Malherbe H: The fate of H^3-norepinephrine in animals. J Pharmacol Exp Ther 132:193–201, 1961.
8. Wurtman RJ: Catecholamines. Boston: Little, Brown, 1966.

9. Kopin IJ: Storage and metabolism of catecholamines: the role of monoamine oxidase. Pharmacol Rev 16:179–191, 1964.

10. Kopin IJ: Biochemical assessment of peripheral adrenergic activity. In: The release of catecholamines from adrenergic neurons, pp. 355–372. Paton DM, ed. Oxford: Pergamon, 1979.

11. Langer SZ, Massingham R, Shepperson NB: Presence of postsynaptic β_2-adrenoceptors of predominantly extrasynaptic location in the vascular smooth muscle of the dog hind limb. Clin Sci 59:225s–228s, 1980.

12. Davis JO, Freeman RH: Mechanisms regulating renin release. Physiol Rev 56:2–56, 1976.

13. Starke K: Action of angiotensin on uptake, release and metabolism of ^{14}C-noradrenaline by isolated rabbit hearts. Eur J Pharmacol 14:112-123, 1971.

14. Philipp T. Brokamp B, Cordes U, Lüth B, Distler A: Sympathikusaktivität und pressorische Wirkung von Noradrenalin bei Patienten mit hypo- und hyperthyreoter Stoffwechsellage. Verh Dtsch Ges Inn Med 85:1047-1049, 1979.

15. Abboud FM, Heistad DD, Mark AL, et al.: Reflex control of the peripheral circulation. Prog Cardiovasc Dis 18:371-403, 1976.

16. Robertson D, Shand DG, Hollifield JW, Nies AS, Frölich JC, Oates JA: Alterations in the responses of the sympathetic nervous system and renin in borderline hypertension. Hypertension 1:118-124, 1979.

17. DiCara LV, Miller NE: Instrumental learning of vasomotor responses by rats: learning to respond differentially in the two ears. Science 159:1485-1486, 1968.

18. Engelman K, Portnoy B, Lovenberg W: A sensitive and specific double-isotope derivative method for the determination of catecholamines in biological specimens. Am J Med Sci 255:259-268, 1968.

19. DaPrada M, Zürcher G: Simultaneous radio-enzymatic determination of plasma and tissue adrenaline, noradrenaline and dopamine within the femtomole range. Life Sci 19:1161–1174, 1976.

20. Peuler JD, Johnson GA: Simultaneous single isotope radioenzymatic assay of plasma norepinephrine, epinephrine and dopamine. Life Sci 21:625–636, 1977.

21. Miura Y, Campese V, de Quattro V, Meijer D: Plasma catecholamines via an improved fluorimetric assay: comparison with an enzymatic method. J Lab Clin Med 89:421-427, 1977.

22. Sever PS: Catecholamines in essential hypertension: The present controversy. In: Circulating Catecholamines and Blood Pressure, pp. 1–10. Birkenhäger WH, Falke HE, eds. Utrecht: Bunge Scientific, 1978.

23. Lake CR, Ziegler MG, Coleman MD, Kopin IJ: Age-adjusted plasma-norepinephrine levels are similar in normotensive and hypertensive subjects. N Engl J Med 296:208-209, 1977.

24. Pedersen EB, Christensen NJ: Catecholamines in plasma and urine in patients with essential hypertension determined by double-isotope derivative techniques. Acta Med Scand 198:373-377, 1975.

25. Sever PS, Osikowska B, Birch M, Tunbridge RDG: Plasma noradrenaline in essential hypertension. Lancet I:1078-1081, 1977.

26. De Champlain J, Cousineau D: Lack of correlation between age and circulating catecholamines in hypertensive patients. N Engl J Med 297:672, 1977.

27. De Quattro V, Chan S: Raised plasma catecholamines in some patients with primary hypertension. Lancet I:806-809, 1972.

28. Wallin BG, Sundlöf G, Eriksson B-M, Dominiak P, Grobecker H, Lindblad LE: Plasma noradrenaline correlates to sympathetic muscle nerve activity in normotensive man. Acta Physiol Scand 111:69-73, 1981.

70

29. De Champlain J, Farley L, Cousineau D, van Ameringen M-R: Circulating catecholamine levels in human and experimental hypertension. Circ Res 38:109–114, 1976.
30. Lake CR, Ziegler MG, Kopin IJ: Use of plasma norepinephrine for evaluation of sympathetic neuronal function in man. Life Sci 18:1315–1326, 1976.
31. Vecht RJ, Gordon D, Sever P: Catecholamines, isometric exercise and left ventricular function. In: Hypertension. Mechanisms and Management, pp. 55–63. Philipp T, Distler A, eds. Berlin: Springer-Verlag, 1980.
32. Jones DH, Allison DJ, Hamilton CA, Reid JL: Selective venous sampling in the diagnosis and localization of phaeochromocytoma. Clin Endocrinol 10:179–186, 1979.
33. De Champlain J: The contribution of the sympathetic nervous system to arterial hypertension. Canad J Physiol Pharmacol 56:341–353, 1978.
34. Haefely W, Hürlimann A, Thoenen H: Relation between the rate of stimulation and the quantity of noradrenaline liberated from sympathetic nerve endings in the isolated perfused spleen of the cat. J Physiol 181:48–58, 1965.
35. Yamaguchi N, de Champlain J, Nadeau R: Correlation between the response of the heart to sympathetic stimulation and the release of endogenous catecholamines into the coronary sinus of the dog. Circulat Res 36:662–667, 1975.
36. Irving MH, Britton BJ, Wood WG, Padgham C, Carruthers M: Effects of β-adrenergic blockade on plasma catecholamines in exercise. Nature (London) 248:531–533, 1974.
37. Distler A, Keim HJ, Cordes U, Philipp T, Wolff HP: Sympathetic responsiveness and antihypertensive effect of beta-receptor blockade in essential hypertension. Am J Med 64:446–451, 1978.
38. de Leeuw PW, Wester A, Willemse PJ, Birkenhäger WH: Patterns of noradrenaline and renin in essential hypertension – effects of stress and therapy. In: Hypertension. Mechanisms and Management, pp. 49–54. Philipp T, Distler A, eds. Berlin: Springer-Verlag, 1980.
39. Romoff MS, Keusch G, Campese VM, Wang M-S, Friedler RM, Weidmann P, Massry SG: Effect of sodium intake on plasma catecholamines in normal subjects. J Clin Endocrinol Metabol 48:26–31, 1978.
40. Bannister R, Sever PS, Gross M: Cardiovascular reflexes and biochemical responses in progressive autonomic failure. Brain: 100:324–344, 1977.
41. Louis WJ, Doyle AE, Anavekar SH: Plasma norepinephrine levels in essential hypertension. N Engl J Med 288:599–601, 1973.
42. Brecht HM, Schoeppe W: Relation of plasma noradrenaline to blood pressure, age, sex and sodium balance in patients with essential hypertension and in normotensive subjects. Clin Sci mol Med 55:81s–83s, 1978.
43. Bertel O, Bühler FR, Kiowski W, Lütold BE: Decreased beta-adrenoceptor responsiveness as related to age, blood pressure, and plasma catecholamines in patients with essential hypertension. Hypertension 2:130–138, 1980.
44. Philipp T, Cordes U, Distler A: Sympathetic nervous system and blood pressure control in essential hypertension. Lancet ii:959–963, 1978.
45. Le Blanc J, Côté J, Jobin M, Labrie A: Plasma catecholamines and cardiovascular responses to cold and mental activity. J Appl Physiol 47:1207–1211, 1979.
46. Weidmann P, Beretta-Piccoli C, Ziegler WH, Keusch G, Glück Z, Reubi FC: Age versus urinary sodium for judging renin, aldosterone, and catecholamine levels: studies in normal subjects and patients with essential hypertension. Kidney Int 14:619–628, 1978.
47. Engelman K, Portnoy B, Sjoerdsma A: Plasma catecholamine concentrations in patients with essential hypertension. Circ Res 26 and 27 (Suppl. I):141–145, 1970.

5. ROLE OF THE RENIN–ANGIOTENSIN SYSTEM AND PROSTAGLANDINS IN BLOOD PRESSURE REGULATION AND SODIUM HOMEOSTASIS

RAINER DUSING and JAMES B. LEE

In addition to its well-known excretory function, the mammalian kidney has important metabolic and endocrine functions such as gluconeogenesis, production of the active compound of the vitamin D system, erythropoietin synthesis and release, and secretion of renin, which ultimately leads to generation of the vasoconstrictor angiotensin II and release of the mineralocorticoid aldosterone. The renin–angiotensin–aldosterone axis, the so-called prohypertensive renal function, together with the sympathetic nervous system, represent at least two of the major known mechanisms for production of an elevated blood pressure. Evidence that activation of prohypertensive renal principles might underlie the etiology of human hypertension received great impetus from the studies of Goldblatt in 1934 [1] which showed that partial renal artery occlusion raised arterial blood pressure – a finding subsequently associated with an increase in the activity of the renin–angiotensin axis.

However, except for a contribution of this prohypertensive axis to the hypertension of advanced renal disease and for a fairly well defined etiological role of renin in the small percentage of patients with renovascular and malignant hypertension, studies so far have not uncovered an etiological role for the renal prohypertensive axis in the genesis of ordinary human essential hypertension.

In addition to the prohypertensive function of the kidney, evidence has also been presented supporting the fact that the kidney is not only the origin of humoral vasopressor substances, but is also the site of potent humoral vasodepressors which may act to lower systemic arterial blood pressure. Thus, arterial blood pressure could be considered as the net result of an antagonistic system in which vasoconstrictive prohypertensive factors, such as the renin–angiotensin system and the activity of the autonomic nervous system, are counteracted by vasodilator antihypertensive substances which decrease peripheral arteriolar resistance and thereby lower blood pressure.

The first evidence that such factors might be present in the kidney was presented by Menéndez and von Euler [2], who demonstrated that removal of both kidneys resulted in sodium-dependent renoprival hypertension, which obviously cannot be ascribed to any excess in renal pressor functions.

Amery, A. (ed.) Hypertensive Cardiovascular Disease: Pathophysiology and Treatment
© *1982, Martinus Nijhoff Publishers. The Hague / Boston / London*
ISBN-13: 978-94-009-7478-4

Although such renoprival hypertension was at first attributed to a nonspecific effect of the uremia accompanying bilateral nephrectomy, it was shown by Grollman and co-workers [3] that anastomosis of the ureters into the inferior vena cava of dogs resulted in the same degree of uremia as the removal of both kidneys, but that renoprival hypertension did not occur. This suggested a specific antihypertensive function of the kidney independent of its excretory function, which may be mediated by one or more humoral vasodepressor substances.

Muirhead and his co-workers [4] presented evidence that the renal factor(s) which prevented renoprival hypertension might reside in the renal medulla, while Hamilton and Grollman [5] suggested the active principle was located in the cortex. In further investigations, Muirhead and his co-workers concluded that a neutral lipid may be the responsible antihypertensive compound, while Lee and co-workers, in their early experiments [6, 7] suggested that more polar compounds, now known to be prostaglandins (PGs), were responsible for the antihypertensive renal endocrine function.

HISTORICAL ASPECTS

The prostaglandins were independently discovered in the early 1930s by Kurzrok and Lieb, and by Goldblatt and von Euler, who demonstrated that extracts of human semen or sheep seminal vesicle possess potent blood pressure lowering and nonvascular, smooth muscle stimulating activity. In 1936, von Euler further characterized the responsible factors as fatty acids and named them prostaglandins [8]. Bergström, Sjövall and their co-workers isolated and identified two main classes of prostaglandins, the PGEs and the PGFs, in the early 1960s [9–11]. In general, prostaglandins are 20-carbon fatty acids with a five-membered cyclopentane ring. Various unsaturations and substitutions may be introduced naturally or synthetically into the hypothetical parent compound called prostanoic acid. Minor changes in the chemical structure of the compounds result in marked alterations in their biological activity. This situation can be compared to the steroids in which minor alterations in the chemical structure of the compound also result in compounds with markedly different biological activities. Moreover, the naturally occurring PGEs and PGFs possess the most diverse and potent biological activities of almost any naturally occurring compounds which have been discovered to date. For instance, depending on the species and the type of prostaglandin, they may dilate or constrict bronchiolar smooth muscle, inhibit gastric hydrochloric acid secretion and experimental peptic ulcer production, produce or inhibit platelet aggregation, induce labor and act as abortifacients, produce bone reabsorption, and act as important mediators of inflammatory and immune responses. While these examples are not the only actions of this ubiquitous class of compounds, they do illustrate their markedly diverse biologic activities.

In the early 1960s, unaware of the early prostaglandin developments, Lee et al. [6], investigating the antihypertensive activity of the kidney, noted that extracts of rabbit renal medulla resulted in a potent blood pressure lowering effect in the normotensive rat. In a series of investigations, three fatty acids were isolated from the rabbit renal medulla, compound 1, compound 2 and medullin [7]. Compound 2 and medullin were shown to be responsible for the blood pressure lowering activity of crude renal medullary extracts. Only medullin, however, had selective cardiovascular effects and was devoid of the nonvascular activities of compounds 1 and 2. Identification of these three compounds [12] revealed them to be $PGF_{2\alpha}$ (compound 1), PGE_2 (compound 2) and the hitherto unknown PGA_2 (medullin). See Figure 1. A further characteristic of the latter compound was that, in contrast to the PGEs and PGFs, it was not metabolized significantly in the pulmonary vascular bed; therefore, PGA_2 could theoretically function as a true circulating hormone. This circulating hormonal role cannot be ascribed to either the PFEs or the pGFs, since they are extensively metabolized by the lungs and probably function as local rather than systemic hormones.

However, nonspecific dehydration of PGE to PGA under acidic conditions has been known to occur from the beginning and numerous studies have failed to delineate an enzymatic synthesis of PGA from either PGE or essential fatty acid precursors. The nonenzymatic dehydration of PGE to PGA has led some investigators [13, 14] to suggest that PGA_2 is simply a dehydration artifact of PGE_2, since it has not been detected by GLC-mass

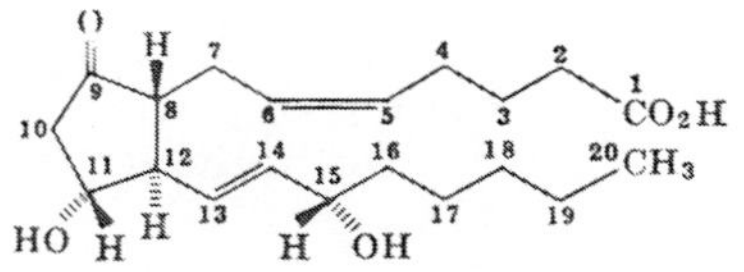

PGE₂ (compound 2)   PGF₂α (compound 1)

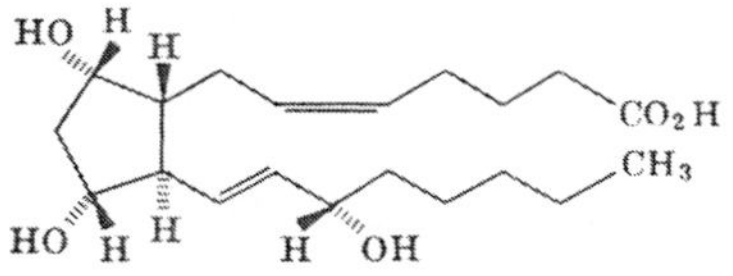

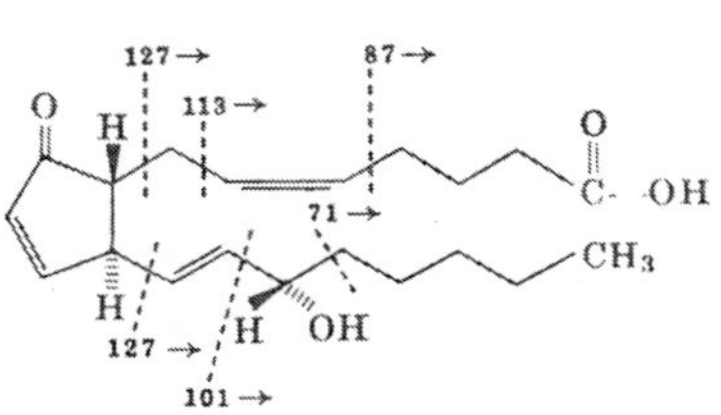

PGA₂ (medullin)

Figure 1. Structures of the renomedullary prostaglandins. Identification of compound 1 as $PGF_{2\alpha}$, compound 2 as PGE_2 and medullin as PGA_2 by massspectrometry. Suggested fragmentation for all three compounds is indicated inthe structure of PGA_2. From [12], with permission of the publisher.

74

spectrometry in either rabbit renal medulla or human plasma. Previous studies in our laboratory also failed to detect significant biosynthesis of PGA$_2$ in rabbit papillary slices in vitro [15].

SYNTHESIS AND METABOLISM

Prostaglandins in general are synthesized ubiquitously from unsaturated fatty acids through intermediate cyclic endoperoxides. This synthesis involving the enzyme conglomerate prostaglandin synthetase has been shown by Flower et al. [16] to be markedly inhibited by aspirin, indomethacin, and other nonsteroidal antiphlogistic agents. This has provided an extremely useful approach for elucidating possible endogenous roles of the prostaglandins in physiologic and pathologic processes. Many of the clinical effects and side effects of aspirin and indomethacin have recently been ascribed to the inhibition of prostaglandin synthesis. This would include their antiinflammatory and antipyrogenic effects as well as peptic ulceration, hyperacidity, elevation in blood pressure and aspirin-induced asthma.

In addition to PGE$_2$ and PGF$_{2\alpha}$, PGD$_2$ has recently been demonstrated in the kidney [17]. Furthermore, the potent vasodilatory and platelet aggrega-

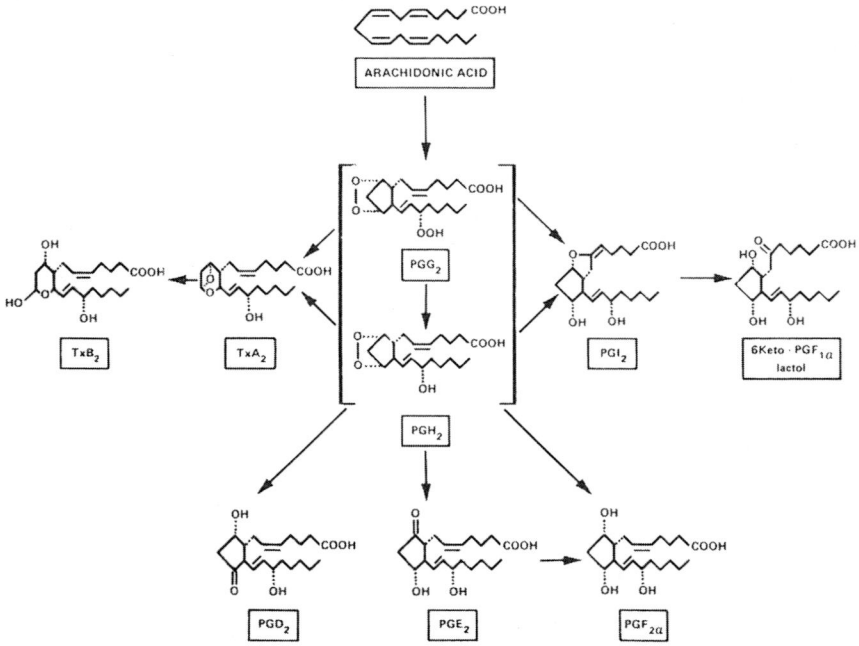

Figure 2. The major pathways of prostaglandin (PG), prostacyclin (PGI$_2$), and thromboxane (TX) formation from arachidonic acid.

tion-inhibiting prostacyclin (PGI$_2$) has been demonstrated in blood vessels [18] and the vasoconstricting, platelet-aggregating thromboxane A$_2$ (TXA$_2$) has been shown to be present in platelets [19]. Whereas in the kidney the classical prostaglandins PGE$_2$ and PGF$_{2a}$ are predominantly produced in the renal medulla and papilla [20, 21], 6-keto-PGF$_{1a}$, the stable hydrolysis product of prostacyclin is formed mainly in the vascular compartment of the renal cortex [22, 23]. Thromboxane biosynthesis may be low or even absent in the kidney under physiologic circumstances, but has been recognized in the hydronephrotic rabbit kidney [24]. The major pathways of arachidonic acid metabolism are demonstrated in Figure 2.

While the distribution of biosynthesis of the 'classical' prostaglandins PGE$_2$ and PGF$_{2a}$ within the kidney is characterized by high PG synthetase activity in the inner medulla with much lower activity in the outer medulla and the renal cortex, PG metabolizing activity is predominant in the renal cortex. In addition to the two primary enzymes, 15-PG dehydrogenase and 13-PG reductase, another potentially important enzyme activity, PGE-9-keto reductase, is present in the kidney converting PGE$_2$ into PGF$_{2a}$ [25]. The lung metabolizes PGEs and PGFs by a combination of oxidation and reduction to 15-keto; 15-keto 13, 14-dihydro; and 13,14-dihydro prostaglandins. They appear to be excreted in the urine as 16-carbon tetranor compounds. However, the pulmonary vascular bed does not inactivate PGI$_2$, since it is equally potent as a vasodilator whether given intravenously or intra-arterially [26]. Therefore, this compound could, in fact, exhibit systemic activity. Since prostacyclin is a major product of arachidonic acid in all vascular tissues studied so far, it would seem unlikely that this substance could represent the antihypertensive endocrine renal function. However, the kidney may be a quantitatively important source of circulating PGI$_2$ activity, so that any impairment in the kidneys' capacity to produce PGI$_2$ would represent a lack of antihypertensive principles eventually leading to changes in arterial blood pressure.

Accumulating evidence supports the hypothesis that renal prostaglandins may be modulators of the renal excretion of sodium and water. Soon after the original description of prostaglandins PGE$_2$, PGF$_{2a}$ and PGA$_2$, in the rabbit renal medulla, it became evident that PGA and PGE were markedly natriuretic when infused into the experimental animal [27, 28]. This increase in renal sodium excretion was accompanied by enhanced total renal plasma flow. The significance and the specificity of this natriuretic effect of prostaglandins of the A and E series, however, have been questioned because of the following: 1) the effect is transitory; 2) it is unlikely that the PGE series can reach the renal arterial circulation to produce its natriuretic effects, since it is effectively degraded by the lung; 3) other nonspecific vasodilators, such as acetylcholine, lead to similar changes in renal function when infused into the renal artery; 4) total intrarenal PGE concentrations in the rat were found to rise under conditions of low salt intake and decrease during chronic salt loading [29] conditions, which is the reverse of what would be expected if renal prostaglandins promoted natriuresis.

On the other hand, contrasting evidence has been presented that the renal prostaglandins could in fact be mediators of renal sodium excretion. In chronic salt-loaded rabbits, administration of the PG synthetase inhibitor indomethacin was followed by a significantly decreased renal salt excretion [30]. Furthermore, during acute saline infusion in conscious rats, concomitant administration of indomethacin led to a marked decrease in urinary volume and renal sodium and potassium excretion [31]. Since in the same study indomethacin had no effect on renal function in non-salt-loaded animals, it was suggested that prostaglandins may play a role in adapting renal function to either an acute or chronic salt load. Studies in man are conflicting, since indomethacin was shown to reduce renal sodium excretion in some, but not in others.

Further support for a role of endogenous renal prostaglandins in regulating the excretory renal function is derived from studies in which endogenous renal prostaglandin systhesis was stimulated by infusion of the PG precursor arachidonic acid. Arachidonic acid led to a dose-dependent increase in urinary flow rate and sodium and potassium excretion, while a parallel infusion of a prostaglandin synthesis inhibitor blunted this effect [32]. Recent studies in isolated portions of the nephron showed that PGE_2 inhibits chloride transport in the isolated medullary thick ascending limb of Henle, suggesting that endogenous prostaglandins, at least under some circumstances, may be natriuretic [33].

In addition to the proposed effects of endogenous renal prostaglandins on electrolyte excretion, evidence has been presented that at least prostaglandins of the E series are also important modulators of renal water excretion. In vitro studies in the toad urinary bladder and the isolated collecting duct have demonstrated that PGE inhibits vasopressin induced water movement in these tissues presumably by inhibiting vasopressin activated adenyl cyclase [34, 35]. In vivo studies in hypophysectomized dogs undergoing a water diuresis demonstrated a marked increase in the renal response to exogenous vasopressin when the animals were pre-treated with a prostaglandin inhibitor [36]. Furthermore, prostaglandin inhibition enhanced urinary osmolality in response to exogenous vasopressin in man [37].

Thus, information so far available strongly supports the hypothesis that renomedullary prostaglandins, most probably those belonging to the E series, play an important role in the regulation of renal water excretion by modulating the effect of vasopressin in the hormone sensitive parts of the nephron. The mechanism of this effect may include alterations of intracellular cyclic-AMP metabolism. Additionally, increased renomedullary biosynthesis of prostaglandin E may increase medullary blood flow and therefore lead to a washout effect with diminished medullary hypertonicity and resultant impairment of the renal concentration ability.

SYSTEMIC ANTIHYPERTENSIVE EFFECTS

Two different theories of how prostaglandins could be involved in the regulation of systemic arterial blood pressure have been described. The first theory arises from the early observations proposing that a circulating vasodepressor substance may exist with its origin in the kidney, most likely the renal medulla. According to the second theory prostaglandins, predominantly those of the E series, as well as the vasodilatory PGI_2, have been shown to be released in arterial walls of different vascular beds and to interfere locally with pressor systems [38, 39]. Vascular PG biosynthesis is stimulated by angiotensin II and prostaglandins attenuate the vasoconstrictor effect of this vasopressor and finally are responsible for long-term tachyphylaxis against this compound [40, 41]. Similarly, PGE and PGI_2 biosynthesis are stimulated by catecholamines and both substances modulate the cardiovascular effects of the autonomic nervous system [42, 43].

The question whether endogenous renal and/or vascular prostaglandins are involved in the regulation of arterial blood pressure has been approached by either pharmacological blockage or stimulation of PG biosynthesis by administration of their fatty acid precursors. Increases in peripheral arteriolar resistance with slight increases in arterial blood pressure have been described following indomethacin in normal volunteers and hypertensive patients [44, 45], while oral administration of PG precursor fatty acids induced a slight decrease in a small group of hypertensive patients [46]. The small degree of the observed changes in blood pressure following inhibition and stimulation of PG synthesis does not exclude a major role of vasodilator prostaglandins in the regulation of arterial blood pressure. PG inhibition not only suppresses biosynthesis of vasodilator PGE_2 and PGI_2, but also affects synthesis of vasoconstrictor PGF and TXA. Moreover, it is accompanied by a suppression of the renin–angiotensin axis and a decrease in circulating plasma norepinephrine concentrations [44, 47, 48]. In contrast, administration of the PG precursor arachidonic acid as well as PGE_2 or PGI_2 have all been shown to stimulate renal renin secretion, thereby activating one of the most potent pressor systems known so far [47, 49, 50].

Radioimmunoassay measurements of urinary PGE_2 excretion which reflect renal PGE_2 production have revealed decreased excretion of PGE_2 in patients with essential hypertension [51, 52]. In addition, urinary PGE_2 excretion is inversely correlated with sodium intake and with activation of enhanced de novo PGE_2 renal biosynthesis under conditions of low salt intake and vice versa [53, 54]. The increased PGE_2 biosynthesis during salt

78

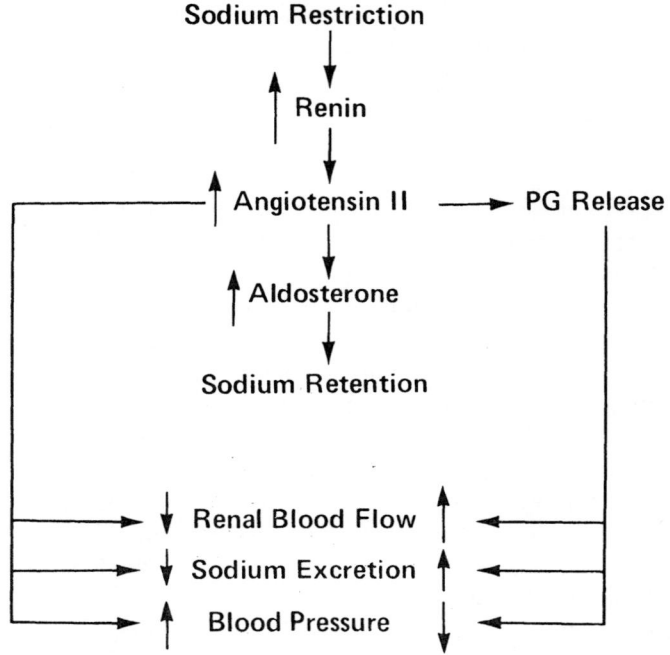

Figure 3. Hypothetical schema of the interaction of the renin–angiotensin–aldosterone axis with the PG system during dietary sodium restriction. From Lee JB: Clin Nephrol 14:159, 1980.

restriction may either function as an antinatriuretic factor stimulating the renin–angiotensin–aldosterone axis or may be directed to maintenance of basal renal blood flow and sodium excretion. In this fashion, the PGEs would function to offset the vasoconstricting and antinatriuretic actions of the renin–aldosterone system. If the latter is the case, it is possible that a primary rise in renin during low salt intake leading to generation of angiotensin II results in a compensatory enhanced PGE_2 production, since angiotensin II is a potent stimulator of PG synthesis [55] and PG synthesis is markedly inhibited by angiotensin blockade with saralasin [56]. Figure 3 summarizes this possible angiotensin–PG interrelationship. In the case of patients with essential hypertension, the decreased urinary PGE_2 raises the question whether impaired renomedullary PG production could play an etiological role in this disorder, or whether this biochemical abnormality reflects a secondary response to the elevation in arterial blood pressure.

To test the hypothesis that impaired renomedullary PG biosynthesis participates in the maintenance of elevated arterial blood pressure, PGA_2 [57] and PGA_1 [58, 59] were administered to patients with essential hypertension. Both substances induced a striking fall in peripheral arteriolar resistance and arterial blood pressure. Of interest is the interrelationship be-

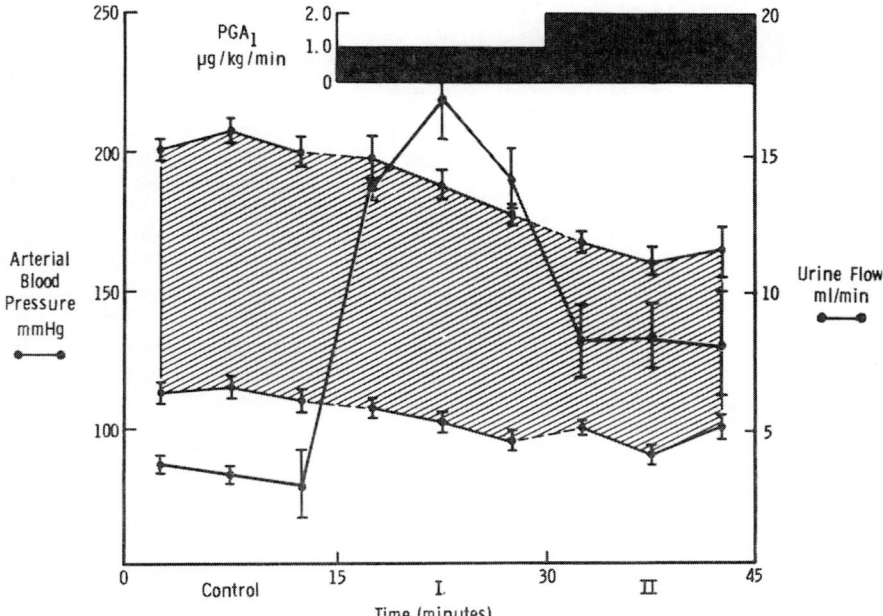

Figure 4. Effect of PGA₁ on blood pressure and urine flow in essential hypertension. Note rise in urine flow before maximal blood pressure decrease (period 1) and return of elevated urine flow toward control values when blood pressure declines (period II). From Westura EE, et al.: Circ Res 27 (Suppl 1): 131, 1970 (With permission of the publisher.)

tween renal function and the decrease in arterial blood pressure following PGA infusion. The earliest effect of PGA administration to patients with essential hypertension is an almost immediate increase in renal blood flow and urine flow (Figure 4). With a subsequent decrease in systemic arterial blood pressure, renal blood flow returns to or toward preinfusion values. This transitory phase of enhanced renal blood flow is also accompanied by an increase in glomerular filtration rate and sodium and potassium excretion. Since total renal function returns to preinfusion values after lowered blood pressure is achieved, prostaglandins of the A series, at least in acute intravenous experiments, act as ideal antihypertensive agents in that they favorably affect blood pressure and renal function. Again, the decrease in arterial blood pressure observed following PGA infusions is even more remarkable since this substance is also capable of stimulating the renin-aldosterone axis [60].

In addition to dietary sodium depletion, some diuretics have also been shown to increase urinary excretion of PGE₂. This stimulation is marked during furosemide administration and occurs almost immediately following administration of the diuretic paralleling a fall in blood pressure and an increase in plasma renin activity [44, 61]. Since the fall in blood pressure

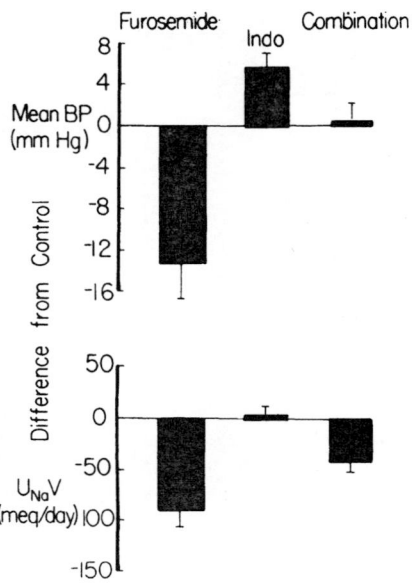

Figure 5. Antagonism of antihypertensive and natriuretic activity of furosemide by indomethacin. Administration of furosemide resulted in expected significant reduction of blood pressure and natriuresis in four normotensive and six hypertensive subjects on a normal sodium intake. The prostaglandin synthetase inhibitor, indomethacin, administered to the same ten subjects, resulted in slight but statistically significant increase in blood pressure with little change in sodium excretion. The combination of furosemide and indomethacin either abolished or markedly diminished the antihypertensive and natriuretic effects of this diuretic suggesting that prostaglandins may mediate such actions. From [44], with permission of the publisher.

cannot be ascribed to changes in salt excretion immediately after furosemide administration, it seems reasonable to speculate that the stimulation of renal and/or vascular prostaglandins might be involved in this effect.

To study further the mechanism of action of diuretics with regard to prostaglandins, Patak et al. [44] administered furosemide alone and indomethacin alone and in combination to normotensive subjects, as well as to patients with essential hypertension on a normal sodium intake. Furosemide alone resulted in a significant reduction of blood pressure, marked natriuresis and elevation of plasma renin, and urinary aldosterone (Figures 5 and 6). Administration of the prostaglandin synthetase inhibitor, indomethacin, to the same human subjects resulted in a uniform rise in blood pressure, unchanged sodium excretion, and a marked decrease in plasma renin activity. However, during combination treatment with furosemide and indomethacin, the antihypertensive and natriuretic effects of furosemide were either completely abolished or markedly diminished. The effects of plasma renin activity were intermediate between the marked inhibition observed with indomethacin alone and the elevation with furosemide.

From these results, it seems obvious that the antihypertensive and natriuretic effect of the diuretic furosemide may be mediated, at least in part, by prostaglandins, possibly renal in origin. Interference with the action of diuretics by prostaglandin inhibitors has also been demonstrated for ethacrynic acid [62], bumetamide [63], and spironolactone [64]. The exact mechanism of how prostaglandins may intervene in the action of diuretics remains unclear to date, but these studies support the hypothesis that pros-

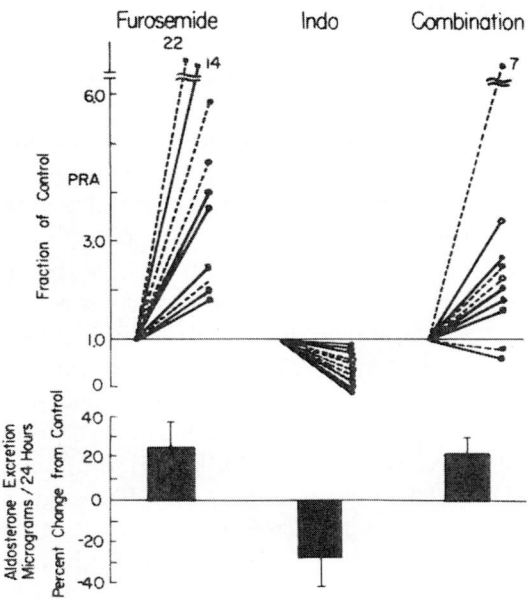

Figure 6. Plasma renin activity and aldosterone excretion. In the same ten subjects discussed in Figure 5, PRA and aldosterone excretion were increased in response to furosemide, and markedly decreased by indomethacin. The combination of furosemide and indomethacin resulted in an intermediate rise in PRA when compared with that of furosemide alone. The interrupted lines denote normotensive subjects and the solid lines, patients with essential hypertension. Plasma renin activity is expressed as fraction of control which indicates the ratio of PRA after furosemide therapy to that before. From [44], with permission of the publisher.

taglandins may mediate the ameliorative effects of low sodium diet and diuretic therapy. The mechanism of stimulation of renomedullary PG biosynthesis seems to be dependent on increased circulating angiotensin II concentrations during salt depletion and diuretic therapy, since furosemide itself does not stimulate PGE_2 biosynthesis when added to rabbit papillary slices in vitro [65].

Thus, there is evidence to support the theory of a renomedullary antihypertensive function in the pathogenesis of essential hypertension, possibly exerted via prostaglandins. The precise biochemical nature of this effect remains unclear, since to date a naturally occurring PGA or PGA-like compound has not been demonstrated. Preliminary data, however, suggest that PGI_2 may also be generated in significant amounts in the human renal medulla [66]. Further studies will be needed to define more precisely how the renomedullary-antihypertensive function is involved in the etiology and/or pathogenesis of human essential hypertension and which biochemical substance may be the mediator of this function.

With regard to the role of vascular PG biosynthesis in essential hypertension, no studies in humans are available to date. However, in vitro studies comparing aortic PG biosynthesis in normotensive rats and in rats with spontaneous hypertension (which serves as a model for human essential hypertension) have provided further insight into the possible role of the vascular prostaglandin system in this disorder. While aortic tissue from normotensive rats converts arachidonic acid into PGE_2, PGF_2 and PGI_2 in similar proportions, tissue from spontaneously hypertensive rats directs this conversion quite specifically to PGI_2 formation, producing approximately four- po fivefold more PGI_2 than aortic tissue from control rats [67]. Since PGI_2 is a more potent vasodilator than PGE_2 [68] and, unlike PGE_2, is not significantly metabolized in the pulmonary circulation, it might be speculated that, if these results are applicable in vivo, directing vascular PG biosynthesis towards increased PGI_2 production might function as an adaptive response in the presence of elevations in arterial blood pressure.

In conclusion, evidence today supports the theory that renal and/or vascular prostaglandins are involved in the pathogenesis of essential hypertension in a secondary way, representing an effort to attenuate elevations in blood pressure. It still remains an open question if a renomedullary prostaglandin mediates the antihypertensive function of the renal medulla and how this function is linked to the etiology and/or the pathogenesis of essential hypertension. To link the vascular and renal prostaglandin system with the multitude of functional and endocrine factors that may be involved in the pathogenesis of human essential hypertension will help to draw a much clearer picture about a possible participation of the role of prostaglandins in blood pressure regulation.

ACKNOWLEDGEMENTS

This work was supported by grants 1453 and K016 from the New York State Health Research Council and grant 400965 from the Saudi Arabian Educational Mission, Houston, Texas. The authors thank Audrey Lee for preparation of the manuscript. This chapter has been reprinted with permission of Resident & Staff Physician 26:99, 1980.

REFERENCES

1. Goldblatt H, Lynch J, Hanzal RF, et al.: Studies in experimental hypertension. 1. The production of persistent elevation in blood pressure by renal ischemia. J Exp Med 59:347, 1934.

2. Braun-Menéndez E, von Euler US: Hypertension after bilateral nephrectomy in the rat. Nature 160:905, 1957.

3. Grollman A, Muirhead EE, Vanatta J: Role of the kidney in pathogenesis of hypertension as determined by a study of the effects of bilateral nephrectomy and other experimental procedures on the blood pressure of the dog. Am J Physiol 157:21, 1949.

4. Muirhead EE, Jones F, Stirman JA: Antihypertensive property in renoprival hypertension of extract from renal medulla. J Lab Clin Med 56:167, 1960.

5. Hamilton JG, Grollman A: The preparation of renal extracts effective in reducing blood pressure in experimental hypertension. J Biol Chem 233:528, 1958.

6. Lee JB, Hickler RB, Saravis CA, Thorn GW: Sustained depressor effect of renal medullary extract in the normotensive rat. Circ Res 13:359, 1963.

7. Lee JB, Covino BG, Takman BH, et al.: Renomedullary vasodepressor substance, medullin: Isolation, chemical characterization and physiological properties. Circ Res 17:57, 1965.

8. von Euler US: On the specific vasodilating and plain muscle stimulating substances from accessory genital glands in man and certain animals (prostaglandin and vesiglandin). J Physiol 81:65, 1936.

9. Bergström S, Sjövall J: The isolation of prostaglandin F from sheep prostate gland. Acta Chem Scand 14:1693, 1960.

10. Bergström S, Sjövall J: The isolation of prostaglandin E from sheep prostate gland. Acta Chem Scand 14:1701, 1960.

11. Bergström S, Ryhage R, Samuelsson B, et al.: The structure of prostaglandin E, F_1 and F_2. Acta Chem Scand 16:501, 1962.

12. Lee JB, Crowshaw K, Takman BH, et al.: The identification of prostaglandin E_2, F_2 and A_2 from rabbit kidney medulla. Biochem J 105:1251, 1967.

13. Larsson C, Änggård E: Mass spectrometric determination of prostaglandins in regions of the rabbit kidney. p. 179. Proceedings of the Int. Conference on Prostaglandins, Florence, Italy (May 26–30), 1975.

14. Frölich JC, Sweetman BJ, Carr K, et al.: Assessment of the levels of PGA_2 in human plasma by gas chromatography–mass spectrometry. Prostaglandins 10:185, 1975.

15. Düsing R, Lee JB: Renomedullary prostaglandin biosynthesis: dependence on extracellular potassium concentration. In: Prostaglandins in Cardiovascular and Renal Function, pp. 123–141. Scriabine R, ed. Philadelphia: Spectrum, 1980.

16. Flower R, Gryglewski R, Herbaczynska-Cedro K, et al.: Effects of anti-inflammatory drugs on prostaglandin biosynthesis. Nature (New Biol) 238:104, 1972.

17. Oelz O, Sweetman BJ, Oates JA, Nies AS, Data J: Prostaglandin D_2, another renal prostaglandin. Pharmacologist 18:163, 1976.

18. Moncada S, Gryglewski R, Bunting S, Vane JR: An enzyme isolated from arteries transforms prostaglandin endoperoxides to an unstable substance that inhibits platelet aggregation. Nature 263:663, 1976.

19. Samuelsson B: Introduction: new trends in prostaglandin research. In: Advances in Prostaglandin and Thromboxane Research, Vol 1, pp. 1–6. Samuelsson B and Paoletti R, eds. New York: Raven, 1976.

20. Janszen FH, Nugteren DH: Histochemical localization of prostaglandin synthetase. Histochemistry 27:159, 1971.

21. Larsson C, Änggård E: Regional differences in the formation and metabolism of prostaglandins in the rabbit kidney. Eur J Pharmacol 21:30, 1973.

22. Whorton AR, Smigel M, Oates JA, Frölich JC: Regional differences in prostacyclin formation by the kidney: prostacyclin is a major prostaglandin of the renal cortex. Biochim Biophys Acta 529:176, 1978.

23. Oliw E: Prostaglandins and kidney function: an experimental study in the rabbit. Acta Physiol Scand (Suppl):461, 1979.

84

24. Morrison A, Nishikawa K, Needleman P: Unmasking of thromboxane A_2 synthesis by ureteral obstruction in the rabbit kidney. Clin Res 25:442A, 1977.
25. Pace-Asciak CR: Biosynthesis and metabolism of prostaglandins in the kidney. In: Renal Prostaglandins. Vol 1, pp. 55–83. Lee JB, ed. Montreal: Eden Press, 1978.
26. Pace-Asciak CR, Carrara KC: Evidence suggesting a systemic antihypertensive role for PGI_2. Prostaglandins 15:704, 1978.
27. Gross JB, Bartter FC: Effects of prostaglandins E_1, A_1 and F_{2-} on renal handling of salt and water. Am J Physiol 225:218, 1973.
28. Vander AJ: Direct effects of prostaglandin on renal function and renin release in anesthetized dog. Am J Physiol 214:218, 1968.
29. Tobian L, O'Donnell M, Smith P: Intrarenal prostaglandin levels during normal and high sodium intake. Circ Res 34, 35 (suppl):83, 1974.
30. Attallah AA, Lee JB: Radioimmunoassay of prostaglandin A. Intrarenal PGA_2 as a factor mediating saline-induced natriuresis. Circ Res 33:696, 1973.
31. Düsing R, Melder B, Kramer HJ: Prostaglandins and renal function in acute extracellular volume expansion. Prostaglandins 12:3, 1976.
32. Tannenbaum J, Splawinski JA, Oates JA, et al.: Enhanced renal prostaglandin production in the dog. Effects on renal function. Circ Res 36:197, 1975.
33. Stokes JB: Effect of prostaglandin E_2 on chloride transport across the rabbit thick ascending limb of Henle: selective inhibition of the medullary portion. J Clin Invest 64:495, 1979.
34. Orloff J, Handler JS, Bergström S: Effect of prostaglandin (PGE_1) on the permeability response of toad bladder to vasopressin, theophylline and adenosine 3'5'-monophosphate. Nature 205:397, 1965.
35. Grantham JJ, Orloff J: Effect of prostaglandin E_1 on the permeability response of the isolated collecting tubule to vasopressin, theophylline and adenosine 3'5'-monophosphate. J Clin Invest 47:1154, 1968.
36. Anderson RJ, Berl T, McDonald KM, et al.: Evidence for an in vivo antagonism between vasopressin and prostaglandin in the mammalian kidney. J Clin Invest 56:420, 1975.
37. Silverstein ME, Feldman RC, Henderson LW, et al.: Effects of indomethacin on human renal clearance of sodium and H_2O (abstract). Clin Res 22:721, 1974.
38. Gimbrone MA Jr, Alexander RW: Angiotensin II stimulation of prostaglandin production in cultured human vascular endothelium. Science 189:219, 1975.
39. Pace-Asciak CR, Rangaraj G: Distribution of prostaglandin biosynthetic pathways in several rat tissues: formation of 6-keto-prostaglandin F_1. Biochim Biophys Acta 486:579, 1977.
40. McGiff JC, Crowshaw K, Itskowitz HD: Prostaglandins and renal function. Fed Proc 33:40, 1974.
41. Aiken JW: Effects of prostaglandin synthesis inhibitors on angiotensin tachyphylaxis in the isolated coeliac and mesenteric arteries of the rabbit. Pol J Phamacol Pharm 26:217, 1974.
42. Hedqvist P: Control by prostaglandin E_2 of sympathetic neurotransmission in the spleen. Life Sci 9:269, 1970.
43. Pace-Asciak CR: Prostaglandin synthetase activity in the rat stomach fundus: activation by L-norepinephrine and related compounds. Biochim Biophys Acta 280:161, 1972.
44. Patak RV, Mookerjee BK, Bentzel CJ, et al.: Antagonism of the effects of furosemide by indomethacin in normal and hypertensive man. Prostaglandins 20:649, 1975.
45. Wennmalm A: Influence of indomethacin on the systemic and pulmonary vascular resistance in man. Clin Sci Mol Med 54:141, 1978.
46. Comberg HU, Heyden S, Hames CG, Vergroesen AJ, Fleichman AI: Hypotensive effect of dietary prostaglandin precursor in hypertensive man. Prostaglandins 15:193, 1978.
47. Larsson C, Weber P, Änggård E: Arachidonic acid increases and indomethacin decreases plasma renin activity in the rabbit. Europ J Pharmacol 28:391, 1974.

48. Düsing R, Gill JR Jr, Bartter FC, Güllner HG: The effect of potassium depletion on urinary prostaglandins in normal man. In: Advances in Prostaglandin and Thromboxane Research, p. 1189. Samuelsson B, Ramwell PW, Paoletti R, eds. New York: Raven, 1980.

49. Werning C, Vetter W, Weidmann P, Schweiker HV, Stiel D, Siegenthaler W: Effect of prostaglandin E_1 on renin in the dog. Am J Physiol 220:852, 1977.

50. Whorton AR, Misono K, Hollifield J, Frölich JC, Inagami T, Oates JA: Prostaglandins and renin release – I. Stimulation of renin release from rabbit renal cortical slices by PGI_2. Prostaglandins 14:1095, 1977.

51. Tan SY, Bravo E, Mulrow PJ: Impaired renal PGE_2 biosynthesis: A specific abnormality in essential hypertension. Clin Res 23:369, 1978.

52. Weber PC, Scherer B, Lange HH, Held E, Schenermann J: Renal prostaglandins and renin release: relationship to regulation of electrolyte excretion and blood pressure. Proc VII Int Congr Nephrol, Montreal, p. 99. Basel: Karger, 1978.

53. Sthal R, Attallah AA, Bloch DL, Lee JB: Stimulation of rabbit renal PGE_2 biosynthesis by dietary sodium restriction. Am J Physiol 237:F344, 1979.

54. Stahl R, Attallah AA, Bloch DL, Lee JB: Stimulation of rabbit renal PGE_2 biosynthesis by dietary sodium restriction. In: Advances in Prostaglandin and Thromboxane Research, Bol 17, pp. 1053–1055. Samuelsson B, Ramwell PW, Paoletti R, eds. New York: Raven, 1980.

55. Zusman RM, Keiser HT: Prostaglandin biosynthesis by rabbit renomedullary interstitial cells in tissue culture: stimulation by angiotensin II, bradykinin and arginine vasopressin. J Clin Invest 60: 215, 1977.

56. Attallah AA, Stahl R, Bloch DL, Lee JB: Furosemide stimulates and saralasin inhibits prostaglandin E_2 biosynthesis. Clin Res 27:599, 1979.

57. Lee JB: Chemical and physiological properties of renal prostaglandins: the antihypertensive effects of medullin in essential human hypertension. Second Nobel Symposium, Prostaglandins, pp. 197–210. Bergström S, Samuellsson B, eds. Stockholm: Almqvist & Wiksell, 1967.

58. Carr AA: Effect of PGA_1 on renin and aldosterone in man. Prostaglandins 3:621, 1973.

59. Lee, JB, McGiff JC, Kannegiesser H, et al.: Prostaglandin A_1: antihypertensive and renal effects. Ann Intern Med 74:703, 1971.

60. Fichman MP, Lettenburg G, Brooker G, et al.: Effect of prostaglandin A_1 on renal and adrenal function in man. Circ Res 31 (suppl II):19, 1972.

61. Scherer B, Weber PC: Time-Dependent changes in prostaglandin excretion in response to furosemide in man. Clin Sci 56:77, 1979.

62. Williamson HE, Marchand GR, Bourland WA, et al.: Ethacrynic acid induced release of prostaglandin E to increase renal blood flow. Prostaglandins 11:519, 1976.

63. Olsen UB, Ahnefelt-Rønne I: Bumetamide induced increase of renal blood flow in conscious dogs and its relation to local renal hormones (PGE, kallikrein and renin). Acta Pharmacol Toxicol 38:219, 1976.

64. Tweedale MG, Ogilvie RI: Antagonism of spironolactone-induced natriuresis by aspirin in man. N Eng J Med 289:198, 1973.

65. Düsing R, Attallah AA, Braselton WE, Lee JB: Antihypertensive effect of volume depletion: interrelation with renal prostaglandins. Contr Nephrol 12:41, 1978.

66. Hassid A, Dunn MJ: In vitro prostaglandin biosynthesis by human kidney, p. 49. Proc 12th Annual Meeting Am Soc Nephrol, 1979.

67. Pace-Asiak CR, Carrara MC, Rangaraj G, Nicolaou KC: Enhanced formation of PGI_2, a potent hypotensive substance, by aortic rings and homogenates of the spontaneously hypertensive rat. Prostaglandins 15:1005, 1978.

68. Pace-Asiak CR, Carrara MC, Nicolaou KC: Prostaglandin I_2 has more potent hypotensive properties than prostaglandin E_2 in the normal and spontaneously hypertensive rat. Prostaglandins 15:999, 1978.

6. ROLE OF KALLIKREIN IN BLOOD PRESSURE REGULATION

Klaus O. Stumpe and Axel Overlack

Kallikreins are proteolytic enzymes that generate vasoactive kinins from plasma a_2-globulin substrates, called kininogens [1]. Kinins are among the most potent vasodilators endogenously produced in man [2]. Several different kallikreins have been characterized, the most extensively evaluated being those found in plasma and those isolated from urine, the latter arising from the kidney rather than from plasma [2-5].

Despite several reports that implicate plasma bradykinin as a vasodilator in various disease states and other studies that imply a role for the renal kallikrein–kinin system in salt and water metabolism [6-8], little is known about the cardiovascular and renal actions of endogenous kinins and the importance of the kallikrein–kinin system in the regulation of systemic arterial blood pressure.

This review will describe some of the studies that are exploring the kallikrein–kinin system and its possible role in blood pressure regulation under physiological conditions.

BIOCHEMISTRY OF THE KALLIKREIN-KININ SYSTEM

All mammals thus far studied have two types of kallikreins: plasma kallikreins and glandular kallikreins.

Plasma kallikrein is formed in the liver and circulates in the blood as an inactive precursor, prekallikrein [9-11]. Conversion of prekallikrein, also known as Fletcher factor [12], to kallikrein is dependent upon activation of the Hageman factor, occurring on certain negatively charged surfaces, e.g. the basement membrane, and requires the presence of high molecular weight kininogen [13]. Thus, activation of plasma kallikrein is closely associated with the intrinsic blood clotting mechanism, the fibrinolysis and the complement sequence [14-16]. This system is also involved in the activation of plasminogen to plasmin [15] and in the organism's response to injury and inflammation.

The glandular kallikreins differ from the plasma enzyme in molecular weight and other physicochemical characteristics, immunologically, enzy-

Amery, A. (ed.) Hypertensive Cardiovascular Disease: Pathophysiology and Treatment
© *1982, Martinus Nijhoff Publishers. The Hague / Boston / London*
ISBN-13: 978-94-009-7478-4

Table 1. Differences between plasma and glandular kallikreins [47]

	Plasma kallikrein	Glandular kallikrein
Molecular weight	100 000	24 000–44 000
Substrate	HMWK	LMWK and HMWK
Kinin released	Bradykinin	Lys-bradykinin
Function	Coagulation Fibrinolysis Inflammation? Blood pressure regulation?	Regulation of local blood flow? Water and electrolyte excretion? Blood pressure regulation?

LMWK = Low molecular weight kininogen
HMWK = High molecular weight kininogen

matically and are affected by various inhibitors. Glandular kallikreins have been highly purified from such organs as the porcine pancreas [17], the guinea pig coagulating gland [18], the rat salivary glands [19] and kidney [4], and such secretions as the urine of horses [20], rats [21, 22] and humans [23, 24]. In general, the glandular kallikreins are acidic glycoproteins with molecular weights from 24 000 to 43 600 daltons. In contrast, human plasma prekallikrein has a molecular weight of ~100 000 daltons (Table 1).

Glandular kallikreins release the decapeptide lysylbradykinin (kallidin) from low and high molecular weight kininogen, in contrast to plasma kallikrein which forms bradykinin [25]. The glandular enzyme cleaves two dissimilar peptide bonds, a methionyl-lysine bond and an arginyl-serine bond within kininogens [26], suggesting that the enzyme may have two different active sites.

Inactivation of kallikreins

Glandular as well as plasma kallikreins are inhibited by protease inhibitors in human plasma but the inactivation of plasma kallikrein is more rapid and complete than that of glandular kallikreins. There are at least four different plasma protein inhibitors of plasma kallikrein, including a_2-macroglobulin, C_1-inactivator, a_1-antitrypsin, and antithrombin III. The inactivation of glandular kallikrein has been mainly ascribed to a_1-antitrypsin [27]. Only one endogenous renal kallikrein inhibitor has been described thus far [28]. However, several natural or synthetic kallikrein inhibitors are just beginning to be used to assess the role of kallikrein in blood pressure regulation [29] and renal function [30]. These include aprotinin (Trasylol®), diisopropyl-fluorophosphate analogues, and several aromatic trisamidines.

Kinin metabolism

Activated plasma kallikrein releases bradykinin, whereas glandular kallikreins release kallidin (lysyl-bradykinin) [9]. Kallidin is rapidly converted to bradykinin by aminopeptidase [9] and also into methionyl-lysyl-bradykinin by a uropepsin, another urinary serine proteinase active at an acid pH.

Both kinins (kallidin and bradykinin) are inactivated by enzymes called kininases which are found in blood and other tissues [31]. The two main kininases have been named kininase I and II. Kininase I is carboxypeptidase and kininase II is a peptidyldipeptide hydrolase also known as angiotensin converting enzyme, because it converts angiotensin I to angiotensin II [32] (Figure 1).

The half-life of bradykinin determined in blood is about 20 s and that of kallidin somewhat longer [33, 34]. The rapid degradation of bradykinin has been ascribed to kininase II [32]. Much of the interest in kininase II is due to the fact that it also converts angiotensin I to angiotensin II and that it may play an essential role in blood pressure regulation.

Localization of kallikrein–kinin system components

The first kallikrein discovered was urinary kallikrein [35]. This enzyme appears to be produced by the kidney, since Nustad and co-workers [4] demonstrated that rat kidney slices synthesized kallikrein. More recently, Roblero et al. [36] have shown that kallikrein is present in urine produced by the isolated rat kidney that has been perfused with fluids not containing

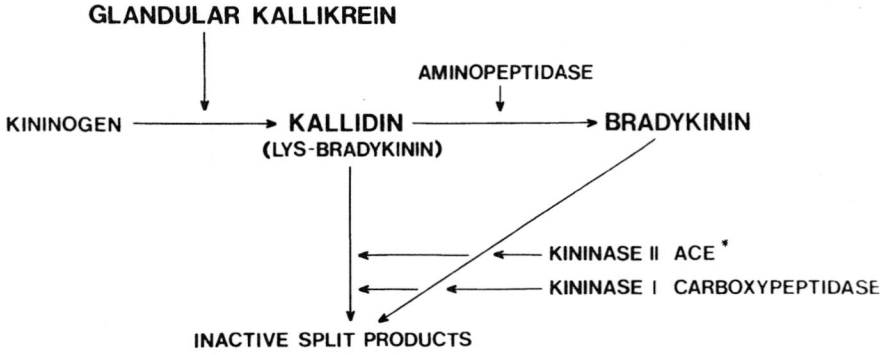

*ACE = Angiotensin I converting enzyme

Figure 1. Production and inactivation of kinins.

either prekallikrein or kallikrein. From the data of Carretero and co-workers [37] it can be derived that over 90% of the renal kallikrein is in the cortex, decreasing from the outer to the inner cortex, with very little kallikrein activity in the medulla and papilla. Using stop-flow techniques it has been shown that kallikrein is incorporated into the urine at the level of the distal tubule [38].

It is not known if the kallikrein produced in the distal tubule is secreted only in the lumen of the nephron or if it is also secreted in the interstitial and vascular space, where it could release kinins and induce hemodynamic changes and, consequently, changes in the renal function. Recent reports indicate that the renal kallikrein could appear in the extracellular and/or the vascular space of the kidney [37, 39, 40]. In a previous study by Geiger and co-workers [41], a glandular kallikrein from human plasma was isolated by immunaffinity-chromatography which appeared to be identical to urinary kallikrein. The possibility of extracting active glandular kallikrein from human plasma and the observation that inhibition of renal kallikrein in human plasma proceeds very slowly [41] may indicate that at least part of the glandular kallikrein is present in plasma as an active enzyme. Thus, glandular kallikrein in plasma could maintain a physiological kinin level throughout in blood and other body fluids by its action on ubiquitously occurring kininogens. This may have implications on the role of the kallikrein–kinin system in the regulation of vascular tone.

The role of the kallikrein–kinin system in blood pressure regulation

The varied physiological and biochemical effects that result from activation of the kallikrein–kinin system are almost universally considered to be the result of the formation of bradykinin or lysyl-bradykinin. Studies in normal human subjects or animals have established that either intravenously or intra-arterially administered kallikrein, bradykinin or kallidin cause reduction in blood pressure and renal arterial vasodilatation [34, 35, 42, 43]. However, the fact that pharmacologic doses of kinins produce vasodilatation does not prove that the kallikrein–kinin system performs this function in situ. Probably, no route of administration of kinins reproduces the effects evoked by release of kinins intrarenally or at local vascular sites, in terms of either concentrations achieved at their sites of action, localization of activity, or the sequence of vascular elements affected [44]. Therefore, it becomes difficult to conclude a priori that the kallikrein–kinin system participates in the regulation of arterial pressure. The issue will probably remain unsettled until the development of specific kinin-receptor blockers, the lack of which has been a great impediment to progress in defining various roles for kallikrein and kinin. Furthermore, although glandular kallikrein can attack kininogen to release lysylbrady-kinin, the processes and factors that regulate the formation and release of kinins by glandular kallikrein have in essence not been described. Such is not the case with respect to the formation and generation of plasma kinins, as mentioned earlier. Nevertheless, some data have been generated which indicate that the extremely powerful vasodilator effect of the kallikrein–kinin system coupled with the fact that the kinins can develop anywhere in the circulatory system with ease, must play important roles in circulatory control.

Basic principles of arterial pressure regulation

The following relationship between mean arterial pressure, cardiac output, and total peripheral resistance bears repeating: pressure = cardiac output × total peripheral resistance. Any factor that increases either the cardiac output or total peripheral resistance or both causes an increase in the mean arterial pressure. Therefore, the body can control mean arterial pressure by changing either the cardiac output or the total peripheral resistance.

There are three different methods by which the arterial pressure is normally regulated, each operating, at least partly, independently of the other two and each having specific capacities in keeping the arterial pressure regulated at a constant value. They are the following:
1) Regulation by the autonomic nervous system
2) Regulation of sodium homeostasis and extracellular fluid volume by the kidneys
3) Regulation by hormones such as renin, angiotensin, aldosterone, the prostaglandins, norepinephrine, and epinephrine.
Previous investigations have provided evidence that there are important interrelationships between these three pressure control mechanisms and the kallikrein–kinin system which are complicated by a mosaic of direct and indirect effects of the various hormones. Therefore, discussion of the role of the kallikrein–kinin system in blood pressure regulation has to consider the various relations between the system and the factors known to be involved in the control of the circulation.

Relation between the kallikrein–kinin system and the autonomous nervous system

Interrelations between the kallikrein–kinin and the autonomous nervous system are not well defined. Kinins release catecholamines from the adrenal medulla in the rabbit, the rat, the cat and the dog [45].

The vasodilator action of bradykinin is potentiated after a-adreno-receptor blockade with phenoxybenzamine, and bradykinin decreases vasoconstriction induced by sympathetic nerve stimulation and by injections of noradrenaline in the isolated perfused kidney of the rabbit.

Streeten and co-workers [46] have described a familial syndrome characterized by orthostatic fall in blood pressure paralleled by an increase in heart rate. These patients had increased bradykinin levels and in some cases subnormal kininase activity in plasma. Phenoxybenzamine produced a slight improvement, whereas β-receptor blockade with propranolol was most effective in alleviating the symptoms. However, there was no evidence of propranolol having any direct action on the kinin system. Carretero and co-workers [47] have shown that chronic beta-blockade with propranolol at doses that significantly decrease the heart rate, does not change urinary kallikrein excretion in the rat. Furthermore, there is no variation in urinary kallikrein excretion with relation to posture, indicating no apparent correlation with sympathetic nervous system activity [48]. Moreover, an increase in sympathetic activity produced by sinoaortic deafferentation does not result in any significant changes in urinary kallikrein excretion in rats. On the other hand, isoproterenol and dopamine infused in the renal artery have been shown to increase urinary kallikrein excretion [8, 49]. This discussion indicates that the autonomous nervous system and the kallikrein–kinin system may be interrelated. However, the interactions between the two systems are complex and could be bidirectional. Their possible physiologic role in blood pressure regulation remains uncertain and needs more extensive examination.

Kallikrein–kinin system activity and regulation of extracellular fluid volume by the kidney

The kidney plays a central role in long-term regulation of arterial blood pressure. One of the most important mechanisms by which the kidney regulates blood pressure chronically is based on the effect of arterial pressure and of neural and hormonal influences on renal excretion of sodium and water. One hormonal system that has been postulated to play a role in regulating renal sodium excretion and arterial pressure is the kallikrein–kinin system.

Several observations have shown that kinins infused into the renal artery result in increased blood flow, diuresis and natriuresis [50–52]. Increased sodium excretion produced by bradykinin infusions was shown to be secondary to increased renal blood flow [50, 52]. Part of the vasodilator effect of kinins in the kidney is mediated through the prostaglandin system since the vasodilator action of kinins is attenuated after the administration of indomethacin, a prostaglandin synthesis inhibitor [53]. There is no convincing evidence available showing that bradykinin has *direct* inhibitory action on tubular electrolyte and water transport, although stop-flow studies in the dog indicate that intra-arterial infusions of bradykinin reduce proximal reabsorption of sodium and water [54]. Other studies have provided evidence that the diuretic and natriuretic effect of kinins is due to their action at the level of the distal nephron [50, 52]. However, it is uncertain if this effect is due to a direct effect of the kinins on distal tubular cells, the vasodilator effect of the peptide, changes in the osmotic gradient of the renal medulla or a combination of these three effects [47].

The role of *endogenously* generated kinins in the regulation of renal blood flow and sodium and water excretion has been studied by using the converting-enzyme and kininase II inhibitor teprotide (SQ 20881, Squibb). This peptide increases the concentration of endogenous kinins by inhibiting kininase II. There were significant increases in urine flow and sodium excretion which were positively correlated with increased levels of kinins in blood and urine, and in renal blood flow [44]. However, the use of teprotide does not allow for differentiation between the potentiation of kinin activity and the inhibition of the conversion of angiotensin I to angiotensin II. The need for specific kinin inhibitors in this type of study is obvious. Mills and co-workers have shown direct correlations between sodium, water and kallikrein excretion in man [55] as well as in rabbits and rats on free salt and water intake [56].

Effects of changes in extracellular fluid volume on kallikrein–kinin system activity

The above mentioned pharmacologic studies and measurements of kallikrein or kinin activity suggest that the system is associated with natriuretic and diuretic processes and by this mode of action may also control arterial blood pressure. However, there are several data which appear inconsistent with the assumption that the endogenous kallikrein–kinin system promotes natriuresis and diuresis. It has been shown that the urinary excretion of kallikrein is increased by low dietary sodium intake in humans and in the rat [57–60]. Furthermore, normal subjects showed a marked decrease in urinary kallikrein when they were changed from a free salt and water intake to a high sodium diet (Stumpe et al., unpublished results; see also Figure 2).

Other indirect evidence suggesting relations between the kallikrein–kinin system and sodium homeostasis is based on the demonstration of decreased plasma kinin levels with saline infusions into normal human subjects and

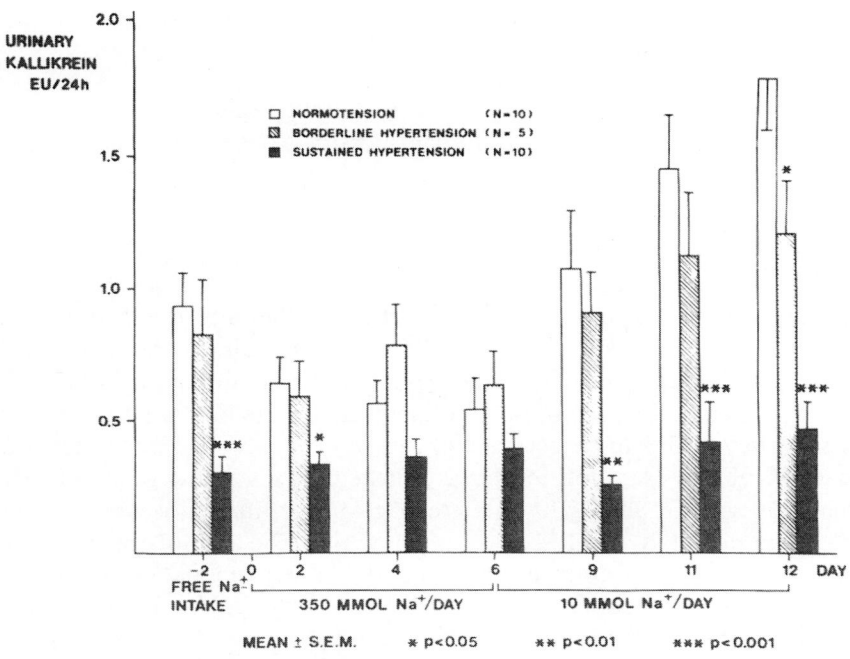

Figure 2. Response of urinary kallikrein excretion in normotensive and hypertensive subjects to different sodium diets.

an increase in plasma kinins during prolonged low dietary sodium intake [61].

The *origin* of kinins in peripheral blood is uncertain; they could be the product of either plasma kallikrein or glandular kallikrein. As mentioned before, some renal kallikrein is secreted into the vascular compartment and continuously forms kinins in the circulating plasma. The physiological significance of the increase in urinary kallikrein activity and in plasma kinins after sodium restriction with regard to blood pressure regulation is not clear. However, it is known that in sodium-depleted man the high plasma levels of angiotensin II are not associated with a rise in blood pressure and, furthermore, that with sodium restriction, the vascular response to angiotensin II is blunted both in man and in the experimental animal [62–65]. A possible mechanism for this phenomenon would be a decreased vascular sensitivity due to an increase in bradykinin levels [61]. It is obvious that, on the basis of the data discussed, the exact role of the kallikrein–kinin system in water or electrolyte homeostasis is as yet unclear. Nevertheless, the findings that the kallikrein–kinin system and the renin–angiotensin system are highly correlated because both respond to changes in extracellular fluid volume, suggest that kinins could play a role in regulating systemic blood pressure by counterbalancing the vasoconstrictive actions of angiotensin II.

INTERACTIONS BETWEEN THE KALLIKREIN–KININ SYSTEM AND
OTHER HORMONAL AND VASOACTIVE SYSTEMS

The biochemical mechanism by which kallikrein–kinin system activity is
influenced by changes in sodium homeostasis or extracellular fluid volume
is unknown.

Interaction between kallikrein and aldosterone

It has been suggested that kallikrein excretion by the kidney is determined,
at least in part, by the effective level of circulating sodium-retaining steroid
hormone, presumably as a consequence of some action of steroids on renal
cells [58]. Thus, administration of fluorocortisone to human subjects, or
desoxycorticosterone or aldosterone to rats or dogs [55, 57, 58, 66] increases
urinary kallikrein excretion, while spironolactone, an aldosterone antagonist, decreases it [57, 58, 67]. It is interesting to note that kallikrein does not
increase immediately, but three or more days after the administration of the
mineralocorticoids. In dogs, in which kallikrein was studied in relation to
the escape phenomenon, Carretero and co-workers [67] have found that urinary kallikrein excretion increased after the dogs escaped from the sodium-
retaining effect of desoxycorticosterone. This suggests that the mineralocorticoids have an indirect effect, perhaps secondary to an increase in extracellular fluid or a decrease in potassium. On the other hand, aldosterone has
been shown to increase the production of kallikrein by kidney cortical cells
in suspension [68]. However, this study is difficult to assess because the
aldosterone concentration used in the incubation medium was extremely
high. Whether the effects of mineralocorticoids are direct or indirect, all of
these studies suggest that aldosterone is one of the factors that controls kallikrein excretion. Also, it has been shown that patients with primary aldosteronism and patients with Bartter's syndrome, both syndromes being characterized by high aldosterone secretion, have high kallikrein excretion [69–
71]. However, high aldosterone is not necessarily accompanied by high kallikrein excretion. Rats with severe, two-kidney renovascular hypertension
(one kidney clipped, the contralateral untouched) have high aldosterone, low
kallikrein excretion, and low tissue kallikrein [47]. Although these findings
indicate that other, as yet unidentified, factors control renal kallikrein excretion, the data show that under various physiologic conditions urinary kallikrein excretion correlates closely with mineralocorticoid activity.

It has been demonstrated that urinary kallikrein excretion can increase,
while plasma kinin levels do not change when mineralocorticoids are
administered or endogenous levels are increased [58, 72]. Thus, urinary kallikrein and blood kinins can vary independently of one another. At present
it is unknown whether renal kallikrein production plays a role in regulating

systemic blood pressure by counterbalancing the sodium-retaining effects of mineralocorticoids.

Interaction between the kallikrein–kinin and the renin–angiotensin system

Renal kallikrein is situated in the cells of the distal convoluted tubule, adjacent to the storage site of renin and its distribution in the kidney parallels that of renin in that it is highest in the cortex and diminishes in the juxtamedullary area [38]. This anatomic proximity of the two enzymes could be of functional significance. Recently, Sealey et al. [73] have reported that human urinary kallikrein converts plasma-inactive renin to active renin and they proposed that kallikrein may be the endogenous renin activator in the kidney. Such a possibility is supported by the findings of Suzuki et al. [74] that urinary kallikrein acts directly on the rat kidney to release renin, probably via proteolytic conversion of prorenin to renin. Furthermore, the observation of a direct relationship between the daily excretion of urinary kallikrein and the proportion of active renin in the circulation points to a functional link between the two systems [75]. It is possible that the two enzymes which produce peptides with diametrically opposing actions could act concurrently at different sites so as to regulate systemic arterial pressure without simultaneously comprising local kidney perfusion [76]. Thus, angiotensin, by arteriolar constriction, would maintain an appropriate pressure level. Such vasoconstriction would normally result in a concomitant renal vasoconstriction and reduced renal blood flow. But, if bradykinin is concurrently formed locally in the kidney, renal perfusion would be protected. Thus, the dual system would work rapidly to maintain a normal renal tissue perfusion while increasing systemic pressure [76] (Figure 3). A positive cor-

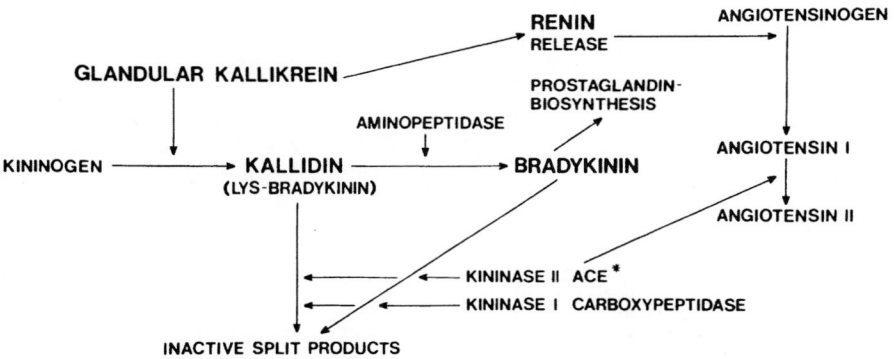

* ACE: Angiotensin I converting enzyme

Figure 3. Interactions between the kallikrein–kinin and the renin–angiotensin system.

relation has been reported in man between renal blood flow and the logarithm of the ratio urinary kallikrein activity to plasma renin activity, suggesting that the opposing effects of the renal kallikrein–kinin system and the renin–angiotensin system on renal blood flow are of physiological importance [77].

Mersey et al. [72] have proposed that plasma kinins correlate best with the activity of the renin–angiotensin system, while urinary kallikrein excretion correlates closely with mineralcorticoid activity, at least in normal man. Even if the regulation of renin is abnormal (e.g. normal renin hypertensives with delayed suppression of plasma renin activity during saline loading) the renin–angiotensin and blood–kinin systems appear to be physiologically related.

A clinical example of blood pressure control by a balance of the renin–angiotensin–aldosterone system, the dilator action of the kallikrein–kinin system and the prostaglandins is Bartter's syndrome. This syndrome consists of hyperreninemia, hyperangiotensinemia, hyperaldosteronism, and hypokalemic alkalosis, but the blood pressure is normal. On the other hand, urinary kallikrein activity and plasma bradykinin levels as well as urinary prostaglandins are increased. Further, these patients have been shown to have juxtaglomerular cell hyperplasia, hyporesponsiveness to angiotensin and decreased reabsorption of chloride in the thick ascending limb of the loop of Henle, the latter alteration probably being the primary cause of the syndrome [78]. When these patients are treated with indomethacin, an inhibitor of prostaglandin synthesis, their elevated levels of urinary prostaglandins fall, as do their sodium excretion, plasma renin activity and urinary aldosterone. At the same time the elevated levels of urinary kallikrein and plasma bradykinin decrease. The blood pressure remains normal. This shows the complex interactions between these potent vasoactive systems.

All of the studies taken together suggest that the kallikrein–kinins could play a role in regulating systemic blood pressure by buffering angiotensin II-induced changes in the vasculature.

Interaction between the kallikrein–kinin system and the renal prostaglandin system

Increasing evidence suggests an intimate link between the renal kallikrein–kinin and prostaglandin systems. Thus bradykinin increases the production of prostaglandins, apparently by activating phospholipase A [79–81]. In addition, blood vessels release prostaglandin E_2, a potent vasodilator, when treated with bradykinin (or angiotensin II) in vitro [82]. Prostaglandins have been suggested as mediating and altering the actions of bradykinin on renal function [80]. Indomethacin reduces the vasodilatory effect of bradykinin infusion in isolated blood-perfused canine kidney [83]. On the other hand, it has been reported that urinary kallikrein excretion is increased when PGE_2 is infused into the renal artery [8]. These observations suggest that there is a functional coupling of the renal kallikrein–kinin and the prostaglandin system. Work needs to be done to see whether vasodilatory prostaglandin I_2 production is altered by kinins. In contrast to prostaglandin E_2 which does not cross the lungs and acts mainly as a local hormone, prostaglandin I_2 is a circulating hormone. Its release by locally acting kinins could produce systemic circulatory effects.

Hypotensive effect of orally administered glandular kallikrein

Previous investigations of the kallikrein–kinin system in essential hypertension have provided evidence that urinary kallikrein is excreted in smaller amounts in hypertensive than in normotensive subjects [71, 77, 60]. Because decreased urinary kallikrein activity may reflect deficiency of vasodepressor kinins, it has been proposed that impaired renal kallikrein activity may contribute to the genesis of hypertension. Recently, we have demonstrated that oral administration of a pure preparation of pig pancreatic kallikrein (600 biological units/day in gastric juice resistant tablets) lowered elevated arterial pressure in essential hypertensive patients [60, 84, 85] and normalized decreased urinary kallikrein activity. The hypotensive action of oral kallikrein, as well as its stimulating effects on renal kallikrein release, suggest that the kallikrein–kinin system is involved in blood pressure regulation and that impaired renal kallikrein activity may be a factor in the maintenance of essential hypertensioin. The mechanism underlying the hypotensive response to oral kallikrein is unclear. Recent observations (Stumpe and Overlack, unpublished data) show that oral kallikrein induces a marked rise in renal prostaglandin E_2 release which was accompanied by an increase in renal blood flow and glomerular filtration rate. Thus, it may be speculated that increased prostaglandin production plays a role in mediating the hypotensive response to kallikrein, possibly via changes in local (renal) blood flow and/or urinary sodium excretion. Whether the effect of kallikrein on prostaglandin release is direct or secondary to a change in kinin production is unclear. A similar increase in renal prostaglandin release with kallikrein treatment was observed in a group of normotensive subjects. However, in these subjects the decrease in blood pressure was only small and not significant.

It could be questioned whether pig pancreatic kallikrein by oral administration produces any effects, because digestion in the gastrointestinal tract would be expected. However, like other proteins such as trypsin [86], chymotrypsin [86] and insulin [87], pig pancreatic kallikrein seems to be absorbed from the gut in small amounts [88, 89], probably in enzymatically active form [88]. In addition, Geiger et al. [90] have shown that human serum has a low inhibitory potential against kallikrein. In the case of pig pancreatic kallikrein only slow inhibition is observed by a_1-antitrypsin [91], the only unequivocally identified inhibitor of glandular kallikreins [92]. Further, the possibility of extracting active glandular kallikrein from plasma by immunaffinity chromatography [41] would strongly indicate that at least part of the glandular kallikrein is present there as active enzyme. The same should hold true for orally administered kallikrein.

Altogether, it seems to be possible that glandular kallikrein may produce systemic vasodilatory effects by maintaining a physiological level of kinins due to ubiquitously occurring kininogens. Whether glandular kallikrein, produced in the parotic gland or in the pancreas, is reabsorbed in sufficient amounts to play a role in the control of arterial blood pressure under physiologic conditions is far from clear.

SUMMARY

Kallikreins are enzymes that generate vasoactive kinins from plasma globulin substrates called kininogens. Kinins are among the most potent vasodilators endogenously produced in man. The role of the kallikrein–kinin system in regulation of systemic blood pressure is uncertain. The fact that intra-arterially administered kallikreins or kinins produce vasodilatation and reduction in blood pressure does not prove that the kallikrein–kinin system performs this function under physiological conditions. Nevertheless, there are important functional interrelationships between the kallikrein-kinin system and the three major control mechanisms of blood pressure regulation, the latter including regulation by the autonomic nervous system, regulation of sodium homeostasis by the kidneys and regulation by hormones such as renin, angiotensin, aldosterone, prostaglandins, norepinephrine and epinephrine. Thus, evidence has been provided that the kallikreinkinin system is associated with natriuretic and diuretic processes and by this mode of action may control arterial blood pressure. Further, renal kallikrein production correlates closely with aldosterone and may control vascular tone by counterbalancing the sodium-retaining effects of mineralocorticoids. Also, there are important links between kallikrein and renin. Kallikrein may be the endogenous activator of renin in the kidney and there are indications that kallikrein–kinin system activity could be involved in blood pressure regulation by buffering vasoconstrictor angiotensin II-induced changes in the vasculature. Intimate functional links between the kallikrein–kinin and the prostaglandin systems have been described and part of the vasodilator effect of kinins appears to be mediated through the prostaglandin system.

Finally, the observation that oral administration of glandular kallikrein lowers elevated blood pressure in essential hypertensive patients and increases glomerular filtration rate and prostaglandin release suggests that glandular kallikrein may produce systemic vasodilatory effects by maintaining physiological levels of kinins and by this mechanism could control blood pressure.

REFERENCES

1. Colman RW: Formation of human plasma kinin. N Engl J Med 291:509–515, 1974.
2. Colman RW, Girey GJD, Zacest R, Talamo RC: The human plasma kallikrein–kinin system. Prog Hematol VII:255–298, 1971.
3. Bagdasarian A, Lahiri B, Talamo RC, Wong P, Colman RW: Immunochemical studies of plasma kallikrein. J Clin Invest 54:1444–1454, 1974.
4. Nustad K, Vaaje K, Pierce JV: Synthesis of kallikreins by rat kidney slices. Br J Pharmacol 53:229–234, 1975.
5. Ole-MoiYoi O, Austen KF, Spragg J: Kinin-generating and esterolytic activity of purified human urinary kallikrein (urokallikrein). Biochem Pharmacol 26:1893–1897, 1977.
6. Stein JH, Congbalay RC, Karsh DL, Osgood RW, Ferris TF: The effect of bradykinin on proximal tubular sodium reabsorption in the dog: evidence for functional nephron heterogeneity. J Clin Invest 51:1709–1721, 1972.
7. Willis LR, Ludens JH, Hook JB, Williamson HE: Mechanism of natriuretic action of bradykinin. Am J Physiol 217:1–5, 1969.
8. Mills IH, MacFarlane NA, Ward PE, Obika LF: The renal kallikrein–kinin system and the regulation of salt and water excretion. Fed Proc 35:181–188, 1976.
9. Webster ME: Kallikreins in glandular tissue. In: Handbook of Experimental Pharmacology, pp. 131–156. Bradykinin, Kallidin and Kallikrein. Erdös EG, ed. Berlin: Springer, 1970.
10. Webster ME, Pierce JV: The nature of the kallidins released from human plasma by kallikreins and other enzymes. Ann NY Acad Sci 104:91–107, 1963.
11. Werle E, Berek U: Zur Kenntnis des Kallikreins. Angew Chem 60A:53, 1948.
12. Saito H, Ratnoff OD, Donaldson VH: Defective activation of clotting fibrinolysis and permeability-enhancing systems in human Fletcher trait plasma. Circ Res 34:641–651, 1974.
13. Jacobsen S: Substrates for plasma kinin-forming enzymes in human, dog and rabbit plasma. Br J Pharmacol 26:403–411, 1966.
14. Waldmann R, Abraham JP, Rebuck JW, Caldwell J, Saito H, Ratnoff OD: Fitzgerald factor: a hitherto unrecognized coagulation factor. Lancet I:949–950, 1975.
15. Waldmann R, Scicli AG, McGregor RK, Carretero OA, Abraham JP, Kato H, Han YN, Iwanaga S: Effect of bovine high molecular weight kininogen and its fragments on Fitzgerald trait plasma. Thromb Res 8:785–795, 1976.
16. Saito H, Ratnoff OD, Waldmann R, Abraham JP: Fitzgerald trait – deficiency of a hitherto unrecognized agent, Fitzgerald factor, participating in surface-mediated reactions of clotting, fibrinolysis, generation of kinins, and property of diluted plasma enhancing vascular permeability (PF-DIL): J Clin Invest 55:1082–1089, 1975.
17. Fiedler F: Pig pancreatic kallikreins A and B. In: Methods in Enzymology-Proteolytic Enzymes, Vol 45, p. 289. Lorand L, ed. New York: Academic Press, 1976.
18. Moriwaki C, Watanuki N, Fujimoto Y, Moriya H: Further purification and properties of kininogenase from the guinea-pig's coagulating gland. Chem Pharm Bull 22:628–633, 1974.
19. Brandtzaeg P, Gautvik KM, Nustad K, Pierce JV: Rat submandibular gland kallikreins: purification and cellular localization. Br J Pharmacol 56:155, 1976.

100

20. Prado ES, Prado JL, Brandi CMW: Further purification and some properties of horse urinary kallikrein. Arch Int Pharmacodyn Ther 137:358–363, 1962.
21. Oza NB, Amin VM, McGregor RK, Scicli AG, Carretero OA: Isolation of rat urinary kallikrein and properties of its antibodies. Biochem Pharmacol 25:1607–1611, 1976.
22. Nustad K, Pierce JV: Purification of rat urinary kallikreins and their specific antibody. Biochemistry 13:2312–2319, 1974.
23. Hial V, Diniz CR, Mares-Guia M: Purification and properties of a human urinary kallikrein (kininogenase). Biochemistry 13:4311–4316, 1974.
24. Matsuda Y, Miyazaki K, Moriya H, Fujimoto Y, Hojima Y, Moriwaki C: Studies on urinary kallikreins – I. Purification and characterization of human urinary kallikreins. J Biochem (Tokyo) 80:671–679, 1976.
25. Pierce JV, Webster ME: Human plasma kallidins: Isolation and chemical studies. Biochem Biophys Res Commun 5:353–358, 1961.
26. Pierce JV: Structural features of plasma kinins and kininogens. Fed Proc 27:52–57, 1968.
27. Fink E, Dietl T, Seifert J, Fritz H: Studies on the biological function of glandular kallikrein. Adv Exp Med Biol 120B:261–273, 1979.
28. Geiger R, Mann K: A kallikrein-specific inhibitor in rat kidney tubules. Hoppe Seylers Z Physiol Chem 357:553–558, 1976.
29. Overlack A, Stumpe KO, Kühnert M, Heck I: Altered blood pressure and renin responses to converting enzyme inhibition after aprotinin-induced kallikrein–kinin-system blockade. Clin Sci 59:129s–132s, 1980.
30. Kramer HJ, Moch T, v. Sicherer L, Düsing R: Effects of kallikrein inhibition with aprotinin on renal hemodynamics and urinary water, electrolyte, and prostaglandin E_2-excretion in conscious rats. Acta Endocrinol (Kbh) 91:Suppl 225, p. 381, 1979.
31. Erdös EG, Yang HYT: Kininase. In: Handbook of Experimental Pharmacology. Bradykinin, Kallidin, and Kallikrein. Vol 25, pp. 289–323. Erdös EG, ed. New York: Springer, 1970.
32. Erdös EG: Conversion of angiotensin I to angiotensin II. Am J Med 60:749–759, 1976.
33. Ferreira SH, Vane JR: Half-lives of peptides and amines in the circulation. Nature 215:1237–1240, 1967.
34. Saameli K, Eskes TKAB: Bradykinin and cardiovascular system: estimation of half-life. Am J Physiol 203:261–266, 1962.
35. Frey EK, Kraut H: Ein neues Kreislaufhormon und seine Wirkung. Naunyn Schmiedeberg's Arch Exp Path Pharmak 133:1–56, 1928.
36. Roblero J, Croxatto H, Garcia R, Corthorn J, De Vita E: Kallikrein-like activity in perfusates and urine of isolated rat kidneys. Am J Physiol 231:1383–1389, 1976.
37. Scicli AG, Carretero OA, Oza NB, Schork NA: Distribution of kidney kininogenase. Proc Soc Exp Biol Med 151:57–60, 1976.
38. Scicli AG, Carretero OA, Hampton A, Cortes P, Oza NB: Site of kininogenase secretion in the dog nephron. Am J Phyciol 230:533–536, 1976.
39. Roblero J, Croxatto HR, Albertini RB: Release of renal kallikrein to the perfusate by isolated rat kidney. Experientia 32:1440–1441, 1976.
40. De Bono E, Mills IH: Simultaneous increases in kallikrein in renal lymph and urine during saline infusion. J Physiol (Lond) 241:127–128, 1974.
41. Geiger R, Clausnitzer B, Fink E, Fritz H: Isolation of an enzymatically active glandular kallikrein from human plasma by immunaffinity chromatography. Hoppe Seylers Z Physiol Chem (in press).
42. Gill JR Jr, Melmon KL, Gillespie L Jr, Bartter FC: Bradykinin and renal function in normal man: effects of adrenergic blockade. Am J Physiol 209:844–851, 1965.
43. Webster MF, Gilmore JP: Influences of kallidin-10 on renal function. Am J Physiol 206:714–718, 1964.

44. Nasjletti A, Colina-Chourio J, McGiff JC: Disappearance of bradykinin in the renal circulation of dogs. Effects of kininase inhibition. Circ Res 37:59–65, 1975.
45. Terragno NA, Terragno A: Release of Vasoactive Substances by Kinins. In: Bradykinin, Kallidin and Kallikrein, Handbook Exp Pharm–XXV Suppl, p. 401. Erdös EG, ed. Heidelberg: Springer Verlag, 1979.
46. Streeten DHP, Kerr CB, Prior JC, Dalakos TH: Hyperbradykinism: a new orthostatic syndrome. Lancet 18:1048–1053, 1972.
47. Carretero OA, Scicli AG: The renal kallikrein–kinin system in human and in experimental hypertension. Klin Wochenschr 56:(Suppl I) 113–125, 1978.
48. Wilcox GM, Hial V, Keiser M, Horwitz D, Pisano JJ: Effects of posture on urokinase and kallikrein excretion in man. Clin Res 23:115A, 1975.
49. Mills IH, Obika LFO: The effect of adrenergic and dopaminereceptor blockade on the kallikrein and renal response to intraarterial infusion of dopamine in dogs. J Physiol (Lond) 263:150P–151P, 1976.
50. Stein JH, Congbalay RC, Karsh DL, Osgood RW, Ferris TF: The effect of bradykinin on proximal tubular sodium reabsorption in the dog: evidence for functional nephron heterogeneity. J Clin Invest 51:1709–1721, 1972.
51. Webster ME, Gilmore JP: Influence of kallidin-10 on renal function. Am J Physiol 206:714–718, 1964.
52. Willis LR, Lundens JH, Hook JB, Williamson HE: Mechanism of natriuretic action of bradykinin. Am J Physiol 217:1–5, 1969.
53. McGiff JC, Itskovits HD, Terragno NA: The actions of bradykinin and eledoisin in the canine isolated kidney: relationships to prostaglandins. Clin Sci Mol Med 49:125–131, 1975.
54. Capelo LR, Alzamora F: A stop-flow analysis of the effects of intrarenal infusion of bradykinin. Arch Int Pharmacodyn Ther 230:156–161, 1977.
55. Adetuyibi A, Mills IH: Relation between urinary kallikrein and renal function, Hypertension, and excretion of sodium and water in man. Lancet 2:203–205, 1972.
56. Mills IH, Ward PE: The relationship between kallikrein and water excretion and the conditional relationship between kallikrein and sodium excretion. J Physiol (Lond) 246:695–699, 1975.
57. Geller RG, Margolius HS, Pisano JJ, Keiser HR: Effects of mineralocorticoids, altered sodium intake and adrenalectomy on urinary kallikrein in rats. Circ Res 31:857–861, 1972.
58. Margolius HS, Horwitz D, Geller RG, Alexander RW, GillJR, Pisano JJ, Keiser HR: Urinary kallikrein excretion in normal man. Relationships to sodium intake and sodium-retaining steroids. Circ Res 35:812–819, 1974.
59. Johnston CI, Matthews PG, Dax E: Effects of dietary sodium, diuretics and hypertension on renin and kallikrein. In:Systemic Effects of Antihypertensive Agents, pp. 323–338. Sambhi MP, ed. New York: Stratton Intercontinental, 1976.
60. Overlack A, Stumpe KO, Ressel C, Kolloch R, Zywzok W, Krück F: Decreased urinary kallikrein activity and elevated blood pressure normalized by orally applied kallikrein in essential hypertension. Klin Wochenschr 58:37–42, 1980.
61. Wong PY, Talamo RC, Williams GH, Coleman RW: response of the kallikrein–kinin and renin–angiotensin systems to saline infusion and upright posture. J Clin Invest 55:691–698, 1975.
62. Hollenberg NK, Soloman HS, Adams DF, Abrams HL, Merrill JP: Renal vascular response to angiotensin and norepinephrine in normal man: the effect of salt intake. Circ Res 31:750–757, 1972.
63. Feruglio FS, Greco F, Cesano L, Indovina D, Sardi G, Chiandussi L: Effect of drug infusion on the systemic and splanchnic circulation – I. Bradykinin infusion in normal subjects, Clin Sci 26:487–491, 1964.

64. De Freitas FM, Faraco EZ, de Azeveda DF: General circulatory alterations induced by intravenous infusions of synthetic bradykinin in man. Circulation 29:66–70, 1964.
65. Strewler GJ, Hinricks KJ, Guiod LR, Hollenberg NK: Sodium intake and vascular smooth muscle responsiveness to norepinephrine and angiotensin in the rabbit. Circ Res 31:758–766, 1972.
66. Nasjletti A, McGiff JC, Colina-Chourio J: Interrelations of the renal kallikrein–kinin system and renal prostaglandins in the conscious rat. Influence of mineralocorticoids. Circ Res 43:799–807, 1978.
67. Marin-Grez M, Oza NB, Carretero OA: The involvement of urinary kallikrein in the renal escape from the sodium-retaining effect of mineralocorticoids. Henry Ford Hosp Med J 21:85–90, 1973.
68. Margolius HS, Chao J, Kaizu T: The effects of aldosterone and spironolactone on renal kallikrein. Clin Sci Mol Med (Suppl) 3:279s–282s, 1976.
69. Halushka PV, Wohltmann H, Privitera PJ, Hurwitz G, Margolius HS: A relationship between urinary prostaglandin E-like material and kallikrein in children with Bartter's syndrome: effects of indomethacin. Ann Int Med 87:281–286, 1977.
70. Lechi A, Cori G, Lechi C, Mantero F, Scuro A: Urinary kallikrein excretion in Bartter's syndrome. J Clin Endocrinol Metab 43:1175–1178, 1976.
71. Margolius HS, Geller R, Pisano JJ, Sjoerdsma A: Altered Urinary kallikrein excretion in human hypertension. Lancet II:1063–1065, 1971.
72. Mersey JH, Williams GH, Emanuel R, Dluhy RG, Wong PY, Moore TJ: Plasma bradykinin levels and urinary kallikrein excretion in normal renin essential hypertension, J Clin Endocrinol Metab 48:642–647, 1979.
73. Sealey JE, Atlas SA, Laragh JH, Oza NB, Ryan JW: Human urinary kallikrein converts inactive to active renin and is a possible physiological activator of renin. Nature (Lond) 275:144–145, 1978.
74. Suzuki S, Franco-Saenz R, Tan SY, Mulrow PJ: Direct action of rat urinary kallikrein on rat kidney to release renin. J Clin Invest 66:757–762, 1980.
75. Sealey JE, Atlas SA, Laragh JH: Activation of prorenin-like substance in human plasma by trypsin and by urinary kallikrein. Hypertension 1:179–184, 1979.
76. Sealey JE, Atlas SA, Laragh JH: Linking the kallikrein and renin systems via activation of inactive renin: new data and a hyothesis. In: Topics in Hypertension pp. 111–121. Laragh JH, ed. New York: Yorke Medical Books, 1980.
77. Levy SB, Lilley JJ, Frigon RP, Stone RA: Urinary Kallikrein and plasma renin activity as determinants of renal blood flow. J Clin Invest 60:129–138, 1977.
78. Gill JR Jr, Frölich JC, Bowden RE, Taylor AA, Keiser HR, Seyberth HW, Oates JA, Bartter FC: Bartter's syndrome: a disorder characterized by high urinary prostaglandins and a dependence of hyperreninemia on prostaglandin synthesis. Am J Med 61:43–51, 1976.
79. Lonigro AJ, Itskovitz HD, Crowshaw K, McGiff JC: Dependency of renal blood flow on prostaglandin synthesis in the dog. Circ Res 33:712–717, 1973.
80. McGiff JC, Itskovitz HD, Terragno A, Wong PYK: Modulation and mediation of the action of the renal kallikrein–kinin system by prostaglandins. Fed Proc 35:175–180, 1976.
81. Needleman P, Kauffman AH, Douglas JR, Johnson EM Jr, Marschall GR: Specific stimulation and inhibition of renal prostaglandin release by angiotensin analogs. Am J Physiol 224:1415–1419, 1973.
82. Tuvemo T, Wide L: Prostaglandin release from the human umbilical artery in vitro. Prostaglandins 4:689–694, 1973.
83. McGiff JC, Itskovitz HD, Terragno NA: The actions of bradykinin and eledoisin in the canine isolated kidney: relationships to prostaglandins. Clin Sci Mol Med 49:125–131, 1975.
84. Overlack A, Stumpe KO, Ressel C, Krück F: Low urinary kallikrein excretion and elevated

blood pressure normalized by orally applied kallikrein in essential hypertension. Clin Sci 57:263–265, 1979.

85. Stumpe KO, Overlack A, Ressel C, Krück F: Impaired renal kallikrein activity and elevated blood pressure normalized by orally applied kallikrein in essential hypertension. Agents Actions 10:349–353, 1980.

86. Götze H, Rothman SS: Enteropancreatic circulation of digestive enzyme as a conservation mechanism. Nature 257:607–609, 1975.

87. Danforth E, Moore RO: Intestinal absorption of insulin in the rat. Endocrinology 65: 118–121, 1959.

88. Fink E, Geiger R, Witte J, Biedermann S, Seifert J, Fritz H: Biochemical, pharmacological, and functional aspects of glandular kallikrein. In: Enzymatic Release of Vasoactive Peptides, pp. 101–113. Gross F, Vogel G, eds. New York: Raven Press, 1980.

89. Moriya H, Moriwaki C, Akimoto S: Studies on kallikreins – II. Passage of ^{131}I-labelled hog pancreatic kallikrein across the rat intestine. Chem Pharm Bull 15:403–407, 1967.

90. Geiger R, Stuckstedte U, Fritz H: Isolation and characterization of human urinary kallikrein. Hoppe Seylers Z Physiol Chem 361: 1003–1009, 1980.

91. Fritz H, Brey B, Schmal A, Werle E: Zur Identität des Progressiv-Antikallikreins mit a_1-Antitrypsin aus Humanserum. Hoppe Seylers Z Physiol Chem 350:1551–1552, 1969.

92. Fritz H, Fink E, Truscheit E: Kallikrein inhibitors. Fed Proc 38:2753–2759, 1979.

7. THE LABILITY OF BLOOD PRESSURE

JOHN S. FLORAS and PETER SLEIGHT

> And as the State of the Blood or Blood Vessels are in these
> Respects continually varying from divers Causes, as Motion,
> Rest, Food, Evacuations, Heat, Cold & c. so as probably never
> to be exactly the same, any two Minutes, during the whole Life
> of an Animal, so Nature has wisely provided, that a consider-
> able Variation in these, shall not greatly disturb the healthy
> State of the Animal.
>
> Stephen Hales: Experiment IX (1733) [1]

1. THE VARIABILITY OF ARTERIAL BLOOD PRESSURE

Stephen Hales inserted into the carotid artery of a mare a brass pipe 'and to
that the Wind-Pipe of a Goose; to the other end of which a Glass Tube was
fixed'. During the course of his investigations he noted that blood pressure
varied from beat to beat, often, but not always, in conjunction with respiration. These variations were attributed either to changes in the blood, or in
the vascular resistance. Variations in arterial pressure occur during the
course of daily activities [2] and sleep [3]. Diehl [4] noted that the variation
in measurements obtained over a period of 6 days in 100 students was
unrelated to their mean systolic blood pressure.
  Correlations of the level of arterial pressure and cardiovascular morbidity
or mortality have relied on resting casual or basal clinic blood pressures [5–
8]. The variance observed in these readings from one clinic visit to the next
makes the clinical decision to treat hypertensive individuals difficult if an
arbitrary dividing line for the definition of hypertension is adopted, e.g.
140/90 mm Hg. This dilemma is compounded by uncertainty as to the ultimate prognosis of those individuals, termed 'labile hypertensives' who were
noted to have cuff pressures which fluctuated about this dividing line. It was
suggested that these patients were in an early stage of essential hypertension,
characterized, in some instances, by a 'hyperkinetic circulation' with an
increased cardiac output and a 'hyperreaction' to stressful stimuli [9, 10].
Many of these patients went on to develop normal cardiac output and an
elevation in their peripheral resistance [11]. The fact that similar fluctua-

Amery, A. (ed.) Hypertensive Cardiovascular Disease: Pathophysiology and Treatment
© *1982, Martinus Nijhoff Publishers. The Hague / Boston / London*
ISBN-13: 978-94-009-7478-4

tions occurred in normal and severely hypertensive subjects, but about different levels of blood pressure, tended to be overlooked. Moreover, there was little evidence to suggest that such patients were indeed 'hyperreactors' to stimuli such as bicycle exercise [12, 13]. Without a method for obtaining larger numbers of observations, a means of quantifying and interpreting these fluctuations in arterial pressure was unavailable. Three techniques have been devised to gather these data: home blood pressure recordings, indirect blood pressure recorders, and direct continuous ambulatory monitoring. Varying degrees of accuracy, continuity, freedom of movement, and physician–patient interaction are afforded with the first two methods. Only the latter allows for continuous direct measurement of arterial blood pressure necessary for the reliable assessment of its beat-to-beat variability. Understandably, it is used less frequently due to its invasive and specialized nature.

1.1. Home blood pressure recordings

Patients have been taught to take their own blood pressure at home without difficulty, using a standard aneroid sphygmomanometer and diaphragm stethoscope [14–16]. Ayman and Goldshine [14] obtained several months of recordings in 34 of their hypertension clinic patients. Home blood pressures were found to be lower than clinic blood pressures in all cases; the difference between the two values was independent of casual cuff pressure, and difficult to predict. Juluis and co-workers [15] found that this difference, absent in their normotensive subjects, was on average 14/4 mm Hg in their borderline hypertensive patients. Borderline hypertensives showed slightly increased lability of their systolic blood pressure (expressed as the standard deviation from the mean of their readings), but not of their diastolic. No consistent factor explained the fluctuation between clinic and home blood pressures.

It can be inferred from the data of Laughlin et al. [16] that greater lability of diastolic pressure is seen in subjects with moderate hypertension as opposed to those with borderline hypertension. This relationship is less clear for systolic pressure.

Cuff methods have a serious disadvantage in the assessment of blood pressure variability, which they share with indirect blood pressure recorders: they provide discontinuous measurements, usually obtained at rest, which may be unable to predict or measure changes in blood pressure during routine activity, exercise, coitus, or sleep. Furthermore, the measurements are noticeable to the subject and therefore at risk of provoking a defence reaction. Gould and his colleagues at Northwick Park Hospital [17] have recently demonstrated the superiority of the continuous intra-arterial methods over cuff blood pressure in reproducibility and in the avoidance of the placebo effect.

1.2. The variability of blood pressure measured with indirect blood pressure recording devices

Richardson et al. [18] described a cuff plethysmographic method of measuring blood pressure discontinuously and indirectly, but automatically. Although the activity of these patients was restricted, a fall in blood pressure during sleep, and a diurnal variation in arterial pressure were nonetheless observed. The range of pressure was used as a rough index of blood pressure variability ('undulatory index'). This was similar in normal and hypertensive subjects, but seemed to increase with age.

An alternative approach pioneered by Sokolow and his colleagues in San Francisco records the Korotkoff sounds on tape, semi-automatically (Remler M-100) [19]. The Del Mar Avionics Pressurometer II [20] is fully automatic and also uses microphones strapped over the brachial artery. These methods are therefore dependent on the position of the microphone, which can be displaced by mild activity; more importantly, they depend on the Korotkoff sounds for the interpretation of arterial pressure. Although a good correlation is observed between indirect and direct blood readings when a large number of recordings are compared, there can be wide discrepancies in a particular individual when measurements are taken simultaneously from the same limb [21]. This particularly applies to diastolic pressure (usually overestimated) and appears to be independent of arm circumference [22]. Finally, semi-automatic recorders which require the patient to activate the machine, have the potential for data selection: the patient may choose to record his blood pressure at times of perceived relaxation, or anxiety. Moreover, they are unable to measure blood pressure during sleep. Sokolow [23] used the Remler recorder to examine the relationship between psychological state and blood pressure and found that 'negative affect' was associated with rises in blood pressure, and 'positive affect' with falls. As might be expected, blood pressure was lower when subjects were engaged in isolated or pleasant activities, and higher when engaged in work or in the presence of strangers. The standard deviation of all systolic or diastolic pressures during the day was used to calculate blood pressure variability [24]. These authors found no significant relationship between the variability and the level of arterial pressure, or the overall severity of an individual's end-organ complications.

The question of blood pressure lability in borderline hypertension was studied by Horan et al. [20] with the Avionics device. Hypertension per se was associated with a greater degree of blood pressure variability than normotension, but borderline hypertensives showed no more lability than fixed hypertensives. These data are difficult to interpret, however, as only a small number of the cardiac cycles occurring during the day were included in the calculation of variability, and fluctuations of blood pressure may have been blunted by the presence of treated patients in the 'fixed' group.

The Arteriosonde®, which uses Doppler ultrasound [25], has been employed in several studies of the range and variability of arterial pressure. Although this technique does not interrupt sleep, it restricts the patients' movement, and thus records a smaller range of variation in arterial pressure than might be present under conditions of uninhibited movement. De Leeuw and his colleagues [26] have studied the variability of arterial pressure in 58 patients using this technique. However, workers from this laboratory have defined the variability of blood pressure as the difference between the maximum and the minimum value divided by the maximum, expressed as a percentage. This estimate only represents the extremes of their observations, not the variation in their measurements; this should be borne in mind when comparing their data to that of other groups. Variability thus defined showed a significant inverse relationship with age. The relationship between variability and arterial pressure was not discussed in this report. Clement [27] demonstrated a linear relationship between blood pressure and its variability, using the same ultrasonic technique.

1.3. The variability of blood pressure as measured by direct ambulatory recording

Ambulatory recording was designed to overcome the limitations of the cuff and indirect methods by measuring blood pressure continuously and directly, throughout the day, in the absence of an observer [28, 29]. The technique involves the percutaneous cannulation of the brachial artery with a teflon Seldecath® cannula, 1 mm in external diameter, and 10 cm long. This is connected via fine Portex tubing to an Oxford blood pressure system: a perfusion pump/recording device (Selig, London) and a Medilog cassette recorder (Oxford Instruments), which have been described in detail [30, 31]. A 24-hour record of blood pressure and the electrocardiogram are obtained. Before the development of semi-automatic computer analysis, the tape was replayed directly onto ultraviolet-light-sensitive paper. Now the cassette is replayed at 25 times real time (Oxford Instruments Replay Unit) into a minicomputer (Date General Eclipse) and analysed either in beat-to-beat histograms (Figure 1) or in a condensed version which plots two-minute means of systolic, diastolic and mean blood pressure and heart rate [32] (Figure 2). With this technique, the ambulatory blood pressure and the electrocardiogram have been studied during driving [33], smoking [34], mictu-

108

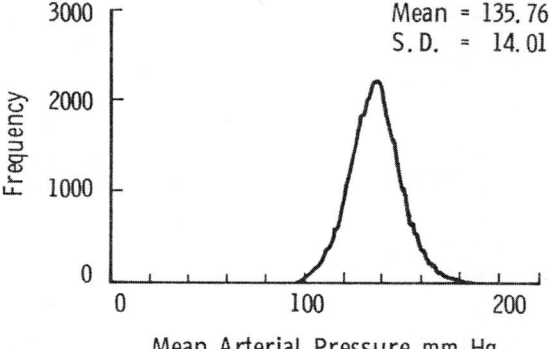

Figure 1. Frequency histogram constructed from all values for mean arterial pressure obtained from a single hypertensive patient during his waking period.

rition and defecation [35], coitus [36] and sleep [37] in normal subjects, and in patients with angina [38], phaeochromocytoma [39] and pre-eclamptic pregnancy [40]. The fluctuation in blood pressure with each of these activities was noted.

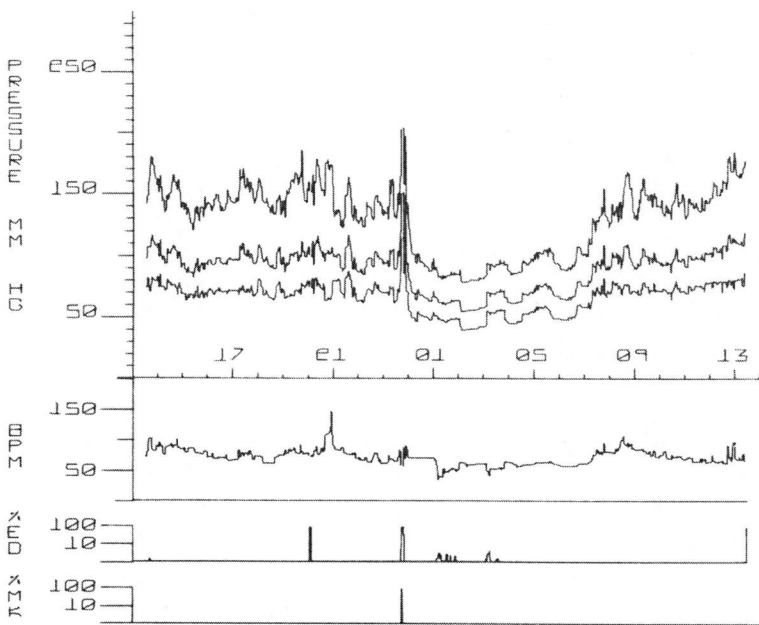

Figure 2. A 24 h blood pressure record from one subject showing systolic mean and diastolic blood pressure (upper tracing) and heart rate (lower tracing) during work (1300–1700 h), driving (1700–1745 h), return to hospital (2000 h), home, resting (2200–2400 h), coitus (2400 h) and sleep (2400–0700 h) (from Floras [44], with permission).

The variation in human activity during day and night is reflected in similar cyclical variations in arterial pressure [41–43]. Blood pressure tends to fall about 25% from waking levels during sleep [44] when this is taken at home, but by about 10% when the subjects sleep in hospital [45]. Preliminary observations with this technique led Pickering [46] to conclude that the range and lability of blood pressure appeared to be similar in normal and hypertensive subjects; these findings supported his thesis that the difference between normal and hypertensive individuals was quantitative rather than qualitative. Several centres have now examined these beat-to-beat variations in blood pressure in a quantitative manner, using direct ambulatory monitoring. Again, the standard deviation about the mean of all blood pressures obtained during the period under observation has been used to define the variability of blood pressure.

Watson et al. [47] found that systolic pressure and its variability were significantly correlated when these were examined under controlled conditions; this was not observed for diastolic pressure. Variability of systolic pressure tended to increase with age as well, but this effect did not appear to be independent of the concomitant increase in arterial pressure as subjects grew older. Mancia et al. [48] looked at small intervals of time rather than at actual beat-to-beat variability, and similarly concluded that the variability of mean arterial pressure expressed in absolute terms increased with age and level of arterial pressure. However, the authors did not examine the independent effects on blood pressure variability of these two factors. Pessina

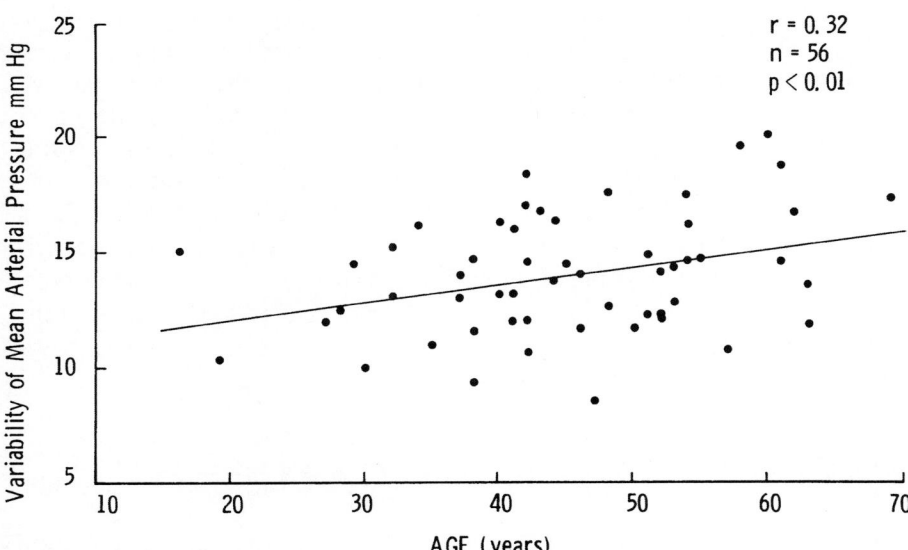

Figure 3. Relationship between beat-to-beat variability of mean arterial pressure and age (n = 56) (from Floras [44], with permission).

110

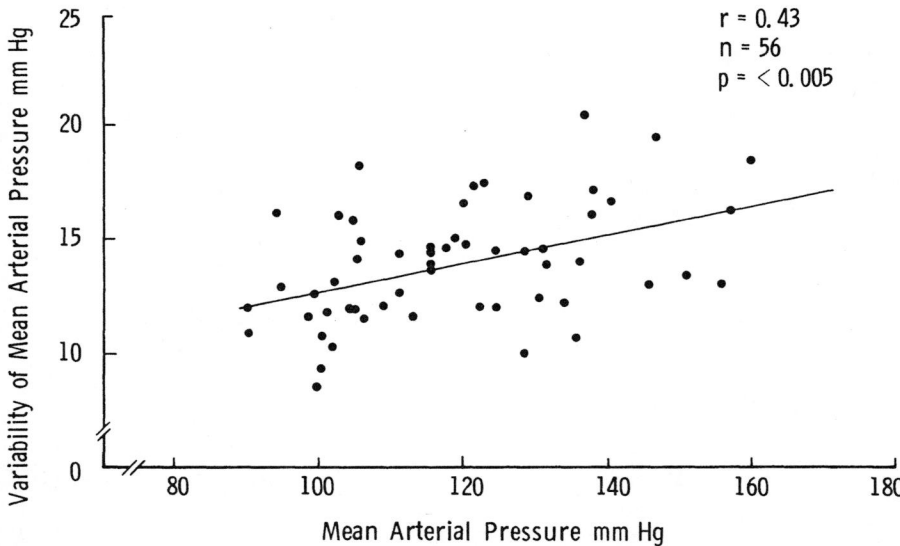

Figure 4. Relationship between beat-to-beat variability of mean arterial pressure and mean arterial pressure (N = 56) (from Floras [44], with permission).

and co-workers [49] noted that the variability of arterial pressure over the waking and sleeping periods of the 24-hour record was greater in 8 'fixed' than 8 'borderline' hypertensive patients; the ages of these individuals are not mentioned.

We examined the variability of mean arterial pressure in 56 subjects, aged 16–69, whose average waking mean arterial pressures ranged from 89.5 mm Hg to 159.5 mm Hg. They were allowed to leave hospital and return to work or home. The variability of mean arterial pressure under these free-ranging conditions increased with advancing age and increasing mean arterial pressure [44] (Figures 3 and 4). None of these studies therefore support the contention that borderline hypertension is associated with an increase in the lability of arterial pressure. We, as others [47], noted differences between clinic cuff pressures and the average ambulatory blood pressure in the majority of our patients. This was not related to the extent of the variation in blood pressure in these patients [50], as might have been anticipated by earlier reports using non-invasive techniques.

2. THE REGULATION OF BLOOD PRESSURE VARIABILITY

Non-invasive techniques have not shed much light on the physiological mechanisms responsible for the control of blood pressure variability, for the reasons mentioned earlier. However, Birkenhäger and Schalekamp [51, 52] did note that blood pressure variability (as defined by them and measured with an oscillometric device) correlated with resting cardiac output and plasma renin concentration. De Leeuw et al. [26] noted that variability measured by Arteriosonde correlated inversely with plasma noradrenaline concentration. Research in this area has concentrated on examining the relationships between blood pressure variability and conventional regulatory systems: the arterial baroreflexes, the sympathetic nervous system, and the renin–angiotensin system. As it is difficult to examine each of these systems alone, independent of the others, in man, most research has correlated these factors without attempting to attribute cause.

There is good evidence from animal experiments, however, to suggest that the baroreceptor reflexes are intimately involved in the regulation of blood pressure variability. Denervation of the sino-aortic baroreceptors in rats and dogs consistently leads to an increase in the beat-to-beat variation in blood pressure or the fluctuations in blood pressure in response to standard stimuli [53–55]. Central interruption of the baroreceptor reflex by lesions to the nucleus tractus solitarii (NTS) produces marked hypertension, sustained tachycardia and blood pressure variability [56]. The latter is pronounced during the day, but not so at night, suggesting a decreased inhibition of the central nervous system's response to routine stimuli and an enhanced sympathetic nervous system following the removal of the tonic inhibition which this reflex normally exerts. More suggestive is the work of Snyder et al. [57] who used 6-hydroxydopamine (6-OHDA) to selectively remove the noradrenergic innervation of the NTS. In doses insufficient to produce hypertension, damage the NTS, or ablate the baroreceptor reflex, a chronic state of increased lability of arterial pressure was produced, manifested by decreased buffering of rises produced by the defence reaction. A threefold increase in variability was associated with a decline in the cardiovagal component of the baroreflex of similar magnitude. This suggested to the authors that the noradrenergic innervation of the NTS tended to modulate baroreflexes; in the absence of this modulation, control of blood pressure lability was diminished.

Similar support for the role of the arterial baroreceptors in the control of blood pressure variability can be found in the work of Watson and his colleagues [47] and in our own laboratory. The sensitivity of the cardiovagal component if the baroreflex was measured, in each instance, by the technique of Smyth et al. [58], with phenylephrine (30–120 µg) substituted for angiotensin as the pressor agent employed. Watson [47] found a significant inverse relationship in 23 subjects between the variability of systolic pressure and baroreflex sensitivity. This correlation was found to be independent of both age and the level of systolic pressure. No such relationship was observed for diastolic pressure. In our series of 55 subjects, a significant inverse relationship was seen between the variability of mean arterial pres-

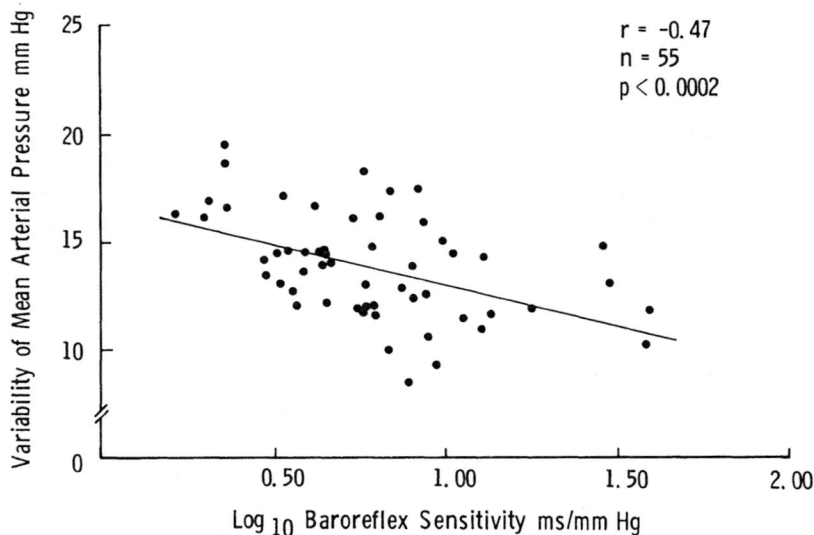

Figure 5. Inverse relationship between beat-to-beat variability of mean arterial pressure and baroreflex sensitivity (n = 55) (from Floras [44], with permission).

sure and baroreflex sensitivity (Figure 5) [59]; this again was independent of the effects of age, and mean arterial pressure on baroreflex sensitivity [60].

Mancia et al. [48] were unable to observe a correlation between their derived value for blood pressure variability and baroreflex sensitivity, calculated either from the reflex change in pulse interval in response to the depressor action of trinitroglycerine, or by the changes in arterial pressure effected by alterations in the pressure exerted on the wall of the carotid sinus by a sealed neck chamber. However, they did note a significant inverse relationship between variability and the baroreflex response following the injection of phenylephrine.

The relationship between heightened sympathetic nervous activity and blood pressure variability is less clear; in man, the former is usually assessed in one of three fashions namely, plasma catecholamine concentrations [61], the blood pressure and heart rate response to standard physical and mental exercises, and the response to pharmacological blockade. Watson et al. [47] were unable to detect a relationship between plasma catecholamines and blood pressure variability, using the direct technique. Clement et al. [62], using the Arteriosonde, also failed to observe a relationship between plasma noradrenaline and blood pressure variability. We did not detect a relationship between plasma noradrenaline at rest and the variability of mean arterial pressure in 44 patients; there was however, a significant relationship between the relative increase in plasma noradrenaline concentrations during bicycle exercise and blood pressure variability in these subjects. The problem in these studies (as in those trying to relate plasma noradrenaline to resting mean arterial pressure) is that plasma levels of catecholamines do not take into account the individual's sensitivity to catechols, nor to the density of adrenocepter sites in the arterial smooth muscle [63]. Wallin and his colleagues in Uppsala using direct recordings from human sympathetic nerves found a positive correlation between nerve discharge and plasma noradrenaline [64].

The pressor response to various physical and psychological manoeuvers has been used in order to predict blood pressure variability. The rise in systolic pressure during a cold pressor test was found to be significantly related to the variability of systolic blood pressure in the same patients [47]; these authors failed to find a similar relationship between blood pressure variability and the rise in arterial pressure during isometric or bicycle exercise. In contrast, we found a significant positive correlation between the variability of mean arterial pressure, and the increase in mean arterial pressure during each of the following activities: mental arithmetic, a reaction time test, isometric exercise, and bicycling [44]. It would therefore seem that a relationship between the level of sympathetic activity and blood pressure lability is present. If a small number of young borderline hypertensive patients with 'labile' blood pressure and increased sympathetic activity [65] does exist, it has yet to be demonstrated with continuous recording techniques.

The interaction between the renin–angiotensin system and central regulation of blood pressure [66] suggests that increased activity of this system may also enhance the lability of arterial pressure, as has been observed following chronic angiotensin infusion into experimental animals [67, 68]. Angiotensin infusion also inhibits the cardiovagal arm of the baroreflex [69]. A relationship between supine plasma renin activity and beat-to-beat blood pressure variability has been observed by Watson et al. [47], when the values for supine PRA are corrected for age. Naturally, it is difficult to isolate this relationship from the effect exerted by the autonomic nervous system on blood pressure variability.

3. SUMMARY

Blood pressure in all individuals fluctuates from minute to minute, depending upon the physical and psychological state of the individual. The most reliable way of assessing these fluctuations is by continuous direct ambulatory monitoring, which can measure the beat-to-beat variation of arterial pressure in a reproducible manner, free of the effect of an observer. The variability of mean blood pressure increases with advancing age and with hypertension. Variability can be roughly predicted in a particular individual

114

from his response to pressor stimuli, whether psychological or physical. The sino-aortic baroreceptor reflexes, the sympathetic nervous system, and the renin–angiotensin system appear to act in concert to regulate these variations in normal and hypertensive man. The extent to which the arterial baroreceptors act as long-term buffers of blood pressure is still controversial [70]. Borderline blood pressure elevation does not appear to be associated with an increase in blood pressure lability; moreover, it would not seem to confer any immunity from subsequent cardiovascular events [71]. We agree with Pickering's view that borderline hypertension represents an arbitrary distinction in a continuously distributed variable.

We similarly believe that the term 'labile hypertension' should be dropped and replaced by a numerical description of the standard deviation of arterial pressure over a defined period and with specified conditions with regard to activity and state of wakefulness.

REFERENCES

1. Hales S: Statistical essays containing haemostatiks. In: Selected Readings in the History of Physiology, 2nd edition, pp. 56–57. Fulton JF, ed. Springfield: Thomas, 1966.
2. Hill L: pressure in man while sleeping, resting working, bathing, J Physiol 22:26P–29P, 1898.
3. Brush LE, Fairweather R: Observations on the changes in blood pressure during normal sleep. Am J Physiokl 5:199–210, 1901.
4. Diehl HS: The variability of blood pressure: morning and evening studies. Arch Int Med 43:835–845, 1929.
5. Miall WE, Oldham PD: Factors influencing arterial blood pressure in the general population. Clin Sci 17:409–444, 1958.
6. Metropolitan Life Insurance Company: Blood Pressure: Insurance Experience and its Implications. New York, 1961.
7. Kannel WB: Role of blood pressure in cardiovascular morbidity and mortality. Prog Cardiovasc Dis 17:5–24, 1974.
8. Smirk FH: Casual, basal and supplemental blood pressures in 519 first degree relatives of substantial hypertensive patients and in 350 population controls. Clin Sci Mol Med 51 (Suppl 3):13s–17s, 1976.
9. Eich RH, Peters RJ, Cuddy RP, Smulyan H, Lyons RH: Hemodynamics in labile hypertension. Am Heart J 63:188–195, 1962.
10. Finkieman S, Worcel M, Agrest A: Hemodynamic patterns in essential hypertension. Circulation 31:356–368, 1965.
11. Eich R, Cuddy Rp, Smulyan H, Lyons RH: Hemodynamics in labile hypertension: follow-up study. Circulation 34:299–307, 1966.
12. Sannerstedt R: Hemodynamic response to exercise in patients with arterial hypertension. Acta Med Scand 180 (Suppl 458):1–83, 1966.
13. Juluis S, Conway J: Hemodynamic study in patients with borderline blood pressure elevation. Circulation 38:282–288, 1968.
14. Ayman D, Goldshine AD: Blood pressure determinations by patients with essential hypertension – I: The difference between clinic and home readings before treatment. Am J Med Sci 200:465–474, 1940.

15. Juluis S, Ellis CN, Pascual AV, Matice M, Hansson L, Hunyor SN, Sandler L: Home blood pressure determination: value in borderline ('labile') hypertension. JAMA 229:663–666, 1974.
16. Laughlin KD, Sherrard DJ, Fisher L: Comparison of clinic and home blood pressure levels in essential hypertension and variables associated with clinic–home differences. J Chron Dis 33:197–206, 1980.
17. Gould BA, Mann S, Davies AB, Altman D, Raftery EB: Does placebo lower blood pressure? Lancet IV: 1377–1381, 1981.
18. Richardson DW, Honour AJ, Fenton GW, Stott FH, Pickering GW: Variation in arterial pressure throughout the day and night. Clin Sci 26:445–460, 1964.
19. Beevers DG, Lim CC, Backhouse CI, Bloxham CA: The Remler M-2000 semi-automatic blood pressure recorder. In: ISAM 1979: Proceedings of the Third, International Symposium on Ambulatory Monitoring, pp. 223–234. Stott FD, Raftery EB, Goulding L, eds. London: Academic Press, 1980.
20. Horan MJ, Kennedy HL, Padgett NE: Do borderline hypertensive patients have labile blood pressure? Ann Int Med 94 (Part 1):466–468, 1981.
21. Raftery EB, Ward AP: The indirect method of recording blood pressure. Cardiovasc Res 2:210–218, 1968
22. Nielsen PE, Jannische H: The accuracy of auscultatory measurement of arm blood pressure in very obese subjects. Acta Med Scand 195:403–409, 1974.
23. Sokolow M: Data obtained with the ambulatory blood pressure recorder. In: Blood Pressure Variability, pp. 19–24. Clement DL, ed. Lancester: MTP Press, 1979.
24. Sokolow M, Werdegar D, Kain HK, Hinman AT: Relationship between level of blood pressure measured casually and by portable recorders and severity of complications in essential hypertension. Circulation 34:279–298, 1966.
25. Kazamias TM, Gander MP, Franklin DL, Ross J Jr: Blood pressure measurement with Doppler ultrasonic flowmeter. J Appl Physiol 30:585–8, 1971.
26. De Leeuw PW, Kho TL, Falke HE, Birkenhäger WH, Wester A: Haemodynamic and endocrinological profile of essential hypertension. Acta Med Scand (Suppl) 622:9–86, 1978.
27. Clement DL: Blood pressure variability in hospitalized patients. Acta Clin Belg 32:163–7, 1977.
28. Bevan AT, Honour AJ, Stott FD: Direct arterial pressure recording in unrestricted man. Clin Sci 36:329–344, 1969.
29. Floras JS, Sleight P: Ambulatory monitoring of blood pressure, In: Scientific Foundations of Cardiology. Sleight P, Jones JV, eds. London: Heineman, 1982 (in press).
30. Littler WA, Honour AJ, Sleight P, Stott FD: Continuous recording of direct arterial pressure and electrocardiogram in unrestricted man. Br Med J 3:76–78, 1972.
31. Stott FD: The Oxford portable blood pressure transducer. In: Blood Pressure Variability. pp. 55–60. Clement DL, ed. Lancaster: MTP Press, 1979.
32. Sleight P, Floras J, Jones JV: Automatic analysis of continuous intra-arterial blood pressure recordings. In: Blood Pressure Variability, pp. 61–66, Clement DL, ed. Lancaster: MTP Press, 1979.
33. Littler WA, Honour AJ, Sleight P: Direct arterial pressure and electrocardiogram during motor car driving. Br Med J 2:273–277, 1973.
34. Cellina GU, Honour AJ, Littler WA: Direct arterial pressure, heart rate and electrocardiogram during cigarette smoking in unrestricted patients. Am Heart J 89:18–25, 1975.
35. Littler WA, Honour AJ, Sleight P: Direct arterial pressure, pulse rate and electrocardiogram during micturition and defaecation in unrestricted man. Am Heart J 88:205–210, 1974.
36. Littler WA, Honour AJ, Sleight P: Direct arterial pressure, heart rate and electrocardiogram during human coitus. J Reproduct Fertil 40:321–331, 1974.

116

37. Littler WA, Honour Aj, Carter RD, Sleight P: Sleep and blood pressure. Br Med J 3:346-8, 1975.
38. Littler WA, Honour AJ, Sleight P, Stott FD: Direct arterial pressure and the electrocardiogram in unrestricted patients with angina pectoris. Circulation 48:125-134, 1973.
39. Littler WA, Honour AJ: Direct arterial pressure, heart rate, and electrocardiogram in unrestricted patients before and after removal of a phaeochromocyoma. Quart J Med (NS) 43:441-449, 1974.
40. Murnaghan GA, Mitchell RH, Raft SC: Blood pressure rhythms in normotensive and pre-eclamptic pregnancy. In: ISAM 1979: Proceedings of the Third International Symposium on Ambulatory Monitoring, pp. 157-166. Stott FD, Raftery EB, Goulding L, eds. London: Academic Press, 1980.
41. Millar Craig MW, Mann S, Balasubramanian V, Raftery EB: Blood pressure circadian rhythm in essential hypertension. Clin Sci Mol Med 55:391s-393s, 1978.
42. Floras JS, Jones JV, Johnston JA, Brooks DE, Hassan MO, Sleight P: Arousal and the circadian rhythm of blood pressure. Clin Sci Mol Med 55:395s-397s, 1978.
43. Rowlands DB, Stallard TJ, Watson RDS, Littler WA: The influence of physical activity on arterial pressure during ambulatory recordings in man. Clin Sci 58:115-117, 1980.
44. Floras JS: Studies on neural regulation of blood pressure in hypertension. D Phil Thesis, University of Oxford, 1981.
45. Bristow JD, Honour AJ, Pickering TG, Sleight P: Cardiovascular and respiratory changes during sleep in normal and hypertensive subjects. Cardiovasc Res 3:476-485, 1969.
46. Pickering G, Stott FD: Ambulatory blood pressure - a review. In: ISAM 1979: Proceedings of the Third International Symposium on Ambulatory Monitoring, pp. 135-145. Stott FD, Raftery EB, Goulding L, eds. London: Academic Press, 1980.
47. Watson RD, Stallard TJ, Flinn RM, Littler WA: Factors determining direct arterial pressure and its variability in hypertensive man. Hypertension 2:333-41, 1980.
48. Mancia G, Ferrari A, Gregorini L, et al.: Blood pressure variability in man: its relation to high blood pressure, age and baroreflex sensitivity. Clin Sci 59:401s-410s, 1980.
49. Pessina AC, Mormino P, Semplicini A, et al.: The Blood pressure in 'labile' and 'established' hypertension: computer analysis of the continuous blood pressure recording. In: ISAM 1979: Proceedings of the Third International Symposium on Ambulatory Monitoring, pp. 253-260. Stott FD, Raftery EB, Goulding L, eds. London: Academic Press, 1980.
50. Floras JS, Jones JV, Hassan MO, et al.: Cuff and ambulatory blood pressures in subjects with essential hypertension. Lancet 3: 107-109, 1981.
51. Birkenhäger WH, Van Es LA, Honwing A, Lamers HJ, Mulder AH: Studies onthe lability of hypertension in man. Clin Sci 35:445-456, 1968.
52. Schalekamp MADH, Schalekamp-Kuyken MPA, Birkenhäger WH: Abnormal renal haemodynamics and renin suppression in hypertensive patients. Clin Sci 38:101-110, 1970.
53. Cowley Jr AW, Liard JF, Guyton AC: Role of the bororeceptor reflex in daily control of arterial blood pressure and other variables in dogs. Circ Res 32:564-576, 1973.
54. Jones JV, Hallbäck M: Cardiovascular reactivity and design in rats with experimental 'neurogenic hypertension'. Acta Physiol Scand 102:41-49, 1978.
55. Ito CS, Scher AM: Hypertension following denervation of aortic baroreceptors in unanaesthetized dogs. Circ Res 42:230-236, 1979.
56. Nathan MA, Reis DJ: Chronic labile hypertension produced by lesions of the nucleus tractus solitarii in the cat. Circ Res 40:72-81, 1977.
57. Snyder DW, Nathan MA, Reis DJ: Chronic lability of arterial pressure produced by selective destruction of the catecholamine innervation of the nucleus tractus solitarii in the rat. Circ Res 43:663-671, 1978.
58. Smyth HS, Sleight P, Pickering GW: Reflex regulation of arterial pressure during sleep in man. Circ Res 24:109-121, 1969.

59. Jones JV, Floras JS, Hassan MO, et al.: Baroreflex regulation of blood pressure variability. In: ISAM 1981: Proceedings of the Fourth International Symposium on Ambulatory Monitoring. London: Academic Press, 1982 (in press).
60. Gribbin B, Pickering TG, Sleight P, Peto R: The effect of age and high blood pressure on baroreflex sensitivity in man. Circ Res 29:424–431, 1971.
61. Lake CR, Ziegler MG, Kopin IJ: Use of plasma norepinephrine for evaluation of sympathetic neuronal function in man, Life Sci 18:1315–1326, 1976.
62. Clement DL, Bogaert MG, Muerman EZ, De Schaepdryver AF: Significance of elevated plasma noradrenaline in patients with essential hypertension. In: Circulating Catecholamines and Blood Pressure, pp. 64-«). Birkenhäger WH, Falke HE, eds. Utrecht: Bunge Scientific, 1978.
63. Philipp T, Distler A, Cordes V: Sympathetic nervous system and blood pressure control in essential hypertension. Lancet 2, 959–963, 1978.
64. Wallin BG, Sundlof G, Eriksson B-H, et al.: Plasma noradrenaline correlates to sympathetic muscle nerve activity in normotensive man. Circulation (in press).
65. Sever PS: Catecholamines in essential hypertension: the present controversy. In: Circulating Catecholamines and Blood Pressure, pp. 1–10. Birkenhäger WH, Falke HE, eds. Utrecht: Bunge Scientific, 1978.
66. Dickinson CJ: Neurogenic hypertension revisited. Clin Sci 60:471–477.
67. Forsyth RD, Hoffbrand BI, Melmon KL: Hemodynamic effects of angiotensin in normal and environmentally stressed monkeys. Circulation 44:119–129, 1971.
68. Cowley Jr AW, DeClue JW: Quantification of baroreceptor influence on arterial pressure changes seen in primary angiotensin-induced hypertension in dogs. Circ Res 39:779–787, 1976.
69. Lumbers ER, McCloskey DI, Potter EK: Inhibition by angiotensin II of baroreceptor-evoked activity in cardiac vagal efferent nerves in the dog. J Physiol (Lond) 294: 69–80, 1979.
70. Sleight P: Arterial Baroreceptors and Hypertension. Oxford: Oxford University Press. 1980.
71. Kannel WB, Sorlie P, Gordon T: Labile hypertension: a faulty concept? Circulation 61:1183–1187, 1980

II. EXPERIMENTAL HYPERTENSION

8. PATHOPHYSIOLOGY OF HYPERTENSION IN GENETICALLY HYPERTENSIVE RATS – ENVIRONMENTAL MODIFICATION AND PREVENTION

YUKIO YAMORI

INTRODUCTION

The establishment of animal models for hypertension and related cardiovascular diseases has made possible studies on the pathophysiology, the pathogenesis and the gene–environment interaction in the initiation of hypertensive diseases, and also the prevention of hypertensive diseases by controlling environmental factors. In addition to the pathophysiological similarities of these hypertensive diseases in man and animals, we confirmed in epidemiological studies some of the experimentally proven environmental effects on hypertension-related diseases. Our experimental and epidemiological studies clarified to a considerable extent the gene–environment interaction in the pathogenesis and the pathophysiology of hypertensive diseases and such is proving to be increasingly important in the prevention of these diseases [1–3].

1. DEVELOPMENT OF VARIOUS MODELS OF HYPERTENSION

Among our animal models established during the past 17 years, *stroke-prone SHR* (SHRSP) [4, 5] were selectively bred from *spontaneously hypertensive rats* (SHR) [6] which had been derived from Wistar-Kyoto rats (WKY). Over 90% of the rats die of stroke, i.e., cerebral hemorrhage and/or infarction [1, 2, 7] (Figure 1). SHRSP quickly develop severe hypertension, over 200 mm Hg at the age of 10 to 15 weeks and maintain this level until most die of stroke, while stroke-resistant SHR (SHRSR) develop hypertension around 200 mm Hg and rarely (less than 5%) die with stroke-lesions.

From among SHRSP, a strain of rats, which developed severe hypertension relatively slowly and usually died of cerebral thrombosis, was developed by selective breeding. This strain is known as *spontaneous thrombogenic rats* (STR) [8, 9].

Additional strains of rats have been developed as models for atherogenesis. These substrains have a greater reactive hypercholesterolemia than do the SHR. This strain was named *arteriolipidosis-prone rats* (ALR) [10–12].

Amery, A. (ed.) Hypertensive Cardiovascular Disease: Pathophysiology and Treatment
© *1982, Martinus Nijhoff Publishers. The Hague / Boston / London*
ISBN-13: 978-94-009-7478-4

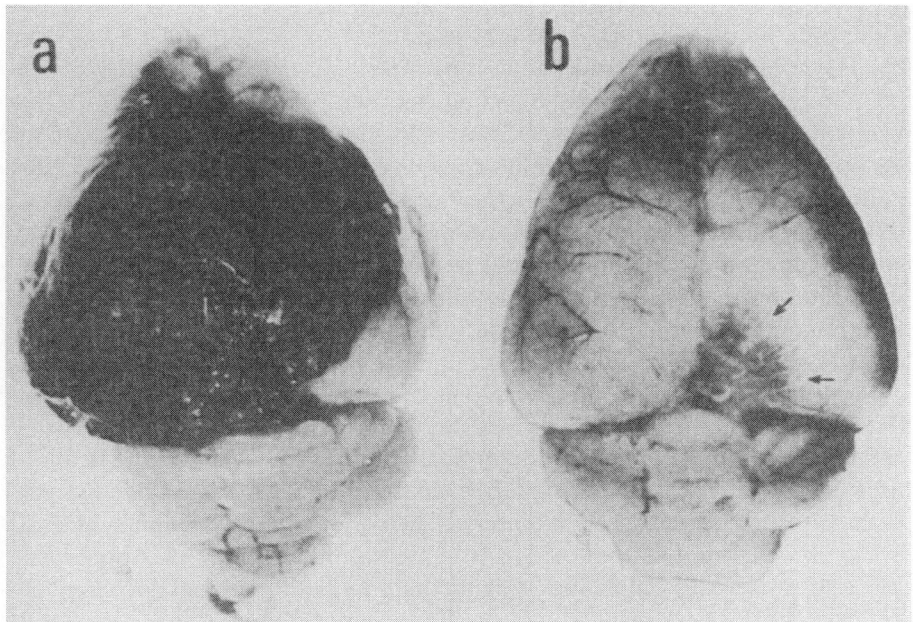

Figure 1. Massive cerebral hemorrhage (a) and infarction (b) in SHRSP.

These rats quickly develop not only hypercholesterolemia, but also arterial fat deposition in small arteries such as cerebrobasal, mesenteric and other arteries within a few weeks when they are fed hypercholesterolemic diets.

Since the combination of atherosclerosis and thrombosis is regarded as being the basic process leading to myocardial infarction, we have selectively bred from the relevant SHR substrains a new substrain which develops ischemic heart disease spontaneously, in a high incidence. Rats of this substrain show typical symptoms of congestive heart failure and die with extensive scattered ischemic lesions in the myocardium [13]. Atherosclerotic vascular lesions with intimal proliferation are frequently noted within a relatively short period when these rats are fed a high fat-cholesterol diet, and thrombosis is also often apparent in the small branches of coronary arteries [14]. Since atheromatous lesions and thrombosis result in scattered fibrosis of the heart in these rats, they have been named *myocardial ischemic rats* (MIR).

The establishment of these models for hypertension, stroke, thrombosis, atherogenesis and myocardial infarction by selective breeding itself indicates the importance of genetic factors. On the basis of these models studies have been carried out not only on the pathophysiology of hypertension-related diseases, but also on gene–environment interaction in the pathophysiological development of these diseases.

2. PATHOGENESIS OF GENETIC HYPERTENSION

The mode of inheritance and the number of major genes of hypertension in SHR were analyzed by cross breeding between SHR and WKY [15]; the results indicated that hypertension was related to genetic factors at rates of 60–90%. As analyzed statistically, three major genes are involved in the additive mode of inheritance. Further, cross-analyses between SHRSP and SHRSR suggested that at least two more major genes were involved in the heredity of severe hypertension and stroke, respectively [16, 17].

On the other hand, environmental factors such as salt and stress leadings were proven to augment hypertension and to aggravate vascular lesions in hypertension [18, 19].

Hypertension mechanisms, which have been proven to be present in SHR, are schematically summarized in Figure 2 [20, 21]. Hypertension is initially caused by an increased peripheral vascular resistance which is functional and of neurogenic origin [22]. Increase in blood pressure and sympathetic vasomotor tone accelerate noncollagen and collagen protein synthesis in the vascular wall to induce adaptive medial hypertrophy and hypertensive arteriosclerosis which finally contribute to nonfunctional increases in the peripheral resistance [20–23]. Close observation of the peripheral branches of the mesenteric arteries in young SHRSP with developing hypertension revealed evidence of vasoconstriction and dilatation which are reversible, but only initially. Such an initial functional stage corresponds to the

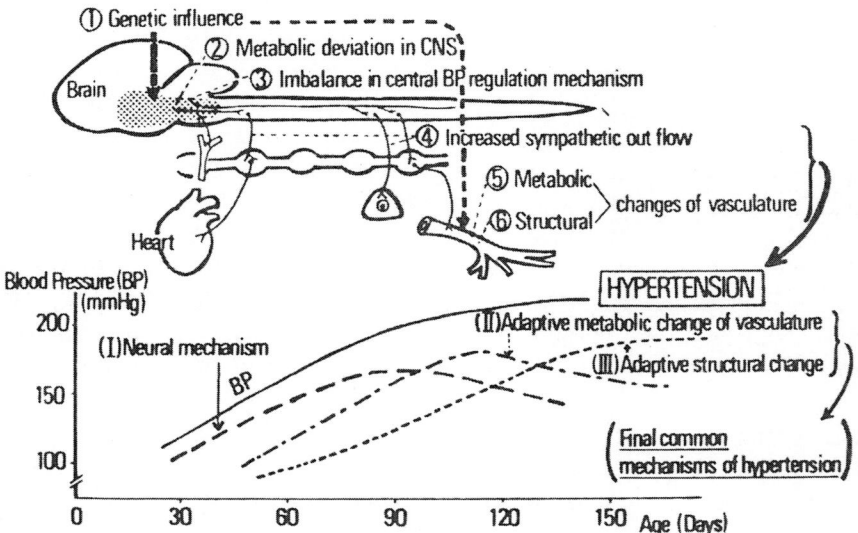

Figure 2. Initiation and maintenance mechanisms of spontaneous genetic hypertension (reproduced from [21]).

neurogenic phase of spontaneous hypertension with increased levels of plasma norepinephrine (NE), accelerated NE turnover of peripheral tissues and increased sympathetic vasomotor discharges [21, 22].

Concomitant with the initial neurogenic rise of blood pressure, the incorporation of labeled amino acids into collagenous and noncollagenous proteins in the vascular wall is accelerated, indicating that the vascular protein synthesis is enhanced, even in the early stage of hypertension [22–24]. Since this enhancement was attenuated by surgical and pharmacological sympathectomy, neural vasomotor tone was thereby proven to stimulate vascular protein synthesis [25]. Our most recent observations on cultured smooth muscle cells obtained by an explant method from the aorta showed that smooth muscle cells from SHRSP and SHRSR grow faster than those from WKY, even under conditions in which the tissue culture is free from physiological and chemical stress, such as blood pressure and NE released from nerve endings [26]. These findings suggest that vascular smooth muscle cells themselves are predisposed to proliferation in genetic hypertension and are more vulnerable to hyperplasia in response to hypertension and neurogenic activation.

Thus, hypertension develops in these models and is maintained mainly by an increased peripheral resistance which is at first due to neurogenic and functional vasoconstriction and later to structural vascular changes induced by accelerated vascular protein synthesis. In severe hypertension such as occurs in SHRSP, regional cerebral blood flow decreases, particularly in brain areas fed by recurrent branches [27, 28]. Mild chronic ischemia increases vascular permeability and induces arterionecrosis. When microaneurysms formed at the necrotic arterial wall rupture, hemorrhage occurs. On the other hand, thrombosis at the necrotic arterial wall or within microaneurysms causes infarction. Thus, stroke in SHRSP has both hemorrhagic and thrombotic elements, and is therefore called arterionecro-thrombogenic stroke [1]. In addition to genetic hypertension, STR have an impairment of the fibrinolytic system and are more liable to develop thrombosis, at the sites of hypertensive vascular lesions. Moreover, ALR genetically develop reactive hypercholesterolemia and arterial fat deposition because of the increased absorption of intestinal cholesterol and the decreased catabolism of cholesterol [11, 12]. The increased incorporation of cholesterol into the arterial wall is due to physical factors such as hypertension and hemodynamic derangements as well as to chemical factors such as lower serum HDL-level (thus, higher atherogenic index – LDL/HDL) and the increased intracellular incorporation of lipoprotein, as seen in liver cells. In the ALR and MIR substrains, atheromatous and thrombotic lesions are relatively much more important and these strains may be useful models for cerebral thombosis and/or myocardial infarction.

3. GENE-ENVIRONMENT INTERACTION IN HYPERTENSION-RELATED DISEASES

Our studies in these animal models clarified the environmental influence on the pathogenesis of genetic hypertension, particularly the effects of excess salt intake and diet on hypertensive disease, i.e., an increased Na/K ratio raised blood pressure, while increased lipid and protein intake decreased blood pressure. Therefore, dietary conditions greatly modify hypertensive diseases; salt intake accelerates arterionecrosis due to hypertension and, thus, increases stroke incidence, while lipid intake induces atherosclerosis due to lipidemia, but decreases stroke incidence because of the attenuation of severe hypertension [1–3, 13].

3.1. Effect of lipid intake on hypertension-related diseases

When SHRSP were fed diets containing 20% fat and various amounts of cholesterol, the development of severe hypertension was attenuated in comparison with the group fed the standard diet. The incidence of stroke was also reduced, presumably because the blood pressure was not so high [1, 2]. These experimental findings are consistent with epidemiological data that show the high incidence of stroke in Japan in areas where the serum cholesterol level is low. However, excess lipid intake leads to atherosclerosis and to myocardial infarction. Thus, differences in lipid intake in various countries in the world well explain the differences in the incidences of stroke and myocardial infarction: high stroke and low myocardial infarction rates in Japan vs. low stroke and high myocardial infarction rates in Western countries [3].

Since a low HDL level and a high ratio of LDL to HDL, i.e., the atherogenic index (AI), were causatively related to atherogenesis, SHRSP fed various high fat-cholesterol diets were examined further for the relation between blood pressure and AI. Since a significant inverse correlation was noted [13], the reduction in blood pressure was obtained at the cost of an increased AI. A further analysis of the mechanism of the reduction of stroke incidence in SHRSP fed a high fat-cholesterol diet showed that the vascular reactivity to the pressor substance norepinephrine in these rats was decreased [29]. This may explain why a high fat diet leads to a reduction in the degree of hypertension.

3.2. Aggravation of hypertension-related diseases by excess salt intake and its mechanisms

We have repeatedly demonstrated that excess salt intake accelerates the development of hypertension in SHR [19], and increases the incidence of stroke. Salt restriction attenuates the development of severe hypertension [30]. Moreover, effect of excess salt intake on blood pressure increase is greater in SHRSP with their genetic disposition to severe hypertension, than in ordinary stroke-resistant SHR or normotensive Wistar-Kyoto rats; thus, a gene–environment interaction was clearly proven [30]. These experimental data together with epidemiological statistics indicate the importance of salt restriction in the prevention of stroke. Our experiments on SHRSP also showed the importance of the Na/K ratio in the development of hypertension; 1% NaCl in drinking water (giving a urinary Na/K ratio over 3.5) augmented hypertension, while 2% KCl in drinking water (giving a urinary Na/K ratio of about 0.1) attenuated the hypertension even within one week of experiment [13, 31]. We found that the Na/K ratio in the erythrocytes had significantly increased in SHRSP even after one week of sodium loading. The intracellular Na/K ratio could be readily modified in these sodium loaded SHRSP but not in normotensive rats, while serum levels of Na and K remained within a normal range[13]. Such findings indicate the possible relation between sodium sensitivity and biomembrane abnormalities [32–38]. As summarized in Figure 3, biomembrane characteristics of erythrocytes noted in SHR and particularly in SHRSP are the increased permeability of Na ions [32], increased osmotic fragility [33–35], increased fluidity [35, 36], increased permeability of lipophilic ions [36–38] and the reduced net Na flux [39]. Biomembrane abnormalities in hypertension are not limited to erythrocytes but are also found in platelets [35], synaptosomes [38, 40] and cultured vascular smooth muscles [26] in SHR and SHRSP, and are commonly noted in humans with essential hypertension [37, 41]. In light of these findings such membrane alterations which lead to accumulation of sodium in the cells should be considered one of the genetic dispositions to hypertension, in animal models, and probably also in man. The accumulation of intracellular sodium ions and the consequent

	Blood Pressure	Na-Ion Permeability	Osmotic Fragility	Fluidity	Lipophilic Ion	Net Na-Flux
WKY	→ (0)	→	→	→	→	→
SHR	↑ (5%)	↑	→	↗	↑	↓
SHRSP	↑↑ (90%)	↑↑	↑	↑	↑↑	↓

( ) : Stroke Incidence

Figure 3. Various biomembrane characteristics of erythrocytes in genetically hypertensive models, SHR and SHRSP.

increase in Na/K ratio would increase the reactivity to neuronal stimuli, accelerate calcium influx to induce contraction in vascular smooth muscle cells and induce the retention of intracellular water. Thus, peripheral vascular resistance increases both functionally and structurally. The cellular mechanism(s) of the acceleration of hypertension by sodium loading seems to be the alteration of intracellular Na/K balance which is more readily induced where there are genetic biomembrane abnormalities such as occur in SHR, especially in SHRSP. This could be regarded as the basic 'cellular' mechanism of the gene–environment interaction in salt-induced or accelerated hypertension.

3.3. Mechanisms of attenuation of hypertension-related diseases by protein intake

The effect of salt was greatly modified by dietary protein intake. SHRSP fed a normal or low protein diet with excess salt quickly developed severe hypertension and all these rats died of stroke within a short period. Without the excess salt intake, 75% died of stroke. In contrast, when SHRSP were fed a high fish protein diet with excess salt, the incidence of stroke was far less. In the group fed a high fish protein diet without excess salt intake, the development of severe hypertension was delayed and there was no incidence of stroke [1–3, 13]. Thus, a high protein diet apparently attenuates the development of severe hypertension and counteracts the adverse effect of salt, at least in rats, and may probably do so in humans, on the basis of our epidemiological studies.

We further analyzed the preventive mechanisms of protein diets and found three major mechanisms: 1) attenuation of hypertension, 2) acceleration of salt excretion and 3) effect on arterial walls [42].

1) Mechanisms of the prophylactic effect of protein were noted to differ depending on the source of the protein. A high fish protein diet containing sulfur amino acids such as methionine and taurine attenuated the development of hypertension, while high soy bean protein diet had no significant effect on blood pressure. Our experimental analysis showed that there were significant inverse correlations between dietary sulfur amino acid contents and blood pressure or stroke incidence in groups of SHRSP fed on different diets [42]. We further confirmed that methionine and taurine administration given in doses of 1–3% in drinking water attenuated the development of severe hypertension and decreased the incidence of stroke down to 30% of the incidence in control SHRSP [42, 43]. We have also studied the acute effects of intraventricular administration of methionine and taurine in SHRSP and found a definite decrease in blood pressure [44]. Moreover, since taurine, the metabolite from sulfur amino acids, had significantly increased in the brainstem of the taurine-treated group of the chronic

experiment [45], taurine may play some role in the modulation of the central regulation of blood pressure. In addition to these sulfur amino acids, we studied the effect of tyrosine given either intraventricularly or intravenously; blood pressure decreased in both cases [46]. This was attributed to the stimulation of central noradrenergic depressor mechanisms, since the turnover of norepinephrine was accelerated in the brainstem of these treated SHRSP. Recently, glutamate has been suggested as a neurotransmitter of baroreceptor afferent nerve fibers [47]. Thus, not only sulfur amino acids, but also tyrosine and glutamate should be considered to attenuate severe hypertension when high protein diets rich in these amino acids are administered.

2) The other mechanism of stroke prevention by dietary protein seems to be related to salt metabolism. Urinary sodium excretion is impaired in SHRSP, and this abnormality is observed even before the development of severe hypertension [48]. Therefore, the salt retention due to a minute renal dysfunction could be one of the causes of severe hypertension in SHRSP. When animals were fed high protein diets, urinary volume and sodium excretion were abruptly increased in normotensive rats and in the SHR and SHRSP [49]. Consequently, increased urinary sodium excretion can be regarded as the main mechanism whereby a high protein diet counteracts the adverse effect of a high salt diet. A similar effect of high protein diet on urinary sodium excretion was recently reported in the case of obese patients treated with a low-caloric high protein diet [50].

3) Soy bean protein diet did not markedly affect blood pressure, but was clearly effective in preventing stroke. No stroke was observed in SHRSP fed a soy bean diet plus 1% NaCl in their drinking water, in spite of severe hypertension, while all in the group fed a normal protein diet plus 1% NaCl in their drinking water died of stroke by the 27th week of age. Since these experimental data indicated a possible alteration of vascular wall characteristics, the stress-elongation curve of the aorta was examined in SHRSP fed high and low protein diets [42]. The maximum stress causing ductile failure of the aorta was less in SHRSP fed a low protein diet than in those on a high protein diet. In other words, vascular walls of rats fed a high protein diet are more elastic than those on a low protein diet. This was confirmed also in cerebral vessels by observing cerebrovascular reactivity in response in CO_2 inhalation [42].

4. ENVIRONMENTAL EFFECTS ON GENETIC HYPERTENSION; ITS RELEVANCE TO HYPERTENSION-RELATED DISEASES IN HUMANS

These experimental findings, especially gene–environment interactions observed in genetically hypertensive models were extrapolated to hypertensive diseases in humans in order to confirm that genetically hypertensive rats could be models for human diseases. Epidemiological evidence for dietary effect on hypertensive diseases was obtained by comparative studies on stroke incidence in farming and fishing villages [51], as well as by observing intracommunity relationships between blood pressure and salt or protein intake [13]. Since one of the great barriers in nutritional surveys of the community is a lack of scientific methodology, we attempted to establish the methodology before initiating the epidemiological studies, and confirmed that sodium excretion and nitrogen or inorganic sulfate excretion in urine over a period of 24 h reflected well the dietary salt or protein intake in healthy volunteer students who, for ten days, had been on high or low protein diets or high or low salt diets, respectively.

The incidence of stroke was clearly different in the farming and fishing villages: the death rate of stroke in the former was twice as high as in the latter. Correspondingly, blood pressure, especially diastolic blood pressure, in adult men and women was significantly higher in the farming than in the fishing village. Urinary sodium and nitrogen excretion were similar in these two villages. However, the urinary excretion of inorganic sulfate (mainly coming from sulfur amino acids) was significantly lower in the farming village. These epidemiological data are consistent with our results obtained in SHRSP, and indicate that stroke incidence and blood pressure are high in populations where protein intake is very low.

Multiple regression analysis indicated that systolic blood pressure and urinary Na/K ratio were significantly correlated in about 1000 inhabitants of the farming village where dietary salt intake was high: Na/K ratio was over 6 on the average, while the ratio was less than 3 in most Western countries. The correlation was highly significant between blood pressure (or the prevalence of hypertension) and Na/K ratio in the aged population. Moreover, systolic blood pressure was correlated not only positively with Na/K ratio, but also negatively with the sulfate (S)/urea nitrogen (N) ratio (as indicated by the following equation: systolic blood pressure $= 1.08(Na/K) - 13.0(S/N) + 0.685 \cdot age + 0.352 \cdot obesity \quad index + 2.47 \cdot sex + 87.8$). Therefore, experimental results in genetically hypertensive models can be consistently extrapolated with respect to cases of human hypertension, so that less salt and a higher protein intake should be the goal for dietary control of hypertension–related diseases in Japan and other Oriental countries where salt intake is high but protein intake is low.

CONCLUSION

In addition to the well-known, spontaneously hypertensive rats (SHR) and the stroke-prone (SHRSP) and stroke-resistant (SHRSR) substrains, we have

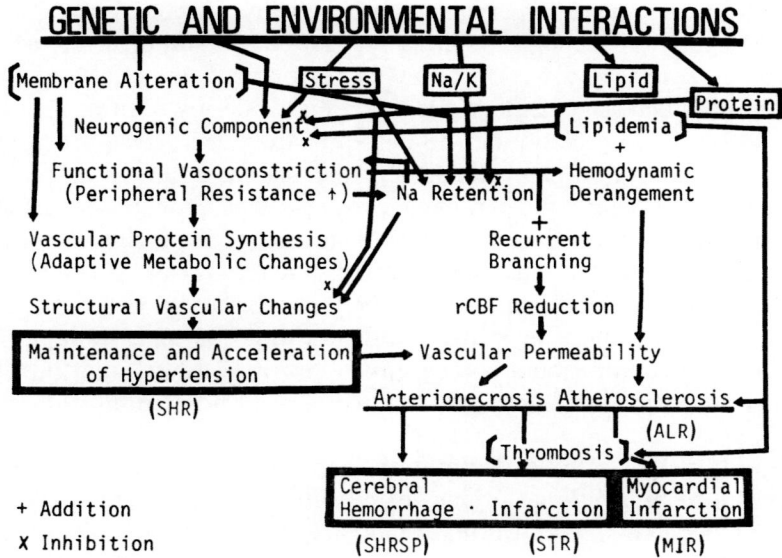

Figure 4. Gene–environment interactions in hypertensive mechanisms of genetically hypertensive rat models.

developed by inbreeding three further strains in relation to hypertensive vascular disease: (1) rats with spontaneous thrombogenesis (STR) which die mainly of cerebral thrombosis; (2) arteriolipidosis-prone rats (ALR) which develop widespread arterial fat deposits when fed lipid-rich diets; (3) rats (MIR) with a high prevalence of ischemic heart disease which occurs spontaneously but worsens when a high cholesterol diet is ingested.

The pathophysiology of hypertensive diseases was studied in these models and we found that gene–environment interaction is important in the pathogenesis of hypertension, stroke and atherosclerosis (Figure 4).

Environmental stress induces hypertension, particularly in some strains of rats or other species predisposed to hypertension. In SHR, which show enhanced cardiovascular responses to environmental stimuli and are regarded as having a greater number of neurogenic components in hypertension, blood pressure becomes elevated in the absence of stress but various forms of stress augment the hypertension and increase the incidence of vascular lesions.

Excess salt intake augments hypertension in SHR and aggravates hypertensive complications, particularly in SHRSP which, with a slight impairment of renal sodium handling and more marked biomembrane abnormalities, are more salt-sensitive than SHRSR.

A protein-rich diet effectively decreases the incidence of stroke and attenuates the adverse effect of salt intake in SHRSP. The preventive mechanisms of stroke by various protein diets have been analyzed; fish protein

128

diets ameliorate severe hypertension probably by affecting central blood pressure regulation through an increased supply of amino acids such as methionine, taurine and tyrosine, and also counteracts the effects of a high salt intake by increasing urinary salt excretion, while soy bean protein diets do not affect blood pressure but do decrease stroke incidence, probably by improving the physical characteristics of the arterial walls.

Hypercholesterolemic diets attenuate hypertension probably by reducing vascular reactivity and decreasing the incidence of hypertensive vascular lesions (arterionecrosis), but they accelerate atherosclerosis.

These nutritional modifications of hypertensive diseases well explain epidemiological differences in stroke incidence which is high in Japan and other Oriental countries and comparatively low in Western countries. Furthermore, our epidemiological studies in fishing and farming villages in Japan suggest that these experimental findings can be extrapolated to humans. Within the farming community, a positive correlation was noted between blood pressure and urinary Na/K ratio, and an inverse correlation between blood pressure and urinary inorganic sulfate to urea nitrogen.

In summary, pathophysiological studies on genetically hypertensive rats indicated that hypertension-related diseases develop under environmental influences such as stress and diet in individuals genetically predisposed to these diseases. Therefore, genetic disposition to hypertensive diseases should be assessed early and hypertension-related diseases may be prevented by controlling environmental factors such as nutrition, particularly in genetically predisposed individuals.

ACKNOWLEDGEMENTS

This review article was based on studies of genetic models of hypertension, and these investigations were supported by grants from the Science and Technology Agency of the Government of Japan, Ministry of Education, Ministry of Public Health and Welfare, Mitsubishi Foundation and Japan Tobacco and Salt Monopoly Public Corporation. M. Ohara kindly helped with the preparation of the manuscript.

REFERENCES

1. Yamori Y, Horie R, Akiguchi I, Nara Y, Ohtaka M, Fukase M: Pathogenetic mechanism of stroke in stroke-prone SHR. In: Progress in Brain Research, 47, Hypertension and Brain Mechanisms, pp. 219–234. De Jong W, ed. Amsterdam: Elsevier, 1977.
2. Yamori Y, Horie R, Handa H, Ohtaka M, Nara Y, Fukase M: Pathogenetic approach to the prophylaxis of stroke and atherogenesis in SHR. In: Spontaneous Hypertension, pp. 269–278. DHEW Publication No. (NIH) 77-1179, 1977.

3. Yamori Y: Experimental models of hypertension as a tool for the control and prevention of clinical hypertension. In: Arterial Hypertension, pp. 209–226. Gross FH, Robertson JIS, eds. Tunbridge Wells: Pitman Medical, 1979.
4. Yamori Y, Nagaoka A, Okamoto K: Importance of genetic factors in hypertensive cerebrovascular lesions; evidence obtained by successive selective breeding of stroke-prone and -resistant SHR. Jpn Circ J 38:1095–1100, 1974.
5. Okamoto K, Yamori Y, Nagaoka A: Establishment of the stroke-prone spontaneously hypertensive rat (SHR). Circ Res 34, 35 (suppl 1):143–153, 1974.
6. Okamoto K, Aoki K: Development of a strain of spontaneously hypertensive rats. Jpn Circ J 27:282–293, 1963.
7. Yamori Y, Horie R, Nara Y, Ikeda K, Kihara M, Ooshima A, Fukase M: Genetics of hypertensive diseases – experimental studies on pathogenesis, detection of predisposition and prevention. In: Advances in Nephrology, pp. 51–74. Hamburger J, Crosnier J, Grunfeld JP, Maxwell MH, eds. Chicago: Year Book Medical publishers, 1981.
8. Yamori Y, Horie R, Ohtaka M, Nara Y, Ikeda K: Genetic and environmental modification of spontaneous hypertension. Jpn Circ J 42:1151–1159, 1978.
9. Yamori Y, Ohta K, Horie R, Ohtaka M, Nara Y, Ooshima A: A new model for cerebral thrombosis and its pathogenesis. Jpn Heart J 20 (Suppl 1):343–345, 1979.
10. Yamori Y: Selection of arteriolipidosis-prone rats (ALR). Jpn Heart J 18:602–603, 1977.
11. Yamori Y, Iritani N, Nara Y, Fukuda E, Kitamura Y: Cholesterol metabolism of arteriolipidosis-prone rats (ALR). Jpn Heart J 20 (Suppl 1):349–351, 1979.
12. Yamori Y, Kitamura Y, Nara Y, Iritani N: Mechanism of hypercholesterolemia in arteriolipidosis-prone rats (ALR). Jpn Circ J 45:1068–1073, 1981.
13. Yamori Y: Environmental influences on the development of hypertensive vascular diseases in SHR and related models, and their relation to human disease. In: New Trends in Arterial Hypertension, Cellular Pharmacology and Physiology, pp. 305–320. Worcel M, Bonvalet JP, Langer SZ, Menard J, Sassard J, eds. Amsterdam: Elsevier/North-Holland Biomedical Press, 1981.
14. Yamori Y, Kihara M, Nara Y, Horie R, Ooshima A: Familial aggregation of myocardial lesions in SHR. Jpn Heart J 22: 503, 1981.
15. Tanase H, Suzuki Y, Ooshima A, Yamori Y, Okamoto K: Genetic analysis of blood pressure in spontaneously hypertensive rats. Jpn Circ J 34:1197–1212, 1970.
16. Yamori Y, Ikeda K, Ooshima A, Fukase M: Inheritance of hypertension in stroke-prone spontaneously hypertensive rats. In: Prophylactic Approach to Hypertensive Diseases, pp. 121–125. Yamori Y, Lovenberg W, Freis ED, eds. New York: Raven Press, 1979.
17. Yamori Y, Ikeda K, Kihara M, Nara Y, Horie R, Ooshima A: Analysis on the heredity of stroke in stroke-prone SHR (SHRSP). Jpn Heart J 21:558, 1980.
18. Yamori Y, Matsumoto M, Yamabe H, Okamoto K: Augmentation of spontaneous hypertension by chronic stress in rats. Jpn Circ J 33:399–409, 1969.
19. Aoki K, Yamori Y, Ooshima A, Okamoto K: Effects of high or low sodium intake in spontaneously hypertensive rats. Jpn Circ J 36: 539–545, 1972.
20. Yamori Y: Pathogenesis of spontaneous hypertension as a model for essential hypertension. Jpn Circ J 41:259–266, 1977.
21. Yamori Y: Interaction of neural and nonneural factors in the pathogenesis of spontaneous hypertension. In:The Nervous System in Arterial Hypertension, pp. 17–43. Julius S, Esler M, eds. Springfield: C.C. Thomas, 1976.
22. Yamori Y: Neural and nonneural mechanisms in spontaneous hypertension. Clin Sci Mol Med 51:431s–434s, 1976.
23. Yamori Y: Contribution of cardiovascular factors to the development of hypertension in spontaneously hypertensive rats. Jpn Heart J 15:194–196, 1974.
24. Ooshima A, Yamori Y, Horie R, Ohtaka M, Fukase M: Vascular protein metabolism in hypertensive models in relation to the prevention of hypertensive diseases. In: Prophylactic

Approach to Hypertensive diseases, pp. 233–240. Yamori Y, Lovenberg W, Freis ED, eds. New York: Raven Press, 1979.

25. Yamori Y, Nakada T, Lovenberg W: Effect of antihypertensive therapy on lysine incorporation into vascular protein of the spontaneously hypertensive rat. Europ J Pharmacol 38:349–355, 1976.

26. Yamori Y, Igawa T, Nara Y, Kihara M, Ooshima A: Characteristics of cultured vascular smooth muscle cells in hypertension. Clin Exp Hypertension 3: 336, 1981.

27. Yamori Y, Horie R, Sato M, Handa H, Fukase M: Pathogenetic similarity of stroke in stroke-prone SHR and humans. Stroke 7:46–53, 1976.

28. Yamori Y, Horie R: Developmental course of hypertension and regional cerebral blood flow in stroke-prone spontaneously hypertensive rats. Stroke 8:456–460, 1977.

29. Yamori Y, Horie R: Vascular reactivity in pathological states. In: Factors Influencing Vascular Reactivity, pp. 268–281. Shibata S, Carrier O, eds. Tokyo: Igaku-Shoin, 1977.

30. Yamori Y, Nara Y, Kihara M, Horie R, Ooshima A: Sodium and other dietary factors in experimental and human hypertension – the Japanese experience. In: Frontiers in Hypertension Research, pp. 46–48. Laragh JH, Bühler FR, Seldin DW, eds. New York: Springer-Verlag, 1981.

31. Yamori Y, Nara Y, Kihara M, Kitamura H: Prophylactic trials for stroke in stroke-prone SHR (6). Alteration of ionic balance in SHR. Jpn Heart J 22:468, 1981.

32. Yamori Y, Nara Y, Horie R: Ion permeability of erythrocyte membrane in SHR. Jpn Heart J 18:604–605, 1977.

33. Yamori Y, Nara Y, Horie R, Ohtaka M: Biomembrane characteristics and chronic effect of tocopheral in models for hypertension and stroke. In: Tocopherol, Oxygen and Biomembranes, pp. 247–256. De Duve C, Hayaishi O, eds. Amsterdam: Excerpta Medica, 1978.

34. Yamori Y, Nara Y, Horie R, Ohtaka M, Ohta K, Mitani F: Biomembrane characteristics in stroke-prone spontaneously hypertensive rats (SHRSP). Jpn Heart J 19:597–598, 1978.

35. Yamori Y, Nara Y, Horie R, Ohtaka M, Ooshima A: Biomembrane characteristics of erythrocytes and platelets in stroke-prone SHR. Tr Soc Path Jpn 68:182–183, 1979.

36. Yamori Y, Horie R, Ohtaka M, Nara Y, Ooshima A, Fukase M: From scientific detection of predisposition to prevention of hypertensive diseases – recent progress in animal models. In: Prophylactic Approach to Hypertensive Diseases, pp. 573–580. Yamori Y, Lovenberg W, Freis ED, eds. New York: Raven Press, 1979.

37. Yamori Y, Nara Y, Horie R, Ooshima A: Abnormal membrane characteristics of erythrocytes in rat models and men with predisposition to stroke. Clin Exp Hypertension 2:1009–1021, 1980.

38. Yamori Y, Nara Y, Kihara M, Horie R, Ooshima A: Is biomembrane abnormality a pathogenic factor or genetic marker of hypertensive diseases? In: Fundamental Fault in Hypertension, Sambhi M, ed, 1981 (in press).

39. De Mendonca M, Grichois M-L, Garay RP, Sassard J, Ben-Ishay D, Meyer P: Abnormal net Na^+ and K^+ fluxes in erythrocytes of three varieties of genetically hypertensive rats. Proc Natl Acad Sci USA 77:4283–4286, 1980.

40. Nara Y, Yamori Y, Horie R, Kihara M, Ooshima A, Lovenberg W: Synaptosomal membrane characteristics in stroke-prone SHR (SHRSP), stroke-resistant SHR (SRHSR) and Wistar -Kyoto rats (WKY). Jpn Heart J 21:559, 1980.

41. Garay RP, Meyer P: A new test showing abnormal net Na^+ and K^+ fluxes in erythrocytes of essential hypertensive patients. Lancet 1:349–353, 1979.

42. Yamori Y, Horie R, Ikeda K, Nara Y, Lovenberg W: Prophylactic effect of dietary protein on stroke and its mechanisms. In: Prophylactic Approach to Hypertensive Diseases, pp. 497–504, Yamori Y, Lovenberg W, Freis ED, eds. New York, Raven Press, 1979.

43. Yamori Y. Horie R, Nara Y, Kihara M, Ikeda K: Experimental prevention of stroke by dietary amino acids in stroke-prone SHR (abstract). In: 8th International Congress of Pharmacology, Tokyo, 1981.

44. Yamori Y, Nara Y, Horie R, Ooshima A, Lovenberg W: Pathophysiological role of taurine in blood pressure regulation in stroke-prone spontaneously hypertensive rats (SHR). In: The Effects of Taurine on Excitable Tissues, pp. 391–403. New York: Spectrum 1981.
45. Nara Y, Yamori Y, Lovenberg W: Effect of dietary taurine on blood pressure in genetically hypertensive rats. J. Biochem Pharmacol 27:2689–2692, 1979.
46. Yamori Y, Fujiwara M, Horie R, Lovenberg W: The hypotensive effect of centrally administered tyrosine. Europ J Pharmacol 68:201–204, 1980.
47. Talman WT, Penone MH, Reis DJ: Evidence for L-glutamate as the neurotransmitter of baroreceptor afferent nerve fibers. Science 209:813–814, 1980.
48. Yamori Y, Horie R, Ohtaka M, Nara Y, Ooshima A: Electrolyte balance in stroke-prone and -resistant SHR. Jpn Heart J 20 (Suppl 1):65–67, 1979.
49. Yamori Y, Horie R, Nara Y, Ikeda K, Ohtaka M, Ooshima A, Sasagawa S: Prophylactic trials for stroke in stroke-prone SHR (4). Mechanism of prevention by dietary protein. Jpn Heart J 20:742, 1979.
50. De Haven J, Sherwin R, Hendler R, Felig P: Nitrogen and sodium balance and sympathetic-nervous-system activity in obese subjects treated with a low-calorie protein or mixed diet. New Eng J Med 302:477–482, 1980.
51. Yamori Y, Tsunematsu T, Note S, Ishikawa S, Fukase M: Nutritional improvement for stroke prevention. In: Prophylactic approach to Hypertensive Diseases, pp. 587–593. Yamori Y, Lovenberg W, Freis ED, eds. New York, Raven Press, 1979.

9. THE PATHOPHYSIOLOGY OF HYPERTENSION: CONTRIBUTIONS OF EXPERIMENTAL PATHOPHYSIOLOGY

J. Carlos Romero, William H. Beierwaltes and Peter C. Houck

INTRODUCTION

The description of the pathogenic events which underly the production of any particular disease is a relatively easy exercise when the etiology of the disease and its symptoms are well established. However, such is not the case with hypertension, for high blood pressure is not itself a disease but merely one of a family of common symptomatic manifestations which develop in response to various pathologies.

This chapter will attempt to describe the current concepts of the pathophysiology of hypertensive disease and the manner in which they interrelate during its evolution. Attention will be given to the principal mechanisms which control the homeostasis of blood pressure, and the ways by which such mechanisms can be disrupted. We believe such a discussion will help the practitioner in interpreting symptomatology and the efficacy of various therapeutic maneuvers by which to treat hypertension.

THE PATHOGENESIS OF HYPERTENSION

Most, if not all, cardiovascular diseases can be generally thought of as some deviation of the normal homeostatic balance of the circulatory system. As such deviations occur, they trigger a variety of compensatory reactions which are designed to return the system to a normal state of balance. However, if the initial pathology or cause is persistent, compensatory reactions may develop a chronically altered condition. This is the result of the system's attempts to achieve as close an approximation to normal homeostasis as possible considering the presence of the pathologic deviation. It is the persistence of these compensating reactions which develop the clinical portrait of the disease. Within this conceptual framework, we may consider the elevation of blood pressure as a secondary deviation produced in response to some primary alteration in cardiovascular homeostasis. The difficulty in analyzing the disease is resolving what initial alteration is responsible for the observable symptoms, and understanding the subsequent compensatory

Amery, A. (ed.) Hypertensive Cardiovascular Disease: Pathophysiology and Treatment
© *1982, Martinus Nijhoff Publishers. The Hague / Boston / London*
ISBN-13: 978-94-009-7478-4

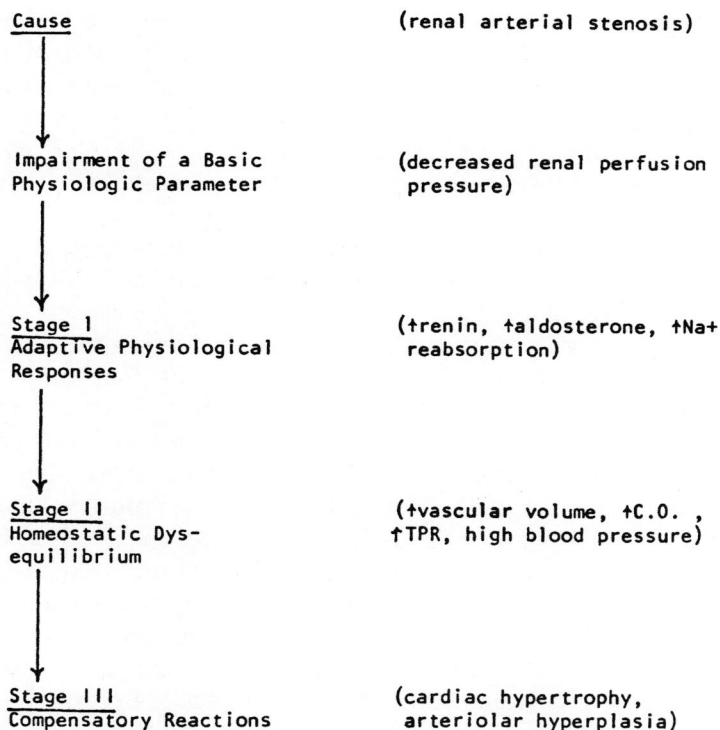

Cause   (renal arterial stenosis)

Impairment of a Basic   (decreased renal perfusion
Physiologic Parameter   pressure)

Stage I   (↑renin, ↑aldosterone, ↑Na+,
Adaptive Physiological   reabsorption)
Responses

Stage II   (↑vascular volume, ↑C.O. ,
Homeostatic Dys-   ↑TPR, high blood pressure)
equilibrium

Stage III   (cardiac hypertrophy,
Compensatory Reactions   arteriolar hyperplasia)

Figure 1. Schematic of the stages in the development of hypertension. Examples from the development of renovascular hypertension are presented to the right in parentheses.

mechanisms which determine the evolution of the disease. It is this understanding which decides the effectiveness of the diagnosis and treatment of hypertension.

Figure 1 is a schematic representation of the development of hypertension. Initially there is some pathology or cause which results in the disturbance or impairment of a physiological parameter. For example, an excessive narrowing of the renal artery (due to fibromuscular dysplasia, atherosclerosis and aneurysm, etc.) results in a decrease of renal perfusion pressure. Because the kidney is no longer confronted by a normal signal from the rest of the circulation, it adjusts for what is interpreted as hypotension. This results in the first stage of the disease, characterized by excessive renin and aldosterone secretion as well as inappropriate retention of sodium. From these inappropriate adaptive responses, a second stage of the disease begins to develop, characterized by abnormal extracellular fluid volume, an increase in cardiac output, and increased peripheral resistance. All of these lead to an increase in blood pressure.

Symptomatically we interpret the high blood pressure as deleterious. However, as a functional adaptation it is an attempt to create within the kidney a normal state of perfusion. As hypertension develops towards a new balance state between pressure and function, the circulatory system attempts to achieve a new homeostasis. Since the original pathology has not been corrected, we may consider this condition a homeostatic disequilibrium (Figure 1).

As the new disequilibrium continues, further morphological reactions must take place in order to protect the system from the newly elevated pressure. Such reactions make up stage 3. Examples of such reactions are cardiac hypertrophy and the arterial hyperplasia seen with sustained hypertension. Although we recognize these medically as deleterious ramifications of the elevated pressure, they are in fact appropriate defense mechanisms.

From the scheme represented in Figure 1 we now see high blood pressure in perspective. It is a secondary event which is a consequence of an alteration in the normal homeostasis. If we are to use an appropriate laboratory test to detect such a disease in the early state, the test must be based on an understanding of what the initiating physiological impairment is. Such a concept has been emphasized in recent experiments directed toward the early detection of hypertension [1]. The same criterion prevails when we consider the efficacy of any therapeutical intervention; the ideal treatment is the reversal of the initiating impairment. In renovascular hypertension, renal arteriogram can indicate a site of arterial stenosis, and surgical repair could correct the defect which caused the disease. However, as in the case of essential hypertension, if the etiology is unknown, then the appropriate treatment is not as obvious. In this case, the most beneficial therapeutic approach is to prevent or minimize the secondary symptoms (such as elevated blood pressure) associated with the disequilibrium state. This approach prevents the development of compensatory reactions (stage 3). However, the initial causative agent still persists, and though the normal progression of the disease has been retarded, a second set of adaptive responses will be initiated. For example, with renovascular hypertension if therapeutic maneuvers decrease renin and aldosterone secretion, or if extracellular fluid volume, cardiac output or resistance are corrected, the occurance of cardiac hypertrophy and vascular hyperplasia will be stopped. However, volume contraction induced by salt restriction or diuretic therapy in some instances of severe renovascular hypertension can further stimulate a vasoconstrictor release, and lead to severe renal insufficiency.

There are two practical concepts which emerge from this discussion of hypertensive disease. Firstly, therapeutic maneuvers which are designed to blunt secondary homeostatic deviations, rather than the direct causative agent, are more effective when they are directed at earlier changes in the sequence of pathogenic events. The sooner the evolution of the disease is arrested, the fewer compensatory reactions will be allowed to occur. Secondly, the variability of physical responses to a given therapy (particularly in essential hypertension) is explained not only by the individual reaction to the drug, but also by the effect such therapy has upon the secondary homeostatic deviations. Essential hypertension may be the consequence of many different causes. Therefore, treatment which is directed only at correcting specific secondary symptoms (i.e., cardiac output, sodium retention) may be more or less effective depending upon the place such a deviation has within the sequence of pathological events.

We have chosen, by convention, renovascular hypertension to illustrate the developmental stages of hypertension because of its known etiology. However, the same scheme outlined in Figure 1 can be applied to other forms of hypertension such as primary aldosteronism, pheochromocytoma or even essential hypertension. Basically, all hypertension can be characterized as a disequilibrium state induced by adaptive physiological responses to some disruptive pathogenic stimulus. Simplistically, this could be elicited by disturbing any of the multiple mechanisms that control blood pressure regulation. However, there are many potent blood pressure control mechanisms, some of which are very transient and act in short duration, while others work in the long term. If a specific pathology is to lead effectively to hypertension, it must primarily alter the long-term controls [2].

Two very potent, but greatly differing, mechanisms which control blood pressure are the sympathetic nervous system and the kidney. Current investigations indicate that, with respect to the regulation of blood pressure, these two mechanisms differ not only in their efficiency to counteract sudden deviations in blood pressure, but also in their effectiveness to sustain such a counteraction during long periods of time. Furthermore, the renal and sympathetic systems do not just operate separately, but each can reciprocally influence the other.

The following sections will discuss the specific roles and the pathophysiologic character of such physiologic mechanisms which act and interact in the evolution of hypertension.

THE ROLE OF NEUROREFLEX MECHANISM AND RENAL MECHANISM IN THE CONTROL OF BLOOD PRESSURE

The arterial baroreceptors, also called the high pressure receptor system, are a specialized network of receptors located in the carotid sinus and in the arch of the aorta. The functional characteristics of this system are illustrated in Figure 2, where the initial arterial pressure reference level is set at 100 mm Hg. A sudden increase in blood pressure to 150 mmHg is followed by activation of arterial baroreceptors, which brings the blood pressure

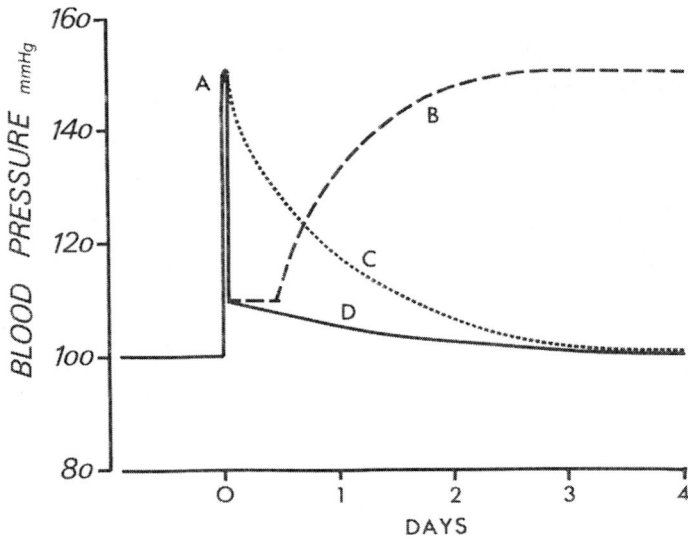

Figure 2. Responses of systemic blood pressure to a 50 mmHg rise in pressure. Curve A represents the pressure rise and the rapid compensation due to baroreceptor reflex. Curve B shows that if the case of the shift is sustained, the baroreceptors adapt allowing pressure to rise again. Curve C depicts the response to the rise in blood pressure due to the action of the kidney. Curve D represents the integrated action of both baroreceptors and the kidney in compensating for the change in blood pressure. (After Guyton et al. [2].)

immediately back down to 110 mm Hg, i.e., only 10 mm above the initial arterial pressure reference level. Thus, the compensatory effect of the baroreceptors is not total but partial. It should be noted here that the same partial compensation occurs if the initial deviation is a decrement rather than an increment of blood pressure.

In Figure 2, curve B illustrates that the counteracting effect of the baroreceptors upon blood pressure deviations does not hold permanently. If the cause of blood pressure change persists, then the baroreceptors adapt, allowing blood pressure to return to its original value. It has been shown by different investigators that baroreceptors reset within 24–48 h [2–6].

Curve C in Figure 2 also depicts what the renal response to a similar increase in blood pressure (up to 150 mm Hg) would be in the absence of the baroreceptors. An increase in renal perfusion pressure of this magnitude will increase exponentially the excretion of sodium (and water) producing a progressive decrease in the extracellular fluid volume and, consequently, in intravascular volume. This action will not cease until blood pressure has reached the initial reference value of 100 mm Hg. This renally mediated compensatory effect upon blood pressure may take anything from three days to three weeks [2]. Such a renal response contrasts with that exerted by baroreceptors in that it completely restores blood pressure to its original value.

Finally, curve D in Figure 2 illustrates the effect of both the compensatory effect of the baroreceptors and the kidney acting simultaneously after blood pressure has been increased from 100 to 150 mm Hg. Such a deviation is primarily counteracted by the baroreceptors, which brings blood pressure to 110 mm Hg. Following this compensation the kidney will continue to reduce blood pressure by decreasing intravascular volume.

From these analyses it becomes apparent that the kidney is the prevailing mechanism in the long-term regulation of blood pressure, whereas the baroreceptors are transient since they are only effective in short-term regulation.

NEURAL INFLUENCE IN THE CONTROL OF VOLUME – THE LOW PRESSURE RECEPTOR SYSTEM

The kidney has the ability to excrete sodium in proportion to renal perfusion pressure [2]. However, doubt has been cast on the validity of this relationship to explain the organism's ability to get rid of an excessive volume load. In fact, it is known that the amount of fluid volume necessary to elevate blood pressure is very large and greatly exceeds the amount which is necessary to increase the urinary excretion of salt and water. Henry and Gauer [7] observed that alterations in atrial pressure could induce significant changes in the secretion of antidiuretic hormones. This observation stimulated a search for some nervous receptor system located in the heart which was capable of detecting minor changes in circulatory volume, and of producing appropriate adaptive renal and vascular responses. These studies have disclosed the existence in the heart and lung of an extensive network of receptors innervated with myelinated and unmyelinated fibers which reach the central nervous system primarily following the pathway of the vagal nerve. Some of these fibers can also reach the central nervous system following the pathway of cardiac sympathetic nerves.

Single-fiber recordings from left atrial receptors with myelinated vagal afferents have shown two different types of neural activity [8]. As is shown in Figure 3, the peak of neural activity was observed in some fibers during the A-wave of atrial pressure, i.e., during systole. A second type of neural activity was recorded in other fibers during the V-wave of the atrial pulse, which is during diastole. Because of these characteristics, the two different kinds of receptors innervated with myelinated fibers are classified as A and B type receptors.

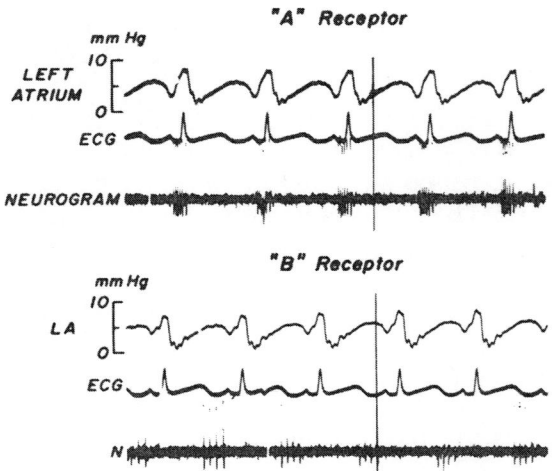

Figure 3. Single fiber recordings of two kinds of atrial receptors; A suring the A-wave of atrial pressure (atrial systole), and B during the V-Wave of atrial pulse (atrial diastole). (After Mancia et al. [8].)

Receptors innervated with unmyelinated vagal fibers are also located in the atria. Under normal conditions these receptors are silent or have a sparse and irregular discharge. However, they can be stimulated mechanically by moderate increments in the left ventricular end diastolic pressure, such as seen during the increase in blood volume after blood transfusion [9].

In summary, there appear to be three different types of receptors in the atria. Two of these are innervated with myelinated fibers, some of which seem to be excited during systole (type A), and others during diastole (type B). The third kind (type C), innervated with unmyelinated fibers, are normally silent and are excited by increases in atrial volume or pressure.

Receptors innervated with myelinated and unmyelinated fibers have also been identified in the ventricles and in the lung [8]. In the ventricle, these receptors produce neural discharges in phase with ventricular systolic pressure and increase the firing rate when ventricular pressures are increased. In the lung, receptors innervated with myelinated and unmyelinated fibers increase neural activity during chemical irritation of the pulmonary airways, during sudden volume changes with lung inflation, or during congestion of the pulmonary circulation. At the present time it is not clear in which manner the central nervous system processes information from cardiopulmonary receptors which are located in the heart or lung. The limited information gathered suggests that collective cardiopulmonary stimulation inhibits adrenergic output from the central nervous system, whereas the opposite occurs when stimulation ceases. Attempts to study the nature of the stimuli and their corresponding reflexes are difficult because the different receptors are spread heterogeneously within the heart and lungs, and because their afferent fibers are not bundled in an independent nerve, but included in the vagus and cardiac sympathetic nerves. Nevertheless, a significant amount of useful information has been accumulated by studying the physiological responses that are obtained by experimental distention of the atria and ventricles. In experimental animals, this is obtained by inflatable balloons which are located within each of the four chambers of the heart. Alternatively, the intracardiac pressure can be altered by different maneuvers such as occlusion of the pulmonary arteries, aorta, pulmonary veins, and jugular veins, or by blood transfusion. In experimental animals, interruption of the nerve traffic from the cardiopulmonary receptors can be obtained by cooling the vagal nerve to 0 °C after the changes in efferent activity of cholinergic fibers have been minimized by a large dose of atropine. In humans, significant changes in the total amount of blood contained in the central circulation (heart and lung) can be obtained by changing body posture from upright to a recumbent position. After assuming a recumbent position, further increments could still be obtained by elevating the lower extremities

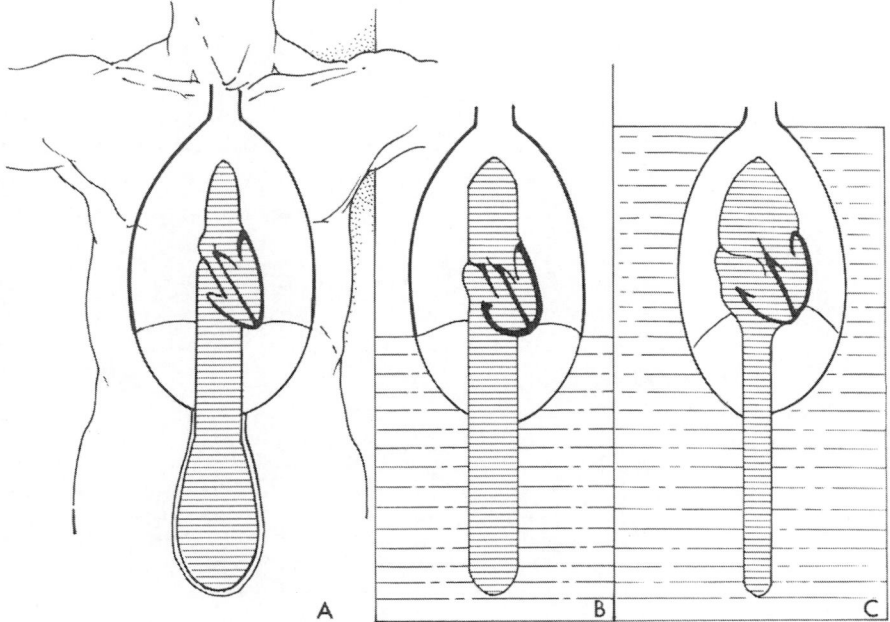

Figure 4. Displacement of blood from the periphery to the chest by immersing the body in water. A progressive shift in blood volume occurs from orthostasis (A) to immersion to the diaphragm (B) and then to the neck (C). The difference in thoracic blood volume has been calculated as 700 ml. (After Gauer and Henry [10].)

140

and the trunk. Furthermore, it has recently been reported that a significant displacement of blood occurs from the periphery to the chest by immersing the body in water [10, 11]. This is due to the compression of the peripheral veins by increased hydrostatic pressure due to a rising water level. The blood was displaced progressively as the body was immersed up to the diaphragm and then up to the neck (Figure 4).

With all these maneuvers it has been found that cardiopulmonary receptors are capable of mediating hemodynamic, humoral and renal responses so as to control the three processes which regulate cardiovascular volume, viz. (a) the excretion of salt and water by the kidney; (b) the distribution of fluids between the interstitial and intravascular compartment; and (c) the secretion of humoral agents which participate in volume control such as antidiuretic hormone and the renin–angiotensin–aldosterone system.

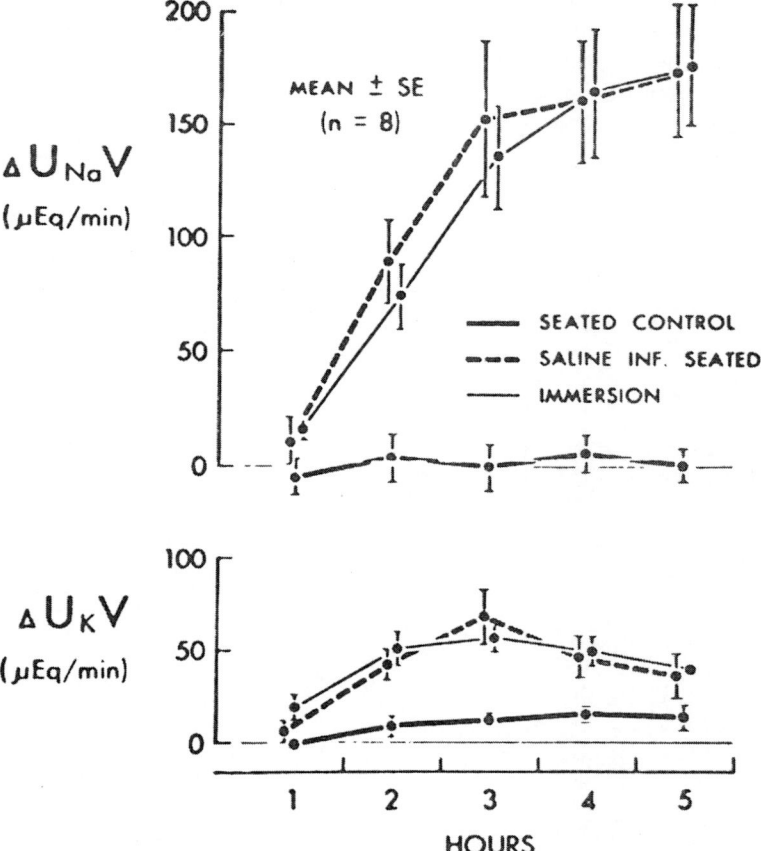

Figure 5. Comparison of the effects in a seated posture of acute saline infusion and immersion upon sodium and potassium excretion.(From Epstein et al. [11].)

(a) *Excretion of salt and water by the kidney*

Epstein et al. [11] studied in humans the effect of whole body immersion on the excretion of sodium and potassium. This was compared with renal excretion of these electrolytes produced by expansion of the extracellular fluid volume with 2 l of saline given over two hours to subjects that were in the same seated position but not immersed in water. Figure 5 shows that the increment in total sodium excretion during immersion was similar to that obtained during saline infusion. Such responses were not observed when the subjects were seated normally (in atmospheric pressure) and did not receive sodium infusion. Interestingly, in such experiments it was also noticed that the kaliuresis during immersion was identical to that obtained during the infusion of saline. No uniform agreement has been obtained on the influence of the low pressor receptor system to alter the renal excretion of sodium and potassium, and other studies have not confirmed the initial observation of Epstein [12, 13].

Evidence has been presented showing that the cardiopulmonary receptors exert a continuous tonic restraint upon the release of renin [14]. Interruption of nerve traffic from the cardiopulmonary receptors to the central nervous system resultes in a 5-fold increase in renin secretion and a concomitant 2.5-fold increase in prostaglandin E-like substance [15]. It has also been shown that the release of renin induced by a non-hypotensive hemorrhage can be suppressed by distension of the cardiopulmonary receptors in the dog or by chemical stimulation of the cardiopulmonary receptors with veratum alkaloids [16].

Recent evidence has shown that cardiopulmonary receptors are involved in the release of renin produced by upright posture or during pooling of blood in lower extremities induced with a pressure cuff [17]. Furthermore, the significant increase in blood volume and the subnormal renin response after cardiac transplantation has been attributed to the lack of afferent vagal input [18].

(b) *Distribution of fluids between the interstitial and intravascular compartment*

The hemodynamic responses which are mediated by the cardiopulmonary receptors consist of vasodilation of vasoconstriction due to withdrawing or enhancing the sympathetic tone, respectively, which has, in turn, been elicited by increments or decrements in the central blood volume.

Figure 6 illustrates the reflex vascular responses mediated by the low pressor receptor system when an increase in intrathoracic blood volume is produced by a change in posture. It can be seen that the elevation of the legs

142

REFLEX VASCULAR RESPONSE TO INCREASE
IN INTRATHORACIC BLOOD VOLUME

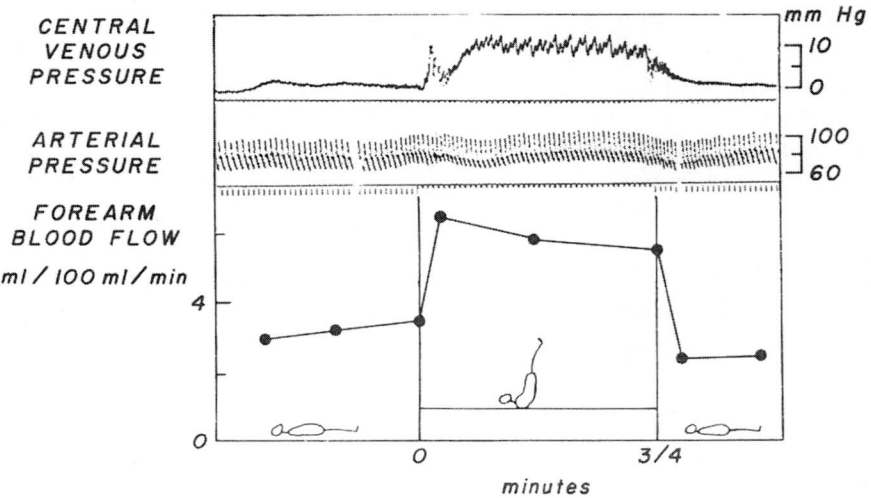

Figure 6. Reflex responses in forearm blood flow during increases in intrathoracic blood volume produced by changes in body posture. (After Roddie et al. [19].)

and trunk produces a significant displacement of blood from the peripheral to the central circulation and is accompanied by a significant increase in central venous pressure. Such a change is followed almost immediately by increases in forearm blood flow with no alteration in systemic arterial pressure. As is shown in this figure, returning the body to recumbent position normalizes the central blood pressure and forearm blood flow to control levels [19]. These observations suggest that the influence of the low pressor receptor system on the resistance of certain vascular compartments does not affect the control of blood pressure, as do the arteriolar receptors, but compensates for changes in central blood volume by facilitating the transfer of fluid from the intravascular to the extravascular compartment or vice versa. This movement of fluids, which occurs during vasoconstriction or vasodilation, can be achieved by changes in the hydrostatic pressure at the capillary level [10]. Therefore, there is a major difference in the 'modus operandi' between high and low pressure receptor system. Changes in sympathetic tone mediated by arterial baroreceptors are generalized to all vascular territories, so that they affect total peripheral resistance and blood pressure. Such responses suggest that baroreceptors primarily modify major deviations in mean systemic pressure. In contrast, changes in the sympathetic tone which are mediated by cardiopulmonary receptors are involved with vascular territories which have little effect upon total peripheral resistance, but are concerned with shifting fluids between vascular compartments. This response maintains the homeostatic equilibrium of the blood volume.

(c) *Secretion of humoral agents which participate in volume control*

The endocrine responses which are affected by the cardiopulmonary receptors involve those hormones which participate in the homeostatic control of fluid volume (i.e., renin, prostaglandins, anti-diuretic hormones). It has already been mentioned that suppression of vagal afferent nerve traffic by cooling to 0 °C is accompanied by significant increase in renal sympathetic tone and the release of both renin and prostaglandins [15].

Evidence suggests that the cardiopulmonary receptors play a major role in controlling the release of antidiuretic hormone (ADH). These actions were first suggested by the experiment of Harry and Gauer [7]. Epstein et al. [20] have found that whole body immersion in water is followed by a 50% decrease in ADH excretion (Figure 7). Share et al. [21] have found that the increments of plasma ADH concentration during slow progressive hemorrhage correlates significantly with a progressive decrease in left atrial pressure rather than with arterial pulse pressure or with systemic arterial pres-

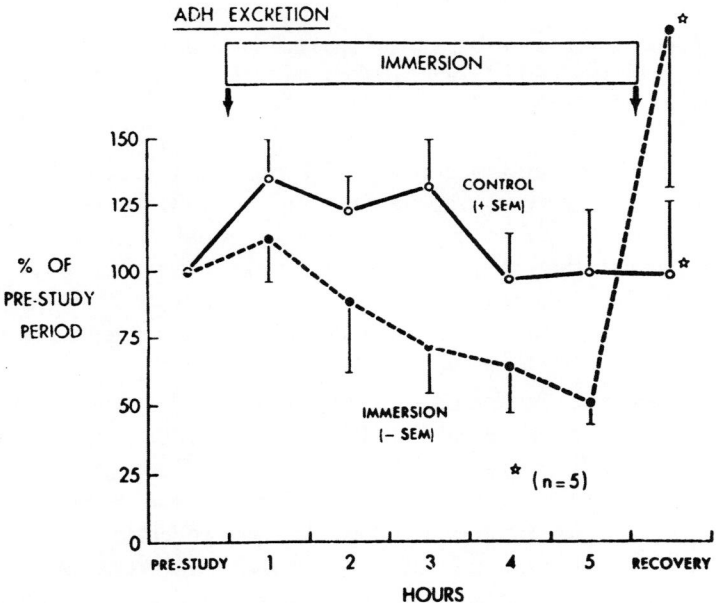

Figure 7. Urinary ADH excretion in dehydrated subjects during 5 h of immersion. (From Epstein et al. [20].)

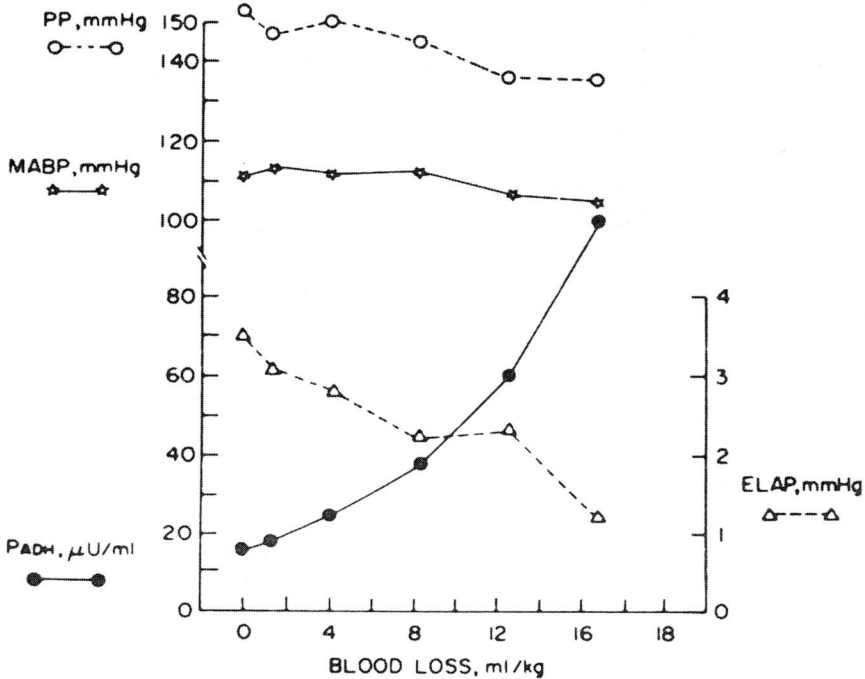

Figure 8. Effect of continuous, slow hemorrhage upon mean arterial blood pressure (MABP), effective left atrial pressure (ELAP), arterial pulse pressure (PP) and plasma ADH concentration (P_{ADH}) in the anesthetized dog. (From Share [21].)

sure (Figure 8). These authors conclude that the cardiopulmonry receptors are located in an ideal anatomical position to detect changes in blood volume before they are reflected in changes in arterial pressure. Gupta et al. [22] have shown that blood volume losses of 10% and 20% (Figure 9) produce a significant decrease in the mean firing rate of atrial receptors, while the firing rate of aortic nerves of the high pressor receptor system is unchanged.

Figure 10 illustrates the anatomical location, afferent pathway and major efferent responses which are mediated by the cardiopulmonary receptors. There is a growing body of evidence which suggest that cardiopulmonary receptors are ideally located to detect changes in volume that occur in the central portion of the circulation before they are reflected in changes of arterial pressure. These changes in neural activity are transmitted to the central nervous system, particularly to the fourth ventricle, by myelinated and nonmyelinated fibers. In the fourth ventricle they may synapse with sympathetic efferents so as to modulate very selectively the renal sympa-

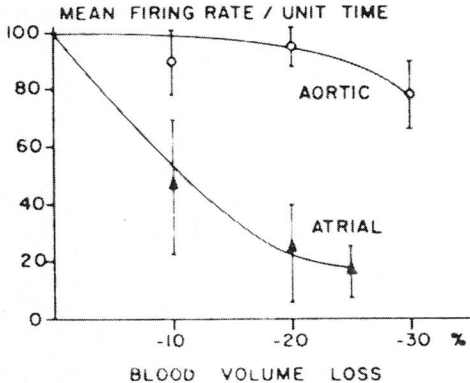

Figure 9. Mean firing rates of aortic and atrial fiber preparations during stepwise reductions in blood volume of 10%, 20% and 30%. (From Gupta et al. [22].)

CARDIOPULMONARY-RENAL REFLEX PATHWAYS

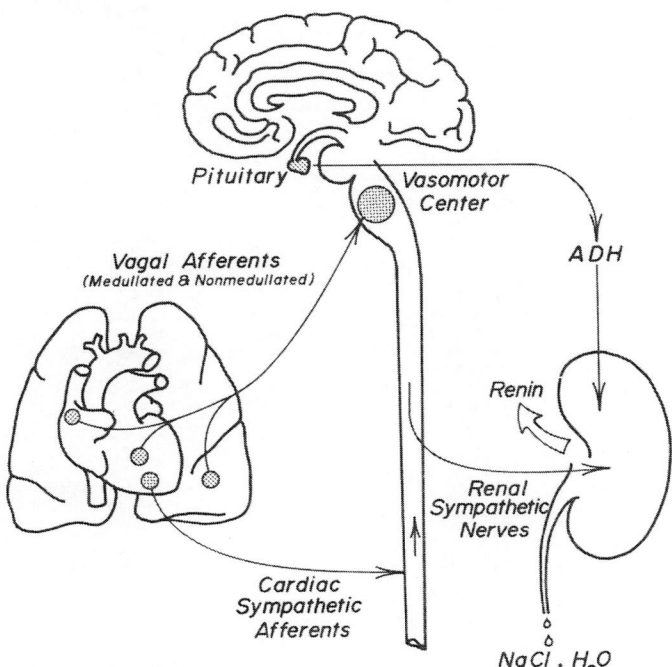

Figure 10. The anatomical location, afferent pathways and the major efferent responses mediated by cardiopulmonary receptors. (From Thames, Fed Proc 37:1978.)

thetic tone and hormonal responses (ADH and renin) which are involved in the control of water and electrolytes.

RENAL INFLUENCE IN THE CONTROL OF CARDIOVASCULAR TONE

Cardiovascular tone is under the strong influence of humoral vasoactive substances which are released from the kidney. The following sections concern these renal hormones.

(a) *The renin–angiotensin system*

The three major mechanisms that control the release of renin have recently been reviewed by Davis and Freeman [23]. They are: (1) the adrenergic system which modulates renin secretion via alpha and beta receptors; (2) renal perfusion pressure which operates by inducing changes in transmural pressure at the level of the glomerular afferent arteriole; and (3) the amount of sodium chloride in the distal nephron delivered to the macula densa.

The release of renin into the circulation results in a cascade of enzymatic reactions that lead to the formation of angiotensin I, angiotensin II and

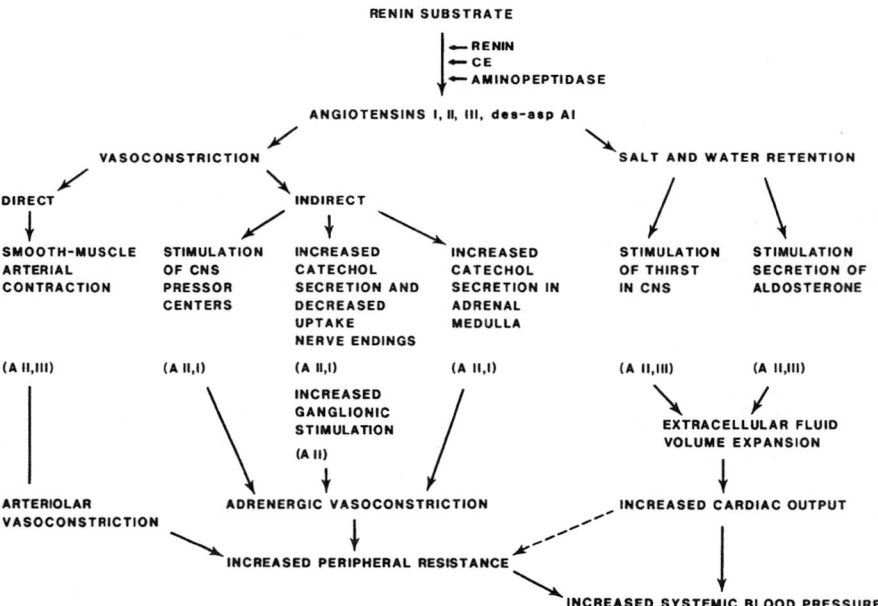

Figure 11. The multiple influences of the renin–angiotensin system in the control of vascular tone and volume. (From Romero and Strong, Pract Cardiol 4:1978.)

other active peptides such as des-Aspertyl angiotensin I (des-Asp-AI) and angiotensin III (des-Asp-AIII). The converting enzyme which forms angiotensin II from angiotensin I and also angiotensin III from des-Asp-AI is also responsible for the metabolism of bradykinin. Therefore, it should be noted that inhibitors of converting enzyme not only diminish pressor activity by blocking the formation of angiotensin II and III, but also enhance the vasodilator property of the kinin system.

Figure 11 summarizes the cascade of events which can be affected by the renin–angiotensin system. Angiotensin can directly increase vascular resistance by its vasoconstrictor properties. Angiotensin II is about 40 times more potent a vasoconstrictor than norepinephrine and 8–10 times more potent than angiotensin III. Angiotensin can also produce vasoconstriction indirectly either by increasing adrenergic tone via the central nervous system at the level of the area postrema (where angiotensin I and II are effective), or by increasing the release of norepinephrine or by decreasing the re-uptake of norepinephrine at the adrenergic nerve terminals. Both angiotensin I and II release catecholamines from the adrenal medulla.

The renin–angiotensin system has a dual role in stimulating a positive balance of sodium chloride and water (Figure 11). Angiotensin stimulates the secretion of aldosterone which induces renal sodium and water conservation, and angiotensin stimulates thirst by acting directly on the central nervous system.

The vasoconstrictor action of the renin–angiotensin system may be the major mechanism in acute development of severe renovascular hypertension, whereas the volume-enhancing component of the renin–angiotensin system may account for the more chronic forms of renovascular and essential hypertension. Some investigators have suggested that such a volume expansion can increase cardiac output and this could trigger an increase in peripheral resistance in an attempt to regulate flow (Figure 11). Either increased cardiac output or increased peripheral resistance will lead to increased blood pressure [24]. For further reference, a comprehensive review of all the biological actions of the renin–angiotensin system has been published by M. Peach [25].

(b) *The prostaglandin system*

Prostaglandins are synthesized (Figure 12) from a major precursor, arachidonic acid, which is released from phospholipids by the action of the enzyme phospholipase A-2. Arachidonic acid is a 20-carbon fatty acid with four double bonds. By the action of fatty acid–cyclo-oxygenase, the arachidonic acid is converted into endoperoxides G_2 and H_2 which exhibit an extremely short half-life (less than 30 s). Subsequently, a peroxidase reduces

148

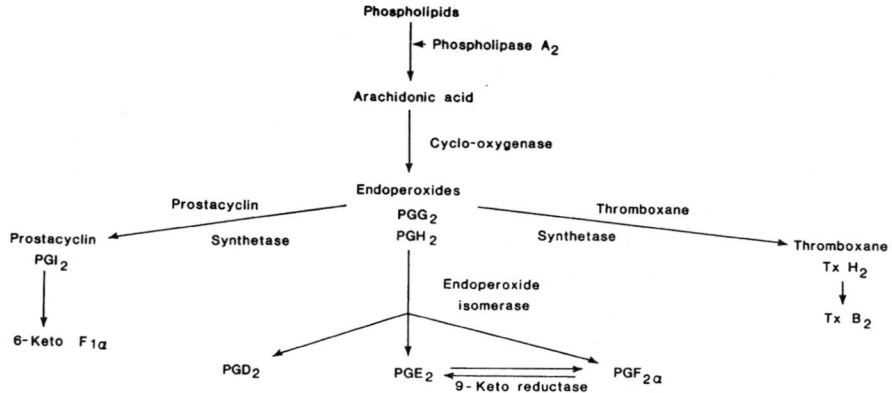

Figure 12. The synthetic pathways of prostaglandins. (After Romero and Strong, Pract Cardiol 4:1978.)

these endoperoxides to either PGF_{2a}, D_2 or E_2. Two other important compounds can also be derived from the endoperoxides prostacyclin (PGI_2) and thromboxane A_2 (TxA_2). Most of the stimuli that trigger the synthesis of prostaglandins, such as decreased renal perfusion pressure, nerve stimulation, angiotensin, norepinephrine, bradykinin and vasopressin, act by stimulating phospholipase A_2. No known stimulus of prostaglandin synthesis acts by stimulating cyclo-oxygenase.

The various prostaglandins have different pharmacological actions. Administration of PGI_2 or PGE_2 into the renal artery is followed by pronounced renal vasodilation, increased renal blood flow and natriuresis, whereas the administration of endoperoxides PGG_2, PGH_2 or thromboxane is followed by renal vasoconstriction and decrease in urine flow.

Administration of arachidonic acid into the renal artery triggers the overall synthesis of renal prostaglandins. This results in a net increase in renal blood flow, urine flow and natriuresis comparable to that elicited by the administration of PGE_2 and PGI_2 given by the same route. This suggests that the vasodilating actions of PGE_2 and PGI_2 overrides the vasoconstrictor effect of the intermediate endoperoxides or thromboxane.

Renal prostaglandins are not stored in the kidney. The release is a reflection of the rate of synthesis. Vane [26] has shown that a number of anti-inflammatory drugs such as indomethacin, meclofenamate, phenylbutazone and aspirin inhibit cyclo-oxygenase activity, thus blocking the formation of all intermediate products and primary prostaglandins. Use of these anti-inflammatory compounds allows assessment of changes in intrarenal function which may be attributed to the lack of prostaglandin synthesis.

The primary prostaglandins PGI_2, PGE_2, PGD_2 and PGF_{2a} have extremely short half-lives in the circulation, probably less than 1 min. They are rapidly converted to 15-keto-13, 14-dehydro metabolites by prostaglandin dehydrogenase. These metabolites have a half-life of about 8 min. Metabolism in the lung probably accounts for the short half-life of primary prostaglandins. This suggests that prostaglandins probably act as local regulators rather than as hormones transported in the circulation to act at the distant target organs. The levels of endogenous primary prostaglandins measured in peripheral circulation may not reflect total endogenous production of prostaglandins in the body. The more accurate index of the increase of the rate of prostaglandin synthesis may be found in the quantitation of the 15-keto-13,14-dehydro metabolites in the serum or the urine.

(c) *Interrelationships between the renin–angiotensin system and the prostaglandin system*

The interrelationships between the renin–angiotensin system and the prostaglandin system are illustrated in Figure 13. A decrease in renal perfusion pressure produced experimentally is followed by an increase in the release of renin and prostaglandins. Blocking the synthesis of prostaglandins decreases the release of renin [27], suggesting that renin release is also influenced by prostaglandins. Recent studies have shown that renin release is stimulated by PGE_2 and PGI_2 and the endoperoxides. In contrast, $PGF_{2\alpha}$ seems to exert an inhibitory action on renin secretion [28]. It has been reported that a high

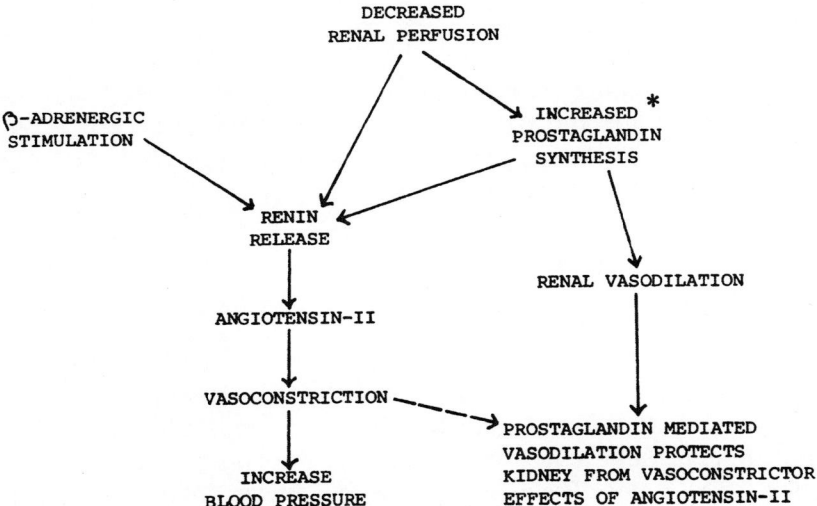

Figure 13. Interactions between the prostaglandin and the renin–angiotensin systems in the control of circulatory homeostasis.
* Abnormal hypersecretion of prostaglandins in Bartter's syndrome; low renin hypertension characterized by abnormally low levels of prostaglandins.

150

sodium diet activates PGE_2-9-keto-reductase (Figure 12), shifting the synthesis of $PGF_{2\alpha}$, whereas the decrease in renin secretion may have been secondary to the reduction of the ratio of PGE_2 to $PGF_{2\alpha}$ [29]. The opposite may occur during low sodium diet. Thus, a low sodium diet stimulates PGE_2 formation and consequently renin secretion, offering another mechanism in the regulation of renin secretion.

The release of renin seems to be under the control of β-adrenergic receptors. Recent in vitro studies [30] of the interrelationship between β-receptor activation and prostaglandin synthesis upon the release of renin suggest that their influence upon renin release is exerted through different and independent metabolic pathways. Hopefully this will lead to an understanding of the conditions under which physiological circumstances dictate whether neural mechanisms or PG mechanisms exert the predominant influence over renin release.

Since renin release depends, at least in part, on the stimulation of prostaglandin synthesis, such a relationship allows the kidney to influence systemic pressure by increasing total peripheral resistance with angiotensin without affecting resistance (Figure 13). The kidney will be protected by the vasodilator action of renal prostaglandins. Aldosterone may also inhibit prostaglandin synthesis and thereby indirectly have a negative-feedback effect upon the release of renin. The importance of the prostaglandins in controlling renal circulatory homeostasis, sodium balance and renin release is supported by the observation that increased prostaglandin synthesis could account for the hypersecretion of sodium, hyperreninemia and hyperaldosteronism characteristic of the Bartter's syndrome. Hypothetically, a deficiency of prostaglandin synthesis could increase renal resistance, produce a subtle decrease in sodium excretion, and suppress plasma renin activity, all of these being features of 'low-renin essential hypertension' [31]. A short review on the role of renal prostaglandins in different forms of hypertension has recently been published [32].

SUMMARY

A systematic analysis of hypertensive disease reveals three basic developmental stages. Understanding these is important in assessing the diagnosis and prognosis, and in determining the efficacy of therapeutic interventions. Initially, some pathologic factor produces a disturbance or impairment of a physiologic parameter. The first stage of the disease involves the body's adaptation to try to compensate for the disturbance. This stage could exist with no apparent clinical manifestations.

If the initial pathology remains, the adaptive response will continue towards a new homeostasis based on the presence of this perturbation. This is the second stage in the evolution of the hypertensive syndrome and it is characterized by the appearance of clinical manifestations.

Finally, a third stage is characterized by the production of undesirable pathological reactions induced by the persistence of the homeostatic disequilibrium. The two most conspicuous complications which can be seen during this stage are arteriolar hyperplasia, leading to a decrease in organ blood perfusion, and cardiac hypertrophy, which subsequently develops into cardiac insufficiency.

There are essentially three basic means by which blood pressure is controlled. These include the high and the low pressure receptor systems, and the kidney. They control resistance through arteriolar tone, and control of cardiac output via the circulating blood. The high and low pressure receptors act through the nervous system. High pressure receptors act primarily in short-term regulation of blood pressure, while the low pressure receptors may act in either short-term or long-term regulation. High pressure receptor systems exert a direct and powerful control of arteriolar tone, but have little influence upon the circulating volume. In contrast, the low pressure receptor systems do not appear to control arteriolar tone but do exert an influence upon the circulation volume.

The kidney plays a major role in long-term blood pressure regulation which is achieved by influencing both arteriolar tone and the circulating volume by means of the renin–angiotensin–aldosterone system and the influence of renal perfusion pressure. As we further understand the role each of these control systems play, we shall be able to develop more effective therapeutical tools to correct early homeostatic deviations as well as to pinpoint the pathology responsible for initiating the pathogenesis of such an important disease as hypertension.

REFERENCES

1. Report of the Hypertension Task Force. National Institutes of Health; Heart, Blood and Lung Institute. Volume 1: General Summary and Recommendations, p. 1628. NIH Publication No. 79, 1979.
2. Guyton AC, Coleman TG, Cowley AW Jr, Manning RD Jr, Norman RA Jr, Ferguson JD: A systems analysis approach to understanding long-range arterial blood pressure control and hypertension. Circ Res 35:159, 1974.
3. Cowley A: Personal communication.
4. McCubbin JW, Green JH, Page IH: Baroreceptor function in chronic renal hypertension. Circ Res 4:205, 1956.
5. Kezdi P, Wennemark J: Baroreceptor and sympathetic activity in experimental renal hypertension. Circulation 17:785, 1958.
6. Krieger EM: Time course of baroreceptor resetting in acute hypertension. Am J Physiol 218:486, 1970.
7. Henry JP, Gauer OH, Reeves JL: Evidence of the atrial location of receptors influencing urine flow. Circ Res 4:85, 1956.

8. Mancia G, Lorenz RR, Shepherd JT: reflex control of circulation by heart and lungs. In: International Review of Physiology, Cardiovascular, Physiology – II, Vol. 9, p. 111. Guyton AC, Cowley AW, eds. Baltimore: University Park Press, 1976.

9. Thorén PN: Characteristic of left ventrivular receptors with non-medullated vagal afferents in cats. Circ Res 40:415, 1977.

10. Gauer OH, Henry JP: Neurohormonal control of plasma volume. In: Cardiovascular Physiology – II, Vol. 9, pp. 145-190. Guyton AC, Cowley AV, eds. Baltimore: University Park Press, 1976.

11. Epstein M, Pins DS, Arrington R, Denunzio AG, Engstrom R: Comparison of water immersion and saline infusion as a means of inducing volume expansion in man. J Appl Physiol 39:66, 1975.

12. Behne HJ, Gauer OH, Kirsch K, Eckert P: Effects of sustained intrathoracic vascular distention on body fluid distribution and renal excretion in man. Pfluegers Arch 313:123, 1969.

13. Gilmore JP, Zucker IM: Failure of left atrial distention to alter renal function in the nonhuman primate. Circ Res 42:267, 1978.

14. Mancia G, Romero JC, Shepherd JT: Continuous inhibition of renin release in dags by vagally innervated receptors in the cardiopulmonary region. Circ Res 36:529, 1975.

15. Mancia G, Romero JC, Strong CG: Neural influences on canine renal prostaglandin secretion. Acta Physiol Lat Am 24:555, 1974.

16. Thames MD: Reflex suppression of renin release by ventricular receptors with vagal afferents. Am J Physiol 233:H181, 1978.

17. Kiowski W, Julius S: Renin response to stimulation of cardiopulmonary mechanoreceptors in man. J Clin Invest 62:656, 1978.

18. Thames MD, Zubair-ul-Hassan, Brackett NC, Lower RR, Kontos HA: Plasma renin responses to hemorrhage after cardiac autotransplantation. Am J Physiol 221:1115, 1971.

19. Roddie C, Shepherd JT, Whelan RF: Reflex changes in vasoconstrictor tone in human skeletal muscle in response to stimulation of receptors in a low-pressure area of the intrathoracic vascular bed. J Physiol 139:369, 1957.

20. Epstein M, Pins DS, Miller M: Suppression of ADH during water immersion in normal man. J Appl Physiol 38:1038, 1975.

21. Share L: The role of cardiovascular receptors in the control of ADH release. Cardiology 61 (Suppl 1):51, 1976.

22. Gupta PD, Henry JP, Sinclair R, von Baumgarten R: Responses of atrial and aortic baroreceptors to nonhypotensive hemorrhage and to transfusion. Am J Physiol 211:1429, 1966.

23. Davis JO, Freeman RH: Mechanisms regulating renin release. Physiol Rev 56:1, 1976.

24. Guyton AC, Cowley AW Jr, Coleman TG, Liard JF, McCaa RE, Manning RD Jr, Norman RA Jr, Young DB: Pretubular versus tubular mechanisms of renal hypertension. In: Mechanisms of Hypertension, pp. 15-29. Sambhi MP, ed. Amsterdam: Excerpta Medica, 1973.

25. Peach MJ: Renin–angiotensin system: biochemistry and mechanisms of action. Physiol Rev 57:313, 1977.

26. Vane JR: Inhibition of prostaglandin synthesis as a mechanism of action for aspirin-like drugs. Nature 231:232, 1971.

27. Romero JC, Dunlap CL, Strong CG: The effect of indomethacin and other anti-inflammatory drugs on the renin–angiotensin system. J Clin Invest 58:282, 1976.

28. Weber PC, Larson C, Anggard E, Hamberg M, Corey EJ, Nicolau KC, Samuelsson B: Stimulation of renin release from rabbit renal cortex by arachidonic acid and prostaglandin endoperoxides. Circ Res 39:868, 1976.

29. Weber PC, Larson C, Scherer B: Prostaglandin E_2-9-keto-reductase as a mediator of salt intake-related prostaglandin–renin interaction. Nature 266:65, 1977.

30. Beierwaltes WH, Schryver S, Olson PS, Romero JC: Interaction of the prostaglandin and renin–angiotensin systems in isolated rat glomeruli. Am J Physiol (in press).
31. Romero JC, Strong CG: Hypertension and the interrelated renal circulatory effects of prostaglandins and the renin–angiotensin system. Mayo Clin Proc 52:462, 1977.
32. Romero JC, Beierwaltes WH: Renal prostaglandins in hypertension. Mineral Water Metab (in press).

III. PATHOGENESIS OF PRIMARY HYPERTENSION

10. ROLE OF CHANGES IN Na^+ TRANSPORT IN CELL MEMBRANES IN THE PATHOGENESIS OF PRIMARY HYPERTENSION

PHILIPPE MEYER

Experimental epidemiological and clinical studies show clearly that there exists a close relationship between primary hypertension and body sodium (Na^+). The fact that the first investigators were oriented towards extracellular Na^+ is not surprising when we consider the high concentration of this ion in the extracellular fluid volume, compared to the intracellular medium, as well the undisputable role of this body fluid compartment in the maintenance of arterial pressure. However, numerous studies have been unable to demonstrate any clear-cut increase in the extracellular fluid volume in essential hypertension, a result that would be expected if an increase in extracellular Na^+ were involved [1].

INTRACELLULAR SODIUM

The possibility that an increase in intracellular Na^+ may be responsible for hypertension was raised by the following two observations. The first was the demonstration by Tobian of an increase in the Na^+ concentration of arterial walls in animals with experimentally induced hypertension (by an excess of Na^+, or of renal origin) [2]. Subsequent studies have specified that the Na^+ accumulates not only in the contractile muscle cells, but also in the interstitial space of the arterial walls, thus complicating the interpretation [3].

The second argument was the demonstration that an increase in the intracellular Na^+ concentration, which results from an inhibition of the Na^+-K^+ ATPase, has a contractor effect: the suppression of extracellular K^+, or the administration of a cardiac glycoside, causes in vitro the contraction of isolated strips of arterial tissue, and in vivo an increase in arterial pressure [4, 5].

The significance of these observations appeared plainly when an Na^+-Ca^{2+} transmembrane-coupled transport was discovered in several excitable tissues (contractile and nervous tissues) of both invertebrates and vertebrates. This transport mechanism is such that the penetration of Na^+ into the cells, which is a downhill movement following the concentration gradient, causes the extrusion of calcium [6].

Amery, A. (ed.) Hypertensive Cardiovascular Disease: Pathophysiology and Treatment
© 1982, Martinus Nijhoff Publishers. The Hague / Boston / London
ISBN-13: 978-94-009-7478-4

Thus, if the intracellular concentration of sodium is increased, then the intracellular penetration of the Na^+ would be reduced, resulting in a reduction of the Ca^{2+} efflux.

According to the kinetic analysis, the stoichiometry of the Ca^{2+}-Na^+ exchange is such that three Na^+ ions entering the cell cause the extrusion of one Ca^{2+} ion. An increase in the intracellular concentration of Ca^{2+} ions has a contractile effect, for it is the Ca^{2+} which triggers off the shortening of the contractile proteins by inducing a sliding of actin molecules onto myosin molecules.

The smooth muscle cells of the arteries are in a permanent state of constriction, a basal tonic state, which implies that the concentration of cytosolic Ca^{2+} is superior to 10^{-7} M. This means that any increase in intracellular Ca^{2+}, such as that secondary to an intracellular sodium increase, will cause a supplementary contraction.

Blaustein, who was the first to underline the interest of the Ca^{2+}-Na^+ coupled transport, calculated that an intracellular Na^+ increase of 0.5 mM causes an increase in Ca^{2+} concentration of 1.5×10^{-7} M to 1.7×10^{-7} M. This small increase appears sufficient to cause an augmentation in the tonus of arterial muscles of up to 50 % [6].

Myocardial contraction also results from an increase in Ca^{2+} concentration, and an Na^+–Ca^{2+}-coupled transport has also been shown to operate at the plasma membrane level in cardiac cells [7].

Thus, we are given to think that primary hypertension, which is hemodynamicly characterized by an increase in peripheral arterial resistance (permanent hypertension), or by an increase in cardiac output (labile hypertension), could be triggered off by an increase in intracellular Na^+. This event in turn affects the intracellular Ca^{2+} concentration which ultimately commands the mechanical activity of contractile cells.

In addition to these events taking place in the contractile tissue, it is possible that comparable phenomena appear in certain neuronal systems. Ouabain, a well-known Na^+-K^+ APTase inhibitor, increases, both in vivo and in vitro, the activity of the catecholaminergic neurones, and also enhances the constrictor effect of noradrenaline, which itself, if produced in excess, can contribute to an increase in peripheral resistance. One of the best illustrations of catecholaminergic hyperactivity triggered off by Na^+, is the increase in the plasma concentration of noradrenaline, occuring in the rat after a long and significant Na^+ load [8].

INTRACELLULAR SODIUM AND HYPERTENSION

Numerous observations support the hypothesis of an intracellular Na^+ increase both in human primary hypertension and in the spontaneous hypertension of the rat. In the course of human hypertension, an increase in the intracellular Na^+ concentration has been clearly demonstrated in those blood cells that are easily accessible: erythrocytes [9, 10], leucocytes [11] and lymphocytes [12]. This increase is nevertheless inconsistent and is only detected in approximately half the subjects.

An increase in the intracellular Na^+ concentration has also been established in the arteries of spontaneously hypertensive rats (S.H.R.) after several weeks of hypertension [13]. Lastly, an acute or chronic Na^+ load, which aggravates the hypertension of S.H.R. [14], increases the intraerythrocyte concentration of Na^+; such a phenomenon does not occur in normotensive rats [15].

The Na^+ transmembrane exchanges put into play a number of mechanisms. Against the passive downhill forces which allow the penetration of Na^+ into the cells, there are numerous opposing active systems, which force back the Na^+ into the extracellular medium (Figure 1).

Compiling the many observations made on genetically hypertensive rats and primary hypertensive humans, cell membrane abnormalities, which can increase the Na^+ intracellular concentration, appear to be constantly present.

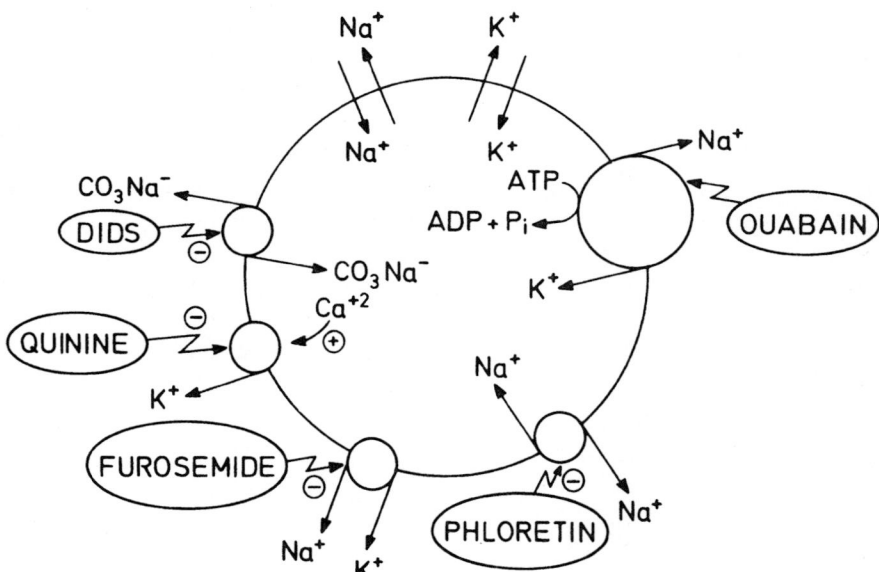

Figure 1. Schematic representation of transmembrane Na^+ fluxes in human erythrocyte. In circles, the names of transport inhibitors. (With kind permission of Garay RP.)

1. Spontaneously hypertensive rats

Recent work performed on the aorta and muscular arteries of S.H.R.s have shown that K^+, Cl^- and Na^+ exchange between the intra- and extracellular compartment is accelerated compared to control normotensive rats [16, 17]. This result, recalling an increase in the passive membrane permeability ('leak'), can perhaps be attributed to a destabilization of the membrane by a reduction of the Ca^{2+}-binding to membrane anionic sites. Further studies to characterize the membrane abnormalities in S.H.R. have been caried out on erythrocytes, which, in contrast to arteriolar cells, are easily accessible.

An increase in passive permeability has been found in erythrocytes using lithium as a marker [18, 19]. It has already been demonstrated that Ca^{2+} fixation to erythrocyte membranes is reduced in the S.H.R. compared with Wistar/Kyoto reference rats [20-22].

It is not possible as yet to establish a relationship between these diverse disturbances and the clear-cut reduction in active Na^+ extrusion, shown recently by De Mendonca et al. [23] in both young S.H.R. (four weeks) and adult S.H.R.

The red blood corpuscles of genetically hypertensive rats (S.H.R., Sabra and Sabra H) present, in all cases, a major abnormality in their tolerance to a Na^+ load. After an intense, chronic dosage of this ion, their intracellular Na^+ concentration is increased, in contrast to that observed in normotensive control rats (like Sabra N - resistant to Na^+), where the intracellular concentration of Na^+ remains strictly normal under identical conditions.

There have been many studies furthering the research into erythrocyte membrane abnormalities. Among the most recent are studies on Ca^{2+} flux abnormalities (increase in passive permeability and reduction of active extrusion) [24], the metabolism of phosphoinositides [25], the Na^+ binding at the internal face of plasma membrane [26], microviscosity and membrane fluidity studied by nuclear electromagnetic resonance [27], and measurement of polarized fluorescence [28]. Lastly, several arguments seem to favor the diffusion of such membrane abnormalities to numerous tissues.

In this way, a diminution of Na^+ extrusion from the leucocytes [11] has been observed, as has a reduction of Ca^{2+} membrane fixation associated with an emission alteration of fluorophore in the plasma membranes of cardiac and hepatic cells, as well as in synaptosomes [29].

Finally, changes of intracellular Ca^{2+} distribution have also been observed in adipocytes [30].

HUMAN HYPERTENSION

Several erythrocyte abnormalities have been found in primary human hypertension. The first is an increase in the flux rate of Na^+ entering and leaving the erythrocyte]21, 34], which suggests an increase in passive membrane permeability. However, this finding has not been confirmed in subsequent studies [33]. Secondly, it is possible that the membrane fixation of Ca^{2+} is reduced, as in the hypertensive rat [22], but this phenomenon seems inconsistent [20]. With the use of lithium, it has also be demonstrated that the Na^+-Na^+ countertransport is increased in essential hypertensive parents [30]. Finally, Garay et al. have shown by measurement of net Na^+ and K^+ fluxes that a major deficiency of essential hypertensives is a deficit in the Na^+-K^+ cotransport, which also appears in 50-57% of hypertensive offspring. The Na^+-K^+ cotransport appears to be markedly low in some black subjects prone to develop hypertension (Garay RP and Meyer P: unpublished data). In secondary hypertension, the Na^+-K^+ cotransport is normal [31-33].

It is not possible at the present time to understand the relationship between the increase in the Na^+-Na^+ countertransport and the decrease in the Na^+-K^+ cotransport.

The mechanism which plays the most important role in the active extrusion of Na^+ is not the Na^+-K^+ cotransport, but the Na^+-K^+ ATPase (sodium pump). A decrease in the activity of the sodium pump was therefore investigated first. Such a decrease was observed by some investigators [35, 36] but was not confirmed by others [32, 37, 38]. In fact, an increase in the Na^+-K^+ ATPase has been reported in the course of moderate and labile hypertension [32] and interpreted as a phenomenon compensating the deficit of the Na^+-K^+ cotransport

The functional activity of the Na^+-K^+ ATPase is so important that 'a priori' one can be doubtful about results suggesting a reduced activity. The enormous intracellular Na^+ retention which would result would cause acute and severe manifestations, very different from the chronic symptomatology of primary hypertension.

Besides erythrocytes, three other cell types have been studied: leucocytes, in which a diminution in Na^+ extrusion has been established [11], blood platelets, which present an abnormality of polarized fluorescence emitted by a fluorophore [28], and adipocytes, where intracellular Ca^{2+} distribution is abnormal [30].

A NEW PATHOGENIC HYPOTHESIS

Thus, in both genetic hypertension of the rat and primary hypertension in man, physiochemical and functional membrane abnormalities exist in several tissues. These abnormalities have certain characteristics which lead us to believe that they may have a determinant role in the mechanism of hypertension.

1) The abnormalities compare well in both rat and man, and appear to be genetically determined and transmitted in direct association with hypertension.

2) These membrane abnormalities appear to be present in several tissues of the organism.

3) The most striking consequence of these abnormalities on a functional basis is an increase in the intracellular Na^+ concentration, which is more marked in man than in animals. The intraerythrocyte Na^+ concentration is increased in more than half of hypertensive subjects. The intraleucocyte Na^+ concentration appears to increase equally. In the genetically hypertensive rat, the intraerythrocyte Na^+ concentration is normal in basal conditions but increases during an Na^+ load. These characteristics give us an idea of the pathogenesis of primary hypertension.

As we have seen, an increase in the intracellular Na^+ concentration in excitable tissues provides a satisfactory explanation for hypertension. This leads us to suggest that the membrane abnormalities originally described in the blood cells (due to their accessibility) are also present in the excitable tissues. One argument, albeit indirect, allows us to think that this may be the case. This argument is based on the demonstration, in plasma membranes of synaptosomes and of cardiac cells, of certain fundamental abnormalities (reduction in Ca^{2+} fixation and biophysical abnormalities of the membrane) previously found in erythrocytes [28, 29]. Hypertension could thus be an illness caused by a genetically transmitted primitive alteration of cell membranes, leading to a possible enrichment of the cells in Na^+. This in turn may result in an enrichment in Ca^{2+} through the Na^+–Ca^{2+} exchange mechanism.

This theory raises several questions. The first is to understand to what extent a dietary sodium excess is harmful. The second is to explain why the membrane abnormalities are expressed functionally only in excitable tissues.

Each dietary Na^+ load tends to increase the transmembrane sodium gradient, which results in a transitory increase in intracellular Na^+ increase. This is rapidly opposed, however, by the active membrane mechanisms assuring the extrusion of Na^+ from the cell.

A deficit in Na^+–K^+ cotransport, such as that which exists in primary human hypertension, could thus cause a temporary intracellular accumulation of Na^+, until Na^+–K^+ ATPase become hyperactive. Such a compensatory phenomenon appears to exist in the moderate hypertension of young subjects where the intracellular enrichment in Na^+ and, consequently, in Ca^{2+} is moderate and transitory, thus explaining the lability of the disease in its early stages. However, Na^+–K^+ ATPase activity appears to return to normal during sustained hypertension, but the reason for this subsequent fall in activity is unknown. It follows that the deficit in Na^+–K^+ cotransport can be plainly expressed and can lead to a chronic increase in the intracellular Na^+ concentration. Because of this, a certain amount of cell water retention takes place, such as has been clearly observed in vascular walls [40, 41] and which forms part of the structural modifications of arteries, contributing to the increase in peripheral resistance [42]. Also, this increase in intracellular Na^+ leads to a permanent increase in intracellular Ca^{2+}, a source of permanent hypercontraction in arteries.

Little is known about the cell topography and functional characteristics of the Na^+–K^+ cotransport which appears to exist in renal tubules. However, one may conceive that a reduction in the activity of this Na^+–K^+ cotransport at the level of the kidney could be involved in the development of primary hypertension and could explain the discrete and ephemeral increase in extracellular Na^+ which comes about at the beginning of the disease.

A further problem concerns an explanation of how a membrane alteration, which affects all cells of an organism, is only expressed in excitable cells. Why, for instance, do hepatic cells, which present membrane abnormalities (reduction of Ca^{2+} fixation) and in which Na^+ concentration is probably increased, not have any particular functional alteration? The simplest explanation is that the functional equipment of excitable and non-excitable cells is different, and that the activity of the latter is not modified by an increase in Na^+ concentration. The research into membrane abnormalities in hypertension thus emerges as an interesting problem of cellular differentiation.

CONCLUSION

Primary hypertension is paradigmatic of polyfactorial diseases stemming from both innate and acquired factors. Dietary sodium is certainly an exogenous factor, but there does seem to exist an individual 'suspectibility' to Na^+ which is genetically transmitted, as shown by Dahl [43], which could be the innate factor of the disease.

The membrane abnormality which enriches cells in Na^+ appears to be genetically transmitted in both animals and man. It is transmitted as a monogenic (or oligogenic) and autosomic factor closely associated with hypertension. If we take into account all its consequences, this membrane abnormality could thus be the innate factor of primary hypertension.

Research carried out in humans has shown these abnormalities to be biochemical markers of hypertension. This could form the basis of a selective prevention of the disease. In reducing the harmful factors of the environment (especially sodium excess) as much as possible in the subjects who show erythrocyte abnormalities, but who are still normotensive, one may indeed hope to diminish the chances of the development of hypertension.

One may expect that similar practical methods can be adopted in the treatment of other polyfactorial diseases which also depend on both innate and acquired factors.

REFERENCES

1. Schalekamp A, Beevers DG, Kolsres G, Lebel M, Froser R, Birkenhäger WH: Body fluid volume in low renin hypertension 2:310–314, 1974.
2. Tobian L, Binion JT: Tissue cations and water in arterial hypertension. Circulation 5:754, 1952.
3. Villamil MF, Matloff J: Changes in vascular ionic content and distribution across aortic coarctation in the dog. Am J Physiol 228:1087–1093, 1975.
4. Leonard E: Alteration of contractile responses of artery strips by a potassium-free solution, cardiac glycosides and changes in stimulus frequency. Am J Physiol 189:185–190, 1957.
5. Mason DT, Braunwald E: Studies on digitalis – Effects of ouabain on forearm vascular resistance and venous tone in normal subjects and in patients in heart failure. J clin Invest 43:532–543, 1964.
6. Blaustein MP: Sodium ions, calcium ions, blood pressure regulation and hypertension: a reassessment and a hypothesis. Am J Physiol 232:c165–c173, 1977.
7. Horackova M, Vassort G: Na–Ca exchange in regulation of cardiac contractility. J Gen Physiol 73:403–424, 1979.
8. Franco-Morselli R, Bauddouin-Legros M, De Mendonca M et al.: Plasma catecholamines in essential human hypertension and in DOCA-salt hypertension of the rat. In: Circulating Catecholamines and Blood Pressure, pp. 27–38. Birkenhäger WH, Falk HE, eds. Utrecht: Bunge, 1978.
9. Gesser von U: Intra- und extrazellulare Electrolyte Veränderungen bei essentieller Hypertonie vor und nach Behandlung. Z Kreislaufforsch 51:177–183, 1962.
10. Losse M, Wehmeyer H, Wessels F et al.: Electrolytgehalt von Erythrocyten bei arterieller Hypertonie. Klin Wochenschr 38:393–395, 1960.
11. Edmondson RPS, Thomas RD, Hilton PJ, Patrick J, Jones NF: Abnormal leucocyte composition and sodium transport in essential hypertension. Lancet 1:1%%:–1005, 1975.
12. Ambrosioni E, Tartagnis F, Montebugnoli L, Costa FV, Magnani B: Intralymphocytic sodium in hypertensive patients. In: Intracellular Electrocytes and hypertension, pp. 78–86. Zumkley H, Losse H, eds. Stuttgart: Georg Thieme, 1980.
13. Nagaoka A, Kinuchi K, Aramaki Y: Participation of tissue electrolytes and water to spontaneous hypertension in rats. Jap Circ Res 34:489, 1980.
14. Dietz R, Harbara M, Schönig H: The role of the kidney in the pathogenesis of spontaneous hypertension of rats. Jap Heart J 20 (suppl 1):52–54, 1979.
15. De Mendonca P, Garay RP, Ben-Ishai D, Meyer P: Abnormal erythrocyte cation transport in primary hypertension: clinical and experimental studies. Hypertension 3: 179, 1981.
16. Jones AW: Altered ion transport in vascular smooth muscle from spontaneously hypertensive rats. Influences of aldosterone, norepinephrine and angiotensin. Circ Res 33:563–572, 1973.
17. Friedman SM: Evidence for enhanced sodium transport in the tail artery of the spontaneously hypertensive rat. Hypertension 1:572–582, 1979.
18. Ben-Ishay D, Aviram A, Viskoper R: Increased erythrocyte sodium efflux in genetic hypertensive rats of the Hebrew University strain. Experientia 31:660–662, 1975.
19. Friedman SM, Nakashima M, McIndoe RA et al.: Increased erythrocyte permeability to Li and Na in the spontaneously hypertensive rat. Experientia 32:476–478, 1976.

20. Gulak PV, Boroskina GM, Postnov YV: Ca^{2+} binding to erythrocyte membrane of hypertensive men and rats: effects of acetylcholine and eserine. Experientia 35:1471–1472, 1979.

21. Postnov YV, Orlov SN, Shevchenko A et al.: Altered sodium permeability, calcium binding and NA^{+} K^{+} ATPase activity in the red cell membrane in essential hypertension. Pfluegers Arch 371:263–269, 1977.

22. Postnov YV, Orlov SN, Poludin N: Decrease of calcium binding in the red blood cell membrane in spontaneously hypertensive rats and in essential hypertension. Pfluegers Arch 379:181–195, 1979.

23. De Mendonca M, Grichois ML, Garay RP et al.: Abnormal net Na^{+} and K^{+} fluxes in erythrocytes of three varieties of genetically hypertensive rats. Proc Nat Acad Sci USA 77:4283–4286, 1980.

24. Devynck MA, Pernollet MG, Nunez AM, Meyer P: Analysis of calcium handling in erythrocyte membranes of genetically hypertensive rats. Hypertension 3: 397, 1981.

25. Boriskina GN, Gulak PV, Postnov YV: Phosphoinositide content in the erythrocyte membrane of rats with spontaneous and renal hypertension. Experientia 34:744, 1978.

26. Urry DW, Trapane DL, Andrews SK, Long MM, Overbeck HW, Oparie S: NMR observation of altered sodium interaction with human erythrocyte membranes of essential hypertensives. Biochem Biophys Res Comm 96:514–521, 1980.

27. Daveloose D, Viret J, Molle D, Grenier F: Mise en évidence par marquage de spin d'une modification structurale de la membrane erythrocytaire du rat génétiquement hypertendu. C R Acad Sci [D] (Paris 290:85, 1980.

28. Montenay-Garestier T, Aragon I, Devynck MA, Meyer P, Helene C: Structural modifications of erythrocyte membranes in spontaneously hypertensive rats. A fluorescence polarization study. Biochem Biophys Res Comm, 100: 660, 1981.

29. Devynck MA, Pernollet MG, Nunez AM, Aragon I, Montenay–Garestier T, Hélène C, Meyer P: Biophysical and biochemical demonstration of a diffuse alteration of plasma membrane in SHR's. In: Rats with Spontaneous Hypertension and Related Studies, Ganten D, ed. Stuttgart: Schattauer Verlag (in press).

30. Postnov YV, Orlov SN: Evidence of altered calcium accumulation and calcium binding by the membranes of adipocytes in the membranes of spontaneously hypertensive rats. Pfluegers Arch 385:85–89, 1980.

31. Canessa M, Adragna N, Solomon HS, Connolly TM, Tosteson DC: Increased sodium–lithium countertransport in red cells of patients with essential hypertension. Engl J Med 302:772–777, 1980.

32. Garay RP, Meyer P: A new test showing abnormal net Na^{+} and K^{+} fluxes in erythrocytes of essential hypertensive patients. Lancet 1:349–353, 1979.

33. Garay RP, Dagher G, Pernollet MG, Devynck MA, Meyer P: Inherited defect in a Na^{+} K^{+} co-transport system in erythrocytes from essential hypertensive patients. Nature 284:281–283, 1980.

34. Garay RP, Elghozi JL, Dagher G, Meyer P: Laboratory distinction between essential and secondary hypertension by measurement of erythrocyte cation fluxes. N Engl J Med 302:769–711, 1980.

35. Wessels VF, Junoe-Hulsing G, Hosse H: Untersuchungen zur Natrium Permeabilität der Erythrozyten bei Hypertonikern und Normotonikern mit familiarer Hochdruckbelastung. Kreislaufforsch 56:374–380, 1967.

36. De Wardener HE, McGregor G: The possible role of a circulating sodium transport inhibitor in the aetiology of essential hypertension. In: Intracellular Electrolytes and Hypertension. Zumkley H, Losse H, eds. Stuttgart: Georg Thieme, 1980.

37. Walter U, Distler A: Effects of ouabain and furosemide on ATPase activity and sodium transport in erythrocytes of normotensives and of patients with essential hypertension. In:

163

Intracellular Electrolytes and Hypertension, pp. 170–181. Zumkley H, Losse H, eds. Stuttgart: Georg Thieme, 1980.

38. Erdmann E, Werdan K, Hegelberger R, Prudiniewski M, St Christe: Determination of the number of $Na^+ K^+$-ATPase molecules, their enzymatic activity and the active $Na^+ K^+$ transport of human erythrocytes in kypokaliemia and in hypertension. In: Intracellular electrolytes and hypertension, pp. 164–169. Zumkley H, Losse H, eds. Stuttgart: Georg Thieme, 1980.

39. Wambach G, Helber A, Bönner G, Hummerich W, Kaufmann W: Na^+ and K^+ concentration in erythrocytes and $Na^+ K^+$-ATPase activity in red cell ghosts in controls and patients with essential hypertension. In: Intracellular electrolytes and hypertension, pp. 158–163. Zumkley H, Losse H, eds. Stuttgart: Georg Thieme, 1980.

40. Webb RC, Bhalla RC: Altered calcium sequestration by subcellular factions of vascular smooth muscle from spontaneously hypertension rats – J. Mol Cell Cardiol 8:651–661, 1976.

41. Friedman SM, Friedman CL: The ionic matrix of vasoconstriction. Circ Res 20–21 (suppl 2):147–155, 1967.

42. Rorive GL, Van Cauwenberg H: Ionic composition of arterial wall in experimental hypertension. Clin Sci Mol Med 45:305s, 1973.

43. Folkow B: The haemodynamic consequences of adaptive changes of the resistance vessels in hypertension. Clin Sci 41:1–12, 1971.

44. Dahl LK, Heine M, Tassinari L: Role of genetic factors in susceptibility to experimental hypertension due to chronic excess salt ingestion. Nature 194:480, 1962.

11. PATHOPHYSIOLOGY OF PRIMARY HYPERTENSION: ROLE OF ADRENOCEPTORS IN THE TRANSFORMATION FROM AN EARLY HIGH CARDIAC OUTPUT INTO A LATER HIGH ARTERIOLAR RESISTANCE PHASE

FRITZ R. BÜHLER

INTRODUCTION

High blood pressure ranks as the main risk factor in cardiovascular disease, which nowadays accounts for almost half the mortality figures. If the pathogenetic mechanisms of essential hypertension and its pathophysiological interrelationships were better understood, it would be easier to take more specific preventive or therapeutic measures.

The likelihood of hypertension developing is closely related to three main factors: psychosocial environmental influences; high dietary intake of salt; possibly, too, hereditary predisposition. The initial and later development of hypertension involves extremely varied mechanisms of circulatory regulation and sodium/volume homoeostasis, which have been accused singly or jointly of being the causes of essential hypertension. Accordingly, various factors and regulatory systems have been discussed:

1) central and peripheral functions of the autonomic nervous system
2) baroreflex influences
3) cardiac output and peripheral arteriolar resistance
4) kidneys and sodium/volume homeostasis
5) renin–angiotensin–aldosterone regulation.

All these systems are interlinked. Moreover, it is difficult to classify them by order of importance, since almost all factors which raise blood pressure are themselves affected by the increased pressure, so that their role in the hypertensive process is masked. However, because of the key role played by the autonomic nervous system in both circulatory regulation and sodium/volume homeostasis, this system might be chiefly responsible for the occurrence of hypertension. Our own clinical research has followed these lines over the last few years. Two aspects in particular will be discussed in this article:

1) The increased activity of the autonomic nervous system is a striking feature, especially in the developmental phase of essential hyperten-

Amery, A. (ed.) Hypertensive Cardiovascular Disease: Pathophysiology and Treatment
© *1982, Martinus Nijhoff Publishers. The Hague / Boston / London*
ISBN-13: 978-94-009-7478-4

sion, but also in the maintenance phase. Other hypertensive mechanisms are subordinated to this adrenergic control function.

2) A new research hypothesis has been drawn up, postulating that a hyperadrenergic, hyperdynamic developmental phase is transformed into a maintenance phase in which adrenergic tone is maintained and in which structural alterations of the arteriolar wall also play a role.

We shall not cover all aspects within the framework of this chapter but shall refer instead to findings which lend weight to this pathophysiological concept.

EPIDEMIOLOGICAL CLUES TO PATHOGENESIS OF HYPERTENSION

Psychosocial environmental influences

The striking frequency of occurrence of hypertension found in industrialised countries has drawn attention to environmental influences affecting blood pressure and to the way in which environmental situations are dealt with mentally. This can be summed up under the term 'psychosocial stress', as defined by Seley's concept of stress [1]. The importance of the environment was already recognised 50 years ago, since hypertension did not then exist, for example, in non-industrialised African tribes in Kenya [2]. Hypertension was increasingly found as certain tribes became urbanised [3]. Moreover, stress over a long period of time – at work [4], in time of war [5], or during natural catastrophes [6] – is linked with high blood pressure. Less surprisingly, in students sitting an examination, an increase in blood pressure can also be found in many cases attaining hypertensive values [7]. Support for the significance of environmental influences has chiefly come from experiments with animals in which communal life engendering conflicts has been related to the development of high blood pressure [8, 9]. These data, based primarily on correlations, do not constitute definite proof that stress can cause hypertension. There have also been contradictory observations [10] and, so far, only a few basic experimental approaches have emerged from the field of ethology [11]. On the other hand, it is almost impossible to separate psychosocial environmental factors from another ubiquitous factor – salt intake in food – since the spread of civilisation goes hand in hand with an increase in salt consumption [10].

Salt

Numerous epidemiological surveys have proven the correlation between salt intake and the height of blood pressure [10, 12]. Hypertension is almost never to be found in primitive tribes who eat a minimal amount of salt [13]. The prevalence of abnormally high blood pressure values only attains a few per cent if salt intake is less than 3 g/day. When salt intake is higher – between 5 and 15 g/day – the prevalence of hypertension rises to 15–20% of the adult population. In Switzerland, for example, where salt consumption averages 10 g/day [14], up to 19% of the population have a diastolic pressure ≥95 mm Hg [15]. Where there is excessive salt intake, e.g. the 25 g/day that can be seen in the north-east of Japan, the prevalence of hypertension rises to 30–40% of the population [16]. Conversely, a fall in blood pressure can be achieved on a low-salt diet, as was earlier achieved on the Kempner rice diet [17, 18]. However, it seems that a drastic reduction in salt intake, down to 1 g/day, would be necessary in order to achieve a marked fall in pressure but, under present-day circumstances, this is hardly feasible [19, 20].

Age

Any discussion of the pathophysiology of hypertension must pay special attention to the influence of age. For example, age is linked to the salt factor. Blood pressure hardly rises with age in people on a low-salt diet [21], whereas on a high-salt diet, which is considered to be 'normal' in our country, blood pressure rises with age not only in hypertensive patients [7, 12, 23], but also in the population as a whole [22]. The influence of age on various hypertensive factors is of major importance and will be discussed below.

Heredity

In man, the significance of hereditary factors with respect to hypertension has not been clearly proven, in spite of the experimental genetic models of hypertension. A rise in blood pressure with age does seem to run in families, and hypertension certainly does [7, 24]. However, this could be favoured or even caused by the same environmental factors being at work within one family. The force of this objection has been undermined by observations carried out on twins, in whom a simultaneous, similar development of severe hypertension has been recorded, despite completely different environments [25]. The observations by Zinner et al. [26] weigh heavily in the balance here, since they found higher pressure readings in children less than 2 years of age who had hypertensive parents. Finally, Biron et al. [27] found no correlation in blood pressure between adopted children of the same age, sex and ethnic group and their stepparents, which limits the significance of the family environment.

Most recently, a hereditary factor has gained new support by the observation that a defect in membrane (erythrocytes) sodium co-transport resulting in increased cellular sodium (and calcium) may be a marker or even causative factor in essential hypertension [28]. This new theory, however, deserves more clarification before it can be regarded as a hereditary defect which might also be present in arteriolar smooth muscle cells.

NEUROGENIC FACTORS IN ESSENTIAL HYPERTENSION

Autonomic nervous system and cardiovascular regulatory mechanisms

The main gates involved in the autonomic control of circulatory regulation are located in the vasomotor centre and the reticular formation in the

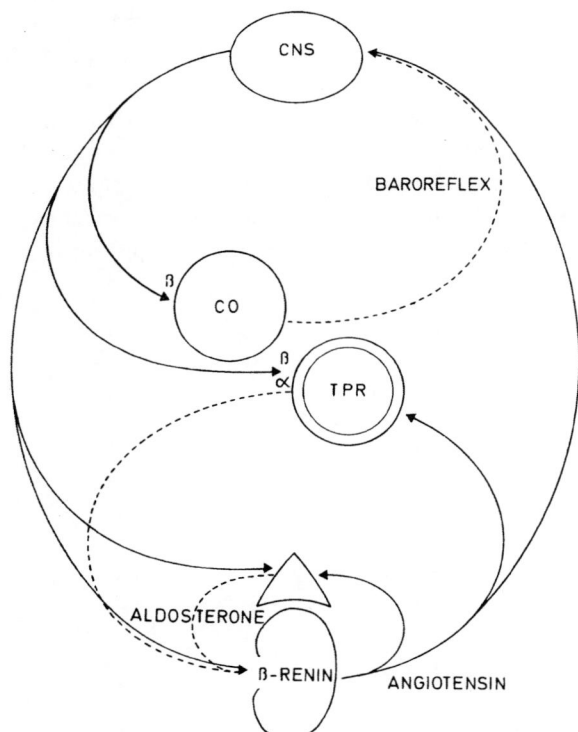

ADRENERGIC AND ANGIOTENSINERGIC CARDIOVASCULAR REGULATION

Figure 1. Adrenergic and angiotensinergic regulation of the circulation. key role of alpha (α) and beta (β) adrenoceptors. CNS = central nervous system. CO = Cardiac output. TPR = total peripheral resistance.

medulla oblongata. This centre is modulated by higher integratory centres located in the hypothalamus and limbic system and by cortical influences. Non-central nervous system influences are provided by afferents of the baroreceptors of the vessels in the vicinity of the heart on the one hand and by angiotensin stimulation of the area postrema and its link with the vaso-motor centre on the other [29].

The integration of all these influences by the vasomotor centre results in a continual adaptation of the mechanisms regulating the circulation, under the control of the autonomic nervous system: efferent parasympathetic fibres inhibit the heart rate; efferent sympathetic fibres activate both the cardiovascular system via postganglionic neurones (the peripheral arterioles being richly innervated by the sympathetic [30]) and the secretion of cate-cholamines by the adrenal medulla via preganglionic neurones [31] (Figure 1).

Noradrenaline lies ready in the storage vesicles of the nerve endings. It is generally formed from dopamine by the action of intravesicular dopamine beta-hydroxylase (DBH). Noradrenaline is converted into adrenaline in the adrenal medulla by phenylethaneamine-N-methyl-transferase. The trans-mitters are released by exocytosis and activate specific receptors. Specific adrenoceptors [32] are responsible for the transformation of the stimulus at the target organ. These adrenoceptors are stimulated by the noradrenaline released by the sympathetic nerve endings or by the circulating adrenaline secreted by the adrenals. Noradrenaline is partly re-uptaken directly by the nerve endings (uptake 1) or diffused in the surrounding tissue (uptake 2). About 10–20% of the noradrenaline released reaches the bloodstream.

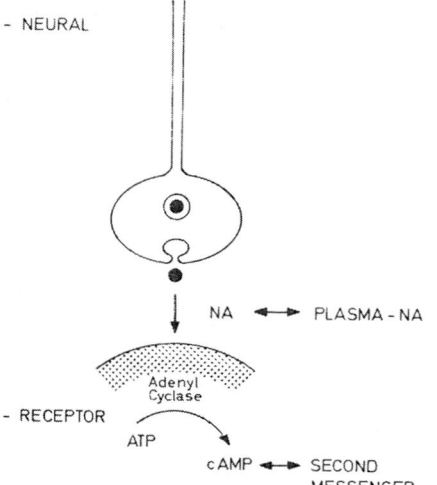

Figure 2. Possibilities for measuring sympa-thetic activity in clinical research: nerve ac-tivity, noradrenaline released and spilled over in plasma, adrenergic receptors and their effects on cyclase system.

Problems in measuring sympathetic activity

The measurement of sympathetic activity in man involves considerable problems of methodology and interpretation. The complexity of the system alone obliges us to take a critical look at the individual variables, if they are not correlated with other functions. An indication of the activity and reactivity of adrenergic functions can be obtained by measuring (Figure 2):

1) the electric potential of adrenergic neurones
2) catecholamines and their metabolites in urine
3) tissue catecholamines
4) plasma dopamine beta-hydroxylase
5) plasma catecholamines
6) reactions to pharmacological interventions
7) the function of the adrenoceptors.

Direct derivation of the potential of adrenergic neurones is difficult in man, since only the skin and muscle nerves are accessible. Nevertheless, Wallin et al. [33] recently reported the first direct proof of increased adrenergic nervous activity in hypertensive patients, based on derivation of the potential of the sural nerve. Determination of catecholamines in the vas deferens, removed on vasectomy, showed slightly elevated values in hypertensive patients, the vas deferens having a rich sympathetic innervation [34]. The long era of measurement of catecholamines and their metabolites in urine has yielded contradictory results. The amount of transmitter excreted only represents a fraction of total turnover. Moreover, noradrenaline is reabsorbed [35] and excreted by the kidneys, depending on renal function [36] and urine volume [37]. However, standardised test procedures have shown increased excretion of noradrenaline, adrenaline, vanillyl mandelic acid or normetanephrine in about 25% of hypertensive patients [36, 37]. Increased urine values [38] are found in a high percentage of younger patients or those with labile forms of hypertension [39]; these patients present a greater rise in catecholamine levels under mental stress [40]. Studies with radioactively labelled neurotransmitter precursors such as DOPA have also shown increased synthesis, release and excretion of noradrenaline in patients with elevated catecholamine values [41]. Great hopes were placed in the determination of plasma dopamine beta-hydroxylase (DBH), since DBH is released by the nerve endings at the same time as noradrenaline [42], diffuses almost entirely in the circulation [43] and moreover would be suitable for use as an adrenergic marker because of its long plasma half-life [44]. However, considerable interindividual, genetically determined variability limits the significance of DBH measurement [45]. It should be noted that there may be an age-dependent increase in plasma concentrations of DBH [46], as well as a relationship between DHB and plasma noradrenaline concentration and between DBH and resting diastolic pressure [47].

Measurement of plasma catecholamines

Plasma catecholamines appear to mirror the activity of the sympathetic nervous system [48, 49]. Newer, sensitive radioenzymatic methods have enabled us to determine catecholamines in a very small amount of plasma, and have made it possible to repeat these measurements as often as we desire [50, 51]. The arrangements for measuring plasma catecholamines are of decisive importance in assessing the results. As far as possible, therefore, the time and the patient's posture at the moment of taking the sample should be standardised, as should emotional environmental factors. Despite these factors of uncertainty, results have been obtained in the last few years which point to the dominant role of the adrenergic nervous system in the genesis of hypertension.

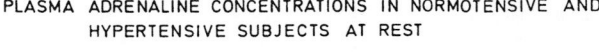

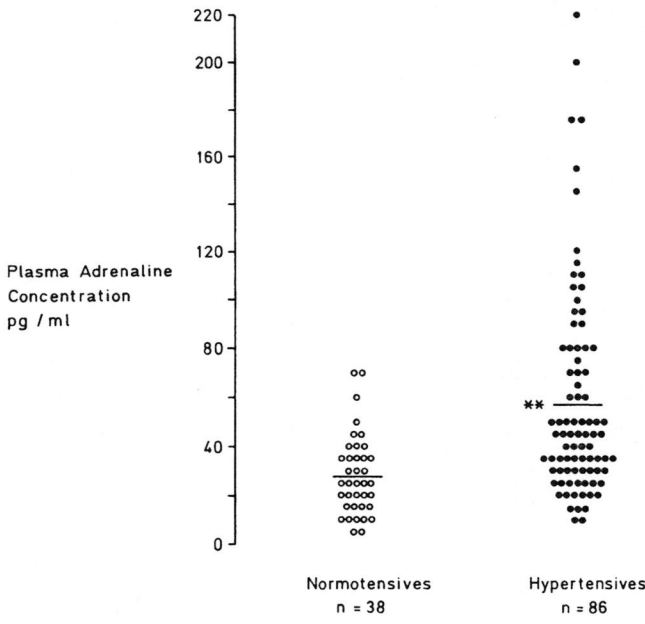

** p < 0.01

Figure 3. Plasmaadrenaline concentrations obtained in the resting recumbent position in normotensive (open circles) and hypertensive individuals (closed circles).

Under standardised conditions, at rest, plasma noradrenaline and adrenaline concentrations are generally slightly elevated in hypertensive patients [52–60]. As shown in Figure 3, about a third of hypertensive patients show elevated adrenaline values. The considerable overlap with the values in normotensive people has been differently described [52, 61]. This is especially true of the plasma noradrenaline concentration, which is elevated in around 30% of cases [53, 55–60]. However, when age is taken into consideration [39, 57, 60, 61], these supranormal values are chiefly to be found in younger patients (Figure 4). The age-dependent increase in noradrenaline observed in normotensive people is disturbed by these values. These results point to increased sympathetic tone, at least in the developmental phase of hypertension. Moreover, the observations show that noradrenaline release from sympathetic nerve endings tends to increase with age, i.e., the slightly increased sympathetic tone in hypertensive patients tends to be maintained rather than fall with age.

Plasma catecholamines and beta-adrenoceptor-mediated functions

Since the significance of single determinations of plasma catecholamines proved rather unconvincing, the next step was to look for relationships with

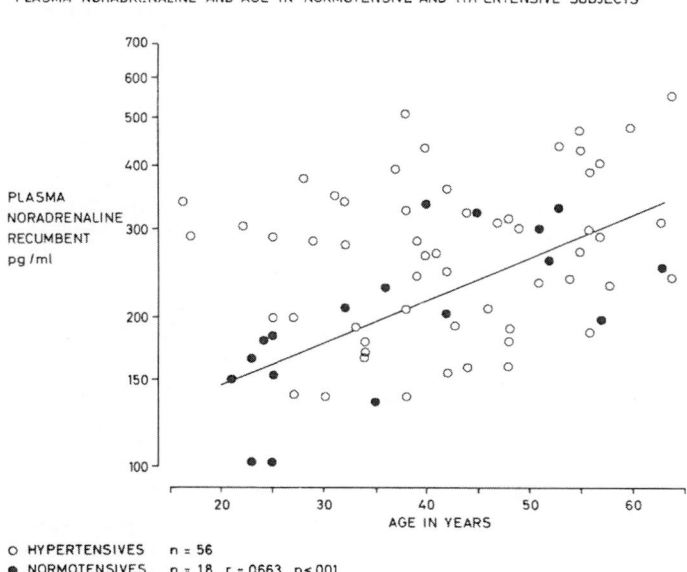

Figure 4. Plasma noradrenaline and age in normotensive and hypertensive subjects.

sympathetically controlled functions which were known to be activated by physical [62] and mental [63] stimulation. De Champlain has described a group of hyperadrenergic patients with elevated noradrenaline levels, together with a shortened systolic time interval and increased heart rate when standing upright. This syndrome also fits hyperdynamic hypertension described by Fröhlich [64]. On the other hand, Esler et al. have linked elevated plasma noradrenaline concentrations to increased renin activity [65].

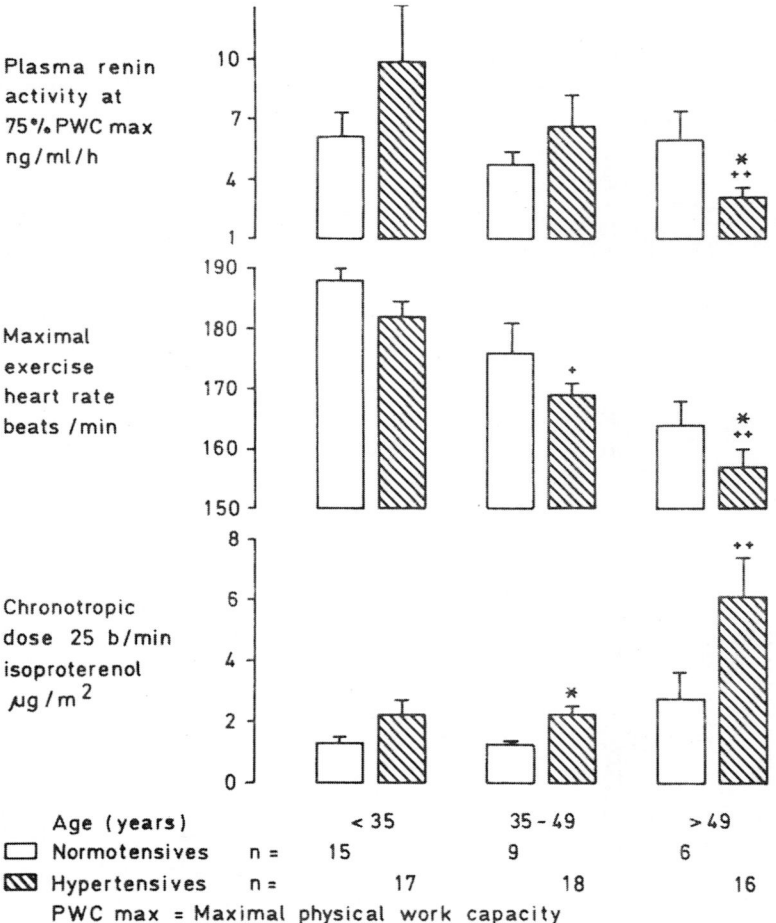

Figure 5. Exercise-stimulated renin and heart rate responses decrease with older age, which tallies with the decreasing isoproterenol sensitivity. These age–related changes are enhanced in the older hypertinsive patients.

Since the sympathetic nervous system is gradually stimulated, while the parasympathetic nervous system is inhibited, as physical effort increases [62] and since this stimulation is paralleled by an increase in plasma catecholamines [48], we studied the sympathetic reaction by means of a dynamic method allowing interindividual comparisons to be made. Plasma noradrenaline and adrenaline concentrations, beta-adrenoceptor mediated increase in heart rate and renin, together with blood pressure, were measured in hypertensive patients before and during, stepped exercises on an ergometer [58].

In the same study, the chronotropic dose of isoproterenol required to cause an increase in heart rate of 25 beats/min was determined (in a dose-response relationship) in order to test beta-adrenoceptor responsiveness pharmacologically [66]. The results of this test packet showed marked age-dependent differences and relationships between the variables. In individual cases, plasma catecholamines, heart rate, renin and blood pressure rose simultaneously. Hypertensive patients taken as a group showed a greater increase in noradrenaline and adrenaline, which became more marked with age. Conversely, the responsiveness of heart rate and renin fell with age (Figure 5).

Despite the somewhat more elevated plasma noradrenaline–adrenaline concentrations found with age and with higher blood pressure, the beta-adrenoceptor mediated response to stimuli was lower. This physiologically reduced beta-receptor sensitivity could also be confirmed pharmacologically. With age and increasing blood pressure, heart rate shows less response to isoproterenol [58] (Figure 5). Conversely, blood pressure is maintained. Blood pressure rises with age and increasing plasma noradrenaline levels. Since the increase in blood pressure on exercise is chiefly due to alpha-adrenoceptor–mediated vasoconstriction, this finding points to impairment of the balance between beta- and alpha-mediated phenomena.

This point of view has been supported by our recent findings, which have shown reduced peripheral vasodilation in response to isoproterenol in older patients (Figure 6) and patients with high diastolic blood pressure [60].

The predominance of beta-adrenoceptor-mediated adrenergic functions in the developmental phase, replaced later by alpha-adrenoceptor-mediated vasoconstriction, constitutes the keystone of our research hypothesis on the pathophysiology of essential hypertension, which is discussed below. A series of other observations fit this concept. Physiologically, the height of maximal exercise tachycardia falls with age [67]. Frohlich [64] found isoproterenol sensitivity to be elevated in a subgroup of labile, borderline-hypertensive patients and, in line with our own results, London et al. [68] found it to be lowered in older patients with higher blood pressure. In both normal [69] and hypertensive [70] people the response to beta blockade falls with age. Moreover, production of the second messenger cAMP is reduced in older

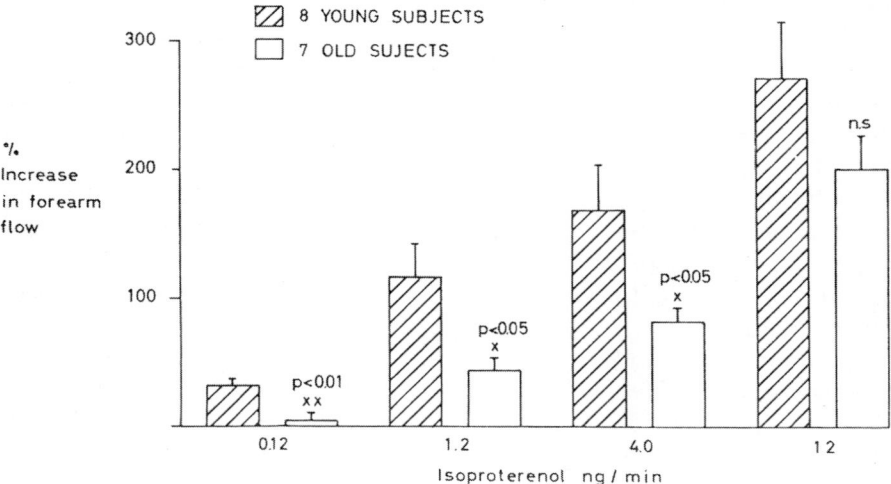

INCREASE IN FOREARM BLOOD FLOW WITH INTRA-ARTERIAL ISOPROTERENOL INFUSION
IN 8 YOUNG AND 7 OLD NORMOTENSIVE SUBJECTS

Figure 6. Greater isoprenalin-induced forearm blood flow response in 8 young as compared with 7 elderly normotensive subjects.

hypertensive patients, which is thought to reflect reduced activation of beta-adrenoceptors [71]. Certain studies show that beta-receptors may possibly change in the same way throughout the organism. These experiments showed that radioactively labelled beta blockers bind less to circulating mononuclear leucocytes in old age ex vivo [72]. However this age-dependent effect was not confirmed by Landmann et al. [73] who found beta-adrenoceptor binding sites on leucocytes to be similar in young and old individuals, pointing to a defect distal to the adrenoceptor site.

Plasma catecholamines, alpha-adrenoceptors and height of blood pressure

Assuming that plasma catecholamine concentrations reflect sympathetic activity and that the latter has something to do with the height of blood pressure, a direct relationship between these two variables can be expected. Several years ago such a relationship had already been described by Louis et al. [55], but this has been denied by others [53, 56]. As shown in Figure 7, we ourselves have recently found a direct correlation between plasma noradrenaline concentration and the height of diastolic pressure [74].

What are the processes which enable plasma noradrenaline concentrations to be confined within normal limits and yet to correlate with blood pres-

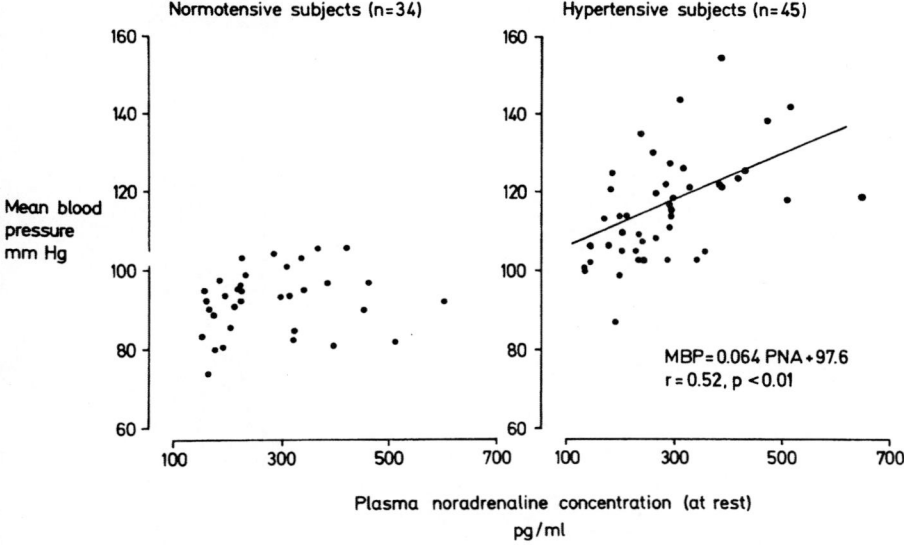

Figure 7. Plasma noradrenaline concentration obtained in the resting recumbent position correlates with the height of mean blood pressure.

sure? Thanks to the basic research done by Langer et al. [75], Rand et
al. [76] and Yamaguchi et al. [77], attention has been called to presynaptic
receptors. Presynaptic beta-receptors facilitate the release of noradrenaline,
which in turn potentiates its own release. If presynaptic beta-receptors also
become less sensitive with age and pressure, a decrease in this positive
feedback could bring neurohumorally released noradrenaline back to 'normal'. Angiotensin's action of amplifying noradrenaline release, which falls
with pressure and age, could also play a role in this process [78]. Finally,
adrenaline could also intervene to facilitate presynaptic noradrenaline release [79] and thereby contribute to the enhanced alpha-adrenoceptor-mediated vasoconstriction observed in patients with essential hypertension [80]
(Figure 8).

Whatever the way in which 'normal' noradrenaline production is regulated, a 'normal' noradrenergic stimulus could cause increased alpha vasoconstriction, either as a result of somewhat reduced beta-adrenoceptor-
mediated vasodilation or because the impaired wall–lumen ratio is responsible for vasoconstriction [81]. Various results point in this direction. For
example, it can be inferred from noradrenaline infusion studies that, with
increasing age, smaller amounts of noradrenaline are necessary in order to
obtain the same rise in pressure [82, 83] and that this reaction is also
favoured by high initial pressure values [83]. Alpha-receptor-mediated platelet aggregation also increases with age [84].

176

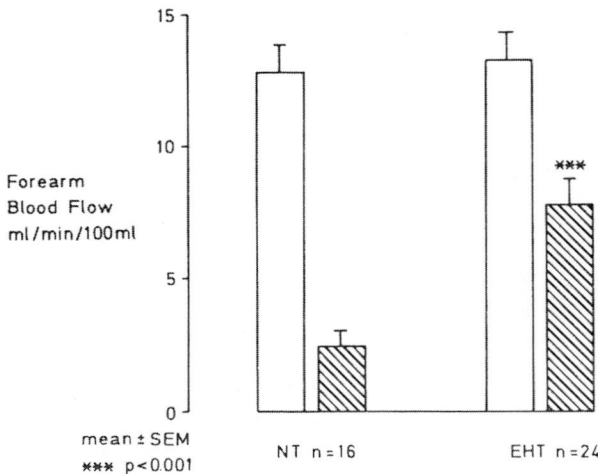

CHANGE IN FOREARM BLOOD FLOW DURING SODIUM NITROPRUSSIDE
(0.6 μg/min/100 ml) AND PRAZOSIN (0.5 μg/min/100 ml) INFUSIONS IN
PATIENTS WITH ESSENTIAL HYPERTENSION (EHT) AND
NORMOTENSIVE SUBJECTS (NT)

Figure 8. Forearm blood flow during nonspecific vasodilator infusion od sodium nitroprusside (0.6 μg/min/100 ml) and during selective postjunctional alpha-adrenoreceptor blockade with prazosin (0.5 μg/min/100 ml) in normotensive (NT) subjects and patients with essential hypertension (EHT). The greater response to prazosin in patients suggests enhanced alpha-adrenoreceptor-mediated vasoconstriction in essential hypertension. Mean ± SEM; *** p<0.001.

The role of the parasympathetic nervous system

The counterweight to the sympathetic nervous system is only too often ignored, one of the main reasons being that acetylcholine-mediated processes are difficult to measure. However, since parasympathetic influences inhibit the release of noradrenaline thanks to presynaptic, muscarinergic receptors [76, 85], inhibition of parasympathetic tone could also stimulate noradrenaline production. Reduced parasympathetic activity has indeed been demonstrated in both labile [86, 87] and sustained [88] essential hypertension. The disappearance of a parasympathetic inhibitory mechanism could therefore reinforce or even trigger off sympathetic activity. An increase in sympathetic activity and inhibition of the parasympathetic fit the classic defence reaction to stress [89].

The contribution of the baroreflex

A possible cause of increased sympathetic and decreased parasympathetic activity could be a disturbance of the afferent or central part of the baroreflex arc, restricted baroreflex sensitivity being held responsible for this [90]. Primarily, a defect in the medullary interneurons, which normally inhibit the vasomotor centre, has been postulated on the basis of experimental stimulation in this area [91]. On the other hand, central disturbances could result from stimulation of the defence area in the hypothalamus. However, it is difficult to say whether these observations are applicable to man. Since the work of McCubbin et al. [92], upward resetting of the baroreceptors in the carotid sinus has also been mentioned, i.e., the carotid receptors are less sensitive and only react at higher levels of blood pressure [93].

The decrease in sympathetic activity induced by an increase in blood pressure due to phenylephrine infusions can be quantified in man by measuring baroreflex-induced bradycardia [94]. The sensitivity of this reflex decreases considerably with increasing age and pressure [95]. This could be the consequence of, e.g., hardening of the vascular walls due to degenerative or arteriosclerotic processes. It is unlikely that a primary defect in the baroreceptors themselves leads to insufficient buffering of the daily fluctuations in blood pressure, thus initiating the development of hypertension, since experiments in which the baroreflex afferents are sectioned have shown that debuffering only leads to transient lability of blood pressure and not to

Table 1. Neurogenic factors in essential hypertension

	Developmental phase	Maintenance phase
Plasma adrenaline	increased	increased
Plasma noradrenaline	increased/normal	normal
Beta-adrenoceptor-mediated functions:		
i) heart rate	increased/normal	increased/normal
ii) exercise tachycardia	normal	reduced
iii) isoproterenol sensitivity	normal/reduced	reduced
iv) production of CAMP	increased	reduced
v) peripheral arteriolar vasodilation	normal/reduced	reduced
vi) renin	high/normal	low
Beta adrenoceptor responsiveness to blockade	increased	reduced
Alpha-adrenoceptor-mediated functions:		
i) peripheral arteriolar vasoconstriction	normal/increased	increased
Parasympathetic tone	reduced	reduced
Baroreflex sensitivity	normal	reduced

sustained hypertension [96]. As shown in the case of renal hypertension, the secondary fall in baroreflex sensitivity resulting from high blood pressure favours increased sympathetic activity [97]. Debuffering at the medullary gates is rather unlikely to be a causal factor in essential hypertension; it is far more likely that the pressure level triggering the baroreflex is reset and that the receptors react less per unit of change of pressure.

This exhaustive discussion of the adrenergic nervous system has regrouped the arguments in favour of increased sympathetic activity, especially in the developmental phase of essential hypertension (Table 1). However, results seem to indicate that later on there is a reorganisation of beta- and alpha-adrenoceptor-mediated effects, themselves determined by the ageing process and the development of high blood pressure. Below we shall attempt to expound these processes, by discussing observations made on the heart, kidneys and renin system.

CARDIAC OUTPUT AND ARTERIOLAR RESISTANCE

Blood pressure is defined as the product of cardiac output and total peripheral resistance. The study of the haemodynamics and pathophysiology of essential hypertension takes this equation as its starting point. Arterial pressure and cardiac output are measured and peripheral resistance is calculated as the product of these two factors.

Experimental observations on animals, especially those made by Ledingham and Cohen in 1963 [98], have shown that there is a transient rise in cardiac output in renal hypertensive rats when blood pressure begins to rise. At first, peripheral resistance is normal, later rising as cardiac output decreases. Ferrario [99] found a similar, transient increase in cardiac output in the initial stage of renal hypertension in the dog, with an increase in peripheral resistance occurring later. This transient increase in cardiac output can be triggered off by stimulation of the stellate ganglion and inhibited by phenoxybenzamine [100]. A hyperdynamic initial stage can be induced by sympathetic activity: this is a primary phenomenon in the genetically hypertensive rat and a secondary phenomenon due to the central excitatory action of angiotensin in renal hypertension [101, 102]. According to Folkow et al. [103], biochemical and morphological changes in the myocardium and arterioles can already be observed after only a few days of high blood pressure.

Cardiac output

Similar stages of development can be found in man. Early haemodynamic studies carried out in patients with essential hypertension showed cardiac pressure as a consequence of increased peripheral resistance [104, 105]. Yet, even 50 years ago increased cardiac output was measured in isolated cases and was assumed to have a causal relationship with hypertension [106, 107]. Several well-controlled studies then confirmed the existence of a group of patients with increased cardiac output compared with normal subjects of the same age [108, 109, 110]. These were mostly younger patients who were in the developmental phase of essential hypertension or in the preliminary phase, referred to as borderline, labile or early hypertension. Although the definition of these disease entities and the patient population studied varied from one investigator to another, common features can nevertheless be found: about 30% of these patients, most of whom were under 45, presented high cardiac output at rest [111], this being due to an increase in heart rate [110, 112] and stroke volume [110].

Some investigators found that these differences are accentuated on exercise [113]. Others found no differences on exericise [114], or a lower rise than normal in cardiac output [115, 116]. The reduced rise in cardiac output on exercise has been interpreted as an indication of the existence of restrictive vascular changes, conflicting with the widespread assumption that peripheral circulation is normal. However, an increase in cardiac output need not occur in every case [112].

In the later maintenance phase of hypertension cardiac output is found to be normal, so that increased resistance is calculated [104, 105]. This is ascribed to functional and/or organic changes in the arterioles. Besides the cross-sectional studies of the various phase of hypertension which we have referred to so far, the first intra-individual longitudinal studies have been made, supplying direct proof of this haemodynamic transformation. For example, in patients with borderline hypertension initially presenting increased cardiac output and normal resistance, Lund-Johansen observed that, 10 years later on average these patients showed a decrease in cardiac output, together with a simultaneous increase in peripheral resistance [117]. As Weiss et al. [118] have recently shown, these changes can be seen already over a period of 4 years, accompanied by a decrease in heart rate. This transformation, which takes place over a relatively short period of time, may explain why cross-sectional studies do not record this phase and why most hypertensive patients present 'normal' cardiac output values. In normal subjects of the same age these haemodynamic variables seem to remain constant over the period of observation mentioned above [118]. The question now is how this transient hyperdynamic syndrome arises and how the counterregulatory mechanisms reduce cardiac output to normal.

Initial factors and counterregulatory mechanisms

The autonomic nervous system seems to play a key role in bringing about increased cardiac output in the initial stage of hypertension. This is evidenced by pharmacological interventions and measurement of plasma catecholamine levels. The fact that increased cardiac output crops more sharply in hypertensive patients following acute beta blockade than it does in normotensive people has also been interpreted as reflecting increased sympathetic activity; yet, cardiac output remains significantly higher than normal in these patients [86]. Additional inhibition of the vagus nerve by means of atropine, thus achieving complete autonomic blockade of the heart, causes a lesser rise in cardiac output in hypertensive patients than it does in normotensive people. This seems to indicate reduced parasympathetic tone during this phase [86]. Increased sympathetic activity coupled with decreased parasympathetic activity is found in the defence reaction described above [89]. Moreover, increased sympathetic activity can be demonstrated by investigating systolic time intervals, especially the pre-ejection period, which is controlled by the sympathetic nervous system. Patients with raised cardiac output have a shortened pre-ejection period; beta blockade lengthens it, significant differences compared to normal controls being observed [65]. Finally, increased plasma noradrenaline concentrations and increased heart rate have been described in this group [59, 65]. In older patients in whom left ventricular hypertrophy has developed, plasma noradrenaline levels are even higher, reflecting a further increase in sympathetic activity; yet, here the pre-ejection period is significantly lengthened as a result of reduced contractility. Increased beta-adrenoceptor sensitivity, as observed by Frohlich et al. [119] by means of isoproterenol infusion tests, could provide a further explanation for a neurogenic origin of increased cardiac output. However, our own work [66] and that of others [120] seem to show that hypersensitivity to isoproterenol is rare and cannot therefore be the sole explanation for raised cardiac output in about 30 % of borderline hypertensives.

An increase in circulating blood volume or cardiopulmonary blood volume could provide an alternative explanation, instead of a neurogenic increase in cardiac output. This would contribute to determining the preload and, via the Frank-Starling mechanism, contractility. Although increased cardiopulmonary volume has occasionally been found in borderline hypertensives [121], it proves to be normal in most cases [122, 123]. Increased cardiopulmonary volume could, it is true, be explained by an increase in venous tone, as has been observed in animal experiments [124] and in borderline hypertensives [125], but it seems hardly likely that an increase in cardiopulmonary volume could lead to a chronically raised cardiac output, for any increase in venous filling of the heart would be corrected within minutes by means of the Starling mechanism (so long as no cardiac insufficiency is present).

Moreover, total circulating blood volume shows no direct relationship

Table 2. Cardiac output and arteriolar resistance

	Developmental phase	Maintenance phase
Cardiac output:	increased/normal	normal
i) heart rate	increased/normal	increased/normal
ii) stroke volume	increased/normal	normal
Arteriolar resistance:	'normal'	increased
i) thickness of vascular wall	normal	increased
ii) beta adrenoceptor mediated vasodilation	normal	reduced
iii) alpha adrenoceptor mediated vasoconstriction	normal/increased	increased
iv) pressor response to noradrenaline	increased	further increased
pressor response to angiotensin	normal	increased

either to cardiac output or to the height of blood pressure [126] and appears therefore to be of less significance as regards the level of cardiac output.

Taken together, these arguments plead in favour of the importance of the sympathetic nervous system as a causal factor in the initial, transient increase in cardiac output. A decline in cardiac beta-adrenoceptor responsiveness could bring about the age-dependent and pressure-dependent transformation and, in doing so, 'normalise' this variable (Table 2).

Peripheral arteriolar resistance

Guyton et al. [127] interpret the increase in peripheral resistance by 'autoregulatory' processes as a throttling hyperperfusion – luxury perfusion – of the tissue. However, since oxygen absorption is normal and not elevated in patients with increased cardiac output [128], this explanation lacks a vital link in the chain.

Other work points more to arteriolar processes, which occur simultaneously with other processes in the developmental phase. For example, Doyle and Fraser [129] found an increased, altered vascular reactivity to noradrenaline in the prehypertensive phase, i.e. in the normotensive children of hypertensive parents.

It could be thought, therefore, that constant or intermittent sympathetic hyperactivity in a patient presenting this vascular response [130], which may be hereditary, leads to excessive vasoconstriction. Brod et al. [131] also found greater vascular resistance in the renal, visceral and cutaneous vascular bed in the initial phase of hypertension, but reduced vascular resistance in the muscles. This regional pattern corresponds to that of the vascular 'defence reflex' [132]. It is heightened by emotional stress, and is more marked in hypertensive patients than in normal subjects [7].

The uneven distribution of vascular resistance makes it more difficult to assess peripheral resistance, particularly in the initial phase of essential hypertension. For example, unlike the 'defence' pattern [133] renal resistance can be reduced; on the other hand, the reduced vascular resistance found in the muscles can be raised by increasing salt intake [134]. However, as hypertension progresses, the vascular bed of the muscles [135, 136] and the kidneys [137] is regularly drawn into the resistance network.

The cause of a stronger vasoconstrictor response is largely unknown. Increased sodium and calcium [138, 139] content, both intracellular and in the vascular wall, seems to offer the first understandable substrate for this increased contraction. However, whether this process is a cause [137] or already the consequence of elevated arterial pressure [140] or sympathetic activity remains to be seen. Higher salt intake also increases sensitivity to angiotensin II [141]. In clinical practice, administration of salt [134] or aldosterone [142] over a short period of time leads to a more marked vaso-constrictor response to noradrenaline in hypertensive patients. Increased intra-arterial pressure and increased sodium content in the vascular wall stimulates new synthesis of proteins and mucopolysaccharides in the vascular musculature [143] and thus also prepares the anatomical substrate for medial hypertrophy [135]. The renin–angiotensin–aldosterone system, which is activated in the initial stage of hypertension [144], sustains the supply of sodium.

Folkow et al. [103] have demonstrated the significance of structural alterations to the vascular wall in the crucial rise in peripheral resistance. Haemodynamic studies on the forearm [135] and the vascular bed of the hand [80] have shown that hypertensive patients have increased peripheral resistance, even with maximum vasodilation. They show a steeper rise in the noradrenaline dose–response curve, for the same threshold dose, and a supranormal response to the administration of a maximum dose of noradrenaline. From the shape of this noradrenaline response curve it may be concluded that the increased vasoconstrictor response is at least in part due to the change in the wall/lumen ration (Table 2).

That the balance between beta-adrenoceptor-mediated (vasodilation) and alpha-adrenoceptor-mediated effects (vasoconstriction) in the develop-

Table 3. Kidneys and sodium/volume homeostatis

	Developmental phase	Maintenance phase
Perfusion	normal/reduced	reduced
Glomerular filtration	normal	normal
Filtration fraction	normal/reduced	increased
Renal arteriolar resistance	normal/increased	increased
Plasma and extracellular fluid volume	normal/decreased	normal/increased

mental phase may be disturbed by a shift from beta- to alpha–effects is borne out by some of our more recent studies. The vasodilator response of forearm flow to isoproterenol is reduced both in older normotensive subjects [145] and in patients with higher blood pressure [146]. As depicted in Figure 8, alpha-adrenoceptor-mediated vasoconstriction, as assessed by postsynaptic alpha-adrenoceptor blockade with prazosin, is enhanced in patients with essential hypertension, a response which correlates with the height of pressure [80].

THE KIDNEYS AND SODIUM VOLUME HOMEOSTASIS

For several decades research has stressed the key role played by the kidneys in the pathophysiology of hypertension. Yet, the crucial question remains unanswered: do the kidneys constitute a primary trigger factor and is essential hypertension of renal origin?; or are the kidneys, as excretory organs, secondarily involved in the maintenance of high blood pressure because of functional and/or structural changes?

The kidneys contribute to circulatory regulation by excreting water and salt and thereby maintaining the homeostasis of extracellular fluid volume. Moreover, they produce vasoactive substances. Kinins and prostaglandins have a local vasodilator action [147, 148], but the pathophysiological relevance of this effect is not yet clear. Via angiotensin, renin has a vasoconstrictor action at the periphery and in the kidneys [149, 150]; at the same time, via aldosterone, it intervenes in sodium homeostasis [151]; moreover, via angiotensin it stimulates central nervous relays [102]. However, renal arteriolar resistance plays a key role. It must be stressed at the outset that all these functions are directly controlled by the adrenergic nervous system (see Figure 1).

The relationship between blood pressure and excretion of sodium – pressure natriuresis [152, 153] – is the most important factor in the long-term regulation of blood pressure [154, 155], which is impaired in essential hypertension. Blood pressure seems to rise to a point where the sodium balance is restored, i.e. pressure natriuresis is reset [155, 156]. An increase in renal vascular resistance and in the filtration fractions is said to be responsible for this. The natriuresis, which results from an increase in peritubular hydrostatic pressure, itself due to high blood pressure, is counterbalanced by an increase in proximal tubular reabsorption of sodium due to the elevated filtration fraction and the consequent increase in peritubular oncotic pressure [155, 156]. Functional and structural influences may increase renal arteriolar resistance, although it should be noted here that renal resistance increases with age in normotensive people [157, 158]. However, in hypertensive patients this process takes place earlier and in a more prominent way.

It is interesting to note that increased renal perfusion can sometimes be found in young, borderline-hypertensive patients [159]. The latest results reported by Bianchi et al. [160] seem to be especially significant here. Renal blood flow was found to be higher in normotensive [aged 14–30] of hypertensive parents, than it was in the comparison group. This could mean that increased renal perfusion is necessary in order to maintain glomerular filtration. Perfusion of the individual nephrons seems to be the key factor here [160, 161]. Prostaglandins [147], kinins [162] and cholinergic vasodilators [163] have all been discussed as possible, but more unlikely causes. In our opinion, beta-adrenoceptor-mediated adrenergic vasodilation could be an alternative cause. However, such patients have normal, not increased cardiac output – perhaps already normalised again [164].

The kidneys during the developmental phase of hypertension

Cross-sectional studies show an increase in renal arteriolar resistance at the expense of renal perfusion in two thirds of young hypertensive patients [159]. Several authors have found that the variability of renal perfusion is doubled or even tripled in this initial phase, indicating active vasoconstriction [159, 165, 166]. The stronger response shown to vasodilator substances also agrees with functionally increased renal vascular tone [163]. This process is still reversible; the relationship between pressure and natriuresis can still be normalised. The adrenergic nervous system appears to play a major part here. Direct evidence was provided by Hollenberg [163] who found that young hypertensive patients showed a greater rise in renal blood flow after intrarenal infusion of alpha blockers. Regional differences in adrenergic activity or increasing responsiveness may well make it possible that general signs of increased sympathetic activity are lacking at this stage [167]. The most important argument demonstrating that the above changes lead to an increase in blood pressure is the result of the examination of the contralateral kidney in unilateral renal artery stenosis, blood pressure having been normalised in the contralateral kidney after the operation. Renal perfusion fell by some 20 % [159], as is the case in young hypertensive patients with reduced renal blood flow.

The kidneys in the maintenance phase of hypertension

Later on, renal perfusion drops, whereas glomerular filtration remains normal [156, 166]. Consequently, vascular resistance and the filtration fraction increase, causing a further rise in blood pressure so as to maintain the sodium/volume balance. How does this transformation come about? Following the initial, functional increase in renal arteriolar resistance, which is probably of adrenergic origin, structural changes to the arterioles take place with time, as a result of the increased pressure. The major change is medial hyperplasia, leading to an increase in the wall–lumen ratio [81]. Moreover, sodium deposits in the vascular wall increase [138], so that sensitivity to vasoconstrictor substances rises [168]. In turn, this provokes increased renal arteriolar resistance, despite normal adrenergic activity.

However, there is a further change that might affect this transformation. Arteriolar dilation could decrease with age and rising blood pressure, as other beta-adrenoceptor-mediated functions do. Alpha-adrenoceptor-mediated vasoconstriction would then tend to predominate.

Severe or malignant forms of hypertension should be dealt with separately in this discussion. Pressure-induced renal changes can lead to severe renal damage, which induces salt loss in the kidneys and excessive renin–angiotensin production. This results in low renal perfusion, a decrease in glomerular filtration and even renal insufficiency. This high renin renal form [70] should be distinguished from high renin essential hypertension (see also Figure 1).

Sodium/volume factor

Epidemiological [10] and experimental [168] data have established beyond doubt that salt makes an essential contribution to all forms of hypertension. Various authors have postulated that a salt/volume factor can play a role in triggering hypertension [10] or have spoken of 'volume-dependent' hypertension and linked this with low renin forms in particular [169]. These theories were mainly derived from forms where the primary factor is increased sodium retention, as in primary aldosteronism or renal insufficiency. In fact, in these clinical forms the sequence of initial sodium retention, increase in extracellular plasma volume and cardiac output, leading to an increase in blood pressure and later to an increase in peripheral arteriolar resistance has been demonstrated [170].

There are two reasons why measurement of volume has contributed little to our understanding of the pathophysiology of hypertension. 'Effective' blood volume, sandwiched between the left ventricle and the arteriolar resistance vessels, cannot be measured although it would be the most pertinent variable. Measurement of volume is subject to considerable methodological difficulties [158] and interindividual fluctuations [171].

For this reason most studies have been unable to show any difference between normotensive and hypertensive subjects as regards plasma and/or extracellular volume. Nor can any increase in plasma volume, which might have initiated the development of hypertension, be found in the prehypertensive phase [160]. Here, too, the question of what is 'normal' arises, since volume must go down in response to pressure natriuresis when blood pressure is high. 'Normal' volume would therefore be too high, in view of the high blood pressure. Finally, other authors have also found a slightly reduced plasma volume in hypertensive patients; especially in cases of great increased diastolic pressure and increased peripheral resistance [172]. It is precisely this inverse relationship between blood volume and the height of blood pressure [172, 173] which has been observed by many authors and can also be found in normal subjects [174], that seems to indicate that pressure determines volume. Relative hypovolaemia seems to occur mainly at night and in the early morning, resulting from mild pressure nycturia and albumin transudation in the interstitial tissue [175]. The accentuated morning low and the diurnal fluctuations in plasma volume in hypertensive patients [171] also fits this picture.

Just as the accentuated nocturnal pressure natriuresis does in hypertensive patients [175], increased hydrostatic capillary pressure with increased transcapillary albumin escape in the morning [175] can reduce plasma volume in relation to interstitial fluid volume and reinforce the trend to increased extracellular fluid volume and total exchangeable sodium [176]. This process would be favoured by increased venular tone. It is quite conceivable that this process be initiated by the morning peak in sympathetic activity. Such a partition is not observed in normal subjects [177].

Different attempts to define the relationship between plasma volume and age have failed [178, 179]. Most recently, Beretta-Piccoli et al. [180] observed a relatively reduced exchangeable sodium in younger hypertensive individuals, but higher values in older ones.

The finding that there is no direct correlation between blood volume and cardiac output [126] is also important. This, too, would be consistent with the view that a predominantly beta-adrenoceptor-mediated hyperdynamic cardiovascular state, resulting in pressure diuresis and a trend towards hypovolemia, is important in the developmental phase, while a sodium factor and alpha-adrenoceptor-mediated vasoconstriction prevail in the maintenance phase of essential hypertension. This short summary shows that the relationship between blood pressure and volume is far more complex than just an 'overfilling of the circulation' triggering off hypertension.

THE RENIN-ANGIOTENSIN-ALDOSTERONE SYSTEM

The renin–angiotensin–aldosterone system constitutes the link between adrenergic regulation of the circulatory system and sodium/volume homeostasis [181, 182], manifested simultaneously. It can be thought of as a long endocrine arm of the sympathetic nervous system, since the renin system directly reflects sympathetic activity, thanks to postganglionic renal neurones and beta-adrenoceptor-mediation in the juxtaglomerular cells [70, 144, 183]. Blood pressure and sodium determine renin secretion, especially in extreme situations, thanks to the baroreceptors in the vas afferens and the sodium receptors in the macula densa. Renin acts on an alpha globulin produced by the liver to split off the decapeptide angiotensin I. Angiotensin I is then de-aminated, mainly by a pulmonary renal and vessel wall converting enzyme and transformed into the biologically active principle angiotensin II. Angiotensin II has various actions. It acts on special arteriolar receptors causing vasoconstriction, which is further reinforced by the simultaneous activation of alpha-adrenoceptors [184]. Moreover, circulating angiotensin II stimulates sympathetic activity in the central nervous system [102]. In addition to its vasoconstrictor role, angiotensin II is responsible for distal tubular reabsorption of sodium thanks to selective stimulation of aldosterone biosynthesis, thus causing blood volume to expand [182]. The resultant increase in blood pressure and therefore, in pressure natriuresis has a twofold effect, viz. reducing renin release and restoring sodium/volume homeostasis.

Two important developments have taken place in the last 10 years. Firstly, radioimmunoassays of the various components of the renin–angiotensin-aldosterone system have given us new insights into the regulation of the system itself and have enabled us to classify hypertensive patients into high, normal and low renin groups [185, 186], thus giving rise to new concepts in pathophysiology, pharmacotherapy and prognosis [70, 146, 187]. Secondly, drugs can be used to suppress renin secretion [178, 189]; they inhibit the conversion of angiotensin [190] or interfere competitively with the binding of angiotensin to its receptors [191], so that the role of the renin system in man can be defined more accurately.

Sympathetic activity and the renin system

Various stimuli applied to the sympathetic nervous system cause increased renin secretion. Animal experiments have shown that electric stimulation of the medulla oblongata [192] or of the renal splanchnic nerve [83] leads to renin release. This is mediated by beta-adrenoceptors [229], whereas the activation of alpha-adrenoceptors [194], like angiotensin itself, suppresses renin. Circulating noradrenaline and adrenaline both stimulate renin secretion [195, 196]. Likewise, physiological stimuli which are accompanied by increased sympathetic activity, such as the sympathetic morning peak [197], upright posture, exercise [198, 199] and cold [200], also stimulate renin secretion. Even after sodium deprivation, some renin secretion occurs due to activation of the sympathetic nervous system [201]. Finally, renin secre-

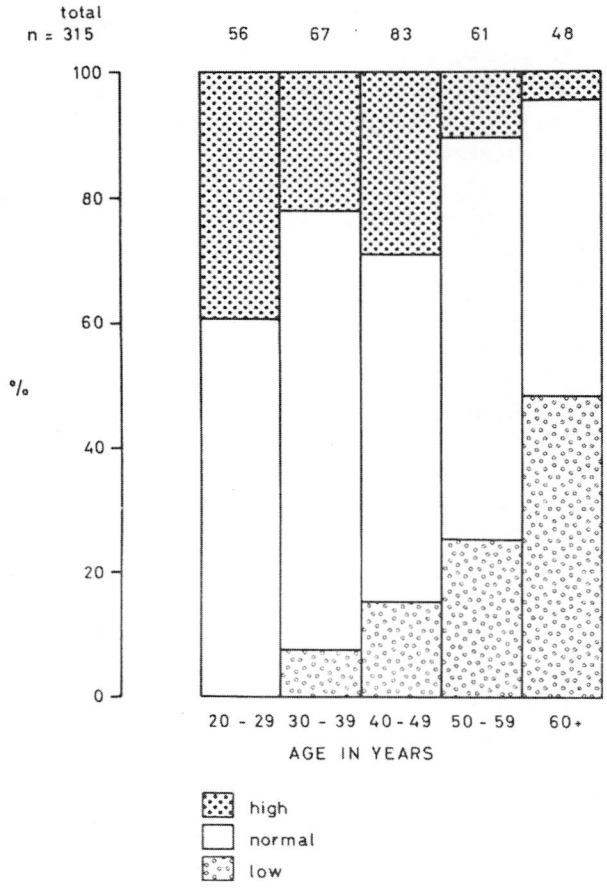

Figure 9a. Percentage distribution of the renin subgroups in essential hypertension by age. The frequency of low renin forms increases with age whilst high renin forms become less frequent. Moreover, high renin patients are numerous in the 40–49 age group, corresponding to the severe forms of hypertension shown in Figure 9b.

tion can be stimulated by isoproterenol [202] and suppressed by beta blockers [189]. These observations allow us to conclude that renin secretion can be stimulated directly, viz. neurally, or indirectly via plasma catecholamines. A reduction in renin secretion may be due to various factors: 1) a reduction in beta receptor influences; 2) stimulation of alpha receptors (or both); 3) an increase in pressure recorded by the baroreceptors; 4) an increase in the sodium load in the macula densa.

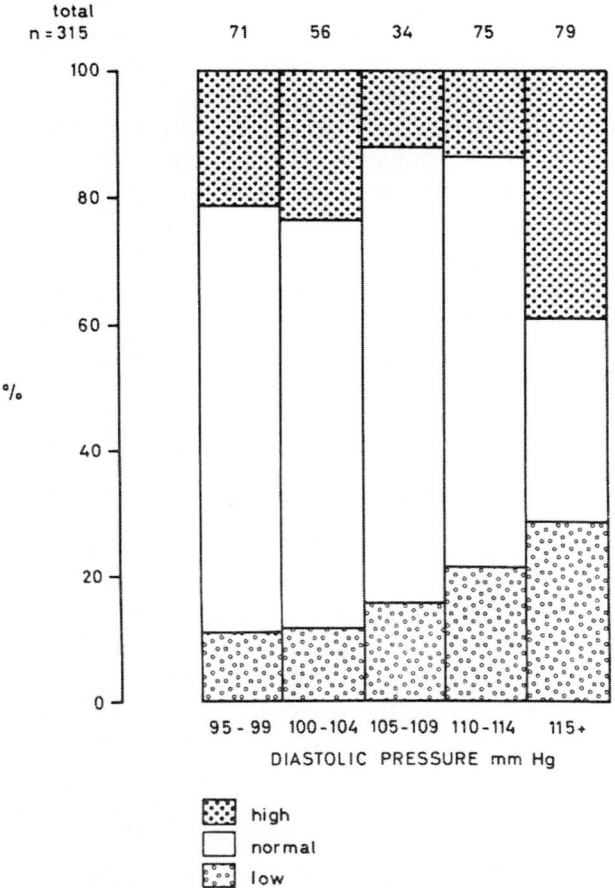

Figure 9b. Percentage distribution of the renin subgroups in essential hypertension by diastolic values.

Age, blood pressure and renin

Plasma renin activity diminishes somewhat with age in normotensive people [203]. If renin activity is related to 24-h urinary excretion of sodium in patients with essential hypertension [185, 186], 20% can be said to have a high renin–sodium index, 60% to have normal values, and (with the help of mild salt depletion [70, 185, 186]) 20% can be said to have a low index. The analysis by age given in Figure 9a shows a relative decline in high renin forms and an increase in low renin forms with age. Besides renin [70, 204], plasma angiotensin II levels also fall with age [205]. Low renin forms become commoner with higher blood pressure values, showing a similar pattern (Figure 9b).

There is, however, an important exception, viz. the fact that patients with severe diastolic hypertension more often have high renin values. These patients, who are often older, frequently present signs of renal damage, which could be partly due to high renin activity [70]. On the other hand, there is an inverse relationship between renin and peripheral arteriolar resistance [206], the latter increasing with age and with diminishing variability of blood pressure [23]. On the basis of these observations, the classification of hypertensive patients into renin subgroups seems to correspond more to passages in the course of a disease which lasts for decades rather than to characterise different, uniform subgroups. Confirming this hypothesis, the biochemical, haemodynamic and pharmacological findings discussed above in relation to the developmental and maintenance phases of hypertension are also found in the various renin groups.

High renin essential hypertension

These patients are generally younger, often with labile or borderline forms of hypertension [207], presenting greater variability of blood pressure, increased heart rate and cardiac output [207, 208], yet tending to have a lower circulating blood volume [166]. Haematocrit and blood urea nitrogen levels are higher in comparison [209]. Peripheral and renal arteriolar resistance are 'normal' [207], meaning that they are too high in relation to the raised blood pressure, since resistance appears to be diminished right at the outset.

Younger patients with elevated plasma noradrenaline concentrations also account for a good share of high renin patients [65, 210, 211, 212]; in addition to hyperreactive renin they also have hyperreactive adrenergic functions [208]. One study [65] also described a particular personality structure in high renin patients, characterised by excessive guilt feelings, self-control, submission and repressed aggressiveness, which was recently confirmed by Perini et al. [213] on the basis of a projective psychological test. Sensitivity to isoproterenol is normal or scarcely diminished [58, 66]; the reaction to beta blockade is especially good [214–217].

Patients with high renin levels, especially those with high renin, severe hypertension and renal damage, respond particularly well to competitive angiotensin receptor blockade with saralasin [191] or to inhibitors of angiotensin I converting enzyme [190]. This also points to the dominant nature of angiotensin's role as a vasoconstrictor in these patients; we talk of angiotensin-dependent hypertension.

Normal renin essential hypertension

With regard to age and adrenergic, biochemical and haemodynamic characteristics, this group of patients lies between high and low renin forms. It may also be that it represents a bridging or transformation stage in which renin activity has become 'normal' as a result of high blood pressure. However, 'normal' renin, 'normal' plasma catecholamines and 'normal' haemodynamics would then be abnormal in relation to the high pressure. If these assumptions are correct, an initial triggering process, for example a neurogenic one, could cause a slight rise in blood pressure, which in turn could lead to suppression of renin secretion. It would not be necessary, therefore, for a high renin stage to be gone through in each case. Likewise, renal arteriolar resistance, which is still 'normal', and 'normal' aldosterone might be respnosible for slight sodium retention, which would be counterbalanced by pressure natriuresis.

Low renin essential hypertension

This type of hypertension is usually found among older patients with less variability in blood pressure and increased peripheral and renal arteriolar resistance [158]. Compared to patients with normal renin levels, with these patients plasma volume and total exchangeable sodium are only increased in isolated cases [218–220] and never diminished. The slight increase in stroke volume is counterbalanced by the low heart rate (Figure 5), so that cardiac ouput remains normal [206, 208]. The less obvious exercise tachycardia and the diminished sensitivity to isoproterenol also fit the picture of hyporeactive renin [146]; the production of cAMP is reduced [71] as is responsiveness to beta blockers [214–217]. Pharmacological interference with angiotensin-induced vasoconstriction does not have any noticeable antihypertensive effect either, which proves that angiotensin plays a subordinate role here. The sodium/volume component is crucial, however, as can be deduced from the fact that salt depletion leads to a fall in blood pressure in cases of low renin hypertension [221], whereas acute excess volume is more rapidly eliminated [179, 222]. Overproduction of a mineralocorticoid has been suggested in this group of patients [224–226] because of the suppressed, hyporeactive renin [223]. On the analogy of what happens in an aldosterone-producing adrenal adenoma, aldosterone has also been accused of being a cause of low renin essential hypertension, especially as plasma potassium levels are generally somewhat lower and abnormally low in a few cases [219]. In low renin patients, aldosterone secretion is generally normal, being slightly elevated in a few cases [226]. However, its characteristic feature is that it is more difficult to suppress during heavy salt loading and less easy to stimulate during salt deprivation [227]. This practically fixed level of aldosterone secretion is always accompanied by very low renin levels. However, since even bilateral adrenalectomy does not lower blood pressure much [228], the importance of aldosterone as a factor maintaining hypertension (and therefore that of other mineralocorticoids) can be doubted. (If another mineralocorticoid were involved, reduced secretion of aldosterone could be expected; this is not the case.) This doubt is reinforced by the fact that an increase in total exchangeable sodium is only found in isolated cases [180, 229]. However, it is possible that a poorly detectable sodium/volume factor is involved, judging from the very good antihypertensive response of these patients to diuretic therapy [219, 230].

Although the possibility of a mineralocorticoid causing hypertension should not be excluded in individual low renin patients, an alternative explanation is needed. Because of its generally close relationship with the height of blood pressure and with age, low renin is far more likely to be a consequence of both these variables. For physical reasons [230], increased renal arteriolar resistance is responsible for increased proximal tubular sodium retention, while aldosterone, which is difficult to suppress if salt intake is high (as it usually is), is also responsible for increased distal tubular sodium retention. The homeostasis of sodium retention is regulated by the raised blood pressure. Since the constellation of low renin and slightly raised aldosterone can also be induced by long-term treatment with beta blockers [215] low renin essential hypertension could be the underlying cause of hypertension-induced, endogenous beta-adrenoceptor insufficiency. Similarly, a beta-defect may also account for postglomerular vasoconstriction and reduced filtration fraction encountered in older hypertensive [156].

Pharmacotherapeutic consequences

With the discovery of renin subgroups, a pattern of response to hypertensive drugs has emerged. Blood pressure can be normalised with a beta-blocker alone in patients with high renin more frequently than in those with normal or low renin [214–217, 232]. The latter may even respond with an increase in blood pressure in some cases [233]. Therapy with beta blockers alone is less successful in older patients [70, 216, 232], which is in line with the correlation between renin and age (Figure 9). On the other hand, diuretics – and not just the aldosterone antagonist spirolactone [230] – are more effective in low renin essential hypertension [219, 229, 230, 232, 233]. It would seem, too, that older patients, who have had hypertension for a long time and who present arteriolar changes, also benefit more frequently from the addition of a vasodilator to a beta blocker/diuretic combination [232]. The better response shown by low renin patients to the postsynaptic alpha blocker pra-

zosin, allows us to confirm an important alpha-adrenoceptor-mediated vasoconstrictor component in these patients [234].

SUMMARY

Primary hypertension is believed to develop through an interaction over a
long period of time between a genetic factor and two external factors –
psychological stress and an excessive salt intake. The key function of the
autonomic nervous system in cardiovascular regulatory mechanisms and
the fact that it also intervenes in the renal mechanisms suggest that it is of
prime importance, at all events, particularly in the initial stages of the disease.

If effects of the sympathetic nervous system are broken down, as in pharmacological experiments, into alpha- and beta-adrenoceptor-mediated
mechanisms, then in the early developmental stages of hypertension, which
are typically associated with a raised cardiac output and high plasma renin
levels, there is predominance of beta-adrenoceptor-mediated effects (Figure
10). In the later stages of the disease, however, when the peripheral resis-

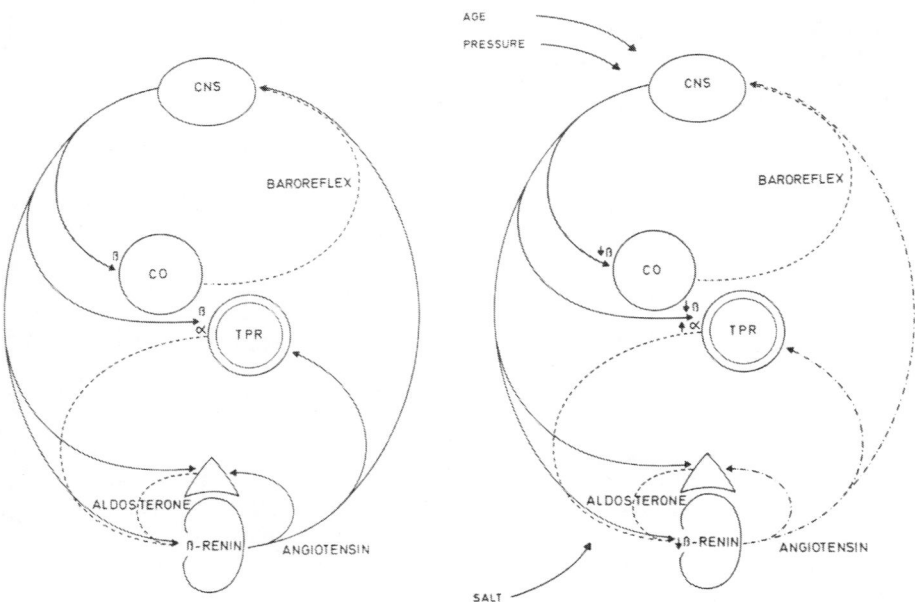

Figure 10. Age, salt and blood pressure per se contribute to the transition from a predominantly
hyperbeta-adrenoceptor-mediated cardiovascular regulation in the *developmental* phase of hypertension (figure left) to a later *maintenance* phase where beta-effects are blunted and alpha-adrenoceptor-mediated vasoconstriction prevails (figure right).

194

tance is raised, there is prevailing alpha–adrenoceptor–mediated vasocon-striction. The elevated sympathetic tone, which manifests itself as a slight increase in plasma adrenaline is accompanied by a reduced parasympathetic tone. Two of the factors influencing the central regulation of these auton-omic efferent pathways are angiotensin and afferent nerves from the baror-eceptors of the carotid sinus.

Structural changes, with an increased deposition of sodium in the vessel wall, contribute to the increased arteriolar resistance. Sodium reabsorption by the kidneys is promoted by aldosterone, the release of which is mediated in the early stages of the disease by renin and angiotensin. The increased vascular resistance leads to reduced renal blood flow, offsetting the relation between the blood pressure and sodium excretion. This pathophysiological concept postulates a hyper- (beta-)adrenergic, hyperdynamic developmental phase which is transformed into a maintenance phase in which sustained adrenergic tone and adaptive changes at the level of adrenoceptors combine with structural alterations of the arteriolar resistance vessels.

ACKNOWLEDGEMENTS

We are indebted to Drs. F. W. Amann, O. Bertel, P. Bolli, E. Bürgisser, P. van Brummelen, C. Hulthén, W. Kiowski, R. Landman, B. E. Lütold and Ch. Perini for their collaboration. Research work was supported by Swiss National Funds Nr. 3.452.74, 3-894.77 and 3.807.80.

REFERENCES

1. Selye H: Stress. Montreal: Acta Med Publ, 1950.
2. Donnison CP: Blood pressure in the African native; its bearing on the etiology of hyper-piesia and arteriosclerosis. Lancet 1:6, 1929.
3. Scotch NA, Geiger JH: Epidemiology of essential hypertension: psychologic and sociocul-tural factors in etiology. J Chronic Dis 16:1183, 1963.
4. Cobb S, Rose RM: Hypertension, peptic ulcer and diabetes in air traffic controllers. JAMA 224:489, 1973.
5. Graham JDP: High blood pressure after battle. Lancet 248:239, 1945.
6. Ruskin A, Beard OW, Schaffer RL: Blast hypertension. Am J Med 4:228, 1948.
7. Pickering GW: High Blood Pressure, 2nd edn. New York: Grune & Stratton, 1968.
8. Henry JP, Meehan JP, Stephens PM: Use of psychosocial stimuli to induce prolonged systolic hypertension in mice. Psychosom Med 29:408, 1967.
9. Benson H, Herd JA, Morse WA, Kelleher RT: Behavioral induction of arterial hyperten-sion and its reversal. Am J Physiol 217:30, 1969.
10. Freis ED: Salt, Volume and the prevention of hypertension. Circulation 53:589, 1976.
11. Forsyth RP: Mechanisms of the cardiovascular responses to environmental stressors. In: Cardiovascular Psychophysiology, pp. 5–32. Obrist PA, Black AH, Brenner J, DiCara LV, eds. Chicago: Aldine, 1974.

12. Dahl LK: Salt and hypertension. Am J Clin Nutr 25:231, 1972.
13. Oliver WJ, Cohen EL, Neel JV: Blood pressure, sodium intake and sodium related hormones in the Yanomamo Indians, a no-salt culture. Circulation 52:146, 1975.
14. Bühler RR, Patel U, Marbet G: Ambulante und stationäre Bestimmung des Renin-Natrium-Index zur Unterteilung und gezielten Behandlung der essentiellen Hypertonie. Schweiz Med Wochenschr 104:1802, 1974.
15. Bühler FR, de Lèche AS, Schüler G, Gutzwiller F, Baumann F, Schweizer W: Das Hypertonieproblem in der Schweiz: analysiert anhand einer Blutdruckuntersuchung bei 21 589 Personen. Schweiz Med Wochenschr 106:99, 1976.
16. Sasaki N: The relationship of salt intake to hypertension in the Japanese. Geriatrics 19:735, 1964.
17. Murphy RJF: The effect of 'rice diet' on plasma volume and extracellular fluid space in hypertensive subjects. J Clin Invest 29:912, 1950.
18. Watkin DM, Fraeb HF, Hatch FT, Gutman AB: Effects of diet in essential hypertension II. Results with unmodified Kempner rice diet in fifty hospitalized patients. Am J Med 9:411, 1950.
19. Corcoran AC, Taylor RD, Page IH: Controlled observations on the effect of low sodium diettherapy in essential hypertension. Circulation 3:1, 1951.
20. Parijs J, Joosens JV, Vander Linden L, Verstreken G, Amery AH: Moderate sodium restriction and diuretics in the treatment of hypertension. Am Heart J 85:22, 1973.
21. Page LB, Danion A, Moellering RC Jr: Antecedents of cardiovascular disease in six Solomon Islands societies. Circulation 49:1132, 1974.
22. Metropolitan Life Insurance CO. Statist Bull 50:1, 1969.
23. Miall WE, Lovell HG: Relation between change of blood pressure and age. Br Med J 2:660, 1967.
24. Miall WE, Oldham PD: The hereditary factor in arterial blood pressure. Br Med J 1:75, 1963.
25. Smirk FH: High Arterial Pressure. Oxford: Blackwell, 1957.
26. Zinner SH, Levy PS, Kass EH: Familial aggregation of blood pressure in childhood. N Engl J Med 284:401, 1971.
27. Biron P, Mongeau JC, Bertrand D: Familial aggregation of blood pressure in 558 adopted children. Can Med Assoc J 23:773, 1976.
28. Garray RP, Elghozi JL, Dagher G, Meyer P: Laboratory distinction between essential and secondary hypertension by measurement of erythrocyte cation fluxes. N Engl J Med 302:769, 1980.
29. Ferrario CM, Dickinson CJ, McCubbin JW: Central vasomotor stimulation by angiotensin. Clin Sci 39:239, 1970.
30. Burnstock G, Gannon B, Iwayama T: Sympathetic innervation of vascular smooth muscle in normal and hypertensive animals. Circ Res 26 and 27 (Suppl 2):5, 1970.
31. Malmejac J: Activity of the adrenal medulla and its regulation. Physiol Rev 44:186, 1964.
32. Ahlquist RP: A study of the adrenotropic receptors. Am J Physiol 163:586, 1948.
33. Wallin BG, Delius W, Hagbarth KE: Comparison of sympathetic nerve activity in normotensive and hypertensive subjects. Circ Res 33:9, 1973.
34. DeQuattro V, Miura Y, Lurvey A, Cosgrove M, Mendez R: Increased plasma catecholamine concentrations and vas deferens norepinephrine biosynthesis in men with elevated blood pressure. Circ Res 36:118, 1975.
35. Overy HR, Pfister R, Chidsey CA: Studies on the renal excretion of norepinephrine. J Clin Invest 46:482, 1967.
36. Ikoma T: Studies on catechols with reference to hypertension. Jpn Circ J 29:1269, 1965.

37. DeSchaepdryver AF, Leroy JG: Urine volume and catecholamine excretion in man. Acta Cardiol 16:631, 1961.
38. Nestel PJ, Doyle AE: Excretion of free noradrenaline and adrenaline by healthy young sugjects and by patients with essential hypertension. Aust Ann Med 17:295, 1968.
39. Pedersen EB, Christensen NJ: Catecholamines in plasma and urine in patients with essential hypertension determined by double-isotope derivative techniques. Acta Med Scand 198:373, 1975.
40. Nestel PJ: Blood pressure and catecholamine excretion after mental stress in labile hypertension. Lancet 1:692, 1969.
41. DeQuattro V: Evaluation of increased norepinephrine excretion in hypertension using l-dopa ^{3}H. Circ Res 28:84, 1971.
42. Weinshilboum RM, Thoa NB, Johnson DB, Kopin KJ, Axelrod J: Proportional release of norepinephrine and dopamine-beta-hydroxylase from sympathetic nerves. Sciences 174:1349, 1971.
43. Axelrod J: Dopamine-beta-hydroxylase. Regulation of its synthesis and release from nerve terminals. Pharmacol Rev 24:233, 1972.
44. Rush RA, Geifen LG: Radioimmunoassay and clearance of circulating dopamine-beta-hydroxylase. Circ Res 31:444, 1972.
45. Weinshilboum R: Dopamine-beta-hydroxylase activity in serum. Life Sci 13:167, 1973.
46. Goldstein M, Freedman LS, Bonnay M: An assay for dopamine-beta-hydroxylase in tissues and serum. Experientia (Basel) 27:632, 1971.
47. Geffen LB, Rush RA, Louis WJ, Doyle AE: Plasma dopamine-beta-hydroxylase and noradrenaline amounts in essential hypertension. Clin Sci 44:617, 1973.
48. Planz G, Wiethold G, Appel E et al.: Correlation between increased dopamine-beta-hydroxylase activity and catecholamine concentration in plasma: determination of acute changes in sympathetic activity in man. Eur J Clin Pharmacol 8:181, 1975.
49. DeChamplain J: Evaluation of the neurogenic component in human hypertension. In: The Nervous System in Arterial Hypertension. pp. 267–300. Julius S, Esler MD, eds. Springfield: Charles C. Thomas, 1976.
50. Da Prada M, Zürcher G: Simultaneous radioenzymatic determination of plasma and tissue adrenaline, Noradrenaline and dopamine within the femtomole range. Life Sci 19:1161, 1976.
51. Lütold BE, Bühler FR, Da Prada M: Dynamik von Plasmakatecholaminen und Beta-Adrenozeptor-Funktionen. Anwendung einer neuen radioenzymatischen Mikromethode. Schweiz Med Wochenschr 106:1735, 1976.
52. Engelman K, Portnoy B, Sjoerdsma A: Plasma catecholamine concentrations in patients with hypertension. Circ Res 26 and 27 (Suppl 1):141, 1970.
53. DeQuattro V, Chan S: Raised plasma catecholamines in some patients with primary hypertension. Lancet 1:806, 1972.
54. Christensen MS, Christensen NJ: Plasma catecholamine in hypertension. Scand J Clin Lab Invest 30:169, 1972.
55. Louis WJ, Doyle AE, Anavekar S: Plasma catecholamine concentrations in patients with hypertension. Circ Res, 1973.
56. Franco-Morselli R, Elghozi JL, Joly E et al.: Increased plasma adrenaline concentrations in benign essentiel hypertension. Br Med J 2:1251, 1977.
57. Sever PS, Owikowska B, Birch M et al.: Plasma noradrenaline in essential hypertension. Lancet 1:1078, 1977.
58. Bertel O, Bühler FR, Kiowski W, Lütold BE: Decreased beta-adrenoceptor responsiveness as related toage, Blood pressure and plasma catevholamines in patients with essential hypertension. Hypertension 2:130, 1980.
59. Cousineau D, Lapointe L, De Champlain J: Circulating catecholamines and systolic time

intervals in normotensive and hypertensive patients with and without left ventricular hypertrophy. Am Heart J, 1978.

60. Bühler FR, Kiowski W, van Brummelen, Amann FW, Bertel O, Landmann R, Lütold BE, Bolli P: Plasma catecholamines and cardiac, renal and peripheral vascular adrenoceptor-mediated responses in different age groups of normal and hypertensive subjects. Clin Exp Hypertension 2:409, 1980.

61. Lake CR, Ziegler MG, Coleman MD et al.: Age-adjusted plasma norepinephrine levels are similar in normotensive and hypertensive subjects. N Engl J Med 296:208, 1977.

62. Robinson BF, Epstein SE, Beiser GD et al.: Control of heart rate by the autonomic nervous system. Studies in man on the interrelation between baroreceptor mechanisms and exercise. Circulat Res 19:400, 1966.

63. Brod J, Fencl V, Heijl Z, Jirka J: Circulatory changes underlying blood pressure elevation during acute emotional stress (mental arithmetic) in normotensive and hypertensive subjects. Clin Sci 18:269, 1959.

64. Frohlich ED, Dustan HP, Page IH: Hyperdynamic beta-adrenergic circulatory state. Arch Intern Med 117:614, 1966.

65. Esler M, Julius S, Zweifel A et al.: Mild high-renin essential hypertension. Neurogenic human hypertension? N Engl J Med 296:405, 1977.

66. Bertel O, Bühler FR, Kiowski W: Isoproterenol sensitivity testing in different age and renin groups of essential hypertension. In: Circulating Catecholamines and Blood Pressure. Birkenhäger WH, Falke HE, eds. Utrecht: Bunge, 1978.

67. Åstrand PO, Rodahl K: Textbook of Work Physiology. New York: McGraw-Hill, 1970.

68. London GM, Safar ME, Weiss YA et al.: Isoproterenol sensitivity and total body clearance of propranolol in hypertensive patients. J Clin Pharmacol 16:174, 1976.

69. Conway J: Effect of age on the response to propranolol. Int J Clin Pharmacol 4:148, 1970.

70. Bühler FR, Burkart F, Lütold BE et al.: Antihypertensive beta-blocking action as related to renin and age: a pharmacological tool to identify pathogenetic mechanisms in essential hypertension. Am J Cardiol 36:653, 1975.

71. Lowder SC, Hamet P, Liddle GW: Contrasting effects of hypoglycemia on plasma renin activity and cyclic adenosine 3', 5'-mono-phosphate (cyclic AMP) in low renin and normal renin essential hypertension. Circulat Res 38:105, 1976.

72. Schocken DD, Roth GS: Reduced beta-adrenergic receptor concentrations in ageing man. Nature 267:856, 1977.

73. Landmann R, Bittiger H, Bühler FR: High affinity beta-2 adrenergic receptors in mononuclear leucocytes: similar density in young and old subjects. Life Sci (in press).

74. Kiowski W, Bühler FR, Van Brummelen P, Amann FW: Plasma noradrenaline concentration and alpha-adrenoceptor-mediated vasoconstriction in normotensive and hypertensive man. Clin Sci 60:483, 1981.

75. Langer SZ, Enero MA, Adler-Graschinsky E, Dubocovich ML, Celuchi SM: Presynaptic regulatory mechanisms for noradrenaline release by nerve stimulation. In: Central Action of Drugs in Blood Pressure Regulation, pp. 133–150. Davies DS, Reid JL, eds. London: Pitman Medical, 1975.

76. Rand MJ, McCulloch MW, Story DF: Prejunctional modulation of noradrenergic transmission by noradrenaline, dopamine and acetylcholine. In: Central Action of Drugs in Blood Pressure Regulation. pp. 94–132. Davies DS, Reid JL, eds. London: Pirman Medical, 1975.

77. Yamaguchi N, De Champlain J, Nadeau RA: Regulation of norepinephrine release from cardiac sympathetic fibres in the dog by presynaptic alpha and beta receptors. Circ Res 41:108, 1977.

78. Starke K: Regulation of noradrenaline release by presynaptic receptor systems. Rev Biochem Pharmacol 77:1, 1977.

198

79. Rand MJ, Majewski H, McCulloch MW, Story DF: An adrenaline mediated positive feedback loop in sympathetic transmission and its possible role in hypertension. Proc IU-PHAR, Paris, 1978.
80. Amann FW, Bolli P, Kiowski W, Bühler FR: Enhanced alpha-adrenoceptor-mediated vasoconstriction in essential hypertension. Hypertension, 1981 (in press).
81. Sivertsson R: The hemodynamic importance of structural vascular changes in essential hypertension. Acta Physiol Scand 1 (Suppl 353), 1970.
82. Gombos EA, Hulet WH, Bopp P et al.: Reactivity of renal and systemic circulations to vasoconstrictor agents in normotensive and hypertensive subjects. J Clin Invest 41:203, 1962.
83. Safar ME, London GM, Weiss YA et al.: Vascular reactivity to norepinephrine and hemodynamic parameters in borderline hypertension. Am Heart J 4:480, 1975.
84. Johnson M, Ramey E, Ramwell PW: Sex and age differences in human platelet aggregation. Nature 253:355, 1975.
85. Levy MN: Sympathetic parasympathetic interactions in the heart. Circ Res 29:437, 1971.
86. Julius S, Pascual AJ, London R: Role of parasympathetic inhibition in the hyperkinetic type of borderline hypertension. Circulation 44:413, 1971.
87. Julius S, Esler M: Autonomic nervous cardiovascular regulation in borderline hypertension. Am J Cardiol 36:685, 1975.
88. Korner RI, Shaw J, Uther JB, West HJ, McRitchie RJ, Richards JG: Autonomic and non-autonomic circulatory components in essential hypertension in man. Circulation 48:107, 1973.
89. Folkow B, Rubinstein EH: Cardiovascular effects of acute and chronic stimulations of the hypothalamic defence area in the rat. Acta Physiol Scand 68:48, 1966.
90. Sleight P: Neural control of the cardiovascular system. In: Modern Trends in Cardiology. Oliver MF, ed. London: Butterworth, 1974.
91. Doba N, Reis DJ: Acute fulminating neurogenic hypertension produced by brainstem lesions in the rat. Circ Res 32:584, 1973.
92. McCubbin JW, Green JH, Page IH: Baroreceptor function in chronic renal hypertension. Circ Res 4:205, 1956.
93. Sleight P, West MJ: The effects of clonidine on the baroreflex arc in man. In: Control Action of Drugs in the Regulation of Blood Pressure. Davies DS, Reid JL, eds. London: Pitman Medical, 1975.
94. Smyth HS, Sleight P, Pickering GW: Reflex regulation of arterial pressure during sleep in man: a quantitative method of assessing baroreflex sensitivity. Circ Res k4:109, 1969.
95. Gribbin B, Pickering TG, Sleight P, Peto R: Effect of age and high blood pressure on baroreflex sensitivity in man. Circ Res 29:424, 1971.
96. Nathan MA, Reis DJ: Chronic labile hypertension produced by lesions of the nucleus tractus solitarii in the cat. Circ Res 40:78, 1977.
97. Liard JF, Cowley AW Jr, McCaa RE, McCaa CS, Guyton AC: Renin, aldosterone, body fluid volumes and the baroreceptor reflex in the development and reversal of Goldblatt hypertension in conscious dogs. Circ Res 34:549, 1974.
98. Ledingham JM, Cohen RD: The role of the heart in the pathogenesis of renal hypertension. Lancet II, 979, 1963.
99. Ferrario CM, Page IH, McCubbin JW: Increased cardiac output as a contributory factor in experimental renal hypertension in dogs. Circ Res 27:799, 1970.
100. Liard JF, Tarazi RC, Ferrario CM, Manger WM: Hemodynamic and humoral characteristics of hypertension induced by prolonged stellate ganglion stimulation in conscious dogs. Circ Res 36:455, 1975.
101. Dickinson CJ, Yu R: Mechanisms involved in the progressive pressor response to very small amounts of angiotensin in conscious rabbits. Circ Res 21 (Suppl 2):157, 1967.

102. Ferrario CM, Gildenberg PL, McCubbin JW: Cardiovascular effects of angiotensin mediated by the central nervous system. Circ Res 30:257, 1972.

103. Folkow B: Central neurohormonal mechanisms in spontaneously hypertensive rats compared with human essential hypertension. Clin Sci 48:205, 1975.

104. Goldring W, Chasis H: Hypertension and hypertensive disease. New York: The Commonwealth Fund, 1944.

105. Fries ED: Hemodynamics of hypertension. Physiol Rev 40:27, 1960.

106. Liljestrand E, Stranström M: Clinical studies on the work of the heart during rest – III. Blood flow in cases of increased arterial blood pressure with observations on the influence of pregnancy on flow. Acta Med Scand 63:142, 1925.

107. Wezler K, Böger A: Die Dynamik des arteriellen Systems. Der arterielle Blutdruck und seine Komponenten. Ergeb Physiol 41:292, 1939.

108. Eich RH, Peters FJ, Cuddy RP, Smulyan H, Lyons, RH: Hemodynamics in labile hypertension. Am Heart J 63:188, 1962.

109. Lund-Johansen P: Hemodynamics in early essential hypertension. Acta Med Scand 183 (Suppl 482):9, 1967.

110. Julius S, Conway J: Hemodynamic studies in patients with borderline blood pressure elevation. Circulation 38:282, 1968.

111. Julius S, Schork MA: Borderline hypertension – a critical review. J Chronic Dis 23:723, 1971.

112. Fouad FM, Tarazi RC, Dustan HP, Bravo EL: Hemodynamics of essential hypertension in young subjects. Am Heart J 96:646, 1978.

113. Lund-Johanssen P: Hemodynamics in essential hypertension. Clin Sci Mol Med 59:343, 1980.

114. Conway J, Julius S, Amery A: Effect of blood pressure level on the hemodynamic response to exercise. Hypertension 16:79, 1968.

115. Lund-Johansen P: Hemodynamic alterations in essential hypertension. In: Hypertension: Mechanisms and Management, p. 43. HRSE: Onset G, Kim UE, Moyer JM, eds. New York: Grune & Stratton, 1973.

116. Sannerstedt R: Hemodynamic findings at rest and during exercise in mild arterial hypertanion. Am J Med Sci 258: 70, 1969.

117. Lund-Johansen P: Beeinträchtigung der Hämodynamik bei Hypertonie: spontane Veränderungen und Auswirkungen einer medikamentösen Therapie. Acta Med Scand (Suppl 1), 1977.

118. Weiss YA, Safar ME, London G, Simon AC, Levenson JA, Milliez PM: Repeat hemodynamic determinations in borderline hypertension. Am J Med 64:382, 1978.

119. Frohlich E, Tarazi RC, Dustan HP: Hyperdynamic beta-adrenergic circulatory state. Increased beta-receptor responsiveness. Arch Intern Med 123:1, 1969.

120. Cleaveland CR, Rangno RE, Shand DG: A standardized isoproterenol sensitivity test. The effects of sinus arrhythmia, atropine and propranolol. Arch Intern Med 130:47, 1972.

121. Tarazi RC, Ibrahim MM, Dustan HP, Ferrario CM: Cardiac factors in hypertension. Circ Res 34 and 35 (Suppl 1):213, 1974.

122. Ellis CN, Julius S: Role of central blood volume in hyperkinetic borderline hypertension. Br Heart J 35:450, 1973.

123. Safar ME, Weiss YA, London GM, Frackowiak RF, Milliez PL: Cardiopulmonary blood volume in borderline hypertension. Clin Sci 47:153, 1974.

124. Ricksten SE, Yao T, Thorén P: Systemic and central vascular compliance in conscious spontaneously hypertensive rats. Clin Sci Mol Med, 1981 (in press).

125. Takeshita A, Mark AM: Decreased venous distensibility in borderline hypertension. (Abstract). Circulation 58:II-166, 1978.

126. Tarazi RC, Dustan HP, Bravo EL: The importance of plasma volume in the treatment of

hypertension. In: Betablockers – Present Status and Future Prospects. Schweizer W, ed. Bern: Huber, 1975.

127. Guyton AC, Coleman TG, Cowley AW Jr, Manning RD Jr, Horman RA Jr, Ferguson JD: A System analysis approach to understanding long-range arterial blood pressure control and hypertension. Circ Res 35:159, 1974.

128. Eich RH, Cuddy RP, Smulyan H, Lyons RH: Hemodynamics in labile hypertension: a following study. Circulation 34:299, 1966.

129. Doyle AE, Fraser JRE: Essential hypertension and inheritance of vascular reactivity. Lancet 2:509, 1961.

130. Pickering Sir George: Personal views on mechanisms of hypertension. In: Hypertension, Physiòpathology and Treatment pp. 598–606. Genest J, Koiw E, Juchel O, eds. New York: McGraw–Hill, 1977.

131. Brod J et al.: Essential hypertension: hemodynamic observations with a bearing on its pathogenesis. Lancet 2:773, 1960.

132. Lindgren P: The mesencephalon and the vasomotor system. Acta Physiol Scand 35 (Suppl 121):5, 1955.

133. Hollenberg NK, Adams DF: Hypertension and intrarenal perfusion patterns in man. Am J Med Sci 261:232, 1971.

134. Mark AL, Lawton WJ, Abboud FM, Fitz AE, Conner WE, Heistad DD: Effects of high and low sodium intake on arterial pressure and forearm vascular resistance in borderline hypertension. Circ Res 36 (Suppl 1):1–194, 1975.

135. Conway J: A vascular abnormality in hypertension. A study of blood flow in the forearm. Circulation 27:520, 1963.

136. Amery A, Bossaert H, Verstracle M: Muscle blood flow in normal and hypertensive subjects. Am Heart J 78:211, 1969.

137. Brod J, Fencl V, Heijl Z, Jirka J, Ulrych M: General and regional hemodynamic pattern underlying essential hypertension. Clin Sci 23:339, 1962.

138. Tobian L, Binion JI: Tissue cations and water in arterial hypertension. Circulation 5:754, 1952.

139. Blaustein MP, Lang S, James-Kracke M: Cellular basis of sodium-induced hypertension. In: Frontiers in Hypertension Research, p. 87. Laragh JH, Bühler R, Selsin DW, eds. New York: Springer, 1981.

140. Constantopoulos BM, Kusumoto JM, Rono. Ortaga P, Granger R, Boucher R, Genest J: Arterial water, cations and norepinephrine in early and late renovascular hypertension. Am J Physiol 228:1415, 1975.

141. Brunner HR, Chang P, Wallach R, Sealey JE, Laragh JH: Angiotensin II vascular receptors: their avidity in relationship to sodium balance, the autonomic nervous system, and hypertension. J Clin Invest 51:58, 1972.

142. Mendlowitz M, Naftchi NE, Bobrow EB, Wolf RL, Gitlow SE: The effect of aldosterone on electrolytes and on digital vascular reactivity – I. 1.Norepinephrine in normotensive, hypertensive and hypotensive subjects. Am Heart J 65:93, 1963.

143. Wissler RW: The arterial medial cell, smooth muscle or multifunctional mesenchyme. Circulation 36:1, 1967.

144. Bühler FR: Essentielle Hypertonie: Adrenerges Kontrollsystem, Renin–Angiotensin–Effektorachse, Niere und Alter, Schweiz Med Wochenschr 106:1798, 1976.

145. Van Brummelen P, Bühler FR, Kiowski W, Amann FW: Age-related decrease in cardiac and peripheral vascular responsibeness to isoproterenol. Clin Sci 60:571, 1981.

146. Bühler FR, Kiowski W, Landmann R, van Brummelen P, amann W, Bolli P, Bertel O: Changing role of beta and alpha adrenoceptor-mediated cardiovascular responses in the transition from a high cardiac output into a high peripheral resistance phase in essential hypertension. In:Frontiers in Hypertension Research, Laragh JH, Buâbühler FR, Seldin DW, eds. New York: Springer, 1981.

147. McGiff JC, Itskovitz HD: Prostaglandins and the kidney. Circ Res 33:479, 1973.
148. Carretero OA, Seidi AG: Renal kallikrein localisation and possible role in renal function. Fed Proc 35:194, 1976.
149. Corcoran AC, Kohlstaedt KG, Page IH: Changes of arterial blood pressure and renal hemodynamics by injection of angiotensin in human beings. Proc Soc Exp Biol Med 46:244, 1941.
150. De Bono E, Lee GJ, Mottram FR, Pickering GW, Brown JJ, Keen H, Peart WS, Sanderson PH: The action of angiotensin in man. Clin Sci 25:123, 1967.
151. Laragh JH, Angers M, Kelly WG, Ueberman S: Hypotensive agents and pressor substances. The effect of epinephrine, norepinephrine, angiotensin II and others on the secretory rate of aldosterone in man. JAMA 174: 234, 1960.
152. Selkurt EG: Effect of pulse pressure and mean arterial pressure modification on renal hemodynamics and electrolyte and water excretion. Circulation 4:541, 1951.
153. Thomson JMA, Dickinson CJ: Relation between pressure and sodium excretion in perfused kidneys from rabbits with experimental hypertension. Lancet 2:1362, 1973.
154. Guyton AC, Coleman TG, Cowley Am, Scheel KW, Manning RA, Norman RA: Arterial pressure regulation. Overriding dominance of the kidneys in long-term regulation and in hypertension. Am J Med 52:584, 1972.
155. Brown JJ, Lever AF, Robertson JIS, Schalekamp MA: Renal abnormality of essential hypertension. Lancet 2:320, 1974.
156. Brown JJ, Fraser R, Lever AF, Morton JJ, Robertson JIS, Schalekamp MADH: Mechanisms in hypertension: a personal view in hypertension, pp. 529–548, Genest J, Koiw E, Kurchel O, eds. New York: McGraw-Hill, 1977.
157. Hollenberg NK, Adams DF, Salomon HS, Rashid A, Abrams HL, Merrill JD: Senescence and the renal vasculature in normal man. Circ Res 34:304, 1974.
158. Birkenhäger WH, Schalekamp MADM: Control Mechanisms in Hypertension. Amsterdam: Elsevier, 1976.
159. Hollenberg NK, Boruchi LJ, Adams DF: The renal vasculature in early essential hypertension: evidence for a pathogenetic role. Medicine 57:167, 1978.
160. Bianchi G, Picotti GB, Bracchi G, Cusi D, Gatti M, Lupi GP, Ferrari PL, Barlussina C, Combo G, Gori D: Familial hypertension and hormonal profile, renal hemodynamics and body fluids of young normotensive subjects. Clin Sci Mol Med 55:3675, 1973.
161. Deen WM, Robertson CR, Brenner BM: Glomerular ultrafiltration. Fed Proc 33:15, 1974.
162. Nasjletti A, Coline-Chowrio J, McGiff JC: Disapearance of bradykinin in the renal circulation of dogs. Circ Res 37:1975.
163. Hollenberg NK, Adams DF, Solomon H, Chenitz WR, Burger BM, Abrams HL: Renal vascular tone in essential and secondary hypertension: hemodynamic and angiographic responses to vasodilators. Medicine 54:29, 1975.
164. Tuck ML, Sullivan JM, Hollenberg NK, Dluhy RG, Williams GH: Hemodynamic and endocrine response pattern in young patients with normal renin essential hypertension. Clin Res 21:505, 1973.
165. Hollenberg NK, Adams DF: The renal circulation in hypertensive disease. Am J Med 60:773, 1976.
166. Schalekamp MADH, Krauss XH, Birkenhäger WH: Renin suppression in hypertension in relation to body fluid volumes, patterns of sodium excretion and renal hemodynamics. Clin Sci Mol Med 45 (Suppl 1):2835, 1973.
167. Tobian L: Salt and hypertension. In: Hypertension, Physiopathology and Treatment, pp. 423–433. Genest J, Koiw E, Juchel O, eds. New York: McGraw-Hill, 1977.
168. Holloway ET, Bohr DF: Reactivity of vascular smooth muscle in hypertensive rats. Circ Res 33:678, 1973.

169. Laragh JH: Vasoconstriction volume analysis for understanding and treating hypertension. The use of renin and aldosterone profiles. In: Hypertension Manual, pp. 823–851, Laragh JH, ed. New York: York Medical, 1973.

170. Man in 't Veld AJ, Schalekamp MADH: Haemodynamics of renoprival hypertension in man: studies during graded fluid withdrawal. Clin Sci Mol Med 59:1655, 1980.

171. Cranston WI, Brown W: diurnal variation in plasma volume in normal and hypertensive subjects. Clin Sci 25:107, 1963.

172. Tarazi RC, Dustan HP, Frohlich ED: Plasma volume in men with hypertension. Engl J Med 278:762, 1968.

173. Julius S, Pacual AV, Reilly X, London R: Abnormalities of plasma volume in borderline hypertension. Arch Int Med 127:116, 1971.

174. Weidmann P, Steffen F, Bühler FR, Reubi FC: The sodium/volume renin product, an important determinant of blood pressure in normal subjects and hemodialyses patients. Clin Res 23:377A, 1975.

175. Parving HM, Rossing M, Jensen HAE: Increase of metabolic turnover rate and transcapillary escape rate of albumin in essential hypertension. Circ Res 35:544, 1974.

176. Tarazi RC, Dustan HP, Frohlich ED: Relation of plasma to interstitial fluid volumein essential hypertension. Circulation 40:357, 1969.

177. Tarazi RC: Hemodynamic role of extra-cellular fluid in hypertension. Circ Res 38 (Suppl II): 73, 1976.

178. Chien S, Usami S, McAllister RL, S.F.F., Gregersen MI: Blood volume and age: repeated measurements of normal men after 17 years. J Appl Physiol 21:583, 1966.

179. Schalekamp MADH, Krauss XH, Schalekamp-Kuyken MPA, Kolsters G, Birkenhäger WH: Studies on the mechanism of hypernatriuresis in essential hypertension in relation to measurements of plasma renin concentration, body fluid compartment and renal function. Clin Sci Mol Med 41:219, 1971.

180. Beretta-Piccoli C, Davies DL, Boddy K, Brown JJ, Cumming AMM, East WB, Fraser R, Lever AF, Padfield PL, Robertson JIS, Weidmann P, Williams E: Abnormal relations of exchangeable and total body sodium to arterial pressure in essential hypertension. Clin Sci Mol Med, 1981 (in press).

181. Gross F, Brunner H, Ziegler M: Renin–angiotensin system, aldosterone and sodium balance. Recent Prog Harm Res 21:119, 1965.

182. Laragh JH, Sealey JE: The renin–angiotensin–aldosterone hormonal system and regulation of sodium, potassium and blood pressure homeostasis. In: Handbook of Physiology – Renal Physiology, p. 831. Orloff J, Berliner RW, eds. Baltimore: Waverly, 1974.

183. Vander AJ, Luciano JR: Neural and humoral control of renin release in salt depletion. Circulat Res 21 (Suppl 2):69, 1967.

184. Starke K, Schümann HJ: Interactions of angiotensin, phenoxybenzamine and propranolol on adrenaline release during sympathetic nerve stimulation. Eur J. Pharmacol 18:27, 1972.

185. Brunner HR, Laragh JH, Baer L, Newton MD, Goodwin FT, Krakoff LR, Bard RH, Büler FR: Essential hypertension: renin and aldosterone, heart attack and stroke. N Engl J Med 286:441, 1972.

186. Laragh JH, Baer L, Brunner HR, Büler FR, Sealey JE, Vaughen ED Jr: Renin, angiotensin and aldosterone system in pathogenesis and management of hypertensive vascular disease. Am J Med 52:633, 1972.

187. Laragh JH: Hypertension manual. New York: Dun-Donelley, 1975.

188. Michelakis AM, McAllister RG Jr: Renin secretion, adrenergic blockade and hypertension. In: Control of Renin Secretion, p. 83. Assaykeen TA, ed. New York: Plenum, 1972.

189. Bühler FR, Baer L, Vaughan ED et al.: Inhibition of renin secretion by propranolol: a specific treatment of renal hypertension? J Clin Invest 51:17a, 1972.

190. Gavras H, Brunner HR, Laragh JH, Sealey JE, Gavras I, Vukovich RA: Angiotensin converting enzyme inhibitor to identify and treat vasoconstrictor and volume factors in hypertensive patients. N Engl J Med 291:817, 1974.
191. Brunner HR, Gavras H, Laragh JH, Sealey JE, Gavras I, Vukovich RA: Hypertension in an: exposure of the renin and sodium components using angiotensin II blockade. Circ Res 34 (Suppl I): 33, 1974.
192. Zanchetti A, Stella A: Neural control of renin release. Clin Sci Mol Med 48:215s, 1975.
193. Winer N, Chokshi DS, Yoon MS, Freedman AD: Adrenergic receptor mediation of renin secretion. J Clin Endocrinol Metab 19:1168, 1969.
194. Pettinger WA, Mitchell HC: Clinical Pharmacology of angiotensin antagonists. Fed Proc 35:2521, 1976.
195. Wathaen RL, Kingsbury WS, Stouder DA, Schneider EG, Rostorfer HH: Effects of infusion of catecholamines and angiotensin II on renin release in anesthetized dogs. Am J Physiol 209:1012, 1965.
196. De Champlain J, Genest J, Veyrat R, Boucher R: Factors controlling renin in man. Arch Intern Med 117:355, 1966.
197. Gordon RD, Wolfe LK, Island DP, Liddle GW: Diurnal rhythm in plasma renin activity in man. J Clin Invest 45:1587, 1966.
198. Gordon RD, Kuchel O, Liddle GW, Island DP: Role of the sympathetic nervous system in regulating renin and aldosterone production in man. J Clin Invest 46:599, 1967.
199. Bühler FR, Marbet G, Patel U, Burkart F: Reninsuppressive potency of various beta adrenergic blocking agents at supine rest and during upright exercise. Clin Sci 48:61s, 1975.
200. Peytremann A, Favre L, Vallotton MG: Effect of cold pressure test and 2-deoxy-d-glucose infusion on plasma renin activity in man. Eur J Clin Invest 2:432, 1972.
201. Brubacher ES, Vander AJ: Sodium deprivation and renin secretion in ananesthetized dogs. Am J Physiol 214:15, 1968.
202. Assaykeen TA, Tanigawa H, Allison DJ: Effect of adrenoceptor blocking agents on the renin response to isoproterenol in dogs. Eur J Pharmacol 26:185, 1974.
203. Weidmann P, De Myttenaeve-Bursztein S, Maxwell MH, De Lima J: Effects of ageing on plasma renin and aldosterone in normal man. Kidney Int 8:325, 1975.
204. Tuck ML, Williams GH, Cain JP, Sullivan JM, Dluhy RG: Relation of age, diastolic blood pressure and known duration of hypertension to presence of low renin essential hypertension. Am J Cardiol 32:637, 1973.
205. Padfield PL, Nelson CS, Beevers DG, Hawthorne VM, Greaves DA, Duncan S, Glyth M, Yong J: Hypertension and the renin–angiotensin system in an unselected population. In: Hypertension – Its Nature and Treatment, p. 19. Burley DM, Birdwood GFB, Fryer JH, Taylor SH, eds. Horsham, Sussex: Ciba Laboratories, 1975.
206. Fagard R, Amery A, Reybrouck T, Lijnen P, Billiet L, Joossens JV: Plasma renin levels and systemic heamodynamics in essential hypertension. Clin Sci Mol Med 52:591, 1977.
207. Dustan HP, Tarazi Rc, Frohlich ED: Functional correlates of plasma renin activity in hypertensive patients. Circulation 41:555, 1970.
208. Burkart F, Bühler FR, Pfister M, Lütold BE, Küng M: Hemodynamic responses to exercise and acute beta-blockade in renin subtypes of essential hypertenaion. Clin Sci 51:493s, 1976.
209. Brunner HR, Sealey JE, Laragh JH: Renin as a risk factor in essential hypertension: more evidence. Am J Med 55:295, 1973.
210. DeQuattro V, Muira Y: Neurogenic factors in human hypertension: mechanism or myth? Am J Med 55: 362, 1973.
211. Kiowski W, Bertel O, Bühler FR: The renin type of essential hypertension and the rela-

tionships between plasma catecholamines, renin and age. In: Central Nervous System and Hypertension. Meyer Ph, ed. Paris: Flammarion, 1978.

212. Bühler FR, Bertel O, Kiowski W: Plasma noradrenaline and adrenaline and beta-adrenoceptor responsiveness in renin subgroups of essential hypertension. Clin Sci 55-57s, 1978.

213. Perini Ch, Rauchfleisch W, Bühler FR: Personality structure and renin type in essential hypertension (submitted).

214. Bühler FR, Laragh JH, Baer L, Vaughan ED Jr, Brunner HR: Propranolol inhibition of renin secretion: a specific approach to diagnosis and treatment of renin.dependent hypertensive diseases. N Engl J Med 286:1209, 1972.

215. Bühler FR, Laragh JH, Vaughan ED Jr, Brunner HR, Gavras H, Baer L: The antihypertensive action of propranolol: specific antirenin responses in high and normal renin essential, renal, renovascular and malignant hypertension. Am J Cardiol 32:511, 1973.

216. Hollified JW, Sherman K, Vander Zwaag R, Shand DG: Proposed mechanisms of propranolol's antihypertensive effect in essential hypertension. N Engl J Med 295:68, 1976.

217. Bühler FR: Antihypertensive actions of betablockers. In: Frontiers in Hypertension Research, p. 423. Laragh JH, Bühler FR, Seldin DW, eds. New York: Springer, 1981.

218. José A, Crout JR, Kaplan NM: Suppressed plasma renin activity in essential hypertension. Role of plasma volume, blood pressure and sympathetic nervous system. Ann Intern Med 72:9, 1970.

219. Distler A, Keim HJ, Philipp Th: Austauschbares Natrium, Gesamtkörperkalium, Plasmavolumen und Blutdruck-senkende Wirkung verschiedener Diuretika bei Patienten mit essentieller Hypertonie und niedrigen Plasmarenin. Dtsch Med Wochenschr 99:864, 1974.

220. Weidmann P, Hirsch D, Beretta-Piccoli C, Reubi FC, Ziegler W: Beziehungen zwischen Blutdruck, Blutvolumen, Plasmarenin und Urinkatecholaminen bei Normalpersonen und bei der benignen essentiellen Hypertonie. Schweiz Med Wochenschr. 106:1741, 1976.

221. Luetscher JA, Weinberger NH, Dowdy AD, Nokes GW, Balikian H, Brodie A, Willoughby S: Effects of sodium loading, sodiumdepletion and posture on plasma aldosterone concentration and renin activity in hypertensive patients. J Clin Endocrinol Metab 29:1310, 1969.

222. Dunn MJ, Tanner RL: Low renin essential hypertension. In: Hypertension: Physiopathology and Treatment, p. 349. Genest J, Koiw E, Kuchel O, eds. New York: Mc Graw-Hill, 1977.

223. Helmer OM, Judson WE: Metabolic studies on hypertensive patients with suppressed plasma renin activity not due to hyperaldosteronism. Circulation 38:965, 1968.

224. Melby JC, Dale SL, Grekin RJ, Gaunt R, Wilson TE: 18-hydroxy-II-seoxycorticosterone (18-OH-DOC) secretion in experimental and human hypertension. Recent Prog Horm Res 28:287, 1972.

225. Sennett JA, Brown RD, Island DP et al.: Evidence for a new mineralocorticoid in patients with low renin essential hypertension. Circ Res 36 (Suppl 1-2-1-9) 1975.

226. Bühler FR, Laragh JH, Sealey JE, Brunner HR: Plasma aldosterone renin interrelationships in various forms of essential hypertension: studies using a rapid assay of plasma aldosterone. Am J Cardiol 32:554, 1973.

227. Williams GH, Rose LI, Dluhy RG et al.: Abnormal responsibeness of the renin aldosterone system to acute stimulation in patients with essential hypertension. Ann Intern Med 72:213, 1970.

228. Gunnnels JC, McGuffin Wl, Robinson RR, Grim CE, Wells S, Silver D, Glenn JF: Hypertension adrenalabnormalities, and alterations in plasma renin activity. Ann Intern Med 73:901-911, 1970.

229. Crane MG, Harris JJ: Effect of spironolactone in hypertensive patients. Am J Med Sci 260:311, 1970.

230. Vaughan ED Jr, Laragh JH, Gavras I, Bühler FR, Gavras H, Brunner HR: The volume factor in low and normal renin essential hypertension. Its treatment with either spironolactone or chlorthalidone. Am J Cardiol 32:523, 1973.
231. Early LE, Daugharty TM: Sodium metabolism. N Engl J Med 281:72, 1969.
232. Bühler FR, Bertel O, Lütold BE: Simplified and age-stratified antihypertensive therapy based on beta-blockers. Cardiovasc Med 3:135, 1978.
233. Drayer JIM, Keim HJ, Weger MA, Case DB, Laragh JH: Unexpected pressor response to propranolol in essenial hypertension. Am J Med 60:897, 1976.
234. Bolli P, Amann FW, Bühler FR: Antihypertensive response to postsynaptic β-blockade with prazosin in low and normal renin hypertension. J Cardiovasc Pharmacol 2:399S, 1980.

12. GENETICS IN HUMAN HYPERTENSION

John M. Ledingham

1. INTRODUCTION

This chapter is in the section devoted to primary hypertension, but it must be remembered that primary hypertension itself is not a clearly defined entity and that in the past sixty years a number of disease processes, including phaeochromocytoma and primary aldosteronism, have been defined and thereby removed from within the category of primary hypertension. This process is likely to continue until all genetic and environmental factors involved in the wide spectrum of disease known as primary hypertension have been discovered. Therefore, before considering the genetics of primary hypertension, brief reference should be made to the inherited factor in secondary hypertension. Thus, phaeochromocytoma may develop in association with von Recklinghausen's disease and as part of a multiple endocrinopathy associated with medullary carcinoma of the thyroid and hyperplasia or multiple adenomata of the parathyroid glands (Sipple's syndrome). Both of these ectodermal dysplasias are inherited as autosomal dominant traits [1, 2]. Although no clear genetic factor has emerged in the case of primary aldosteronism due to an adrenal adenoma, the situation is more complex in the case of primary aldosteronism associated with adrenal hyperplasia and the suggestion has been made that this represents one end of the spectrum of primary hypertension [3].

Congenital adrenal hyperplasia due to 11-hydroxylase [4] or 17-hydroxylase deficiency [5] results in hypertension and here autosomal recessive inheritance is involved. Lastly, mention should be made of certain forms of renal disease, including polycystic disease and the hereditary nephropathies, which have an important genetic basis and which may result in hypertension. A large number of causes of secondary hypertension, in which there is evidence of Mendelian inheritance, have been listed [6].

With these considerations in mind, attention will now be given to the hereditary factor in what is conventionally termed primary hypertension.

Amery, A. (ed.) Hypertensive Cardiovascular Disease: Pathophysiology and Treatment
© *1982, Martinus Nijhoff Publishers. The Hague / Boston / London*
ISBN-13: 978-94-009-7478-4

2. EVIDENCE FOR INVOLVEMENT OF A GENETIC FACTOR IN PRIMARY HYPERTENSION

For very many years clinicians have been aware that hypertension tends to run in families. This, by itself, does not establish the existence of a genetic component to hypertension, since families tend to share the same environment and may pass from one generation to the next patterns of behaviour, including those relating, for example, to diet and to exercise, which theoretically could be responsible. Such considerations apply to studies of the correlation between the blood pressure of propositi and their first degree relatives and may influence the interpretation of the significance of differences observed in the degree of concordance of blood pressure within monozygotic and dizygotic twinships.

Studies have been made of the correlation between the blood pressures of hypertensive propositi and their first degree relatives [7, 8] and between randomly selected individuals and their first degree relatives [9–14]. For the latter group linear regression analysis revealed a correlation coefficient of between 0.13 and 0.34 for systolic and rather less for diastolic pressure, there being little difference between parent–child and sib–sib correlations. Taking a figure of 0.25, the variance of blood pressure for an individual which is accounted for by both parents is 0.5, which implies that at least 50 % of the variance of the blood pressure of an individual must be attributable to factors other than hereditary. The correlation for systolic and diastolic pressure between spouses has been reported to be either statistically insignificant [8, 15] or weakly positive [12]. Furthermore, no correlation was found between the blood pressure of parents and their adopted children and a significant, but weak correlation between natural and adopted sibs within the same family [16, 17].

Studies of the correlation between the blood pressure in twins [13, 18–20] revealed close concordance for monozygotic twins with correlation coefficients of 0.55 and 0.58 for systolic and diastolic pressures respectively, and in the case of dizygotic twins the correlation coefficient was approximately half and similar to that between first degree relatives, excluding twins [13]. Although it is probably true to say that dizygotic twins do not share so precisely the same environment as monozygotic twins, this finding strongly supports the hypothesis that these correlations mainly represent an important genetic factor. The full interpretation of these many correlations lies beyond the scope of this chapter, but the reader may be referred to a recent survey by Feinleib [21].

The total variance of the blood pressure is composed of factors:

1) between individuals:
    i) genetic variance.
    ii) environmental variance.

2) within individual:

    intra-person variance, which includes measurement error and short-term temporal variation in blood pressure from multiple undefined causes, including circadian rhythms.

Unfortunately, this is an oversimplification, since genetic and environmental variances cannot be clearly separated on account of genetic–environmental interactions. Thus the apparent genetic variance estimated for one population could differ from another if the environments differed in such a manner as to alter the degree of genetic–environmental interaction.

When correlations are obtained for blood pressure between specified pairs of individuals, such as monozygotic or dizygotic twins, it cannot be concluded that the correlation exclusively represents the genetic variance, since it inevitably includes an element of shared environment and this is likely to be of more importance in monozygotic than in dizygotic twins. The influence of shared environment depends not only on the length of time of sharing and therefore on the age when the comparison is made, but also on the period of life over which the environment is shared. Thus the absent or low correlation observed between spouses suggests that the influence of environment in adult life is small; this is supported by the observation that, whereas there is no correlation between parent and adopted child, there is an undoubted, albeit low, correlation between adopted and natural children in the same family, who share the same environment at a younger age.

Another problem is that it is customary to regard the genetic variance to be additive, between generations, with half the variance deriving from each parent. However, it is more than likely that dominance occurs in relation to some genes and that interaction between genes (epistatic interactions) is also present which would result in a lower correlation between parent and child than between siblings.

Feinleib [21] concludes with the estimate that in the National Heart and Lung Institute Twin Study in the U.S.A. about 50% of the population variance of blood pressure may be attributed to genetic factors, the remainder being due to a combination of environmental and intraperson variance.

3. THE MODE OF INHERITANCE IN PRIMARY HYPERTENSION

In the previous section, the evidence for a hereditary factor in the aetiology of essential hypertension has been presented and it has been assumed that multiple genes are involved. We must now consider more closely the mode of inheritance and the evidence that this is indeed polygenic.

Controversy has featured frequently in the history of this subject, which reached its peak some twenty years ago in the form of a series of papers and letters from Platt and his supporters, on the one hand, who favoured a single specific dominant gene and Pickering and his supporters, on the other, who favoured polygenic inheritance. Pickering's hypothesis was based on studies of the frequency distribution of blood pressure in an out-patient hospital population [8]. It was shown that both systolic and diastolic blood pressure rose with age and that the range progressively widened; at no time were the distribution curves bimodal.

Pickering claimed, justifiably, that there was no evidence of a dividing line separating those in the lower range from those in the higher pressure range and thereby destroyed the concept of essential hypertension as a dis-

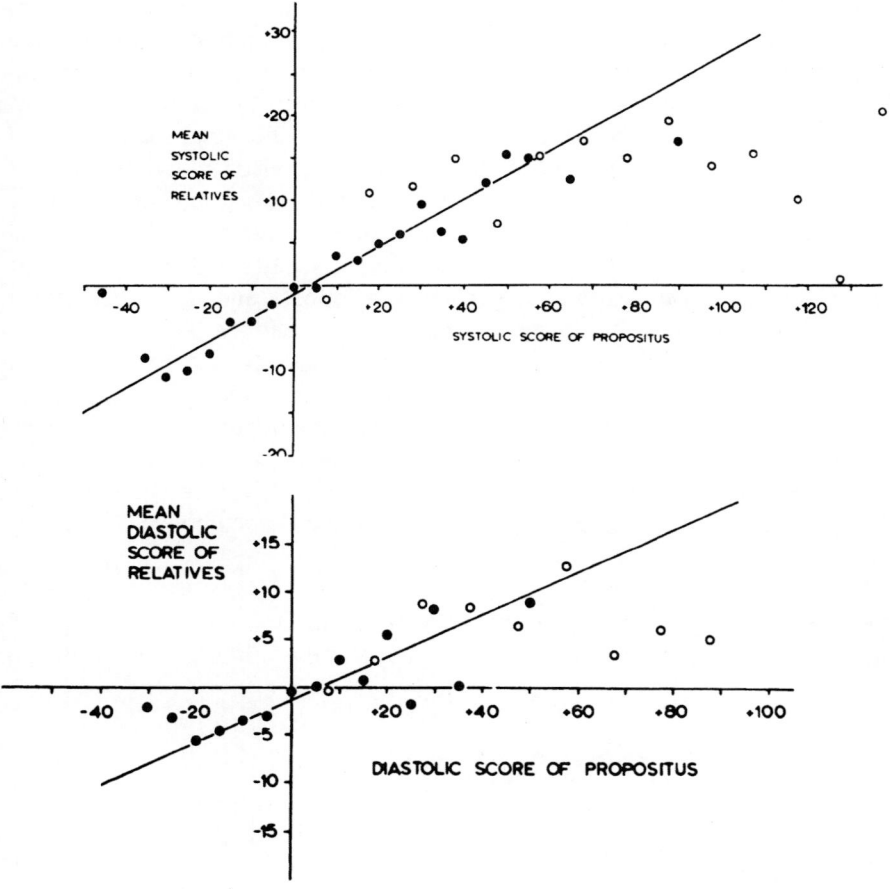

Figure 1. The relationship between mean systolic (upper) and diastolic (lower) Scores of first degree relatives and those of propositi: general population in Welsh study (●), compared with hospitalised hypertensives' families (○). Data for latter from cases of essential hypertension provided by Pickering and Platt (personal communications). The regression line is drawn for the Welsh study. (Figure reproduced from Miall [24] by courtesy of New York Academy of Sciences.)

ease entity, naturally rather than arbitrarily, demarcated from the rest of the population. Miall and Oldham [22, 23] confirmed these findings in a randomly selected population and demonstrated a linear regression of blood pressure of first degree relatives on that of the propositi (Figure 1, data for general population) [24], but in order to do so they had to make use of age- and sex-adjusted blood pressure scores. This finding strongly supported the multifactorial mode of inheritance. Platt questioned the validity of the use of age- and sex-adjusted scores and examined the frequency distribution of blood pressure in the sibs of hypertensive propositi all within a narrow age range; using his and the data of Sobye et al. [7], he claimed that the frequency distribution curve for the sibs was bimodal with a sharp dip at 150 mm Hg systolic and 90 mm Hg diastolic, suggesting that in this group a single dominant gene was involved [25]. Pickering criticised the interpretation of these distribution curves and failed to confirm bimodality [26]. Subsequent studies have supported Pickering's [9, 10] rather than Platt's [27, 28] hypothesis, and it is now agreed that, in general, raised blood pressure is inherited polygenically. However, the possibility remains that for extremely high blood pressure, inheritance may be by one or possibly more, powerful dominant genes. It has been pointed out [29] that, although the regression line relating blood pressure of hypertensive propositi and their first degree relatives is linear over the lower ranges of hypertension it becomes discontinuous for more severe hypertension in the propositi (Figure 1, data for hospitalised hypertensives), which implies two qualitatively different populations and the possibility of a single dominant gene operating at this level. The question of the mode of inheritance for all degrees of severity of hypertension has not yet been fully resolved and will have to await the definition of the nature of the many genotypically determined biochemical abnormalities.

Attempts have been made to estimate the number of gene loci involved in determining the level of blood pressure using different methods [30] and figures of between six and ten obtained, but these are likely to be underestimates.

4. BIOCHEMICAL GENETICS OF BLOOD PRESSURE CONTROL SYSTEMS THOUGHT TO BE INVOLVED IN PATHOGENESIS OF ESSENTIAL HYPERTENSION

The pathogenesis or pathological physiology of essential hypertension is still a matter of great debate and is largely unsolved. Thus, it is still uncertain what part is played by derangements within the sympathetic nervous sytem in essential hypertension, nor do we know the precise nature of any alteration in renal function involved in its development. Faced with these major uncertainties, it is extremely hard to know in which direction to search for genetic determinants of steps in this complex pathogenetic chain. The procedure has been to select a known blood pressure control system, which may or may not be primarily or secondarily involved in essential hypertension, and then to search for genetic polymorphisms within this system. The phenotypes are then defined in terms of specific biochemical variables and the pattern of inheritance of each variable determined by pedigree analysis in families identified as possessing segregating alleles. If it can then be shown that genetically controlled phenotypes possess significantly different blood pressures, a causal role for the particular genes is established [31]. Examples of this approach in the case of the sympathetic nervous system have been made in regard to plasma dopamine-β-hydroxyglase (DBH) [32], red cell catechol-O-methyltransferase (COMT) [33] and platelet monomamine oxidase (MAO) [34]. Although clear evidence of the heritability of these enzymes has been obtained, as yet these studies have been unrewarding in regard to their relevance to essential hypertension. No significant correlation of DBH with blood pressure in randomly selected subjects has been found [35], and information on the correlation of red cell COMT and platelet MAO with blood pressure is lacking.

The genetic basis for other blood pressure regulating systems, which may be implicated in essential hypertension, has not been explored through studies of familial aggregation. However, the kallikrein–kinin system is now thought to be involved in renal vasodilatation and sodium excretion and thereby in blood pressure regulation. Familial aggregation in childhood has been demonstrated in this system. Furthermore, families with the lowest urinary kallikrein were found to have a significantly higher blood pressure than those with the highest urinary kallikrein [36]. The findings were reproducible at a follow-up study three to four years later [37].

The role of intracellular sodium and potassium in the pathogenesis of essential hypertension is still controversial; recently the hypothesis has been advanced that a linked calcium–sodium exchange system exists across cell membranes and that when sodium concentration increases within the cell, calcium concentration does likewise. If this process takes place in the smooth muscle of vascular tissue, it could be responsible for an increase in tone and so for an increase in arterial resistance [38]. The smooth muscle cell of arteriolar wall is not easily amenable to study, but in leucocytes from patients with essential hypertension an increase in cell sodium has been reported and has been attributed to a reduction in the sodium efflux rate constant [39]. In erythrocytes which have been subjected to preliminary sodium loading and potassium depletion, the ratio of the rate of sodium efflux to that of potassium influx during recovery has been shown to be depressed in essential hypertension and in about 50% of young normotensive children of hypertensive parents [40]. This observation suggests the possibility of a genetically determined abnormality in cell sodium and potassium transport which could be involved in the pathogenesis of essential hypertension.

5. ASSOCIATION OF GENETIC TRAITS NOT KNOWN TO BE DIRECTLY INVOLVED IN BLOOD PRESSURE REGULATION, WITH ESSENTIAL HYPERTENSION

In the ABO blood group system, an association has been described between higher blood pressure and greater incidence of blood group O and lesser incidence of group A [41, 42]. In the MN system, NN has been reported to be associated with higher and MM with lower blood pressure [43], but this has not been confirmed [44] and in the MNS system as a whole, S has been reported to be significantly less and s more frequent in essential hypertensive than in normotensive white subjects. Neither of these two blood group systems has a recognised relationship with any system which is known to be implicated in blood pressure regulation, but if the population under study were in linkage equilibrium, it must be postulated that some cause and effect relationship exists between these two variables.

6. THE SEARCH FOR HEREDITARILY DETERMINED RESPONSES TO POSSIBLE ENVIRONEMENTAL FACTORS INVOLVED IN ESSENTIAL HYPERTENSION

There have been a number of studies of the responses of hypertensive individuals to various external stimuli, such as cold, psychological stress, exercise stress and salt loading. Usually, the responses in the hypertensive individuals have been compared with those in normotensive control subjects and it has not been possible to conclude whether any abnormal response is a possible cause, as opposed to a consequence, of the hypertension. More recently attention has been directed to such studies in the children of hypertensive parents, before clinically recognised hypertension has developed. A comparison of the response in such children with that in children of normotensive parents can give a clue to possible interactions between genetic and hereditary factors involved in the development of hypertension.

The effect of the stress of mental arithmetic on blood pressure and heart rate has been studied in adolescents with and without a family history of hypertension [45]. Those with a family history of hypertension exhibited a greater and more protracted elevation of systolic and diastolic pressure and heart rate and a higher poststress plasma catecholamine level. The adolescents with a family history of hypertension were arbitrarily placed in subgroups according to the resting level of blood pressure and the response to stress, but no clear evidence of a natural aggregation into these subgroups emerged. Nonetheless, the findings strongly support the concept that an accentuated sympathetic response to mental stress may be a factor in the development of hypertension and represent gene–environment interaction.

After an intravenous infusion of Ringer lactate, the maximum rate of urinary sodium excretion was greater in normotensive sons of hypertensive than of normotensive parents, suggesting a gene–environment interaction in regard to sodium handling which could be relevant to the development of hypertension [46]. A similar study involving an older group of normotensive first degree relatives of hypertensives, showed that over the 24-h period following infusion, actually less sodium was excreted than by normotensive relatives of normotensives [47]. A prolonged increased dietary intake of sodium raises blood pressure in both normal and hypertensive subjects [48], the rise being somewhat greater in the latter.

7. CONCLUSION

The elucidation of the genetic factors involved in determining the level of blood pressure in an individual in any given population is still only in its earliest stages. New models for the analysis of quantitative inheritance in man have recently been developed [49, 50]. These involve the sampling of family sets comprising an index case, a sibling, a first cousin and two persons having an environmental connection, one being the spouse and the other an unrelated person matched to the index case. Using these methods, it should be possible to resolve genetic and environmental effects, including gene–environment interactions, and to partition the genetic variance into additive, dominant, epistatic, X-linked and autosomal components.

The overwhelming importance of gene–environment interactions is only now being recognised from the observations that in certain unacculturated populations blood pressure does not rise with age [51]; yet when individuals of such populations either emigrate or become exposed to patterns of social life practised by the so-called advanced societies [52, 53] their blood pressure rises with age in a manner similar to that seen in those societies. Gene–environment interaction in one developed country, Japan, has been estimated, from a study of concordance rate in hypertensive twins exposed to the same or different environments, to contribute 9 % to the total variance of blood pressure [30].

REFERENCES

1. Crowe FW, Schull WJ, Neel JV: A Clinical Pathological and Genetic Study of Multiple Neurofibromatosis, Springfield, Ill: Charles C Thomas, 1956.

214

2. Catalone WJ, Engelman K, Ketcham AS, Hammond WG: Familial medullary thyroid carcinoma, phaeochromocytoma and parathyroid adenoma (Sipple's syndrome). Study of a kindred. Cancer 28:1245–1254, 1971.

3. Brown JJ, Lever AF, Robertson JIS, Beevers DG, Alison MM, Cumming DL, Davies R, Fraser R, Mason P, Morton JJ, Tree M: Are idiopathic hyperaldosteronism and low-renin hypertension variants of essential hypertension? Ann Clin Biochem 16:380–388, 1979.

4. Eberlein WR, Bongiovanni AM: Plasma and Urinary corticosteroids in the hypertensive form of congenital adrenal hyperplasia. J Biol Chem 223:85–94, 1956.

5. Biglieri EG, Herron MA, Brust N: 17-hydroxylation defiency in man. J Clin Invest 45:1946–1954, 1966.

6. Murphy EA: Genetics in hypertension. Circ Res 32, 33 (Suppl 1):129–137, 1973.

7. Sobye P: Heredity in Essential Hypertension and Nephrosclerosis. Copenhagen: Ejnar Munksgaard, 1948.

8. Hamilton M, Pickering GW, Fraser Roberts JA, Sowry GSC: The aetiology of essential hypertension-4. The role of inheritance. Clin Sci, 13:273–304, 1954.

9. Miall WE, Oldham PD: The hereditary factor in arterial hypertension. Br Med J 1:75–80, 1963.

10. Ostfeld AM, Paul O: The inheritance of hypertension. Lancet 1:575–579, 1963.

11. Johnson BC, Epstein FH, Kjelsberg MU: Distribution and familial studies of blood pressure and serum cholesterol levels in a total community – Tecumseh, Michigan. J Chron Dis 18:147–160, 1965.

12. Hayes CG, Tyroler HA, Cassel JC: Family aggregation of blood pressure in Evans County, Georgia. Arch Int Med 128:965–975, 1971.

13. Feinleib M, Garrison MS, Borhani MD, Rosenman R, Christian J: Studies of hypertension in twins. In: Epidemiology and Control of Hypertension, pp. 3–17. Paul O, ed. New York: Stratton Intercontinental, 1975.

14. Kass E, Zinner SH, Margolius HS, Lee YH, Rosner B, Donner A: Familial aggregation of blood pressure and urinary kallikrein in early childhood. In: Epidemiology and Control of Hypertension, pp. 359–374. Paul O, ed. New York: Stratton Intercontinental, 1975.

15. Miall WE, Heneage P, Khosal T, Lovell HG, Moore F: Factors influencing the degree of resemblance in arterial pressure of close relatives. Clin Sci 33:271–283, 1967.

16. Biron P, Mongeau J, Bertrans D: Familial aggregation of blood pressure in 558 adopted children. Can Med Asso J 115:773–774, 1976.

17. Biron P: Pediatric aspects of hypertension. In: Genetic Analysis of Common Diseases, pp. 195–199. Alan R. Liss, 1979.

18. Hines EA, McIlhaney M, Gage R: A study of twins with normal blood pressure and with hypertension. Trans Ass Am Physicians 70:282–287, 1957.

19. Mathers JA, Osborne RH, De George FV: Studies of blood pressure, heart rate and the electrocardiogram in adult twins. Am Heart J 62:634–642, 1961.

20. Vandermulen R, Brewer G, Honeyman MS: A study of hypertension in twins. Am Heart J 79:454–457, 1970.

21. Feinleib M, Robert PH, Garrison RJ: The contribution of family studies to the partitioning of population variations of blood pressure. In: Genetic analysis of Common Diseases, pp. 653–673. New York: Alan R Liss, 1979.

22. Miall WE, Oldham PD: A study of arterial blood pressure and its inheritance in a sample of the general population. Clin Sci 14:459–488, 1955.

23. Miall WE, Oldham PD: Factors influencing arterial blood pressure in the general population. Clin Sci 17:409–444, 1958.

24. Miall WE: Genetic considerations concerning hypertension. Ann NY Acad Sci 304:18–27, 1978.

25. Platt R: The nature of essential hypertension. Lancet 2:55–57, 1959.

26. Oldham PD, Pickering G, Roberts JAF, Sowry GSC: The nature of essential hypertansion. Lancet 1:1085–1093, 1960.
27. Morrison SL, Morris JN: Epidemiological observations on high blood pressure without evident cause. Lancet 2:864–870, 1959.
28. Platt R: Heredity in hypertension. Lancet 1:899–904, 1963.
29. Morrison SL, Morris JN: The nature of essential hypertension. Lancet 2:829–832, 1960.
30. Miyao S, Furusho T: Genetic study of essential hypertension. Jpn Circ J 42:1161–1186, 1978.
31. Weinshilboum R: Hypertension, a biochemical genetic approach. In: Genetic Analysis of Common Diseases: Applications to Predictive Factors in Coronary Disease, pp. 157–181. New York: Alan R Liss, 1979.
32. Weinshilboum RM, Raymond FA, Elveback LR, Weidman WH: Serum Dopamine-β-hydroxylase activity: sibling–sibling correlation. Science 181:943–945, 1973.
33. Weinshilboum RM, Raymond FA, Elveback LR, Weidman WH: Correlation of erythrocyte catechol-O-methyltransferase activity between siblings. Nature 252:490–491, 1974.
34. Murphy DL, Donnelly CH: Monoamine oxidase in man: enzyme characteristics in platelets, plasma and other human tissues. Adv Biochem Psychopharmacol 12:71–85, 1974.
35. Weinshilboum RM, Schrott HG, Raymond FA, Weidman WH, Elveback LR: Inheritance of very low serum dopamine-β-hydroxylase activity. Am J Hum Genet 27:573–585, 1975.
36. Zinner SH, Margolius HS, Rosner B, Keiser HR, Kass EG: Familial aggregation of urinary kallikrein concentration in childhood: relation to blood pressure, race and urinary electrolytes. Am J Epidemiol 104:124–132, 1976.
37. Zinner SH, Margolius HS, Rosner B, Kass EH: Eight-year longitudinal Study of blood pressure and urinary kallikrein in childhood. Clin Res 25:266A, 1977.
38. Blaustein M: Sodium ions, calcium ions, blood pressure regulation and hypertension: a reassessment and a hypothesis. Am J Physiol 232:C.165–C.173, 1977.
39. Edmondson RPS, Thomas RD, Hilton PJ, Patrick J, Jones NF: Abnormal leucocyte composition and sodium transport in essential hypertension. Lancet 1:1003–1005, 1975.
40. Garay RP, Elghozi J-L, Dagher G, Meyer P: Laboratory distinction between essential and secondary hypertension by measurement of erythrocyte cation fluxes. N Engl J Med 302:769–771, 1980.
41. Perera GA, Adler G: ABO groups in the accelerated form of hypertension. Ann Intern Med 53:84–86, 1960.
42. Nance WE, Krieger H, Azevedo E, Mi MP: Human blood pressure and the ABO blood group system: an apparent association. Hum Biol 37:238–244, 1965.
43. Cruz-Coke R, Nagel R, Etcheverry R: Effects of locus MN on diastolic blood pressure in human population. Ann Hum Genet 28:39–48, 1964.
44. Miller JZ, Grim CE, Conneally PM, Weinberger MH: Association of blood groups with essential and secondary hypertension: a possible association with the MNS system. Hypertension 1:493–497, 1979.
45. Falkner B, Onesti G, Angelakos ET, Fernandes M, Langham C: Cardiovascular response to mental stress in normal adolescents with hypertensive parents. Haemodynamics and mental stress in adolescents. Hypertension 1:23–30, 1979.
46. Wiggins RC, Basar I, Slater JDH: Effect of arterial pressure and inheritance on the sodium excretory capacity of normal young men. Clin Sci 54:639–647, 1978.
47. Grim CE, Luft FC, Miller JZ, Brown PL, Gannon MA, Weinberger MH: Effects of sodium loading and depletion in normotensive first-degree relatives of essential hypertensives. J Lab Clin Med 94:764–771, 1979.
48. Sullivan JM, Ratts TE, Taylor JC, Kraus DH, Barton BR, Patrick DR, Reed SW: Haemodynamic effects of dietary sodium in man. Hypertension 2:506–514, 1980.

49. Nance WE, Corey LA: Genetic models for the analysis of data from the families of identical twins. Genetics 83:811–826, 1976.
50. Harburg E, Erfurt JC, Schull WJ, Schlork MA, Colman R: Heredity, Stress and blood pressure, a family set method – I. Study aims and sample flow. J Chron Dis 30:625–647, 1977.
51. Oliver WJ, Cohen EL, Neel JV: Blood pressure, sodium intake and sodium related hormones in the Yanomamo Indians, a 'no-salt' culture. Circulation 52:146–151, 1975.
52. Cruz-Coke R, Etcheverry R, Nagel R: Influence of migration on blood pressure of Easter Islanders. Lancet 1:697–699, 1964.
53. Ward RH, Chin PG, Prior IAM: Tokelau island migrant study: effect of migration on the familial aggregation of blood pressure. Hypertension 2 (Suppl I):43–54, 1980.

13. PSYCHOPHYSIOLOGIC EVIDENCE FOR THE ROLE OF THE NERVOUS SYSTEM IN HYPERTENSION

STEVO JULIUS

As early as 1905, the same year that Korotkoff described a practical method for measurement of the diastolic blood pressure, Geisböck [1], using the old method of finger occlusion plethysmography, stated that among patients with systolic hypertension 'one finds an unusual frequency of those who as directors of big enterprises had a great deal of responsibility and who after a long period of psychic overwork, became nervous.' This hypothesis, that nervous tension somehow causes the disease of arterial hypertension, caught the imagination of many investigators but 75 years after the original suggestion, the question is still wide open. There are a few reasons for this. First are the methodological difficulties of behavioral research. If one is to prove that certain personality characteristics or behavioral patterns are typical of patients with essential hypertension, the methods used should be objective, reproducible, easily applicable to unselected patients, and most of all comparable from study to study. Unfortunately, behavioral research is dominated by conceptual thinking, which influences both the instruments of measurement and the interpretation to such a degree that it is frequently impossible to compare various studies. The second problem is the lack of a suitable animal model. Whereas it is relatively easy to create experimental hypertension by renal arterial stenosis, mineralocorticoids and by genetic inbreeding, attempts to create neurogenic experimental chronic hypertension have failed. The underlying principle of the theory of neural genesis of hypertension, viz. that repeated acute neurogenic pressor episodes lead to sustained hypertension, has not been demonstrated experimentally. Acute elevations of the blood pressure can be elicited by direct stimulation of the defense area [2], or by more complex behavioral paradigms [3], but chronic hypertension could not be caused by prolonged stimulation of the defense area [4], by operant conditioning of monkeys [5], by baroreceptor debuffering [6] or by destruction of the nucleus tractus solitarius [7]. The closest to a successful model are the hypertensive socially naive mice placed into crowded colonies developed by Henry [8], but the complexities of the 'social stress' in these experiments becloud the interpretation.

The third problem relates to difficulties of assessing autonomic nervous

Amery, A. (ed.) Hypertensive Cardiovascular Disease: Pathophysiology and Treatment
© *1982, Martinus Nijhoff Publishers. The Hague / Boston / London*
ISBN-13: 978-94-009-7478-4

function in human beings. The total physiologic effect of alterations in sympathetic function depends on the prevailing tone, the characteristics of the receptor population and the responsiveness of the organ. The issue is even more complicated by the fact that the discharge from the central nervous system is not uniform so that, if methods of assessing the regional sympathetic tone [9] were to become available, the results in one area may not be representative of the overall pattern of discharge. Similarly, measuring the plasma catecholamine levels is not necessarily useful in assessing sympathetic tone in a specific area. Mancia et al. [10] have shown that large changes of vascular resistance can be induced without a noticeable change in catecholamine levels. Furthermore, catecholamine levels depend on a number of factors unrelated to the tone [11–13]. Recent development of specific autonomic receptor agonist and antagonist has provided new information about the net autonomic drive to various organ systems. However, the interpretation of these results is complex for the receptor sensitivity and responsiveness as well as the specific functional and anatomic properties of the responding organs must all be taken into account.

In spite of these methodological difficulties, a clearer picture of the role of the nervous system in human essential hypertension has slowly emerged over the past few decades. The overall impression is that an abnormality of the autonomic nervous function may well be present in very mild hypertension. There is also good evidence for an autonomic overactivity in normotensive offspring of hypertensive parents. As hypertension advances, it is harder to demonstrate a strong autonomic nervous component in the disease. Whereas such a state of affairs could be well explained within the Folkow concept [14], viz. that neurogenic factors initiate and structural factors sustain hypertension, a number of questions remain open, and there is a real possibility that mild neurogenic hypertension is a separate entity whose natural history is different from that of other forms of hypertension. To the extent that this is possible from the existing literature, I will address some of these questions in the present review.

1. PERSONALITY AND REACTIVITY TO MENTAL STRESS

I will review only that portion of research on personality in hypertension where investigators obtained information by application of an objective instrument of measurement. These instruments are either questionnaires or predetermined check lists of observed behavior. Even when such instruments are used, the conceptual framework is often so disparate as to preclude a study-to-study comparison. Therefore, I have purposely chosen to review only those studies that have used a common sense nomenclature of observed or self-described behavior. Scales that use such factors as 'neuroticism,' 'kinesthetic perception,' 'structured versus unstructured neurosis' and 'chronic anxiety' could be useful only if there were a widely prevailing conceptual agreement as to what these terms mean. After such a *subjective* preselection of the available literature, there emerge two wide areas of agreement. The first is that patients with hypertension appear to have difficulties with assertiveness. Ayman, in 1933 [15], described his patients as being 'sensitive' and 'given to inner excitement,' and 'shy and easily offended.' In 1942, Hamilton [16] described the patients as submissive, less assertive, less self-confident and somewhat introverted. Harris et al. in 1953 [17] and Kalis et al. in 1957 [17] found their hypertensives to be egocentric and easily offended. We have performed three independent studies of personality patterns in patients with hypertension [19–21]. These studies were performed with the same instrument in two different cultures: in Yugoslavia (for English description see [22]) and in the United States [20]. Eleven years elapsed between the first [20] and second [21] U.S. study, and the populations in these studies were quite different. Nevertheless, in different populations across different cultures and over a wide span of time, we obtained reasonably consistent results. In essence, the patients described themselves as submissive and having difficulties expressing anger. These findings are much in line with personality descriptions of hypertensives in the large Detroit-area study on psychosocial aspects of hypertension [23]. In that study, the hypertensives were described as 'keeping anger in when attacked' and 'feeling guilt when expressing anger.'

The second area of agreement is that this characteristic personality pattern is found in *mild* hypertension. Even in those studies where the frame of reference does not allow comparison, more abnormality has been found in mild as opposed to more severe hypertension [24, 25]. If one assumes that these personality patterns are prone to inner conflict or to increased awareness in processing external stimuli, this could lead to a heightened autonomic alertness akin to a chronic 'fight or flight' reaction [26] or to enhanced 'coping stress' [27]. Consequently, because of their personality, patients with mild hypertension should be prone to enhanced emotional cardiovascular reactivity, manifested as an increase of blood pressure and heart rate variability. Conceptually, summation of frequent and repeated pressor episodes could lead to hypertension. As earlier indicated, such a sequence, where repeated pressor episodes lead to sustained hypertension, could not be demonstrated in the majority of animal experiments. Nevertheless, the concept is still a viable one, particularly in view of the suggestion that mental stress may lead to hypertension if stresses are applied to animals genetically prone to hypertension [28, 29].

It is therefore appropriate to review whether this presumed cardiovascular hyperreactivity to mental stress can in fact be demonstrated in patients with mild hypertension, or in those individuals who, based on their family background, have a tendency to develop hypertension. On the whole, the literature provides good evidence for increased cardiovascular reactivity to mental stress in such patients. There is strong suggestion in the older literature that patients with hypertension, irrespective of severity, tend to be hyperresponsive to mental stress [26]. However, the specificity of this response could be questioned, as in more severe hypertension structural arteriolar changes tend to increase the pressor responsiveness. In mild and borderline hypertension, the overall pressor responsiveness is normal. These patients have a normal response to cold pressor stress [30], static exercise [31], dynamic exercise [32–34] and infusion of dextran [34, 35]. Whereas the majority of them has a normal blood pressure response to tilting [36], there appears to be a subgroup of hyperresponders to tilt [37, 38]. The experiments with mental stress in mild hypertension are in contrast with this apparently normal blood pressure response to physical stresses. Nestel [39] used mental arithmetics and found his patients to be hyperresponsive. The increase in blood pressure and increase in catecholamines were well correlated. These observations have recently been strengthened even more by the important work of Falkner and her group [40]. In their study, adolescents with borderline hypertension, adolescents with normal blood pressure but a positive family history, and normotensive adolescents without a genetic background for hypertension were compared. During and after the stress of mental arithmetics, subjects with borderline hypertension had a higher and prolonged increase of systolic and diastolic blood pressure and of the heart rate. Normotensive subjects with a positive family background had a response pattern which fell between those borderline hypertensives and normotensives without the family history. Posttest catecholamines were elevated in both borderline hypertensives and genetically predisposed subjects. Similar results, but with a different experimental approach, were gathered by Light and Obrist [41]. They categorized the subjects by baseline blood pressures and by the heart rate responsiveness to various experimental stresses. Heart rate hyperresponders to stress also had a higher blood pressure response and higher baseline blood pressure. Most interestingly in this study, again, hyperresponders had a more prevalent family history of hypertension. It should be emphasized that in both of these studies there was a strong association between tendency toward a higher blood pressure and a faster heart rate response. Recent work by Hollenberg et al. [42], in addition to blood pressure and heart rate, also deals with the response of the renal vasculature to mental stress. In this study, patients with 'hypertension' are compared to normotensive subjects with and without a family history of hypertension. The mean intra-arterial blood pressure in the hypertensive patients was 98 ± 3.8 mm Hg, an average rather similar to our patients with borderline hypertension [32, 35]. When challenged with a nonverbal IQ test and with Raven's Progressive Matrices, these patients, as in two other studies, exhibited an increased heart rate and blood pressure responsivenss.

Finally, Hollenberg demonstrated a sustained decrease in renal blood flow in such patients. Normotensive subjects with a positive family history reacted to the mental stress with a renal vascular response which was less pronounced, but clearly in the same direction as hypertensive patients.

2. HEMODYNAMIC, HUMORAL AND PHARMACOLOGIC EVIDENCE ABOUT THE BASELINE NEUROGENIC TONE IN HYPERTENSION

All of the above mentioned studies [40–42] show not only higher but also *prolonged* responses to mental stress in mild hypertension and in subjects with a genetic predisposition for hypertension.

Does this prolonged emotional responsiveness lead to an increased sympathetic discharge also in the 'baseline state' of the 'resting' but alert patient with essential hypertension? The answer could be given only in the negative; if there were no signs of increased sympathetic tone in the baseline state, one could not support the concept of hyperreactivity carrying over into the resting state. However, the evidence is positive and consistent with the suggestion.

I do not propose to review all of the evidence on plasma catecholamines in hypertension. For this the reader is referred to other chapters of this book and to the recent authoritative and careful review of the topic [43]. After submitting all evidence to a thorough analysis, Goldstein concluded that elevation of resting plasma norepinephrine is characteristically present in a proportion of young patients with essential hypertension. Essential hypertension at younger ages is also synonymous with borderline hypertension. At the University of Michigan, we have had repeated opportunity to screen young students [age 18–28] for hypertension [44, 45] and found less than 0.5% to have sustained hypertension, whereas about 20% of all screened subjects had borderline hypertension. This then means that out of 100 patients with 'hypertension' found on screening of young subjects, 97.5% will have borderline hypertension.

Catecholamine data point to increased sympathetic activity in young patients with mild hypertension. Similarly, mental stress data show that increased blood pressure and heart rate responsiveness are most easily found in young patients with mild hypertension. Data on 'resting' hemodynamics are not different. Again, an increased heart rate is typical for young patients with borderline hypertension. This 'hyperkinetic state' of a high cardiac output and a fast heart rate has repeatedly been reported in such patients [32–34, 46–49]. The elevation of heart rate in these subjects is associated with an elevation of plasma norepinephrine [50]. We have shown that this elevation of heart rate and cardiac output is neurogenic, since it can be abolished by pharmacologic blockade of the cardiac autonomic control [51]. These experiments have also demonstrated that elevation of the resting heart rate stems from an increased sympathetic drive and decreased parasympathetic inhibition to the sinus node. We concluded that such a reciprocal change in the sympathetic and parasympathetic autonomic tone of the heart must emanate from an abnormal *central* nervous integration of the autonomic control, presumably in the integration centers in the medulla oblongata. An examination of afferent inputs into these centers revealed normally functioning arterial baroreceptors [52]. Our research into personality characteristics of these subjects [20, 21] suggested that input descending on the medullary centers from higher areas in the brain may be responsible for this abnormal integration of the autonomic discharge. The characteristic personality pattern of submissiveness and controlled anger could be conducive to a chronic alertness and a chronic 'defense reaction.' An increased sympathetic discharge and a decreased vagal inhibition [53] have been described in the course of acute defense reaction.

When one blocks the sympathetic and parasympathetic transmission to the heart and thereby brings the cardiac output into the normal range, the blood pressure does not become normal [35]. Since, at this point, the only remaining effective sympathetic discharge is to alpha-adrenergic receptors, it was logical to give additional alpha-adrenergic blockade to these beta-adrenergically and vagally blocked subjects [54]. With the addition of phentolamine 15 mg to these patients, all of the autonomic transmission was blocked. If the blood pressure elevation was neurogenic, this elevation should be abolished after autonomic blockade. However, after full autonomic blockade, the vascular resistance and blood pressure was abolished only in roughly one-third of the patients. These were patients with a high plasma renin level, elevated plasma catecholamines and with an abnormal personality profile [21].

Our evidence, then, is that some patients with borderline hypertension have an entirely neurogenic hypertension, that the abnormality is of central nervous origin and that the most likely explanation for the increased central sympathetic discharge is in the personality-specific emotional influences on the integrative centers of the autonomic control. These conclusions are in contrast to a recent report by Esler et al. [13], who suggest that patients with high-renin borderline hypertension may have a defective neuronal uptake of norepinephrine as the cause of sympathetic overactivity. Whereas, of necessity, their method measures only peripheral neuronal uptake it is conceivable that a similar primary abnormality in the central nervous system norepinephrine uptake may be responsible for the abnormalities of central nervous discharge observed in these patients. Further research to clarify these points is needed.

3. IS THERE A TRANSITION FROM NEUROGENIC BORDERLINE HYPERTENSION TO SUSTAINED HYPERTENSION? WHAT COULD BE THE MECHANISM OF THE TRANSITION?

Safar and his colleagues have produced a series of convincing papers which indicate there is good evidence for an increased neurogenic tone or for a 'neurogenic factor' in borderline hypertension, whereas in established hypertension such neurogenic factors are not recognized [55–57]. They suggested that in the course of hypertension the initially important neurogenic factors are replaced by a much more important role of volume factors. Although some of these suggestions have been based on cross-sectional data, they have recently completed a longitudinal study to support this contention. However, we were unable to confirm that these alterations in the hemodynamic picture, which also occur in our patients, are not necessarily associated with a *progression* from borderline to sustained hypertension [58].

There is, however, some indirect evidence that the hyperkinetic state may indeed precede the development of sustained hypertension. The best evidence is epidemiological. A number of studies have shown that the heart rate, independent of blood pressure, is a predictor of future hypertension [59–61]. Thus the rapid heart rate so characteristic of patients with borderline hypertension is not innocent; it is rather a marker of future hypertension. By inference, then, the hyperkinetic state, which has been shown in various laboratories to be neurogenic in origin, may indeed lead to later established hypertension.

The other line of evidence that such a transition from borderline to sustained hypertension may occur is from cross-sectional analysis of pathophysiologic similarities between borderline and sustained hypertension. If these two groups share some pathophysiologic similarities, and knowing that borderline hypertension tends to progress to sustained hypertension [62], it would be reasonable to assume that some of these patients with sustained hypertension may have undergone a phase of neurogenic borderline hypertension. Such similarities indeed exist, particularly in the high-renin types of borderline and sustained hypertension. Another example of similarity supporting the concept that such a transition occurs is shown in Figure 1. If the transition occurs, then patients with borderline hypertension but a normal cardiac output and a slower heart rate should be one step closer to the development of sustained hypertension. Such patients still show some degree of increased sympathetic drive to the heart and have a similar decrease of vagal inhibition as the hyperkinetic patients. Korner et al. [63] studied patients with sustained hypertension by similar means and their data suggest that such patients are one step further; there is no evidence for increased sympathetic stimulation but the decreased vagal inhibition is still demonstrable.

224

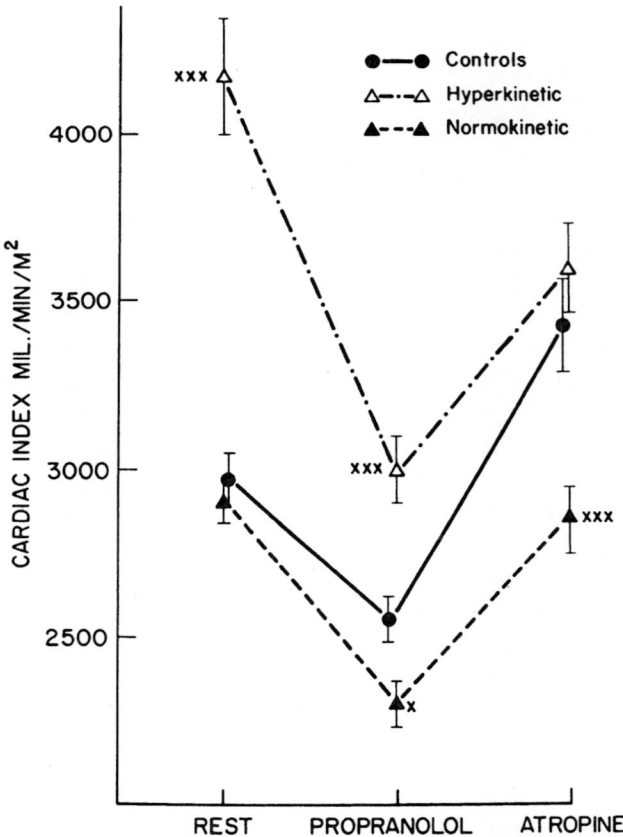

Figure 1. Effect of propranolol (0.2 mg/kg iv) and atropine
(0.04 mg/kg iv) on the cardiac index in normotensive control
subjects (n = 24), patients whose cardiac index was two standard deviations outside the normal mean ('hyperkinetic',
n = 18) and the rest of patients (n = 26). All patients had borderline hypertension. All subjects were age-matched (18–35
years). Asterisks denote the difference from control group:
* p<0.05, ** p<0.02, *** p<0.001. Bars denote standard error of
the mean. Changes after propranolol symbolize sympathetic
drive to the heart; a larger decrease means more sympathetic
drive. After atropine the amount of increase is proportional to
vagal inhibition of the heart. Note that both the 'hyperkinetic'
and 'normokinetic' groups show more sympathetic drive and
less parasympathetic inhibition than control subjects.

How could such a transition occur? Why do the signs of increased sympathetic stimulation in the evolution of sustained hypertension disappear?
These questions are difficult to answer, but it is my personal belief that an
important part in this transition might be in the alteration of the respon-

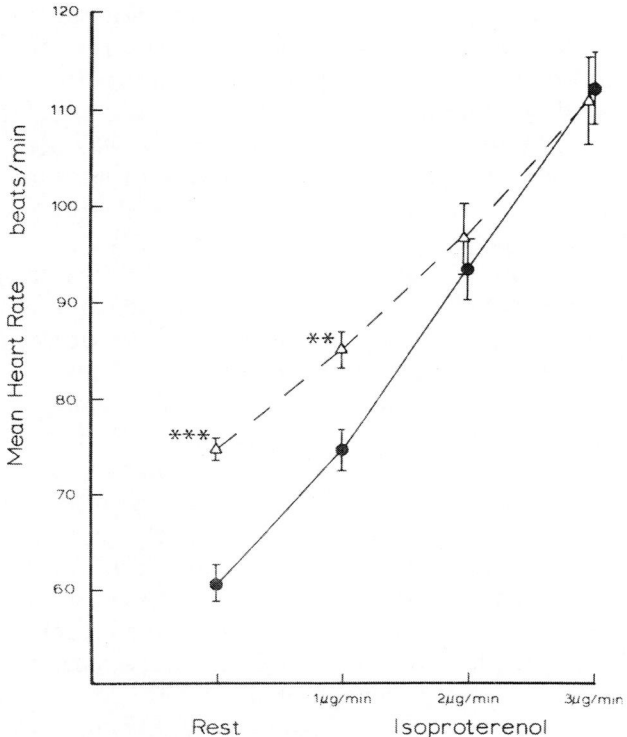

Figure 2. Infusion of increasing dose of isoproterenol. Each infusion step lasted four minutes and results at the fourth minute are shown. Hyperkinetic subjects with borderline hypertension (n = 5) are compared with normotensive controls (n = 18). Symbols as in Figure 1. Note that hyperkinetic patients had a lesser response to increasing doses of isoproterenol. Reproduced from [52], by permission of the Charles C Thomas Company, Publishers.

siveness to sympathetic stimuli. The key evidence for this concept can be found in Figure 2. Sympathetic receptors are subject to 'down regulation,' that is to a decreased sensitivity if they have been exposed to more sympathetic tone [64]. Thus a prolonged exposure to higher sympathetic tone in patients with neurogenic borderline hypertension should lead to a decreased responsiveness of sympathetic receptors. As can be seen from Figure 2, this seems to be the case in patients with hyperkinetic borderline hypertension. We also found the same decreased responsiveness to isoproterenol infusion in patients with 'normokinetic' borderline hypertension [65]. The Paris group has also reported a decreased sensitivity of beta-adrenergic receptors in patients with established hypertension [57]. There are two apparent objections to this concept that receptor 'down regulation' is responsible for the transition from hyperkinetic borderline hypertension to a normal cardiac output and less elevated heart rate in sustained hypertension. First, if 'hyperkinetic' and 'normokinetic' subjects with borderline hypertension show the same decreased chronotropic responsiveness, why does one group have an elevated heart rate and cardiac output whereas the other does not? The cardiac output differences can be explained by differences in stroke volume. Hyperkinetic patients respond with an exaggerated stroke volume due both to an increased inotropic state and a tighter peripheral venous compartment which favors a distribution of blood from the peripheral to the cardiopulmonary space resulting in a larger end-diastolic stretch [57]. In normokinetics, the decreased stroke volume is probably due to a decreased cardiac compliance [65]. It is much more difficult to explain why the heart rate is set back to a lower level in one group and not in the other. Jose suggested that, as the cardiac function changes, the intrinsic rate of firing of the sinus node also tends to change [66]. Whether this mechanism in fact occurs in the course of hypertension is not clear. The other apparent discrepancy regarding the concept that down regulation of sympathetic receptors is important in the transiton from hyperkinetic borderline to sustained hypertension is that of the vascular resistance and blood pressure increase as hypertension progresses. If in borderline hypertension a generalized sympathetic overdrive exists, then the vascular alpha-receptors should also be subject to 'down regulation.' The end result should be a decreased arteriolar sympathetic responsiveness, lower vascular resistance and normalization of the blood pressure. The responsiveness to sympathetic stimulation depends not only on the receptor sensitivity but also on the intrinsic property of the responding cells as well as on the structural properties of the organ. In the case of alpha-adrenergic responsiveness of arterioles, I believe that the decreased sensitivity of alpha-receptors is compensated by a large increase in the responsiveness of the arterioles due to the changes in the wall: lumen ratio as proposed by Folkow [14]. That such a change in responsiveness occurs in humans and that it parallels the severity of hypertension has been amply demonstrated [67].

The proposed mechanism of transition is hypothetical. Discordant with the concept is the finding that catecholamine elevation is more difficult to find in established hypertension [43] and also that the personality abnormality cannot be as well-documented in established hypertension. This could simply reflect the 'dilution' effect. I do not believe that all patients with hypertension start out as the neurogenic hyperkinetic subtype. If the smaller proportion of neurogenic hypertension merges with a large pool of patients with essential hypertension of other pathophysiologies, it will be more difficult to find evidence of autonomic abnormality in an unselected group of patients with established essential hypertension. Alternatively, it is possible that a true downward resetting of the sympathetic *tone* and also alterations of behavior occur in the course of hypertension. An attractive hypothesis is that there may be changes in the sensitivity of the central nervous adrenergic receptors.

SUMMARY

The case for a neurogenic component in human hypertension is strongest for patients with mild or borderline hypertension and for normotensive offspring of hypertensive parents. In these subjects there is evidence for a peculiar personality which may make them prone to inner conflict and to a permanent increased state of mental alertness, both leading to increased emotional blood pressure variability. There is also good humoral and pharmacologic evidence that the sympathetic tone is increased in these patients while in the resting 'basal' state. The case for a neurogenic hypertension is best documented in patients with mild or borderline hypertension who also have an elevated plasma renin activity. As the hypertension advances, it is harder to demonstrate the neurogenic component. This may be due to the dilution of the smaller number of originally neurogenic hypertensives into a larger pool of patients with established hypertension whose blood pressure elevation is not neurogenic. We hypothesize that it is equally feasible to postulate that the 'disappearance' of a neurogenic factor in established hypertension is secondary to changes in sensitivity of adrenergic receptors combined with structural cardiovascular changes in the course of hypertension.

REFERENCES

1. Geisböck W: Die Bedeutung der Blutdruckmessung für die Praxis. Dtsch Arch Klin Med 83:363–374, 1905.
2. Eliasson S, Folkow B, Lundgren P, Unvos B: Activation of sympathetic cholinergic vasodilator nerves in cats during hypothalamic stimulation. Acta Physiol Scand 23:333–351, 1951.
3. Zanchetti A, Baccelli C, Mancia G: Cardiovascular effects of emotional behavior. In: Cardiovascular Regulation, pp. 17–32. Bartorelli C, Zanchetti A, eds. Milan: Cardiovascular Research Institute, 1961.
4. Folkow B, Rubinstein EH: Cardiovascular effects of acute and chronic stimulation of the hypothalamic defense area in the rat. Acta Physiol Scand 68:48–57, 1966.
5. Herd JA: The physiology of strong emotions: Cannon's scientific legacy re-examined. Physiologist 15:5–16, 1972.
6. Cowley AW Jr, Liard JF, Guyton AC: Role of the baroreceptor reflex in daily control of arterial blood pressure and other variables in dogs. Circ Res 32:564–576, 1973.
7. Nathan MA, Reis DJ: Chronic labile hypertension produced by lesions of the nucleus tractus solitarii in the cat. Circ Res 40:72–81, 1977.

228

8. Henry JP, Ely DL, Stephens PM: The role of psychosocial stimulation in the pathogenesis of hypertension. Verh Dtsch Ges Inn Med 80:1724–1740, 1974.
9. Wallin BG, Sundlöf G: A quantitative study of muscle nerve sympathetic activity in resting normotensive and hypertensive subjects. Hypertension 1:67–77, 1979.
10. Mancia G, Leonetti G, Picotti GB, Ferrari A, Galva MD, Gregorini L, Parati G, Pomidossi G, Ravazzani C, Sala C, Zanchetti A: Plasma catecholamines and blood pressure responses to the carotid baroreceptor reflex in essential hypertension. Clin Sci 57:165s–167s, 1979.
11. Nicholls MG, Kiowski W, Zweifler AJ, Julius S, Schork MA, Greenhouse J: Plasma norepinephrine variations with dietary sodium intake. Hypertension 2:29–32, 1980.
12. Lake CR, Ziegler MG, Coleman MD, Kopin IJ: Age-adjusted plasma norepinephrine levels are similar in normotensive and hypertensive subjects. N Engl J med 296:208–209, 1977.
13. Esler M, Jackman G, Bobik A, Leonard P, Kelleher D, Skews H, Jennings G, Korner P: Norepinephrine kinetics in essential hypertension. Defective neuronal uptake of norepinephrine in some patients. Hypertension 3: 149–156, 1981.
14. Folkow B: Role of vascular factor in hypertension. Contr Nephrol 8:81–94, 1977.
15. Ayman D: Personality type of patients with arteriolar essential hypertension. Am J Med Sci 186:213–223, 1933.
16. Hamilton JA: Psychophysiology of blood pressure – I. Personality and behavior ratings. Psychosom Med 4:125–133, 1942.
17. Harris RE, Sokolow M, Carpenter LG, Friedman M, Hunt S: Response to psychologic stress in persons who are potentially hypertensive. Circulation 7:874–879, 1953.
18. Kalis BL, Harris RE, Sokolow M, Carpenter LG Jr: Response to psychological stress in patients with essential hypertension. Am Heart J 53:572–578, 1957.
19. Julius S: Psihosomatske znacajke studenata s povisenim sistolickim tlakom. Sc. D. thesis, University of Zagreb, Yugoslavia, 1964.
20. Harburg E, Julius S, McGinn NF, McLeod J, Hoobler SW: Personality traits and behavioral patterns associated with systolic blood pressure levels in college males. J Chronic Dis 17:405–414, 1964.
21. Esler M, Julius S, Zweifler A, Randall O, Harburg E, Gardiner H, De Quattro V: Mild high-renin essential hypertension: Neurogenic human hypertension? N Engl J Med 296:405–411, 1977.
22. Julius S: The psychophysiology of borderline hypertension. In: Brain, Behavior and Bodily Disease, pp. 293–303. Weiner H, Hofer MA, Stunkard AJ, eds. New York: Raven 1981.
23. Harburg E, Erfurt JC, Hauenstein LS, Chape C, Schull WJ, Schork MA: Socio-ecological stress, suppressed hostility, skin color, and black-white male blood pressure: Detroit. Psychosom Med 35:276–296, 1973.
24. Richter-Heinrich E: Psychophysiological personality patterns of hypertensive and normotensive subjects. Psychother Psychosom 18:332–340, 1970.
25. Safar ME, Kamieniecka HA, Levenson JA, Dimitriu VM, Pauleau NF: Hemodynamic factors and Rorschach testing in borderline and sustained hypertension. Psychosom Med 40:620–630, 1978.
26. Brod J, Fencl V, Hejl Z, Jirka J: Circulatory changes underlying blood pressure elevation during acute emotional stress (mental arithmatic) in normotensive and hypertensive subjects. Clin Sci 18:269–279, 1959.
27. Light KC, Obrist PA: Cardiovascular response to stress: effects of opportunity to avoid shock experience and performance feedback. Psychophysiology 17:243–250, 1980.
28. Hallbäck M, Jones JV, Bianchi G, Folkow B: Cardiovascular control in the Milan strain of spontaneously hypertensive rat (MHS) at 'rest' and during acute mental 'stress.' Acta Physiol Scand 99:208–216, 1977.
29. Friedman SM, Friedman CL: Cell Permeability, sodium transport, and the hypertensive process in the rat. Circ Res 39:433–441, 1976.

30. Cuddy RP, Smulyan H, Keighley JF et al.: Hemodynamic and catecholamine changes during a standard cold pressor test. Am Heart J 71:446–454, 1966.
31. Sannerstedt R, Julius S: Systemic haemodynamics in borderline arterial hypertension: Response to static exercise before and under the influence of propranolol. Cardiovasc Res 6:398–403, 1972.
32. Julius S, Conway J: Hemodynamic studies in patients with borderline blood pressure elevation. Circulation 38:282–288, 1968.
33. Sannerstedt R: Hemodynamic response to exercise in patients with arterial hypertension. Acta Med Scand Suppl 458:1–83, 1966.
34. Lund-Johansen P: Hemodynamics in early essential hypertension. Acta Med Scand (Suppl 482:1–105, 1967.
35. Julius S, Pascual A, Sannerstedt R, Mitchell C: Relationship between cardiac output and peripheral resistance in borderline hypertension. Circulation 43:382–390, 1971.
36. Sannerstedt R, Julius S, Conway J: Hemodynamic response to tilt and beta-adrenergic blockade in young patients with borderline hypertension. Circulation 42:1057–1064, 1970.
37. Frohlich ED, Tarazi RC, Ulrych M, Dustan HP, Page IH: Tilt test for investigating a neural component in hypertension. Circulation 36:387–393, 1967.
38. Hull DH, Wolthuis RA, Cortese T, Longo MR Jr, Triebwasser JH: Borderline hypertension versus normotension: differential response to orthostatic stress. Am Heart J 94:414–420, 1977.
39. Nestel PJ: Blood pressure and catecholamine excretion after mental stress in labile hypertension. Lancet 1:692–694, 1969.
40. Falkner B, Onesti G, Angelakos ET, Fernandes M, Langman C: Cardiovascular response to mental stress in normal adolescents with hypertensive parents. Hemodynamics and mental stress in adolescents. Hypertension 1:23–30, 1979.
41. Light KC, Obrist PA: Cardiovascular reactivity to behavioral stress in young males with and without marginally elevated casual systolic pressures. Comparison of clinic, home, and laboratory measures. Hypertension 2:802–808, 1980.
42. Hollenberg NK, Williams GH, Adams DF: Essential hypertension: abnormal renal vascular and endocrine responses to a mild psychological stimulus. Hypertension 3:11–17, 1981.
43. Goldstein DS: Plasma norepinephrine in hypertension. A study of the studies. Hypertension 3:48–52, 1981.
44. Julius S, McGinn NF, Harburg E, Hoobler SW: Comparison of various clinical measurements of blood pressure with the self-determination technique in normotensive college males. J Chronic Dis 17:391–396, 1964.
45. Julius S, Ellis CN, Pascual AV, Matice M, Hansson L, Hunyor SN, Sandler LN: Home blood pressure determination: Value in borderline ('labile') hypertension. JAMA 229:663–666, 1974.
46. Widimsky J, Fejfarová MH, Fejfar Z: Changes of cardiac output in hypertensive disease. Cardiologia 31:381–389, 1957.
47. Eich RH, Peters RJ, Cuddy RP, Smulyan H, Lyons RH: The hemodynamics in labile hypertension. Am Heart J 63:188–195, 1962.
48. Frohlich ED, Kozul VJ, Tarazi RC, Dustan HP: Physiological comparison of labile and essential hypertension. Circ Res 26 (Suppl I):55–69, 1970.
49. Safar ME, Weiss YA, Levenson JA, London GM, Milliez PL: Hemodynamic study of 85 patients with borderline hypertension. Am J Cardiol 31:315–319, 1973.
50. Esler M, Zweifler A, Randall O, Julius S, DeQuattro V: Agreement among three different indices of sympathetic nervous system activity in essential hypertension. Mayo Clin Proc 52:379–382, 1977.
51. Julius S, Pascual AV, London R: Role of parasympathetic inhibition in the hyperkinetic type of borderline hypertension. Circulation 44:413–418, 1971.

52. Julius S: Neurogenic component in borderline hypertension. In: The Nervous System in Arterial Hypertension, pp. 301–330. Julius S, Esler M, eds. Springfield, IL: Charles C Thomas, 1976.

53. Hilton SM: Inhibition of baroreceptor reflexes on hypothalamic stimulation. J Physiol (Lond) 165:56–57, 1963.

54. Esler MD, Julius S, Randall OS, Ellis CN, Kashima T: Relation of renin status to neurogenic vascular resistance in borderline hypertension. Am J Cardiol 36:708–715, 1975.

55. Alexandre JM, London GM, Chevillard C, Lemaire P, Safar ME, Weiss Y: The meaning of dopamine β-hydroxylase in essential hypertension. Clin Sci Mol Med 49:1–7, 1975.

56. Weiss YA, Safar ME, London GM, Simon AC, Levenson JA, Milliez PM: Repeat hemodynamic determinations in borderline hypertension. Am J Med 64:382–387, 1978.

57. Safar ME, Weiss YA, London GM, Frackowiak RF, Milliez PL: Cardiopulmonary blood volume in borderline hypertension. Clin Sci Mol Med 47:153–164, 1974.

58. Julius S, Quadir H, Gajendragadkar S: Hyperkinetic state: a precursor of hypertension? A longitudinal study of borderline hypertension. In: Perspectives in Cardiovascular Research. Prophylactic Approach to Hypertensive Diseases, pp. 309–314. Yamori Y, Lovenberg W, Freis ED, eds. New York: Raven, 1979.

59. Levy RL, White PD, Stroud WD, Hillman CC: Transient tachycardia: Prognostic significance alone and in association with transient hypertension. Jama 129:585–588, 1945.

60. Stamler J, Berkson DM, Dyer A, Lepper MH, Lindberg HA, Paul O, McKean H, Rhomberg P, Schoenberger JA, Shekelle RB, Stamler R: Relationship of multiple variables to blood pressure. Findings from four Chicago epidemiologic studies. In: Epidemiology and Control of Hypertension, pp. 307–352. Paul O, ed. Miami, Symposia Specialists, 1975.

61. Paffenbarger RS Jr, Thorne MC, Wing AL: Chronic disease in former college students – VIII. Characteristics in youth predisposing to hypertension in later years. Am J Epidemiol 88:25–32, 1968.

62. Julius S, Schork MA: Borderline hypertension – a critical review. J Chronic Dis 23:723–754, 1971.

63. Korner PI, Shaw J, Uther JB, West MJ, McRitchie RJ, Richards JG: Autonomic and nonautonomic circulatory components in essential hypertension in man. Circulation 48:107–117, 1973.

64. Lefkowitz RJ: β-Adrenergic receptors: recognition and regulation. N Engl J Med 295:323–328, 1976.

65. Julius S, Randall OS, Esler MD, Kashima T, Ellis CN, Bennett J: Altered cardiac responsiveness and regulation in the normal cardiac output type of borderline hypertension. Circ Res 36–37 (Suppl I):I-199–I-207, 1975.

66. Jose AD, Taylor RR: Autonomic blockade by propranolol and atropine to study intrinsic myocardial function in man. J Clin Invest 48:1019–2031, 1969.

67. Sivertsson R: The hemodynamic importance of structural vascular changes in essential hypertension. Acta Physiol Scand 79 (Suppl 343):3–56, 1970.

14. INTERACTION BETWEEN FUNCTIONAL AND STRUCTURAL ELEMENTS IN PRIMARY HYPERTENSION

BJÖRN FOLKOW and MARGARETA HALLBÄCK-NORDLANDER

A. INTRODUCTION

Hardly more than a century after William Harvey's monumental discovery and soon after Rev. Stephen Hales performed the first arterial pressure measurement known to history in his mare, a young professor of medicine in Berlin, Samuel Schaarschmidt, who died prematurely in 1747, had identified and even treated a clinical condition defined as 'spastic constriction of the arteries'. His posthumously published writings reveal that he had a surprisingly good grasp of what we now call 'essential' or 'primary' hypertension [1]. His treatment was no less astonishing, as it anticipated modern therapeutic principles by some 200 years. Thus, he prescribed elimination of mentally stressful influences, nitrites and venesection, which at least here was a rational use as it reduced venous return. In other words, his scheme of treatment served to depress sympathetic activity, dilate arterioles and veins and reduce cardiac output, which is precisely what modern hypotensive drugs aim at.

Further, the morphological foundations of what will be the main theme below were actually discovered before arterial pressure was ever measured in man, insofar as Richard Bright in 1836 and George Johnson in 1968 showed that chronic 'Bright's disease' was characterized by wall hypertrophy in heart, arteries and arterioles. Despite the fact that these are perhaps the most obvious and consistent of all changes in chronic hypertension, their *hemodynamic* consequences remained largely unknown for a century or so [2]. True enough, 'nothing is really new under the sun', but it can certainly take time before major implications of early discoveries are fully understood.

Since these early highlights, a steadily growing mass of scientific contributions has made primary hypertension perhaps the most studied item in cardiovascular research. The present survey aims at illustrating how an individually varying *interaction* between 1) genetic, 2) environmental 'functional' influences, and 3) a per se 'normal' structural adaptation of major cardiovascular compartments is necessary for the initiation and maintenance of primary hypertension [2] rather than any single cardinal 'pressor' influence, as was earlier commonly believed.

Amery, A. (ed.) Hypertensive Cardiovascular Disease: Pathophysiology and Treatment
© *1982, Martinus Nijhoff Publishers. The Hague / Boston / London*
ISBN-13: 978-94-009-7478-4

B. PRINCIPAL PATHOGENETIC ELEMENTS

1. Genetic predisposition

In contrast with the situation in secondary hypertension, where pressure is raised because of some specific interference in cardiovascular control, primary hypertension depends on an intricate interaction between several major components. Although most investigators have their 'pet' hypotheses concerning its exact background, they generally agree that this disorder of regulation can be traced back to a *poly*genetically linked predisposition. This is the case both in man [3, 4] and in the different varieties of primary hypertension in rats [5–10]. It means that even the initiation of primary hypertension must be quite complex, as it derives from different combinations of predisposing genes, and for that reason cannot represent any uniform disturbance.

As a result, several cardiovascular control mechanisms and/or effector functions may well be simultaneously affected. Also, these deviations may vary both in nature and extent between individuals when it comes to man, and between strains in the pure-bred variants of rat primary hypertension. Furthermore, some of these genetic elements may only be 'latent', in the sense that they exert significant hemodynamic influences when environmental influences are also present to precipitate overt effects.

2. Environmental influences

Certain environmental influences can be considered as facilitating the effects of a given predisposition and may, as mentioned, sometimes also precipitate a hypertensive state if the genetic predisposition alone is not strong enough. Among such 'triggering' environmental influences *psycho-emotional responses* to a mentally hectic, and sometimes even stressful life, which convey more or less intermittent sympatho-hormonal excitatory effects on the cardiovascular system, have often been considered, as will be further dealt with below [11–13].

In addition, *the extent of salt intake* is also considered an important 'environmental' factor [4, 9, 14]. For example, the Dahl strain of hypertension-sensitive rats (HSR) is largely normotensive on ordinary salt intake, but severe hypertension ensues upon salt loading [7]. With respect to man, when a similar type of genetic predisposition is at hand, an excess of salt intake may likewise help gradually to induce hypertension by causing sodium and water retention and thereby a modest blood volume increase. This, in turn, has been considered to cause hypertension due to an elevation of cardiac output with subsequent 'whole body autoregulation' [14, 15]. However, sodium retention might also cause an altered ionic balance across vascular smooth muscle cell membranes for example, whereby myogenic activity and responsiveness to extrinsic stimuli are affected. There is mounting evidence that one key genetic deviation in primary hypertension expresses itself as an increased sodium permeability in cell membranes in general, both in man and SHR, though more or less compensated for by increased active sodium transport [16]. If, however, this active out-transport is suppressed by a generally acting natriuretic hormone [16], perhaps released as a reflex action after sodium and volume loading, a consequent cellular dysbalance of sodium might also considerably increase smooth muscle and autonomic nerve responsiveness. This is at present an intensely studied topic, though with many unknowns and open questions. To these two alternatives may be added other, so far less well-known, environmental influences that might in other ways affect the development of primary hypertension.

3. Structural cardiovascular adaptation

Regardless of the way in which the combined genetic and environmental influences are arranged in terms of their interaction and relative roles, they will in different ways induce functional 'pressor' effects, though these may well, at least initially, be quite mild, gradual and even intermittent in nature.

However, even fairly mild additions to the ordinary excitatory influences on the cardiovascular system tend to induce per se normal structural adjustments of heart and vessels, as is the case with any tissue exposed to increased load where skeletal muscle offers an obvious example. In those parts of the cardiovascular system which are directly exposed to increased average load, this initially quite marginal adaptation in design is therefore from the *local* point of view quite appropriate. For example, in dependent veins, which in the upright position are exposed to raised transmural pressures, the induced proportional media thickening implies an efficient structural compensation which helps to counteract peripheral pooling of blood [17]. Likewise, in the left heart, large arteries and precapillary resistance vessels in early hypertension, and gradually also for the venous side, the same principle of proportional hypertrophic wall thickening occurs, which in the resistance vessels is associated with a modest luminal narrowing [2, 18–20].

Though this adaptation is appropriate for the individual muscle cell or vessel by adjusting its contractile power and performance to meet the increased work load, it will in the long run have deleterious consequences on the thick-walled resistance vessels when, as in hypertension, the *entire* systemic circulation is simultaneously so affected. The reason is that the additional, at first very mild, increase in wall/lumen ratio (w/r_i) implies proprotionally exaggerated luminal reduction to given smooth muscle contraction. In this way intensified resistance and hence pressor responses to functional excitatory influences are induced on a purely structural basis, where the raised w/r_i acts as an 'amplifying lever'.

Furthermore, since the average pressure load constitutes the main stimulus for adaptive wall thickening, further resistance vessel hypertrophy is triggered as long as the initial excitatory drive remains, which is likely to be the case when as here it derives from a genetic predisposition as facilitated by more or less ordinary environmental influences. This, in turn, results in additional exaggeration of both the functional luminal reductions and the consequent pressor effects, and so on, because a positive-feedback interaction is now introduced at this key point of circulatory control. In other words, by being generalized to all resistance vessels, a per se normal and initially mild secondary structural adaptation opens the way for a vicious circle which tends to aggravate the functional impact of perhaps quite mild, though more or less steadily present genetic–environmental pressor influences, which *alone* might have remained fairly harmless.

For studies of such complex interactions between 'initiating' and 'secondary' elements the access to various strains of genetically hypertensive rats has been of the greatest value [7]. By prolonged inbreeding it has here been possible to 'purify' their respective genetic combinations so that they regularly cause specific, uniform types of primary hypertension. These strains, with mutually different genetic combinations, vary therefore considerably with respect to the onset and nature of the cardiovascular disturbance, as well as in sensitivity to the various environmental influences. They are of principal interest also because they clearly demonstrate how primary hypertension can indeed be initiated in several different ways.

C. INTERACTION OF GENETIC AND ENVIRONMENTAL 'TRIGGER' INFLUENCES

1. The situation in rat primary hypertension

a) *The Kyoto 'spontaneously hypertensive rat' (SHR)*, developed by Okamoto and Aoki in Japan [5, 6], is, with respect to cardiovascular function, mainly characterized by an enhanced central neuro-hormonal influence emanating from limbic-hypothalamic levels. This is, among other things, expressed as a hyper-reactivity to environmental psychogenic stimuli, which results in an accentuated nervous and hormonal drive on the circulatory system. Thus, hormonal mechanisms are also involved, since hormonal

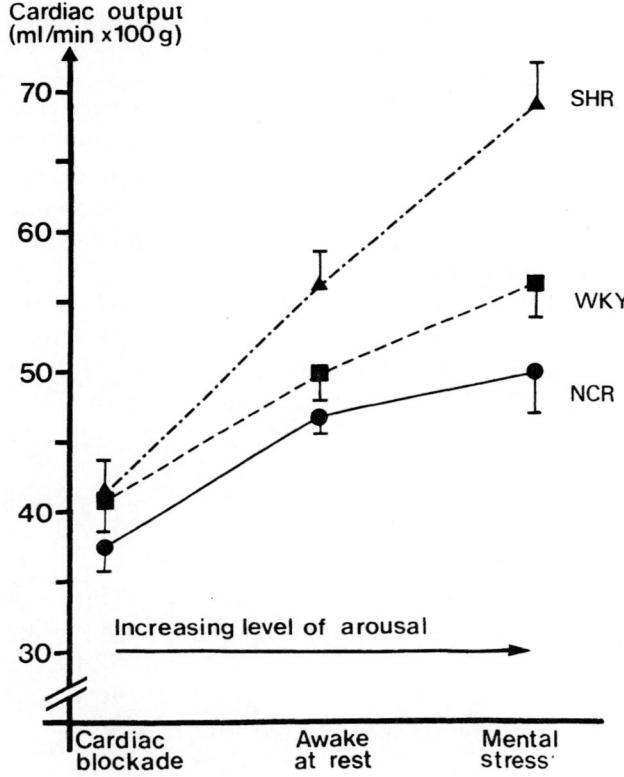

Figure 1. Changes in cardiac output in 6 week old male SHR
(▲), ordinary Wistar normotensive control rats, NCR (●) and
Wistar-Kyoto normotensive rats, WKY (■), during increasing
levels of arousal. The combination of methylscopolamine and
propranolol during pentobarbitone anesthesia is considered to
cause complete inhibition of nervous control to the heart, i.e.,
'cardiac blockade'. Environmental stimuli will become increasingly important in determining the neurogenic control of
the heart during the awake state, i.e., 'awake at rest' and particularly during short-lasting 'mental stress' (high noise and a
jet of air for 30 s). Vertical bars indicate SEM. (from [21]).

control is at these CNS levels closely linked with autonomic-nervous components influencing the circulation and forming highly differentiated neurohormonal patterns [11, 13]. For example, SHR respond with exaggerated
and prolonged 'defence reactions' to mild environmental stimuli [7, 21–23].
For such reasons, early phases of SHR hypertension are more or less 'hyperkinetic' in hemodynamic balance, as is typical when the central neurogenic drive on the circulation is moderately enhanced, as shown in Figure 1.

However, this early 'hyperkinetic' stage is gradually transformed towards a normalized or even reduced cardiac output, though with a correspondingly raised systemic resistance once the established phase of SHR hypertension is reached around 3–4 months of age. In all these hemodynamic respects SHR appear to closely simulate the perhaps most common variant of human primary hypertension [4, 11, 12]. This makes it likely that also in man central neurohormonal influences constitute a common and major 'triggering' influence as an expression of the genetic predisposition interacting with environmental influences [11–13].

b) *The New Zealand 'genetically hypertensive rat' (GHR)*, developed by Smirk and his group in Dunedin [7, 8], also seems to have a dominant engagement of the sympathetic nervous system, though probably not organized exactly as in SHR. The initiation of hypertension in both these hypertensive strains seems not to depend on any increase in plasma and blood volumes ('volume' hypertension), since they show normal or even slightly subnormal plasma and blood volumes throughout the developing phase of their primary hypertension. This is also commonly the case in most variants of early primary hypertension in man [3, 4, 12, 24].

c) *The Brookhaven 'hypertension-sensitivive rat' (HSR)*, developed by Dahl and his group [7, 9], has a quite different genetic background. This strain is actually hypertension-*prone* rather than overtly hypertensive, but is easily provoked into severe hypertension by mild salt-loading. Here it contrasts with another genetic variant developed in parallel, the hypertension-resistant rat (HRR), which is unusually resistant to salt-loading. The sensitivity to salt in HSR is to a great extent dependent on their kidney function. Thus, transplantation of an HSR kidney to HRR will render this genetically hypertension-resistant rat hypertensive. In addition to their renal abnormality, HSR appear to display some deviation of the adrenal corticoid secretion. An interesting observation in HSR, which in all likelihood reflects the important consequences of an early structural adaptation also in this type of primary hypertension, is that if salt-loading is continued for more than a few weeks, but is then interrupted, the hypertensive state usually remains. Some other component must then have taken over the maintenance of hypertension, and the time course and other characteristics strongly suggest a dominant influence of secondary structural adaptation, as further described below.

d) *The 'Milan spontaneously hypertensive strain' (MHS)*, developed by Bianchi and co-workers [7, 10], represents a fairly mild 'renal' type of hypertension. Here, a significant volume component may really contribute decisively to the initiation. Also in MHS hypertension follows the kidneys when cross-transplantations are performed between normo- and hypertensive animals. It seems as if MHS for genetic reasons have a slightly lowered glomerular filtration capacity when related to the tubular reabsorption capacity, resulting in a modest retention of sodium and water. The result is an early plasma volume expansion, whereby cardiac output becomes elevated thanks to the increased venous return. As suggested by both Guyton's and Ledingham's groups [14, 15], this would be followed by 'whole body autoregulation'. The consequent pressure elevation would normalize glomerular filtration and thereby blood volume, though now at a higher arterial pressure equilibrium. Probably this suggested chain of events is too simplified since the sodium chloride retention might, as mentioned, involve also other changes, e.g. in ionic balance across cell membranes [16], in turn affecting mechanisms like precapillary myogenic activity, etc.

Quite likely there are possibilities for alternative genetic combinations that may initiate a hypertensive state by primary involvements of cardiovascular control mechanisms other than those so far known and here mentioned.

2. The situation in human primary hypertension

In contrast to the situation in pure-bred hypertensive rats, the genetic constellations responsible for primary hypertension in human beings are probably far more variable, as a natural result of man's randomized habits of reproduction. For such reasons, the genetic combinations contributing to primary hypertension in man are likely more to resemble those obtained when the various pure-bred hypertensive rat strains are allowed to cross-breed freely. Thus, in primary hypertension in man *individually variable* patterns of genetically predisposing elements are likely to prevail and they may therefore allow for a whole spectrum of hypertension variants. This by no means denies that some genetic constellations may be more common and/or more efficient in eliciting high blood pressure than others. For example, it appears from several studies as though enhanced neurogenic influences are fairly common in early human primary hypertension [4, 11–13, 24]. However, in others neurogenic influences hardly dominate but, instead, there may be signs of, for instance, increased mineralcorticoid activity and/or 'inherent' renal deviations in the handling of sodium chloride [4, 14, 24].

Thus, most authorities seem to agree that both salt intake and environmental psycho-emotional influences can be of importance in the initiation of human primary hypertension as well. For example, in several isolated groups of human populations, the incidence of high blood pressure is quite low, but seems to increase rapidly when confronted with the mixed blessings of western civilization with its easy access to salt and its hectic, technological way of life [4]. However, in man it is quite difficult to analyse in detail how these environmental influences interact with hereditary predisposing

238

elements. Therefore, studies of the mentioned rat strains, where both environment and type of genetic predisposition can be well defined and where life span is far shorter, serve to clarify some general principles concerning this important interaction between inherent predisposition and environmental infuences.

3. Differences in responsiveness between hypertensive rat strains, with parallels to man's situation

Concerning environmentally elicited psychogenic influences, SHR primary hypertension is greatly aggravated by enhanced 'mental stress' [5–7], while deprivation of normal social contacts, with elimination of the trivial daily confrontations and stimuli that this implies, attenuates the development of hypertension in SHR [23]. This inherent central hyper-reactivity to environmental 'arousal' stimuli in SHR is not present in MHS as shown in Figure 2, as they have a quite different genetic background [25]. It has already been mentioned how increased access to sodium chloride can virtually precipitate

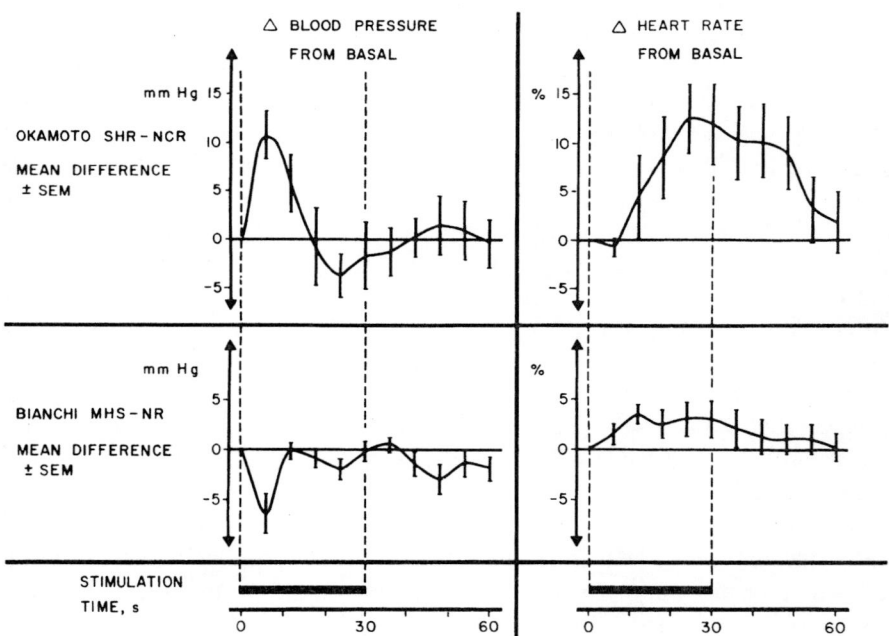

Figure 2. Mean difference ($\pm$ SE) in blood pressure (left) and heart rate (right) responses to 'stress' stimulation (sudden loud noise for 30 s) between 9 pairs of the Okamoto SHR and their controls, NCR, and between 18 pairs of MHS rats and their controls, NR (lower panel). Changes in heart rate are expressed as per cent from resting heart rate. (From [25]).

hypertension in HSR, which is fairly insensitive to 'mental' stress [7, 9], while the initiation of hypertension in SHR and GHR is not crucially dependent on the level of salt intake [7, 8]. This does not deny, of course, that more advanced stages of SHR hypertension, when kidney function becomes increasingly affected, can be definitely sensitive to salt intake.

These examples from rats illustrate how sensitivity to environmental factors is dependent to a great extent on the nature of genetical predisposition. This is likely to hold also for man, though here the patterns of genetic elements are for natural reasons more variable than in pure-bred rat strains, which may also be the case with regard to sensitivity to environmental factors. These various combinations of genetic and environmental elements constitute a complex of functional triggering influences for the cardiovascular system. Such influences would, however, perhaps only exceptionally in themselves be able to create a truly chronic hypertension worthy of the name. In order to maintain and, in part, even to initiate this disorder of regulation, the structural adaptation of heart, vessels and barostat functions seems to play a major role.

D. INTERACTION BETWEEN FUNCTIONAL 'TRIGGER' INFLUENCES AND SECONDARY STRUCTURAL ADAPTATION

1. Resistance vessel adaptation, with hemodynamic consequences

While the presence of media hypertrophy in arterioles during hypertension was shown more than 100 years ago, the functional relevance of this particular structural change remained largely unrecognized until the 1950s. Experimental analyses in man were then started to explore the hemodynamic influence of an increased w/r_i in the resistance vessels [18, 19]. Following these initial studies in hypertensive man, further and extensive studies have been carried out in SHR and in renal hypertensive rats in comparison with normotensive control rats (NCR) [2, 20].

Nature of change. Both in hypertensive man and rats, resistance to flow is increased in virtually all systemic vascular beds, even at complete vascular smooth muscle relaxation. In this situation, only the structurally set dimensions of the resistance vessels determine resistance to flow at any given distending pressure. Thus, in hypertension there is a clear structural luminal reduction at the precapillary resistance level, besides hypertrophic wall thickening [2, 20]. Furthermore, when smooth muscle contraction is initiated by constrictor agents, including the adrenergic transmitter noradrenaline, hypertensive vascular beds consistently exhibit greater resistance increases than normotensive ones (Figure 3), and vice versa if dilator agents are given at any present level of vascular tone. However, smooth muscle

COMPILED EXPERIMENTAL RESULTS

PERFUSION PRESSURE, mm Hg
(PROPORTIONAL TO FLOW RESISTANCE)

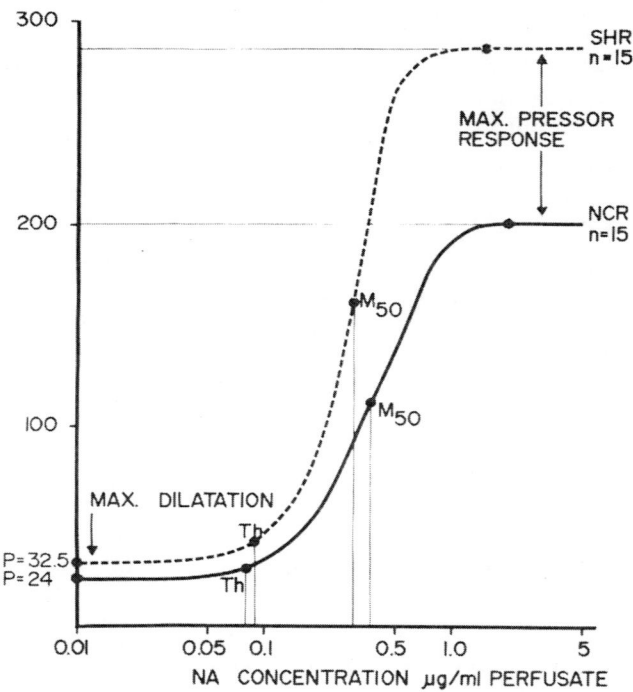

Figure 3. Mean dose–response 'resistance curves' from paired, constant-flow perfusion experiments on the hindquarter vascular beds of 15 SHR and 15 NCR, relating log noradrenaline concentration to perfusion pressure (i.e., to flow resistance). Note the increased resistance at maximal dilatation, increased steepness of the resistance curve and increased maximal pressor response of the SHR. There is, however, no difference in threshold sensitivity to NA between groups. The minor difference in 'M_{50}' is a consequence of the increased w/r_i in SHR precapillary resistance vessels. (From [20]).

sensitivity to NA appears to be largely unchanged, in both man and SHR. Thus, hypertensive resistance vessels display an unspecific *vascular* hyper-reactivity as a consequence of their altered design with increased w/r_i. The reason for this vascular hyper-reactivity is that upon vascular smooth muscle activation, which is normally initiated from the outer layer as the vaso-constrictor fibres only make direct contacts with this layer, a greater bulk of tissue is forced towards the lumen.

In this way amplified luminal reductions, and hence increases in resistance, are established as a geometric consequence of the increased w/r_i in hypertensive precapillary resistance vessels. As a further result of the media hypertrophy, hypertensive resistance vessels display reduced wall distensibility, as well as an increased maximal contractile strength, illustrated in Figure 3 as a greater pressor response at maximal smooth muscle activation. These changes are largely confined to the *pre*capillary resistance vessels and they are closely proportional in extent to the arterial pressure rise. They may therefore be denoted as a '*structural autoregulation*', as a long-term analogue to the 'functional autoregulation' also induced locally, though now acutely, to pressure increases [2].

The results from such detailed hemodynamic analyses of entire vascular beds in hypertensive rats are in close agreement with recent direct morphometric measurements [26]. On the other hand, strips of small arteries from normotensive and hypertensive human subjects, a procedure which eliminates the geometric impact of an increased w/r_i on the luminal reduction, show a largely normal contractile strength in the hypertensive arteries per unit transverse section area, and also a fairly normal sensitivity to noradrenaline [27, 25].

When taken together, these results suggest that it is the *structurally* increased arteriolar w/r_i, rather than any greatly enhanced smooth muscle activity, that, in the 'resting equilibrium', is responsible for the raised systemic resistance in established primary hypertension, and also for the characteristic vascular hyper-reactivity that in the long run tends further to aggrevate the situation. Furthermore, the gradually more pronounced alteration in resistance vessel design and behavior is the result of a long-term interaction between per se fairly mild excitatory functional influences and the natural tendency of tissues under load to adapt their structure accordingly, which at this point of the vascular bed unfortunately happens to introduce a positive-feedback effect.

Rate of change. Concerning *rate* of development, the mentioned hypertrophic adaptation of cardiac, arterial and arteriolar design can be established so rapidly that it must contribute even to the initiation of hypertension. Thus, muscle hypertrophy of the left heart and systemic resistance vessels can be fully completed in rats in less than 2–3 weeks after a drastic pressure rise [29]. In man, with a slower rate of metabolism, such processes should be correspondingly slower and rather a matter of months than of weeks, which is still a very short period of time in these matters. For example, observations on young military conscripts in the first early phases of primary hypertension indicate that structural vascular changes had already then started [30]. This means that the functional triggering mechanisms and the structural adaptation of heart and precapillary vessels will be so intertwined in time that they both contribute to hypertension, almost from the very start of the pressure rise. Because of this early interaction between functional trigger mechanisms and structural adaptation, it is almost meaningless to distinguish them as in *time* separated primary and secondary elements. Admittedly, the functional triggering influences are presumably 'first on the scene', to the extent that they are part of the genetic code. It should be realized, however, that the secondary structural adaptation also may well be part of the genetic predisposition [2, 19, 20]. For example, one factor predisposing to hypertension might be that cardiovascular effector cells tend to respond with a slightly accentuated structural adaptation to a given load. This would be achieved if some key enzymatic link involved in protein synthetis were genetically altered so as to facilitate this cellular growth process, or so stimulated by some increased 'trophic' influence of a hormonaltransmitter nature as a consequence of, for example, an inherent CNS hyper-responsiveness to stimuli, as in SHR. Thus, the extent of resistance vessel adaptation and left ventricular hypertrophy in SHR seems to be significantly greater than in genetically normotensive rats provoked to secondary renal hypertension of about the same duration and severity as in SHR [2, 29]. Furthermore, in young SHR where arterial pressure is barely above normal, there are already significant structural changes in the left heart and signs of resistance vessel hypertrophy [31].

Upon drastic and sustained pressure reduction, by pharmacological or other means, more or less complete regression of the hypertrophic changes can occur in rats in 2–3 weeks [29], at least after fairly short-lasting hypertension. However, if hypertension has been of such long duration as to allow for other structural changes than pure smooth muscle hypertrophy, regression is far more difficult to achieve [29]. Thus, in time vascular smooth muscles gradually add collagen and other interstitial material [32], which increasingly contributes to wall thickening in chronic hypertension. Regression of collagen elements is much poorer than that of muscle hypertrophy following pressure reduction [32] which probably explains why it is increasingly difficult to produce true reversal the longer primary hypertension lasts [32]. From such a point of view, hypotensive therapy should start before such wall infiltration with interstitial material contributes more substantially to vascular and cardiac adaptation.

2. Cardiac structural adaptation, with hemodynamic consequences

Left ventricular hypertrophy in hypertension forms a natural part of the overall structural adaptation, because it allows for improved systolic work performance and hence for coping better with the raised afterload [18, 31, 34]. However, it inevitably also affects the diastolic properties of the heart. Thus, according to Laplace's law, increased left ventricular wall

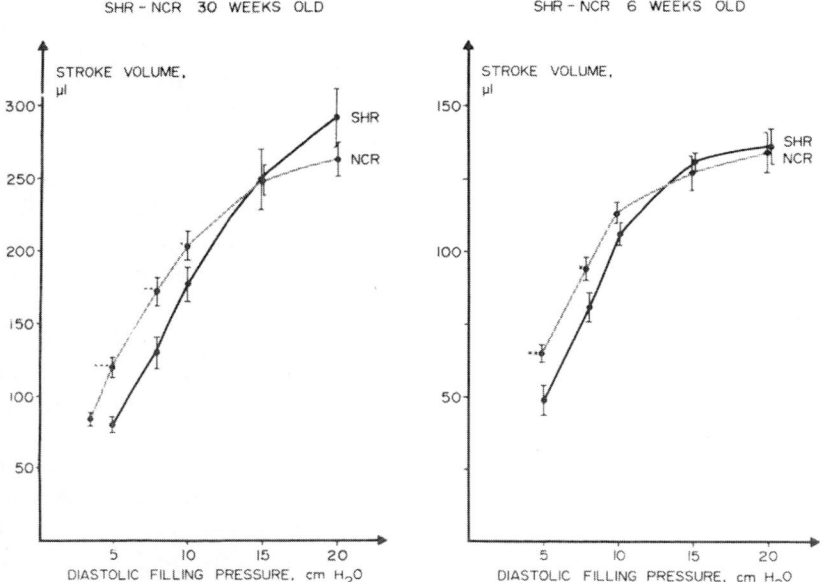

Figure 4. Left. Relation between left ventricular diastolic filling pressure and stroke volume (Frank–Starling relation) for isolated hearts from 30 week old rats (SHR) and normotensive controls (NCR), the left ventricle working against an afterload of 50 mmHg. *Right.* The same relation for hearts from 6 week old SHR and NCR. The vertical bars indicate ± standard error; ** = probability (p<0.01); *** = p<0.001. (from [34]).

thickness implies for the *average* myocardial fibre a lower degree of diastolic 'prestretch' at given levels of end-diastolic pressure. Since it is the degree of prestretch rather than the end-diastolic pressure per se that determines the force of contraction, the Frank-Starling curve of hypertrophied hypertensive hearts tends to be displaced towards the right of that of normotensive ones, at least in the lower curve range, though 'crossing over' in terms of contractile power occurs once optimal degrees of prestretch are reached. As illustrated in Figure 4 on isolated perfused left hearts from SHR and normotensive controls (NCR), the extent of the rightward curve shift is largely proportional to the degree of wall hypertrophy [34].

This rightward displacement of the Frank-Starling curve in these situations is, however, by no means a sign of a 'failing' myocardium, though myocardial degeneration or lesions may, of course, be superimposed, particularly in advanced stages of hypertension. This is clear from the fact that if SHR and NCR hearts are compared at pre- and afterloads producing similar degrees of diastolic prestretch and intrinsic 'homeometric autoregulation' (Anrep effect) in relation to respective ventricular wall thicknesses, the hypertrophic ventricle displays an increased contractile strength that well matches the degree of myocardial thickening.

Another aspect concerning the functional consequences of a thicker myocardial wall is that inner wall layers tend to become more unloaded during systole and may thereby contribute relatively less to the contraction, particularly at lower degrees of filling. This, and the tendency towards a reduced diastolic prestretch at established cardiac hypertrophy, would lead to reductions in stroke volume compared with controls, if there were no compensations. However, such compensation seems to be at hand in the form of an increased left cardiac filling pressure, to judge from direct measurements in awake SHR, in which left atrial pressure is about twice as high as in normotensive controls [35].

This, in turn, would call for increased venous capacitance involvement as hypertension progresses, in order to produce an adequate filling pressure for the hypertrophying heart. Actually, the venous 'low-pressure' side also displays signs of structural adaptation, with reduction in wall distensibility at a largely unchanged 'unstressed' volume, implying that venous pressure would always be somewhat higher in hypertensive cardiovascular systems compared with controls at equal degrees of filling and smooth muscle engagement [36].

3. Structural 'resetting' of barostat functions

a) *Renal 'long-term barostat' function.* Structural autoregulation of systemic precapillary vessels is a generalized process insofar as it takes place wherever pressure is increased, and it therefore includes also the preglomerular section of the renal vascular bed [37]. It has often been pointed out that a hypertensive state cannot be maintained in the presence of an entirely unaltered kidney function [14] but there are, of course, many ways by which kidney function can be reset. A particularly efficient way is simply to increase the preglomerular resistance in proportion to the arterial pressure rise. It has actually been shown in SHR that the pressure-exposed preglomerular resistance vessels adapt structurally like other systemic precapillary vessels, thereby raising the preglomerular resistance and the ratio between the pre- and postglomerular resistances even at maximal dilatation [37]. Thereby, the glomerular filtration pressure can remain normal despite an increased systemic arterial pressure and particularly since the preglomerular vessels display a media thickening and vascular hyper-reactivity as well as a modest luminal reduction. This is illustrated in Figure 5 as a right-hand, parallel displacement of the pressure–filtration curve for maximally dilated, perfused SHR kidneys compared with normotensive ones. The curve displacement is marked in established SHR hypertension, but is only marginal in early borderline phases, indicating that it represents a 'secondary' structural autoregulation, though with efficient renal barostat resetting, and *not*

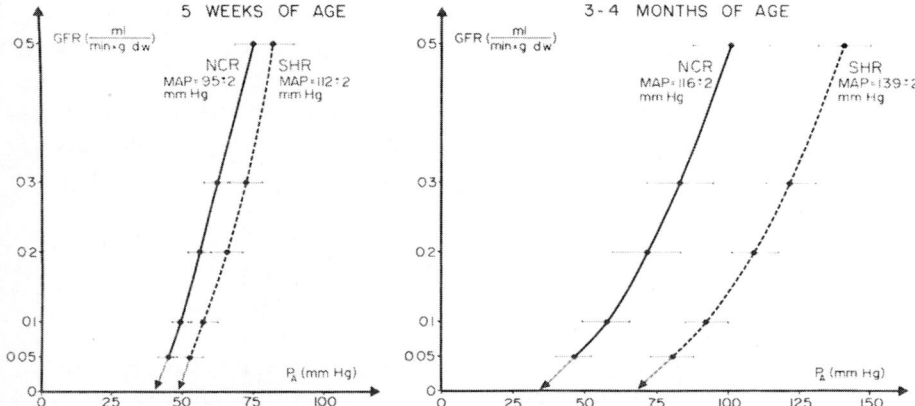

Figure 5. The relationship between perfusion pressure (P_A) and glomerular filtration rate (GFR) in the maximally vasodilated, artificially perfused kidney from young (left part) and adult (right part) SHR and NCR. Note the righthand, parallel shift of this relationship in adult SHR, indicating a structurally based increase of the ratio between the pre- and postglomerular vascular resistances. (From [37]).

any 'primary' hypertension-inducing element, at least not in the SHR variant of primary hypertension. The parallel curve displacement further indicates that glomerular filtration capacity is not reduced compared to controls, because then the SHR curve would also have been less steep than the NCR one.

b) *'Short-term barostat' functions.* This terminology, introduced by Guyton [14], denotes the effects of cardiovascular homeostatic reflexes, as initiated from low-pressure ('volume') mechanoreceptors in heart and central veins and from high-pressure ('baro-') mechanoreceptors in carotid arteries and aortic arch.

With respect to the former receptor group, the structural changes in the left heart contribute to the resetting of the cardiac mechanoreceptors, where those with unmyelinated afferents produce reflex vagal bradycardia and generalized sympathetic inhibition, which particularly involves renal sympathetic control. In SHR these cardiac afferents are clearly reset towards higher diastolic pressures in SHR [38], which at least in part is due to structurally altered wall distensibility.

As for the arterial baroreceptors, essentially the same process of structural vascular adaptation contributes to the resetting of their range of operation to a higher pressure level by reducing wall distensibility also in larger arteries [39]. Therefore, the structural vascular adaptation in hypertension contributes importantly not only to the increase of systemic resistance but also to the resetting of homeostatic mechanisms, which operate via renal control of cardiovascular filling as well as via low-pressure and high-pressure receptor control of efferent sympathetic and vagal influences on heart, resistance and capacitance vessels. In other words, the simple process of local tissue adaptation to changes in average load has most important and far-reaching consequences in hypertension, and its early involvement makes it one of the really important initiating mechanisms when it comes to chronically raising the arterial pressure equilibrium.

E. GENERAL CONCLUSIONS CONCERNING STRUCTURAL CARDIOVASCULAR ADAPTATION IN PRIMARY HYPERTENSION

The principle of adaptive muscle hypertrophy, common to all types of muscle exposed to increased load, seems greatly to affect the hemodynamic situation in hypertension throughout the high-pressure cardiovascular sections, i.e., left cardiac dynamics, barostat functions, systemic resistance control, kidney function and, indeed, the venous capacitance side as well. As hypertension and this structural process advances, stroke volume and cardiac output gradually tend to become lower in association with increasing systemic resistance. Both short-term and long-term barostats 'accept' the raised pressure equilibrium, while the positive-feedback interaction at the resistance level seems gradually to aggravate the situation, at least as long as an even marginally accentuated functional drive prevails. Considering these deleterious consequences of a per se normal type of tissue adaptation to load, it is, in a way, more surprising that some 80% of the population manage to stay fairly normotensive throughout life, than the fact that around 20% become hypertensive with age.

REFERENCES

1. Backer M: Essential Hypertension: the birth of its concept two hundred years ago. Angiology 4:207–209, 1953.
2. Folkow B: Cardiovascular structural adaptation; its role in the initiation and maintenance of primary hypertension. The Fourth Volhard Lecture. Clin Sci Mol Med 55:3–22, 1978.
3. Pickering G: High Blood Pressure. London: JA Churchill, 1968.
4. Genest J, Koiw E, Kuchel O: Hypertension. New York: McGraw-Hill, 1977.
5. Okamoto K: Spontaneous hypertension in rats. Int Rev Exp Pathol 7:227–270, 1969.
6. Okamoto K: Spontaneous Hypertension. Its Pathogenesis and Complications. Tokyo: Igaku Shoin, 1972.
7. Folkow B, Hallbäck M: Physiopathology of Spontaneous Hypertension in Rats. In: Hypertension, pp. 507–522. Genest J, Koiw E, Kuchel O, eds. New York: McGraw-Hill, 1977.
8. Simpson FO, Phelan EL, Clark DWJ, Jones DR, Gresson CR, Lee DR, Bird DL: Studies on the New Zealand strain of genetically hypertensive rats. Clin Sci Mol Med 45:15–21, 1973.
9. Dahl LK, Heine M, Thompson K: Genetic influence of the kidneys on blood pressure.

247

Evidence from chronic renal homografts in rats with opposite predispositions to hypertension. Circulat Res 34:94–101, 1974.

10. Bianchi G, Fox U, Di Francesco GF, Bardi U, Radice M: The hypertensive role of the kidney in spontaneously hypertensive rats. Clin Sci Mol Med 45:135–139, 1973.

11. Folkow B: Central neurohormonal mechanisms in spontaneously hypertensive rats compared with human essential hypertension. Clin Sci Mol Med 48:205–214, 1975.

12. Julius S, Esler M: The Nervous System in Arterial Hypertension. Springfield, IL: Charles C Thomas, 1976.

13. Henry JP, Stephens PM: Stress, Health and the Social Environment. New York: Springer Verlag, 1977.

14. Guyton AC, Granger HJ, Coleman TB: Autoregulation of the total systemic circulation and its relation to control of cardiac output and arterial pressure. Circulat Res 28 and 29 (Suppl 1):93–97, 1971.

15. Ledingham JM, Cohen RD: Changes in extracellular fluid volume and cardiac output during the development of experimental renal hypertension. Canad Med Ass J 90:292–294, 1964.

16. Zumkley H, Losse H: Intracellular Electrolytes and Arterial Hypertension. Stuttgart: Georg Thieme, 1980.

17. v. Kügelgen A: Über das Verhältnis von Ringmuskulatur und Innendruck in menschlichen grossen Venen. Zellforsch 43:168–183, 1955.

18. Folkow B: Structural, myogenic, humoral and nervous factors controlling peripheral resistance. pp. 163–174. In: Hypotensive Drugs. Oxford: Pergamon Press, 1956.

19. Folkow B, Grimby G, Thulesius O: Adaptive structural changes of the vascular walls in hypertension and their relation to the control of the peripheral resistance. Acta Physiol Scand 44:255–272, 1958.

20. Folkow B, Hallbäck M, Lundgren Y, Sivertsson R, Weiss L: Importance of adaptive changes in vascular design for establishment of primary hypertension, studied in man and in spontaneously hypertensive rats. Circulat Res 32 and 33 (Suppl 1):2–16, 1973.

21. Hallbäck, M: Interaction between central neurogenic mechanisms and changes in cardiovascular design in primary hypertension. Acta Physiol Scand (Suppl 424), 1975.

22. Lundin S, Hallbäck-Nordlander M: Background of hyperkinetic circulatory state in young spontaneously hypertensive rats. Cardiovasc Res 14:561–567, 1980.

23. Hallbäck M: Consequence of social isolation on blood pressure, cardiovascular reactivity and design in spontaneously hypertensive rats. Acta Physiol Scand 93:455–465, 1975.

24. Birkenhäger WH, Schalekamp MADH: Control Mechanisms in Essential Hypertension. Amsterdam: Elsevier Scientific, 1976.

25. Hallbäck M, Jones JV, Bianchi G, Folkow B: Cardiovascular control in the Milan strain of spontaneously hypertensive rat (MHS) at 'rest' and during acute mental 'stress'. Acta Physiol Scand 99:208–216, 1977.

26. Warshaw DW, Mulvany MJ, Halpern W: Mechanical and morphological properties of arterial resistance vessels in young and old spontaneous hypertensive rats. Circulat Res 45:250–259, 1979.

27. Horwitz D, Clineschmidt BV, Buren JM, Ommaya AK: Temporal arteries from hypertensive and normotensive man. Circulat Res 34 and 35 (Suppl 1):109–115, 1974.

28. Thulesius O, Gjöres JE: Arterielle Hypertonie und Funktionsänderungen in der Endstrombahn. In: Hypertonie, Risikofaktor in der Angiologie, pp. 27–31. Zeitler, ed. Baden-Baden: Witzstock, 1975.

29. Lundgren Y: Adaptive changes of cardiovascular design in spontaneous and renal hypertension. Acta Physiol Scand (Suppl 408), 1974.

30. Sannerstedt R, Sivertsson R, Lundgren Y: Hemodynamic aspects of the early stages of human arterial hypertension. In: Proc. Symp. on The Arterial Hypertensive Disease, Liège 1975. Rorive, van Cauwenberge, eds. Paris: Masson, 1976.

248

31. Hallbäck-Nordlander M, Lundin S: Cardiovascular reactions in young spontaneously hypertensive rats. In: Hypertension in the Young and Old, pp. 107–119. Onesti G, Kim KE, eds. New York: Grune & Stratton, 1981.
32. Wolinsky H: Long-term effects of hypertension on the rat aortic wall and their relation to concurrent ageing changes. Circulat Res 30:301–309, 1972.
33. Weiss L: Aspects of the relation between functional and structural cardiovascular factors in primary hypertension. Acta Physiol Scand. (Suppl 409), 1974.
34. Hallbäck-Nordlander M, Noresson E, Thoren P: Hemodynamic consequences of left ventricular hypertrophy in spontaneously rats. Am J Cardiol 44:986–993, 1979.
35. Noresson E, Ricksten S-E, Thoren P: Left arterial pressure in normotensive and spontaneously hypertensive rats. Acta Physiol Scand 197:9–12, 1979.
36. Haraldsson B, Nilsson H, Folkow B: Structurally reduced distensibility of cardiovascular 'low-pressure' compartments in primary hypertension, as studied in spontaneously hypertensive rats (SHR). Acta Physiol Scand 112:473–480, 1981.
37. Folkow B, Göthberg S, Lundin S, Ricksten S-E: Structural 'resetting' of the renal vascular bed in spontaneously hypertensive rats (SHR). Acta Physiol Scand 100:270–272, 1977.
38. Thoren P, Noresson E, Ricksten S-E: Resetting of cardiac C-fibre endings in spontaneously hypertensive rats. Acta Physiol Scand 107:13–18, 1979.
39. Aars H: Relationship between aortic diameter and aortic baroreceptor activity in normal and hypertensive rabbits. Acta Physiol Scand 75:406–414, 1969.

15. ROLE OF THE KIDNEY IN THE PATHOGENESIS OF PRIMARY HYPERTENSION

GIUSEPPE BIANCHI

1. INTRODUCTION

Theoretically, in primary hypertension the kidney might be a cause of the hypertension or might be a target organ damaged by the hypertension. The possibility that hypertension might cause kidney damage that in turn would contribute to the maintenance of hypertension is now widely recognized [1–4], and will not be discussed further in this chapter. However, it is important to keep in mind that the ability of hypertension to damage the kidney also depends upon many others factors that favour the development of arteriosclerotic lesions, so that the duration and the degree of hypertension necessary to produce a kidney damage cannot be easily established. Theoretically, it is never possible to exclude, even in a patient with a mild hypertension of recent unset, that any given modification in kidney function is secondary to the raised blood pressure per se. For these reasons, the question of a causal role of the kidney in primary hypertension cannot be established directly in patients already hypertensive and I have been looking for an answer to this question along the following three main lines of approach:
1) Evaluation of what we know at present about hypertension caused by renal lesions and the degree to which this is compatible with the hypothesis that primary hypertension may also be renal in origin.
2) Review of the data on the role of the kidney in rats with a primary type of hypertension, the so-called genetic or spontaneous hypertension.
3) Evaluation of the data available on renal pressor mechanisms in rats or humans with primary hypertension in order to see whether they are similar or differ, especially during the phases preceding or accompanying the development of hypertension.

The reasons behind this particular sequence of topics is clear. We would like to know, first, whether or not the changes caused by a known renal lesions that produces hypertension are like those found in primary hypertension. Next, does the kidney have a causal role in 'primary' hypertension of rats? If so, we may have a model for studying the renal mechanisms that produce primary hypertension. Finally, we want to know whether the results ob-

Amery, A. (ed.) Hypertensive Cardiovascular Disease: Pathophysiology and Treatment
© *1982, Martinus Nijhoff Publishers. The Hague / Boston / London*
ISBN-13: 978-94-009-7478-4

tained in the rat model may prove useful for studying renal machenisms in human hypertensives. This will clearly depend upon the similarities between rats and humans during the stages preceding or accompanying the development of hypertension.

Two major problems arise in this type of approach: one is the probable heterogeneity of the genetic mechanisms functioning in humans with essential hypertension, who are compared with rats selected genetically for presumably a single mechanism. This problem cannot be solved, and the only thing we can do is to see 'a posteriori' whether one subgroup of patients has more similarities than other subgroups.

The other problem is to define the prehypertensive stage in humans. Since it is known that children of hypertensive parents have a much higher probability of developing hypertension later in life than children of normotensive parents [5] we can compare these two groups of children.

2. RENAL HYPERTENSION

Goldblatt [6] was the first to suggest that, since there are many similarities between 'primary hypertension and experimental renal hypertension', the former might be caused by renal lesions that were not detectable with the available diagnostic tests. Since he made this suggestion, a tremendous amount of work in both humans and animals has failed to prove or disprove this suggestion.

In 1966, we developed a device for the constriction of the renal artery in the conscious dog. The device could be placed on a renal artery two weeks before the experiment, while removing one kidney. After complete recovery of the animal from the operation, the effect of renal artery constriction on factors involved in blood pressure regulation could be studied without interference from anaesthesia and surgery. This experiment [7] showed that the sequence of events following renal artery constriction to a single remaining kidney could be divided into three phases if the hypertension was benign:

1st phase: within a few minutes after constriction, plasma renin, blood pressure and total peripheral resistance increased and, in the first hours, the amount of renin present in the plasma was sufficient to account for the rise in blood pressure, as could be assessed by comparison with data obtained after intravenous infusion of exogenous renin into the same dogs a few days before.

2nd phase: this phase lasted a few days, during which renal sodium retention and expansion of extracellular and plasma volumes occurred simultaneously with the increase in cardiac output.

3rd phase: all the factors mentioned above returned to normal and the only abnormalities left were the increases in blood pressure and peripheral resistance.

This sequence of events has been confirmed by different groups of investigators [8-10] using the same experimental procedure, i.e. observation of the events following renal artery constriction in the conscious dog without any other kind of manipulation. Guyton and Coleman [11] obtained similar changes when they simulated renal artery constriction in their computer model and postulated the hypertensive mechanisms to be an increase in renin secretion and renal retention of sodium and water. The main message of these experiments is that, even when well-known renal mechanisms of hypertension are triggered by renal lesions, the regulatory systems of the body are powerful enough to mask these mechanisms and in the steady state the systemic pattern of renal experimental hypertension is similar to that of 'essential' hypertension as was suggested by Goldblatt [6] many years ago. Different types of experimental conditions can alter this sequence of events [12, 13], but whatever physiological significance one gives to these findings, they do not contradict the conclusions derived from data obtained in normal and undisturbed animals with all their regulatory mechanisms intact.

3. SPONTANEOUS OR PRIMARY HYPERTENSION IN RATS

It has been claimed that rats are the best animal model for human primary hypertension. Even though this claim has not yet been proved, we have no better model for primary hypertension in humans. In view of the findings on dogs mentioned in the previous section, it is important to see whether the changes that occur during the development of hypertension in these rats are compatible with a renal pressor mechanism.

This review is limited to the results obtained in Milan Hypertensive Strain (MHS), Dahl Salt-Sensitive Strain (DS), Spontaneously Hypertensive Rat Strain (SHR), Genetically Hypertensive Strain (GH) rats, since these are the strains in which the kidney factors have been studied most extensively. Although MHS have almost the same blood pressures as controls at weaning, they differ from the controls in having higher water consumption, urinary output and plasma volume, lower Hct and plasma renin activity, total and single nephron GFR and kidney weight to body weight ratio. The renal blood flow in absolute values is not significantly different in the two strains, but when expressed as a percentage of cardiac output (CO) it is significantly higher in MHS [14-18]. Over a period of 2-3 weeks the blood pressure of MHS increases by about 40-50 mm Hg, simultaneously with renal retention of sodium and the differences present at weaning disappear. Table 1 shows the main differences between MHS and controls before and after the devel-

Table 1. Differences between MHS and MNS (↑ or ↓, higher or lower in MHS)

	Before	After (Development of hypertension in MHS)
Body weight	=	=
Liver weight	=	=
Heart weight	=	↑
Adrenal glands weight	=	=
Total body sodium and water	=	=
Extracellular fluid volume	=	=
Plasma aldosterone	=	=
Number of glomeruli	=	↓
Kidney weight	↓ ↓	↓
GFR (total and single nephron)	↓	=
Glomerular permability	↓	=
Filtration fraction	↓	=
Urine osmolality	↓	=
Plasma renin and vasopressin	↓ ↓	↓
Urine kallikrein	↓	↓
24 h urinary output	↑	
24 h water intake	↑	=
Renal excretion Na load	↑	↑
Blood volume	↑ ↑	↑

opment of hypertension. It is clear that after the development of hypertension the differences between MHS and controls are those that can also be seen when humans with primary hypertension are compared with appropriate controls. The overall pattern of changes seen here is compatible with a renal origin of hypertension and in fact kidney function seems to be depressed before and normalized after the development of hypertension. The key role of the kidney in the hypertension of MHS was demonstrated clearly by kidney cross-transplantation between MHS and controls. It was demonstrated that the hypertension could be transplanted into normotensive controls by kidney transplantation and, vice versa, hypertensive rats may become almost normotensive when they are given a kidney from a control [19, 20]. This kidney effect is present even before the development of hypertension, so any secondary mechanism may be excluded [21].

Dahl et al. [22] derived two strains of rats from the same Sprague Dawley strain by selective inbreeding based on their different blood pressure responses to a high salt diet: one strain develops hypertension (DS) and the other remains normotensive (DR). It was then shown that their pressor responses to other hypertensinogenic stimuli also differ. There is no difference in whole-kidney function between DS and DR before or after the development of hypertension, but the susceptibility of the DS strain for developing hypertension on high salt diet could be 'transplanted' to the DR strain with a transplanted kidney. Vice versa, DS rats can become resistant when a DR kidney is transplanted and their own kidneys are removed [23]. When the single nephron dynamics of the DS kidney are compared to those of the DR kidney some differences appear [24, 25]. The single nephron of the DS has higher blood flow, filtration rate and intracapillary hydrostatic pressure. In spite of these differences, the whole-kidney blood flow and GFR are similar in the two strains because there are fewer nephrons in the DS. The renin level is lower both in the renal tissue and in the peripheral circulation of DS.

In the Kyoto strain of spontaneously hypertensive rats (SHR) the role of the kidney is much less clear than in the two strains described above. Kidney transplantation experiments showed that it is possible to 'transplant' a portion of hypertension with the kidney [26]. However, these experiments were performed in animals already hypertensive and, therefore, secondary kidney changes caused by the hypertension cannot be excluded as possibly contributing to the differences in the kidney pressor effect. When renal function was measured in anaesthetized 17–18-week-old hypertensive and normotensive rats, the following results were obtained [27]: total and single nephron GFR, kidney weight, total number of glomeruli, glomerular capillary hydrostatic pressure, net ultrafiltration pressure. Tubular pressure and peritubular capillary pressure were similar in the two strains, while afferent and efferent arteriolar resistances and filtration fraction were higher and glomerular blood flow was lower in hypertensive rats. Unfortunately, we cannot evaluate the primary role of the kidney in blood pressure regulation in these rats from these results because they were obtained with already hypertensive animals. However, important differences from the MHS and Dahl strains can be detected when hypertensive animals are compared to appropriate controls. In MHS and Dahl rats, hydrostatic glomerular capillary pressure and single nephron GFR are higher and the number of glomeruli is smaller in the hypertensive animals, while in SHR rats these factors do not differ in hypertensive and normotensive animals. Even though we do not know the meaning of these differences at present, they do demonstrate that the interaction between the kidney and blood pressure can differ in animals with different genetic backgrounds sustaining the primary hypertension.

In Genetically Hypertensive rats (Dunedin) (GH) neither kidney transplantation nor measurement of single nephron dynamics has been carried out. However, there is some indirect evidence indicating that modification of kidney function is most likely not a part of the pathogenesis of this type of hypertension [28]. Plasma volume and extracellular fluid volume tend to be lower in hypertensive animals. In no phase of the development of hypertension is there an increase in exchangeable body sodium and plasma renin is always definitely lower in hypertensive rats. Renal blood flow is lower in hypertensive rats but similar to that of controls during the developmental phase of the hypertension. Hypertensive rats excreted a saline load less quickly than normotensive rats. This finding, which is just the opposite of what happens in patients with essential hypertension, suggests that there is some kind of kidney function impairment in hypertensive rats, but other explanations cannot be excluded.

4. COMPARISON OF RATS AND HUMANS WITH PRIMARY HYPERTENSION

The experimental data for rats with different types of primary hypertension reviewed in the previous section clearly demonstrate that the kidney may have a causative role in some of these types of hypertension, but in spite of this, when whole-kidney function is measured in adult hypertensive rats they do not differ from control rats. This may explain why we have not yet obtained definitive data about the role of the kidney in humans with primary hypertension. In this section we will discuss the similarities in kidney function between rats and humans, examining the individual aspects of this function in parallel in the two species during the phases preceding or accompanying development of hypertension.

4.1. Renal blood flow

In MHS, DS, SHR and GH rats renal blood flow is similar to that of controls, during the early hypertensive phase when expressed in absolute values [29–35]. During the prehypertensive phase in MHS, RBF expressed as a percentage of cardiac output is higher than in controls, indicating selective vasodilatation [17]. I am unaware of any study in the other strains in which cardiac output and RBF were measured simultaneously in the prehypertensive stage.

In children with both parents hypertensive RBF, measured by PAI clearance, is higher than in children of normotensive parents, while the cardiac output is equal in the two groups of subjects and average BP is only 3 mm Hg higher in the children of hypertensive parents [36]. The overall pattern suggests that in this group there is a selective renal vasodilatation as in the prehypertensive stage in MHS. Since it has been demonstrated that renal extraction of PAI is similar in hypertensive and normotensive subjects [37], there is no reason to believe that the differences in RBF between the two groups of subjects are influenced by differences in renal PAI extraction. I am unaware of any other RBF measurements in humans made before the development of hypertension. However, many reports describe the RBF values obtained in patients with essential hypertension at different stages and compared to matched controls [38–46]. These results many be summarized as follows: in the early stages of hypertension, RBF may be similar or slightly lower in hypertensive subjects. At this stage, there seems to be evidence that there may be a subgroup in which the RBF is definitely higher than in controls, but with current methods no valid subdivisions can be made. In the later stages of hypertension, renal blood flow is definitely lower in hypertensive subjects. The GFR remains similar to that of controls for a longer period of time than the RBF as hypertension progresses, due to a progressive increase the filtration fraction.

4.2. Na^+ balance and renal excretion of Na load

In MHS there is a mild renal sodium retention during the development of hypertension. Total exchangeable sodium, though slightly higher in MHS, is not statistically different from controls [14], while in GH rats total exchangeable sodium tends to be lower [28]. In humans, no difference between hypertensive and normotensive subjects has been demonstrated in total exchangeable sodium or extracellular fluid volume.

In MHS, DS and SHR rats, differences in sodium handling by the kidney can be demonstrated after acute loading only when appropriate experimental conditions are used such as conscious and undisturbed rats, loaded with moderate amounts of isotonic saline [15, 47–49]. Under other conditions [18, 47, 48, 50–52], this difference may disappear. These findings, which are also demonstrable before the development of hypertension in MHS and DS rats or in SHR rats still with normal hydrostatic pressure in the renal microvasculature [49], suggest that this phenomenon is not due to the increase in hydrostatic pressure per se.

In humans, adult hypertensive patients excrete sodium faster [53–55]. It has recently been found that children of hypertensive parents excrete sodium faster than children of normotensive parents [56]. Another group [57] of investigators, using a different technique, got opposite results. As in rats, the difference between the two groups of subjects studied by the different investigators may be present only under appropriate experimental conditions. For instance, the second group of investigators studied this phenomenon in subjects free to move around, and it is known [58] that standing may mask the exaggerated natriuresis of hypertensive patients.

4.3. Renin

In the GH, DS and MHS strains, plasma renins are lower than in the controls [14, 28, 29]. In MHS, plasma renin is much lower before the development of hypertension than after, kidney renin secretion is also lower in young MHS [59]. In SHR, plasma renin similar to, lower or higher than that of controls has been found by different investigators [60–66]. At present it is not possible to explain these discrepancies, though we may assume that differences in the source of the animals and in the methodology used to take the blood and to measure renin are implicated.

In humans, the natural history of the relationship of plasma renin to the development of primary hypertension is not clearly established. Children of hypertensive parents may have renin levels similar to [36, 56] or higher [57] than those in children of normotensive parents. However, the subjects within the first group that have higher RBF [36] and sodium excretion after loading [57] tend to have lower plasma renin than the other subjects of the first group or of the second group. In previously untreated adult patients, plasma renin seems to be lower than in their appropriate controls [67, 68]. The relationships between plasma renin, renal blood flow, sodium excretion and the stages of hypertension have been widely debated in the past. The two main different positions can be summarized as follows: one [69–72] suggests that plasma renin and renal blood flow may decrease as hypertension and age progress, as the result of the secondary kidney changes caused by the hypertension. On the other hand, in young patients with mild and recent onset of hypertension or still normotensive children of hypertensive parents, the relationships between these factors seem to go in the opposite direction. Subjects with low renin seem to have higher renal blood flow [36, 39–41, 43], faster sodium excretion [73, 74] and, when hypertensive, a greater fall in blood pressure on diuretic treatment [69, 75, 76] or on sodium restriction [77, 78] than their corresponding controls. This pattern is consistent with the hypothesis that there is a subgroup within the entire group of patients with primary hypertension which can be recognized mainly in the early stages, before the appearance of the kidney changes secondary to hypertension. In these patients the kidney functions differently from that in the other patients. As hypertension and age progress, all these differences may be smoothed out into a uniform pattern of kidney function, due to the effects of the high blood pressure on the kidney.

4.4. Kidney transplantation

As stated in the previous section, in the MHS and DS strains the susceptibility for developing hypertension goes with the transplanted kidney. In the SHR, too, a portion of hypertension can be transplanted with the kidney, but, because these experiments were carried out in adult animals, the influence of secondary kidney changes cannot be excluded.

In humans, the kidney transplantation program may provide us with the possibility of evaluating whether the results obtained in rats are also applicable to man. The influence of the donor's familial hypertension on the blood pressure and antihypertensive therapy requirements of the recipients was evaluated by us in 36 patients, selected by rigid criteria from a total of 340 kidney transplants carried out in Milan over a period of 8 years [79]. These recipients were divided into two groups well-matched for age, sex, body surface area, familial hypertension, duration of haemodialysis before transplantation and original kidney disease. In one group, all the members of the donor's family had diastolic blood pressures below 90 mm Hg, while in the other group at least one parent of the donor had a diastolic blood pressure equal to or above 95 mm Hg. Discriminant analysis and analysis of variance of the values for blood pressure, prednisone and antihypertensive therapy requirements, plasma creatinine and number of rejection crisis recorded during the first year after transplantation revealed a significant difference ($p<0.05$) in the greater antihypertensive therapy requirement during the first four months after transplantation of the recipients of kidneys removed from donors with familial hypertension. From 5–12 months after transplantation, the differences in antihypertensive therapy requirement were not significant. All the other factors were almost the same in the two groups of recipients.

5. CONCLUSIONS

The main conclusions that can be drawn from this review are:
1) In dogs with renovascular hypertension, the characteristic changes caused by the kidney lesion disappear during the early stages and, at the steady state, with a benign form of hypertension, the haemodynamics, hormonal and body fluid systemic parameters are similar to those found in primary hypertension. This is consistent with the hypothesis that not yet discovered kidney lesion may well be responsible for a type of hypertension indistinguishable from human primary hypertension.
2) In two of four strains of rats with types of primary hypertension, the role of the kidney was studied in cross-transplantation experiments. In these two strains, hypertension goes with the kidney. But, more relevant for human primary hypertension, the characteristic changes that suggest kidney involvement in one of these strains (MHS) were present only before or during the very early phase, while in the adult hypertensive animals the differences from the control strains were very similar to those found when patients with primary hypertension are compared to controls.
3) The functional renal abnormality tht might be responsible for these changes and for the subsequent development of hypertension has been discussed in detail elsewere [80, 16, 36]. In brief, the sequence of events in

MHS and in some humans appears to be the following: a reduction of glomerular ultrafiltration coefficient and single nephron GFR may cause, on the one hand, a retention of sodium and water leading to hypertension and, on the other hand, decreased delivery of salt and water to the macula densa leading, through the tubular glomerular feedback mechanism, to a reduction of renin secretion and glomerular vasodilatation. Development of hypertension or an increase in renal blood flow may correct the lower GFR. According to this sequence, the exaggerated natriuresis in the prehypertensive stage could be due either to the renal vasodilatation [81, 82], or to the lower delivery of fluid and salt to the thick ascending limb, causing impairment of the kidney concentrating capacity [80, 16].

Although all these events have been demonstrated to occur in MHS, in humans not all findings are in agreement with the hypothesis. In children of hypertensive parents, the GFR tends to be higher than that in children of normotensive parents [36], even though the difference is not statistically significant. Moreover, recent findings about abnormalities of ion transplant through the cellular membranes both in rats and in humans [83–90] suggest that the tubular reabsorption of ions and water might also be altered in individuals prone to develop primary hypertension, and this could be an alternative explantation for the exaggerated natriuresis in these subjects [91]. Future investigators of the pathophysiology of hypertension should attempt to study the relationship between abnormalities of kidney function and cellular membrane transport present before and during the development of hypertension, in order to see to what extent the former are consistent with the latter. In this way, we may be able to define the place of the kidney within the framework of the relationship between hereditary factors, cellular membrane permeability and consequent changes in cell and organ function that lead to hypertension.

ACKNOWLEDGEMENTS

I am indebted to Miss P. Protasoni (Farmitalia Dept. Nerviano) for the secretarial assistance.

REFERENCES

1. Pickering D: High Blood Pressure, 2nd edn, pp. 236–290. London: Churchill,
2. Koletsky S, Rivera-Velez JM: Factors determining the success or failure of nephrectomy in experimental renal hypertension. J Lab Clin Med 76:54–65, 1970.
3. Ljungquist A: Intrarenal vascular alterations and the persistence of experimantal hypertension. Acta Pathol Microbiol Scand 76:561–574, 1969.
4. Wilson C, Byrom FB: The vicious circle in chronic Bright's disease. Experimental evidence from the hypertensive rat. J Med 10:65–93, 1941.

5. Ayman D: Heredity in arteriolar (essential) hypertension: a clinical study of blood pressure of 1524 members of 277 families. Arch Intern Med 53:792–802, 1934.

6. Goldblatt H: Experimental renal hypertension. Mechanisms of production and maintenance. Circulation 17:642–647, 1958.

7. Bianchi G, Tenconi LT, Lucca R: Effect in the conscious dog of constriction of the renal artery to a sole remaining kidney on haemodynamics, sodium balance, body Fluid volumes, Plasma renin concentration and pressor responsiveness to angiotensin. Clin Sci 38:741–766, 1970.

8. Ferrario CM: Contribution of cardiac output and peripheral resistance to experimental renal hypertension Am J Physiol 226:711–717, 1974.

9. Schultze G, Kirsch K, Preu K, Lohmann FW, Stolpmann HJ, Gotzen R, Dibmann TH: Hämodynamik, Flussigkeitshaushalt, Plasmarenin und Plasmakatecholamine in unterschiedlichen Phasen der renovaskularen Hypertonie des Schafes. Verh Dtsch Ges Kreislaufforsch 38:1–11, 1973.

10. Liard JF, Cowley AW, McCaa RE, McCaa C, Guyton AC: Renin, aldosterone, body fluid volumes, and the baroreceptor reflex in the development and reversal of Goldblatt hypertension in conscious dogs. Circ Res 34:549–560, 1974.

11. Guyton AC, Coleman TG: Quantitative analysis of the pathophysiology of hypertension. Circ Res 24 (Suppl 1):1–19, 1969.

12. Freeman RH, Davis JO, Watkins BE: Development of chronic perinephritic hypertension in dogs without volume expansion. Am J Physiol 233:F278–F281, 1977.

13. Stephens GA, Davis JO, Freeman RH, DeForrest JM, Early DM: Hemodynamic, fluid, and electrolyte changes in sodium-depleted, one kidney renal hypertensive dogs. Circ Res 44:316–321, 1979.

14. Bianchi G, Baer PG, Fox U, Duzzi L, Pagetti D, Giovanetti AM: Changes in renin, water balance, and sodium balance during development of high blood pressure in genetically hypertensive rats. Circ Res 36, 37 (Suppl 1):1–153,–I–161, 1975.

15. Bianchi G., Baer PG, Fox U, Pagetti D: Kidney function and blood pressure in a genetic type of hypertension. 6th Congr Nephrol, Florence, 1975, pp. 274–283. Basel: Karger, 1976.

16. Baer PG, Bianchi G, Duzzi L: Renal micropuncture study of normotensive and Milan Hypertensive rats before and after development of hypertension. Kidney Int 13:452–466, 1978.

17. Bianchi G, Varavaggi AM, Cusi D, Barlassina C, Lupi GP, Duzzi L, Gatti M, Ferrari P, Velis O: Is an abnormal kidney development involved in the pathogenesis of essential hypertension? Proc Int Symposium Juvenile Hypertension, Parma. New York: Raven, 1980. In press.)

18. Bianchi G, Baer PG: Characteristics of the Milan Hypertensive strain (MHS) of rat. Clin Exp Pharmacol Physiol (Suppl 3):15–20, 1976.

19. Bianchi G, Fox U, Di Francesco GF, Bardi U, Radice M: The hypertensive role of the kidney in spontaneously hypertensive rats. Clin Sci Mol Med 45 (suppl 1):135s–139s, 1973.

20. Bianchi G, Fox U, Di Francesco GF, Giovanetti AM, Pagetti D: Blood pressure changes produced by Kidney cross-transplantation between spontaneously hypertensive rats and normotensive rats. Clin Sci Mol Med 47:435–448, 1974.

21. Fox U, Bianchi D: The primary role of the kidney in causing the blood pressure difference between the Milan Hypertensive strain (MHS) and normotensive rats. Clin Exp Pharmacol Physiol (Suppl 3):71–74, 1976.

22. Dahl LK, Heine M, Tassinari L: Effects of chronic excess salt ingestion. J Exp Med 115:1173, 1962.

23. Dahl LK, Heine M, Thompson K: Genetic influence of the kidneys on blood pressure.

Evidence from chronic renal homografts in rats with opposite predispositions to hypertension. Circ Res 34:94, 1974.

24. Azar S., Limas C, Iwai J, Weller D: Single nephron dynamics during high sodium intake and early hypertension in Dahl. Jpn Heart J 20 (Suppl 1):138–140, 1979.

25. Azar S, Johnson MA, Iwai J, Bruno L, Tobian L: Single nephron dynamics in 'post-slat' rats with chronic hypertension. J Lab Clin Med 91:156–166, 1978.

26. Kawabe K, Watanabe TX, Shiono K, Sobake H: Role of the kidney in the pathogenesis of SHR, and other hypertensive rats determined by renal isografts. Jpn Heart J 20 (Suppl 1):87–89, 1979.

27. Azar S, Johnson MA, Scheinman J., Bruno L, Tobina L: Regulation of glomerular capillary pressure and filtration rate in young Kyoto hypertensive Rats. Clin Sci 56:203–209, 1979.

28. Simpson FO, Phelan EL, Jones DR, Butt TJ, Young PL, Ledingham JM: Pathogenesis of hypertension in the New Zealand strain of genetically hypertensive (GH) rats. Jpn Heart J 20 (suppl 1):58–60, 1979.

29. Iwai J, Dahl LK, Knudsen KD: Genetic influence on the renin–angiotensin system. Circ Res 32:678–684, 1973.

30. Arendshorst WJ, Beierwalters WH: Renal tubular reabsorption in spontaneously hypertensive rats. Am J Physiol 237:F-38-F-47, 1979.

31. Nishiyama A, Frohlich ED: Regional blood flow in NR and rats. Am J Physiol 230:691–698, 1976.

32. Ben-Ishay D., Knudsen KD, Dahl LK: Renal function studies in the early stage of salt hypertension in rats. Proc Soc Exp Biol Med 125:515–518, 1967.

33. Tobia AJ, Walsh GM, Tadepalli AS, Lee J: Unaltered distribution of cardiac output in the conscious young spontaneously hypertensive rat: evidence for uniform elevation of regional vascular resistances. Blood Vessels 11:287–294, 1974.

34. Fink GD, Brody MJ: Renal vascular resistance and reactivity in the SHR. Am J Physiol 237:F128–F132, 1979.

35. Butt TJ, Jones DR, Wallis AT, Simpson OF: Intrarenal blood flow fistribution in the genetically hypertensive rat. Nephron 26:49–52, 1980.

36. Bianchi G, Cusi D, Gatti M, Lupi FP, Ferrari P, Barlassina C, Picotti GB, Bracchi G, Colombo G, Gori D, Velis O, Mazzei D: A renal abnormality as a possible cause of 'essential' hypertension. Lancet 173–177, 1979.

37. Reubi FC, Weidmann P: Relationship between sodium clearance, plasma renin activity, Plasma aldosterone, renal hemodynamics and blood pressure in essential hypertension. Clin Exp Hyper 2:593–612, 1980.

38. Birkenhager WH, Krauss XH, Schalekamp MADH, Kolsters G, Zaal GA: Consecutive haemodynamic patterns in essential hypertension. Lancet II:450–564, 1972.

39. Blaufox MD, Fromowitz A, Lee HB, Chien-Hsing Meng, Elkin M: Renal blood flow and renin activity in renal venous blood in essential hypertension. Circ Res 27:913–919, 1970.

40. Grundfeld JP, Raphael JC, Bankir L: Intrarenal distribution of blood flow. In: Advances in Nephrology. Hamburger J, Crosnieer J, Maxwell MH, eds. Chicago Year Book.

41. Hollenberg NK, Epstein M, Basch RI, Conch NP, Merril JP, Hickler RB: Renin secretion in essential and accelerated hypertension. Am J Med 47:855–859, 1969.

42. Kioschos JM, Kirkendall WM, Valenca MR, Fitz AE: Unilateral renal hemodynamics and characteristics of dye-dilution curves in patients with essential hypertension and renal disease. Circ. 35:229–248, 1967.

43. Hollenberg NK, Hollenberg NK, Adams DF: The renal circulation in hypertensive disease. Am J Med 60:773–784, 1976.

44. Hollenberg NK, Borucki LJ, Adams DF: The renal vasculature in early essential hypertension: evidence for a pathogenetic role. Medicine 57:167–178, 1978.

45. Reubi FC, Weidmann P, Hodler J, Cottier PT: Changes in renal function in essential hypertension. Am J Med 64:556–563, 1978.
46. Hollenberg NK, Merrill JP: Intrarenal perfusion in the young 'essential' hypertensive: a subpopulation resistant to sodium restriction. Trans Am Assoc Phys 83:93–101, 1970.
47. Ben-Ishay D, Knudsen KD, Dahl LK: Exaggerated response to isotonic saline loading in genetically hypertension-prone rats. J Lab Clin Med. 82:597–604, 1973.
48. Willis LR, Williams C, Hollingsead P: Natriuretic responses of spontaneously hypertensive rats to intragastric and intravenous saline loads. J Lab Clin Med 94:42–51, 1979.
49. Di Bona GF, Rios LL: Mechanism of exaggerated diuresis in spontaneously hypertensive rats. Am J Physiol 235:F409–F416, 1978.
50. Arenshorst WJ, Beierwalters WH: Renal tubular reabsorption in spontaneously hypertensive rats. Am J Physiol 237:F38–F47, 1979.
51. Farman N, Bonvalet JP: Abnormal relationship between sodium excretion and hypertension in spontaneously hypertensive rats. Pfluegers Arch 354:39–53, 1975.
52. Vandewalle A, Farman N, Bonvalet JP: Renal handling of sodium in Kyoto-Okamoto rats: a micropuncture study. Am J Physiol 235:F394–F402, 1978.
53. Cottier PT, Weller JM, Hoobler SW: Effect of an intravenous sodium chloride load on renal hemodynamics and electrolyte excretion in essential hypertension. Circ 17:750–760, 1958.
54. Lowenstein J, Beranbaum ER, Chasis H, Baldwin DS: Intrarenal pressure and exaggerated natriuresis in essential hypertension. Clin Sci 38:359–374, 1970.
55. Schalekamp MADH, Krauss XH, Schalekamp-Kuyken MPA, Kolsters G, Birkenhager WH: Studies on the mechanism of hyper-natriuresis in essential hypertension in relation to measurements of plasma renin concentration, body fluid compartments and renal function. Clin Sci 41:219–231, 1971.
56. Wiggins RC, Basar I, Slater JDH: Effect of arterial pressure and inheritance on the sodium excretory capacity of normal young men. Clin Sci Mol Med 54:639–647, 1978.
57. Grim CE, Luft FC, Miller JZ, Brown PL, Gannon MA, Weinberger MH: Effects of sodium loading and depletion in normotensive first-degree relatives of essential hypertensives. J Lab Clin Med 94:764–771, 1979.
58. Van Statius EPS. LW, Birkenhager WH, Stertefeld t: De invloed van de lichaamshouding op de 'hypernatriurese' bij lijders aan hypertensie. Ned Tijdschr Geneeskd 106:623–628, 1962.
59. Caravaggi AM, Duzzi L, Bianchi G: Renin secretion in Milan Hypertensive Rats. (In preparation.)
60. De Jong W, Lovenberg W, Sjoerdsma A: Increased plasma renin activity in the spontaneously hypertensive rat. Proc Soc Exp Biol Med 139:1213–1216, 1972.
61. Sen S., Smeby RR, Bumpus FM: Renin in rats with spontaneous hypertension. Circ Res 31:876–880, 1972.
62. Freeman RH, Davies JO, Varsano-Aharon N, Ulick S, Weinberger MH: Control of aldosterone secretion in the spontaneously hypertensive rat. Circ Res 37:66–71, 1975.
63. Shiono K, Sokabe H: Renin–angiotensin system in spontaneously hypertensive rats. Am J Physiol 231:1295–1299, 1976.
64. Czyzewski LB, Pettinger WA: Failure of feedback suppression of renin release in the spontaneously hypertensive rat. Am J Physiol 225:234–239, 1973.
65. Forman BH, Mulrow PJ: Effect of propranolol on blood pressure and plasma renin activity in the spontaneously hypertensive rat. Circ Res 35:215–221, 1974.
66. Berglund G, Lundin S, Herlitz H, Sven-Erik R, Gotberg G, Aurell M, Hallback-Nordlander M: Sodium balance, renin and aldosterone during development of hypertension in SHR. Jpn Heart J 20 (Suppl 1):153–155, 1979.
67. Thomas GW, Ledingham JGG, Beilin LJ, Norman-Stott a, Yeates KM: Reduced renin activity in essential hypertension: a reappraisal. Kidney Int 13:513–518, 1978.

68. Berglund G, Aurell M, Wikstrand J, Wallentin I: Plasma renin activity and hypertensive organ manifestations in 50-Year-old males. Acta Med Scand 199:243–249, 1976.
69. Dunn MJ, Tannen RL: Low renin in hypertension. Kidney Int 5:317–325, 1974.
70. Birkenhager WH, Schalekamp MADH, Krauss XH, Kolsters G, Schalekamp-Kuyken MPA, Kroon BJM, Teulings FAG: Systemic and renal haemodynamics, body fluids and renin in benign essential hypertension with special reference to natural history. Eur J Clin Invest 2:115–122, 1972.
71. Brown JJ, Lever AF, Robertson JIS, Schalekamp MADH: Renal abnormality of essential hypertension. Lancet:320–323, 1974.
72. Birkenhager WH, Schalekamp MADH: Elsevier Scientific, p. 107, 1976.
73. Kraboff LR, Goodwin FJ, Baer L, Torres M, Laragh JH: The role of renin in the exaggerated natriuresis of hypertension. Circ 42:335–345, 1970.
74. Luft FC, Grim CE, Willis LR, Higgins JT, Weinberger MH: Natriuretic response to saline infusion in normotensive and hypertensive man. Circ 55:779–784, 1977.
75. Marks AD, Marks DB, Kanefsky TM, Adlin VE, Channick BJ: Enhanced adrenal responsiveness to Angiotensin II in patients with low renin essential hypertension. J Clin Endocrinol Metab 48:266–270, 1979.
76. Spark RF, O'Hare CM, Regan RM: Low-renin hypertension. Arch Intern Med. 133:205–211, 1974.
77. Kawasaki T, Delea CS, Bartter FC, Smith H: The effect of high-sodium and low-sodium intakes on blood pressure and other related variablesin human subjects with idiopathic hypertension. Am J Med 64:193–198, 1978.
78. Longworth DL, Drayer JIM, Weber MA, Laragh JH: Divergent blood pressure responses during short-term sodium restriction in hypertension. Clin Phar Ther 27:544–546, 1980.
79. Guidi E, Bianchi G, Dallosta V, Cantalupi A, Vallino F, Polli E: The influence of familial hypertension of the donor on the blood pressure and antihypertensive therapy of kidney graft recipients. Nephrology. (in print.)
80. Bianchi G., Baer PG, Fox U, Guidi E: The role of the kidney in the rat with genetic hypertension. Postgrad Med J 53 (Suppl 2):123–135, 1977.
81. Early LE, Friedler RM: The effects of combined renal vasodilatation and pressor agents on renal hemodynamics and the tubular reabsorption of sodium, J Clin Inv 45:1668–1685, 1966.
82. Daugharty TM, Belleau LJ, Martino JA, Early LE: Interrelationship of physical factors affecting sodium reabsorption in the dog. Am J Physiol 215:1442–1447, 1968.
83. Postnov YV, Orlov S, Gulak P, Shevchenko A: Altered permeability of the erythrocyte membrane for sodium and potassium ions in spontaneously hypertensive rats. Pfluegers Arch 365:257–263, 1976.
84. Postnov YV, Orlov SN, Shevchenko A, Adler AM: Altered sodium permeability, calcium binding and Na, K-ATPase activity in the red blood cell membrane in essential hypertension. Pfluegers Arch 371:263–269, 1977.
85. De Mendoca M, Grichois ML, Garay Rp, Ben-Ishay D, Sassard J, Bianchi G, Caravaggi AM, Meyer P: Abnormal net sodium and potassium fluxes in erythrocytes of four varieties of genetically hypertensive rats. In: Int. Symposium on Intracellular Electrolytes and Arterial Hypertension. Stuttgart: Thieme, 1980.
86. Garay RP, Meyer P: A new test showing abnormal net Na^+ and K^+ fluxes in erythrocytes of essential hypertensive patients. Lancet 1:349–353, 1979.
87. Canessa M, Adragna N, Solomon HS, Connolly TM, Tosteson DC: Sodium–lithium countertransport is increased in red cells of patients with essential hypertension. N Engl J Med, 1980. (in press.)
88. Editorial: Hypertension and the red cell. N Engl J Med 302:804, 1980.
89. Postnov YV, Orlov SN, Pokudin NI: Decrease of calcium binding by the red blood cell

membrane in spontaneously hypertensive rats and in essential hypertension. Pfluegers Arch 379:191–195, 1979.

90. Ambrosioni E, Tartagni F, Montebugnoli L, Magnani B: Intralymphocytic sodium in hypertensive patients: a significant correlation. Clin Sci 57:325s–327s, 1979.
91. Taylor A, Windhager EE: Possible role of cytosolic calcium and Na–Ca exchange in regulation of transepitheliai sodium transport. Am J Physiol 236:F505–F512, 1979.

NOTE

Recent, yet unpublished measurements of whole kidney GFR both in MHS and MNS, using an Inutest® plasma concentration much lower than in the published experiments, demonstrate that the former have higher values than the latter when GFR was expressed per 1 g of kidney weight, while the difference between the two strains was not seen when GFR was expressed per 100 g of body weight.

16. ROLE OF SODIUM IN THE PATHOGENESIS OF IDIOPATHIC HYPERTENSION

Frederic C. Bartter

INTRODUCTION

The role of sodium in idiopathic or 'primary' or essential hypertension has been the subject of controversy ever since medicine emerged from its primitive origins and began to acquire respectability as a science.

Whereas much of the controversy continues, there is general agreement that sodium plays a role in the hypertension of some patients; as regards that of others, there is still no consensus. In a larger sense, it may be that the question cannot be answered adequately while the terms 'essential' and 'primary' remain. The implication that all (presumably) non-endocrine hypertension has a single cause (a conclusion now definitively refuted for the rat) persists in much current thinking. The concept of 'salt-sensitive' as opposed to 'non-salt-sensitive' hypertension is being clarified, but few studies have explored the possibility that 'normal' people may be salt-sensitive (salt loads inducing hypertension) or 'non-salt-sensitive' (no blood pressure rise with salt).

It is not, of course, surprising that prospective studies in man have not been designed or attempted. The firmer one's belief that long-term ingestion of large amounts of sodium may induce sustained high blood pressure, the more reluctant one would be to attempt to verify this experimentally in man. Short-term studies, on the other hand, give equivocal results whose applicability to the long-term situation is very poorly understood. Progress in this area has of necessity depended upon retrospective studies of populations and sub-populations in man, from extensive studies of the effects of long-term sodium loading in the rat and rabbit, from genetic studies in rats, and from extensive studies of cardiovascular response to salt in normal animals, especially the dog.

Although it was not possible to study the effect of long-term sodium loads in man, it was, of course, readily possible to study the effect of salt deprivation in hypertensive human beings. These studies have left little doubt that removal of body sodium leads to a decrease in blood pressure in all subjects in whom it can be effectively carried out. As regards interpretation, there remain many questions as to whether such maneuvers counteract an

Amery, A. (ed.) Hypertensive Cardiovascular Disease: Pathophysiology and Treatment
© *1982, Martinus Nijhoff Publishers. The Hague / Boston / London*
ISBN-13: 978-94-009-7478-4

element in the primary, etiologic, mechanism or simply overwhelm those pathophysiologic mechanisms that produce the high blood pressure in the first place.

In any event, the notion that there is a relationship of high blood pressure to sodium intake or to the steady-state total body sodium is firmly entrenched in current thinking and in current practice, because of the enormous success of diuretic therapy in the treatment of idiopathic hypertension.

A role for dietary sodium in blood pressure control in man has been inferred, then, from studies of populations and sub-populations, and from studies of the effects of dietary restriction or pharmacologically induced renal loss of sodium on blood pressure in hypertensive patients. More recently, the physiological effects of short-term sodium loading in normals have been studied. Several controlled studies on the effects of sodium loading in hypertensive subjects have been reported. A role for sodium has also been inferred by analogy with rat studies in which genetic factors and sodium intake have been separately controlled.

Finally, recent studies of the various 'sodium pumps' in erythrocytes, and of the ouabain-sensitive sodium pump of renal cells, granulocytes, and smooth-muscle cells have suggested that there are genetically determined factors that suggest correlation of the activity of such pumps with the arterial blood pressure. Whether such correlations serve only as genetic markers of idiopathic hypertension, as, e.g., in erythrocytes, or may be related to blood pressure by their action on intracellular sodium, as, e.g., in vascular smooth muscle, has not been resolved.

THE STUDY OF POPULATIONS AND SUB-POPULATIONS

As opposed to those primitive populations in which blood pressure is normal and does not rise with advancing age, in other populations a high incidence of hypertension is found even in the young and blood pressure rises progressively with age, to constitute a major cause of illness and death. One such population is found in the Akita Prefecture in Northern Japan: this population stands out as one in which daily salt intake is extremely high [1, 2]. Dahl had concluded from studies on rats that sodium intake is an important factor in the pathogenesis of idiopathic hypertension. He plotted the incidence of hypertension in samples from this and various other populations against the average daily sodium intake estimated for these same samples [3]. The result (Figure 1) showed a high degree of positive correlation ($r = 0.98$) between average sodium intake and the incidence of hypertension. This and similar studies provide strong circumstancial evidence for an etiologic relationship between sodium intake and elevated blood pressure.

266

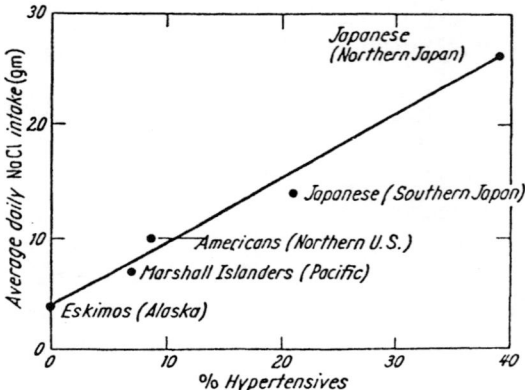

Figure 1. Correlation of average daily sodium chloride intake with prevalence of hypertension in different geographic areas. Printed with permission from [3].

The concept of a role for dietary sodium in blood pressure control has been reinforced from studies of sub-populations derived genetically from primitive, hypertension-free populations. In all such studies, the sub-populations were analyzed during the process of 'acculturation' involved in the transition from the original, primitive culture to one which required adjustment to the complexity of a more highly structured culture in the process of urbanization and the social organization required for nonagricultural existence, trade, competition and defense [4, 5]. The acculturating sub-populations showed rising blood pressure with age, a phenomenon which occurred in women more rapidly than in men. In this situation, the role of genetic factors in the physiological changes observed in the acculturating sub-populations could, of course, be ruled out because of their known origins from the original, isolated stock. As noted, sodium intake in the primitive stock has often been relatively or extremely low. In all cases, the process of acculturation brought with it a substantial increase in sodium intake. Accordingly, the rise in blood pressure was often attributed to the increase in sodium intake. The difficulty with such studies is clear. Whereas an increase in salt intake is indeed involved in the process of acculturation, it is clearly but one of a host of factors to which urbanization and 'civilization' subject the individual. The evidence, then, is circumstantial and must be interpreted with extreme caution.

EXPERIMENTAL DATA IN THE RAT

Further and stronger circumstantial evidence derives from studies of salt-feeding in rats. In 1953 Meneely showed that blood pressure rose with increasing sodium intake in a large proportion of his Sprague Dawley rats [6]. In examining this phenomenon further on a much larger sample of Sprague Dawley rats, Dahl found that some of them showed little or no rise of blood pressure with increasing dietary loads of salt [7]. He selected and inbred these 'salt-resistant' rats and compared them with a similarly inbred group of rats chosen for a very high response of blood pressure to sodium loads (salt-sensitive rats). Derivative generations of the inbred strains retained their non-responsiveness and responsiveness to dietary sodium loads. As expected, sodium-loaded resistant rats showed no increase in mortality with long-term feeding of high-sodium diets, whereas sodium-loaded salt-sensitive rats showed a progressive rise of mortality with increases in dietary sodium. From these results, a genetic basis for the relationship of dietary sodium to blood pressure appeared established – a finding that greatly strengthened the belief of similar genetic control of this relationship in man.

Another important result emerged from these studies: in the salt-sensitive strain, it was found that for any given sodium intake, the average rise of blood pressure and the consequent increase in mortality rate could be ameliorated by increasing the potassium intake [8, 9]. As we shall see, this finding has important implications for current concepts of the mechanism of salt-induced hypertension.

A second important group of studies was made possible by the availability of Dahl's salt-sensitive and salt-resistant strains of rat. It became possible by careful transplants of the kidneys of salt-sensitive rats to nephrectomized, salt-resistant rats to make the salt-resistant recipients salt-sensitive. When the transplant was carried out in the reverse direction by grafting the kidneys of salt-resistant rats to nephrectomized, salt-sensitive ones, the salt-sensitive recipients became salt-resistant [10].

With isolated organ perfusion, Tobian showed that the kidneys from salt-resistant rats could excrete more sodium (at given perfusion pressures) than those from salt-sensitive rats. In further studies, he found evidence that the inability of the kidney from the salt-sensitive donors to excrete sodium was related to a lower renal medullary plasma flow in the salt-sensitive as opposed to the salt-resistant donors [11, 12].

The evidence for relative sodium retention of renal origin as the primary mechanism or for the genetically controlled sensitivity of blood pressure to salt in the salt-sensitive rats was thus considerably strengthened.

Perhaps the most important of the results derived from the study of Dahl's salt-sensitive and salt-resistant rats was achieved by the use of parabiosis [13]. In a now classic paper, bearing the subtitle 'Evidence for a humoral factor' [13], it was shown that renal artery constriction with contralateral nephrectomy produced hypertension in the unoperated parabiotic partner only if the operated rat was of the salt-sensitive strain. They speculated that a humoral pressor agent, whose production in the salt-sensitive rats was stimulated by renal artery constriction, could cross the parabiotic junction to produce hypertension in the partner. Further, they speculated that the pressor substance was identical to a salt-losing substance in the plasma of salt-loaded salt-sensitive rats [14].

SODIUM DEPLETION

In 1920 Allen began a series of studies of the effect of drastic reduction of sodium intake on the blood pressure of hypertensive patients [15–17]. He concluded from these studies that sodium intake and blood pressure are etiologically related. In 1944, Kempner began his well-known studies on the effect of the 'rice, fruit diet' on the treatment of vascular disease, especially hypertension [18]. The effect of this regimen in lowering blood pressure was unequivocally established. The mechanism for the effect was not clarified in these studies. The inevitable weight loss and, probably of greater importance, the high potassium content of the fruit could also have played a part. The effects of such variables are confounded in these studies. Upon further analysis of the results, and from experiments of his own, Dahl concluded that the effect of weight loss per se probably played a minor role in the fall of blood pressure with the rice, fruit diet [19]. The effect of the high potassium content of the diet on blood pressure, on the other hand, was strongly supported by the rat studies of Meneely [8] and of Dahl [9].

With the introduction and subsequent widespread use of the oral diuretics, a role for sodium depletion in the lowering of blood pressure was established beyond a reasonable doubt.

SODIUM LOADING IN NORMAL MAN

A number of studies undertook a prospective study of the effect of dietary sodium in normal man with the use of short-term sodium loading under controlled metabolic conditions [20, 21]. Some of them revealed that an adequate increase in sodium intake produced a corresponding rise in blood pressure, while suppressing plasma renin activity, aldosterone and catecholamines, pressor agents whose role in salt-induced hypertension was thus effectively ruled out, providing that the short-term study is similar to the real-life situation.

Whereas these studies of sodium loading in normal individuals have been interpreted as supporting, in some measure, a role for salt in idiopathic hypertension, there are important reservations. In the first place, in all cases a rise of blood pressure is accompanied by a rise in cardiac output and no rise, or actually a fall, in peripheral resistance. In established 'essential' hypertension, on the other hand, it is clear that cardiac output is normal, and peripheral resistance is elevated. Secondly, the evidence is still only circumstantial.

SODIUM LOADING IN HYPERTENSIVE SUBJECTS

Whereas the applicability of experimental sodium loading in normal subjects to the study of hypertensive subjects is open to question – as must be all 'acute' studies – the possible value of sodium loading in known hypertensives remains to be explored. In two series of subjects recently diagnosed as hypertensive, in whom known causes of hypertension had been ruled out, we studied the effects of sodium loading and of moderate sodium deprivation on blood pressure and on certain variables known or thought to be related to blood pressure control [22, 23].

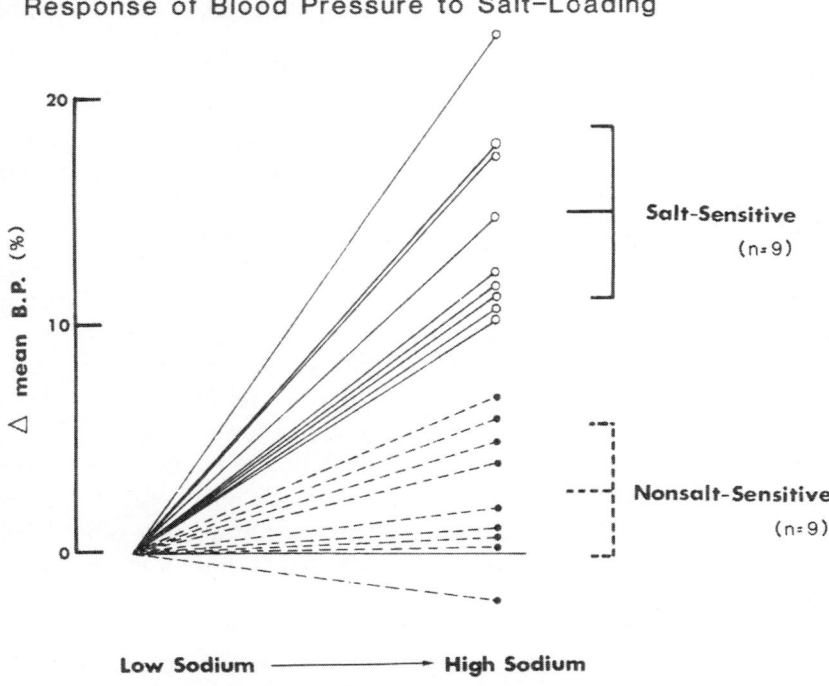

Figure 2. The effect of high-sodium intake on the change in mean blood pressure in 18 patients with idiopathic hypertension. The salt-sensitive and the non-salt-sensitive groups differ in their blood pressure response to a high-sodium load (p<0.001). Reprinted with permission from [22].

Subjects on strict metabolic regimen were studied for seven control days and then for seven days on a low-sodium diet, followed by seven days on a high-sodium diet. The dosage of sodium chosen for the high-sodium diet was one (250 mEq, or about 15 g of sodium chloride per day) that has been shown [20, 21] to have no effect on blood pressure or on cardiac output in normal subjects. With certain unavoidable exceptions (vide infra) all variables were measured at intervals no more than 4 hours apart (day and night), so that the average daily values provide an estimate of the mesor (rhythm-adjusted mean). Blood pressure was measured at half-hour intervals. Besides providing a first 'correction' for circadian variation, this method greatly increases the sensitivity of the measurements. Thus, a significant fall of blood pressure was observed in all groups when the average-sodium diet (109 mEq a day) was changed to a low-sodium diet.

In most of the subjects, the daily average of mean blood pressure rose with the salt loading; in half of them, the rise was by 10% or more of the low-salt values (Figure 2). For purposes of analysis, the subjects were arbitrarily divided into two groups, those with a rise of 10% or more in blood pressure ('salt-sensitive hypertensives') and those with a smaller or no rise ('non-salt-sensitive hypertensives'). The groups were analyzed for a number of variables.

In two independent, consecutive studies, half of the patients fell into the salt-sensitive, and half into the non-salt-sensitive group: this fraction has now been found in a third series of non-selected hypertensives. The salt-sensitive patients consistently retained more sodium with the sodium loads than the non-salt-sensitive ones, and gained more weight. From analysis of each day's values, the difference in sodium retention and weight gain could be shown to appear on day 3 of the 7-day protocol. On day 3, the non-salt-sensitive subjects 'escaped' from the sodium load (urinary sodium exceeding intake) and, pari passu, ceased to gain weight (Figure 3).

Plasma renin activity and aldosterone concentration, which had increased more with the low-sodium regimen in the non-salt-sensitive groups, fell to the same low values with the high-salt regimen in both groups.

Urinary prostaglandin E_2 (PGE_2) rose to a higher value with the low-salt regimen in the non-salt-sensitive patients. With the high-sodium regimen, urinary PGE_2 decreased to the same low values in both groups. Since PGE_2, a vasodilator, under some circumstances increases both plasma renin activity and urinary sodium, the results suggest that the greater rise of PGE_2 in the non-salt-sensitive patients contributed to the increase in plasma renin activity and aldosterone in that group and may also have played a part in the resistance of blood pressure to the sodium loads in the non-salt-sensitive groups.

In one group, cardiac output was measured by a non-invasive, echo-cardiographic technique, before and during the salt-loading (Figure 4). Car-

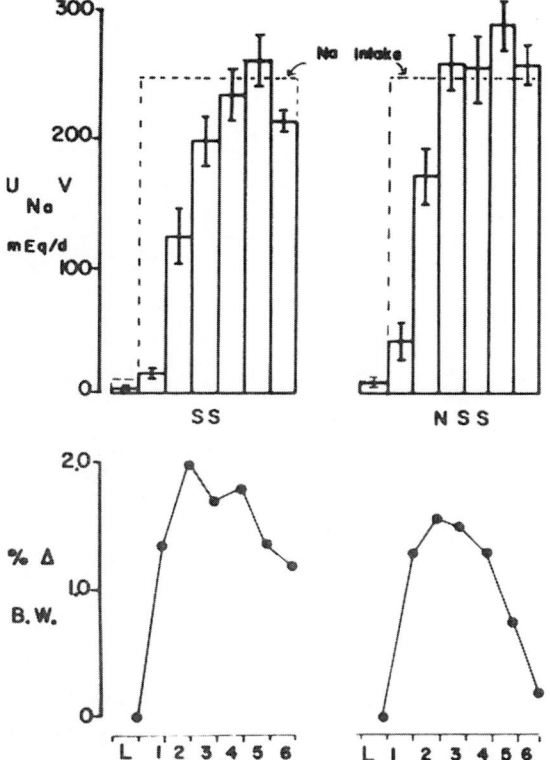

Figure 3. Sodium excretion ($U_{Na}V$) and percent changes of body weight (' B.W.) with the high-sodium intake in salt-sensitive (SS) and non-salt-sensitive (NSS) patients with hypertension. L = sixth day of low-sodium intake. Reprinted with permission from [23].

diac output increased with the sodium loads in the salt-sensitive, but not in the non-salt-sensitive patients. Peripheral resistance tended to decrease in the salt-sensitive patients; whereas this decrease was not statistically significant, it clearly suggests that there was no rise in peripheral resistance.

Plasma norepinephrine, which could not for technical reasons be studied at frequent intervals in each patient, was measured on the low-sodium regimen and on days 3 and 4 of the high-sodium regimen. These days were chosen because it was known that 'escape' occurs on day 3 in the non-salt-sensitive patients, and because of the known relationship of norepinephrine not only to blood pressure, but also to urinary excretion of sodium [24, 25]. In all subjects, plasma catecholamines decreased during the first three days of sodium loading. By day 4, however, plasma norepinephrine had risen significantly ($p < 0.01$) in the salt-sensitive patients, but had not changed in the non-salt-sensitive patients. Thus, a rising plasma nore-

272

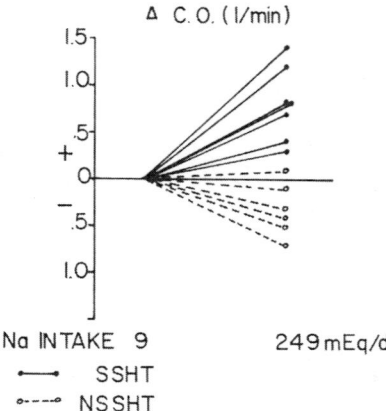

Na INTAKE 9   249 mEq/d
●——● SSHT
○----○ NSSHT

Figure 4. The effect of high-sodium intake
on cardiac output in saltsensitive (SS) and
non-salt-sensitive (NSS) patients with hypertension. The difference in cardiac output between the two groups is significant
at p<0.001.

pinephrine in the salt-sensitive patients may have contributed, not only to
the greater rise of blood pressure in these patients, but also to their inability
to excrete the sodium load as rapidly as the non-salt-sensitive patients.

These studies support a role for sodium intake in idiopathic hypertension.
They may also shed some light on the difference of blood pressure response
to sodium between the salt-sensitive and the non-salt-sensitive patients.

They do not explain the discrepancy, mentioned above, between the picture (increased peripheral resistance, normal cardiac output) reported for a
large number of patients with 'established' idiopathic hypertension and that
observed with salt loads in our hypertensive patients.

COMPARISON OF SODIUM-INDUCED TO 'ESTABLISHED' IDIOPATHIC
HYPERTENSION

The role of 'volume expansion' in the development of raised blood pressure
has been explored in numerous physiologic studies. The animal 'models'
used include the rat, the rabbit, and the sheep, but the great majority of
studies has been carried out in the dog. In virtually all these studies, 'acute'
sodium loading has been shown to produce increases of blood pressure and
of cardiac output.

These, of course, are the changes produced by sodium in our salt-sensitive
subjects. Long-term expansion of body fluids in the dog, on the other hand,

reproduces the pattern reported for idiopathic hypertension, i.e., increased blood pressure with normal cardiac output. From an elegant 'systems analysis' of long-term results in the dog, Guyton and his colleagues [26] have concluded that the progression from the 'acute' to the 'chronic' situation results from 'total body autoregulation', which, in turn, is a response to the increases in cardiac output and in tissue perfusion. The mechanism by which this comes about requires further explanation. This form of autoregulation is clearly not analogous to the well-known autoregulation by which, for example, the kidney responds with vasoconstriction to an increase in perfusion pressure, a phenomenon whose time constant is measured in seconds, whereas the phenomenon of rising peripheral resistance with rising cardiac output and consequent rising tissue perfusion may not appear before as long as 90 min. Indeed, it may not reach a plateau for a period of days [27]. A growing body of evidence suggests that a circulating pressor agent is responsible for this form of 'autoregulation'.

EVIDENCE THAT DAHL'S SALT-LOSING PRESSOR AGENT MAY CAUSE HYPERTENSION BY INHIBITION OF Na–K ATPase

In 1976, Haddy and Overbeck reviewed the evidence that so-called volume-expanded hypertension (such as that caused by massive increase of body sodium by diet or infusion) is generally associated with a decreased activity of the electrogenic ouabain-sensitive sodium 'pump' in vascular smooth muscles [28]. They speculated that expansion of extracellular volume stimulated production by the body of an inhibitor of this pump and, further, that this inhibitor is the same as that produced by Dahl's salt-sensitive rats. (In the parabiotic pairs, renal artery constriction in the salt-sensitive partner produced the volume-expanded hypertension in that rat, and the inhibitor could cross the parabiotic junction to produce hypertension in the partner.)

This hypothesis could explain why the inhibitor was salt-losing: if Na–K ATPase in the kidney is inhibited, sodium reabsorption by the tubules will be diminished. Blaustein proposed an explanation of the ability of the inhibitor to raise blood pressure [29]. Since vascular smooth muscle is stimulated to contract by intracellular calcium, and calcium enters and is extruded from the cell by a Na–Ca 'pump' which can function in both directions, an increase of intracellular sodium with inhibition of Na–K ATPase would tend to force this Na–Ca pump to function to extrude sodium, and thus to admit calcium ions.

The hypothesis may serve to explain the phenomenon, known since Meneely's early studies, that potassium loading clearly lowers blood pressure in salt-induced hypertension [8]. This would be expected if the added potas-

274

sium, by facilitating entry of potassium into cells, partially overcomes the inhibition of Na–K ATPase, allowing more sodium to be extruded by this pump, and thus relatively more of the intracellular calcium to be extruded by the Na–Ca pump.

There remains the task of identification of the postulated inhibitor. A number of investigators have made considerable progress in this area. Buckalew and Gruber [30] obtained evidence that the inhibitor cross-reacts with antibodies raised against ouabain, the established inhibitor of Na–K ATPase. De Wardener and his associates have explored the properties of a low-molecular-weight (<500 daltons) substance, found in plasma and urine of expanded subjects, which appears to qualify as 'the' substance [31]. Viskoper and associates, on the other hand, have studied a high-molecular-weight-substance (>10 000 daltons) found in the urine [32].

GENETIC MARKERS FOR IDIOPATHIC HYPERTENSION

Two possible genetic 'markers' for idiopathic hypertension have recently been proposed. Garay and associates [33] reported that sodium–potassium cotransport, by which coupled extrusion of potassium and sodium from the cell is effected, is below normal in erythrocytes of patients with idiopathic hypertension. This 'pump' is inhibited by ethycrinic acid but not by ouabain. Canessa and associates [34] reported that sodium–lithium counter transport, by which external sodium or lithium ions are exchanged for internal sodium or lithium ions, is above normal in the erythrocytes of patients with idiopathic hypertension. This 'pump' is inhibited by phloretin but not by ouabain. Since both groups reported the same defects in erythrocytes of normotensive, first-degree relatives of the hypertensives, it is unlikely that these abnormalities are related to the mechanism for the hypertension itself.

REFERENCES

1. Fukuda T: Investigation on hypertension in farm villages in Akita Prefecture. J Chiba Med Soc (Jpn) 29:490–496, 1954.
2. Sasaki N: High blood pressure and the salt intake of the Japanese. Jpn Heart J 3:313–324, 1962.
3. Dahl LK: Possible role of salt intake in the development of essential hypertension. In: Essential Hypertension, pp, 53–65. Bock KD, Cottier PT, eds. Berlin: Springer-Verlag, 1960.
4. Page LB, Damon A, Moellering RC: Antecedents of cardiovascular disease in six Solomon Islands Societies, Circulation 49:1132–1146, 1974.
5. Prior IAM, Grimley-Evans J, Harvey HPB, Davidson F, Lindsey M: Sodium intake and blood pressure in two Polynesian populations. N Engl J Med 279:515–520, 1968.

6. Meneely GR, Tucker RG, Darby WJ, Auerbach SH: Chronic sodium chloride toxicity in albino rat – II. Occurrence of hypertension and syndrome of edema and renal failure. J Exp Med 98:71–80, 1953.

7. Dahl LK, Heine M, Tassinari L: Effects of chronic excess salt ingestion. Evidence that genetic factors play an important role in susceptibility to experimental hypertension. J Exp Med-115:1173–1190, 1962.

8. Meneely Gr, Ball COT, Youmans JB: Chronic sodium chloride toxicity: Protective effect of added potassium chloride. Ann Intern Med 47:263–273, 1957.

9. Dahl LK, Leitl G, Heine M: Influence of dietary potassium and sodium/potassium molar ratios on the development of salt hypertension. J Exp Med 136:318.328, 1972.

10. Tobian L, Coffee K, McCrea P, Dahl L: A comparison of the antihypertensive potency of kidneys from one strain of rats susceptible to salt hypertension and kidneys from another strain resistent to it. J Clin Invest 45:1080, 1966.

11. Tobian L, Johnson MA, Lange J, Magraw S: Effect of varying perfusion pressures onthe output of sodium and renin and the vascular resistance in kidneys of rats with 'post-salt' hypertension and Kyoto spontaneous hypertension. Circ Res 36, 37 (suppl 1):162–172, 1974.

12. Tobian L: Salt and Hypertension in Hypertension, pp. 423-433. Genest J, Koiw E, Kuchel O, eds, New York: McGraw-Hill, 1977.

13. Iwai J, Knudsen KD, Dahl LK, Heine M, Leitl G: Genetic influence on the development of renal hypertension in parabiotic rats. Evidence for a humoral factor. J Exp Med 129:507–522, 1969.

14. Dahl LK, Knudsen KD, Iwai J: Humoral transmission of hypertension: evidence from parabiosis: Circ Res 24, 25:I-21-I-33, 1969.

15. Allen FM: Arterial hypertension. JAMA 74:652, 1920.

16. Allen FM: Treatment of arterial hypertension. Med Clin North Am 6:475, 1922.

17. Allen FM, Sherril JW: The treatment of arterial hypertension. J Metab Res 2:429–435, 1922.

18. Kempner W: Treatment of hypertensive vascular disease with rice diet. Am J Med 4:545–552, 1948.

19. Dahl LK, Silver L, Christie RW: The role of salt in the fall of blood pressure accompanying reduction in obesity. N Engl J Med 258:1186–1192, 1958.

20. Kirkendall WM, Connor WE, Abboud F, Rastogi SP, Anderson TA, Fry M: The effect of dietary sodium chloride on blood pressure, body fluids, electrolytes, renal function, and serum lipids of normotensive man. J Lab Clin Med 87:418–434, 1976.

21. Murray RH, Luft FC, Block R, Weyman AE: Blood pressure responses to extremes of sodium intake in normal man. Proc soc Exp Bio Med 159:432–436, 1978.

22. Kawasaki T, Delea CS, Bartter FC, Smith H: The effect of high-sodium and low-sodium intakes on blood pressure and other related variables in human subjects with idiopathic hypertension. Am J Med 64:193–198, 1978.

23. Fujita T, Henry WL, Bartter FC, Lake CR, Delea CS: Factors influencing blood pressure in salt-sensitive patients with hypertension. Am J Med 69:334–344, 1980.

24. Gill JR Jr, Mason DT, Bartter FC: Adrenergic nervous system in sodium metabolism: effects of guanethidine and sodium-retaining steroids in normal man. J Clin Invest 43:177–184, 1964.

25. Gill JR Jr, Bartter FC: Adrenergic nervous system in sodium metabolism – II. Effects of guanethidine on the renal response to sodium deprivation in normal man. N Engl J Med 275:1466–1471, 1966.

26. Cowley AW, Guyton AC: Baroreceptor reflex effects on transient and steady-state hemodynamics of salt-loading hypertension in dogs. Circ Res 36:536–546, 1975.

27. Coleman TG, Bower JD, Langford HG, Guyton AG: Regulation of arterial pressure in the anephric state. Circulation 42:509–514, 1970.

28. Haddy FJ, Overbeck HW: The role of humoral agents in volume expanded hypertension. Life Sci 19:935–948, 1976.
29. Blaustein MP: Sodium ions, calcium ions, blood pressure regulation, and hypertension: a reassessment and a hypothesis. Am J Physiol 232:C165–C173, 1977.
30. Gruber KA, Whitaker JM, Buckalew VM: Endogenous digitalis-like substance in plasma of volume-expanded dogs. Nature 287:743–745, 1980.
31. Poston L, Sewell RB, Wilkinson SP, Richardson PJ, Williams R, Clarkson EM, MacGregor GA, de Wardener HE: Evidence for a circulating sodium transport inhibitor in essential hypertension. Br Med J 282:847–849, 1981.
32. Viskoper JR, Czaczkes JW, Schwartz N, Ullman TD: Natriuretic activity of a substance isolated from human urine during the excretion of a salt-load. Nephron 8:540–548, 1971.
33. Garay RP, Dagher G, Pernollet M-G, Devynck M-A, Meyer P: Inherited defect in a Na^+, K^+-cotransport system in erythrocytes from essential hypertensive patients. Nature 284:281–283, 1980.
34. Canessa M, Adragna N, Solomon HS, Connolly TM, Tosteson DC: Increased sodium–lithium countertransport in red cells of patients with essential hypertension. N Engl J Med 302:772–776, 1980.

17. ROLE OF OBESITY IN THE PATHOGENESIS OF PRIMARY HYPERTENSION

H. E. ELIAHOU

> He is fat and scant of breath.
> *Hamlet*, V, 2, 298.

In the past, the obese have been considered to be of jovial and easy-going character. Yet, they seem to pay heavily for these social qualities as far as their physical health is concerned. Obesity was dismissed as a contributor to disease [1], due to the lack of a direct cause-and-effect relationship and because the association of obesity with disease was largely epidemiological. In this context, Mann [1] distinguishes between causation and association, and claims that obesity is an inevitable and incurable condition, at least in western society. He maintains that treatment is so ineffective that its influence on any disease process cannot be evaluated. Berger [2], in his review at the 3rd International Congress on Obesity, claimed that the higher mortality rates in obesity were only associated with an overweight which exceeded the ideal body weight by at least 25–30%. Van Itallie, however, found that even 10% over the ideal weight was associated with higher mortality rates [3]. He compared mortality rates according to variations in body weight in three separate studies: the Build and Blood Pressure Study [4], The American Cancer Society Study [5] and the Build Study [4]. From their tables it can be seen that at 10% overweight, the mortality percentage is 113, 107 and 111 respectively for males and 109, 108 and 107 respectively for females. At 30% overweight these figures increase to 142, 137 and 135 respectively for males and 130, 138 and 125 respectively for females.

There is ample evidence to implicate obesity as the cause of many diseases, or at least in bringing certain incipient conditions into the open. We are all too familiar with the technical problems experienced in hospital wards with the sick obese patient in whom access to blood vessels is difficult and anesthesia problematic. Cardiovascular disease [3, 6–8], diabetes mellitus [4, 6], hypertension [9], hyperlipidemia [10] and respiratory disorders [11], especially sleep apnea, are clinical conditions known to be associated with obesity. Other conditions which are associated with obesity include: hyperuricemia [12], cholelithiasis [13, 14], osteoarthritis of weight-bearing joints [15], increased frequency of obstetrical complications, re-

Amery, A. (ed.) Hypertensive Cardiovascular Disease: Pathophysiology and Treatment
© *1982, Martinus Nijhoff Publishers. The Hague / Boston / London*
ISBN-13: 978-94-009-7478-4

duced fertility and menstrual irregularities and psychosocial adjustment problems [3]. Even mortality from cancer was found to be significantly higher in severely obese patients [5] who were more than 40% above their ideal body weight. In summary, obesity cannot be taken lightly as if it were a benign condition causing only esthetic and social inconveniences.

The association of overweight with hypertension has been observed on many occasions and is already well established [16, 17]. In the Build and Blood Pressure Study of 1959, overweight was the condition most frequently found in hypertension and the elevations in blood pressure were highly correlated with increase in body weight [18]. As early as 1940 hypertension was reported to be 3 to 6 times as frequent in obese men and women as in individuals of normal weight [17]. In the Framingham Study, the prevalence of hypertension was more commonly observed in the obese, increasing with the degree of overweight [9]. The highest correlation with blood pressure was the relative weight, which is the weight of each subject as compared to the median weight of his cohorts having the same height. A relative weight of over 114 in men aged 50–59 years had a prevalence of 47% of definite hypertension (160/95 mm Hg or more) as compared with only 22% in the group with a relative weight of 85–99. In women of the same age group, the figures were 46% as compared to 27%. In the younger age group of 30–39 years these differences were even more striking. For men, a relative weight of 114 or more was associated with 27% hypertension as compared to 14% in a relative weight of 85–99. For women these figures were 17% as compared to only 1%. However, the fact that there was a certain delay in the subsequent development of hypertension in the already obese normotensive subjects led the authors to believe that the relationship is neither simple nor direct. This lack of a direct relationship between overweight and hypertension actually explains the low order of correlation between body weight and hypertension [9], indicating that there may be other factors involved, such as hereditary traits. The correlation coefficients between relative weight and systolic blood pressure was 0.31 for the ages of 20–29 and 0.37 for the ages of 30–39, whereas for the diastolic blood pressure it was 0.24 for the ages 20–29 and 0.34 for the ages of 30–39 years [19]. Despite these findings, which linked overweight and hypertension, some doubts were expressed by Epstein [20] as well as by Mann [1] as to the effect of avoiding obesity or treating it on the observed hypertension. Yet a number of reports were published claiming that reduction in body weight is associated with reduction in blood pressure, especially in patients with moderate hypertension [17]. Excluding the non-compliant patients whose percentage reached 58%, in a follow-up averaging 8.2 months an average loss of 23.5 pounds in weight decreased blood pressure in 72% of the patients.

A short term follow-up was made on three groups of overweight patients with uncomplicated essential hypertension, who were placed on a weight-reducing diet of 800–1000 calories per day and who were encouraged to eat salt freely. Group 1 consisted of patients on a weight-reducing program not receiving any antihypertensive drug therapy. Group 2a consisted of patients on a weight reducing program and on regular antihypertensive drug therapy. Group 2b consisted of patients not on diet but receiving regular antihypertensive drug therapy. Obviously, in the latter 2 groups this therapy was inadequate to control blood pressure. In group 1 there was a 13.5 ± 6.3 reduction in percent overweight representing 8.8 ± 4.3 kg. This was associated with a reduction of 25.7 ± 16.8 mm Hg for the systolic and 20.0 ± 10.5 mm Hg for the diastolic blood pressure. In group 2a the mean reduction in weight was 14.9 ± 5.3 in percent overweight, representing 9.8 ± 3.8 kg. This was associated with a reduction of 37.4 ± 21.3 mm Hg and 23.3 ± 11.6 mm Hg for the systolic and the diastolic blood pressures respectively. Group 2b showed a reduction of only 1.2 ± 2.2 in percent overweight $(0.7 \pm 1.3$ kg$)$ and a decrease in blood pressure of only 6.9 ± 23.2 and 2.5 ± 10.4 mm Hg for the systolic and diastolic blood pressures respectively. The authors concluded that weight control without salt restriction is a potent tool in the control of hypertension in overweight patients, whether or not they were on antihypertensive drug therapy [21]. In a long-term follow-up of 30 patients with overweight and essential hypertension, it was observed that the reduction in blood pressure, which was associated with reduction in overweight, can be maintained as long as the reduction in body weight was maintained. The follow-up of these patients is presented in Table 1.

The slopes of quantitating every patient's reduction in blood pressure in relation to loss in percent overweight showed marked individual variations. Thus, every individual is expected to follow his own particular slope which is unknown beforehand. It is tempting to assume that genetic factors determine these individual variations.

However, the major problem with weight control, as a therapeutic approach to the overweight-hypertensive patient, is that of long-term compliance. The difficulty in achieving and, even more so, in maintaining body weight within the normal range is obvious. Out of 212 overweight hypertensive patients initiated on a low calorie diet, 40 abandoned the follow-up after four or less visits to the clinic, and 49 were unable to follow their diet so that the reduction in their overweight, if present, was less than 5 %, giving a total non-compliance of 42 % [22]. These figures are similar to those presented by Adlesberg et al. [17] and Ramsay et al. [23]. In a weight-reduction clinic, Linet et al. [24] reported even higher drop-out rates after one year, of 68 % for the individually treated and 59 % for those who had group therapy for behavior modification.

Normal blood pressure was obtained in most overweight hypertensive patients, however, when they had lost only half of their percent overweight.

Table 1. Patients' data, their follow-up periods, body weights and blood pressures

Number	30		
Follow-up period (months):			
Range	20–45		
Mean ± SD	33.12±7.8		
Number of visits:			
Total	256		
Range/patient	6–15		
Mean/patient	8.5		
Males	17		
Females	13		
Age (years):			
Range	25–67		
Mean ± SD	54.2±9.7		
	initial	*at minimal weight within first 6 months*	*at last follow-up visit*
Body weight (kg)	83.1± 9.7	74.7± 8.9	77.6±10.2
Percent overweight	24.5±14.6	12.1±13.6	18.2±16.2
Systolic blood pressure mmHg	181.6±28.0	138.9±16.9	151.3±22.4
Diastolic blood pressure mmHg	114.3±13.6	91.3± 9.8	95.3±13.0
Combined blood pressure categories			
Normal:up to 140 systolic and 90 diastolic	0	12	9
Mild: 141–160 systolic or 91–104 diastolic or both	2	12	10
Moderate: 161–180 systolic or 105–114 diastolic or both	13	6	7
Severe: more than 180 systolic or 114 diastolic or both	15	0	4

In 46 such patients not on any antihypertensive drugs, 82% actually attained normal blood pressure during their follow-up, while most of them were still with an excess in body weight of >10% [25]. Even after a weight reduction of 10% only, 44% of the patients attained a normal systolic blood pressure of 140 mm Hg and 32% attained a diastolic blood pressure of 90 mm Hg or less.

There are many speculations as to the pathogenesis of hypertension in obesity. There is no question as to the influence of heredity on the basal level of blood pressure and the tendency towards hypertension. Various other factors play a role too, one of them being obesity. Chiang et al. [26]

eloquently stated that weight gain constitues one kind of environmental stress that brings a genetic predisposition toward hypertension into the open. The possible pathogenetic mechanisms of high blood pressure in the overweight patient are the following.

Hemodynamic changes

Kaltman and Goldring [27] demonstrated some hypervolemia, increased cardiac output and central circulatory congestion in obesity. They also found that the left ventricular end-diastolic pressure (LVEDP) was in the upper limit of normal at rest, rising immediately to significantly high levels after the smallest effort such as raising a leg. This large rise in LVEDP following a small rise in central blood volume was interpreted to indicate reduced distensibility of the central vessels in obesity. Further support is obtained from the fact that this phenomenon is reversible following weight reduction. The latter was accompanied by a decrease in central blood volume and by the restoration of the response of the LVEDP to exercise to normal.

However, Dustan [28] concluded that there is no characteristic hemodynamic pattern in obesity, since the cardiac index and the total peripheral resistance were the same in the obese and in the non-obese hypertensive. However, since mean arterial pressure = cardiac output × total peripheral resistance, it follows that the responsible entity for the raised blood pressure in obesity is the absolute increase in cardiac output together with an increased aortic wall stiffness or increased aortic impedence.

Insulin and carbohydrate intolerance

De Fronzo et al. [29] as well as Kolanowski et al. [30] found that insulin increases sodium reabsorption in the renal tubule. De Fronzo has shown that insulin affects sodium transport as indicated by an increase in the short-circuit current in the toad-bladder and by a fall in FE_{Na} and C_{Na} in the experimental animal without change in GFR following intrarenal arterial infusion of insulin. These findings, in clinical medicine, are expressed as starvation natriuresis and edema of refeeding and sodium wasting in the diabetic. Furthermore, it has already been shown that in obesity there is a raised plasma insulin, possibly due to resistance to insulin and intolerance to glucose. These changes were shown by Sims [31] to occur in volunteers who deliberately gained weight. These changes were also found to be reversible upon loss of excess weight. De Fronzo [32] suggested that the development of hypertension in obesity in the genetically prone patient may be due to the renal sodium retention secondary to the high insulin levels. This hypothesis was also put forth by Krotkiewski et al. [33] who suggested that hypertension in the overweight patient is secondary to the sodium-retaining effect of the high insulin levels in obesity.

Salt.

The relation of salt to hypertension is still controversial. From his study on eight patients who were given a low calorie diet keeping salt intake normal, Dahl concluded categorically that salt restriction rather than weight loss is the responsible factor for the reduction in blood pressure [34]. However, in Dahl's data two of his eight patients did reduce their blood pressure considerably with their weight loss. Since the upper 95 % confidence limit for the proportion of two in a sample of eight is 65 %, his conclusion should have been that in overweight hypertension weight reduction can reduce blood pressure in 65 % of patients with normal salt intake.

Epidemiological studies in isolated communities demonstrated a strong correlation between high sodium intake and the prevalence of hypertension [35] leading to the obvious conclusion that salt intake is a major determinant in the development of hypertension. Takahashi et al. [36] found that in Akita, Japan, death rates from strokes increased when daily sodium chloride intake exceeded 360 mEq. Shaper [37] followed herdsmen who were drafted into the Kenyan army. They increased their daily intake of salt from about 50 mEq to about 300 mEq. Though their blood pressure did not rise significantly in the first year, there was a progressive rise during the second and the third years. But there was also a considerable early rise in body weight following their recruitment, which again interferes with a clear-cut conclusion that the chronic salt intake per se might have been the responsible factor for their raised blood pressure. Observations which favor the hypothesis that salt restriction reduces blood pressure satisfactorily relate to drastic reductions in sodium intake [38, 39]. According to Page, patients with essential hypertension do not respond with a satisfactory reduction in blood pressure when placed on a very low sodium diet. He claimed that he has yet to see a completely convincing study of sequential sodium balance during the development of hypertension [40].

In our studies we observed that the salt excretion in the groups of overweight essential hypertension who reduced blood pressure following body weight loss, were similar to that in patients who were not on a weight reduction program [21]. Furthermore, 34 patients who were on a low energy diet with unrestricted salt intake and who reduced blood pressure following body weight loss, showed high urine sodium excretion, as can be seen in Table 2.

Further support is obtained from the data of Dornfeld et al. [41] who had two groups of overweight hypertensives placed on 300 calories daily, one group with 40 mEq and the other with 210 mEq sodium a day. The decrease in diastolic blood pressure was similar in both groups following weight loss.

Nevertheless, a genetic proneness for the blood pressure to respond to sodium load or withdrawal is obvious in experimental animals. Hyperten-

Table 2. The 24-h urine sodium in overweight patients with essential hypertension not on anti-hypertensive or diuretic therapy, but on low energy diet

	At start of low energy diet	During weight loss	After reduction in both weight and blood pressure
Number of patients	34*	34*	11
24-h urine sodium (mEq)	118±64.5	168±64.2	137±66.4

* Mean of two different groups.

sion is readily induced in Dahl 'S' rats by oral NaCl loading. Isolated perfused kidneys from the 'S' rats excrete about 50% less sodium than 'R' rat kidneys. The 'S' rats not on thiazide showed a prompt rise of blood pressure while on an 8% NaCl diet. The 'R' rats not on thiazide did not increase their blood pressure (Figure 1) [42]. This might be due to an intrinsic shift in the pressure–natriuresis curve. Kidneys from 'R' rats favor rapid natriuresis at lower pressures, while kidneys from 'S' rats favor a slower natriuresis, thus causing salt retention and a rise in blood pressure.

Norepinephrine turnover and overfeeding.
Searching for a more sensitive parameter than plasma levels of norepinephrine to assess sympathetic nervous system activity, Landsberg [44] used ³H.norepinephrine turnover rates in sympathetic nerve endings in small animals. The turnover rate is represented by the disappearance of the labelled norepinephrine at the nerve endings where it is initially taken up. It was found that during fasting this rate markedly diminishes, probably as the result of an adaptive process to decrease metabolism, but in sucrose overfeeding it markedly increases. He concluded that fasting suppresses sympathetic nervous system activity, whereas overfeeding stimulates it. This increase in sympathetic tone in obesity can in itself facilitate the rise in blood pressure. A less likely explanation is the increase in tubular sodium reabsorption caused by the increased turnover of the norepinephrine.

Physical exercise.
Lack of physical training has certain obvious correlations with obesity, especially with regard to glucose intolerance and insulin blood levels [45]. The lack of physical exercise may enhance an increase in blood pressure; it is suggested by Horton's data that physical training reduces blood pressure measured at rest and at mild work loads [46]. Krotkiewski et al. [33] gave physical training in a gymnasium to 27 normotensive women with varying degrees of obesity, for 6 months. Their blood pressures, both systolic and diastolic, were significantly reduced at rest as well as after mild work loads

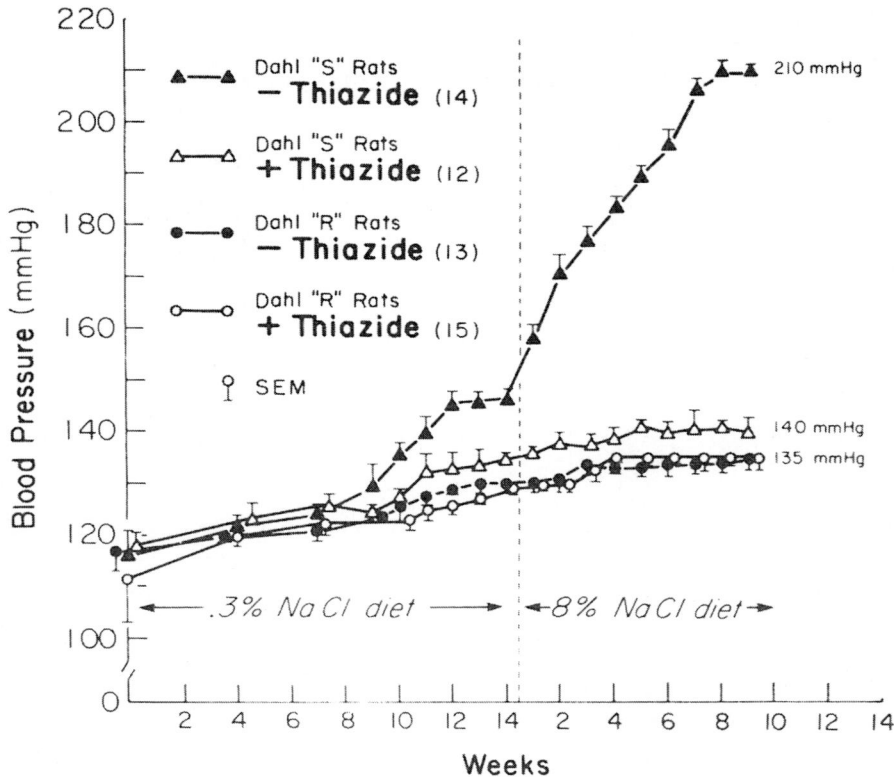

Figure 1. Blood pressure response to high and to low sodium diets and to treatment with thiazides in the Dahl 'S' and 'R' rats, clearly indicating an inherent, most probably genetically determined, difference of blood pressure response. (from Tobian et al. [42], with permission of Hypertension, American Heart Association, Inc., Dallas, TX, U.S.A.).

even though there was no change in the body weight of the total group. The blood pressures at rest were as follows: systolic 134 ± 4 mm Hg before and 125 ± 4 mm Hg after training; diastolic 87 ± 2 mm Hg before and 80 ± 2 mm Hg after training.

Thyroid hormones.

The finding of Danforth et al. [47] that overfeeding increases triiodothyronine (T_3), the active form of the thyroid hormone, and decreases the inert reverse T_3, prompted Sims et al. [48] to associate the thyroid hormone with the pathogenesis of hypertension in obesity. In the hyperthyroid state there is evidence of a high sympathetic nervous system activity as indicated by the increased number of beta-adrenergic receptors. The number of these receptors in the myocardium in rats is increased after thyroxine [49, 50]. It decreases during the chronic administration of propyl-thiouracyl in rats [51] or following beta-adrenergic agonists in humans [52]. It seems likely therefore, that overfeeding increases T_3 to such an extent that it results in a meaningful increase in the number of beta-adrenergic receptors, causing an increase of vascular sensitivity. It is logical that the combination of an increased number of cardiac beta-adrenergic receptors and the presence of a high norepinephrine turnover will result in a high inotropic effect, high cardiac output and increase in blood pressure. There are no data, however, on the influence of thyroxine on the sympathetic nervous system at the periphery, i.e. at the vascular walls. The only clinical finding so far is that there are no changes in the number of beta-adrenergic receptor sites in the circulating mononuclear cells in patients with hyperthyroidism [53]. The mechanism by which the thyroid hormones increase blood pressure needs further investigation.

The red-cell sodium–potassium pump.

In the obese patients, the red blood cells were found to have a significantly reduced number of sodium–potassium ATPase units as measured by ouabain binding capacity of their membranes when compared with red cells from individuals with normal body weight. As a matter of fact, a significant negative correlation was found between maximal ouabain binding capacity (i.e. number of Na–K ATPase units) and the percentage of ideal body weight [54]. Since considerable energy is used by the sodium–potassium pump, reduction in its activity, i.e. reduction of Na–K ATPase units, may be the cause of reduced cellular thermogenesis, resulting in reduced energy expenditure, making it available to produce overweight and obesity. Furthermore, the decreased activity of the sodium–potassium pump in obesity allows a higher concentration of sodium in the cell. Indeed, a 35 % increase in red cell sodium concentration was observed in the obese population.

On the other hand, in patients with essential hypertension, Garay et al. [55] found an abnormally low Na/K net flux ratio, i.e. a high net sodium influx into the red cells. In other words there is a low ratio of sodium extrusion to potassium uptake. They attributed their finding to an inherited defect in the Na–K co-transport system which they thought is genetically associated with hypertension [56]. Sodium–lithium counter-transport was found to be increased in red cells of patients with essential hypertension, again indicating a defect in the cell-membrane sodium transport in this condition [57]. In his review, Haddy [58] finds storng evidence for an increased ouabain-insensitive rubidium-86 uptake in blood vessels of experimental animals with genetic models of hypertension. Since this uptake reflects passive transport into the cells, it seems that in genetic hypertension there is an increase in passive penetration of sodium into the cells. Furthermore, he also finds evidence for an increased ouabain-sensitive rubidium-86 uptake, suggesting an increased activity of the Na–K pump. He concludes that in genetic hypertension, there is an icreased passive permeability of the cell membranes, i.e. to sodium, which in itself stimulates the Na–K pump from the inside.

This increased cellular permeability to sodium in hypertension has the same effect as the decreased Na–K pump activity of the obese, both tending to increase cellular sodium. The implication is that this transmembrane disorder of sodium extrusion in red cells and of increased passive permeability to sodium in cells of blood vessel walls in hypertension might be present in all cells responsible for an increase in arteriolar tone, leading to the tendency of developing hypertension. However, it should be emphasized that the interrelationships of these mechanisms have not been clearly elucidated as yet and calls for further interesting and, most probably, rewarding investigations.

High PRA state.

In the course of our studies we have compared the plasma renin activity (PRA) in overweight with that in non-overweight patients with essential hypertension. In a group of 43 overweight hypertensive patients the mean PRA at rest was 1.45 ± 0.19 ng/ml/h and after ambulation 3.38 ± 0.39 ng/ml/h. In 61 non-overweight hypertensive patients (matched for sex, age ± 3 years and 24-h urine sodium ± 10 mEq/day), the PRA values were 1.06 ± 0.07 ng/ml/h and 2.41 ± 0.16 ng/ml/h respectively. The differences are significant with $p < 0.01$. Normotensive controls had PRA levels of 0.64 ± 0.33 and 1.6 ± 0.8 ng/ml/h at rest and after ambulation respectively. This finding has not yet been confirmed by others and its importance is still not clear. It could be a reactive rather than a causative process, secondary to the 'low distensibility' of the larger central vessels in obesity, simulating and therefore signalling a 'low volume' state.

In summary overweight predisposes to hypertension, depending upon the genetic background of the individual. Reduction in body weight by a low calorie and an unrestricted salt diet reduces the high blood pressure. It seems that the increase in body weight causes an inherited tendency towards hypertension to come out into the open. The pathogenetic mechanisms for this have not been clearly defined. The possible factors which help in the development of hypertension in overweight include high cardiac output and blood volume in the presence of decreased distensibility of the arterial wall, higher insulin levels which encourage sodium reabsorption at the renal tubules, possible accumulation of salt which might result in higher vascular wall sensitivity to vasoconstrictive processes, a higher norepinephrine turnover, lack of physical exercise, a facilitating effect of triiodothyronine which is known to increase in overfeeding, a higher plasma renin activity and a decrease in the amount of sodium–potassium ATPase units resulting in higher intracellular sodium content, possibly sensitizing the cells to the vasoconstrictor responses.

REFERENCES

1. Mann GV: The influence of obesity on health. N Engl J Med 291:178–185, 226–232, 1974.
2. Klesse R, Berchtold P, Dannehl K, Gebler S, Greiser E, Berger M, Jörgens V, Gries FA, Zimmermann H: Mortality of obese patients: the Dusseldorf mortality study. 3rd International Congress of Obesity. Alim Nutr Metab 1:291, 1980.
3. Van Itallie TB: Obesity: adverse effects on health and longevity. Am J Clin Nutr 32:2723–2733, 1979.
4. Build and blood pressurestudies 1957. vol. 1. Chicago: Society of Actuaries, 1959.
5. Lew EA, Garfinkel L: Variations in mortality by weight among 750,000 men and women. J Chronic Dis 32:563–576, 1979.
6. Richards R, DeCasseres M: The Problem of Obesity in developing countries: its prevalence and morbidity. In: Obesity Symposium, pp. 74–84. Burland WL, Samuel PD, Yudkin J, eds. Edinburgh: Churchill Livingstone, 1974.
7. Kannel WB, Gordon T: Obesity and cardiovascular disease: the Framingham Study. Clin Endocrinol Metab 5:367–75, 1976.
8. Berchtold P, Bergman M, Greiser M, Dobse M, Irmscher K, Gries FA, Zimmerman H: Cardiovascular risk factors in gross obesity. Int J Obesity 1:291, 1977.
9. Kannel WB, Brand N, Skinner JJ, Dawber TR, McNamare PM: The relation of adiposity to blood pressure and development of hypertension. Ann Intern Med 67:48–59, 1967.
10. Pelkonen R, Nikkila EA, Koskinin S, Penttinen K, Sarna S: Association of serum lipids and obesity with cardiovascular mortality. Br Med J 2:1185–1187, 1977.
11. Zwillich CW, Sutton FD, Pierson DJ, Creagh EM, Weil JV: Decreased hypoxic ventilatory drive in the obesity-hypoventilation syndrome. Am J Med 59:343–348, 1975.
12. Kannel WB, Gordon T: Obesity and cardiovascular disease: the Framingham Study. In: Obesity Symposium,pp. 24–51. Burland WL, Samuel PD, Yudkin J, eds. Edinburgh: Churchill Livingstone, 1974.
13. Miettinen TA: Cholesterol production in obesity. Circulation 44:842–850, 1971.
14. Friedman GD, Kannel WB, Dawber TR: The epidemiology of gallblader disease: observations in the Framingham Study. J Chr Dis 19:273–292, 1966.
15. Leach RE, Baumgard S, Broom J: Obesity: its relationship to osteoarthritis of the knee. Clin Orthop 93:217, 1973.
16. Pickering GW:High Blood Pressure. London: Churchill, 1955.
17. Adlesberg D, Colcher HR, Laval J: Effect of weight reduction on course of arterial hypertension. J Mount Sinai Hosp (N.Y.) 12:984–992, 1946.
18. Lew EA: High blood pressure, other risk factors and longevity. The insurance view point. Am J Med 55:281–294, 1973.
19. Epstein FH, Francis T, Hayner NS, Johnson BC, Kjelsberg MO, Napier JA, Ostrander LD, Payne MW, Dodge HJ: Prevalence of chronic diseases and distribution of selected physiological variables in a total community, Tecumseh, Michigan. Am J Epidemiol 81:307–322, 1965.
20. Epstein FH: Estimating the effect of preventing obesity on total mortality and hypertension. Int J Obesity 3:163–166, 1979.
21. Reisin E, Abel R, Modan M, Silverberg DS, Eliahou HE, Modan B: Effect of weight loss

without salt restriction on the reduction of blood pressure in overweight hypertensive patients. N Engl J Med 298:1–6, 1978.

22. Iaina A, Goldfarb D, Gaon T, Shochat J, Eliahou HE: Low energy diet in the essential hypertension patient. Third International Congress on Obesity. Rome, 8–11 Oct., 1980.

23. Ramsay LE, Ramsay MH, Hettiarchi J, Davies DL, Winchester J: Weight reduction in a blood pressure clinic. Br Med J 2:244–245, 1978.

24. Linet OI, Metzler CM, Vantasset M: Evaluation of a 'free' weight control clinic. Obesity/Bariatric Med 8:152–157, 1979.

25. Eliahou HE, Iaina A, Gaon T, Shochat J, Modan M: Body Weight reduction necessary to attain normotension in the overweight hypertensive patient. Obesity and Hypertension, Satellite Symposium tothe Third International Congress on Obesity in Rome. Florence, 6–7 Oct., 1980.

26. Chiang BN, Perlman LV, Epstein FH: Overweight and hypertension. A review. Circulation 39:403–421, 1969.

27. Kaltman AJ, Goldring RM: Role of circulatory congestion in the cardiorespiratory failure of obesity. Am J Med 60:645–653, 1976.

28. Dustan HP: Hemodynamics in obesity. Obesity and Hypertension, Satellite Symposium to the Third International Congress on Obesity. Florence, 6–7, Oct., 1980.

29. De Fronzo RA, Cooke CR, Andres R, Faloona GR, Davis PJ: The effect of insulin or renal handling of sodium, potassium, calcium and phosphate in man. J Clin Invest 55:845–855, 1975.

30. Kolanowski J, Salvador G, Desmecht P, Henquin JC, Crabbe J: Influence of glucagon on natriuresis and glucose-induced sodium retention in the fasting obese subject. Eur J Clin Invest 7:167–175, 1977.

31. Sims EAH, Danforth E, Horton ES, Bray GA, Glennon JA, Salans LB: Endocrine and metabolic effects of experimental obesity in man. Recent Prog Horm Res 29:457–496, 1973.

32. De Fronzo RA: Effect of insulin and glucagon on electrolytes and blood pressure in experimental animals. Obesity and Hypertension, Satellite Symposium to the Third International Congress on Obesity. Florence, 6–7 Oct., 1980.

33. Krotkiewski M, Mandroukas M, Sjöström L, Sullivan H, Witterquist H, Björntorp P, Wilhelmsen L: Effects of long-term physical training on body fat, metabolism and blood pressure in obesity. Metabolism 28:649–658, 1979.

34. Dahl LK, Silver L, Cristie RW: Role of salt in the fall of blood pressure accompanying reduction in obesity. N Engl J Med 258:1186–1192, 1958.

35. Tobian L: The relationship of salt to hypertension. Am J Clin Nutr 32:2739–2748, 1979.

36. Takahashi E, Sasaki N, Takeda J, Ito H: The geographic distribution of cerebral hemorrhage and hypertension in Japan. Hum Biol 29:139, 1957.

37. Shaper AG: Cardiovascular disease inthe tropics – III. Blood pressure and hypertension. Br Med J 3:805–807, 1972.

38. Kempner W: Treatment of kidney disease and hypertensive vascular disease with rice diet. N Carolina Med J 5:125–133, 1944.

39. Murphy RFJ: The effect of 'rice diet' on plasma volume and extracellular fluid space in hypertensive subjects. J Clin Invest 29:912–917, 1950.

40. Page IH: Some regulatory mechanisms of renovascular and essential arterial hypertension. In: Hypertension, pp. 576–587. Genest J, Koiw E, Kuchel O, eds. New York: McGraw.Hill, 1977.

41. Dornfeld LS, Kushiro T, Yanagava N, Waks AU, Vertes V, Maxwell MH: Blood pressure changes in obese subjects during rapid weight reduction. Third International Congress on Obesity. Rome 8–11 Oct., 1980. Alim Nutr Matab 1:254, 1980.

42. Tobian L, Lange J, Iwai J, Hiller K, Johnson MA, Goossens P: Prevention with thiazide of NaCl-induced hypertension in Dahl 'S' rats. Hypertension 1:316–323, 1979.

43. Fujita T, Henry WL, Barther FC, Lake CR, Delea CS: Factors influencing blood pressure in salt-sensitive patients with hypertension. Am J Med 69:334–343, 1980.

44. Landsberg L: Nutrition and regulation of the sympathetic nervous system and its relation to hypertension. Obesity and Hypertension, Satellite Symposium to the Third International Congress on Obesity. Florence, 6–7 Oct., 1980.

45. Sims EAH: Mechanisms of hypertension in the syndromes of obesity. An overview. Obesity and Hypertension, Satellite Symposium tothe Third International Congress on Obesity. Florence, 6–7 Oct., 1980.

46. Horton ES: The role of exercise inthe treatment of hypertension in obesity. Obesity and Hypertension, Satellite Symposium to the Third International Congress on Obesity. Florence, 6–7 Oct., 1980.

47. Danforth E Jr, Horton ES, O'Connell M, Sims EAH, Banger AG, Ingbar SH, Braverman L, Vagenakis AG: Dietary-induced alterations in thyroid hormone metabolism during overnutrition. J Clin Invest 64:1336–1347, 1979.

48. Sims EAH, Phinney SD, Vaswani A: The management of hypertension associated with obesity. Int J Obesity 2:215, 1978.

49. Williams LT, Lefkowitz RJ, Watanabe AM, Hathaway DR, Besch HR Jr: Thyroid hormone regulation of β-adrenergic receptor number. J Biol Chem 252:2787–2789, 1977.

50. Williams LT, Lefkowitz RJ, Watanabe AM, Hathaway DR, Besch HR Jr: Thyroid hormone regulation of β-adrenergic receptor number: possible biochemical basis for the hyperadrenergic state in hyperthyroidism. Clin. Res. 25(3):458A, 1977.

51. Ciaraldi T, Marinetti GV: Thyroxine and propylthiouracyl effects in vivo on α and β-adrenergic receptors in rat heart. Biochem Biophys Res Commun 74:984–991, 1977.

52. Galant SP, Duriseti L, Underwood S, Insel PA: Decreased β-adrenergic receptors on polymorphonuclear leukocytes after adrenergic therapy. N Engl J Med 299:933–936, 1978.

53. Williams RS, Guthrow CE, Lefkowitz RJ. β-adrenergic receptors in human lymphocytes are unaltered by hyperthyroidism. J Clin Endocrinol Metab 48:503–505, 1979.

54. Dre Luise M, Blackburn GL, Flier JS: Reduced activity of the red-cell sodium-potassium pump in human obesity. N Engl J Med 303:1017–1022, 1980.

55. Garay RP, Elghozi JL, Dagher G, Meyer P: Laboratory distinction between essential and secondary hypertension by measurement of erythrocyte cation fluxes. N Engl J Med 302:769–771, 1980.

56. Garay RP, Dagher G, Pernollet MG, Devynck MA, Meyer P: Inherited defect in a Na^+-K^+ co-transport system in erythrocytes from essential hypertensive patients. Nature 284:281–283, 1980.

57. Canessa M, Adragna N, Solomon HS, Connolly TM, Tosteson DC: Increased sodium-lithium counter transport in red cells of patients with essential hypertension. N Engl J Med 302:772–776, 1980.

58. Haddy FJ: Mechanism, prevention and therapy of sodium-dependent hypertension. Am J Med 69:746, 1980.

18. ROLE OF CATECHOLAMINES IN THE PATHOGENESIS OF PRIMARY HYPERTENSION

P. W. DE LEEUW and W. H. BIRKENHÄGER

INTRODUCTION

As illustrated elsewhere in this book, the autonomic nervous system plays a major role in blood pressure control by modulating venous capacity, heart rate and contractility and arteriolar resistance. The intensity of sympathetic stimulation varies greatly with posture, activity, physical conditioning and emotional state.

From a clinical point of view, excess sympathetic stimulation appears to be a highly likely mechanism for the elevation of blood pressure. Suggestive features of early hypertension are an increased heart rate, enhanced myocardial contractility, and the combination of a high cardiac output and an inappropriately elevated systemic vascular resistance. The activity of the sympathetic system is difficult to assess and only indirect methods are available. One approach which is used frequently, is the measurement of catecholamines under various conditions.

INVESTIGATIONAL PROBLEMS

The quantification of adrenergic activity poses enormous methodological problems. Although it is generally assumed that increased activity of the sympathetic nervous system is associated with greater entry of noradrenaline into the blood stream, most of neurotransmitter released from sympathetic nerve endings is subject to re-uptake and local degradation. Furthermore, when an impulse reaches the nerve terminal, the amount of noradrenaline liberated, will be greatly influenced by presynaptic receptor mechanisms which may either enhance or inhibit subsequent release of the hormone.

Estimation of noradrenaline output by studying urinary excretion of this compound and its metabolites is complicated not only by the strong minute-to-minute variations in adrenergic activity, but also by the influence of renal function. Since renal hemodynamics are disturbed in primary hypertension to a varying degree, one can have serious doubts about the use of

Amery, A. (ed.) Hypertensive Cardiovascular Disease: Pathophysiology and Treatment
© 1982, Martinus Nijhoff Publishers. The Hague / Boston / London
ISBN-13: 978-94-009-7478-4

urinary excretion of catecholamines as a reliable parameter of sympathetic activity.

On the other hand, plasma levels of catecholamines are generally below 1 μg/l both in normotensive and hypertensive subjects. Therefore, sensitive and specific techniques are required for reliable assessment of plasma concentrations. The development of radio-enzymatic methods and adequate separation procedures has now set the stage for such assessments.

A question which is still unsettled is whether it is justified to equate circulating noradrenaline levels with net transmitter overflow and to equate the latter again with the intensity of sympathetic nerve traffic. However, despite wide inter-subject differences a positive relationship between systolic blood pressure and plasma noradrenaline has been found during short-term increases in sympathetic activity [61]. Although this suggests a dynamic relationship between plasma noradrenaline levels and sympathetic activity, it still does not prove whether such a relationship exists under basal conditions.

CATECHOLAMINES IN ESSENTIAL HYPERTENSIVES AT REST

Early studies on the excretion of catecholamines and their metabolites in patients with essential hypertension frequently gave results which were within or slightly above the normal range. On the other hand, elevated urinary catecholamine excretion was described in patients with 'borderline' hypertension [44]. In established essential hypertension urinary excretion of catecholamines usually is normal [3, 38], only a number of patients showing an increase [36]. As stated before, such data on urinary excretion of catecholamines have to be interpreted with caution.

After sensitive methods became available to measure plasma catecholamines, a large number of studies has been devoted to the neurohumoral aspects of essential hypertension. Engelman et al. [21] measured total plasma catecholamines in 32 resting normal adults and 18 patients with essential hypertension. Average values were 0.24 (range 0.10–0.34) μg/l in the normals and 0.45 (range 0.20–0.78) μg/l in the hypertensives, which was significantly higher. In both groups noradrenaline constituted 80% of the plasma catecholamines.

DeQuattro and Chan [18] reported a smaller but still significant difference between the average total catecholamine concentrations of 25 normotensive subjects and 27 patients with hypertension. In 10 patients with sustained hypertension, total catecholamine level was 0.387 μg/l, in 17 patients with labile hypertension 0.334 μg/l and in 25 normotensive controls 0.273 μg/l. In 7 of the hypertensives, plasma catecholamines were clearly raised. Subsequently, many authors demonstrated increased levels of catecholamines in hypertensive patients [5, 7, 9, 10, 12, 19, 22, 23, 31, 39, 40, 43, 48, 55, 56], although this could not always be confirmed [2, 8, 16, 30, 32–34, 37, 46, 59]. When present, however, differences in distribution pattern between normotensives and hypertensives appear to be rather subtle [56]. More recently, attention has been paid to adrenaline levels, which were found to be elevated in most studies [1, 2, 23, 25, 29], but normal in others [51, 65].

In order to permit an accurate appraisal of plasma catecholamines in primary hypertension, several factors need consideration. They will be described below.

DETERMINANTS OF PLASMA CATECHOLAMINES IN HYPERTENSION

Choice of control population

In order to conclude that plasma catecholamines are raised in primary hypertension, one has to know the normal range for these hormones. In most studies healthy laboratory personnel or volunteer subjects, who may be medical or paramedical staff, were selected as controls. This may be inappropriate, however, because these subjects usually are preconditioned to investigative procedures and show less anxiety, fear or stress, all of which could influence plasma noradrenaline.

Probably, the problem is rooted even more deeply, because the human condition of hypertensives and normotensive controls is basically different. The awareness of having hypertension and being studied for that very reason, is likely to induce a state of expectancy which will be far more intensive and persistant than the mere 'needle reflex' in control subjects. This is illustrated in the study by Jones et al. [33], who measured plasma noradrenaline concentrations in normotensive and hypertensive outpatients as well as in laboratory control subjects. The normotensive outpatients were evaluated for symptoms such as headache, tiredness, chest discomfort or abdominal pain. Noradrenaline concentrations were found to be similar in both groups of outpatients, but significantly lower in laboratory control subjects. The latter group also exhibited lower values for blood pressure and heart rate. The authors considered these data to be suggestive of decreased sympathetic nervous activity in the volunteers. Moreover, they speculated that both outpatient groups had not attained the same 'basal' level of sympathetic discharge as the volunteers. Although it cannot be excluded that the time period allowed for resting before withdrawal of blood samples was too short, the data presented do not support the hypothesis of excessive sympathetic nervous activity in primary hypertension. A similar conclusion was reached by DeLeeuw et al. [16] who took as controls patients who were hospitalized for diagnostic tests or who were in the reconvalescent phase of a 'minor' illness. The latter included healed uncomplicated duodenal ulcer, which still may not be appropriate since in the active phase of this disease, plasma noradrenaline is raised [4].

Age, sex and race

With a few exceptions [13, 16], most authors agree that noradrenaline physiologically tends to rise with age [2, 37, 46, 55, 56, 64]. Jones et al. [32] observed such a relationship in white males only. In hypertensives the rise of noradrenaline with age is usually less clear or even absent. Although the effect of age on the plasma level of catecholamines has not yet been completely settled, available data demand that control populations have to be carefully matched for age. On that basis a subgroup of young hypertensives with raised noradrenaline levels has been identified [2, 27, 56].

Plasma adrenaline levels tend to fall slightly with age in both normotensives [25, 65] and hypertensives [2].

Another factor to be taken into account is the sex distribution of study groups, since hypertensive women appeared to have higher plasma levels of noradrenaline than hypertensive men [26]. The latter study shows that hypertensive women also had higher noradrenaline values than normal women, but this could be due to differences in age. Evidence has also been presented that genetic influences on basal noradrenaline levels exist in normal man [42]. In view of the inheritable nature of essential hypertension, such influences may occur in hypertensives as well, although this remains to be established. There is no evidence that catecholamines differ between blacks and whites [57].

Time and site of sampling

Standardisation of sampling time closely relates to the question whether a diurnal rhythm exists for plasma catecholamines. Indeed, both noradrenaline and adrenaline peak in the late morning and early afternoon and reach lowest values at night during sleep [50, 60]. Therefore, Zadik et al. [67] measured 24-h integrated concentrations of noradrenaline and adrenaline in normal subjects and in patients with mild essential hypertension. No significant difference could be found between levels in the hypertensives and in the controls. Although these data suggest that sympathetic activity is normal in hypertension, they show that sampling time should be taken into account when single samples have been drawn.

For reasons of convenience, blood samples for plasma catecholamines are usually drawn from a forearm vein. It has been reported that catecholamine levels at that site do not differ significantly from those at several other vascular sites [62], although they are usually lower in the hepatic vein [34]. Planz and coworkers [49] measured catecholamine levels in blood from renal and suprarenal veins in five normal subjects and four patients with essential hypertension. As expected, noradrenaline and adrenaline levels were far higher in suprarenal venous blood than elsewhere. The ratio between adrenaline and noradrenaline was above 1 in the suprarenal and renal vein, but fell below 1 in the inferior vena cava. Similar values were found in the hypertensives and in the controls. From these data one would conclude once again that adrenergic activity is not enhanced in primary hypertension.

In our own laboratory, we took blood samples simultaneously from the renal artery and vein of hypertensive patients and found significantly higher levels of noradrenaline in the renal vein [15, 17]. Inasmuch as renal noradrenaline release reflects local sympathetic activity, these data may indicate that peripheral venous levels of catecholamines are only a weak reflection of what is going on at the level of a particular organ. Indeed, when we compared data from an untreated hypertensive population to those obtained in propranolol-treated hypertensives, marked differences in renal noradrenaline release were found, despite similar peripheral venous plasma levels [17].

Effect of physical and mental activity

In most studies cited above, plasma catecholamine levels have been measured not only at rest, but also during a variety of challenge procedures such as postural change, static exercise (e.g. isometric handgrip), dynamic exercise (e.g. bicycle ergometry) and mental stress. Although all these manoeuvres increase the plasma level of catecholamines, quantitatively the response may differ between hypertensives and controls and has often been found to be larger in the former.

There is frequent dissociation, however, between the effects of different stimuli on noradrenaline and adrenaline [53] which may confound interpretation of available data. Thus far the results of various studies indicate that in a number of, mainly younger, patients with essential hypertension, the increment of plasma catecholamines during exercise or postural stimulation is larger than in normals. Whether this reflects abnormally-increased sympathetic activity or enhanced neurotransmitter release upon normal nerve traffic, remains conjectural.

Diet

It has been almost unanimously observed that plasma catecholamines rise in response to sodium restriction. Sodium loading or high dietary salt intake lowers catecholamines, although they may rise again at a sodium intake beyond 200 mmol per day [45].

In normal subjects plasma noradrenaline varies inversely with nocturnal sodium secretion and directly with nocturnal potassium excretion. The latter relationship is lost in patients with essential hypertension [41]. These recent observations call for strict dietary control when comparing catecholamines between hypertensives and control subjects. There is evidence to suggest that the dietary influence is demonstrable also during challenge studies [53].

In conclusion, it can be stated that many external conditions may affect plasma catecholamines. Yet, these conditions vary greatly between different investigations and it is only recently that some factors have been controlled. Therefore, the controversy about whether catecholamines are increased in hypertension still cannot be solved. To take away some of the uncertainties, one could approach the problem in a slightly different way, namely by relating the prevailing level of catecholamines to parameters of blood pressure control.

CATECHOLAMINES AND BLOOD PRESSURE CONTROL MECHANISMS IN ESSENTIAL HYPERTENSION

If catecholamines play a primary role in causing hypertension, one would anticipate a relationship between these hormones and blood pressure. A direct relationship between plasma noradrenaline and blood pressure has indeed been found in several studies [5, 19, 39, 40], but was absent in others [9, 16, 32, 43]. Chobanian et al. [6] found such a relationship only in male patients. Kiowski et al. [35] found a weak relationship between noradrenaline and blood pressure in hypertensive patients but not in normals, even though both groups had similar noradrenaline levels. Franco-Morselli et al. [25] described a direct relationship between systolic blood pressure and plasma adrenaline. However, this relationship was rather weak and only present when normotensives, labile hypertensives and sustained hypertensives were lumped together. In another study [29] no relationship between blood pressure and adrenaline was found.

It should be noted that in the studies where a relationship between catecholamines and blood pressure has been found, a rather wide range of blood pressures was needed for this relationship to become apparent. Furthermore, it has to be borne in mind that any relationship between catecholamines and blood pressure may be lost should cardiac (beta-) receptors or vascular (alpha-) receptors be stimulated preferentially. There is, however, a paucity of data on the relationship of catecholamines with the hemodynamic determinants of blood pressure. In the study of Miura et al. [43] values of plasma noradrenaline were shown to correlate significantly with total peripheral vascular resistance, a relationship which was more obvious in labile than in sustained hypertension. On the other hand, the group of DeChamplain has published several reports from which it appears that increased levels of catecholamines are associated with enhanced cardiac contractility and elevated heart rate [10, 12]. In these studies hypertensive patients were divided into a 'normo-adrenergic' (catecholamine concentration within normal range) and a 'hyperadrenergic' (concentrations above normal range) subgroup. The latter showed increased heart rates and shorter pre-injection periods. However, from all those studies one cannot fully escape the conclusion that the results are influenced by the inclusion of subjects who may have been rather tense during the investigations. If this were the case, then the results might reflect a mechanism of anxiety rather than a mechanism of essential hypertension (although these are not necessarily mutually exclusive). In our laboratory, where patients were studied under basal conditions, while their salt intake was controlled, we were unable to find a relationship between noradrenaline and cardiac output or systemic vascular resistance.

On the other hand, regional hemodynamic patterns might be more revealing. In essential hypertension, the distribution of the cardiac output is diverted away from visceral organs and the skin and this pattern certainly is compatible with a sympathetic mechanism. It is surprising, therefore, that only a few data are available that relate biochemical indices of adrenergic activity to organ blood flow.

Clement et al. [9] compared skin and muscle blood flow in hypertensives with high and low values of plasma noradrenaline. There was no difference in skin blood flow and, although patients with high noradrenaline levels tended to have a lower muscle blood flow, the difference was not significant.

Kiowski et al. [35] infused the alpha-adrenoceptor blocking agent phentolamine into the brachial artery of hypertensive patients and found that the increase in forearm blood flow produced by this drug correlated with the plasma noradrenaline concentration at rest. Also, a positive correlation was observed between mean blood pressure at rest and the increase in forearm blood flow induced by phentolamine. In the normotensives such relations were absent. On the basis of these data the authors concluded that the resting level of plasma noradrenaline can be considered to be a marker of alpha-adrenoreceptor-mediated vasoconstriction, which, in part, also determines the height of the blood pressure.

Since phentolamine in hypertensive subjects also increases renal blood flow [28], we studied the relationship between sympathetic activity and renal perfusion. Although we expected to find a relationship between plasma noradrenaline and renal vascular resistance, this was virtually absent. How-

UNTREATED

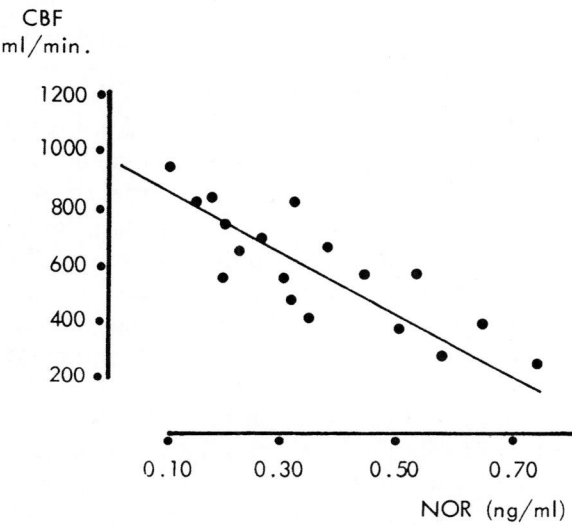

Figure 1. Relationship between renal cortical blood flow (CBF) and plasma noradrenaline levels in hypertensive subjects ($r = -0.76$; $p<0.05$).

ever, in a subgroup of sixteen patients, we assessed outer cortical blood flow using the ^{133}Xe-washout technique and, as shown in Figure 1, in this subgroup we found a significant inverse relationship between plasma noradrenaline and cortical perfusion [17]. This would seem to indicate that vascular resistance, when assessed very selectively, is indeed dependent on sympathetic activity. Failure to demonstrate such a relationship on a larger scale may be due to differences in end-organ responsiveness and the balance between alpha- and beta-stimulation as discussed below.

Both in our study and in the one by Kiowski et al. [35] plasma noradrenaline levels were normal, yet a relationship was found with renal blood flow and blood pressure, respectively. Thus the activity of the sympathetic nervous systesm per se cannot be the only factor responsible for the increase in vascular resistance and two theories have emerged to explain these findings. As a first possibility enhanced vascular smooth muscle responsiveness to neurogenic stimulation seems an attractive hypothesis. This theory is supported by many studies which show exaggerated responses to exogenous catecholamines in hypertensive patients. However, increased vascular reactivity is not always demonstrable and may occur also in normotensive offspring of hypertensive patients [20]. Safar et al. [54] even found the pressor dose of noradrenaline to be increased in patients with borderline hypertension. Some of this controversy may be eliminated when vascular reactivity to noradrenaline is related to the circulating level of noradrenaline, as has been done by Philipp et al. [47]. These investigators infused noradrenaline in normotensive and hypertensive subjects and determined vascular reactivity from the reciprocal value of the dose needed to increase blood pressure by 20 mm Hg. When reactivity was plotted against the circulating level of stimulated noradrenaline (the latter being obtained during dynamic exercise), a hyperbolic inverse relationship was observed in the normotensives. This relationship was present also in the hypertensives, but with increasing blood pressure progressively shifted to the right. In other words, at any given level of noradrenaline (or for that matter: sympathetic drive) vascular responsiveness is increased in patients in whom resting blood pressure is higher. As the same study did not show an alteration of the response to angiotensin II in hypertension, the authors suggested that functional rather than structural alterations were responsible for their findings.

An inappropriate association between normal adrenergic activity and increased pressor responsiveness to noradrenaline was also described by Weidmann et al [66], who found this association to be present already in subjects with borderline hypertension. However, it remains to be established whether these abnormalities are primary or secondary to the hypertensive process.

A somewhat alternative hypothesis was put forward by the group of Bühler. These investigators measured sympathetic activity at rest and during dynamic exercise and in addition assessed beta-adrenoceptor sensitivity with bolus injections of isoproterenol [2]. Both in normotensives and in hypertensives, older age appeared to be associated with diminished exercise tachycardia and increased blood pressure response to exercise. In addition, isoproterenol sensitivity decreased with age, while noradrenaline levels rose. In hypertensive patients these patterns were more pronounced and from that the authors concluded that an increase in blood pressure and age is accompanied with a progressive reduction in beta-adrenoceptor sensitivity and/or reactivity. As a corollary, defective beta-receptor-mediated responses may then result in unopposed alpha-receptor-mediated vasoconstriction and thereby contribute to the hypertensive process. Increased pressor responsiveness to noradrenaline can thus be explained by an imbalance between arteriolar alpha- and beta-receptor-mediated effects.

Although the hypotheses seem attractive, they have to account for an impairment of baroreceptor functioning. This in itself may already lead to an increase in plasma noradrenaline: when hypertensive patients were subjected to a standard dynamic exercise, those with poor baroreflexes responded with a greater increase in blood pressure and in the plasma noradrenaline levels than those with good reflexes [58]. If an impairment of baroreceptor function would be a primary event in essential hypertension, then enhanced alpha-adrenergic vasoconstriction with increases in plasma noradrenaline and adaptive down-regulation of beta-receptors could result as secondary phenomena. However, thus far no data are available to show that changes in adrenergic activity (and the development of hypertension) follow a primary disturbance in baroreceptor functioning. The latter, on the other hand, may be related to the lability of blood pressure, although there is no evidence that blood pressure variability is directly related to catecholamine levels [9, 63]. Conversely, in our laboratory we observed an inverse relationship between the 'pressor range' (i.e. the maximal amplitude of upward diurnal blood pressure excursions from basal blood pressure) and plasma noradrenaline. Although the relationship was weak in untreated persons (presumably due to the time of blood sampling), subsequent treatment with propranolol strengthened this inverse relationship [14]. This implies that sympathetic traffic is governed by alterations in vessel wall tone, which in turn may effect baroreceptor tuning. In this view, the basic fault again is situated at the level of the vascular wall.

In discussing the effects of adrenergic activity on vascular smooth muscle dynamics, one has to bear in mind that the renin–angiotensin system may also be involved. It is known that sympathetic stimulation and catecholamines can increase renin secretion [11] and angiotensin may exert a positive feed-back on the central nervous system [24]. In hypertensive patients the relationship between basal levels of noradrenaline and renin has been reported to be positive, negative and absent. The lack of agreement on this topic probably reflects differences in patient selection and lack of standardization procedures. As yet, no definite conclusions can be drawn on the interaction of the sympathetic system and angiotensin in the elaboration of essential hypertension.

SUMMARY AND CONCLUSION

There is general agreement that plasma catecholamines are increased in some hypertensive patients. Plasma noradrenaline seems to be normal more often than plasma adrenaline. Results of different studies have to be interpreted with caution since many variables, like age, sex, sodium intake, level of activity and method of sampling may affect the results. Moreover, the choice of a control population is important, since the psychology of hypertensives and normotensive controls with respect to the investigative procedure may be fundamentally different.

Plasma catecholamines and blood pressure are related in only part of the studies reviewed. In the final analysis, however, catecholamines and noradrenaline in particular should be associated with vascular resistance and indeed in one study this has been found. On the other hand, relationships have been found between noradrenaline and regional hemodynamic measurements in forearm and kidney. The mechanisms whereby neurogenic vascular tone could be increased, are still open to dispute, but several hypotheses have been put forward. Among these are an enhanced vascular smooth muscle response to sympathetic stimulation, an imbalance between vascular alpha- and beta-receptors and malfunctioning of the baroreceptor reflex. It is conceivable that other pressor mechanisms, like the renin–angiotensin system interact with sympathetic activity, but no conclusive data are available to support such a statement. Presently the most that can be claimed for the sympathetic system is that it plays a permissive role in the maintenance of essential hypertension. The possibility of an initiating role, however plausible from a clinical point of view, awaits further confirmation.

REFERENCES

1. Beretta-Piccoli C, Weidmann P, Meier A, Grimm M, Keusch G, Glück Z: Effects of short-term norepinephrine infusion on plasma catecholamines, renin and aldosterone in normal and hypertensive man. Hypertension 2:623, 1980.
2. Bertel O, Bühler FR, Kiowski W, Lütold BE: Decreased beta-adrenoceptor responsiveness as related to age, blood pressure, and plasma catacholamines in patients with essential hypertension. Hypertension 2:130, 1980.
3. Bing RF, Harlow J, Smith AJ, Townshend MH: The urinary excretion of catecholamines and their derivatives in primary hypertension in man. Clin Sci Mol Med 52:319, 1977.
4. Brandsborg O, Brandsborg M, Løogreen NA, Christensen NJ: Increased plasma noradrenaline and serum gastrin in patients with duodenal ulcer. Eur J Clin Invest 8:11, 1978.
5. Brecht HM, Schoeppe W: Relation of plasma noradrenaline to blood pressure, age, sex and sodium balance in patients with stable essential hypertension and in normotensive subjects. Clin Sci Mol Med 55 (Suppl 4):81s, 1978.
6. Chobanian AV, Gavras H, Melby JC, Gavras I, Jick H: Relationship of basal plasma noradrenaline to blood pressure, age, sex, plasma renin activity and plasma volume in essential hypertension. Clin Sci Mol Med 55 (Suppl 4):93s, 1978.
7. Chodakowska J, Nazar K, Wocial B, Jarecki M, Shórka B: Plasma catecholamines and renin activity in response to exercise in patients with essential hypertension. Clin Sci Mol Med 49:511, 1975.
8. Christensen MS, Christensen NJ: Plasma catecholamines in hypertension. Scand J Clin Lab Invest 30:169, 1972.
9. Clement DL, Bogaert MG, Moerman EZ, De Schaepdrijver AF: Significance of elevated plasma noradrenaline in patients with essential hypertension. In: Circulating Catecholamines and Blood Pressure. Birkenhäger WH, Falke HE, eds. Utrecht: Bunge Scientific, 1978.
10. Cousineau D, DeChamplain J, Lapointe L: Circulating catecholamines and systolic time intervals in labile and sustained hypertension. Clin Sci Mol Med 55 (Suppl 4):65s, 1978.
11. Davis JO: The control of renin release. Am J Med 55:333, 1973.
12. De Champlain J, Farley L, Cousineau D, Van Ameringen MR: Circulating catecholamine levels in human and experimental hypertension. Circ Res 38:109, 1976.
13. DeChamplain J, Cousineau D: Lack of correlation between age and circulating catecholamines in hypertensive patients. N Engl J Med 297:672, 1977.

14. DeLeeuw PW, Falke HE, Kho TL, VanDongen R, Wester A, Birkenhäger WH: Effects of beta-adrenergic blockade on diurnal variability of blood pressure and plasma noradrenaline levels. Acta Med. Scand 202:389. 1977.
15. DeLeeuw PW, Falke HE, Punt R, Birkenhäger WH: Noradrenaline secretion by the human kidney. Clin Sci Mol. Med 55 (Suppl 4):85s, 1978.
16. DeLeeuw PW, Wester A, Punt R, Falke HE, Birkenhäger WH: Noradrenaline levels in essential hypertensives and normotensive controls. Neth J Med 22:145, 1979.
17. DeLeeuw PW, Punt R, Birkenhäger WH: Renal blood flow and noradrenaline secretion during treatment with propranolol. Clin Sci 59 (Suppl 6):477s, 1980.
18. DeQuattro V, Chan S: Raised plasma-catecholamines in some patients with primary hypertension. Lancet i:806, 1972.
19. DeQuattro F, Miura Y, Lurvey A, Cosgrove M, Mendez R: Increased plasma catecholamine concentrations and vas deferens norepinephrine biosynthesis in men with elevated blood pressure. Circ. Res 36:118, 1975.
20. Doyle AE, Fraser JRE: Essential hypertension and inheritance of vascular reactivity. Lancet ii:509, 1961.
21. Engelman, K, Portnoy B, Sjoerdsma A: Plasma catecholamine concentrations in patients with hypertension. Circ Res 26/27 (Suppl 1):141, 1970.
22. Esler MD, Nestel PJ: High catecholamine essential hypertension: clinical and physiological characteristics. Aust. N.Z.J. Med 3:117, 1973.
23. Esler M, Julius S, Zweifler A, Randall O, Harburg E, Gardiner H, DeQuattro V: Mild high-renin essential hypertension. N Engl J Med 296:405, 1977.
24. Ferrario CM, Dickinson CJ, McCubbin JW: Central vasomotor stimulation by angiotensin. Clin Sci 39:239, 1970.
25. Franco-Morselli R, Elghozi JL, Joly E, Diginilio S, Meyer P: Increased plasma adrenaline concentrations in benign essential hypertension. Br Med J 2:1251, 1977.
26. Henry DP, Luft FC, Weinberger MH, Fineberg NS, Grim CE: Norepinephrine in urine and plasma following provocative maneuvers in normal and hypertensive subjects. Hypertension 2:20, 1980.
27. Hofman A, Boomsma F, Schalekamp, MADH, Valkenburg HA: Raised blood pressure and plasma noradrenaline concentrations in teenagers and young adults selected from an open population. Br Med J 1:1536, 1979.
28. Hollenberg NK, Adams DF, Solomon H, Chenitz WR, Burger BM, Abrams HL, Merrill JP: Renal vascular tone in essential and secondary hypertension. Medicine 54:29, 1975.
29. Hong Tai Eng FW, Huber-Smith M, McCann DS: The role of sympathetic activity in normal renin essential hypertension. Hypertension 2:14, 1980.
30. Ibsen H, Christensen NJ, Hollnagel H, Leth A, Kappelgaard AM, Giese J: Plasma noradrenaline concentration in hypertensive and normotensive 40-year-old individuals: relationship to plasma renin concentration. Clin Sci 57 (Suppl 5):181s, 1979.
31. Jiang NS, Stoffer SS, Pikler GM, Wadel O, Sheps SG: Laboratory and clinical observations with a two-column plasma catecholamine assay. Mayo Clin Proc 48:47, 1973.
32. Jones DH, Hamilton CA, Reid JL: Plasma noradrenaline, age and blood pressure: a population study. Clin Sci Mol Med 55 (Suppl 4):73s, 1978.
33. Jones DH, Hamilton CA, Reid JL: Choice of control groups in the appraisal of sympathetic nervous activity in essential hypertension. Clin Sci 57:339, 1979.
34. Jones DH, Allison DJ, Hamilton CA, Reid JL: Selective venous sampling in the diagnosis and localization of phaeochromocytoma. Clin Endocrinol 10:179, 1979.
35. Kiowski W, Van Brummelen P, Bühler FR: Plasma noradrenaline correlates with α-adrenoceptor-mediated vasoconstriction and blood pressure in patients with essential hypertension. Clin Sci 57 (Suppl 5):177s, 1979.
36. Kuchel O: Autonomic nervous system in hypertension: clinical aspects. In: Hypertension-

302

physiopathology and treatment. Genest J, Koiw E, Kuchel O, eds. New York: McGraw-hill, 1977.

37. Lake CR, Ziegler MG, Coleman MD, Kopin IJ: Age-adjusted plasma norepinephrine levels are similar in normotensive and hypertensive subjects. N Engl. J Med 296:208, 1977.

38. Lorimer AR, McFarlane PW, Provan G, Duffie T, Lowrie TD: Blood pressure and catecholamine responses to 'stress' in normotensive and hypertensive subjects. Cardiovasc. Res 5:169, 1971.

39. Louis WJ, Doyle AE, Anavekar S: Plasma norepinephrine levels in essential hypertension. N Engl J Med 228:599, 1973.

40. Louis WJ, Doyle AE, Anavekar SN, Johnston CI, Geffen LB, Rush R: Plasma catecholamine, dopamine-beta-hydroxylase and renin levels in essential hypertension. Circ Res 34/35 (Suppl 1):57, 1974.

41. Luft FC, Weinberger MH, Grim CE, Henry DP, Fineberg NS: Nocturnal urinary electrolyte excretion and its relationship to the renin system and sympathetic activity in normal and hypertensive man. J Lab Clin Med 95:395, 1980.

42. Miller JZ, Luft FC, Grim CE, Henry DP, Christian JC, Weinberger MH: Genetic influences on plasma and urinary norepinephrine after volume expansion and contraction in normal men. J Clin Endocrinol Metab 50:219, 1980.

43. Miura Y, Kobayashi K, Sakuma H, Tomioka H, Adacki M, Yoshinago K: Plasma noradrenaline concentrations and haemodynamics in the early stage of essential hypertension. Clin Sci Mol Med 55 (Suppl 4):69s, 1978.

44. Nestel PJ, Doyle AE: The excretion of free noradrenaline and adrenaline by healthy young subjects and by patients with essential hypertension. Aust Ann Med 17:295, 1968.

45. Nicholls MG, Kiowski W, Zweifler AJ, Julius S, Schork MA, Greenhouse J: Plasma norepinephrine variations with dietary sodium intake. Hypertension 2:29, 1980.

46. Pedersen EB, Christensen NJ: Catecholamines in plasma and urine in patients with essential hypertension determined by double-isotope derivative techniques. Acta Med Scand 198:373, 1975.

47. Philipp T, Distler A, Cordes U: Sympathetic nervous system and blood pressure control in essential hypertension. Lancet ii:959, 1978.

48. Planz G, Gierlichs HW, Hawlina A, Planz R, Stephany W, Rahn KH: A comparison of catecholamine concentrations and dopamine-beta-hydroxylase activities in plasma from normotensive subjects and from patients with essential hypertension at rest and during exercise. Klin Wochenschr 54:561, 1976.

49. Planz G, Planz R, Persigehl M, Bundschu HD, Heintz R: Adrenaline and noradrenaline concentration in blood of suprarenal and renal vein in man with normal blood pressure and with essential hypertension. Klin Wochenschr 56:1109, 1978.

50. Prinz PN, Halter J, Benedetti C, Raskind M: Circadian variation of plasma catecholamines in young and old men: relation to rapid eye movement and slow wave sleep. J Clin Endocrinol Metab 49:300, 1979.

51. Rahn KH, Henquet JW, Kho T, Schols M, Thijssen H: Plasma catecholamine levels and the renin–angiotensin-system in subjects with borderline hypertension. In: Hypertension–Mechanisms and Management. Philipp T, Distler A, eds. Berlin: Springer-Verlag, 1980.

52. Robertson D, Johnson G, Robertson RM, Nies AS, Shand DG, Oates JA: Comparative assessment of stimuli that release neuronal and adrenomedullary catecholamines in man. Circulation 59:637, 1979.

53. Robertson D, Shand DG, Hollifield JW, Nies AS, Frölich JC, Oates J: Alterations in the response of the sympathetic nervous system and renin in borderline hypertension. Hypertension 1:118, 1979.

54. Safar ME, London GM, Weiss YA, Milliez PI: Vascular reactivity to norepinephrine and hemodynamic parameters in borderline hypertension. Am Heart J 89:480, 1975.

55. Sever PS, Binch M, Osikowska B, Tunbridge RDG: Plasma-noradrenaline in essential hypertension. Lancet i:1078, 1977.
56. Sever PS: Catecholamines in essential hypertension: the present controversy. In: Circulating Catecholamines and Blood Pressure. Birkenhäger WH, Falke HE, eds. Utrecht: Bunge Scientific, 1978.
57. Sever PS, Peart WS, Davies IB, Tunbridge RDG, Gordon D: Ethnic differences in blood pressure with observations on noradrenaline and renin – 2. A hospital hypertensive population. Clin Exp Hypertension 1:745, 1979.
58. Sleight P, Floras JS, Hassan MO, Jones JV, Osikowska BA, Sever P, Turner KL: Baroreflex control of blood pressure and plasma noradrenaline during exercise in essential hypertension. Clin Sci 57 (Suppl 5):169s, 1979.
59. Taylor AA, Pool JL, Lake CR, Ziegler MG, Rosen RA, Rollins DE, Mitchell JR: Plasma norepinephrine concentrations – no differences among normal volunteers and low, high or normal renin hypertensive patients. Life Sci 22:1499, 1978.
60. Thurton MB, Deegan T: Circadian variations of plasma catecholamine, cortisol and immunoreactive insulin concentrations in supine subjects. Clin Chim Ach 55:389, 1974.
61. Watson RDS, Hamilton CA, Reid JL, Littler WA: Changes in plasma norepinephrine, blood pressure and heart rate during physical activity in hypertensive man. Hypertension 1:341, 1979.
62. Watson RDS, Page AJF, Littler WA, Jones DH, Reid JL: Plasma noradrenaline concentrations at different vascular sites during rest and isometric and dynamic exercise. Clin Sci 57:545, 1979.
63. Watson RDS, Stallard TJ, Flinn RM, Littler WA: Factors determining direct arterial pressure and its variability in hypertensive man. Hypertension 2:333, 1980.
64. Weidmann P, Hirsch D, Beretta-Piccoli C, Reubi FC: Interrelations among blood pressure, blood volume, plasma renin activity and urinary catecholamines in benign essential hypertension. Am J Med 62:209, 1977.
65. Weidmann P, Beretta-Piccoli C, Ziegler WH, Keusch G, Glück Z, Reubi FC: Age versus urinary sodium for judging renin, aldosterone, and catecholamine levels: studies in normal subjects and patients with essential hypertension. Kidney Int 14:619, 1978.
66. Weidmann P, Grimm M, Meier A, Glück Z, Keusch G, Minder I, Beretta-Piccoli C: Cardiovascular pressor reactivity as related to plasma catecholamines: role in the pathogenesis of essential hypertension and in the antihypertensive mechanism of diuretic treatment. In: Hypertension – Mechanisms and Management. Philipp T, Distler A, eds. Berlin: Springer-Verlag, 1979.
67. Zadik Z, Hamilton BP, Kowarski AA, Lukas K: Integrated concentration of epinephrine and norepinephrine in normal subjects and in patients with mild essential hypertension. J Clin Endocrinol Metab 50:842, 1980.

19. ROLE OF RENIN IN THE CONTROL OF THE CIRCULATION IN HYPERTENSIVE DISEASE AND IN HEART FAILURE

EDGAR HABER

That renin plays an integral role in blood pressure homeostasis and in the pathogenesis of hypertension has been appreciated since its discovery by

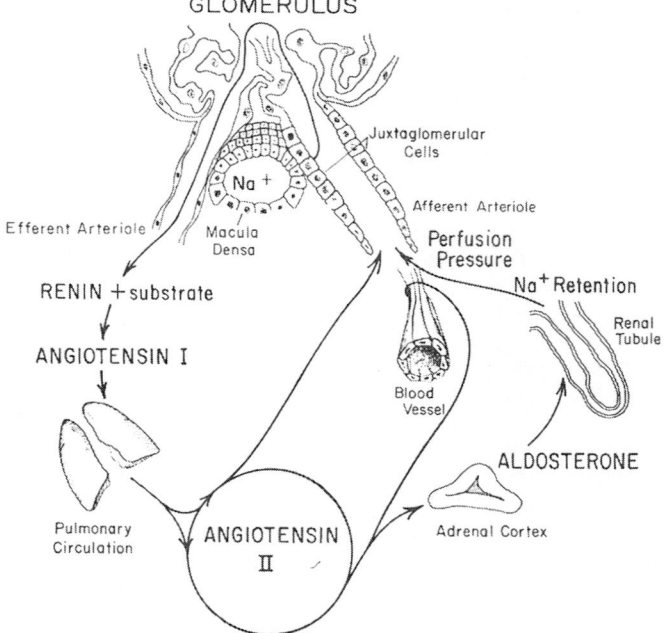

Figure 1. Renin is produced in the juxtaglomerular cells (modified smooth muscle cells of the afferent arterioles of the kidney). It is released into the plasma in response to a drop in renal perfusion pressure. The macula densa is composed of cells of the distal convoluted tubule that lie directly adjacent to the afferent arteriole. These epithelial cells may transmit fluctuations in the sodium concentration of the tubular fluid to the afferent arteriolar cells, thereby exerting a control over renin release. Adrenergic neurons innervate the juxtaglomerular cells and so influence renin release. The functional unit composed of the juxtaglomerular cells and the macula densa is called the juxtaglomerular apparatus. Reprinted with permission of the Massachusetts Medical Society [2].

Amery, A. (ed.) Hypertensive Cardiovascular Disease: Pathophysiology and Treatment
© *1982, Martinus Nijhoff Publishers. The Hague / Boston / London*
ISBN-13: 978-94-009-7478-4

Tigerstedt and Beman at the turn of the century. The specific role of renin in the production of various forms of hypertension remains a subject of lively debate [1–3].

Renin is a proteolytic enzyme produced in the kidney by modified afferent arteriolar smooth muscle cells located in the juxtaglomerular apparatus (Figure 1). Although other anatomic sites containing renin-like enzymes have been identified, their physiologic role in blood pressure regulation has not been documented.

BIOCHEMISTRY AND PHYSIOLOGY OF THE RENIN SYSTEM

Once released into the circulation, renin acts on renin substrate, an alpha globulin synthesized in the liver, to release angiotensin I, a decapeptide without apparent physiologic effect. Angiotensin I, in a single passage through the pulmonary circulation, is cleaved by the membrane-bound converting enzyme to produce angiotensin II, the most potent vasoconstrictor known. This substance is also a primary stimulus for adrenocortical production of aldosterone, a mineralocorticoid that promotes the reabsorption of

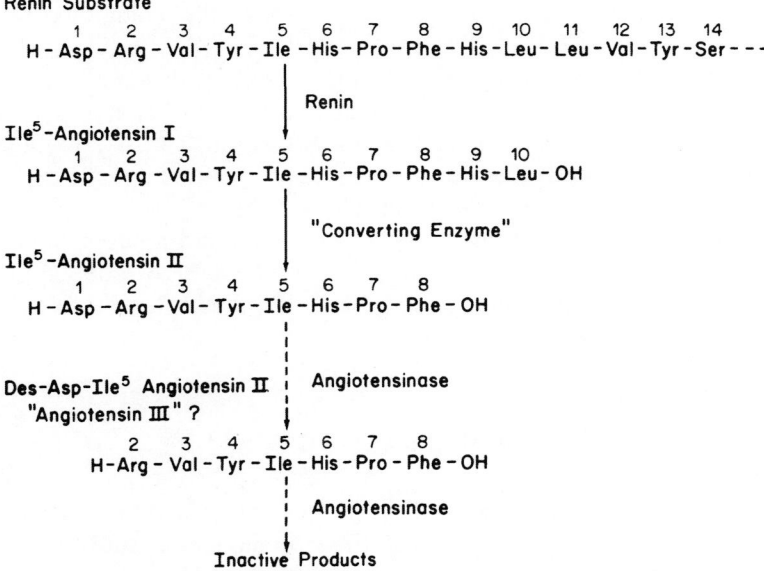

Figure 2. Biochemistry of the renin–angiotensin system. Ile⁵-angiotensin contains isoleucine in the 5 position and is the form of peptide that occurs in man. The existence of des-Asp¹-angiotensin II as an intermediate in the pathways has not been definitely established. Reprinted with permission of the Massachusetts Medical Society [2].

sodium and water by the renal tubules. This biochemical sequence has been termed the renin–angiotensin–aldosterone (RAA) system (Figure 2).

Renin release is subject to an intricate control system, the chief components of which are usually identified as renal perfusion pressure, sodium concentration, and beta-adrenergic stimulation. The net effect of these physiologic controls is to render renin production inversely proportional to effective blood volume. Therefore, anything that decreases effective blood volume stimulates renin, and anything that increases effective blood volume suppresses renin. For example, hemorrhage or rapid diuresis stimulates renin release by a decrease in effective blood volume. Production of angiotensin II and aldosterone results, so that hypotension is corrected, both by direct vasoconstriction and by fluid retention. Effective blood volume is restored and renin release is stopped by negative feedback.

Renin measurement

Human renin has recently been purified by Slater and co-workers [4], and this advance should lead to the eventual ability to measure renin directly. Until then, renin must be quantified by measuring the rate of generation of the product of renin's action, angiotensin I, using a radioimmunoassay [5]. Plasma renin activity (PRA) is expressed as nanograms of angiotensin I per ml/h.

PRA is exquisitely sensitive to variations in sodium balance and to posture. The commonly used antihypertensive drugs also alter PRA. Thus, PRA is customarily measured when the patient is on a normal diet and not receiving antihypertensive medication. Although a more accurate definition of the patient's renin status can be obtained either by simultaneous measurement of 24-h urine sodium or by a stimulated and a suppressed renin value, it is now generally agreed that the stimulated PRA value alone can serve as a simple and sufficient screen for renin-related forms of secondary hypertension [6–8].

Determinants of renin secretion in normal man

In the normal unstressed individual, the major determinants of renin secretion are posture, sodium intake, and time of day. In a study of normal controls [9], very low levels of both renin activity and plasma aldosterone concentration are observed at the highest sodium intake, 240 mEq/day (Figure 3). There seemed to be little variation during the course of the day. At 100 mEq sodium intake, renin activity was low during sleep but rose by a factor of nearly ten, reaching a maximum by the middle of the day. By

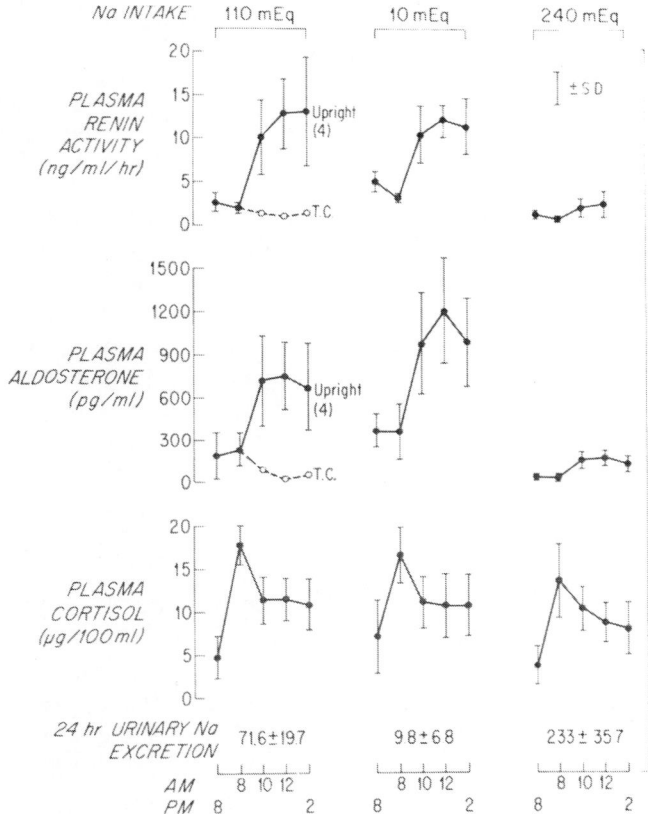

Figure 3. Diurnal and dietary variations in plasma aldosterone, renin activity, and cortisol in five normal subjects. The values for subject T.C. are plotted separately in the left-hand column for both aldosterone and renin activity but are included with the other data in the two other columns. Reprinted with permission of Academic Press [9].

20:00, it had declined to early morning levels, even though the subjects remained upright at normal activity throughout this period. Plasma aldosterone levels followed renin activity faithfully. At a low sodium intake, 10 mEq/day, night time levels of both renin and aldosterone were higher and plasma aldosterone seemed to peak at a still higher level. On the other hand, plasma cortisol, which reflects ACTH secretion, followed a different and independent diurnal pattern. Cortisol peaked at 08:00 and gradually fell during the course of the day. Its cycle was not at all correlated with either renin or aldosterone, and the magnitude of peak plasma concentration was independent of sodium intake. If normal individuals were kept in bed for 24 hours, diurnal cycles of renin secretion could still be observed, but the height of the peaks was considerably blunted [10, 11].

Inhibitors of the renin–angiotensin system

The ability to measure renin activity and angiotensin II concentration by radioimmunoassay proved to be most helpful to the physiologist and clinical investigator in understanding the response of the renin–angiotensin system to a variety of interventions. However, it was not until specific inhibitors were available that it became possible to define precisely the role of renin in any given physiologic or pathologic situation. Inhibitors may: (a) interfere with the action of renin on its substrate; (b) block converting enzyme in its action on angiotensin I to produce angiotensin II; (c) compete in the interaction of angiotensin II with its receptor site in blood vessels or in the adrenal cortex (Figure 4).

Renin inhibitors
Antirenin antibody was the earliest inhibitor used in physiologic studies [12–14]. The removal or inactivation of renin from the circulation with a specific antibody should also remove whatever physiologic consequences its presence might engender. Antirenin antisera lowered blood pressure in experimental renovascular hypertension, but the specificity of the antibody, and consequently the interpretation of the results, was uncertain.

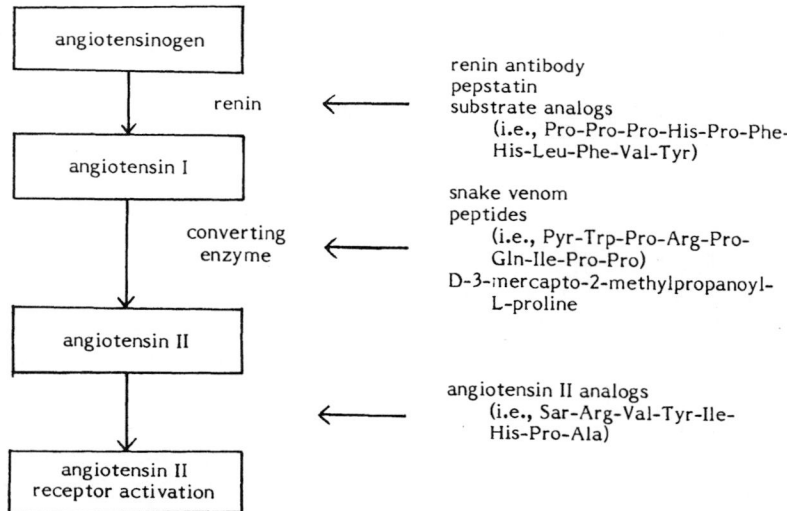

Figure 4. Sites of action of inhibitors of the renin–angiotensin system.

Most recently Dzau and co-workers [15] fully purified canine renin and elicited mono-specific antibodies. These antibodies proved to be both highly effective and highly specific inhibitors of renin in the unanesthetized dog.

Pepstatin is a non-specific acid protease inhibitor which also inhibits renin [16]. Conflicting data in earlier experiments cast doubt on its efficacy in vivo [17]. Most recently, Menard et al. [18] have solubilized pepstatin by the addition of hydrophilic residue to the C-terminal part of the molecule. This resulted in a 100-fold increase in water solubility. Solubilized pepstatin also proved to be an effective inhibitor when utilized in certain in vivo preparations.

A new class of competitive renin inhibitors based on substrate structure has now been synthesized [19, 20]. Skeggs et al. [21, 22] reported that the first peptide shown in Table 1, a small portion of renin substrates sequence, was sufficient as substrate for renin and also could be shown to be competitive. A number of analogs were synthesized by Burton and his colleagues [23] that exhibited stronger inhibitory effects than the parent octapeptide. The most successful of these (Table 1) was a highly effective inhibitor when used in vivo in the unanesthetized monkey [24].

Converting enzyme inhibitors
A series of peptides originally isolated from snake venom are effective inhibitors of angiotensin-converting enzyme [25]. They act to block cleavage of angiotensin I and thereby prevent the formation of angiotensin II [26]. The synthetic nonapeptide Pyr-Trp-Pro-Arg-Phe-Gln-Ile-Pro-Pro, based on the structure of one of the natural snake venom peptides [27], has now been used in both animal and human studies which will be described in detail subsequently.

More recently, a new inhibitor of converting enzyme has become available for clinical use. Ondetti et al. reported the synthesis of D-3-mercapto-2-methylpropanoyl-L-proline (Captopril), a relatively low molecular weight compound which inhibits angiotensin-converting enzyme after oral administration [28]. The application of this material in several clinical studies will be detailed later.

Table 1.

	Renin cleavage site ↓
Minimal renin substrate	His-Pro-Phe-His-Leu-Leu-Val-Tyr
Renin inhibitor	Pro-His-Pro-Phe-His-Phe-Phe-Val-Tyr-Lys

Competitive inhibitors of angiotensin II

Sarcosine[1]-alanine[8]-angiotensin II (saralysin) [29] is an example of a series of effective and specific inhibitors [30] that compete with angiotensin II at its receptor sites. These peptides are based on variants of the structure on angiotensin II. The critical site of amino acid substitution, which determines the efficacy of an inhibitor, is the carboxy-terminal position. Substitutions at the amino-terminal position serve to enhance activity. These compounds have found both experimental and clinical application [31, 32] but have been superseded by Captopril.

Renin and sodium balance

The intravenous infusion of converting enzyme inhibitor (CEI) has no discernible effect either on blood pressure or PRA in a normal experimental animal maintained on adequate sodium intake [33–35]. The angiotensin II competitive inhibitor saralysin results in a brief pressor response in the normal animal, followed by prompt return of blood pressure to normal levels even though infusion of the drug may continue [36, 37].

Sodium deprivation, however, uncovers an altered response [35]. On a normal intake of sodium (50–60 mEq/day), CEI did not lower blood pressure. However, on an intake of 10 mEq Na/day, very different results were obtained. Baseline blood pressure levels were within the normal range. The animal was alert and manifested normal activity and behavior. PRA was moderately elevated. Upon administration of saralysin, blood pressure levels first rose 25 mm Hg and then fell 27 mm Hg below control levels. These hemodynamic changes were associated with a striking rise in PRA. Blood pressure soon returned to control levels coincident with a fall in renin activity. The subsequent administration of CEI resulted in a prompt fall in blood pressure to the same degree without the initial rise noted when saralysin was used. Renin activity also rose coincidentally with the hemodynamic change in response to both inhibitors.

These experiments have now been confirmed utilizing two more specific renin inhibitors. In the unanesthetized sodium-depleted dog, renin-specific antibody caused a precipitous fall in blood pressure [15] (Figure 5). The unanesthetized monkey responded in a similar manner to the specific renin blocker based on substrate structure [24].

Studies in normal human subjects

Does the renin–angiotensin system come into play only at the extremes of extracellular fluid volume depletion, or does it also play a role in blood

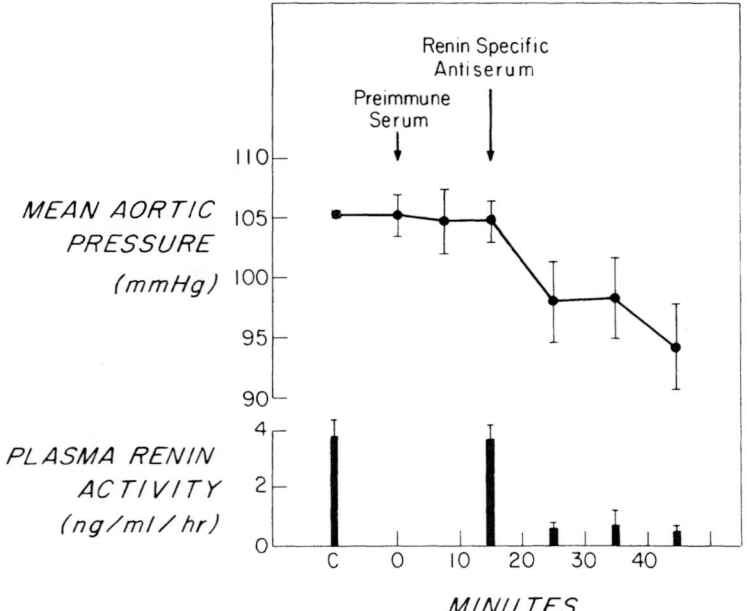

Figure 5. A fall in blood pressure in a sodium-depleted animal consequent to blockade of the action of renin by two very different methods suggests that, in the presence of a limited extracellular fluid volume, the hormone plays a major role in blood pressure maintenance. Reprinted with permission of the American Association for the Advancement of Science [15].

pressure regulation at lesser degrees of physiologic stress? Studies in human subjects have addressed this question [38]. Four normal young subjects were in sodium balance on a 110 mEq intake. They were first studied in the supine position, then tilted upright to 70 degrees before and after administration of CEI. The nature and duration of the tilting stress was judiciously chosen so that none of these normal subjects would become either hypotensive or faint. During the study, heart rate and blood pressure were monitored and frequent blood samples were obtained for plasma renin activity and aldosterone concentration.

As can be seen from Figure 6, prior to the administration of CEI, upright tilting resulted in little hemodynamic change, a minimal narrowing of pulse pressure, and a slight tachycardia. However a rise in both plasma renin activity and plasma aldosterone concentration occurred. The administration of CEI did not result in significant hemodynamic changes either in the supine position or on tilting. Renin activity increased both in the supine position and on tilting, but no corresponding rise in aldosterone concentration was apparent; after sodium depletion, either by diet or after the admin-

312

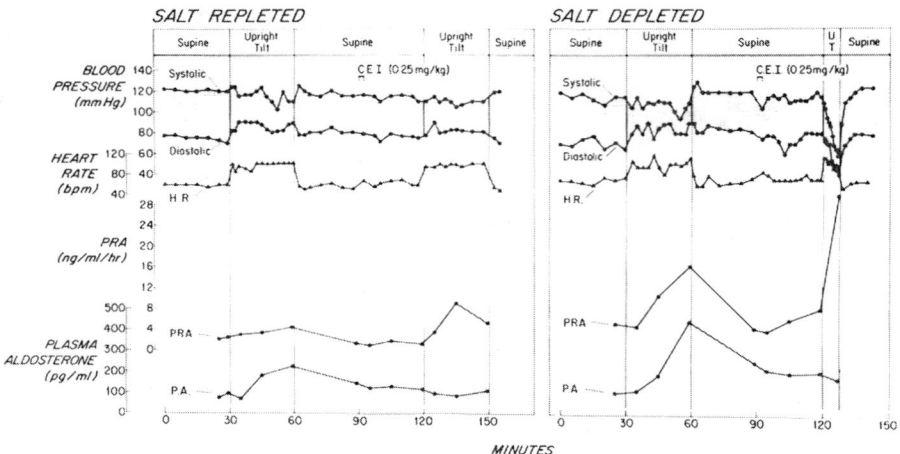

Figure 6. Representative example of a subject (J.C.) in group I examined in the supine posture and during tilting while sodium-repleted and sodium-depleted prior to and subsequent to the administration of converting enzyme inhibitor (CEI). HR: heart rate; PRA: plasma renin activity; PA: plasma aldosterone; UT: upright tilt. Reprinted with permission of the American Heart Association [38].

istration of a diuretic, an average weight loss of 2.6 kg was observed. Supine renal and aldosterone plasma values were higher during the control period; the hemodynamic response to tilting was somewhat more marked than on the higher sodium intake. After administration of CEI, tilting was associated with a striking fall in blood pressure to hypotensive levels accompanied by an even greater elevation in renin activity; there was, remarkably, no change in plasma aldosterone concentration.

These observations in normal man extend and reinforce the conclusions of earlier experiments in sodium-depleted animals. A marked fall in blood pressure and a rise in heart rate on tilting in sodium-depleted, but not in sodium-repleted subjects, indicate that angiotensin I is an essential element of blood pressure control, even in states of only modest extracellular fluid volume depletion. The rise of plasma renin activity in the supine position subsequent to CEI, in the absence of a fall in blood pressure, suggests that angiotensin II exerts direct feedback control on renin secretion. The absence of the expected rise in plasma aldosterone after CEI, both on tilting or sodium depletion in the presence of an exaggerated renin activity, suggests that angiotensin II is the primary stimulus to aldosterone secretion in response to sodium depletion and postural change.

PATHOPHYSIOLOGY OF THE RENIN SYSTEM

Experimental renovascular hypertension

The importance of renin in the genesis and maintenance of renovascular hypertension has been subject to conflicting interpretations and, at times, apparently irreconcilable experimental data. An elevation in renal vein renin has proven to be a most useful diagnostic test for curable unilateral renal artery stenosis. Yet, in chronic experimental or clinical renovascular hypertension, plasma renin activity is often normal.

Acute experimental studies are difficult to interpret because anesthesia, surgical trauma, and blood loss all modify the response of the renin–angiotensin system. To circumvent some of these problems, studies were performed on trained, conscious animals appropriately prepared and studied at least two weeks after surgery.

A substantial gradient was established between the aorta and the renal artery and was maintained at a constant level by adjustment of a constrictor cuff [34]. A rapid rise in mean aortic pressure to hypertensive levels occurred and was associated with an early elevation of PRA. The administration of CEI and later renin-specific antibody resulted in a prompt fall in blood pressure to near-normotensive levels. These observations indicated that the renin–angiotensin system was responsible for the initial rise in systemic blood pressure that results from renal artery hypotension. Blockade of the system promptly reduced blood pressure to normal.

When renal artery constriction is maintained over a long period, persistent hypertension results, but PRA remains elevated for only a few days, returning to control levels as sodium and water retention occur [39]. If angiotensin II levels are prevented from rising by continuous administration of CEI after renal artery constriction, blood pressure does not rise over a 4-day period in a conscious one-kidney dog with renal artery constriction [35]. Once hypertension is established, however, inhibitors have little effect, indicating that angiotensin II may not play a significant role in the maintenance of chronic hypertension in the one-kidney experimental preparation [29, 40–42]. The decreasing effectiveness of CEI and angiotensin II antagonists in lowering blood pressure in chronic renovascular hypertension suggests that over time other factors begin to play an increasingly important role in the maintenance of elevated blood pressure.

What are these contributing factors? Tobian et al. [43] and Buyton et al. [44] have stressed the importance of sodium and water retention in the maintenance of the elevated blood pressure of chronic renovascular hypertension. Rocchini and Barger [45] produced reversible renal artery stenosis in trained, unanesthetized dogs maintained on a diet containing less than 10 mEq of sodium/day [20]. Renal artery perfusion pressure was reduced to

314

60–70 mm Hg, blood pressure rose 37 ± 4 mm Hg within 1 h of constriction and remained at this level throughout the 14 days of the experiment. Presumably because of the low sodium intake, fluid and sodium retention did not occur. At the end of 14 days, the animals were exquisitely sensitive to CEI. In contrast to animals on an *ad libitum* sodium intake, which are unresponsive to CEI, blood pressure fell to normal within 5 min of an intravenous bolus injection of the drug. Thus, unlike the experimental models in which a normal sodium intake is permitted, one-kidney renovascular hypertension is characterized by a persistently elevated renin activity when sodium and fluid accumulation is prevented by dietary sodium restriction. Thus, the evidence seems to point to sodium and water retention as the principal factors in the maintenance of persistent hypertension in the animal with renal artery constriction.

There seem to be two phases of renovascular hypertension: initially, elevated blood pressure is maintained by the direct pressor actions of angiotensin II; during a later chronic phase, blood pressure is maintained largely as a result of hypervolemia, mediated by sodium and water retention.

The renin–angiotensin system in experimental congestive heart failure

The role that the renin–angiotensin system plays in congestive heart failure remains uncertain. Early experiments of Deming and Leutscher [46] demonstrated sodium-retaining activity in the urine of patients with cardiac failure. Davis et al. [47] later suggested that increased circulating angiotensin II levels were responsible for hypersecretion of aldosterone in experimental heart failure.

Watkins et al. [48] addressed this question directly by employing CEI in a congestive failure model in the conscious dog. Either the thoracic inferior vena cava or the pulmonary artery were compressed by an externally controlled inflatable cuff. As either of the cuffs was inflated, blood pressure fell and PRA and plasma aldosterone levels rose rapidly. Sodium excretion fell to nearly zero; plasma volume and body weight increased. When ascites and edema were manifest, blood pressure was gradually restored. Upon hemodynamic compensation, PRA and aldosterone fell to control levels and sodium excretion rose. A new equilibrium was established in a volume-expanded animal. However, if CEI was administered while PRA was elevated and prior to the development of volume expansion, a 25–30 mm Hg drop in blood pressure occurred. Chronic infusion of CEI prevented the establishment of the new equilibrium. Plasma aldosterone concentration did not rise, volume expansion did not occur, and hypotension persisted.

Thus, congestive heart failure appears to be analogous in a number of ways to renovascular hypertension. The renin–angiotensin–aldosterone system is essential in the initiation of compensatory adjustments that are the hallmark of this pathophysiologic state, particularly the increase in plasma volume and consequent development of edema.

RENIN IN HUMAN DISEASE

Levels of PRA in a variety of disease states can be predicted from knowledge of the physiology of the renin system (see Table 2).

Renal artery stenosis raises PRA by decreasing renal perfusion pressure. Hypertension is then mediated either by the direct vasoconstrictive effect of angiotensin II, by fluid retention secondary to aldosterone released by the adrenal cortex, or by a combination of both vasoconstrictor and volume factors. Both PRA and aldosterone levels are usually elevated.

In primary hyperaldosteronism (Conn's syndrome, or idiopathic hyperaldosteronism), the autonomous secretion of aldosterone induces sodium retention, an expanded plasma volume, and resultant hypertension. Renin is suppressed, and PRA is usually undetectable.

Rarely, renal tumors or cysts can mimic renal artery stenosis by extrinsic compression of the renal vasculature, resulting in an elevated PRA. They are distinguished from stenotic lesions by arteriography. Tumors that secrete renin are exceedingly rare.

A renin-deficiency syndrome characterized by hyperkalemia, postural hypotension, subnormal PRA, and subnormal aldosterone levels in the face of otherwise normal adrenal function has been described recently [49]. Patients

Table 2. Renin and aldosterone levels in several disease states

Disease state	Renin level	Aldosterone level	Confirmation of diagnosis
Renovascular hypertension	↑ or −	↑ or −	Differential venous renin measurements Angiography
Primary aldosteronism	0	↑	Aldosterone determination Venography
Renal tumors, cysts	↑	↑	Angiographic appearance of lesion
Essential hypertension	↑ or − or ↓	↑ or − or ↓	
Low-renin state	↓	↓	↓ Creatinine clearance Clinical setting
Bartter's syndrome	↑	↑	Patient normotensive Clinical setting

with this disorder tend to be elderly; they have evidence of prior renal disease and diminished creatinine clearance. Diabetics, especially those with longstanding disease, may also exhibit features of this syndrome [50]. The cause of the deficiency is thought to be an acquired abnormality of the juxtaglomerular apparatus. Salt repletion and, if necessary, mineralocorticoid administration are effective in treatment.

Bartter's syndrome is characterized by juxtaglomerular cell hyperplasia, hyperreninemia, hyperaldosteronism, hypokalemia, and normal blood pressure. Responsiveness to infused angiotensin II or norepinephrine is subnormal, and proximal tubular reabsorption of sodium by the kidney is diminished. It is probable that all these defects, including the hyperreninemia, are mediated through the synthesis of prostaglandin E_2 (PGE_2) in the kidney [51, 52]. The traditional therapy of propranolol, spironolactone, and potassium supplements may eventually be replaced by agents that are capable of suppressing PGE_2 synthesis, such as indomethacin, aspirin, ibuprofen, or naproxen [53, 54].

Renin in essential hypertension

In 1972, Laragh and associates classified patients with essential hypertension on the basis of PRA [55]. Of the hypertensive patients studied, 16% had abnormally high PRA levels, 57% had normal levels, and 27% had suppressed renin activity. It was suggested that the cause of essential hypertension was related to these differences in PRA and that the incidence of complications of hypertension appeared dependent on the level of PRA; the higher the renin level, the greater the incidence of 'vasculotoxic' events. This latter observation has not been confirmed by other investigators, who feel that prognosis is dependent on level and duration of hypertension regardless of the renin status [56]. Since this original report, many authors have criticized the classification of essential hypertension on the basis of PRA by arguing that it imposes arbitrary divisions on a continuous spectrum of renin values [57]. On the basis of evidence to date, we agree that it is not necessary to classify every hypertensive patient on the basis of PRA [58, 59]. If a renin-related form of secondary hypertension is suspected, however, PRA should serve as a valuable screening test, helping to identify those patients with both renovascular disease and primary hyperaldosteronism.

There is also considerable controversy about the value of PRA as a guide to the selection of drugs in initial antihypertensive therapy [60–66]. For the most part, patients cannot be classified simply as vasoconstrictive or volume-dependent hypertensives with regard to their response to therapy [63]. Thus, it is generally agreed that initial diuretic treatment will be effective in most patients with essential hypertension regardless of their renin status. However, renin typing is of value in facilitating selection of the most effective therapeutic regimen in the following groups of patients: (a) those who have severe disease, (b) those who respond poorly to empiric therapy despite good compliance, and (c) those patients in whom rapid and rigorous control of hypertension is mandatory.

Renal artery stenosis

The role of the renin–angiotensin–aldosterone system in the pathogenesis of experimental renovascular hypertension has already been described. Anatomically, renal artery stenosis arises either from fibroplasia of arterial tissue or from atherosclerosis. Fibroplasia is seen predominantly in female patients aged 20–30 years, whereas atherosclerosis of the renal arteries generally appears in patients over 45 years of age who have evidence of diffuse atherosclerosis. Physical examination of the patient with renal artery stenosis is unremarkable except for the inconstant presence of an abdominal bruit, which is heard in 50% of these patients as opposed to 10% of patients without the disease [67]. Candidates for screening for renal artery stenosis should be less than 30 or more than 45 years of age at the onset of hypertension, and they should be considered eligible for surgical correction. A negative family history for hypertension or presence of an abdominal bruit favors a possible diagnosis of renal artery stenosis.

There is no simple reliable screening protocol for renal artery stenosis as there are for other forms of secondary hypertension. A suppressed or stimulated PRA is most often markedly elevated in renal artery stenosis, but it can be normal [67].

If stenosis is strongly suspected on the basis of clinical presentation of difficult-to-control hypertension, even if screening tests are negative, combined differential renal venous catheterization and renal artery arteriography must be performed. The diagnostic accuracy of differential renal venous sampling is increased in patients by maximally stimulating PRA by the use of diuretics, salt restriction, or blocking agents such as saralysin or converting enzyme inhibitor. Stimulation of PRA enhances specificity and does not introduce false positive results [68]. If renal artery constriction is demonstrated on arteriography, if the PMA ratio between the two renal venous samples is greater than 2:1, and if the PRA from the uninvolved renal venous effluent is suppressed, the probability of surgical cure is high [2, 68–70]. Renovascular hypertension may, of course, be caused by bilateral renal artery stenoses. The diagnosis and potential for surgical cure are far more difficult to ascertain under these circumstances.

The optimal surgical treatment is arterial repair or bypass rather than

318

nephrectomy. Risk is high in the elderly patient who shows evidence of compromised cardiac or renal function and in individuals of all ages with bilateral lesions. Because pharmacologic control of this form of hypertension is often possible, the risks of surgery must be carefully weighed against the problems of lifelong pharmacologic therapy and potential deterioration of renal function, when deciding whether or not to operate.

Revascularization for left renal artery stenosis now appears to be most appropriately performed by means of the splenorenal arterial anastomosis. Autogenous tissue is employed and only a single anastomosis is required. The spleen continues to be nourished by the short gastric arteries. This technique minimizes the incidence of postoperative renal failure by obviating the need for aortic cross clamping and avoids the difficulties often encountered when grafting to an atherosclerotic aorta is required [71].

Percutaneous balloon catheter dilatation angioplasty to remove either atherosclerotic or fibromuscular obstruction of the renal artery has been attempted at specialized centers with initial success [72]. This technique has also been useful in the relief of peripheral vascular occlusions [73]. A major limitation of the technique is that the lesion must be patent enough to allow catheter passage in order for dilatation to proceed. Thus far, complications have been similar to those of percutaneous angiography. Unknown is the duration of the arterial patency provided by angioplasty.

PRIMARY ALDOSTERONISM

High blood pressure that develops as a result of increased aldosterone production is the classic example of volume-related hypertension. Aldosterone promotes renal sodium retention while increasing urinary loss of potassium and hydrogen ions, which results in hypokalemic alkalosis. Hypokalemia can in turn produce insulin resistance with glucose intolerance, renal tubular damage with polyuria, muscle weakness, and cardiac arrhythmias. Although hyperaldosteronism leads to salt and water retention, the ultimate mechanism that sustains hypertension is unknown [74].

Primary aldosteronism results either from a benign adrenal adenoma (Conn's syndrome) or from bilateral adrenal hyperplasia (idiopathic hyperaldosteronism). Conn's syndrome occurs approximately four times more frequently than idiopathic hyperplasia does. Because hyperkalemia will eventually appear in almost all patients with primary aldosteronism, screening for this disease need be undertaken only in those patients who exhibit either unprovoked or significant diuretic-induced hypokalemia despite dietary sodium restriction [75]. Screening tests include stimulated PRA, which yields a very low result in primary aldosteronism, and a 24-h urine determination is 30 or more mEq K^+ in the face of hypokalemia when the disease is present. The definitive diagnosis of hyperaldosteronism is made by demonstrating elevated aldosterone levels that do not decline or decline only very slightly after sodium loading.

Approximately 25% of essential hypertensives have low PRA levels and low or normal aldosterone levels. In a very small fraction of these low-renin hypertensives, mineralocorticoid excess due to a compound other than aldosterone has been demonstrated [76]. In the majority, however, mineralocorticoid excess has not been found. Clear differentiation in the pathogenesis of such patients from that of patients with mineralocorticoid excess requires determination of mineralocorticoid levels in addition to renin.

Inhibition of the renin–angiotensin system in therapy: Captopril

Ondetti and his colleagues at Squibb have synthesized an orally absorbed converting enzyme inhibitor, Captopril. This compound is the first of a class of drugs (several others are now under development by other drug companies) that act, in part, by inhibiting the enzyme that is responsible for converting angiotensin I to angiotensin II. This drug has now been cleared by the U.S. Food and Drug Administration for prescription in otherwise treatment-resistant hypertension. Hemodynamically, the drug appears to reduce peripheral resistance without changing cardiac index, an effect that suggests a combination of arteriolar and venous dilatation.

Hypertension

Captopril has been markedly successful in reducing blood pressure in refractory hypertensives. Experience has now accumulated in more than 3000 patients. It is of interest that the effectiveness of the drug is not directly related to pre-treatment plasma renin activity. Indeed, hypertensive patients with normal renin parameters and even low renin patients have responded well to Captopril. This observation suggests that the drug may have effects additional to angiotensin-converting enzyme blockade. It is of additional interest that patients who are not responsive may become so after the addition of a diuretic to their program.

Side effects have included rash or pruritus (sometimes associated with fever) in 14% of patients, proteinuria in 1.2% and granulocytopenia in 0.7%. Nearly all patients who developed granulocytopenia were concomitantly receiving other drugs that might be incriminated. All instances of granulocytopenia and most instances of proteinuria reversed when Captopril was discontinued. In a few patients, however, pathologic evidence of membranous glomerulonephritis was demonstrated. Patients receiving this drug should be closely monitored with respect to hematologic and renal function parameters. Dosage should not exceed 450 mg/day.

It may well be that renin inhibitors will simplify the treatment of hypertension. While Captorpil has proven to be moderately toxic in some patients, it is likely that its successors will be less so and that inhibition of the renin–angiotensin system will be a major treatment modality in the future.

Congestive heart failure

Severe congestive heart failure (CHF) activates neural and humoral mechanisms. These mechanisms increase systemic vascular resistance to maintain arterial pressure in the face of low cardiac output. Increased activity of the renin–angiotensin system has been suspected because of the demonstration of increased PRA in some instance of experimental and clinical heart failure [48, 77, 78] and profound effects of renin blockade in experimental heart failure have been detailed earlier in these notes. Formation of excess levels of angiotensin II could contribute to vasoconstriction [79, 80] and to stimulation of aldosterone secretion [81, 82].

Because vasoconstriction may further depress left ventricular performance in CHF, vasodilator therapy has been used acutely to interrupt this cycle [83–85] and chronically in an effort to improve out-patient management of CHF [86–88]. The encouraging preliminary results with the use of nonspecific vasodilators such as nitrates, hydralazine and prazosin has led to interest in using agents that inhibit the conversion of angiotensin I to II (CEI). Not only could the drugs be effective therapeutically as vasodilators, but they might also provide insight into the role of the renin–angiotensin system in CHF.

The availability of an orally effective CEI [89], Captopril, has made it possible to assess the response to chronic inhibition of the renin–angiotensin system in CHF.

Several promising reports have now appeared. Levine et al. [90] administered Captopril to 11 patients with severe CHF. Peak effect was observed at 1.5 h after administration. At peak effect right atrial pressure fell from 3.4 to 0.0 mm Hg, pulmonary capillary wedge pressure (PCW) fell from 22.7 to 12.3 mm Hg, mean arterial pressure (MAP) fell from 79.5 to 62.1 mm Hg, systemic vascular resistance (SVR) fell from 1989 to 1370 dyn-sec-cm [76], pulmonary vascular resistance fell from 843 to 523 dyn-sec-cm [76], and cardiac index (CI) rose from 1.96 to 2.43 l/min/m^2. These were all statistically significant. Control PRA was elevated (25.9 ng/ml/h) and correlated with resting PCW ($r = 0.65$). The acute hemodynamic response was related to PRA: a fall in MAP ($r = 0.74$), a fall in PCW ($r = 0.80$), a fall in SVR ($r = 0.45$) and a rise in CI ($r = 0.45$). Eight patients were placed on chronic Captopril therapy. After two or more months, their exercise time was significantly increased from 6.8 to 11.7 min. Their cardiothoracic ratios showed a significant decrease, from 0.55 to 0.52, and most patients reported symptomatic improvement. Chronic response was not predicted by acute hemodynamic response. Captopril is therefore a vasodilator with both arterial and venous effects that are at least partially caused by inhibition of the renin–angiotensin system.

Dzau et al. [91] used Captopril in seven patients with severe congestive heart failure refractory to conventional therapy, including vasodilators. All had dyspnea, edema, elevated pulmonary wedge pressure $(28.0 \pm 2.6$ mm Hg), low CI $(1.1 \pm 0.1$ l/min/m^2), and elevated levels of serum creatinine $(2.3 \pm 0.2$ mg/dl $[203.3 \pm 17.7$ µmol of urea per liter]), PRA $(21 \pm 7$ ng of angiotensin I/ml/h), plasma angiotensin II $(271 \pm 51$ ng/ml), and plasma aldosterone $(65 \pm 14$ ng/dl). After one week of therapy, all indexes improved. Creatinine and p-aminohippurate clearances were also increased $(P<0.01)$. Improvement was sustained (more than six months) and was associated with a statistically significant increase in cardiac ejection fraction $(12 \pm 3$ to $26 \pm 7\%)$.

With a mean follow-up of seven months, the New York Heart Association Functional Class has been reduced from IV to II, and the number of days of hospitalization to less than 10% of that before Captopril therapy.

Thus Captopril reduces afterload in advanced CHF and induces sustained improvements in clinical status and renal function. These observations, in addition to providing a new insight into the role of renin in contributing to the unfavorable homeostatic changes in advanced CHF, provide a potentially useful avenue of therapy.

REFERENCES

1. Hypertension – the chicken and the egg (editorial). Lancet 1:345, 1976.
2. Oparil S, Haber E: The renin–angiotensin system (pts 1 and 2). N Engl J Med 291:389, 446, 1974.
3. Haber E: The renin–angiotensin system and hypertension.Kidney Int. 15:427, 1979.
4. Slater EE, Cohn RC, Dzau VJ et al.: Purification of human renal renin. Clin Sci Mol Med 55:117S, 1978.
5. Haber E, Koerner T, Page LB et al.: Application of a radioimmunoassay for angiotensin I to the physiologic measurements of plasma renin activity in normal human subjects. J Clin Endocrinol Metab 29:1349, 1969.
6. Wallach L, Nyarai I, Dawson KG: Stimulated renin: a screening test for hypertension. Ann Intern Med 82:27, 1975.
7. Kaplan NM, Kem DC, Holland DB et al.: The intravenous furosemide test: a simple way to evaluate renin responsiveness. Ann Intern Med 84:639, 1976.
8. Swales JD: The hunt for renal hypertension. Lancet 1:577, 1976.
9. Poulsen k, Sancho J, Haber E: A simplified radioimmunoassay for plasma aldosterone employing an antibody of unique specificity. Clin Immunol Immunopathol 2:273, 1974.
10. Sancho J, Re RN, Kliman B, Haber E: Diurnal variation of plasma aldosterone in low renin hypertension. Circulation 50 (Suppl 3):202, 1974.
11. Vagnucci AH, McDonald RH Jr, Drash AL, Wong AKC: Intradian changes of plasma

aldosterone, cortisol, corticosterone, and growth hormone in sodium restriction. J Clin Endocr 38:761, 1974.

12. Deodhar SD, Haas E, Goldblatt H: Production of antirenin to homologous renin and its effect on experimental renal hypertension. J Exp Med 119:425, 1964.

13. Romero JC, Hoobler SW, Kozak TJ, Warzynski RJ: Effect of antirenin in blood pressure of rabbits with experimental renal hypertension. Am J Physiol 225:810, 1973.

14. Wakerlin GE: Antibodies to renin as proof of the pathogenesis of sustained renal hypertension. Circulation 16:653, 1958.

15. Dzau VJ, Kopelman RI, Barger AC et al.: Renin specific antibody for study of cardiovascular homeostasis. Science 207:1091, 1980.

16. Gross F, Lazar J, Orth H: Inhibition of the renin–angiotensinogen reaction by pepstatin. Science 175:656, 1972.

17. Kokubu T, Hiwada K, Nagasaka Y, Yamamura Y: Effect of several proteinase inhibitors on renin reaction. Jpn Circulat J (En) 38:955, 1974.

18. Menard J, Gardes J, Kreft C, Evin G, Castro B, Corvol P: Soluble pepstatin: a new approach in the in vivo blockade of the renin–angiotensin system. In. Proceedings of the 5th Meeting of the International Society of Hypertension, 1978. Clin Sci Mol Med 55 (Suppl 4):167s, 1978.

19. Burton J, Poulsen K, Haber E: Competitive inhibitors of renin: Inhibitors effective at physiological pH. Biochemistry 14:3892, 1975.

20. Poulsen K, Burton J, Haber E: Competitive inhibitors of renin. Biochemistry 12:3877, 1973.

21. Skeggs LT Jr, Kahn JR, Lentz KE, Shumway NP: The preparation, purification and amino acid sequence of a polypeptide renin substrate. J Exp Med 106:439, 1957.

22. Skeggs LT, Lentz KE, Kahn JR, Hochstrasser H: Kinetics of the reaction of renin with nine synthetic peptide substrates. J Exp Med 128:13, 1968.

23. Haber E, Burton J: Inhibitors of renin and their utility in physiologic studies. Fed Proc 38:2768, 1979.

24. Cody RJ Jr, Burton J, Herd JA, Haber E: Specific inhibition of renin by an angiotensinogen analog: studies in sodium depletion and renin dependent hypertension. Proc Natl Acad Sci USA 77:5476, 1980.

25. Ferreira SH: A bradykinin-potentiating factor (BPF) present in the venom of Bothrops Jararca. Br J Pharmacol 24:163, 1965.

26. Bakhle YS: Inhibition of angiotensin I converting enzyme by venom peptides. Br J Pharmacol 43:252, 1971.

27. Ondetti MA, Williams NJ, Sabo EF, Pluscec J, Weaver ER, Kocy O: Angiotensin converting enzyme inhibitors from the venom of Bothrops jararca: isolating elucidation of structure and synthesis. Biochemistry 10:4033, 1971.

28. Ondetti MA, Rubin B, Cushman DW: Design of specific inhibitors of angiotensin converting enzyme: new class of orally active antihypertensive agents. Science 196:441, 1977.

29. Pals DT, Masucci FD, Sipos F, Denning GS Jr: A specific competitive antagonist of the vascular action of angiotensin II. Circ Res 29:664, 1971.

30. Khosla MC, Smeby RR, Bumpus FM: Structure-activity relationships in angiotensin II analogs. In: Angiotensin, p. 126. Page H, Bumpus FM, eds. Berlin: Springer Verlag, 1974.

31. Johnson JA, Davis JO, Spielman WS, Freeman RH: The role of the renin–angiotensin system in experimental renal hypertension in dogs. Proc Soc Exp Biol 147:387, 1974.

32. Streeten GHP, Anderson GH, Freiberg JM, Dalakos TG: Use of an angiotensin II antagonist (saralysin) in the recognition of 'angiotensinogenic' hypertension. N Engl J Med 292:657, 1975.

33. Bianchi A, Evans DB, Cobb M, Peschka MT, Schaeffer TR, Laffan RJ: Inhibition by

SQ20881 of vasopressor response to angiotensin I in conscious animals. Eur J Pharmacol 23:90, 1973.

34. Miller ED Jr, Samuels AI, Haber E, Barger AC: Inhibition of angiotensin conversion in experimental renovascular hypertension. Science 177:1108, 1972.

35. Miller ED Jr, Samuels AI, Haber E, Barger AC: Inhibition of angiotensin conversion and prevention of renovascular hypertension. Am J Physiol 228:448, 1975.

36. Gavras H, Brunner HR, Vaughan ED Jr, Laragh JH: Angiotensin–sodium interaction in blood pressure maintenance of renal hypertensive and normotensive rats. Science 180:1369, 1973.

37. Johnson JA, Davis JO: Effects of a specific competitive antagonist and angiotensin II on arterial pressure and adrenal steroid secretion in dogs. Circ Res 32 (Suppl 1):159, 1973.

38. Sancho J, Re RM, Burton J, Barger AC, Haber E: The role of the renin–angiotensin–aldosterone system in cardiovascular homeostasis in normal human subjects. Circulation 53:400, 1976.

39. Tagawa H, Gutmann FD, Haber E, Miller ED Jr, Samuels AI, Barger AC: Reversible renovascular hypertension and renal arterial pressure. Proc Soc Exp Biol Med 146:975, 1974.

40. Brunner HR, Kirshman JD, Sealey JE, Laragh JH: Hypertension of renal origin: evidence of two different mechanisms. Science 174:1344, 1971.

41. Krieger EM, Salgado HC, Assan CJ, Greene LLJ, Ferreira SH: Potential screening test for detection of overactivity of renin–angiotensin system. Lancet 1:269, 1971.

42. Skeggs LT, Kahn JR, Levine M, Dorer FE, Lentz KE: Chronic one-kidney hypertension in rabbits. III. Renopressin, a new hypertensive substance. Circulation Res 40:143, 1977.

43. Tobian L, Coffee K, McCrea P: Contrasting total exchangeable sodium levels in rats with two different types of Goldblatt hypertension. J Lab Clin Med 66:1027, 1965.

44. Guyton AC, Coleman TG, Granger HJ: Circulation: overall regulation. Annu Rev Physiol 34:13, 1972.

45. Rocchini AP, Barger AC: Renovascular hypertension in sodium-depleted dogs: role of renin in carotid sinus reflex. Am J Physiol (in press).

46. Deming QB, Leutscher JA: Bioassay of desoxycorticosterone-like material in urine. Proc Soc Exp Biol Med 73:171, 1950.

47. Davis JO, Hartroft PM, Titus EO, Carpenter CCJ, Ayers CR, Speigel HE: The role of the renin–angiotensin system in the control of aldosterone secretion. J Clin Invest 41:378, 1962.

48. Watkins L Jr, Burton JA, Haber E, Cant JR, Smith FW, Barger AC: The renin–angiotensin–aldosterone system in congestive failure in conscious dogs. J Clin Invest 57:1606, 1976.

49. Schambelan M, Stockigt JR, Biglieri EG: Isolated hypoaldosteronism in adults: a renin-deficiency syndrome. N Eng J Med 287:573, 1972.

50. DeLeiva A, Christlieb AR, Melby JC et al.: Big renin and biosynthetic defect of aldosterone in diabetes mellitus. N Engl J Med 295:639, 1976.

51. Gill JR, Frolich JC, Bowden RE et al.: Bartter's syndrome: a disorder characterized by high urinary prostaglandins and a dependence of hyperreninemia on prostaglandin synthesis. Am J Med 61:43, 1976.

52. McGiff JC: Bartter's syndrome results from an imbalance of vasoactive hormones. Ann Intern Med 87:369, 1977.

53. Norby L, Lentz R, Flamenbaum W et al.: Prostaglandins and aspirin therapy in Bartter's syndrome. Lancet 2:604, 1976.

54. Katz FH, Bortz AI: Treatment of Bartter's syndrome with naproxen. N Engl J Med 299:100, 1978.

55. Brunner HR, Laragh JH, Baer L et al.: Essential hypertension: renin and aldosterone, heart attack and stroke. N Engl J Med 286:441, 1972.

56. Kaplan NM: The prognostic implications of plasma renin in essential hypertension. JAMA 231:167, 1975.
57. Thurston H, Swales JD: Low renin hypertension: a distinct entity. Lancet 2:930, 1976.
58. When to measure renin? (Editorial). Lancet 1:783, 1975.
59. Kaplan NM: Renin profiles: the unfulfilled promises. JAMA 238:611, 1977.
60. Drayer JI, Keim HJ, Wever MA et al.: Unexpected pressor responses to propranolol in essential hypertension: an interaction between renin, aldosterone, and sympathetic activity. Am J Med 60:897, 1976.
61. Buhler FR, Burkart F, Lutold BE et al.: Antihypertensive beta-blocking action as related to renin and age: a pharmacologic tool to identify pathogenetic mechanisms in essential hypertension. Am J Cardiol 36:653, 1975.
62. Buhler FR, Bertel P, Lutold BE: Simplified and age-stratified antihypertensive therapy based on beta blockers. Cardiovasc Med 3:135, 1978.
63. Woods JW, Pittman AW, Pulliam CC et al.: Renin profiling in hypertension and its use in treatment with propranolol and chlorthalidone. N Engl J Med 294:1137, 1976.
64. Laragh JH: Symposium on hypertension: vasoconstriction-volume analysis for understanding and treating hypertension: the use of renin and aldosterone profiles. Am J Med 55:261, 1973.
65. Vaughan ED Jr, Laragh JH, Gavras I et al.: Symposium on high blood pressure: volume factor in low and renin essential hypertension: treatment with either spironolactone or chlorthalidone. Am J Cardiol 32:523, 1973.
66. Drayer JI, Loppenborg PW, Festen J et al.: Intrapatient comparison of treatment with chlorthalidone. spironolactone and propranolol in normoreninemic essential hypertension. Am J Cardiol 36:716, 1975.
67. Simon N, Franklin SS, Bleifer KH et al.: Clinical characteristics of renovascular hypertension (cooperative study). JAMA 200:1209, 1972.
68. Re R, Novelline R, Escourrou M-T et al.: Inhibition of angiotensin-converting enzyme for diagnosis of renal-artery stenosis. N Engl J Med 298:582, 1978.
69. Marks LS, Maxwell MH: Renal vein renin: value and limitations in the prediction of operative results. Urol Clin North Am 2:311, 1975.
70. Vaughan ED Jr, Buhler FR, Laragh JH et al.: Renovascular hypertension: renin measurements to indicate hypersecretion and contralateral suppression, estimate renal plasma flow, and score for surgical curability. Am J Med 55:402, 1973.
71. Brewster DC, Darling RC: Renal artery reconstruction. Surgical Rounds 1(3):18, 1978.
72. Gruntzig A, Vetter W, Meier B et al.: Treatment of renovascular hypertension with percutaneous transluminal dilation of the renal-artery stenosis. Lancet 1:801, 1978.
73. Gruntzig A: Die perkutane transluminale Rekanalisation chronischer Arterienverschluesse mit einer neuen Dilatationstechnik. New York: Verlag Gerhad Witzstrock, 1977.
74. Tarazi RC, Ibrahim MM, Bravo EL et al: Hemodynamic characteristics of primary aldosteronism. N Engl J Med 289:1330, 1973.
75. Brown JJ, Chinn RH, Davies DL et al.: Plasma electrolytes, renin, and aldosterone in the diagnosis of primary hyperaldosteronism: with a note on plasmacorticosterone concentration. Lancet 2:55, 1968.
76. Sambhi MP, Crane MG, Genest J: UCLA conference: essential hypertension: new concepts about mechanisms. Ann Intern Med 79:411, 1973.
77. Merrill AJ, Morrison JL, Brannon ES: Concentration of renin in renal venous blood in patients with chronic heart failure. Am J Med 1:468, 1948.
78. Turini GA, Brunner HR, Ferguson RK, River JL, Gavras H: Congestive heart failure in man hemodynamics, renin, and angiotensin II blockade. Br Heart J 40:1134, 1978.
79. Haddy FJ, Molner JI, Borden CW, Texter EC Jr: Comparison of direct effects of angiotensin and other vasoactive agents on small and large blood vessels in several vascular beds. Circulation 25:239, 1962.

80. Johnson JA, Davis JO: Angiotensin II: Important role in the maintenance of arterial blood pressure. Science 179:906, 1973.
81. Ganony WF, Biglieri EG, Murlow PJ: Mechanisms regulating adrenocorticoid secretion of aldosterone and glucocorticoids. Recent Prog Horm Res 22:381, 1966.
82. Boyd GW, Adamson AR, James VHT, Peart WS: The role of the renin–angiotensin system in the control of aldosterone in man. Proc R Soc Med 62:1253, 1969.
83. Guiha NH, Coh JN, Mikulic E, Franciosa JA, Limas CJ: Treatment of refractory heart failure with infusion of nitroprusside. N Engl J Med 291:587, 1974.
84. Franciosa JA, Mikluic E, Cohn JN, Jose E, Fabie A: Hemodynamic effects of orally administered isosorbide dinitrate in patients with congestive heart failure. Circulation 50:1020, 1974.
85. Franciosa JA, Pierpont G, Cohn JN: Hemodynamic improvement after oral hydralazine in left ventricular failure: a comparison with nitroprusside infusion in 16 patients. Ann Intern Med 86:388, 1977.
86. Franciosa JA, Cohn JN: Sustained hemodynamic effect during long term nitrates without tolerance in heart failure. Circulation 58 (Suppl II):II-28, 1978.
87. Chatterjee K, Ports T, Rubin S, Massies B, Arnold S, Brundage B, Parmley W: Sustained beneficial hemodynamic effects during long-term hydralazine therapy in patients with chronic heart failure. Circulation 58 (Suppl II):II-28, 1978.
88. Awan NA, Miller RR, Miller MP, Specht K, Vera Z, Mason DT: Clinical pharmacology and therapeutic application of prazosin in acute and chronic refractory congestive heart failure: balanced systemic venous and arterial dilatation improving pulmonary congestion and cardiac output. Am J Med 65:146, 1978.
89. Murtley VS, Waldron TL, Goldberg ME, Vollmer RR: Inhibition of angiotensin converting enzyme by SQ 14,225 in conscious rabbits. Eur J Pharmacol 46:207, 1977.
90. Levine TB, Franciosa JA, Cohn JN: Acute and long-term response to oral-converting enzyme inhibitor, Captopril, in congestive heart failure. Circulation 62:35, 1980.
91. Dzau VJ, Colucci WS, Williams GH et al.: Sustained effectiveness of converting-enzyme inhibition in patients with severe congestive heart failure. N Engl J Med 302:1373, 1980.

20. BLOOD PRESSURE IN THE FIRST YEARS OF LIFE

Michael de Swiet, Elliot Anthony Shinebourne and Peter Fayers

ABSTRACT

Because of methodological difficulties it has only been possible to measure blood pressure accurately and non-invasively in a large number of infants and small children in the last ten years. Studies at the Brompton Hospital and elsewhere show that blood pressure in children is related to wakefulness and weight as it is in adults. Blood pressure rises rapidly with age between four days and two weeks and then more slowly until age six weeks. There is then little change through age four years. One of our purposes in making these measurements has been to determine at what age children develop blood pressures that may be representative of those that they will have in adult life. Although it is possible to demonstrate statistically significant correlations in serial blood pressure measurements before one year, the correlation coefficients are low ($r<0.2$). After one year, serial correlation coefficients become stronger so that the coefficient between measurements made at ages three and four years is 0.47. This is approaching the magnitude of serial correlation coefficients in adults. This therefore suggests that children are tracking for blood pressure with increasing strength from the age of one year onwards.

1. INTRODUCTION

Few doctors routinely measure blood pressure when examining sick or healthy children. This is partly because of difficulties of measurement in small children, partly because normal standards of blood pressure have not been available, and partly because the significance of elevated blood pressure measurements in childhood is uncertain. These deficits are being remedied.

Amery, A. (ed.) Hypertensive Cardiovascular Disease: Pathophysiology and Treatment
© *1982, Martinus Nijhoff Publishers. The Hague / Boston / London*
ISBN-13: 978-94-009-7478-4

2. BLOOD PRESSURE MEASUREMENT

It is not possible to use conventional sphygmomanometry in the small arms of infants and children younger than about five years old. Therefore, we currently use the Parks Doppler ultrasound system [1]. This has the advantages over other ultrasound systems that it is relatively inexpensive and that the sensor is very small and separate from the sphygmomanometer cuff. The Parks Doppler system detects red cell and blood vessel wall movements by the frequency shift that they induce in the reflected ultrasound waves. To use the system, we first locate the brachial artery at the elbow with the sensor. After a sphygmomanometer cuff is inflated in the usual way above systolic blood pressure, red cell and blood vessel wall movements cease in the arm distal to the sphygmomanometer cuff. As the cuff is deflated, blood flow occurs when the systolic pressure is reached, and is detected by hearing the rhythmical Doppler tones.

Thus the Parks Doppler system only measures systolic blood pressure but this is superior to diastolic blood pressure for epidemiological purposes [2], and perfectly adequate for most clinical use. It is claimed that other instruments measure diastolic blood pressure, but for some the correlation between diastolic blood pressure and intra-arterial blood pressure is not so good as for systolic blood pressure [3]. For epidemiological purposes, we also use the Random Zero sphygmomanometer which has a zero muddling device to reduce observer bias [4]. A conventional sphygmomanometer and the Parks system would be suitable for measuring the blood pressure of an individual child for clinical purposes.

Cuff size is crucial if the cuff pressure is to be accurately transmitted to the brachial artery. We employ cuffs with inflation bags 4×13.5 cm and 7.6×15.5 cm using the larger cuff wherever possible. We have found that these give accurate blood pressures in children up to the age of eight years with arm circumferences up to 22 cm [5]. Disposable cuffs are also available and these too appear to give satisfactory results if the correct size is chosen [6].

3. NORMAL VALUES

Values for blood pressure are available in older children and these have been reviewed and published in percentile form from age two years by the American Task Force for Blood Pressure Control [7] (see Figure 1). However, in this publication, even the figures for the age group from two to five years were taken from a study group of only 100 children. Until recently, there were no figures for blood pressure in a large group of younger, normal children. We have selected a group of 2000 children born consecutively in

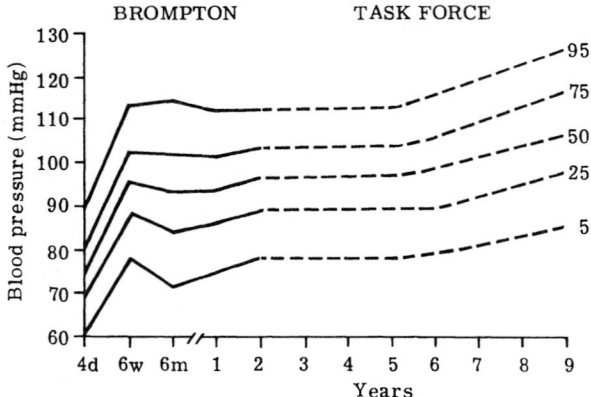

Figure 1. Percentile distribution of systolic blood pressure et
age four days to two years (the Brompton study) and as compiled from two years to nine years by the American task Force
for Blood Pressure Control in Children [7]. With permission of
the American Academy of Pediatrics, Grune and Stratton Inc.,
New York, U.S.A.

one hospital and followed their blood pressures from age four days (the
Brompton study) [5, 8]. The percentile distribution of systolic blood pressure from this study between four days and two years is also given in Figure
1. In this study blood pressure was originally measured around the ages of
four days and six weeks. Blood pressure rises rapidly between the ages of
four and six weeks. In order to determine the time course of this rise more
accurately, we therefore studied another 100 babies born in Farnborough
Hospital, measuring blood pressure more frequently in the first six weeks, to
determine just when this rise in blood pressure occurred [9]. The systolic
blood pressure rose from a mean of 70 mm Hg at the age of two days to a
mean of 84 mm Hg at two weeks in babies awake. There was a further rise
of 9 mm Hg to 93 mm Hg by the age of six weeks. The majority of the
increase, i.e. 14 mm Hg therefore took place in the first two weeks of life.
The mean blood pressure of infants who were asleep when their blood pressure was measured was lower at all ages, but rose in a similar manner.

The mechanism of the early physiological rise in blood pressure in the
neonatal period has not been determined in humans. Studies in sheep have,
however, demonstrated that cardiac output is falling at this time, parallel
with the rise in systolic pressure, implying a marked rise in peripheral resistance during the neonatal period [10]. If this were also the case in man, it
would indicate that in addition to the sudden increase in peripheral vascular
resistance which occurs at delivery with cord clamping and lung expansion,
the total peripheral vascular resistance continues to rise during the first six

weeks of life. A non-invasive method of measuring cardiac output is necessary to confirm this.

4. OTHER STUDIES OF BLOOD PRESSURE IN INFANCY

There are few other large population studies of blood pressure in the first year of life. The Task Force on Blood Pressure Control in Children did not present data in children younger than two years. Other studies of blood pressure measured by indirect techniques in the neonatal period have usually been made in small groups of selected infants. Kirkland and Kirkland [11] also used the Parks Doppler ultrasound system and studied 42 neonates who were both 'resting and sucking'. They did not define the level of activity of the babies any further. However, the range of blood pressure (67–79 mm Hg) found by Kirkland and Kirkland between days three and seven is similar to our data at these ages (68–92 mm Hg) [5]. We did not make measurements while the infants were sucking, because we had previously found that blood pressure was more variable during feeding and sucking than when the neonates were asleep or awake, but not sucking [12]. Zinner and his colleagues in Boston studied 837 infants of varied ethnic origins age one to six days, and found a systolic blood pressure between 69 and 83 mm Hg, depending on the age and level of consciousness [13], values which are about 5 mm Hg higher than those of the Brompton study (68–77 mm Hg) [5]. They used the Arteriosonde, a different Doppler system, in which the cuff is more rigid and also contains the transducer.

In the Miami study, Hennekens and colleagues studied 43 infants from black families [14]. They also used the Arteriosonde and found much higher blood pressures of 78 mm Hg at two days and 103 mm Hg at one month. In the Brompton study the blood pressure was 72 and 68 mm Hg (awake and asleep) at three days, and 86 and 87 mm Hg at six weeks. Apart from using the Arteriosonde device, Hennekens did not specify level of consciousness and made measurements exclusively in a hospital environment. These factors could well account for the difference in blood pressures between the Miami and Brompton studies. The infants of the Miami study were also black. The Brompton study does not include sufficient black infants to analyse the effect of race. However, previous studies have shown no difference in blood pressure between black and white children [13, 15, 16].

5. FACTORS AFFECTING BLOOD PRESSURE IN INFANCY

5.1. Weight and sex

Although the correlation coefficients are low, there is a statistically significant correlation between infants' blood pressures and weights at all ages that we have studied from four days to four years [5, 8]. In the first year of life boys have slightly higher blood pressures than girls. The difference is no greater than 1.5 mm Hg. However, at birth, boys are heavier than girls [17] and, after adjusting for weight, we found that the difference in blood pressure was largely eliminated. The correlation between blood pressure and weight has been noted previously in neonates [18], children [19], and adults [20–22]. In the Bogalusa study, Voors [23] found that the ratio weight/height [3] gave a better prediction of blood pressure than did age in children between the ages of five and fourteen years. He suggested that the increase in body mass is the major determinant of the increase in blood pressure associated with age in the age group five to fourteen years. Height was not measured in the present study, but even making estimates of likely body length we did not find that the ratios of weight/height [2] or weight/height [3] gave better predictions of blood pressure than the relationship with weight alone.

5.2. Wakefulness

Infants awake have higher blood pressures than those asleep (Table 1). At the age of four days, the mean blood pressure was 5.1 mm Hg greater in infants awake than in infants asleep, and at age six weeks the blood pressure was 7.0 mm Hg greater in infants awake than in those asleep. The blood pressure was also higher in infants awake than in infants asleep on each day within the three- to seven-day period on which the nominal four-day measurements were made. Thus, the effect of wakefulness can be demonstrated even in the youngest neonates and is independent of age [5]. We categorised infants as awake if their eyes were open, and asleep if their eyes were closed at the onset of blood pressure measurements [12], and on this basis found

Table 1. Mean blood pressure and 95th percentile at ages four days to three years (figures denote mmHg)*

		4 days	6 weeks	6 months	1 year	2 years	3 years
Mean blood pressure ± SD	Awake	76±9 (171)	96±11 (1135)	93±13 (865)	94±11 (1341)	96±11 (1322)	97±10 (1218)
	Asleep	71±8 (1566)	89±11 (506)	—	—	—	—
95th percentile	Awake	95	113	111	112	114	113
	Asleep	86	106	—	—	—	—

* Number of infants in parenthesis.

higher blood pressure in babies awake, as we [8], and others [18, 24], have previously reported. Indeed, whenever the effect of wakefulness has been examined, the blood pressure has always been found to be higher in babies awake than in those asleep. Any reports of blood pressure should therefore be related to the level of consciousness. It is possible to subdivide the infant's level of consciousness further [25], but we have previously found that such further subdivision does not appreciably reduce blood pressure

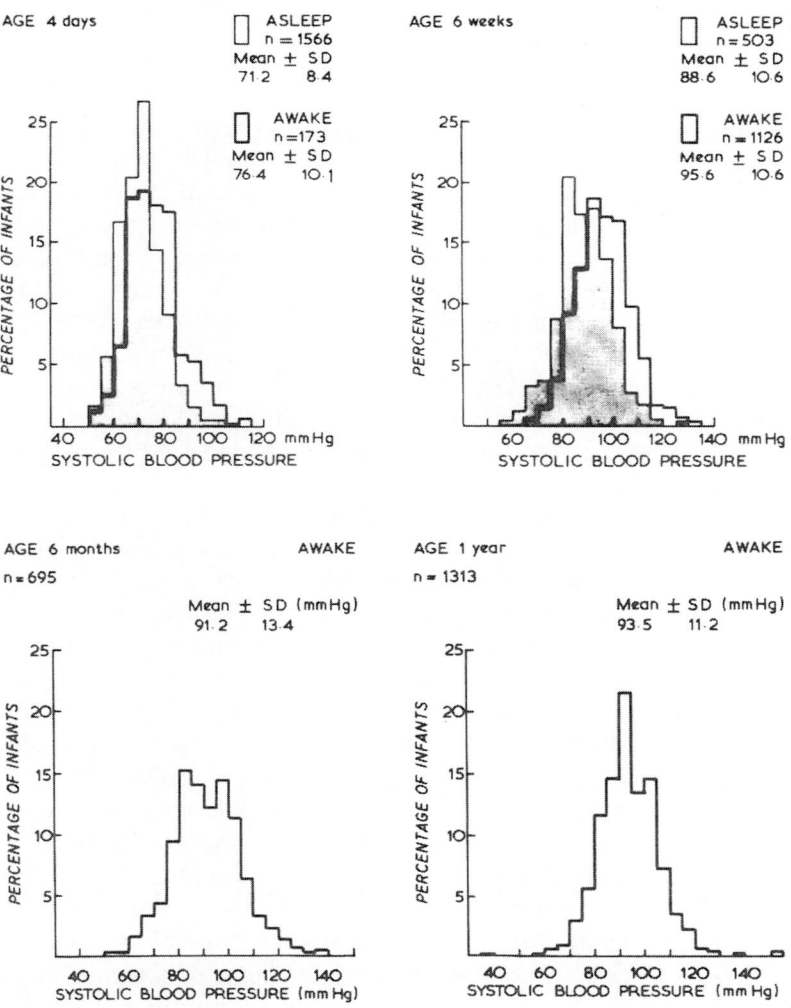

Figure 2. Distribution of systolic blood pressure in infants awake and asleep at ages four days and six weeks, and awake at ages six months and one year (the Brompton Study). With permission of British Medical Journal, British Medical Association, London.

variance in the neonatal period from one occasion to another [12]. It is still possible that blood pressure is related to subdivisions of level of consciousness which differ from those that we employed in the previous study, but we have not explored this further.

6. THE SIGNIFICANCE OF ELEVATED BLOOD PRESSURE IN EARLY CHILDHOOD

6.1. What is hypertension in the first years of life?

Blood pressure is nearly normally distributed in children as it is in adults (Figure 2). Any division of the population into normotensive and hypertensive is therefore arbitrary, although it has recently been suggested that the best definition of hypertension in an adult population is the level of blood pressure at which treatment with hypotensive drugs shows a statistically significant improvement in mortality or morbidity. Such population data is not available in young children and, for the reasons discussed below, it is unlikely that it ever will be. Some individual children do have symptomatic hypertension, usually secondary to renal or endocrine causes or to coarctation of the aorta. These children are very rare; they should only be managed in specialist tertiary referral units, and there were none in the 2000 infants of the Brompton study.

Table 1 summarises the changes in blood pressure that we have found with age (Brompton study) and indicates the 95th percentile for blood pressure at four days, six weeks, six months, and one to three years. These levels of blood pressure are arbitrary levels above which children might be considered hypertensive, if, at the time of measurement, they are awake but neither crying nor feeding. It must be emphasised that comparisons between individual children's blood pressures and those shown in Table 1 should only be made if the same measurement technique is used (Parks Doppler Ultrasound). Published values do vary, as discussed previously, and the most obvious cause of variability is different methodology. The choice of the 95th percentile as the dividing level for hypertension is arbitrary. As stated above, all the children with blood pressures above the 95th percentile in this study were asymptomatic. They were therefore not investigated, and we do not know whether they have any secondary cause for their hypertension. It is certainly unlikely that the 95th percentile is too low a criterion for hypertension, at least in adults. Many physicians would consider a casual blood pressure in excess of 160 mm Hg systolic or 95 mm Hg diastolic as representing hypertension. Using this definition, the National Health Survey has demonstrated that 15–20% of adults in the U.S.A. have hypertension [26].

6.2. At what age does a single systolic blood pressure recording in excess of the 95th percentile have any relevance for prediction of blood pressure in adult life?

Casual measurements showing elevated blood pressures in adults are of considerable significance, and a potent risk factor for cardiovascular disease. They usually continue to be elevated when the blood pressure is measured on subsequent occasions. The correlation coefficient of repeated blood pressure measurements in adults is between 0.6 and 0.7 [27]. Zinner et al., comparing blood pressure measurement four to eight years apart, have shown that such a correlation coefficient is achieved at about 18 years [28]. Although we found significant correlations in blood pressure in a group of infants between ages four days and six weeks, the correlation coefficient was weak (r = 0.2) [29]. We have therefore continued to make blood pressure measurements in this group to determine at what age the correlations may become stronger [8]. At the time of each measurement a child was categorised as ill if taking medicine prescribed by a doctor, and the measurement was excluded since illness might have affected the blood pressure.

Table 2 is the correlation matrix for blood pressures adjusted for level of consciousness in children at the ages of four days, six weeks, six months and one to four years. Although there are statistically significant correlations between blood pressures measured at ages less than one year and later mea-

Table 2. Serial correlations in children's blood pressure, corrected for weight and level of consciousness, between the ages of four days and four years

	4 days	6 weeks	6 months	1 year	2 years	3 years	4 years
4 days		0.17[3] (1594)	0.09[2] (845)	− 0.01 (1303)	−0.05 (1265)	−0.04 (797)	0.10 (287)
6 weeks			0.04 (807)	0.05 (1244)	0.02 (1212)	0.10[2] (765)	0.18[3] (280)
6 months				0.12 (704)	0.12[1] (652)	0.18[3] (766)	−0.03 (274)
1 year					0.26[3] (1056)	0.27[3] (679)	0.23[3] (223)
2 years						0.35[3] (710)	0.32[3] (250)
3 years							0.47[3] (259)

The numbers in parenthesis are the numbers of paired observations compared at each age.
[1] $p<0.05$,
[2] $p<0.01$
[3] $p<0.001$

surements, none of the correlation coefficients is greater than 0.2. However, blood pressure at one year is correlated with all subsequent measurements with coefficients greater than 0.2, and the strongest correlation coefficient (0.47) is between blood pressure measured at three and four years.

6.3. Familial correlations

It is established that there is a significant correlation in blood pressure in adults within families, i.e. hypertension tends to run in families. We therefore looked for this familial correlation in the children of the Brompton study, since, if it occurred, it would be further evidence of the children developing blood pressures related to those that they will have as adults. Although the correlation between mother and child reaches conventional significance levels at ages six months and six weeks, the coefficients are low and not maintained as the children grow older. There is no significant correlation between father's blood pressure and the children's blood pressure. The correlation coefficients were about 30% greater if adjustments were not made for weight. This is because the child's weight is related to the weight of the parent. We are therefore unable to find any marked correlation between the blood pressure of children up to age two years and either of their parents. Similar results have been found by Schachter [30]. However, we do not yet have data analysed from all the parents, and it is possible that when these are available, family correlations will be more meaningful.

Zinner [31] showed a significant familial aggregation of blood pressure in a group of children ages two to fourteen years, and this appeared to be present from the age of two years. However, they also included the contribution of siblings to familial aggregation which we did not. In a selected group of 43 poor, black families, Hennekens [14] showed that inclusion of the infant's systolic or diastolic blood pressure at age one month reduced between-family variability, whereas this effect could not be demonstrated for neonates aged two days. They interpreted this as familial aggregation starting by the age of one month, and, once again, the inclusion of sibling blood pressures and the special characteristics of the population may account for the difference between this study and ours.

6.4. 'Tracking' for blood pressure

The tendency of individuals to maintain their relative position within the distribution of blood pressure as a function of age has been defined as tracking. We would suggest from the evidence of the serial correlations that children start tracking for blood pressure at the age of about one year, and that the tracking is stronger by four years. We originally reported the correlation in blood pressure between four days and six weeks as evidence of tracking [29], but this has not been confirmed as the children grow older. Blood pressure at four days is not correlated with blood pressure measured subsequently [8]. Levine has also reported significant tracking in the first year of life with a correlation coefficient of 0.34 between the ages of six months and one year [32]. However, this publication did not include measurements made in children older than one year.

Schachter has also shown tracking for systolic and diastolic blood pressure in infants from six to fifteen months, but not before six months [30]. In older children, Rosner et al. have demonstrated tracking from the age of five years [27]. They have shown that the correlation coefficient of blood pressure measurements repeated at 4-year intervals between the ages of 5 and 75 years, rises with age from 0.25 to about 0.65 [27]. In the Muscatine Study, Clarke reported a 2-year correlation in repeated blood pressure measurements of 0.27 to about 0.35, (males and females) from five to seven years of age [19]. Our 2-year correlations at one and two years are similar, 0.23 and 0.32 respectively. We therefore believe that tracking can be demonstrated before four years, that it starts at about 1 year, and that by 4 years the correlation coefficient in repeated blood pressure measurements of 0.47 is approaching the adult value of 0.65. Further follow-up studies are still necessary to show to what degree of confidence these data can be used to predict adult blood pressures and therefore adults at risk from hypertension at the time when tracking starts between one and four years.

The most meaningful relationship which may never be proved (because of methodological difficulties and probable intervention) would be to show that elevated blood pressure in childhood is related to outcome in terms of longevity, or the development of cardiovascular disease in adult life.

7. CONCLUSION: THERAPEUTIC IMPLICATIONS

At present, antihypertensive therapy is only used in those children who have marked hypertension (usually secondary) with symptoms or evidence of target organ damage. Although the correlation coefficients of repeated blood pressure are highly significant, they are relatively low and there remains much variability in children's blood pressure in the early years of life.

If one could establish with confidence which asymptomatic children who have elevated blood pressures will continue to have elevated blood pressures in adult life, it would be reasonable to consider antihypertensive therapy in these patients. It is possible that in these circumstances even a short period of antihypertensive treatment might enable an individual to 'jump the tracks' and change to pursuing the 50th percentile rather than the 95th. There is evidence that this occurs in the spontaneously hypertensive rat, treated with antihypertensive drugs during the period of development [33]. However, at present there is too much variability in individual blood pressure measurments to warrant this approach, and we do not yet have the evidence that children with relatively high blood pressures will become adults with hypertension.

ACKNOWLEDGEMENTS

The Brompton study has been supported by the Medical Research Council and the British Heart Foundation. We are indebted to the children and their parents for their cooperation, and to the nurses involved for making the measurements: Julia Mitchell, Betty Szewvzyk, Francis Smith and Doreen Terry. We are also most grateful to Susan Cowley who prepared this manuscript.

REFERENCES

1. Elseed AM, Shinebourne EA, Joseph MC: Assessment of techniques for measurement of blood pressure in infants and children. Arch Dis Child 48:932–936, 1973.
2. Kannel WB, Gordon T, Schwartz MJ: Systolic versus diastolic blood pressure and risk of coronary heart disease: the Framingham Study. Am J Cardiol 27:335–346, 1971.
3. Whyte RK, Elseed AM, Fraser CB, Shinebourne EA, de Swiet M: An assessment of Doppler Ultrasound to measure systolic and diastolic blood pressures in infants and young children. Arch Dis Child 50:542–544, 1975.
4. Wright BM, Dore CF: A random zero sphygmomanometer. Lancet i:337–338, 1970.
5. de Swiet M, Fayers P, Shinebourne EA: Systolic blood pressure in a population of infants in the first year of life: the Brompton study. Pediatrics 65:1028–1035, 1980.
6. Steinfeld L, Dimich I, Reder R, Cohen M, Alexander H: Sphygmomanometry in the pediatric patient. J Pediatr 92:934-938, 1978.
7. Report of the Task Force on Blood Pressure Control in Children: Pediatrics 59(Suppl: 797–820, 1977.
8. de Swiet M, Fayers P, Shinebourne EA: Value of repeated blood pressure measurements in children: the Brompton study. Br Med J 280:1567-159, 1980.
9. Earley A, Fayers P, Ng S, Shinebourne EA, de Swiet M: Blood pressure in the first six weeks of life. Arch Dis Child 55:755–757, 1980.
10. Klopfenstein HS, Rudolph AM: Postnatal changes in the circulation and responses to volume loading in sheep. Cir Res 42:839, 1978.
11. Kirkland Rebecca T, Kirkland JL: Systolic blood pressure measurement in the newborn infant with the transcutaneous Doppler method. J Paediatr 80:52–56, 1972.
12. de Swiet M, Fancourt R, Peto J: Systolic blood pressure variation during the first 6 days of life. Clin Sci Mol Med 49:557–561, 1975.
13. Zinner SH, Lee YH, Rosner B, Oh W, Kass EH: Factors affecting blood pressure in newborn infants. Hypertension 2:1999–2101, 1980.

14. Hennekens CH, Jesse MJ, Klein BE, Gourley JE, Blumenthal S: Aggregation of blood pressure in infants and their siblings. Am J Epidemiol 103:457–463, 1976.
15. McDonough JR, Garrison GE, Hames CG: Blood pressure in hypertensive disease among negroes and whites: a study in Evans County, Georgia. Ann Intern Med 61:208, 1974.
16. Londe S, Gollub SW, Goldring D: Blood pressure in black and white children. J Pediatr 90:93, 1977.
17. Thomson AM, Billewicz WZ, Hytten FE: The assessment of fetal growth. J Obstet Gynaecol 75:903–916, 1968.
18. Lee Y, Rosner B, Gould JB, Lowe EW, Kass EH: Familial aggregation of blood pressures of newborn infants and their mothers. Pediatrics 58:722–724, 1976.
19. Clarke WR, Schrott HG, Leaverton PE, Conner WE, Lauer RM: Tracking of blood lipids and blood presure in school-age children: the Muscatine study. Circulation 58:626–634, 1978.
20. Miall WE, Oldham PD: A study of arterial blood pressure and its inheritance in a sample of the general population. Clin Sci 14:459–488, 1955.
21. Johnson AL, Cornoni JC, Cassel JC, Tyroler HA, Heyden S, Hames CG: Influence of race, sex and weight on blood pressure behaviour in young adults. Am J Cardiol 35:523–530, 1975.
22. Oberman A, Lane NE, Harlan W, Graybiel A, Mitchell RE: Trends in systolic blood pressure in the thousand aviator cohort over a twenty-four year period. Circulation 36:812–822, 1967.
23. Voors AW, Webber LS, Frerichs RR, Berenson GS: Body height and body mass as determinants of basal blood pressure in children: the Bogalusa heart study. Am J Epidemiol 106:101–108. 1977.
24. Gupta JM, Scopes JW: Observations on blood pressure in newborn infants. Arch Dis Child 40:637–644, 1965.
25. Prechtl H, Beintema D: The Neurological Examination of the Fullterm Newborn Infant, p. 6. London: William Heinemann Medical, 1964.
26. Hypertension Study Group: Guidelines for the detection, diagnosis and management of hypertensive populations. Circulation 44:263, 1971.
27. Rosner B, Hennekens CH, Kass EH, Miall WE: Age-specific correlation analysis of longitudinal blood pressure data. Am J Epidemiol 106:306–313, 1977.
28. Zinner SH, Margolius HS, Rosner B, Kass EH: Stability of blood pressure rank and urinary kallikrein concentration in childhood: an eight-year follow-up. Circulation 58:908–915, 1978.
29. de Swiet M, Fayers P, Shinebourne EA: Blood pressure survey in a population of newborn infants. Br Med J ii:9, 1976.
30. Schachter J, Kuller LH, Perkins JM, Radin ME: Infant blood pressure and heart rate: relation to ethnic group (black or white) nutrition and electrolyte intake. Am J Epidemiol 110:205-218, 1979.
31. Zinner SH, Levy PS, Kass EH: Familial aggregation of blood pressure in childhood. N Engl J Med 284:401–404.
32. Levine RS, Hennekens CH, Klein B, Gourley J, Briese FW, Horason J, Gelbano A, Jesse MJ: Tracking correlations of blood pressure levels in infancy. Paediatrics 61:121–125, 1978.
33. Freis ED, Ragan D, Pilsbury III H, Mathews M: Alteration of the course of hypertension in the spontaneously hypertensive rat. Circ Res 31:1–7, 1972.

21. CHILDHOOD HYPERTENSION

Ellin Lieberman

The importance of hypertension in individuals from 1 day to 19 years is no longer disputed. Despite the progress of the past 10 years, information related to this age group is often fragmentary; accordingly, the clinician must extrapolate from experience related to adults, or must rely on clinical judgment with frequent observations. This chapter focuses on primary hypertension in children and adolescents. Other chapters in this text deal with various forms of secondary hypertension and with hypertensive crises.

PRIMARY HYPERTENSION

The prevalence of primary hypertension in children and adolescents throughout the world has not been established. Several circumstances contribute to the difficulty in the establishment of an adequate data base. The numbers that signify hypertension for different ages, both sexes and different races are disputed. The problem is further compounded by the data from well-established epidemiological surveys in the United States of America which have examined tracking phenomena of children. The issue has not yet been resolved as to whether or not children with blood pressure levels in the highest quintiles actually have, or are destined for, primary hypertension [1–7]. Finally, observations from clinical settings which are separate from hospitals have not been collected so that the tracking behavior of blood pressure of free living children and adolescents is not available.

DIAGNOSTIC EVALUATION

Inherent in any discussion of primary hypertension are the biases which physicians bring to the diagnostic evaluation of children and adolescents with elevated blood pressure levels. The published literature in this area of pediatrics is so scant [5, 8–11] that each physician appears to make decisions based on anecdotal experience or extrapolation from studies concern-

Amery, A. (ed.) Hypertensive Cardiovascular Disease: Pathophysiology and Treatment
© *1982, Martinus Nijhoff Publishers. The Hague / Boston / London*
ISBN-13: 978-94-009-7478-4

ing adults. The diagnosis of primary hypertension in the pediatric age group is based on integration of historical data, findings from the physical examination and results of diagnostic tests. Family history is positive for primary hypertension or its complications in up to 50% of affected children and adolescents [10, 12]. The majority of children and adolescents is asymptomatic; their identification as hypertensives may have resulted from incidental recordings of blood pressure. Occasionally, a transient stimulus such as stress or use of a pressor agent may produce symptoms which resolve when the stimulus is withdrawn. In symptomatic individuals, headache is the most frequent complaint. It has been found in up to 30–40% of all pediatric hypertensive patients [12, 13]. It is less common in those with primary hypertension than in patients with elevated blood pressure due to secondary causes. Headaches in children and adolescents are usually frontal in location, variable in severity and in response to analgesics. Epistaxis, dizziness, visual complaints, or syncopal episodes are rarely encountered. Physical examination may be entirely normal. However, in pediatrics there is an association between body mass and blood pressure. Children and adolescents whose body mass is high as compared with their peers have higher blood pressure levels [5, 13–18]. This is true if height exceeds the 95th percentile, if weight is great in proportion to height or if excess weight is due to increased muscle mass or adipose tissue.

Blood pressure levels should be recorded in the standing, sitting and supine positions and in all four limbs at the initial evaluation. At Childrens Hospital of Los Angeles (CHLA) for subsequent visits the right upper arm, sitting position pressure with the three heart sounds (I/IV and V Korotkoff sounds) as recommended by the American Heart Association in 1967 has been adopted [19]. Recording of blood pressure levels in this manner and indicating which cuff size was used allows an accurate comparison of blood pressure levels obtained on different occasions. The pulse rate should be noted and may be rapid in patients with primary hypertension.

Examination of the fundi rarely reveals any abnormality unless hypertension is of moderate severity and of several months duration. The most common finding is arteriolar tortuosity. Arterio-venous nicking or arteriolar spasm is not seen unless blood pressure elevation is severe. The remainder of the physical examination is oriented to the systematic search for any evidence of conditions associated with secondary forms of hypertension (Table 1). The percentage of secondary forms of hypertension in pediatrics is greater than in internal medicine. Clues to these diagnoses in terms of specific organ system involvement or in terms of specific entities are usually present. The need for an exhaustive investigation for all possible causes of secondary forms of hypertension should be thoughtfully analyzed based on the expected yield of diagnostic testing in the absence of reliable signs and symptoms of specific diseases [4, 8, 9, 11, 13]. Accordingly, for asymptomat-

340

Table 1. Secondary causes of hypertension in pediatrics

1) Cardiovascular
Coarctation of the thoracic or abdominal aorta
Hypoplasia of the abdominal aorta
Takayasu's disease (pulseless disease)

2) Renal
Acute acquired renal disorders
  Acute renal failure with hypervolemia
  Acute glomerulonephritis
  Hemolytic uremic syndrome
  Interstitial nephritis
  Obstructive uropathy
  Renal trauma
  Renal vein thrombosis
Chronic acquired renal disorders
  Chronic glomerulonephritis
  Chronic pyelonephritis
  Chronic renal disease
  Hemolytic uremic syndrome
  Radiation nephritis
  Renal trauma
Tumors
  Wilms'
  Renin secreting tumors
Congenital or genetic renal disorders
  Alport's syndrome (familial nephritis)
  Ask Upmark (renal hypoplasia)
  Asymmetric renal disease
  Cystic dysplasia
  Polycystic kidney disease (dominant or recessive types)
  Single cyst
Renal vascular abnormalities
  Neurofibromatosis (von Recklinghausen's disease)
  Post-transplant arterial abnormalities
  Post-umbilical artery catheterization in neonates
  Renal arterial disease: stenosis of main or branches of renal artery
Renal vein thrombosis

3) Endocrine
Adrenal
  Adrenal cortical defects (of unclear origin)
  Cushing's disease
  11 and 17-hydroxylase deficiencies
  Liddle's syndrome
  Neuroblastoma
  Pheochromocytoma
  Primary aldosteronism
Diabetes mellitus
Gonadal dysgenesis (Turner's syndrome)
Parathyroid
  Hyperparathyroidism

Table 1. (continued)

---

4) Connective tissue disorders
Dermatomyositis
Ehlers Danlos syndrome
Juvenile rheumatoid arthritis
Mixed connective tissue disease
Scleroderma
Systemic lupus erythematosus

5) Central nervous system disorders
Dysautonomia
Guillain Barre syndrome
Meningitis
Poliomyelitis
Space-occupying lesions

6) Nephrotoxins and drug related
Drug-withdrawal hypertension (clonidine, methyl dopa, minoxidil, propranolol)
Interstitial nephritis
Oral contraceptives
Phencyclidine (P C P)
Poisoning (lead, mercury)
Steroids (corticosteroids, mineralocorticoids)
Sympathomimetics

7) Orthopedic injuries and procedures
Leg lengthening
Harrington rod placement for scoliosis
Trauma

8) Metabolic
Hypercalcemia (idiopathic, secondary to hypervitaminosis D, metastatic disease, sarcoidosis)
Porphyria

9) Miscellaneous
Stevens Johnson syndrome

---

ic prepubertal children whose blood pressure levels are consistently elevated, the recommended minimal laboratory studies include: blood urea nitrogen (or blood urea) or creatinine and urinalysis with or without urine culture. The Task Force on Blood Pressure Control in Children [20] also included in its recommendations roentgenograms of the chest and an electrocardiogram. At CHLA these studies have generally neither been helpful in terms of diagnosis nor in terms of monitoring clinical status. Echocardiography is now being used to define the existence and magnitude of left ventricular hypertrophy and of septal hypertrophy. However, data supporting the use of the echocardiogram as a non-invasive means to estimate cardiac function in children and adolescents with primary hypertension are unavailable. This technique currently offers an excellent tool with which an initial assessment can be made as well as an innocuous means for long term follow-up to determine whether or not target organ damage has occurred, is occurring, and, most importantly, is reversible with good blood pressure control.

In prepubertal children renal disease is a significant cause for elevation of blood pressure. Many disorders associated with parenchymal renal disease will be reflected by an abnormal urinalysis with or without an abnormal serum creatinine. However, children with asymmetric renal disease, i.e. a small unilateral kidney with a contralateral hypertrophied kidney, or with renal arterial abnormalities may have normal urinalyses and normal renal function studies. If the index of suspicion is high because of a moderately elevated blood pressure, a fixed diastolic elevation, the presence of symptoms associated with hypertension, the presence of hypertensive retinopathy and in our experience at CHLA a thin child, an intravenous pyelogram is warranted to search for these conditions. As reported by Fry and associates and Korobkin and coworkers [21–23], many young children with significant arterial lesions have normal rapid sequence intravenous pyelograms and therefore renal vein renin levels and aortography with selective angiograms may still be needed.

Other screening studies for secondary causes of hypertension, such as urinary vanylyl mandelic acid (VMA), urinary or serum aldosterone levels, peripheral renin activity etc., are not routinely indicated for prepubertal hypertensive patients. These tests currently are still being evaluated in investigative protocols and are not necessary for patient management. The concept of low-renin, normal-renin, and high-renin primary hypertension has not been widely applied to pediatrics. A few reports of children with low-renin (presumably primary) hypertension have been published [24, 25]. These patients appear clinically indistinguishable from those with primary hypertension without depressed renin levels.

The arguments for and against obtaining intravenous pyelograms, serum electrolytes and other diagnostic studies in adolescents have not been resolved. The advocates of detailed testing contend that, even if one study in a hundred is positive, a surgically remediable condition may be diagnosed. The opponents of this view argue that a yield of 1 % is too low to be cost-effective. Several studies of adolescent hypertensives report a low incidence of secondary causes of hypertension [4, 8, 9, 11, 13]. The general way the controversy is being handled in most large American centers is to obtain detailed studies on only those adolescents who have some feature(s) of secondary hypertension. Otherwise, because the incidence of secondary causes is lower in adolescents than in younger children, a course of treatment employing nonpharmacologic [12, 20] and, when needed, pharmacologic therapy is often begun. The youngster must remain under continuing medical care so that the response to treatment can be assessed. If the patient is regarded as compliant but treatment does not result in the anticipated response of normalization of blood pressure over a specified period of time, usually 3 months, then the entire case should be reviewed in terms of the appropriateness of primary hypertension as the diagnosis and the need to exclude other forms of hypertension.

All children and adolescents with a diagnosis of primary hypertension should have fasting lipids measured and serially monitored, whether or not they have received anti-hypertensive drugs. Offspring of parents who have sustained a premature cardiovascular event (i.e. under the age of 50 years) such as stroke, dissecting aneurysm, myocardial infarction or renal failure of unknown origin are at greater risk for hyperlipidemia and should be studied as early as feasible. Glueck and associates [26] have recently outlined the management of hyperlipidemia in childhood.

MANAGEMENT

Identification of young children and adolescents as having primary hypertension carries with it the burden of informing a youngster who is not yet mature that he is abnormal and that he is different from his peers. Communication of such information requires sensitivity as to the developmental stages of childhood and adolescence, knowledge of the child's and family's cultural belief system in terms of health and disease, and patience on the part of the provider in assisting the family to deal with the diagnosis, its evaluation and treatment. Often the most difficult part of patient management is the transmission of information that, although the child is asymptomatic, he needs treatment and, at the present time, once treatment is begun it may be lifelong.

The initial step in treatment is a nutritional assessment to determine whether or not the intake of sodium and/or of calories is excessive. Reduction in either or both of these nutrients may be all that is required for control of blood pressure. Changing the dietary habits of children and their family members is often difficult, time-consuming, a source of friction and frustration and ultimately may lead to hostility among all involved. In many children, about one year is required for alteration of acquired salt appetites, even under optimal circumstances. In those instances where nutritional intervention becomes more burdensome than hypertension itself, it is more prudent to start with the simplest regimen of antihypertensive therapy. In others, nutritional and pharmacological therapy may provide optimal results.

Published results of treatment of pediatric patients with primary hypertension consist of reports of small series of patients not followed for many years [3]. The long-term consequences of oral antihypertensive therapy of young people are unknown [27]. Metabolic complications related to hypertension and/or exaccerbated by decades of thiazide therapy might include hyperuricemia, glucose intolerance, or hyperlipidemia. The impact on central nervous system functions of long-term alpha- and beta-blocking agents which cross the blood brain barrier has not been examined. Will peripheral receptor activity be adversely affected? Do any agents directly or indirectly alter sexual and reproductive functions? Information from treatment of mature men and women suggests that these concerns may be unwarranted. However, these issues must be considered when treating any developing individual for an indefinite period of time.

The pharmacologic treatment of primary hypertension in children that is advocated by the Task Force on Blood Pressure Control in Children [20] as well as by others [12, 28] is that of the stepped care approach. Detailed discussions of therapy are available in several pediatric reviews [12, 13] and in this text (see chapters   ) and therefore will not be reviewed in detail. The general principles outlined in Table 2 are to use the safest drug, in the lowest dosage, with the longest duration of action that is available. Side effects in an asymptomatic child or adolescent may defeat the whole management program. Information about anticipated drug reactions should be carefully presented so as to preserve the child's and the family's trust. Studies evaluating the impact of educating the child and family as to the risks and benefits of hypertension and its treatment have not been published.

Although it has long been customary in the United States to prohibit any child or adolescent with elevated blood pressure from participation in competitive sports, this recommendation is not supported by experts in pediatric hypertension. Acute elevations of both systolic and diastolic pressure have been documented in adolescents with dynamic exercises [29]. Nevertheless, unless the individual has experienced significant cardiac damage or is receiving an agent which alters cardiac function, these children are now being advised to participate in dynamic exercises. Some physicians prefer to test their patients on a treadmill before permitting them to play. Studies of treadmill tests of hypertensive young athletes are not available.

Table 2. Criteria for drug selection for therapy of pediatric hypertension

1) Has been extensively studied in animals and man.
2) Has been used widely for a considerable number of years.
3) Is known to be effective.
4) Has a wide margin of safety.
5) Has the longest possible duration of action.
6) Has minimal side effects, toxicity and drug interactions.
7) Is inexpensive.
8) Is least likely to lead to or require polypharmacy for effectiveness.

SUMMARY

Primary hypertension is well recognized in children and adolescents, but its prevalence has not yet been ascertained because of lack of agreement as to what blood pressure levels indicate hypertension for various ages and because the extent to which blood pressure tracks in childhood and adolescence has not been established. Nonetheless, the diagnosis can be made by careful attention to family and personal history, by diligent physical examination to exclude signs suggesting secondary causes of hypertension and by stepwise laboratory and other testing. In some prepubertal individuals more extensive evaluation may be warranted to rule out a renal or renovascular etiology for elevated blood pressure levels. Adolescents rarely require extensive studies; blood urea nitrogen, creatinine, urinalysis, chest roentgenograms and electrocardiogram and/or echocardiogram are usually sufficient. All pediatric patients diagnosed as having primary hypertension should be screened for and monitored for hyperlipidemia.

Management of primary hypertension in children and adolescents involves sensitive communication of the diagnosis and its meaning. Treatment includes nutritional and other nonpharmacological counseling and, when necessary, antihypertensive agents are prescribed with the understanding that long term effects in children are unknown. The question of involvement in competitive sports is not settled, but experts in the care of young hypertensives are recommending dynamic exercises if there is no evidence of cardiac damage and the patient is not receiving any drug that alters cardiac function.

REFERENCES

1. Fixler DE, Laird WP, Fitzgerald V, Stead S, Adams R: Hypertension screening in schools: results of the Dallas study. Pediatrics 63:32–36, 1979.
2. Levine RS, Hennekens CH, Klein B, Ferrer PL, Gourley J, Cassady J, Gelband H, Jesse MJ: A longitudinal evaluation of blood pressure in children. Am J Public Health 69:1175–1177, 1979.
3. Lieberman E: Pediatric hypertension. In: Hypertension update: Mechanisms Epidemiology Evaluation Management. Hunt JC, Cooper T, Frohlich ED, Gifford RW Jr, Kaplan NM, Laragh JH, Maxwell MH, Strong CG, eds, pp. 95–106. Bloomfield: Health Learning Systems, 1980.
4. Londe S, Goldring D, Gollub SW, Hernandez A: Blood pressure and hypertension in children: studies, problems, and perspectives. In: Juvenile Hypertension. New MI, Levine LS, eds, pp. 13–24. New York: Raven Press, 1977.
5. Rames LK, Clarke WR, Connor WE, Reiter MA, Lauer RM: Normal blood pressures and the evaluation of sustained blood pressure elevation in childhood: the Muscatine study. Pediatrics 61:245–251, 1978.
6. Voors AW, Webber LS, Berenson GS: Time course study of blood pressure in children over a three-year period. Bogalusa heart study. Hypertension 2 (Suppl I):I-102–I-108, 1980.

346

7. Zinner SH, Margolius HS, Rosner B, Kass EH: Stability of blood pressure rank and urinary kallikrein concentration in childhood: an eight-year follow-up. Circulation 58:908–915, 1978.
8. Aschinberg LC, Zeis PM, Miller RA, John EG, Chan LL: Essential hypertension in childhood. JAMA 237:322–324, 1977.
9. Levine LS, Lewy JE, New MI: Hypertension in high school students. Evaluation in New York City. NY State J Med 76:40–44, 1976.
10. Londe S, Bourgoignie JJ, Robson AM, Goldring D: Hypertension in apparently normal children. J Pediatr 78:569–577, 1971.
11. Silverberg DS, van Nostrand C, Juchli B, Smith ESO, van Dorsser E: Screening for hypertension in a high school population. Can Med Assoc J 113:103–113, 1975.
12. Lieberman E: Blood pressure and primary hypertension in childhood and adolescence. In: Current Problems in Pediatrics. Gluck L, ed. pp. 1–35. Chicago: Year Book, 1980.
13. Leumann EP: Blood pressure and hypertension in childhood and adolescence. Adv Intern Med Pediatr 43:109–183, 1979.
14. Cornoni-Huntley J, Harlan WR, Leaverton PE: Blood pressure in adolescence. The United States health examination survey. Hypertension 1:566–571, 1979.
15. Harlan WR, Cornoni-Huntley J, Leaverton PE: Blood pressure in childhood. The national health examination survey. Hypertension 1:559–565, 1979.
16. Higgins M, Keller J, Moore F, Ostrander L, Metzner H, Stoch L: Studies of blood pressure in young people and its relationship to personal and familial characteristics and complications of pregnancy in mothers. Am J Epidemiol 111:142–155, 1980.
17. Miller RA, Shekelle RB: Blood pressure in tenth-grade students. Results from the Chicago Heart Association pediatric heart screening project. Circulation 54:993–1000, 1976.
18. Voors AW, Webber LS, Frerichs RR, Berenson GS: Body height and body mass as determinants of basal blood pressure in children – the Bogalusa heart study. Am J Epidemiol 106:101–108, 1977.
19. Kirkendall WM, Burton AC, Épstein FH, Freis ED: Recommendations for human blood pressure determination by sphygmomanometers. Circulation 36:980–988, 1967.
20. National Heart, Lung, and Blood Institute: Report of the Task Force on Blood Pressure Control in Children. Pediatrics 59 (Suppl):797–820, 1977.
21. Fry WJ, Ernst CB, Stanley JC, Brink B: Renovascular hypertension in the pediatric patient. Arch Surg 107:692–698, 1973.
22. Korobkin M, Perloff DL, Palubinskas AJ: Renal arteriography in the evaluation of unexplained hypertension in children and adolescents. J Pediatr 88:388–393, 1976.
23. Korobkin M, Pick RA, Merten DF, Perloff DL, Palubinskas AJ: Etiologic radiographic findings in children and adolescents with nonuremic hypertension. Radiology 110:615–625, 1974.
24. Gruskin AB, Linshaw M, Cote ML, Fleisher DS: Low-renin essential hypertension– another form of childhood hypertension. J Pediatr 78:765–771, 1971.
25. Leumann EP, Nussberger J, Vetter W: Low renin essential hypertension in a child. Helv Paediatr Acta 30:357–363, 1975.
26. Glueck CJ, McGill HCJr, Shank RE, Lauer RM: Value and safety of diet modification to control hyperlipidemia in childhood and adolescence. Circulation 58:381A–385A, 1978.
27. Blumenthal S, Lauer RM: Where are children's blood pressures headed? Hypertension 3:46–47, 1981.
28. Rance CP, Arbus GS, Balfe JW, Kooh SW: Persistent systemic hypertension in infants and children. Pediatr Clin North Am 21:801–824, 1974.
29. Nudel DB, Gootman N,Brunson SC, Stenzler A, Shenker IR, Gauthier BG: Exercise performance of hypertensive adolescents. Pediatrics 65:1073–1078, 1980.

22. HYPERTENSION IN ELDERLY

F. Forette, J. F. Henry, M.P. Hervy, R. Fagard, P. Lijnen, J. Staessen and A. Amery

1. DEVELOPMENT OF ARTERIAL BLOOD PRESSURE WITH AGE

Blood pressure increases with age in most people. Being more marked for systolic pressure, this increase leads to an increase in pressure amplitude. This is illustrated by Figure 1 which shows the systolic and diastolic blood pressures of a representative sample of a Belgian village [1]. There is no certainty, however, that this phenomenon continues at an extremely advanced age. Cross-sectional studies are contradictory in this respect. In the 1753 subjects over 60 years old in Edwards' study [2] the systolic pressure shows a quasilinear rise up to the age of 70 and then starts to decrease, while diastolic blood pressure remains stable after the age of 60. In Masters' study as well, systolic and diastolic blood pressure in 5757 subjects over 65 years old decreased in women and became stabilized in men after the age of 75 years [3].

Some studies revealed more marked differences between the sexes. In the American National Health Survey study [4] systolic blood pressure decreased in women after the age of 75, while it increased in men after the age of 18 until the age of 79. In both sexes diastolic blood pressure tended to stabilize around the age of 60. On the whole these data are opposite to those of Hamilton [5] which suggest that arterial blood pressure increases steadily with age. The differences in the research material (exclusion of subjects with any heart disease in the Masters study, small population in the Hamilton study, no subjects over 80 years old in the National Health Survey statistics) make it difficult to reach a general conclusion which underlines the importance of longitudinal studies.

The Framingham study showed a constant increase in systolic blood pressure in both sexes until the age of 60 but the data on older subjects have not yet been published. Diastolic pressure decreases after the age of 50 [6]. Most of these cross-sectional or longitudinal studies have shown that arterial blood pressure, which is lower in women than in men during the first half of their lives, increases after the age of 50. The Framingham longitudinal study showed the same findings for systolic pressure but not for diastolic pressure, which was consistently lower in women.

Amery, A. (ed.) Hypertensive Cardiovascular Disease: Pathophysiology and Treatment
© *1982, Martinus Nijhoff Publishers. The Hague / Boston / London*
ISBN-13: 978-94-009-7478-4

In the same vein, the recent study carried out by the 'Hypertension Detection and Follow-up Program Cooperative Group' showed that arterial blood pressure is lower in women at all ages and attributed this peculiarity to the greater consumption of antihypertensive drugs by the female population [7]. It should be emphasized that the age-related increase in blood pressure is not a universal phenomenon. Among some primitive populations, blood pressure is stable throughout life [8].

Various factors have been investigated in an attempt to explain this phenomenon, such as lower salt consumption, stress-free life, genetic factors, physical activity, absence of obesity. A recent study [9] made among Navajo Indians, showed that blood pressure did not change with age in men. It increased moderately in women but remained markedly lower than in American women of the same age. The only factor that seemed correlated to high blood pressure in these populations was body weight. We know that the weight–blood pressure correlation persists even at a very high age [10]. Possibly, the absence of weight gain with age in some subjects accounts for the stable blood pressure of certain population.

One may wonder whether the high blood pressure found in the Western world is real or whether it could be an artifact of blood pressure measurement by cuff due to the reduced elasticity of the arteries. However, several investigators verified their findings by checking intra-arterial pressure: Berliner [11] showed that direct intra-arterial pressure was rather higher in elderly subjects than indirect blood pressure measured by cuff.

In addition, Julius and Amery [12, 13] found a significant increase in intra-arterial systolic pressure from the age of 20 to the age of 70, which refutes the possible bias of indirect blood pressure measurement.

2. VARIATIONS IN BLOOD PRESSURE

The clinical impression of the marked variability of blood pressure in the aged, which is familiar to every physician, is confirmed when this variability is made the subject of an exact study.

In a study made in 1972 [14] among 35 subjects aged 65 to 102, we measured blood pressure at 7 and 11 a.m., and at 3 and 6 p.m. once a week for eight weeks and basic pressure at 7 a.m. over two different periods of 15 consecutive days each. The analysis showed that in none of the subjects the maximum range of systolic blood pressure was less than 40 mm Hg and in two-thirds of the cases was between 70 and 100 mm Hg.

A very extensive study on the variability of blood pressure published in 1978 [15] by the 'Hypertension Detection and Follow-up Program Cooperative Group' and conducted in 159 000 men and women between 30 and 69 years old showed that intra-individual variability increases with age and is, in addition, correlated with sex (higher in men), race (higher in blacks), history of hypertension, and antihypertensive treatment.

Obviously, this variability may lead to errors in estimating the incidence of hypertension if only a single casual blood pressure measurement is considered. Colandrea and Friedman [16] found that hypertension had been overestimated by 10% in a population with an average age of 60. In our older population (average age of 80) the incidence of hypertension is overestimated by 20%. We should therefore have several blood pressure readings (at least three), including one at rest, before making a diagnosis of permanent hypertension.

3. PREVALENCE OF HYPERTENSION

Even after eliminating the bias of variability in blood pressure, the prevalence of hypertension is high above the age of 60; we have estimated the prevalence of hypertension in our long-term hospitalized female population at 46.4%, 31.2% having both systolic and diastolic hypertension (systolic ≥160 and diastolic ≥90) and 15.2% purely systolic hypertension (systolic pressure ≥160) [17].

Our findings from specifically old population (average age of 80) all agree with the studies carried out in large ambulatory populations: Masters [3], National Health Survey [4], Froment [18] (Table 1). Nearly all studies confirm that hypertension is more common in women than in men: 40–50% in women, 30–40% in men (Figure 1).

Table 1.

	Number of subjects	Age	Degree of HTA (mm Hg)	Prevalence (%)
Masters et al. (1950)	5757	>65	150/100	35
National Health Survey (1964)	6672	65–74	≥160 and/or ≥90	Females: 49.9 Males: 31.8
		75–79	≥160 and/or ≥90	Females: 45.9 Males: 41.6
Forette et al. (1975)	224	65–102	≥160/90 ≥160/<90	Females: 31.2 Females: 46.4
Froment et al. (1977)	680	60–64	≥160 and/or ≥94	Females: 39 Males: 25

350

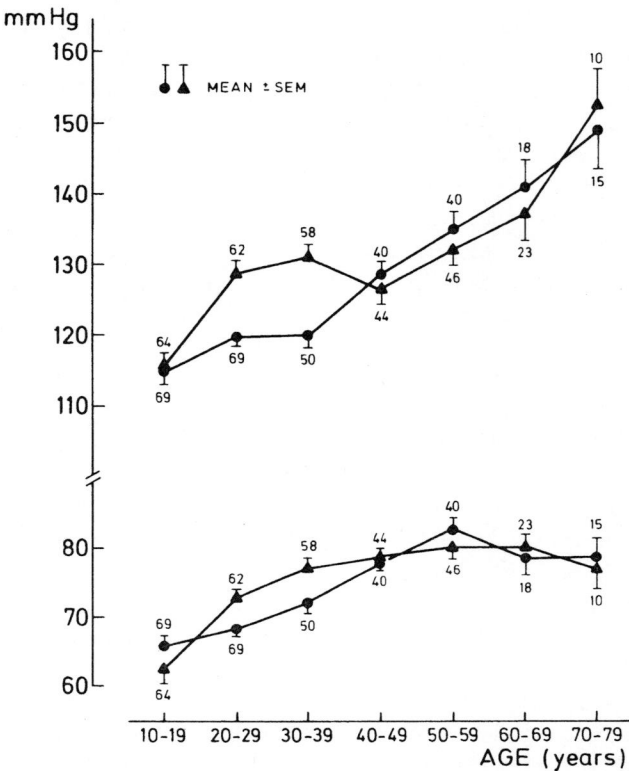

Figure 1. Systolic and diastolic blood pressure (mean ± standard error) according to age in males (▲) and females (●). The number of subjects in each age group is given for both sexes. From Staessen et al. [1].

4. EFFECTS OF HYPERTENSION

Given this prevalence, the problem obviously is to know if morbidity in this hypertensive population is higher than in the normotensive population of the same age. Comparing a population of 70 subjects with systolic and diastolic hypertension with a control population of 55 normotensive subjects of the same age [17], we found a significantly higher prevalence of cardiovascular diseases in the hypertensive subjects: twice as many cerebrovascular accidents (24% vs. 9%), twice as many cases of ischemic cardiopathy (14% vs. 1.8%), and thirteen times as many alterations of the ocular fundus. These data came from a cross-sectional study. We supplemented this study with a longitudinal study aiming to demonstrate that hypertension represents a major risk, even at an extremely advanced age, in terms of cardiovascular illness [10]. A longitudinal survey over a 10-year period (1968-1978) of 191 female subjects hospitalized for a long period showed again that cerebrovascular accidents were twice as common in hypertensive subjects than in normotensive subjects of the same age (20.6% vs. 9.8%). At the beginning of the study blood pressure in subjects who later had cerebrovascular accidents was significantly higher than in subjects who had not (172/88 vs. 158/82, p<0.01). Also, the 10-year incidence of myocardial infarction was three times higher in hypertensive subjects (27.8% vs. 7.8%, p<0.01). At the beginning of the study, blood pressure of subjects who later had a myocardial infarction was significantly higher than that of subjects who had not (178/91 vs. 155/81, p<0.001).

The multivariate analysis showed that hypertension was the only predictive factor for cardiovascular or cerebrovascular diseases, for age, body weight, blood sugar and cholesterol levels did not appear to be cardiovascular risk factors in this study. It should be emphasized that risk increased in relation to moderate blood pressure increase. Moderate, almost exclusively systolic hypertension is, at that age, the great 'purveyor' of cardiovascular accidents.

Shekelle et al. [19], in a large prospective study involving 2772 subjects between the ages of 65 and 74, 42% of whom were hypertensives (blood pressure over 160/95), found a significantly higher incidence (p<0.001) of cerebrovascular accidents (4.2% vs. 2.4%) in the hypertensive subjects. Similarly, a recent report from the Framingham study confirms and reinforces previously published data. In 1970 results in subjects then between 38 and 69 years old showed that hypertension increased the risk of atherothrombotic cerebrovascular accidents fourfold [20]. In 1976, 18 years after the beginning of the longitudinal study in these 5209 subjects, the analysis carried out in subjects aged 45-74 showed that the risk of cerebrovascular accidents was seven times higher in the hypertensive subjects and increased with age [21]. In this study it was found the risk was not limited to cerebral pathology. Kannel [22] has shown that the risk extends to all vascular pathology and increases with age as well as with blood pressure levels in both sexes. Also, the correlation between mortality and blood pressure level has been very clearly demonstrated by this longitudinal study over 30 years, which allowed a comparison between mortality rate of hypertensives and that of normotensives in the same area during the same period of observation by identical methods, which was not the case in other studies such as Fry's [23]. Although it is true that the relative mortality rate of male hypertensives compared with that of normotensives diminishes with age, dropping from 277% at 45-54 years of age to 207% at 65-74 years of age, we must note that it remains twice as high in hypertensives over 65 than in normotensives of the same age. A recent Scandinavian study [29] confirms these data on the basis of a survey over 13.5 years of 855 male subjects born

352

in 1913, showing a strong correlation between the level of blood pressure at the beginning of the study and cardiovascular morbidity and mortality.

Taken as a whole, these studies show that, although hypertension is common in the aged, it remains an unfavorable condition above the age of 60 because of the correlation that exits, even at that age, between level of blood pressure and incidence of vascular complications. The data also show that accidents happen at near-normal diastolic blood pressure levels and at relatively moderately elevated systolic blood pressure levels. There is thus no evidence to support the theory that systolic hypertension in the aged is a 'necessity' to ensure normal circulation through narrowed blood vessels. There is also no support for the theory that systolic hypertension only reflects vascular rigidity without the normal consequences of hypertension. Here again, Kannel demonstrated that pulse pressure, considered as proof of vascular rigidity, is not correlated to vascular accidents more closely than systolic pressure and that its 'influence' on vascular pathology does not increase with age [22].

It is thus obvious that there is no justification for modifying and increasing the WHO criteria (160/95) to define hypertension above the age of 60 since, even at that age, a higher blood pressure is the most important factor contributing to an increase in the incidence of vascular illness. We know that this is an artificial limit since the risk gradient is continuous from the lowest to the highest values; Kannel showed that, from 109 to 190, any elevation of 10 mm Hg in systolic pressure carries a 30% higher risk of atherothrombotic cerebrovascular accidents [21]. This level defines the 20% of the population in whom 60% of cerebrovascular accidents occur. It is useful for determining whether a subject at risk should be systematically monitored and possibly treated. There is no indication, in any case, that this blood pressure level should change after the age of 60.

5. SECONDARY HYPERTENSION

The prevalence of secondary hypertension in the aged is not precisely known because the available data are inadequate. The tests necessary to trace etiology are rarely made in patients over 60, because it is unusual at that age to find a causal condition that is curable. However, there have been reports of pheochromocytomas [25] and primary hyperaldosteronism in subjects over 60 [26].

Only one particular causal condition in the aged deserves to be singled out: atheromatous stenosis of the renal artery. The prevalence of such atheromatous stenoses is high, 9.5% in 800 autopsies performed by Berthaux et al. [27], but their role is difficult to define. While such stenoses are not necessarily associated with hypertension, the latter occurs more frequently in subjects with stenosis than in the general population of the same age (61 % vs. approximately 40 %). In addition, stenosis of the renal artery is often responsible for the rare case of very severe hypertension in elderly persons which is resistant to treatment and develops very rapidly toward irreversible renal insufficiency. The hypertension, usualy diagnosed long ago, evolves in this accelerated manner when a practically complete stenosis on one side is complicated by thrombosis on the opposite side.

In general, stenosis of the renal artery in the aged is left surgically untreated. Some authors, however, such as Ernst [28] and Kotchen [29], suggest revascularization when renal function is normal and there are no multiple atheromas. In their population of 66 patients, 19 of them over 60, in whom revascularization was performed, the prognosis of the operation seemed to depend not on age but on whether the atheromatous stenosis was single and localized.

6. ESSENTIAL HYPERTENSION

Most cases of hypertension in the aged are of the so-called essential type. Some parameters of the syndrome are now being studied and defined but too many data are still missing.

6.1. Hemodynamic parameters

A progressive reduction in cardiac output with age was observed as early as 1955 by Brandfonbrener and Shock [30]. Their data were confirmed by Julius and Amery who showed that from the age of 20–70 the cardiac index diminishes by an average of 15 ml, or 0.4 % per year [31].

Terasawa [32] compared 42 hypertensive subjects having a mean age of 73 with 23 normotensive subjects of the same age and showed that this reduction in cardiac index with age was more marked in elderly hypertensive subjects (3.24 ± 0.13 vs. 3.74 ± 0.28). It seems then that hypertension in the aged means hypertension with low cardiac output and high peripheral resistance. There has been no report of hypertension in the aged at a high cardiac output, but few studies have yet been made on this subject.

According to Simon and Safar [33], the hemodynamic mechanism of systolic hypertension is entirely different in young and old patients. In young subjects, arterial compliance is normal, while in the aged it is significantly reduced and is negatively related to arterial blood pressure. These data could be important for the selection of an antihypertensive therapy.

354

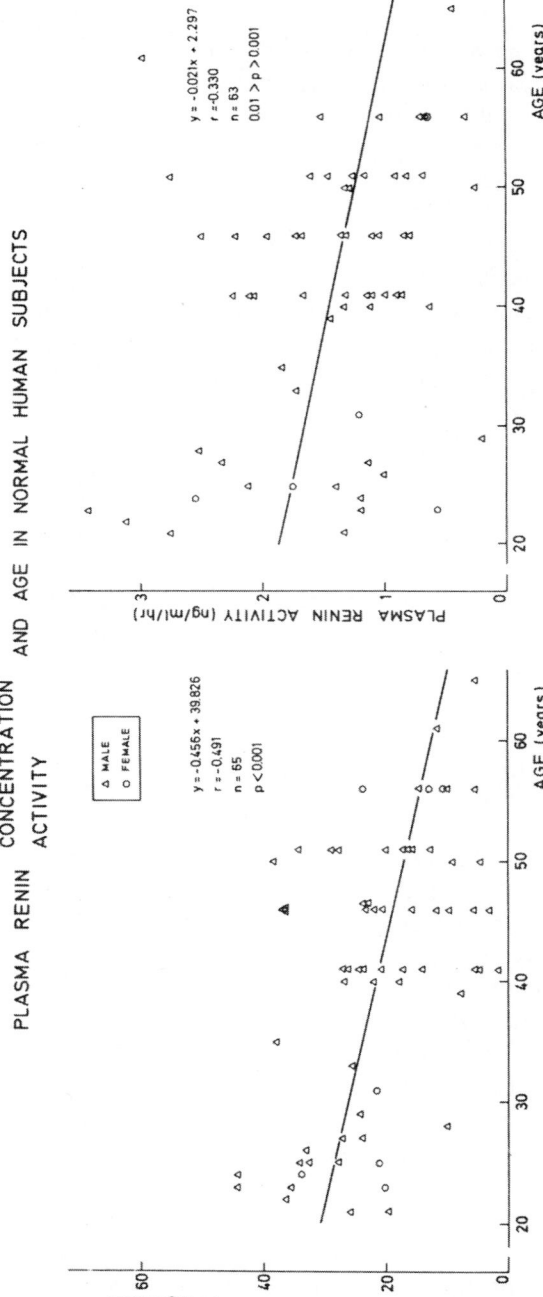

Figure 2. Relative significance of plasma renin activity and concentration in physiologic and pathophysiologic conditions. From Lijnen et al. [38].

6.2. Plasma renin activity (PRA)

According to most studies [34-41], plasma renin activity (PRA) or renin concentration seems to diminish progressively with age in hypertensive patiens. However, the data come from subjects over 60 and none over 80 (Figure 2). This is why we measured plasma renin activity in 126 subjects, being 65-102 years of age (mean age: 82), including 79 hypertensive patients (mean blood pressure: 180/95) and 47 controls (mean blood pressure: 140/80). Readings were taken in standing position after one hour of ambulation, on a diet of normal sodium content. Analysis of the results yielded the following findings [42]:
1) Plasma renin activity in the elderly hypertensive subjects was identical to that of the normotensive elderly subjects (1.28 ng/ml/h vs. 1.22 ng/ml/h, difference not significant). The distribution of the values is comparable, and the histograms coincide.
2) The values are significantly below those obtained in normal adults by Menard and Corvol by the same technique [43] and under the same conditions [44] (1.74 ng/ml/h) ($P<0.03$).

These data contradict those of Tuck [45] and Schalekamp [35] who suggest that PRA does not decrease with age in the normal subject, and who believe that hypertension is definitely related to the decrease in plasma renin activity.

This decrease in PRA with age has not yet been satisfactorily explained, and there is no real evidence of an excess of mineralocorticoids. Crane [46] showed that plasma and urine aldosterone decrease with age. Flood also reported decreased aldosterone secretion and metabolic clearance in aged subjects [47].

6.3. Catecholamines

Are there any peculiarities in the catecholamine metabolism of the aged? Studies of the question have shown that the plasma norepinephrine level increases progressively in normal subjects. According to Lake et al., the levels pass from 0.2 ng/ml at the age of 10 to 0.4 ng/ml at the age of 70 [48, 49]. This increase could be related to the decrease with age of the catecholamine urinary excretion. It does not necessarily mean an increased adrenergic activity, since the baroreceptor sensitivity could be lowered in elderly subjects [50].

Franco-Morselli et al. [51] have found that norepinephrine levels increase with age in normotensive subjects, but that the plasma epinephrine tends to decrease. In hypertensive subjects, however, there is no decrease in epinephrine levels with age. The levels are higher than in normotensives, particularly in older individuals. These data obviously do not indicate whether the changes in the sympathetic nervous system of the elderly hypertensive are linked primarily or secondarily to the elevation of blood pressure.

7. TREATMENT OF HYPERTENSION IN THE AGED

Although there is no denying that there is a risk of arterial hypertension at an advanced age, the problem remains whether antihypertensive treatment can eliminate this risk.

7.1. Present status

Controlled therapeutic trials in adults designed to compare an actively treated hypertensive population with a control population treated with a placebo have shown that the treatment of certain types of hypertension has significantly reduced morbidity and mortality among hypertensive patients.

The Veterans Administration study involved 81 patients over 60 years old [52]. In this elderly population, Fries found a 28.9% rate of complications in the treated group as compared with 62.8% in the placebo group, which showed that the reduction in morbidity brought about by the treatment persisted with age. Review of the complications was also revealing: 10 subjects over 60 treated with a placebo suffered a cerebrovascular accident as compared with only three in the actively treated group. Nine control subjects were found to suffer from congestive heart failure, but none of the treated subjects did. On the other hand, the treatment was found to have had no effect on coronary complications.

The Australian Therapeutic Trial in Mild Hypertension also reported a reduction in mortality in the actively treated group compardd to the placebo treated group. A similar trend was observed in the elderly patients (60–69 years) [53].

The H.D.F.P. study observed a 16.4% difference inthe patients who were 60–69 years of age in the five year mortality between the 'stepped care' group and the 'referred care group', but the analysis of these results is difficult since the 'control' group received a treatment [54].

In contrast with this data in favor of antihypertensive treatment two studies failed to show clearly a better prognosis in the treated groups [55, 56]. Although these data justify a certain amount of optimism with regard to the belated benefits of antihypertensive treatment in the aged, there is no strong evidence for them because the small number of patients over 60 prevented

the differences from attaining statistical significance. This is why a clinical trial specifically designed for elderly subjects was carried out in a much larger number of patients. The E.W.P.H.E. (European Working Party on Hypertension in the Elderly), coordinated by Amery and De Schepdryver, carried out this study [57-60]. This was a longitudinal, randomized, double-blind multicenter study aimed at demonstrating the effect of antihypertensive treatment on the morbidity and mortality of elderly hypertensive patients. After randomization, half the patients received one or two capsules of 25 mg hydrochlorothiazide and 50 mg triamterene, plus 0.50-2 g of methyldopa, depending on the blood pressure. The other half of the patients received a placebo. Six hundred patients have now been included in the study, which has already led to the following findings:
1) Arterial hypertension can be treated, even in the long term, in elderly subjects: some patients have been followed for more than five years.
2) The treatment does affect the blood pressure, for the blood pressure of the treated subjects had been normalized (148/79) whereas the placebo subjects remained hypertensive (174/95) (Figure 3).
3) A well-administered and well-monitored treatment causes no significant electrolyte abnormalities and no serious sideeffects that would necessitate its discontinuation.
4) Most important, treatment does not provoke an increased incidence of cardiovascular or cerebrovascular complications when initiated, as practitioners had feared. On the other hand, an increase in serum creatinine and uric acid levels as well as a moderate change of glucose tolerance were noted [61].

It is hoped that the treatment will favorably influence the patiens' prognosis because of the lowering of blood pressure and the absence of major complications. This can only be proved, however, by statistically significant differences between the two groups in terms of cardiovascular or cerebrovascular accidents. This will take a long time because the patients are enrolled progressively. We must hope that this delay in enrollment will not produce a bias in this important study. As of now we may conclude from this study that antihypertensive treatment of elderly subjects is possible, effective and safe. It is, however, too early to say if it will significantly reduce mortality and morbidity in elderly hypertensive subjects.

7.2. Indications for treatment

While this information is still lacking, the indications for treatment remain to be determined. They are relatively easy to determine for two categories of patients:
1) Patients in whom hypertension, even if moderate, has already had some

358

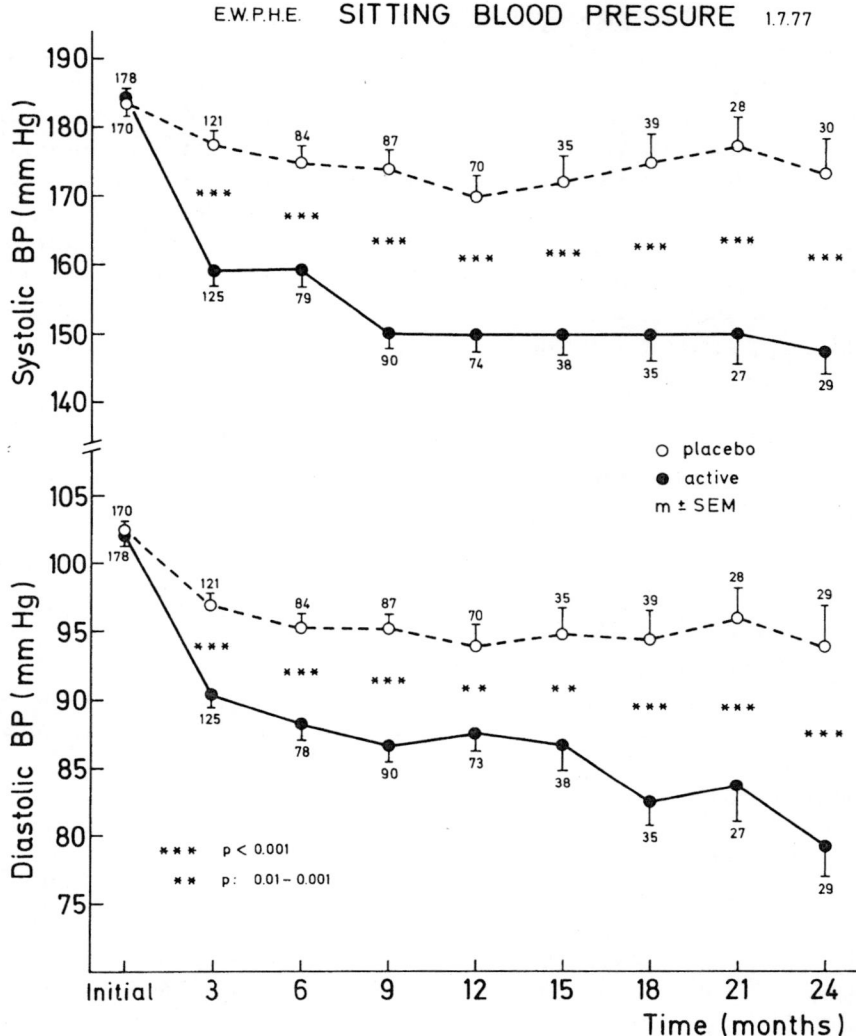

Figure 3. Antihypertensive therapy in the elderly patients. Pilot trial of the European Working Party on High Blood Pressure in the Elderly. From Amery et al. [58].

effect that can be attributed to it such as: left ventricular hypertrophy, cardiac insufficiency, retinopathy, cerebrovascular hemorrhage, etc.

2) Patients with very severe hypertension with diastolic values of 110 mm Hg or higher.

In the other patients, whose hypertension is moderate and asymptomatic, the indication for treatment depends on the point of view of the practising physician.

7.3. Modalities of treatment

Once the difficult problem of indications has been solved, conduct of the treatment in the elderly is relatively easy and only has to meet a few simple conditions:
1) Never routinely prescribe rest or tranquilizers to individuals over 65 years of age. These measures tend to reduce activity in the elderly and thus compromise their independence.
2) Never prescribe a strictly salt-free diet, which frequently leads to anorexia at that age with often catastrophic results in terms of protein or vitamin deficiencies. One should of course advise elderly hypertensive patients not to add salt to food after cooking and generally to avoid food of high salt content (cold cuts, marinated food, etc.).
3) Advise weight reduction in cases of overweight since a positive correlation between body weight and hypertensive exists even at a very advanced age. Weight reduction (often difficult to achieve) alone sometimes normalizes the blood pressure.
4) Always start any medication at half the normal adult dose. The dose should always be increased in stages of at least three weeks.
5) Rigourously monitor the treatment with regular clinical (check for orthostatic hypotension), biological and electrocardiographic tests according to the medication selected: every two weeks at the beginning of treatment, later on once a month, and then every three months once the efficacy and safety of the treatment have been well established.

7.4. Antihypertensive treatment

7.4.1. Single drug regimens
Diuretics are still the most effective single drugs in the elderly. They are relatively well tolerated by subjects over 60 on three conditions:
1) Use diuretics with a gentle, gradual effect, such as thiazide derivatives. Furosemide, on the other hand, should be reserved for certain special indications (urgent need, renal insufficiency, etc.).
2) The diuretics selected should be given routinely in combination with a potassium-sparing drug such as Aldactone®, amiloride (Modamine®), or triamterene (Teriam®). These special combinations of a diuretic and a potassium-sparing agent are particularly useful in the aged because the ease of administration overcomes resistance to intake at that age (Aldactazine®, Moduretic®, Cycloteriam®, Dytenside®). Treatment should be initiated at half the adult dose per day, depending on weight. If the blood pressure reduction is insufficient after three weeks (blood pressure $\geqslant 160/90$), the dose should be doubled. If the effect is still insufficient, the adding of another antihypertensive should be considered.

3) Regular biological monitoring to ensure the safety of the diuretic treatment in the elderly patient. Ion levels (possibly limited to serum sodium and potassium) should be measured every other week at the beginning of treatment, and every month if no electrolyte abnormalities have been found.

The addition of a potassium-sparing drug to the diuretic nearly always prevents hypokalemia and preempts the need for potassium salts, which are often poorly tolerated by the elderly patient. Regular monitoring of electrolyte levels will permit timely detection of hyponatremia, which can develop in some sensitive patients and which always requires immediate discontinuation of treatment.

Beta blockers are theoretically the ideal single drugs (and the only alternative to diuretics) for the following reasons:

1) Most of time they are well tolerated by the elderly patient.
2) If their contraindications are heeded (cardiac insufficiency, AV block, arteritis, respiratory insufficiency, asthma, etc.), the rate of side-effects is no higher than that found in adults generally [62].
3) They are particularly indicated when hypertension is associated with angor or disorders of cardiac rhythm.
4) On the other hand, their relatively low effectiveness when given alone, as compared with their efficacy in younger adults, is a serious drawback.

For these reasons diuretics still seem to us to be the drugs of first choice in the elderly patient. If their effect is insufficient, concomitant use of a beta blocker often produces a remarkable normalization.

7.4.2. Combinations

In most cases, therefore, beta blockers still represent a second choice, for use in combination with diuretics. Other drug combinations are needed when the highest diuretic dose (two tablets per day), reached in two to three months, fails to lower the blood pressure adequately (blood pressure <160/90). The combination of a diuretic and an antihypertensive drug helps avoid salt retention which can be induced by some antihypertensive agents used alone.

Nearly all antihypertensive drugs can be administered to the elderly patients if sideeffects are watched very carefully. Methyldopa (Aldomet®) is very well tolerated but the possible onset of depressive symptoms, which are more common in the aged, should be monitored carefully. Clonidine (Catapres®) can be used provided somnolence is no more marked than in younger adults. However, Catapres is contraindicated in patients known for poor compliance because abrupt withdrawal of this drug can lead to very marked blood pressure rises. They are particularly poorly tolerated by patients over 60. Hydralazine can be used when the hypertension is resistant to other forms of treatment in combination with Beta-blockers to avoid aggravation of latent or unknown angina. Reserpine and its numerous derivatives should definitely be left out of the arsenal of antihypertensive weapons for the elderly because of the incidence of the depressive syndrome at that age. One should avoid reserpine-containing drugs and always verify the composition of combination products.

As far as the newer antihypertensive drugs on the market are concerned, one should be very careful in prescribing them to elderly subjects and await long-term studies in adults to determine the side effects of each of these products. If these elementary precautions are taken, antihypertensive therapy can be administered to elderly hypertensives in the hope that it will prevent cardiovascular accidents, which nearly always result in a permanent deterioration in the condition of elderly individuals and to loss of their self-sufficiency.

REFERENCES

1. Staessen J, Bulpitt C, Fagard R, Joossens JV, Lijnen P, Amery A: Salt and blood pressure in Belgium. (to be published).
2. Edwards F, McKeown T, Whitfield AGW: Arterial pressure in men over sixty. Clin Sci 18:289–300, 1959.
3. Master AM, Lasser RP, Jaffe HL: Blood pressure in white people over 65 years of age. Ann Intern Med 48:284–299, 1958.
4. National Health Survey: Vital and Health Statistics, USA: blood Pressure of adults by age and sex, p. 9. U.S. Government printing Office, 1964.
5. Hamilton M, Pickering GW, Frazer-Robert JA, Sowry GSC: The aetiology of essential hypertension – I. The arterial pressure in the general population. Clin Sci 13:11–35, 1954.
6. Kannel WB: In: Cardiology in Old Age. p. 160. Caird FI, Dall, JLC, Kennedy RD, eds. New York: Plenum Press, 1976.
7. Hypertension Detection and Follow-up Program Cooperative Group: Blood pressure studies in 14 communities. A two-stage screen for hypertension. JAMA 237:2385–2391, 1977.
8. Lowenstein WG: Blood pressure in relation to age and sex in the tropics and subtropics. Lancet i:389–399, 1961.
9. Se Stephano F, Coulehan J, Kennethwiant M: Blood pressure survey onthe Navajo Indian Reservation. Am J Epidemiol 109:335–345, 1979.
10. Forette F, De La Fuente J, Golmard JL, Henry JF, Hervy MP: elderly Hypertension as a Risk Factor. Current Concepts in Hypertension and Cardiovascular Disorders – 1980. I:7–10.
11. Berliner K, Hujry H., Lee DH, Yildiz M. Garnier B: Blood pressure measurement in obese persons – comparison of intra-arterial and auscultatory measurements. Am J Cardiol 8:10–17, 1961.
12. Julius S, Amery A, Whitlock S, Conway J: Influence of age on the haemodynamic response to exercise. Circulation 36:222–230, 1967.
13. Amery A, Bossaert H, Verstraete M: Muscle blood flow in normal and hypertensive subjects. Influence of age exercise and body position. Am Heart J 78:211–216, 1969.
14. Berthaux P, Forette F, Laurent M, Sebban C: Etude des variations spontanées de la pression artérielle chez les personnes âgées. Influence de l'orthostatisme. 9th International Congress of Gerontology, 1972, 2:352–354.

362

15. Hypertension Detection and Follow-up Program Cooperative Group: Variability of Blood Pressure and the result of screening in the hypertension detection and follow-up program. J Chron Dis 31:651–667, 1978.
16. Colandrea MA, Friedman FD, Nichaman MZ, Lynd CN: Systolic hypertension in the Elderly – An epidemiologic assessment Circulation 41:239–245, 1970.
17. Forette F, Henry JF, Forette B, Berthaux P: Hypertension artérielle du sujet agé – prévalence en milieu long séjour. Nouv Presse Méd 4:2997–2998, 1975.
18. Froment A: Hypertension artérielle: envisager le problème médical à l'échelle de la population. Arch Mal Cœur 70:37–46, 1970.
19. Shekelle RB, Ostfeld AM, Klawans HF Jr: Hypertension and risk of stroke in an elderly population. Stroke 5:71–75, 1974.
20. Kannel WP, Wolf PA, Vertes J, McNamara PM: Epidemiologic assessment of the role of blood pressure in stroke – The Framingham Study. JAMA 214:301–310, 1970.
21. Kannel WB, Dawber TR, Sorlie P, Wolf PA: Components of blood pressure and risk of atherothrombotic brain infarction – The Framingham Study. Stroke 7:327–331, 1976.
22. Kannel WB, Gordon T: Evaluation of cardiovascular risk in the elderly – The Framingham Study. Bull NY acad Med 54:573–591, 1978.
23. Fry J: Natural history of hypertension. A case for selective non-treatment. Lancet, ii:431–433, 1974.
24. Svardsudd K, Tibblin G: Mortality and Morbidity during 13.5 years' follow up in relation to blood pressure. Acta Med Scand 205:483–484, 1979.
25. Gifford RW, Kvale WF, Maher FT, Roth GM, Priestley JM: Clinical features, diagnostis and treatment of pheochromocytoma. A review of 76 cases. Mayo Clin Proc 39:281–302, 1964.
26. Conn JW, Knopf RF Nesbit RM: Clinical characteristics of primary aldosteronism from an analysis of 145 cases. Am J Surg 107:159–172, 1964.
27. Berthaux P, Beck H, Polet D, Bouchon JP, Vignalou J: Les sténoses de l'artère Rénale chez le vieillard. Sem Hop 61:3451–3454, 1962.
28. Ernst CB, Stanley JC, Marshall FF, Fry WJ: Renal revascularization for arteriosclerotic renovascular hypertension: pronostic implications of focal renal arterial over generalized arteriosclerosis. Surgery 73:859–867, 1973.
29. Kotchen TA, Ernst CB: Detecting and treating arteriosclerotic renovascular hypertension. Geriatrics 31:83–89, 1976.
30. Brandfonbrener M, Landowne M, Shock NW: Changes in cardiac output with age. Circulation 12:557–566, 1955.
31. Amery A, Julius S, Whitlock L, Conway J: Influence of hypertension on the hemodynamic response to exercise. Circulation 36:231–237, 1967.
32. Terasawa F, Kuramoto K, Ying LH, Suzuki T, Kuramochi M: The study on the Haemodynamics in old hypertensive subjects. Acta Gerontol. Jpn 56:47–55, 1972.
33. Simon AC, Safar ME, Kheder AM, Levenson JA, London GM, Weiss YA: Systolic hypertension: hemodynamic mechanisms and choice of antihypertensive treatment. Am J Cardiol 45:505–511, 1979.
34. Buhler FR, Burkart F, Lutold BE et al.: Antihypertensive beta-blocking action as related to renin and age: a pharmacologic tool to identify pathogenetic mechanisms in essential hypertension. Am J Cardiol 36:653–669, 1975.
35. Schalekamp MADH, Birkenhager WH, Zaal GA, Kolsiers G: Haemodynamic characteristics of low-renin hypertension. Clin Sci Mol Med 52:405–412, 1977.
36. Sambhi MP, Crane MG, Genest J: Essential hypertension – new concepts about mechanisms. Ann Intern Med 79:411–424, 1973.
37. Oparil S, Haber E: The renin-angiotension system. N Engl J Med 292:389–401, 1974.
38. Lijnen PJ, Amery AK, Fagard RH, Reybrouck TM: Relative significance of plasma renin

activity and concentration in physiologic and pathophysiologic conditions. Angiology 29:354–366, 1978.

39. Schalekamp MADH, Kraus XH, Schalekamp Kuyken MPA, Kolster G, Birkenhager V: Studies on the mechanism of hypernatriuresis in essential hypertension in relationship to measurements of plasma renin concentration, body fluid compartment and renal function. Cli Sci 41:219–231, 1971.

40. Dallochio M, Clementy J, Choussat A, Broustet JP, Bricaud H: Risque vasculaire et activité rénine dans l'hypertension artérielle essentielle. Ann Cardiol Angeiol 24:141–147, 1975.

41. Weidmann P, De Myttenaere-Bursztein S, Maxwell MH, Lima JD: Effect of aging on plasma renin and aldosterone in normal man. Kidney Int 8:325–333, 1975.

42. Forette P, Menard J, Forette B, Henry JF, Berthaux P: L'activité rénine plasmatique du sujet âgé normal et hypertendu. Ann Med Intern 129:399–403, 1978.

43. Menard J, Corvol P et al: Mesure de l'activité rénine plasmatique de l'homme par le dosage radio-immunologique de l'angiotensine I, p. 459. Techn Radioimmunol Paris: Inserm, 1972.

44. Corvol P, Houde M, Menard J, Milliez P: Le système rénine angiotensine aldostérone chez les patients hypertendus. Nouv Presse Med 6:2483–2487, 1977.

45. Tuck ML, Williams GH, Cain JP, Sullivan JM, Dluhy RG: Relation of age, diastolic blood pressure and known duration of hypertension to presence of low renin essential hypertension. Am J Cardiol 32:637–642, 1973.

46. Crane MG, Harris JJ, Johns VJ: Hyporeninemic Hypertension. Am J Med 52:457–466, 1972.

47. Flood C, Gherondache C, Pinus C, Tait JF, Tait SAS, Willoughby S: The metabolism and secretion of aldosterone in elderly subjects. J Clin Invest 46:960–966, 1967.

48. Lake CR, Ziegler MG, Kopin IJ: Use of plasma norepinephrine for evaluation of sympathetic neuronal function in man. Life Sci 18:1315–1326, 1976.

49. Lake CR, Ziegler MG, Coelman MD, Kopin IJ: Age-adjusted plasma norepinephrine levels are similar in normotensive and hypertensive subjects. N Engl J Med 296:208–209, 1977.

50. Vestal RE, Wood AJJ, Shand DG: Reduced beta-adrenoceptor sensitivity in the elderly. Clin Pharmacol 26:181, 1979.

51. Franco-Morselli R, Elghozi JL, Joly E, Digiuillio S, Meyer P: Increased plasma adrenaline concentrations in benign essential hypertension. Br Med J 2:1251–1254, 1977.

52. Veterans Administration cooperative study Group on Antihypertensive Agents: Effect of treatment on morbidity in hypertension – III. Influence of age, diastolic pressure and prior cardiovascular disease. Further analysis of side effects. Circulation 45:991–1004, 1972.

53. The Australian therapeutic trial in mild hypertension. Report by the Management Committee. Lancet I:1261–1267, 1980.

54. Hypertension Detection and Follow-up Program Cooperative Group: Five-year findings of the Hypertension Detection and follow-up Programm[1]. Reduction in mortality of persons with high blood pressure, including mild hypertension – II. Mortality by race, sex and age[2]. JAMA 242:2562–2571[1], 2572–2577[2], 1979.
55. Hypertension Stroke Cooperative Group: Effects of antihypertensive treatment on stroke recurrence. JAMA 229:409–418, 1974.
56. Carter AB: Hypotensive therapy in old age. New York: plenum Press, 1976.
57. Amery A De Schaepdryver A: European Working Party on High Blood Pressure in Elderly: EWPHE: Organisation of a double blind multicenter trial on antihypertensive therapy in elderly patients. Clin. Sci Mol Med 45:71–73, 1973.
58. Amery A, Berthaux P, Birkenhager W, Bulpitt C, Clement D, De Schaepdryver A, Dollery C, Ernould H, Fagard R, Forette F, Hellemans J, Kho T, Lund-Johansen P, Meurice J. Pierquin L: Antihypertensive therapy in the elderly patients. Pilot trial of the European Working Party on High Blood Pressure in Elderly. Gerontology 23:426–437, 1977.

59. Amery A, Berthaux P, Birkenhager W, Boel A, Brixko P, Bulpitt C, Clement D, Deruyttere M, De Schaepdryver A, Dollery C, Fagard R, Forette F, Henry JF, Hellmans J, Lasser U, Lund-Johansen P, Mac Farlane J, Malling T, Mutsers A, Nissinen A, Ohm OJ, Pelemans J, Suchettkaye AI, Tuomilehio J, Willems J: Antihypertensive therapy in patients above age 60. Third interim report of the European Working Party on High Blood Pressure in Elderly EWPHE). Acta Cardiol 33:113–134, 1978.

60. Amery A, Berthaux P, Birkenhager W, Boel A, Brixko P, Bulpitt C, Clement D, De Padua F, Deruyttere M, Deschaepdryver A, Dollery C, Fagard R, Forette F, Porte J, Henry JF, Hellemans J, Koistinen A, Laaser U, Lund-Johansen P, Mac Farlane J, Miguel P, Mutsers A, Nissinen A, Ohm OT, Pelemans W, Suchett-Kaye A, Tuomilehto J, Willems J, Willemse P: Antihypertensive therapy in patients above the age of 60.Forth Interim report of the European Working Party on High Blood Pressure in Elderly (EWPHE). Clin Sci Mol Med 55:263s–270s, 1978.

61. Amery A, Berthaux P, Bulpitt C, Deruyttere M, De Schaepdryver A, Dollery C, Fagard R, Forette F, Hellemans J, Lund-Johansens P, Mutsers A, Tuomilehto J: Glucose intolerance during diuretic therapy. Results of trial by the European Working Party on High Blood Pressure in Elderly. Lancet I:681–683, 1978.

62. Forette F, Henry JF, Hervy MP, Forette B, Berthaux P: Traitement de l'H.T.A. du sujet âgé par un Bêta-Bloquant: l'Acebutolol. Nouv Presse Med 8:2881–2884, 1979.

23. BORDERLINE BLOOD PRESSURE ELEVATION

Michel E. Safar and Yves A. Weiss

Borderline hypertension is a condition in which a subject's blood pressure is above the normal range, but the readings are not sufficiently high to warrant early treatment [1, 2]. It is generally accepted that borderline hypertension carries an excess of overall mortality and specific cardiovascular morbidity [1, 2]. However, in the absence of results of appropriate therapeutic trials, the exact contribution of borderline hypertension in cardiovascular morbidity and mortality remains to be confirmed. In contrast, the role of borderline hypertension as an early prediction of future-established hypertension has been amply demonstrated [1]. For this reason, the present review is devoted to the problem of borderline hypertension as an initial stage of the hypertensive vascular disease. A peculiar attempt has been made to the underlying hemodynamic mechanisms. Some of the results have been previously described [1, 2] or reported elsewhere [3].

DEFINITION

According to the World Health Organization (WHO), an adult with normal blood pressure has a systolic arterial pressure inferior to 140 mm Hg and a diastolic arterial pressure inferior to 90 mm Hg. Sustained hypertension occurs when systolic pressure is superior to 160 mm Hg and/or diastolic pressure is superior to 95 mm Hg. The term 'borderline hypertension' refers to the systolic and diastolic pressure ranges which are between 140 and 160 mm Hg and between 90 and 95 mm Hg respectively. From this definition it appears that borderline hypertension concerns a condition of elevated blood pressure where readings are not sufficiently high to warrant early treatment. In clinical practice it is clear that the WHO definition requires some operational criteria. For instance the term borderline hypertension is used for patients who at times demonstrate a normal diastolic arterial pressure (less than 90 mm Hg) and at other times (at least on two separate occasions) demonstrate elevated diastolic pressure (in excess of 90 mm Hg) [1, 2].

Since the definition refers to a minimal blood pressure elevation above an

Amery, A. (ed.) Hypertensive Cardiovascular Disease: Pathophysiology and Treatment
© *1982, Martinus Nijhoff Publishers. The Hague / Boston / London*
ISBN-13: 978-94-009-7478-4

arbitrarily fixed upper limit of normal blood pressures, there still remains some confusion about terminology. Firstly, in view of the standard deviation from the mean of several pressure measurements, an excessive variability of blood pressure can exist in some patients with borderline hypertension but does not exactly meet the definition of the disease [4]. Such fluctuations of blood pressure are also observed in patients with sustained hypertension. Secondly, despite the existence of subgroups with increased blood pressure responsiveness to several conditions such as exercise, tilt test or mental exercise, patients with borderline hypertension on the whole never exhibit hyper-responsiveness to pressor stimuli [1]. Finally, the definition of the disease is not restricted to young subjects but also affects older patients [1]. For these reasons, it is more appropriate to use the term 'borderline hypertension' than the somewhat misleading terms 'labile' or 'juvenile' hypertension.

THE HEMODYNAMIC PATTERN

Cardiac output

Most investigators have found that cardiac output, measured at rest in the supine position, was elevated in young patients with borderline hypertension (see review in [1]). The increase in cardiac output was related to an increase in stroke volume, or in heart rate, or both [1–3]. Despite some discrepancies, the elevated cardiac output was found to be caused by a dominant increase in muscle blood flow, while renal and hepatic blood flow remained within normal ranges [5–7].

The high cardiac output in subjects with mild blood pressure elevation needs some comment. The cardiac index is elevated at rest but this point is discussed in sitting or tilting positions or during exercise [1]. In these conditions, most authors have found normal values. Further, the cardiac output in relation to oxygen consumption is always normal, both at rest and during exercise [8–10]. This suggests that the control mechanisms of cardiac output rather than the level of output itself would be the most important aspect in patients with borderline hypertension.

There are three mechanisms for increasing cardiac output: 1) increase in total blood volume, 2) redistribution of blood in the capacitance system, causing a volume shift from peripheral veins to the pulmonary capacitance bed, and 3) enhanced cardiac performance. Since total blood volume is never increased in borderline hypertension [2, 11, 12], the first possibility can be easily excluded. Several methodologic problems have obscured the study of redistribution of blood volume in patients with borderline hypertension. Firstly, redistribution of blood volume cannot be inferred easily from the curve relating cardiac output to cardiopulmonary blood volume (CPBV), since CPBV is calculated from cardiac output [13]. Secondly, all investigators [11, 12, 14, 15] found normal values of CPBV when expressed in ml/kg or in ml/m^2. However, body weight and body surface area are increased in borderline hypertension [16]. Thus, the references to body size are misleading for the evaluation of CPBV [11, 12, 14, 15]. CPBV is better expressed as a fraction of total blood volume (TBV). In men with borderline hypertension [11, 15], but not in groups consisting of both men and women [14], the CPBV/TBV ratio has been found to be elevated, indicating a relative shift of blood from peripheral veins to the pulmonary capacitance bed. Such a finding suggests a decreased venous distensibility in patients with borderline hypertension, a point which has been recently confirmed [17]. In association with the redistribution of blood volume, an increased cardiac performance has also been observed in patients with minimal blood pressure elevation [14]. Enhanced cardiac function is suggested on the basis of reduced pre-ejection periods and increased ratios between cardiac output and CPBV [14, 18]. A more direct approach to the cardiac function is provided by the study of echocardiographic dimensions. A high incidence of asymetric septal hypertrophy has been reported in the disease and related to the classical haemodynamic abnormalities, such as the elevated cardiac output and the reduced systolic time intervals [19, 20]. Thus, both increased venous return and enhanced cardiac performance are involved in the mechanism of the elevated cardiac output of young patients with borderline hypertension.

Total peripheral resistance

At rest in supine position, total peripheral resistance (TPR) is elevated in patients with normal cardiac output and normal or low in patients with increased cardiac output [1, 21]. In the latter group, TPR is elevated both in tilting position and during exercise [21]. From these observations, it has been suggested that TPR was either elevated or inappropriately adjusted to the increased cardiac output in patients with borderline hypertension [1, 2]. However, such results must be interpreted cautiously. According to the basic physiology, the resistance of the vessels represents the slope of the curve relating blood pressure to blood flow[22]. Since the linearity of the curve through zero has not been clearly demonstrated in men, the ratio between mean arterial pressure and cardiac output is only an indirect approach to evaluate the resistance of the vessels and, consequently, the degree of dilatation of the small arteries in men [22]. Further, the calculated TPR does not give any information about the relative contribution of the neurohumoral factors and the structural changes acting on the observed abnormalities of the vessels. In patients with borderline hypertension, structural changes are certainly important in some parts of the body, as suggested by the studies of the forearm vascular resistance at maximal dilatation [23, 24].

THE NEUROGENIC HYPOTHESIS

The presence of a wide range of physiologic abnormalities in borderline hypertension confirms the epidemiologic experience that borderline hypertension cannot be regarded as an innocuous state of only minimal blood pressure elevation. Several mechanisms, including hyperactivities of the renin–angiotensin and the prostaglandin systems [1, 2, 25], have been proposed to explain the observed aberrations. However, most of the abnormalities can be explained on the basis of a dominant neurogenic disorder [2]. In the present study the proposed arguments for the role of the nervous system in borderline hypertension are reviewed.

Biochemical indexes

Increased levels of plasma and urinary catecholamines have been reported in subgroups of patients with borderline hypertension (see review in [2]). Since a multiplicity of factors can potentially influence the epinephrine and norepinephrine levels [2], the validity of these observations as the sole explanation of sympathetic nervous activity in clinical practice remains an open question. For this reason, in the present report only the biochemical results which are related to the haemodynamic abnormalities of borderline hypertension will be presented.

Excessive catecholamine responsiveness to mental stress and to postural stimulation has been reported in borderline hypertension [26, 27]. Diastolic orthostatic hypertension, a characteristic haemodynamic feature [21, 28], has been related to an exaggerated increase of plasma and urinary catecholamines during tilt. However, the interpretation of these findings of 'increased sympathetic responsiveness' is difficult. As shown by the study of patients with pheochromocytoma [29], the noradrenergic responsiveness in acute situations cannot be clearly related to the state of long-term sympathetic nervous activity at rest.

Since dopamine-beta-hydroxylase is not submitted to local reuptake into the sympathetic nerve terminal after release, the plasma concentration of this enzyme has been proposed as a better index of sympathetic nervous system activity than plasma norepinephrine concentration [2]. In most studies, dopamine-beta-hydroxylase plasma concentration has been found to be normal in borderline hypertension [2]. However, even when normal, the plasma levels have been found to be positively correlated to the cardiac output and the diastolic pressure measured at rest [30]. Since no comparable results were observed in normal subjects and in patients with sustained hypertension [30], the correlations clearly suggest some long-term status of sympathetic nervous hyperactivity in patients with borderline hypertension.

Receptor sensitivity and vascular reactivity

The sensitivity of beta-adrenergic cardiac receptors in borderline hypertension has been evaluated on the basis of the rise in heart rate with short-term infusion of isoproterenol [2]. A beta-adrenergic hypersensitivity has been observed in small subgroups of selected patients [31]. In the overall population of patients with borderline hypertension, beta-adrenergic sensitivity is clearly decreased [32]. The reduced response to isoproterenol is not restricted to patients with borderline hypertension, but can also be observed in patients with sustained hypertension. In the overall population of hypertensives, the isoproterenol response is positively related to age and to the level of blood pressure [32, 33].

Vascular reactivity in borderline hypertension has been studied based on the rise in blood pressure observed with graded doses of norepinephrine and angiotensin [11, 34]. In contrast with patients with sustained hypertension, vascular reactivity to norepinephrine is clearly decreased (and not increased) in patients with borderline hypertension [11]. Such a result excludes the dominant role of adaptive vascular changes in the observed responses and points to the avidity of the receptor sites to norepinephrine in patients with borderline hypertension [11]. This observation has been confirmed by the fact that an inverse relationship has been found between plasma catecholamines and vascular reactivity to norepinephrine in subjects with normal resting blood pressure [35].

In patients with borderline hypertension, the pressordose of norepinephrine (i.e. the inverse of vascular reactivity) has been found to be positively correlated with cardiac output and the ratio between cardiopulmonary and total blood volumes, a result which cannot be observed with the pressor dose of angiotensin [11]. Since no comparable results can be observed in normal subjects and in patients with sustained hypertension [11], the study of vascular reactivities points to a specific norepinephrine-like mechanism in patients with borderline hypertension [11, 15].

Pharmacological agents

After beta-adrenergic blockade with propranolol, cardiac output decreases more in patients with borderline hypertension than in controls [2, 36].

Although the firstpath effect of propranolol could partly obscure this observation [32, 37, 38], the result suggests sympathetic overactivity in patients with borderline hypertension. In addition to the sympathetic hyperactivity, changes in parasympathetic function have also been reported in the disease [39]. Beta-adrenergic blockade alone is not sufficient to decrease cardiac output toward normal values. Cardiac output falls into the normal range only after a total autonomic blockade due to propranolol plus atropine [2, 39]. Such a role of the parasympathetic system has been confirmed by the study of the baroreflex cardiac slowing consecutive to a transient rise in arterial pressure [40] according to the method of Smyth et al. [41]. The dose of atropine required to suppress the reflex is lower in borderline hypertensives than in controls, indicating a decrease in parasympathetic tone [40].

The latter results suggest than both the sympathetic and the parasympathetic systems are involved in the elevation of cardiac output of patients with borderline hypertension. The reciprocal relationship between increased sympathetic discharge and decreased parasympathetic inhibition suggests some abnormality in the central control of the autonomic system [2]. In animals, the experimental evidence of chronic hypertension due to a lesion of the nucleus tractus solitariis could confirm this possibility [42, 43]. In men, the findings of impaired baroreflex mechanisms [44, 45] and/or of psychosomatic disorders [46, 47] could also suggest the validity of this hypothesis. However, the difficulties in methodology are such that the basis of an altered integration of autonomic control in borderline hypertension can still not be ruled out.

REPEAT HAEMODYNAMIC STUDIES IN BORDERLINE HYPERTENSION

Since cardiac output is elevated in borderline hypertension and normal in sustained hypertension, the cross-sectional studies of hypertensive patients suggest that over the years there could be a change in the central haemodynamics, with a fall in cardiac output and an increase in resistance more marked than what is seen in normal subjects [48]. Over the past few years some longitudinal studies have been performed in men to confirm this possibilty.

Central haemodynamic pattern in longitudinal studies

From the longitudinal studies of patients with essential hypertension it appears that most of them are difficult to interpret because of the great variety of age, the small number of patients, the existence of previous treatments and/or of secondary hypertension [3, 49, 50]. Lund-Johansen investigated 28 young males with untreated mild essential hypertension at rest and during exercise [51]. The duration of the follow-up was between 8 and 10 years. Weiss et al. [52] studied 37 young men with borderline hypertension during 47 ± 3 months (±1 standard error of the mean). Blood pressures at the initial examination were lower than those reported in the Lund-Johansen study.

In both investigations [51, 52], a primary increase in cardiac output was followed with time by a secondary increase in total peripheral resistance, while cardiac output decreased. Diastolic pressure did not change [51, 52], but systolic and mean arterial pressure increased significantly in the study of Weiss et al. [52]. The decrease in cardiac output was due to a decrease in either heart rate [52] or stroke volume [51]. In the study of Weiss et al. [52] blood volume decreased. In addition, the diastolic orthostatic hypertension initially observed disappeared during the follow-up of the patients.

Such findings could not be related to age. Several cross-sectional studies in healthy normotensive subjects have shown that aging from twenty to forty years involves no or only negligible changes in cardiac performance [10, 48, 51]. This is in clear contrast to what happens in the patients with borderline hypertension who had deteriorated their cardiovascular system more than expected from aging alone [51, 52].

Studies of the correlations of cardiac output during the follow-up

Lund-Johansen [48] has shown that, during the follow-up, cardiac output remained adapted to the oxygen consumption and, therefore, to the metabolic needs of the tissue. However, this author observed also that the haemodynamic patterns were different at rest and during exercise. At rest the curve relating cardiac ouput to oxygen consumption was the same at the initial examination of the patients and ten years later [48]. In contrast, during exercise the slope of the curve relating cardiac output to oxygen consumption was possibly shallower at the end than at the beginning of the follow-up study [10, 51]. Thus, at least during exercise, a higher oxygen consumption was required at the end of the long-term follow-up in order to reach the same cardiac output level as that at the initial examination of the patients. The result could indicate that some impairment of the relationship between cardiac output and oxygen consumption could occur during the follow-up study.

Such a change in the regulation of cardiac output during the evolution of the disease has been emphasized by the repeat studies of Weiss et al. [52]. At the beginning of the follow-up, the correlation between heart rate and cardiac output was significant, whereas the blood volume – cardiac output correlation was not, suggetsting a dominant neurogenic mechanism. On the other hand, at the end of the survey the blood volume – cardiac output correlation was significant, whereas the heart rate – cardiac output correlation was no longer present, suggesting that, at this period, volume factors played a major role. Such results clearly show that important changes in the regulation of cardiac output could occur during a relatively short-term follow-up period in young patients with borderline hypertension.

In cross-sectional studies [3, 53, 54], it has been shown that, for the same level of cardiac output, important differences in the cardiac output control were observed according to the level of blood pressure in patients with hypertension. Neural mechanisms, as expressed by the correlation between heart rate and cardiac output, were predominant in normotensive and borderline hypertensive ranges, whereas volume mechanisms, as expressed by the correlation between blood volume and cardiac output, were predominant in hypertensive ranges. Thus, the cross-sectional and the longitudinal studies give similar results: the control of cardiac output is different in patients with borderline hypertension and in patients with sustained essential hypertension. In borderline hypertension, increased cardiac function and venous return are due to the modulation of predominant neurogenic influences. In sustained hypertension, the long-term neurogenic mechanisms are less important, while 'volume' mechanisms take place, causing new adjustments between pre-load, post-load and cardiac performance [3].

Auto-regulation of blood flow in human hypertension

In sustained essential hypertension, cardiac output is normal and adapted to the metabolic needs of the tissues. Thus, homeostasis of blood flow exists in human hypertension. In addition, since borderline hypertension with high cardiac output may be an early stage in the natural history of sustained hypertension with normal cardiac output, it can be assumed that some form of autoregulation of blood flow occurs in human essential hypertension.

Based on animal experiments, a sequence of haemodynamic events called 'total body autoregulation' has been described in experimental hypertension [55, 56]. During the development of hypertension, an increase of cardiac output beyond the metabolic needs of the tissue was followed by a rise in peripheral resistance and return of output toward normal values. This sequence of haemodynamic events suggested that autoregulation of blood flow in hypertension was due to the secondary increase in total peripheral resistance.

Since the methodological approaches are quite different in animals from those in men, the differences between autoregulation in human hypertension and autoregulation in experimental hypertension must be discussed and clarified.

This problem has recently been examined after the introduction of clinical data in computer models of the cardiovascular system [54]. Models of the circulation are composed of several blocks that characterize one or several components of the cardiovascular homeostasis. Each block corresponds to one equation and each equation is characterized by one or several coefficients, called regulation coefficients (for instance a and b in $y = ax + b$). When clinical data are put in the computer model, somes changes of the regulation coefficients are necessary to obtain a compatibility between the clinical data and the characteristics of the model. Following this procedure, the elevated cardiac output of borderline hypertensive patients and the normal cardiac output of sustained hypertensive patients have been introduced in the 1967 Guyton-Coleman model [54]. In these conditions, important changes occur in the model. These changes affect mainly the resistance of the vessels. It can be shown that an increase in the destruction process and a decrease in the creative process of the resistance vessels are required for the maintenance of a normal cardiac output in patients with sustained essential hypertension [3, 54].

In conclusion, haemodynamic studies have shown that homeostasis of blood flow exists in human hypertension but that the mechanisms of homeostasis are different from those observed in normal subjects. The introduction of clinical data in cardiovascular models gave a more precise insight in these mechanisms: after the transient increase in cardiac output observed in patients with borderline hypertension, structural changes of the vascular network [23] are necessary to maintain a normal blood flow in men with sustained essential hypertension.

CONCLUSION

In the present study, the haemodynamic mechanisms of borderline hypertension as a potent predictor of future hypertension have been emphasized. In clinical practice, it must be stressed that, although the risk of future sustained hypertension among patients with borderline hypertension is higher than in the general population, the majority of patients will not necessarily develop hypertension [1, 2]. In other words, patients with borderline hypertension cannot be viewed as a uniform population of excessive morbidity. Thus, it is important to identify among them a subgroup of future hypertensive patients who can then be considered for treatment.

Many provocative tests as cold pressor, mental stress, physical exercise and administration of vasoactive agents have been proposed for identifying future hypertensive patients [1, 2]. However, the basic assumption of these tests, that repeated pressor episodes lead to established hypertension, has never been clearly demonstrated in man. Among the possible predicators of future hypertension, the most important parameters remain both the level of blood pressure as such and the existence of an elevated resting heart rate, of a rapid weight gain and of a positive family history for hypertension [1, 2, 57]. Unfortunately, in the literature the quantitative contribution of each of these predictors has still not been clarified. For this reason, the therapeutic management of borderline hypertension cannot be defined and requires further studies including epidemiologic and therapeutic trials.

ACKNOWLEDGMENTS

This study was performed with a grant from the Institut National de la Santé et de la Recherche Médicale (INSERM), the Association pour l'Utilisation du Rein Artificiel (AURA) and the Délégation Générale de la Recherche Scientifique et Technique (DGRST) Paris. We thank Mrs Christine Crespo for her secretarial assistance.

REFERENCES

1. Julius S, Schork MA: Borderline hypertension – a critical review. J Chronic Dis 23:723–754, 1971.
2. Julius S, Esler M: Autonomic nervous cardiovascular regulation in borderline hypertension. Am J Cardiol 36:685–695, 1975.
3. Safar ME, Weis YA, London GM, Simon ACh, Chau NP: Hemodynamic changes in mild early hypertension. In: Hypertension in the Young and the Old. Onesti G, Kim KE, eds. New York: Grune & Stratton, 1981, pp. 19–28.
4. Kannel WB, Sorlie P, Gordon T: Labile hypertension: a faulty concept? The Framingham Study. Circulation 61:1183–1187, 1980.
5. Amery A, Bossaert E, Verstraete M: Muscle Blood flow in normal and hypertensive subjects. Influence of age, exercise, and body position. Am Heart J 78:211–216, 1969.
6. Conway J: A vascular abnormality in hypertension. A study of blood flow in the forearm. Circulation 27:520–529, 1963.
7. Temmar MM, Safar ME, Levenson JA, Totomoukouo JM, Simon ACh: Regional blood flow in borderline and sustained essential hypertension. Clin Sci Mol Med 60:653–658, 1981.
8. Julius S, Conway J: Hemodynamic studies in patients with borderline blood pressure elevation. Circulation 38:282–296, 1968.
9. Sannerstedt R: Hemodynamic response to exercise in patients with arterial hypertension. Acta Med. Scand (Suppl) 458:1–83, 1966.
10. Lund-Johansen P: Hemodynamics in early essential hypertension. Acta Med. Scand (Suppl) 482:1–105, 1967.
11. Safar ME, London GM, Weiss YA, Milliez PL: Vascular reactivity to norepinephrine and hemodynamic parameters in borderline hypertension. Am Heart J 89:480–486, 1975.
12. Ellis CN, Julius S: Role of central blood volume in hyperkinetic borderline hypertension. Br Heart J 35:450–455, 1973.
13. Yu PN: Pulmonary Blood Volume in Health and Disease. pp. 88–122, Philadelphia: Lea & Febiger, 1969.
14. Tarazi RC, Ibrahim MM, Dustan HP, Ferrario CM: Cardiac factors in hypertension. Circ Res 34, 35 (Suppl I):213–221, 1974.

15. Safar ME, Weiss YA, London GM, Frackowiak RF, Milliez PL: Cardiopulmonary blood volume in borderline hypertension. Clin Sci Mol Med 47:153-164, 1974.
16. Chiang BN, Perlam LV, Epstein PH: Overweight and hypertension. Circulation 39:403-421, 1973.
17. Takeshita A, Mark AL: Decreased venous distensibility in borderline hypertension. Hypertension 1:202-206, 1979.
18. Ibrahim MM, Tarazi RC, Dustan HP, Bravo EL, Gifford RW: Hyperkinetic heart in severe hypertension: a separate clinical hemodynamic entity. Am J Cardiol 35:667-674, 1975.
19. Lehner JP, Safar ME, Dimitriu VM, Simon ACh, Carrez JP, Plainfosse Mt: Systolic time intervals and echocardiographic findings in borderline hypertension. Eur J Cardiol 9/4:319-331, 1979.
20. Safar Me, Lehner JP, Vincent Me, Plainfosse MT, Simon ACh: Echocardiographic dimensions in borderline and sustained hypertension. Am J Cardiol 44:930-935, 1979.
21. Safar M, Weiss Y, Levenson J, London G, Milliez P: Hemodynamic study of 85 patients with borderline hypertension. Am J Cardiol 31:315-319, 1973.
22. Noble MIM: The Cardiac Cycle, pp. 163-165. Oxford: Blackwell Scientific, 1979.
23. Folkow B, Grumby G, Thuleslus O: Adaptive structural changes of the vascular wall in hypertension and their relationship to control of the peripheral resistance. Acta Physiol. Scand 79 (Suppl 343):3-56, 1970.
24. Folkow B, Hallback M, Lundgen M, Silvertsson R, Weiss L: Importance of adaptive changes in vascular design for establishment of primary hypertension, studied in man and in spontaneously hypertensive rats. Circ Res 32, 33 (Suppl 1):2-13, 1973.
25. Hornych A, Gaux JC, Guyene TT, Safar M, Bariety J, Milliez P: Renal venous prostaglandins in different forms of hypertension. In: Secondary Forms of Hypertension: Current Diagnosis and Management. Blaufox MC, Bianchi C, eds. New York: Grune & Stratton 1981, pp. 73-88.
26. Esler MD, Nestel PJ: Renin and sympathetic nervous system responsiveness to adrenergic stimuli in essential hypertension. Am J Cardiol 32:643-649, 1973.
27. Cuche JL, Kuchel O, Barbeau A, Langlois Y, Boucher R, Genest J: Autonomic nervous system and benign essential hypertension in man - II. Circulatory and hormonal responses to upright posture. Circ Res 35:290-298, 1974.
28. Hull DH, Wolthuis RA, Cortese T, Longo MR, Trievwasser JH: Borderline hypertension versus normotension: Differential response to orthostatic stress. Am J Cardiol 94:414-420, 1977.
29. Levenson JA, Safar ME, London GM, Simon ACh: Haemodynamics in patients with phaechromocytoma. Clin Sci Mol Med 58:349-356, 1980.
30. Alexandre JM, London GM, Chevillard C, Lemaire P, safar M, Weiss Y: The meaning of DBH in essential hypertension. Cli Sci Mol Med 49:573-579, 1975.
31. Frohlich ED, Dustan HP, Page IH: Hyperdynamic beta-adrenergic circulatory state. Arch. Intern Med 117:614, 1966.
32. London GM, Safar ME, Weiss YA, Milliez PL: Isoproterenol sensitivity and total body clearance of propranolol in hypertensive patients. J Clin Pharmacol 16:174-182, 1976.
33. Bertel O, Buhler FR, Kiowski W, Lutold B: Decreased beta-adrenoreceptor responsiveness as related to age, blood pressure, and plasma catecholamines in patients with essential hypertension. Hypertension 2:130-138, 1980.
34. Wallace JM: Hemodynamic lesions in hypertension. Am J Cardiol 36:670-684, 1975.
35. Philip TH, Distler A, Cordes U: Sympathetic nervous system and blood-pressure control in essential hypertension. Lancet 4:959-963, 1978.
36. Julius S, Esler MD, Randall OS: Role of the autonomic nervous system in mild human hypertension. Cli Sci Mol Med 48:243s-252s, 1975.
37. Weiss YA, Safar ME, Chevillard C, Frydman A, Simon A, Lemaire P, Alexandre JM:

Comparison of the Pharmacokinetics of intravenous dl-Propranolol in borderline and permanent hypertension. Eur J Clin Pharmacol 10:387–393, 1976.

38. Weiss YA, Safar ME, Lehner JP, Levenson JA, Simon A, Alexandre JM: (+)-Propranolol clearance, an estimation of hepatic blood flow in man. Br J. Clin Pharmacol. 5:457–460, 1978.

39. Julius S, Pascual AV, London R: Role of parasympathetic inhibition in the hyperkinetic type of borderline hypertension. Circulation 44:413–418, 1971.

40. Simon ACh, Safar ME, Weiss YA, London GM, Milliez PL: Baroreflex sensitivity and cardiopulmonary blood volume in normotensive and hypertensive patients. Br Heart J 39:799–805, 1977.

41. Smyth HS, Sleight P, Pickering BW: Reflex regulation of arterial pressure during sleep in man: a quantitative method of assessing baroreflex sensitivity. Circ Res 25:109–121, 1969.

42. Doba N, Reis D: Role of central and peripheral mechanisms in neurogenic hypertension produced by brain stem lesions in rats. Circ Res 34:293, 1974.

43. Schmitt H, Laubie M: Destruction of the nucleus tractus solitarii in dogs: acute effects on blood pressure and hemodynamics; chronic effects of blood pressure. In: Importance of the nucleus for effects of drugs, in nervous system and hypertension, p. 172. Meyer P, Schmitt H, eds. New York: John Wiley, 1979.

44. Takeshita A, Tanaka S, Kuroiwa A: Reduced baroreceptor sensitivity in borderline hypertension. Circulation 51:738–742, 1975.

45. Eckberg DL: Carotid baroreflex function in young men with borderline blood pressure elevation. Circulation 59:632–636, 1979.

46. Harburg E, Julius S, McGinn NF: Personality traits and behavioral patterns associated with systolic blood pressure levels in college males. J Chronic Dis 17:405–414, 1964.

47. Safar ME, Kamieniecka HA, Dimitriu VM, Levenson JA, Pauleau NF: Hemodynamic factors and Rorscharch testing in borderline and sustained hypertension. Psychosom Med 8:620–625, 1978.

48. Lund-Johansen P: Hemodynamic alterations in hypertension – spontaneous changes and effects of drug therapy. A review. Acta Med. Scand. (Suppl) 603:1–12, 1977.

49. Eich RH, Cuddy RP, Smulyan H: Hemodynamics in labile hypertension: a follow-up study. Circulation 34:299–307, 1966.

50. Birkenhager WH, Schalekamp MADH, Krauss WH, Kolsters G, Zaal GA: Consecutive haemodynamic patterns in essential hypertension. Lancet 1:560–568, 1972.

51. Lund-Johansen P: Spontaneous changes in central hemodynamic in essential hypertension – a 10 year follow-up study. In: Hypertension Determinants, Complications and Intervention, pp. 201–209. Onesti G, Kim KE, eds. New York: Grune & Stratton, 1978.

52. Weiss YA, Safar ME, London GM, Simon ACh, Levenson JA, Milliez PL: Repeat hemodynamic determinations in borderline hypertension. Am J Med 64:382–387, 1978.

53. Chau NPh, Safar ME, Weiss YA, London GM, Simon ACh, Milliez PL: Relationship between cardiac output, heart rate and blood volume in essential hypertension. Clin Sci Mol Med 54:175–180, 1978.

54. Chau NPh, Safar ME, London GM, Weiss YA: Essential hypertension: an approach to clinical data by the use of models. Hypertension 2:87–97, 1979.

55. Guyton AC, Granger HJ, Coleman TG: Autoregulation of the total systemic circulation and its relation to control of cardiac output and arterial pressure. Circ Res 28, 29 (Suppl I):93–97, 1971.

56. Coleman TG, Samar RE, Murphy WR: Autoregulation versus other vasoconstrictors in hypertension – a critical review. Hypertension 1:324–330, 1979.

57. Payen DE, Safar ME, Levenson JA, Totomoukouo JA, Weiss YA: Repeat hemodynamic studies in borderline hypertension: predictive value of tilt test and weight gain. Am Heart J, 1982 (in press).

24. HEMODYNAMICS OF PRIMARY HYPERTENSION

PER LUND-JOHANSEN

INTRODUCTION

Few doctors will reflect about the mechanisms responsible for the increased blood pressure when they find a patient with hypertension. The diagnostic work-up will concentrate on etiology and cardiovascular complications, so why bother with hemodynamics?

Hemodynamic studies demonstrate the mechanisms behind the pressure elevation in various stages of hypertension. They also disclose functional abnormalities in the heart and the resistance vessels – often even at an early stage – and show how these disturbances develop during the course of the hypertension. Furthermore, the hemodynamic response to various antihypertensive drugs might be studied and valuable information obtained.

BASIC HEMODYNAMICS

The blood pressure is mainly determined by the cardiac output and the total peripheral resistance. Other factors, like the viscosity of the blood, play a minor role. In hemodynamic studies in man the arterial blood pressure is recorded intra-arterially and the cardiac output usually measured by dye dilution technique. The total peripheral resistance is calculated by dividing the mean arterial pressure by the cardiac output. This calculation, $TPR = MAP/CO$ is valid only for laminar flow in straight, rigid tubes, but although it means a rough approximation to apply this equation to the complicated vessel system in man, it is currently used in clinical cardiology and found useful. To correct for differences in body size, index values, $CI = CO/BSA$ and $TPRI = MAP/CI$ are often used (BSA = body surface area, CI = cardiac index, TPRI = total peripheral resistance index).

CENTRAL HEMODYNAMICS AT REST

The first studies on central hemodynamics in hypertensives were performed during rest situation in subjects with hypertension of long duration. The

Amery, A. (ed.) Hypertensive Cardiovascular Disease: Pathophysiology and Treatment
© *1982, Martinus Nijhoff Publishers. The Hague / Boston / London*
ISBN-13: 978-94-009-7478-4

common finding was an increased total peripheral resistance and a normal cardiac output, as long as heart failure was not present. The increased resistance was mainly located in the arterioles and considered to be caused by humoral or nervous mechanisms.

However, systematic studies over the last 15 years have shown that the hemodynamic pattern in primary hypertension differs and depends at least upon the age of the subject and the stage of the hypertensive disorder (reviews in ref. 1–3) (Figure 1).

Early hypertension

Studies from all over the world have shown that in groups of young adults (18–29 years) with borderline or mild hypertension the cardiac index at rest supine is usually increased compared to age-matched normotensive controls. The heart rate is also increased and the stroke index usually normal. The left ventricular ejection rate is increased. The calculated total peripheral resistance is numerically normal. Individual variations are great, however, and a continuous spectrum of cardiac outputs from high to low might be found. In the latter situation the total peripheral resistance is increased.

Systematic invasive studies in younger subjects are few, but recently a high cardiac index and high heart rate have been demonstrated also in a large proportion of children and adolescents with mild labile primary hypertension. A few subjects with high resistance were found also in this age.

The increased cardiac output and heart rate in what is usually supposed to be the starting phase of primary hypertension, has been considered to repre-

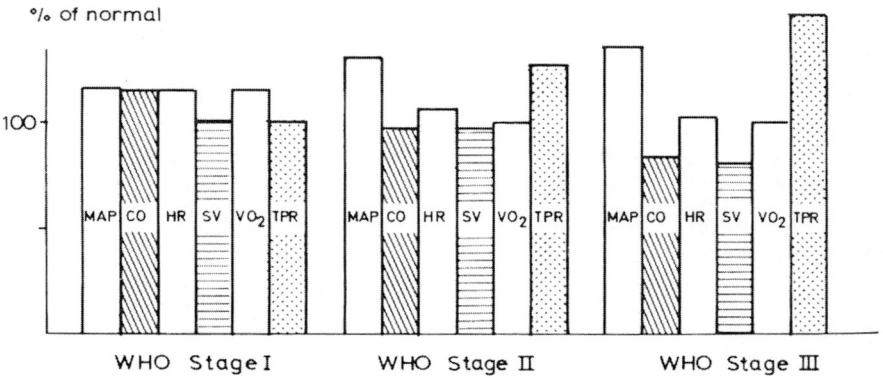

Figure 1. Diagramatic presentation of central hemodynamics during rest in primary hypertension at different stages.
MAP: mean arterial pressure, CO: cardiac output, HR: heart rate, SV: stroke volume, TPR: total peripheral resistance, VO_2: oxygen consumption [10].

sent a 'luxurious' blood flow (more blood to the tissues than what is needed according to the metabolism). This increased blood flow was supposed to induce an increase in arteriolar resistance in order to protect the tissues from overirrigation. In this way the total peripheral resistance increased, maintaining the high blood pressure when the cardiac output fell at a later stage. It should be stressed, however, that the oxygen uptake is also increased in young subjects with primary hypertension and the cardiac output is normal when related to the oxygen consumption. Thus 'autoregulation' can not explain why total peripheral resistance increases in primary hypertension over the years (see below).

In elderly subjects with mild hypertension the cardiac output is usually low, but exceptions are seen.

Late hypertension

Although increased blood pressure imposes a strong burden on the heart, it is usually able to perform its pump function for decades before the patient develops symptoms of heart failure, thanks to various compensatory mechanisms. Hemodynamic studies unveil abnormalities many years before symptoms of heart failure are present. In adults with moderate essential hypertension of several years duration but still in WHO stage I or II, the total peripheral resistance is increased associated with a normal or subnormal cardiac output during rest. The stroke volume is usually somewhat reduced and the heart rate normal or slightly increased. When left ventricular hypertrophy is present (diagnosed by ECG or echocardiography), reduced filling rate and reduced ejection fraction might be seen [4].

Severe hypertension

In patients with severe hypertension (WHO stage III) the total peripheral resistance is usually markedly increased and the cardiac output decreased. The stroke volume tends to be very low. In patients who suffer a myocardial infarction the blood pressure sometimes drops to normal levels, but the resistance remains increased.

When left ventricular strain is present on ECG and when heart failure is present, very low cardiac output and very high total peripheral resistance have been reported. In the final stage increased pressures in the pulmonary circulation and in the left ventricle during diastole are also found. At this stage left ventricular ejection rate is reduced and so is the circumferential fiber shortening [5].

REGIONAL CIRCULATION DURING REST

The increased total peripheral resistance in established primary hypertension is not shared equally in all parts of the body. The renal vascular resistance is usually increased, and also in the splanchnic area the resistance is increased. The resistance in the hand vessels during maximal vasodilatation has been found increased in young subjects with mild hypertension and low cardiac output, but normal when the cardiac output was increased.

In the skeletal muscles the resistance seems to become increased later than in the skin and in the kidneys. Of great interest is of course the coronary circulation. Recently it has been shown that the coronary reserve (defined as the difference between the coronary blood flow during rest and during maximal vasodilatation) is reduced in patients with hypertension already at an early stage. In more severe hypertension a great reduction in coronary blood flow and increase in coronary vascular resistance have been demonstrated. In the cerebral circulation the resistance is usually increased [5-7].

Pulmonary circulation

For many years it has been known that when hypertension is associated with heart failure, the pressures in the pulmonary circulation will increase. In recent years, it has been demonstrated that also in patients without signs or symptoms of heart failure, the pressures in the pulmonary circulation are somewhat increased. This is due to an increase in the pulmonary resistance. A reduced ejection fraction of the right ventricle has been demonstrated in subjects supposed to be in the relatively early stage of hypertension. Thus, also the pulmonary circulation seems to be affected at an early stage of primary hypertension [8].

HEMODYNAMICS DURING DYNAMIC EXERCISE

Muscular exercise represents the most severe type of physiological stress on the circulatory system. The systolic and, to a lesser extent, the diastolic pressure will increase during dynamic exercise. When in the sitting position, the normal heart will increase its stroke volume and rate and the cardiac output might increase to 20 l/min or more. The total peripheral resistance will drop, preventing excess rise in the blood pressure.

When patients with borderline and mild hypertension perform dynamic exercise, the cardiac output tends to be slightly below normal and the high cardiac output pattern, seen so often during rest, disappears. This is due to an insufficient increase in stroke volume, heart rate remaining slightly above normal. Recently, by the gated-pool isotope technique, a reduced filling rate during diastole has been found also in patients with mild and moderate hypertension. Such a reduced filling rate could explain why stroke volume is too small when heart rate is increased. Exercise studies also reveal that the total peripheral resistance is abnormal at an early stage in primary hypertension. The resistance does not fall to the same low levels as in normotensive age-matched controls. The rise in blood pressure is parallel to the rise in controls (Figure 2).

Patients in WHO stage II with left ventricular hypertrophy on ECG (or diagnosed by echocardiography) have abnormally low cardiac output during

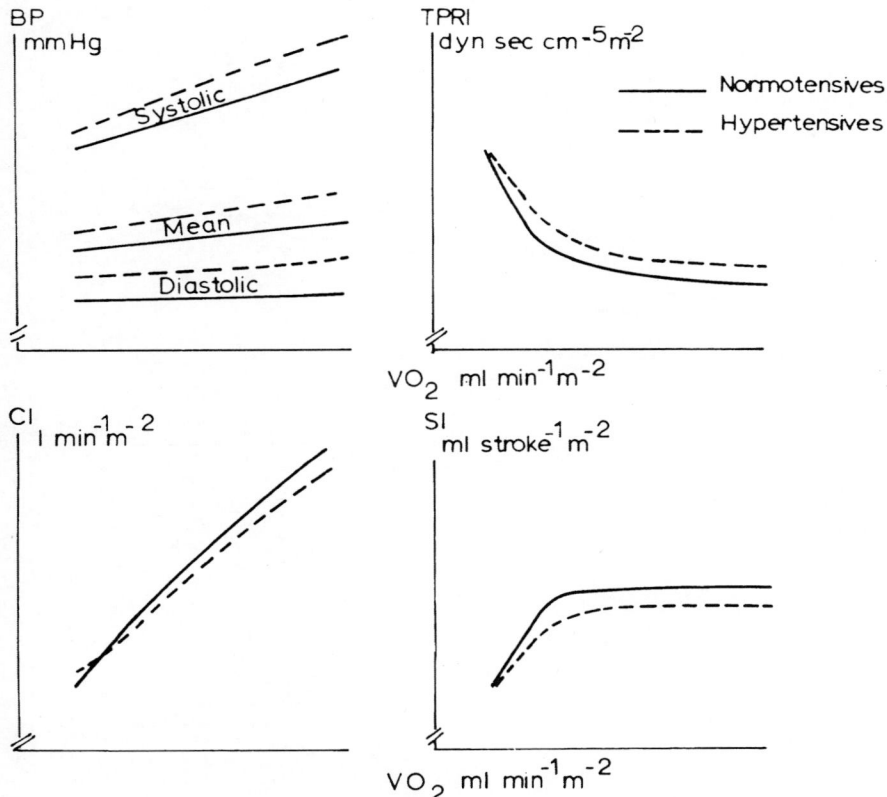

Figure 2. Central hemodynamics during rest sitting and exercise in young subjects with mild and moderate hypertension and in normal controls. Note the subnormal stroke volume during exercise and insufficient decrease in total peripheral resistance during exercise. Also note that the blood pressure rise during exercise is parallel to the normal rise. Figure based on mean values from ref. 3, 4 and 10.

exercise, also due to insufficient increase in stroke volume. The total peripheral resistance is increased. In such subjects the rise in blood pressure is often steeper than in normotensives and systolic blood pressures of 300 mm Hg or more are often seen.

In patients in WHO stage III with severe heart damage exercise studies are relatively few. The cardiac output during even mild exercise is often very much lower than normal due to insufficient rise in stroke volume. A decrease in stroke volume during exercise is then sometimes seen [3, 4, 9].

LONG-TERM CHANGES IN CENTRAL HEMODYNAMICS

Based on cross-sectional data it is usually assumed that the hemodynamic pattern in primary hypertension will change over the years from a 'hyper-

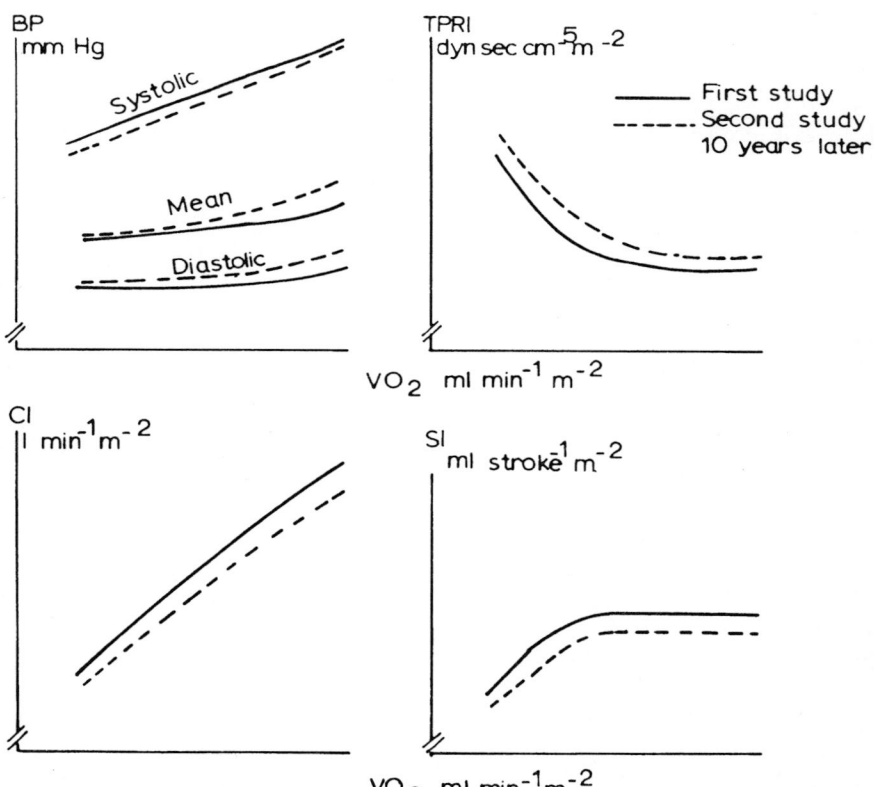

Figure 3. Spontaneous changes in central hemodynamics in mild hypertension. Mean values from 10-year follow-up studies. Age group I and II combined (17–39 years) [10].

kinetic' circulatory system in early age towards a 'low flow–high resistance' pattern in older age.

There have been relatively few systematic follow-up studies on central hemodynamics in untreated hypertensives. In our studies 77 patients who had been investigated hemodynamically from 1964 to 1966 were restudied clinically and 33 of the 34 untreated patients also hemodynamically after about 10 years. The blood pressure at rest in sitting position was 150/92 mm Hg on average in age group I (17–29 years) and 160/99 mm Hg in group II (30–39 years) in the first study. The follow-up study demonstrated surprisingly small changes in the blood pressure during rest. Individual data showed that the blood pressure increase was mainly seen in a few patients who had high total peripheral resistance in the first study. During exercise, however, there was a significant increase in diastolic and mean arterial pressure in both age groups. In spite of the small changes in the arterial pressure there were considerable changes in cardiac output and total peripheral resistance over the 10-year period. At rest the cardiac output had decreased by 15% and 23% in age group I and II respectively. During exercise the decrease was 15% and 14% respectively. The total peripheral resistance had increased at rest as well as during exercise in both groups. Thus the expected changes had indeed occurred (Figure 3).

In the first study, in patients one decade older (40–49 years) showing elevated total peripheral resistance a rise in blood pressure was found due to a marked increase in total peripheral resistance.

Whether the changes in flow and resistance are mainly due to the effects of aging or to the effects of hypertension is still not known. Probably both factors will contribute to the change in the hemodynamic pattern [10].

PATHOPHYSIOLOGICAL MECHANISMS INDUCING AND MAINTAINING THE HEMODYNAMIC ALTERATIONS

The sympathetic nervous system

The increased cardiac output, heart rate and oxygen consumption during rest in patients with early primary hypertension could be due to an overactivity in the sympathetic nervous system. To demonstrate such an overactivity has been difficult. An imbalance between the sympathetic and the parasympathetic nervous system has been suggested. The sympathetic nervous system is described in a previous chapter and will not be discussed any further [11, 12].

The blood volume and the capacitance vessels

Increase in cardiac preload and contractility could be important factors to maintain high or normal cardiac output in hypertension. An increase in the cardiopulmonary blood volume could facilitate the filling of the heart and contribute to maintenance of normal cardiac output and stroke volume when the afterload is high. It is generally agreed that the total blood volume is not increased in mild hypertension and in more severe hypertension it is often abnormally low. However, several investigators have demonstrated an increase in the cardiopulmonary blood volume, indicating a shift of the blood pool from the peripheral veins to the pulmonary capacitance bed. A positive correlation between the cardiopulmonary blood volume and the cardiac output has been demonstrated. The mechanisms behind this shift of the blood are not understood. A reduced venous distensibility could play a role, but the mechanism behind the suspected reduced distensibility is unknown. A reduced venous distensibility in the forearm in patients with primary hypertension has been demonstrated supporting this theory, but unfortunately no correlation between the reduced distensibility and hemo-dynamic parameters was demonstrated, so that this area is still poorly understood [13].

Structural changes in the left ventricle and in the resistance vessels

Studies in the spontaneously hypertensive rats have shown that left ventri-cular hypertrophy occur at a very early stage. The hemodynamic abnormal-ities seen during exercise in man with primary hypertension could be due to increased wall thickness and reduced compliance in the left ventricle and to increased wall thickness in the arterioles. By echocardiography it has been demonstrated that increased wall thickness in the left ventricle is found also in a large fraction of patients with mild hypertension. Increased thickness of the intraventricular septum has been demonstrated in patients even with borderline hypertension.

Obviously, it is more difficult to document early structural changes in the resistance vessels. Here the evidence has to be indirect. Lack of complete normalization of total periheral resistance after alpha-blockade by phento-lamine or after combination of heating and exercise during ischeia has been interpreted as a sign of structural changes. Increase in total peripheral resis-tance with time in untreated patients could reflect the same changes.

In summary, apart from studies by echocardiography evidence for struc-tural alterations in early primary hypertension is only indirect. At later stages, autopsy studies have demonstrated left ventricular hypertrophy and also increased thickness of the arteriolar wall [14, 15].

REGRESSION OF HEMODYNAMIC ALTERATIONS BY DRUG
TREATMENT

Although treatment of hypertension belongs to other chapters in this book, it could be of interest to know whether antihypertensive agents are able to normalize central hemodynamics in subjects with mild and moderate primary hypertension [16].

In relatively young subjects with secondary hypertension due to renal artery stenosis it has been demonstrated that after operation of the stenotic kidney, a marked decrease in total peripheral resistance and normalization of central hemodynamics at rest and during exercise might be seen. So, in this type of hypertension the systemic circulation might revert back to normal, judged from hemodynamic studies.

In primary hypertension conventional drug therapy induces different hemodynamic responses. We have studied more than 200 males with mild to moderate hypertension before and after one year of treatment with one of the commonly used antihypertensive agents. Hydrochlorothiazide reduced blood pressure by about 15% at rest and also during exercise. The pressure reduction was associated with a decrease in total peripheral resistance and there were no changes in heart rate, stroke volume or cardiac output. Thus a partial correction of the hemodynamic abnormalities was achieved.

Seven different beta-blockers all induced dramatic hemodynamic changes. The heart rate at rest and during exercise was decreased by about 25-30%. With some beta-blockers there was a slight compensatory increase in the stroke volume during exercise. Consequently, the cardiac output was reduced a little less than the heart rate, but still a 20-25% reduction in cardiac output at rest and during exercise was common. Total peripheral resistance rarely fell below pretreatment values. Prolongation of beta-blocker treatment for three to five years did not alter the hemodynamic picture seen after one year. Thus, disappointingly there were no signs of a gradual normalization of stroke volume and total peripheral resistance. The beta-blockers rather replaced the 'normal flow–high pressure system' by a 'low flow–normal pressure' system. However, the reduction in the cardiac output was usually well tolerated. To compensate for the reduction in cardiac output with unchanged oxygen consumption, the arteriovenous oxygen difference increased. Since both heart rate and blood pressure were reduced, a marked reduction in the work load on the heart was achieved.

More recently alpha-receptor blockers have been introduced in long-term antihypertensive treatment. Prazosin, a postsynaptic alpha-blocker induced a significant and consistent decrease in total peripheral resistance at rest as well as during exercise. The stroke volume increased and the posttreatment cardiac output was increased, particularly during muscular exercise. Thus, prazosin was able to induce normalization of central hemodynamics.

386

When prazosin and a beta-blocker were combined, a marked reduction in blood pressure was obtained through a combination of reduction in resistance and in cardiac output. During exercise the reduction in cardiac output was moderate and the pressure reduction mainly due to reduction in total peripheral resistance. A similar pattern was seen on labetalol, a relatively new drug with both alpha- and beta-blocking properties [16, 17].

CONCLUSION

This review has shown that the hemodynamic pattern behind the increased blood pressure in a human in his twenties and a human in his sixties is usually very different. With the same pressure the total peripheral resistance might be twice as high in the older patient as in the younger, and the blood flow only half as high. When primary hypertension is left untreated, there is usually a gradual change in the hemodynamic situation towards the high resistance–low flow system found at later stages, possibly due to progressive structural alterations. Pressure rise is probably most marked after the age of 50 years.

Antihypertensive agents correct the hemodynamic disorders to various extents. Relatively few drugs are able to change all hemodynamic parameters in the direction of normal values. In special patients, selection of the most suitable drug is important from a hemodynamic point of view. When it comes to the ordinary patient with mild hypertension, it is still not known which of the available agents will give the best clinical prognosis.

REFERENCES

1. Frohlich ED, Tarazi RC, Dustan HP: Re-examination of the hemodynamics of hypertension. Am J Med Sci 257:9–23, 1969.
2. Birkenhäger WH, Schalekamp MADH: Control mechanisms in essential hypertension. Amsterdam: Elsevier Scientific, 1976.
3. Lund-Johansen P: Haemodynamics in essential hypertension. Clin Sci (Suppl) 59:343s–354s, 1980.
4. Lund-Johansen P: Hemodynamics in late hypertension. In: Phasic Pressor Mechanisms: Hypertension in the Young and the Old. pp. 239–249 Onesti G, Kim KE, eds. New York: Grune & Stratton, 1981.
5. Strauer B-E: Ventricular function and coronary hemodynamics in hypertensive heart disease. Am J Cardiol 44:999–1006, 1979.
6. Brod J: Regional blood flow in essential hypertension. In: Hypertension: Mechanisms and Management, pp. 37–41. Onesti G, Kim KE, Moyer JH, eds. New York: Grune & Stratton, 1973.
7. de Leeuw PW, Kho TL, Falke HE, Birkenhäger WH, Wester A: Haemodynamic and endocrinological profile of essential hypertension. Acta Med Scand (Suppl) 622:1–86, 1978.
8. Ferlinz J: Right ventricular performance in essential hypertension. Circulation 61:156–162, 1980.

9. Amery A: Hemodynamic changes during exercise in hypertensive patients. Mal Cardiovasc 10:227–245, 1969.
10. Lund-Johansen P: Haemodynamic observations in mild hypertension. In: Mild Hypertension: Natural History and Management, pp.102–115. Gross F, Strasser T, eds. Bath: Pirman Medical, 1979.
11. Julius S: Abnormalities of autonomic nervous control in borderline hypertension. Schweiz Med Wochenschr 106:1698–1705, 1976.
12. Weidmann P: Recent pathogenic aspects in essential hypertension and hypertension associated with diabetes mellitus. Klin Wochenschr 58:1071–1089, 1980.
13. Safar ME, Weiss YA, London GM, Simon AC, Chau PN: Hemodynamic changes in mild early hypertension versus sustained hypertension. In: Phasic Pressor Mechanisms: Hypertension in the Young and the Old. pp. 19–27. Onesti G, Kim KE, eds. New York: Grune & Stratton, 1981.
14. Folkow B: Cardiovascular structural adaptation; its role in the initiation and maintenance of primary hypertension. Clin Sci Mol Med 55:3s–22s, 1978.
15. Savage DD, Drayer JIM, Henry WL, Mathews EC Jr, Ware JH, Gardin JM, Cohen ER, Epstein SE, Laragh JH: Echocardiographic assessment of cardiac anatomy and function in hypertensive subjects. Circulation 59:623–636, 1979.
16. Lund-Johansen P: Haemodynamic effects of antihypertensive agents. In: The Treatment of Hypertension, pp. 61–92. Freis ED, ed. Lancaster: MTP Press, 1978.
17. Lund-Johansen P: The effect of beta-blocker therapy on chronic hemodynamics. Primary Cardiology (Suppl) 1:20–28, 1980.

IV. REPERCUSSIONS OF HIGH BLOOD PRESSURE

25. HYPERTENSION AND THE BRAIN

AUSTIN E. DOYLE and GEOFFREY A. DONNAN

INTRODUCTION

The brain is a major target organ for the effects of high blood pressure. Even moderate elevation of blood pressure increases the risk of stroke substantially [1]. This is because increases in blood pressure induce pathological changes in the arteries and arterioles supplying the brain. The type of vascular pathology, and its site influences the extent and location of brain ischaemia and these in turn lead to the clinical manifestations of stroke. However, although hypertension is of great importance, it is only one of the factors which induce vascular disease in the cerebral circulation. As will become evident, certain types of vascular disease are almost exclusively the result of hypertension, whereas in other types hyertension may be an aggravating rather than the sole pathogenetic factor.

The introduction of the newer diagnostic techniques, in particular computerized axial tomography (CT) and angiography, has allowed a much clearer definition of the pathological basis of the various stroke syndromes. The use of such techniques will allow a more precise evaluation of the role of hypertension in the pathogenesis of stroke.

Much of the data presented in this chapter is derived from observations made by one of us (G.A. Donnan) in the Stroke Unit at the Austin Hospital, Melbourne on the first 350 patients admitted with stroke. The data give an idea of the relative frequency of the various stroke syndromes and their pathological causes.

Table 1 shows the numbers of the various types of stroke syndromes admitted in the years 1977–1979 and shows that cortical infarction was the most frequent pathological basis for stroke. These syndromes are discussed in more detail below.

CORTICAL INFARCTION SYNDROMES

Infarction of the cortical region of one cerebral hemisphere results from occlusion of a major artery. It may be due to thrombosis in the common or

Amery, A. (ed.) Hypertensive Cardiovascular Disease: Pathophysiology and Treatment
© *1982, Martinus Nijhoff Publishers. The Hague / Boston / London*
ISBN-13: 978-94-009-7478-4

Table 1. The incidence of various stroke syndromes 1977–1979

	Female	Male	Total
Cortical Infarction	119 (34%)	59 (16.9%)	178 (51%)
Capsular Infarction	53 (15.1%)	17 (4.9%)	70 (20%)
Cerebral Haemorrhage	5 (2.0%)	10 (2.8%)	17 (4.0%)
Posterior Circulation	33 (9.5%)	8 (2.3%)	41 (11.8%)
Miscellaneous (migraine, cerebral tumour, psychogenic, other)	17 (4.9%)	27 (7.6%)	44 (12.5%)
Total	229 (654%)	121 (34.6%)	350 (100%)

internal carotid artery or one of its major cerebral branches, or to embolism, either arising from the heart, or from non-obstructing lesions within the carotid artery.

Thrombosis within large arteries appears to be most common within the common or internal carotid artery. Mohr et al. [2] classified the patients in the Harvard Stroke Registry into thrombotic, haemorrhagic or embolic groups. Two hundred and thirty three patients had a final diagnosis of thrombosis of a large artery. Of these, 138 occurred within the carotid territory. One hundred and two of these were studied by carotid angiography and carotid stenosis or occlusion was demonstrated in all of these. The frequency with which the major cerebral branches of the carotid system show arterial thrombosis in the cerebral arteries is rather uncertain. Hicks and Warren [3] reported that arterial thrombosis in the cerebral arteries in cases of cerebral infarction occurred in less than 10% of cases. It seems from the data from the Harvard Stroke Registry [2] that stenosis or occlusion within the carotid artery rather than in cerebral arteries accounts for the majority of cases of cortical infarction due to arterial thrombosis.

The other major cause of cortical infarction is embolism. The source of the emboli may be fibrillating atria, mural thrombi following myocardial infarction, the mitral or aortic valve in patients with bacterial endocarditis or from the mitral valve in patients with abnormal valves. In the Harvard Stroke Registry the cardiac risk factors for embolism outlined above were present in 170 patients or 25% of the whole population; 112 of those were thought to have had cerebral embolism.

The other major source of embolism is the carotid artery. Gunning, Pickering, Robb-Smith and Ross Russell [4] have provided evidence that embolism may be the result of thrombus formation on atheromatous plaques or ulcers within the carotid arteries. In the report of Mohr et al. [2] 88 patients with cerebral embolism had angiograms and of these 33 (37.5%) had atheromatous lesions in the ipsilateral carotid artery. Thus, cortical infarction, which accounts for about 50% of all stroke syndromes is apparently due in about 80% of cases to disease of the internal carotid arteries with the remainder due to embolism from cardiac causes.

Atheromatous disease of the carotid arteries is common in hypertension. In the Austin Hospital Stroke Unit, a prospective study of 102 patients with cortical infarction demonstrated by CAT scan, had carotid angiography. Of these, 18 had ipsilateral carotid occlusion, 60 had carotid atheromatous lesions and 22 had artrial fibrillation. Two had normal angiograms. Of the patients with carotid disease 50% had a past history of treatment for hypertension and 11% were newly found to be hypertensive, giving an incidence of hypertension of about 50% in these patients with stroke due either to embolism or large vessel thrombosis. Prineas and Marshall [5] found that patients with diastolic pressures less than 110 mm Hg generally had clinical evidence of cortical infarction associated with a high incidence of demonstrable disease in the larger arteries.

Although atheromatous lesions occur in non-hypertensive patients, there is a quantitative increase in the frequency and severity of these lesions in the cerebral and extracranial vessels in hypertension [6]. The other well-known risk factors of hypercholesterolaemia, diabetes and cigarette smoking are also important in the pathogenesis of carotid and cerebral vascular disease.

Clinical Features

The characteristic feature of cortical infarction is the development of a hemiplegia, accompanied by features of cortical involvement such as dysphasia, dyspraxia or hemianopia. Combined sensory and motor symptoms, particularly in a brachiofacial distribution is very suggestive of cortical ischaemia. The pattern of onset may be sudden or gradual, or may involve bursts of hemiplegia, which may resolve completely within hours (T.I.A.). Embolic activity is suggested by the presence of chest pain, amaurosis fugax or palpitations. Cortical infarction may induce headache, occasionally seizures, coma and confusion.

The fully developed syndrome of cortical infarction consisting of hemiplegia, dysphasia, dyspraxia and hemianopia is usually quite evident clinically, although cerebral haemorrhage may induce similar symptoms. However, such cortical signs are by no means invariable. In our series of 178 cortical infarctions, 36 (20.2%) had dysphasia and hemiparesis, 13 (7.3%) had amaurosis fugax and 7 (3.9%) had homonymous hemianopia; 44 patients (24.7%) in the whole group had at least one of these cortical symptom indicators. Similarly, of the 178 patients only 27 (15.2%) had ipsilateral carotid bruits and 24 (13.5%) had atrial fibrillation.

Special Investigations

The E.E.G. may be helpful in diagnosis. Marked asymmetry is suggestive of cortical rather than capsular infarction and occurred in almost 40% of the series of Prineas and Marshall [5]. However, by no means all patients have such features.

The use of computerized axial tomography has proved extremely valuable in the diagnosis of cortical infarction, which can be seen as an area of reduced density (Figure 1).

In an early study, Paxton and Ambrose [7] showed that of 55 patients with occlusive vascular disease, 38 had CT scans which were abnormal. Other early reports [8-11] also demonstrated that CT scanning was useful in stroke diagnosis. Davis et al. [8] made a thorough study of the time of appearance of cerebral infarcts. He found that 16 of 32 cerebral infarcts (50%) were demonstrated when scanned in the 8 to 28 day period and 47 of 55 infarcts (85.5%) after 28 days. Gado et al. [12] found that 55% of recent cerebral infarcts were CT positive. Christie et al. [13] suggested that positive findings on occlusive cerebrovascular disease were most likely in the first 7 days (70%) while positive findings diminish to about 50% in cases one to

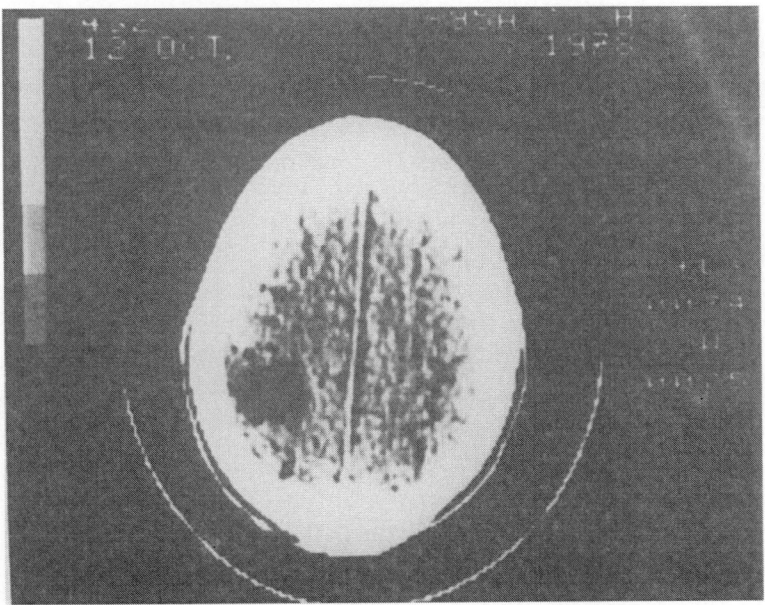

Figure 1. CT Scan of a patient showing a left parieto-occipital infarct. Presentation was with a transient motor weakness with some paraesthesia affecting right face, arm and leg with no speech disturbance. EEG and Neuropsychological testing were unremarkable.

three weeks post infarction. Later studies attempted to correlate duration of the clinical deficit with likelihood of finding an infarct on CT. Kinkel et al. [14] found abnormalities in only 2 of 32 patients with transient ischaemic attacks, while 57 of 58 patients with cerebral infarction had abnormal scans. Constant et al. [15] found infarcts in only 2 of 16 patients with transient ischaemic attacks, 17 of 25 patients with 'rapidly regressing' strokes, 65 of 66 patients with 'serious infarcts without improvement'. Campbell et al. [16] performed the most comprehensive study on the time with one scan as near to the ictus as possible and the next scan 7 days later, he found that, of 141 patients with, 66% of infarcts could be detected by this method. Between the first and second examination 20% of scans became positive and the peak detection times were the 10th and 11th days post infarction. Masdeu et al. [17] also performed a study with serial scans to study the features of infarction in 20 patients. Some mass effect was shown by 70% of cerebral infarcts and enhancement after injection of intravenous contrast was demonstrated by 63%. However, Norton et al. [18] found only 31% of cases enhanced in a similar study and showed that, in some cases, enhancement may be the only manifestation of infarction and may be seen in the range of one day to nine months.

Wing et al. [19] found enhancement in 60% of cases and mass effect in 22%. Alcala et al. [20] found in an autopsy study that the low CT density in

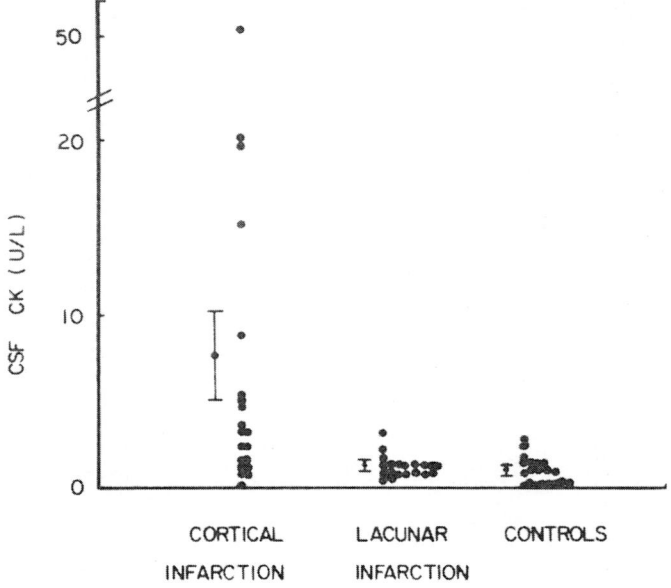

Figure 2. CSF CK levels in 20 patients with cortical infarction and 20 patients with lacunar infarction compared to 20 control patients.

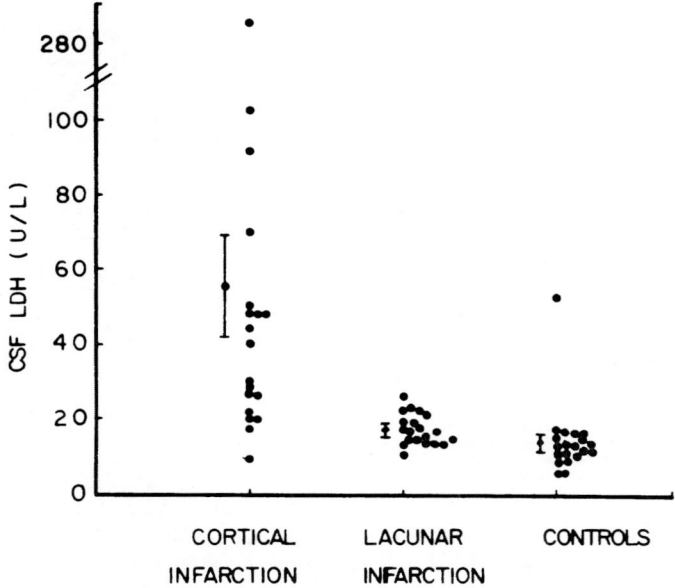

Figure 3. CSF LDH levels in 20 patients with cortical infarction and 20 patients with lacunar infarction compared to 20 control patients.

acute infarcts was due to the accumulation of fluid, whereas in chronic infarcts it was due to cavitation and the presence of lipids.

It is clear that although CT scanning is a useful method of defining cortical infarctions, it does not invariably show these and changes may not become apparent for some time following infarction, and other methods may be useful.

After demonstrating an elevation of AST in the CSF in dogs in which cerebral infarction had been experimentally induced, Fleisher and Wakim [21] showed an elevation of CSF AST in humans after stroke. Their findings were confirmed by other workers [22, 23]. LDH was also shown to rise in the CSF in the presence of cerebral infarction [24]. In one study [23], three enzymes were measured simultaneously and in 30 cases of cerebral infarction, 27 (90%) were found to have elevation of at least one or more of the enzymes CPK, AST or LDH. However, some authors [25] suggested that CSF CPK values lacked diagnostic value.

Recently it has been reported that lumbar puncture may be of value in distinguishing cortical from capsular infarction. Donnan [26] has reported elevation of both creatinine phosphokinase (CPK) and lactate dehydrogenase (LDH) in the CSF of patients with cortical infarction in the first week to ten days after the clinical event (Figures 2, 3 and 4). By contrast, patients with capsular infarction had no enzyme elevation. A finding of considerable

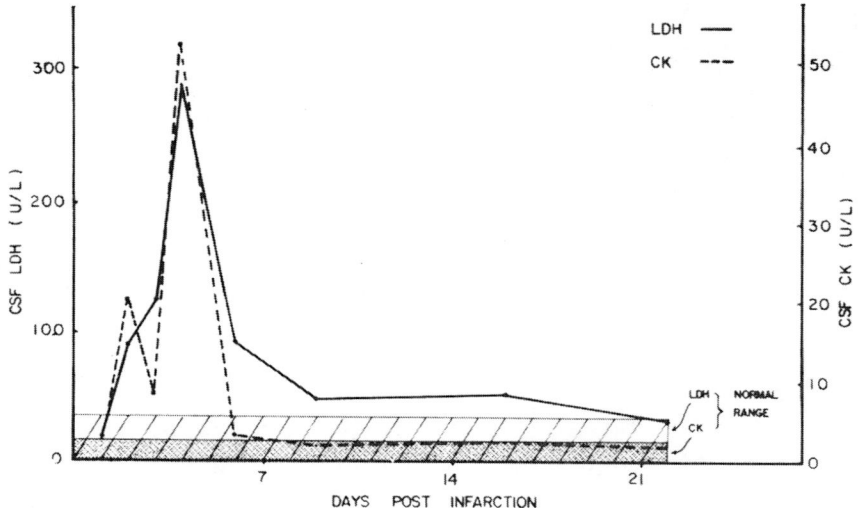

Figure 4. CSF levels of LDH and CK in a patient who had a large cortical infarction at day 0. CSF samples were drawn on days 0, 1, 2,13, 5, 8, 15 and 21.

interest in this study was the close correlation between CSF enzyme level and cortical infarct size as seen on CT scan, while little correlation occurred between enzyme level and clinical deficit. Similarly, there was a very poor correlation between the size of infarct seen on CT scan, and clinical deficit. Hence, marked elevation CSF enzyme levels in the presence of a small neurological deficit may reflect more extensive cerebral damage than is clinically apparent. An awareness of the extent of this damage may alter management in terms of timing of cerebral angiography and subsequent carotid endarterectomy or the use of anticoagulants.

CAPSULAR INFARCTION

In 1901 Marie [27] reported 50 cases of lacunar infarction, although the term 'lacune' had been coined earlier by Durand-Fardel in 1843 [28]. Marie recognized the typical lacunar cavity as a healed infarction resulting from 'rupture or obliteration' of a perforating artery or one of its branches. The same group reported that each lacune contained a centrally placed artery, which, though not occluded was assumed to have been so initially. Hughes, Dodgson and Maclellan [29] described infarction in the basal ganglia and internal capsule in 51 hypertensive patients. Fisher [30] in an autopsy study of 1042 consecutive adult postmortem examinations reported the presence of 376 lacunes in 114 patients of whom 111 had been hypertensive. The lacunes were predominantly situated in the region of the internal capsule and the pons. Significantly, the carotid arteries were examined in each case and a source of embolism was never found.

The pathological basis for these lesions appears to be the arterial abnormalities originally described by Charcot and Bouchard in 1868 [31], and rediscovered by Ross-Russell in 1963 [32]. These lesions appear to occur almost exclusively in the brain of hypertensive patients; they are found most frequently in the putamen, thalamus, pons, cerebellum and subcortex. The pathological basis of these lesions appears to be fibrinoid necrosis, although numerous other pathological names have been attached to the lesion [33, 34]. These vascular changes seem most likely to be responsible for the deep infarcts or lacunes [30] and for the occurrence of intracerebral haemorrhage.

Clinical Features

The description of 'pure motor hemiplegia of vascular origin' by Fisher and Curry [35] is the classical description of the clinical features of lacunar infarction in the internal capsule or pons. The features described were 'paralysis complete or incomplete of the face, arm and leg and one side, unaccompanied by sensory signs, visual field defect, dysphasia or apractagnosia'. The same authors reported that 44 of their 50 cases had either premonitory transient episodes or a stepwise onset. Headache was present in only two cases and 'preservation of mental activity in the presence of a massive hemiplegia was a remarkable feature'. Although this syndrome is the commonest clinical presentation of lacunar infarction, cerebellar features are present additionally in some cases (ataxic hemiparesis, Dysarthria clumsy hand syndrome) and a few cases of purely sensory stroke have been described. The diagnosis, therefore depends on the clinical recognition of these syndromes and on the lack of such cortical signs as dysphasia, neglect, dyspraxia or hemianopia.

It is important to recognize capsular, as distinct from cortical infarction, since the pathological basis of the two syndromes is quite different. In the presence of cortical infarction attention needs to be focussed on a cardiac source of emboli, or in the ipsilateral carotid artery, and although hypertension is commonly an accompanying feature, immediate management needs to be directed towards the underlying pathological cause. This may involve carotid angiography, and when the neurological deficit is transient or slight, carotid endarterectomy needs to be seriously considered.

By contrast, the presence of capsular infarction implies the presence of small arterial disease, which has a hypertensive aetiology in most instances. Recognition of the presence of capsular infarction obviates the need for carotid angiography in almost all cases, and can be regarded as an indication for immediate antihypertensive therapy.

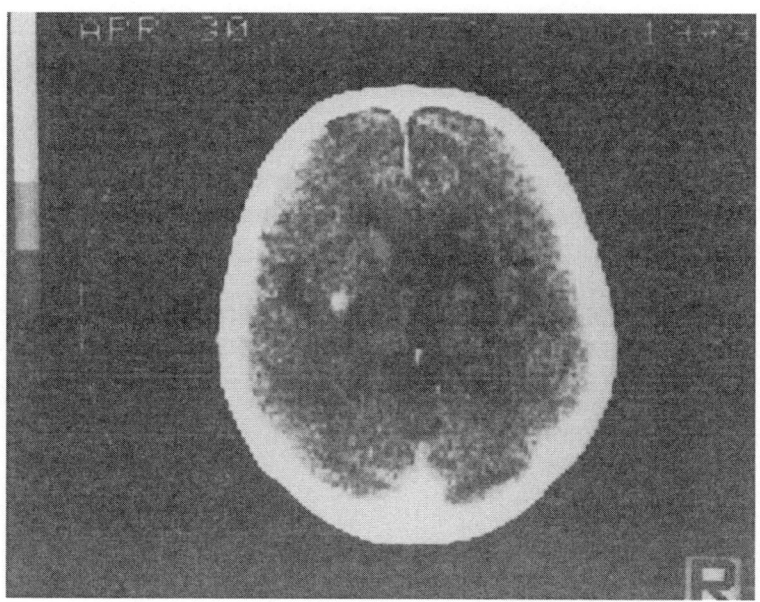

Figure 5. Enhancement shown on CT scan in a lacunar infarction in the region of the internal capsule.

Special Investigations

As mentioned above, carotid angiography is not indicated. Although the electro-encephalograph rarely shows distinguishing features, this relative normality suggests, but does not prove the absence of cortical infarction.

CT scanning has been found to demonstrate the presence of infarction in the region of the internal capsule (Figure 5). Slow scans (5 min) were carried out on slices containing the basal ganglia internal capsules and corona radiata, using a Mark II EMI 1007 head scanner. Eight slices were taken with a line between the external auditory meatus and the lateral angle of the eye acting as a reference line for the first and lowest slice (1A) which was 3 cm above this reference line (Figure 6). In 80 consecutive patients considered to

Table 2. Sequential CI scan study: CI findings in 80 consecutive patients

CT findings	No. of patients	%
Capsular infarction	52	65.0
No lesion demonstrated	23	28.7
Cortical infarction	5	6.3
Total	80	100.0

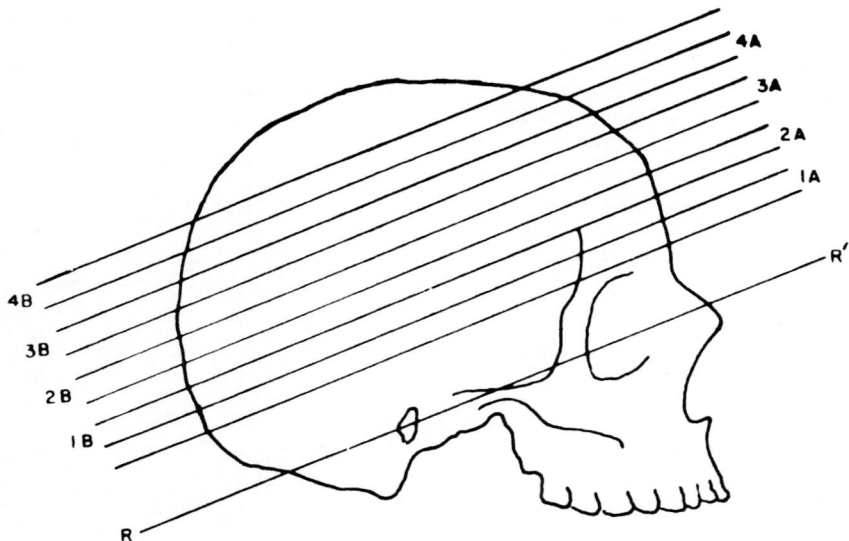

Figure 6. A lateral view of the skull showing the position of 8 slices taken by CT scan with line R-R[1] acting as reference line.

have capsular infarction on clinical criteria, capsular infarction was confirmed in 52 (65%), no lesion was seen in 29% (Table 2) and 5 (6%) had cortical infarction either in the frontal or in the parieto-occipital region (Figure 1). In the whole series, 69 cases of clinically relevant lacunar infarctions were diagnosed clinically and confirmed by CT scan.

The mean diameter of the infarction area was 12.84 mm. The sites of the infarction are shown in Table 3. The most common site of infarction was in the corona radiata and the zone immediately between the corona and the internal capsule.

TRANSIENT ISCHAEMIC ATTACKS

Transient ischaemic attacks consist of transient episodes of focal brain ischaemia. Most are in the distribution of the carotid circulation. These may be cortical, due to small emboli from carotid occlusion or carotid disease or cardiac causes, but may also be capsular, due to small blood vessel disease. The incidence of the various types of syndromes in the Austin Hospital series is shown in Table 4. The clinical features vary according to the site of the ischaemic involvement but the pattern of events is remarkably uniform between each attack. The onset is usually sudden and the deficit increases in severity over a few minutes. The attack usually terminates within 2–4 h. Cortical syndromes due to embolism may be characterized by dysphasia,

398

Table 3. CT findings in 69 cases of clinically relevant lacunar infarction diagnosed clinically and confirmed on CT scan

Site of infarction	No. of patients	Total (%)
Corona radiata/junctional zone		
Corona and junctional zone alone	17	
Posterior limb, corona and junctional zone	8	
Lentiform, corona and junctional zone	2	
Genu, anterior limb and corona	4	
Total	31	44.9
Posterior limb		
Anterior one third	3	
Middle third	9	
Posterior one third	11	
Total	23	33.3
Lentiform and posterior limb	9	13.1
Anterior limb and genu	4	5.8
Giant lacune involving all the above structures	2	2.9
	69	100.0

hemiplegia or amaurosis fugax, while the commonest mode of presentation of the capsular syndrome is that of pure motor hemiplegia. Combined sensory and motor symptoms, particularly in a brachiofacial distribution, suggest a cortical rather than a capsular lesion.

A history of repeated clinical events is commonly obtained in patients with carotid occlusion associated with a long intraluminal clot [36] or in capsular infarction [27, 35]. By contrast repetition of embolic episodes due either to carotid disease or to arterial fibrillation is usually relatively uncommon.

Table 4. Transient ischaemic attacks and stroke as a proportion of each syndrome group

	No. of patients					
	Stroke [1]	(%)	T.I.A. [2]	(%)	Total	(%)
Anterior circulation						
Cortical	127	71.4	51	28.6	178	100
Lacunar	44	62.9	26	37.1	70	100
Posterior circulation	27	65.9	14	34.1	43	100
Cerebral haemorrhage	17	100.0	0	0.0	17	100
All groups	215	70.3	91	29.7	306	100

[1] Neurological deficit of greater than 24 h duration.
[2] Neurological deficit of 24 h duration or less.

Investigation

The presence of transient ischaemic attacks of cortical type require both CT scan, and carotid angiographs and oculoplethysmography. In transient ischaemic attacks due to emboli the CT scan may be normal, although in some instances extensive infarction may be seen (Figure 1). In such instances, the infarction is presumably in a relatively silent area, usually either frontal or parieto-occipital, with temporary involvement of the motor areas. Oculoplethysmography may reveal a lower pressure on the appropriate side and carotid angiography may reveal either carotid occlusion or carotid stenosis or ulceration.

Transient ischaemic attacks due to capsular lesions show evidence of capsular infarction in about half the patients studied (Table 5). When multiple events have been present, about 80% of patients show evidence of capsular infarction.

As with completed strokes, the distinction between transient ischaemic attacks due to embolism or carotid occlusion and those due to hypertensive small blood vessel disease is of major importance in management.

CEREBRAL HAEMORRHAGE

Intracerebral haemorrhage, previously a common complication of hypertension is now a comparatively rare disease. The common sites of cerebral haemorrhage are the region of the internal capsule, the pons and the subcortical areas, a similar area of distribution to that of lacunar infarction. The underlying pathological lesion appears to be Charcot-Bouchard Aneurysm or fibrinoid necrosis of small cerebral arteries. Cerebral haemorrhage occurs most frequently in hypertensive patients whose blood pressure has not been well controlled. Hodge and Smirk [37] noted that onset of cerebral haemorrhage often occurred in patients being treated with ganglion blocking drugs

Table 5. CT scan changes of capsular infarction and duration of neurological deficit

Duration of deficit	No. of patients	No of patients with positive scans	No. of patients with negative scans	% positive
Less than 24 hours	25	13	12	52.0
Less than 1 week	8	6	2	75.0
Less than 6 months	16	13	3	81.2
More than 6 months	26	20	6	76.9
Total	75	52	23	69.3

shortly before a dose was due and concluded that they were the result of the rise in pressure. They also reported a large reduction in the incidence of cerebral haemorrhage following the introduction of ganglion blocking drugs.

Clinical Features

The onset is usually slow, with a progressive development of hemiplegia, clouding of consciousness and coma. The presence of intracerebral haemorrhage is readily confirmed by CT scan. Blood pressure following cerebral haemorrhage often rises still further, presumably due to the raised intracranial pressure. The prognosis is poor, mortality being high and residual deficit usually extensive in survivors.

Cerebellar haemorrhage is an important, although unusual variety of intracerebral bleeding. It may be diagnosed by the use of CT scanning. Its importance is that surgical intervention, with evacuation of the haemorrhage may be life saving, and may be followed by little disability.

HYPERTENSIVE ENCEPHALOPATHY

Although the term hypertensive encephalopathy is often used to describe focal episodes of neurological disability, it is probably best reserved for the unusual syndrome of very severe hypertension, accompanied by fits and loss of consciousness in the absence of definite neurological localizing signs.

Most patients with this syndrome have renal failure and malignant hypertension [38]. The syndrome also occurs in acute nephritis and eclampsia and is probably due to cerebral oedema as the result of a combination of a fall in cerebral blood flow due to severe hypertension [39] and overhydration. Since the introduction of effective antihypertensive drug therapy, the syndrome has become very rare.

HEADACHE

Headache is common in hypertensive patients and is particularly common in those with severe hypertension of recent onset. Headaches are often occipital in site, are classically present on wakening and are almost invariably relieved by effective reduction of blood pressure. Nevertheless, in many patients, whether hypertensive or not, headache is often not due to any discernible cause. Clarke and Murphy [37] found an incidence of headache in 77% of their 73 cases of malignant hypertension. The symptom is much less common in less severe hypertension.

PSEUDO-BULBAR PALSY

Severe hypertension may be associated with a syndrome consisting of bilateral pyramidal signs associated with an organic dementia. There is usually dyarthria, akinesia, and marked emotional lability, associated with memory defects and behavioural disturbances. This syndrome was comparatively common in severe hypertensives 20–30 years ago, but is now not often encountered [29, 37].

The underlying pathological lesion appears to be multiple lacunar infarction due to hypertensive disease of small arteries. Its present comparative rarity presumably results from the widespread early use of antihypertensive drug treatment.

EFFECTS OF ANTIHYPERTENSIVE DRUG TREATMENT

Soon after antihypertensive drug treatment became available in 1950–51, it became apparent that effective control of blood pressure reduced the risk of cerebral haemorrhage, and there was suggestive evidence that the incidence of all types of stroke was reduced. In the first controlled trial of antihypertensive drug treatment, carried out by Hamilton et al. [40], reduction in mortality and morbidity in the treated group was clearly related to the effectiveness of blood pressure control and was particularly due to the lower incidence of stroke in the treated group. In the Veterans' Administration Cooperative Study [41] haemorrhagic stroke occurred in 19 control patients but in only 6 of the treated group. Patients under 60 years of age and those with diastolic pressures above 105 mm Hg seemed to benefit most; these may well have been at risk from small vascular lesions. However, even in persons with mild hypertension, the incidence of stroke or transient ischaemic attacks is reduced by drug treatment. The number of such events was 25 in the placebo treated group as compared to 12 in the actively treated group in the Australian National Blood Pressure Study [1]. A similar reduction in the incidence of stroke was reported in the stepped care group as opposed to the referred care group in the High Blood Pressure Detection and Follow-up Programme [42]. There is some evidence that antihypertensive drug treatment also helps to prevent recurrence of strokes in hypertensive patients. Carter [43] reported the results of a prospective controlled trial in 97 hypertensive survivors of stroke. After 2–3 years, the total mortality was 46% in the control group and 26% of the control group but in 14% of the treated group. Benefit was largely confined to patients aged less than 65 at the onset of the study. However, in the large Hypertension Stroke Cooperative Study [44], no decrease in the incidence of recurrence of stroke was recorded between placebo and treated groups.

None of the studies relating the effects of antihypertensive drugs to stroke incidence have made any clear distinction between cortical infarction, due either to thrombotic events in major arteries or to embolism, and lacunar infarction, due in the main to hypertensive small blood vessel disease. The fact that younger patients with higher blood pressures have been found to be the group apparently having the greatest reduction in risk of stroke, suggests that antihypertensive drug treatment is particularly useful in preventing lacunar infarction.

The observations of Breckenridge et al [45] are of interest. These workers found a comparatively high incidence of stroke in patients who had commenced antihypertensive drug treatment up to one year previously, whereas stroke became much less common in patients who had been given antihypertensive drug treatment for two or more years. This observation suggests either that reduction of blood pressure may occasionally precipitate stroke in the early months of treatment, or that it may take some time for hypertensive vascular disease to respond to treatment.

Since hypertension is a major risk factor for arteriosclerotic lesions in large arteries it is reasonable to suppose that this type of vascular disease might also be prevented or delayed by effective treatment, provided this is given before arterial lesions have occurred. Future studies, based on more precise anatomical localisation of brain lesions will be necessary before the influence of antihypertensive treatment on the various types of vascular lesion can be evaluated fully.

REFERENCES

1. The Australian Therapeutic Trial in Mild Hypertension. Report by the Committee of management. Lancet 1, 1261, 1980.
2. Mohr JP, Caplan LR, Melski JW, Goldstein RJ, Duncan GW, Kistler JP, Pessin MS, Bleich HL: The Harvard Cooperative Stroke Registry: A prospective registry. Neurology (Minneap) 28:754–762, 1978.
3. Hicks SP, Warren S: Infarction of the brain without thrombosis. An analysis of one hundred cases with autopsy. Arch Pathol 52:403–412, 1951.
4. Gunning AJ, Pickering GW, Robb-Smith, Ross-Russell RW: Mural thrombosis of the internal carotid artery and subsequent embolism. Quart J Med 33:155–195, 1964.
5. Prineas J, Marshall J: Hypertension and cerebral infarction. Br Med J 1:14, 1966.
6. Baker AB, Resch JA, Lowenson, RB: Hypertension and cerebral atherosclerosis. Circulation 39:701, 1969.
7. Paxton R, Ambrose J: The EMI Scanner. A brief review of the first 650 patients. Br J Radiol 47:530–565, 1974.

8. Davis KR, Traveras JM, New PFJ, Schnur JA, Roberson GH: Cerebral infarction diagnosis by computerized tomography. Analysis and evaluation of findings. Am J Roentgenol 124:643–660, 1975.

9. Baker HL, Cambell KJ, Houser WD, Reese DF, Sheedy PF, Holman CB, Kurland RL: Computer assisted tomography of the head – an early evaluation. Mayo Clin Proc 49:17–27, 1974.

10. Baker HL, Houser WD, Cambell JK, Reese DF, Holman CB: Computerized tomography of the head. JAMA 233:1304–1308, 1975.

11. New PFJ, Scott WR, Schnur JA, Davis KR, Trevaks JM: Computerized axial tomography with the EMI scanner. Radiology 110:109–123, 1974.

12. Gado MH, Coleman RE, Merlis AL, Alderson PO, Lee KS: Comparison of computerized tomography and radionuclide imaging in 'Stroke'. Stroke 7:109–113, 1976.

13. Christie JH, Mori H, Go RT, Cornell SH, Schapiro RL: Computed tomography and radionuclide studies in the diagnosis of intracranial disease. Am J Roentgenol 127:171–174, 1976.

14. Kinkel WR, Jacobs L: Computerized axial transverse tomography in cerebrovascular disease. Neurology (Minneap) 26:924–930, 1976.

15. Constant P, Renou AM, Caille JM, Verniet J, Dop A: Cerebral ischemia with computerized tomography. Comput Tomogr 1:235–248, 1977.

16. Cambell JK, Houser OW, Stevens JC, Wahner HW, Baker HL, Folger WN: Computed tomography and radionuclide imaging in the evaluation of ischemic stroke. Radiology 126:695–702, 1978.

17. Masdeu JC, Azar-Kia B, Rusino FA: Evaluation of recent cerebral infarction by computerized tomography. Arch Neurol 34:417–421, 1977.

18. Norton GA, Kishore PRS, Lin J: CT contrast enhancement in cerebral infarction. Am J Roentgenol 131:881–885, 1978.

19. Wing SD, Norman D, Pollock JA, Newton TH: Contrast enhancement of cerebral infarcts in computed tomography. Radiology 121:89–92, 1976.

20. Alcala H, Mokhtar G, Torack RM: The effect of size, histologic elements, and water content on the visualization of cerebral infarcts. A computerized cranial tomographic study. Arch Neurol 35:1–7, 1978.

21. Flaisher GA, Wakim KG, Goldstein P: Glutamine oxalacetic transaminase and lactic dehydrogenase in merum and cerebrospinal fluid of patients with neurologic disorders. Mayo Clin Proc 32:188–197, 1957.

22. Green JB, Oldewurthe HA, O'Doherty S, Forster FM: Cerebrospinal Fluid transaminase and lactic dehydrogenase activities in neurologic disease. Arch, Neurol Neurosurg Psychiatry 80:148–156, 1958.

23. Wolinz AH, Jacobs LD, Christoff N, Solomon M, Chernik N: Serum and cerebrospinal fluid enzymes in cerebrovascular disease. Arch Neurol 20:54–61, 1969.

24. Wroblewski F, Decker B, Wroblewski R: Activity of lactic dehydrogenase in spinal fluid. Am J Clin Pathol 28:269–271, 1957.

25. Lisak RP, Craig FA: Lack of diagnostic value of creatinine phosphokinase assay in spinal fluid. JAMA 199:750b–751, 1967.

26. Donnan GA: Enzyme changes in cerebro-spinal fluid as a means of distinguishing cortical and capsular infarction. Aust NZJ Med (in press).

27. Marie P: Des Foyers lacunaires de disentegration. Rev Med 21: 281–298, 1901.

28. Durand-Fardel M: traite du ramolissiment du cerveau. Paris, Baillière, 1843.

29. Hughes W, Dodgson MCH, MacLennan DC: Chronic cerebral hypertensive disease. Lancet 2:770, 1954.

30. Fisher CM: Lacunes: small, deep cerebral infarcts. Neurology 15:774, 1965.

31. Charcot JM, Bouchard C: Nouvelles recherches sur la pathogenie de l'hemorrhagie cerebrale. Arch Physiol Norm Pathol (Paris) 1:110, 1868.

32. Ross-Russell RW: Observations on intracerebral aneurysms. Brain 86:425, 1963.
33. Fisher CM: The arterial lesions underlying lacunes. Acta Neuropathol (Berl) 12:1, 1969.
34. Fisher CM: Cerebral miliary aneurysms in hypertension. Am J Pathol 66:313, 1972.
35. Fisher CM, Curry HB: Pure motor hemiplegia of vascular origin. Arch Neurol 13:30, 1965.
36. Donnan GA, Bladin PF: The stroke syndrome of long intraluminal clot with incomplete vessel obstruction. Clin Exper Neurol 1979.
37. Hodge JW, Smirk FH: The effect of drug treatment of hypertension on the distribution of deaths from various causes. A study of 173 deaths among hypertensive patients in the years 1959 to 1964 inclusive. Am Heart J 73:441, 1967.
38. Clarke E, Murphy EA: Neurological manifestations resulting from malignant hypertension. Br Med J 2:1319, 1956.
39. Byrom FB: The pathogenesis of hypertensive encephalopathy and its relation to the malignant phase of hypertension. Experimental evidence from the hypertensive rat. Lancet 2:201, 1954.
40. Hamilton M, Thompson EN, Wisniewski TKM: The role of blood pressure control in preventing complications of mild hypertension. Lancet 1:235, 1964.
41. Veterans Cooperative Study Group on Antihypertensive Agents: Effects of treatment on morbidity in hypertension. Results in patients with diastolic blood pressures averaging 115 through 129 mmHg. JAMA 202:1028, 1967.
42. Hypertension Detection and Follow-up Program Cooperative Group. Five year findings of the hypertension detection and follow-up program. I. Reduction in mortality of persons with high blood pressure including mild hypertension. JAMA 242:2562, 1979.
43. Carter AB: Hypotensive therapy in stroke survivors. Lancet 1:485, 1970.
44. Hypertension–Stroke Cooperative Study Group: Effect of antihypertensive treatment on stroke recurrence. JAMA 229:409, 1974.
45. Breckenridge A, Dollery CT, Parry EHO: Prognosis of treated hypertension. Quart J Med 39:411, 1970.

26. THE OCULAR FUNDUS AND HYPERTENSION

DAVID G. COGAN

The ocular fundus is a prime site for evaluation of the microvasculature in systemic vascular disease. The retinal blood vessels or, more precisely, their contained columns of blood can be visualized without the interposition of extraneous tissue. Extravasation of blood and serum into the retina indicates their functional incompetence and methods for their examination are conveniently at hand. The aims of the present chapter are to describe these

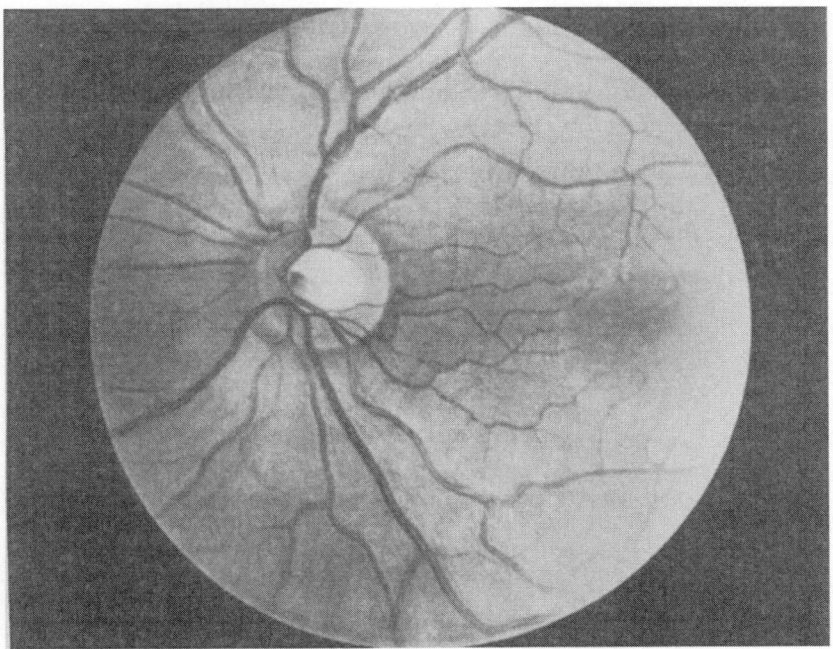

Figure 1. Normal left fundus. The artery emerging from the disc bifurcates supertiorly and inferiorly to supply each quadrant. The veins, Recognizable by their large diameter and darker color, follow a similar distribution. The disc is sharply demarcated and contains, in this case, a large physiologic cup. The macular area on the extreme right is characterized by a slightly darker background, somewhat larger than the disc, and surrounded by a faint light reflex from the surface of the retina.

Amery, A. (ed.) Hypertensive Cardiovascular Disease: Pathophysiology and Treatment
© *1982, Martinus Nijhoff Publishers. The Hague / Boston / London*
ISBN-13: 978-94-009-7478-4

vessels and other relevant structures in the eye, to indicate how they may be clinically evaluated, and to document the changes which occur with hypertension.

ANATOMIC AND PHYSIOLOGIC CONSIDERATIONS

The major retinal vessels comprise an artery and vein entering and exiting through the nerve head (Figure 1). With a maximal diameter no more than 0.1 mm the retinal artery belongs to the category of arterioles. The magnification of direct ophthalmoscopy gives the erroneous impression of a larger vessel. As the retinal artery branches to leave the disc, it loses the elastica and most of its muscle wall. With further subdivision the ultimate branches of the retinal artery consist of precapillary arterioles emerging in rectilinear fashion from the main trunk with diameters not much greater than those of the capillaries which it supplies. Trypsin digest preparations illustrate the

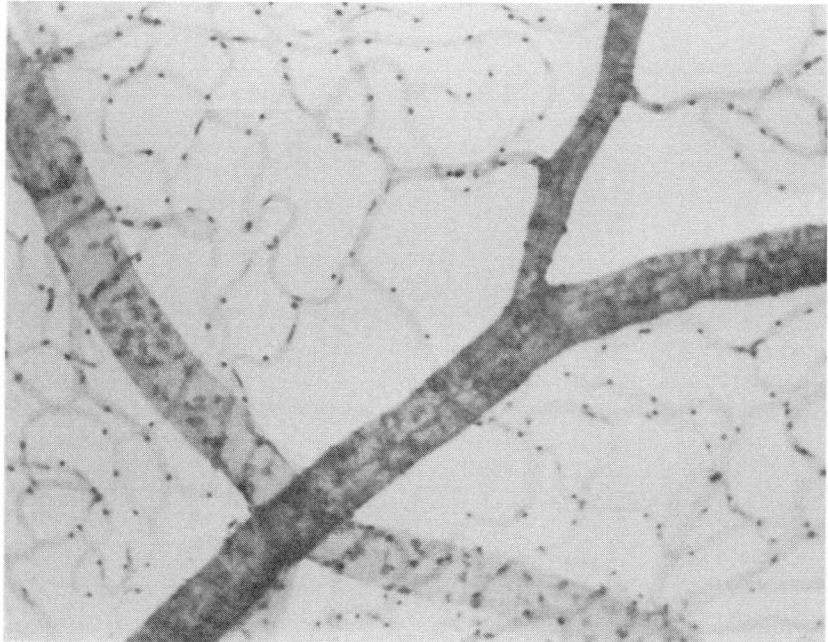

Figure 2. Trypsin digest of normal vessels. The artery courses obliquely upward toward the right and the vein obliquely up to the left. A small vessel emerging from the artery at right angles supplies the maze of capillaries. The capillaries are supplied with two types of cells: endothelial cells having pale staining ellipsoid nuclei and mural cells having darkly staining round nuclei. The former provide an inner lining for the capillaries and the latter presumably provide contractile functions. PAS stain; obj. 16; oc. 10.

task that these precapillary arterioles have in maintaining a constant circulation through a large capillary bed (Figure 2). To regulate the flow the retinal capillaries are provided with intramural cells presumed to have contractile properties analogous to that of vessels elsewhere. They are probably under hormonal as well as local control.

The retinal veins or venules measuring about half again larger than the diameter of the arteries have an overall distribution similar to that of the arteries. Transporting reduced hemoglobin and therefore appearing darker than the arteries they exit from the eye through the nerve head. At the points of arteriovenous crossing and again in the nerve head the vessels frequently share a common adventitia.

Pulsation of the vein on the nerve head, i.e., at the low point of venous pressure, is a normal phenomenon. It is secondary to pulsatile increase in intraocular pressure with each cardiac cycle and has no clinical significance. On the other hand, pulsation of the retinal artery is significant. It means either a pathologically low diastolic pressure in the artery or a pathologic elevation of the intraocular pressure (glaucoma).

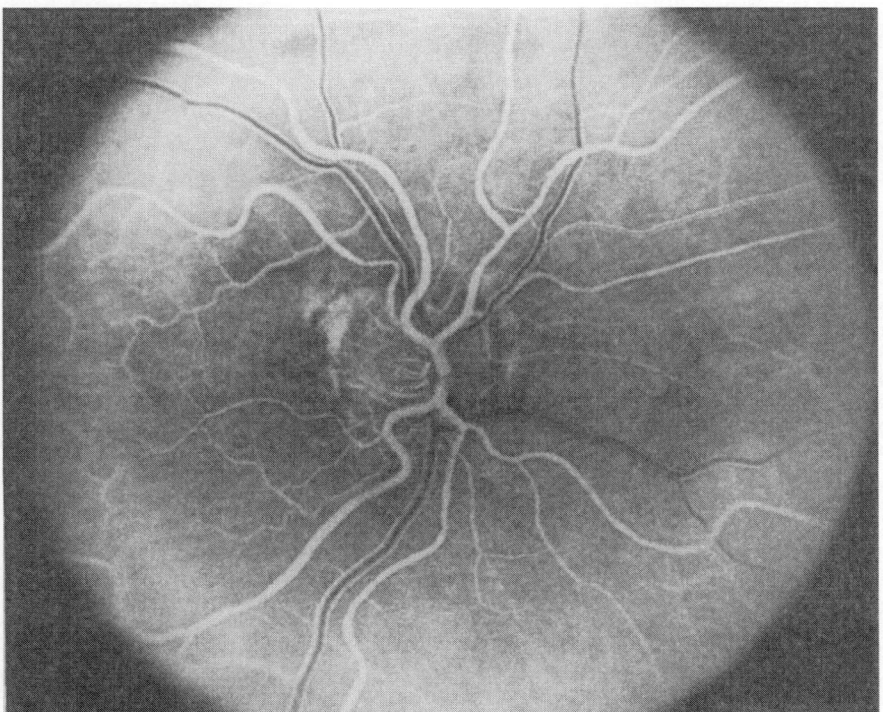

Figure 3. Fluoroangiogram in the arterial phase. The retinal arteries are brightly fluorescent while the veins are just beginning to show laminar flow.

In addition to these main retinal arteries and veins which traverse the center of the nerve head, one or more vessels may enter or leave the eye at the edge of the nerve head and connect with the choroidal vessels. Thus cilioretinal arteries and, to a less extent, optociliary veins are relatively common variants on the temporal side of the disc. By supplying a portion of the retina between the macula and disc some vision may be preserved in cases of obstruction of the central retinal artery.

One further anatomic feature relevant to the subsequent interpretation of clinical signs is the predominantly superficial position of the larger retinal vessels and the relatively deep position of the capillary networks. The main retinal arteries and veins are situated almost exclusively in the nerve fiber layer and in places fuse with the internal limiting membrane, whereas the capillaries interlace the interstitial layers of the retina. On the other hand, the outermost layers comprising the rods, cones, and their nuclei are devoid of blood vessels deriving their nutritional support from the choroid.

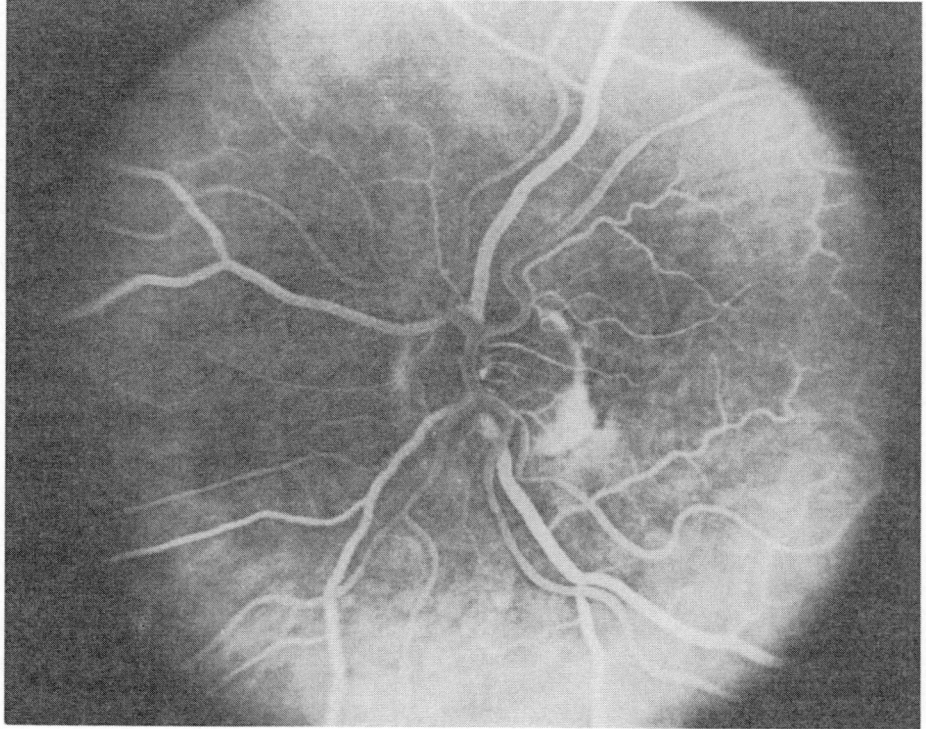

Figure 3b. Fluoroangiogram in the venous phase. The veins are now brightly fluorescent while the arteries are almost devoid of fluorescence.

CLINICAL METHODS OF EXAMINATION

Two methods of ophthalmoscopy are commonly employed, viz. the direct and the indirect method. Direct ophthalmoscopy is the usual method in which a hand-held ophthalmoscope permits examination of the disc area and central fundus with a magnification of approximately $15 \times$. It provides a real image and enables views easiest to interpret by non-ophthalmologists. Dilatation of the pupil is necessary for visualization of the periphery. Indirect ophthalmoscopy, indicated for panoramic views of the fundus, consists of an illuminating system affixed to the examiner's head band and a consensing lens (usually 13 diopters) held between the subject's eye and the examiner. This method has the advantage of a large field, but the disadvantages of a magnification limited to approximately $5 \times$ and an inversion of the (virtual) image. It usually requires a dilated pupil and considerable practice. A further method of examination requiring even further sophistication is the use of slit-lamp biomicroscopy with special lenses on, or close to, the eye. This permits detailed examination of minute details in limited areas.

Fluoroangiography is a method for evaluating circulatory dynamics in the retina (Figure 3a and b). A bolus of fluorescein is injected, usually into the brachial vein. Its entrance and course through the retinal vessels is then monitored in suitably filtered light and recorded by serial photographs. Entering the eye in approximately 10–12 s after the injection the fluorescein first lights up the retinal arteries (the arterial phase) and then causes a laminar illumination of the veins (the venous phase). Full fluorescence of the vein then follows with gradual disappearance after a few minutes from all the vessels. Lighting up of the choroid occurs concomitantly providing a fluorescent background that varies considerably according to the person's complexion. Fluoroangiography is valuable in delineating vessel morphology but more especially for detecting leaks, obstruction to flow, and vasoproliferation.

Ophthalmodynamometry is a method for measurement of blood pressure in the retinal arteries. The test method consists of gradual increase in the intraocular pressure by a calibrated piston or suction device while an examiner observes the retinal arteries ophthalmoscopically. The initial pulsation of the artery occurs at the diastolic pressure whereas the maintained collapse of the artery corresponds to the systolic pressure. Usually the diastolic pressure only is determined and this is normally about half the brachial pressure. Significant lowering of the pressure or differences between the two eyes of more than 20% suggests severe carotid obstructive disease. Ophthalmodynamometry usually contributes little to the study of hypertension; yet in one of our patients with absence of detectable pulses elsewhere it was the only place where the blood pressure could be determined to establish the diagnosis of hypertensive encephalopathy.

Other methods for the study of retinal vessel dynamics, such as the Doppler effect and radiographic wash-outs, are too experimental at present to warrant further description.

THE NORMAL FUNDUS AND AGE-RELATED CHANGES

The retinal vessels have a uniformly diminishing caliber of their lumina with progressive branching. Their walls are invisible. Insofar as they bulge the internal limiting membrane forward they will be capped by a linear light reflex. This and other light reflexes from the surface of the retina move with directional changes of the ophthalmoscope and afford little confusion on ordinary ophthalmoscopic examination but may be a source of confusion in photographs. These retinal reflexes are prominent in young persons but fade in adult eyes leaving only prominent reflexes from the vessels.

Evaluating the diameter of the vessels requires sophisticated judgment. Normally the artery on the nerve head is $\frac{1}{10} - \frac{1}{20}$ the breadth of the disc. In the hyperopic eye the vessels appear small but so does the disc; thus, the proportions remain constant. When the artery branches before surfacing on the disc the several arteries will be proportionately smaller than a single emergent artery.

The background orange or orange-brown color of the fundus is due to the combined effect of the vascular choroidal bed and the overlying pigment epithelium. This latter imparts a dark hue that varies with the individuals' complexion. Unlike the retina the choroid contains arteries with prominent elastica and substantial muscularis. The veins are extraordinarily abundant and communicate with the arteries through a superficial layer of capillary sinuses, the choriocapillaris, beneath the pigment epithelium.

With age, the light reflex from the retinal vessels broadens and often assumes a burnished hue (copper wire). Significant changes occur at the sites of arteriovenous crossing. Whereas in the young this crossing is obliquely angulated and the wall is invisible, in later life the crossing tends toward a right angulation and the wall becomes manifest as a veil silhouetted against the column of blood. At times this veil may become a distinct opacity extending some distance on either side of the crossing and completely hiding the underlying structures. This is commonly referred to as arteriosclerosis, but the evidence that it has anything to do with arteriosclerosis in large vessels is questionable. What is certain, however, is that these sites of arteriovenous crossing with or without opacification of the walls predisposes the veins to obstruction. The portion of the vein peripheral to this site may be relatively distended and occasionally occluded. In the presence of a common adventitia arterial changes may jeopardize the venous flow (see subsequent section on Retinal Vascular Accidents).

Another change which occurs frequently with age, but is even more pronounced with certain diseases, is a tesselated appearance of the background due to attenuation of the pigment epithelium. The interstitial choroidal pigment stands out conspicuously forming an interlacing pattern with the choroidal vessels. This appearance, prominent in darkly pigmented persons, occurs with age but is especially marked in such conditions as retinitis pigmentosa and should not be interpreted as evidence of arteriosclerosis.

THE HYPERTENSIVE FUNDUS

The one reliable sign of hypertension in the fundus is narrowing of the arteries. This may be diffuse and is then non-specific, or focal and has a high degree of specificity. The focal narrowing is often interpreted as spasm but without clear-cut distinction from structural changes. Such focal narrowing and consequent irregularity of the lumina is seen typically in young hypertensives. In older persons the hypertensive abnormalities in the vesssels are less obvious.

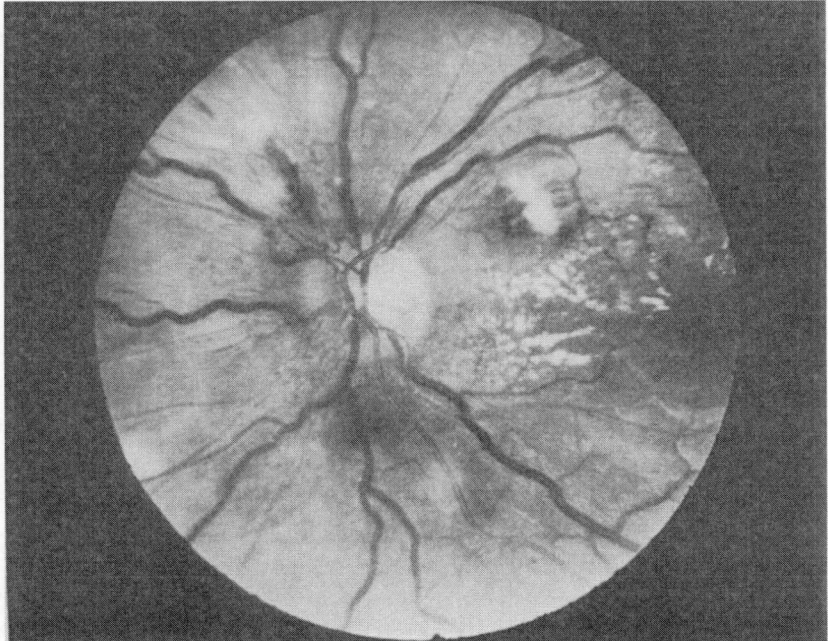

Figure 4. Hypertensive retinopathy. All the arteries are diffusely and segmentally narrow. The splotchy area beneath the superior temporal vessels consists of a cotton-wool spot and a flame-shaped hemorrhage. The more punctate and coalesced spots in the central area represent true exudate. The veins are mildly engorged and tortuous.

Secondary changes include hemorrhages, cotton-wool spots, yellowish-white dots coalescing into masses, papilledema, and detachment of the retina (Figure 4). The hemorrhages are non-specific. They may be flame-shaped when situated in the horizontally coursing nerve fiber layer or they may be punctate when situated in the deeper layers demarcated by the vertically coursing Muller fibers. The cotton-wool spots which are also non-specific occur exclusively in the posterior fundus and represent micro-infarcts of the nerve fiber layer with consequent local obstruction of axoplasmic flow. The term 'soft exudates' for these spots is a misnomer. The yellow-white spots and coalesced masses represent transudate, or resultant lipid, in the middle and deep layers of the retina. Papilledema of hypertensive origin occurs only with severe disease and then usually with hypertensive encephalopathy. Similarly, detachment of the retina secondary to hypertension occurs only in severe disease; it is then bilateral and situated in the dependent portions of the eye. Unlike the common form of retinal detachment associated with a hole in the retina (the rhegmatogenous type) that due to hypertension is a serous type and spontaneously reversible with adequate control of the blood pressure.

The effect of hypertensive retinopathy on vision is too variable to be a reliable index of severity of the retinal changes. The visual acuity may be normal despite extensive retinopathy so long as the macula is neither obscured by hemorrhage nor detached. If either of these occur, the visual loss may be profound.

Although none of these secondary abnormalities are exclusively characteristic of hypertension, some differential points are suggestive. By comparison, diabetic retinopathy shows more of the yellowish, coalesced masses and punctate red dots (microaneurisms and deep hemorrhages) instead of the cotton-wool spots and flame-shaped hemorrhages. Diabetic retinopathy also tends to be more confined to the posterior portions of the fundus and to be accompanied by proliferation of vessels into the vitreous. The retinopathy of the collagenoses, on the other hand, tend to have more cotton-wool spots and fewer hemorrhages so long as hypertension is not also present. The features of retinal vascular accidents as distinct from hypertensive retinopathy will be dealt with in a subsequent section.

CLASSIFICATION OF HYPERTENSIVE RETINOPATHY

Numerous attempts have been made to classify hypertensive retinopathy. The most popular has been the following four categories of Keith, Wagner, and Barker [1].

Grade I: Minimal narrowing of the retinal vessels.

Grade II: Widened light reflex; arteriovenous crossing phenomena; and focal narrowing.

Grade III: Retinal edema, cotton-wool spots, hemorrhages and narrowing of arteries.

Grade IV: Papilledema in addition to the foregoing signs.

This classification leaves much to be desired [2]. Types I and II do not clearly distinguish between hypertensive changes and age-related ('arteriosclerotic') changes [3]. The categories do not differentiate the hypertensive changes in the young and old [4]. The criteria are so ill-defined that different observers come up with quite different typing [5]. Most serious, it seems to me, is the tendency to automatically classify patients into Type III if they have hemorrhages and other retinopathy, and into Type IV if they have papilledema. Hemorrhagic retinopathy may result from an anticoagulative tendency or vascular abnormality occurring incidentally in a patient with mild hypertension. Similarly, papilledema may be only coincidentally related to the hypertension and not a valid basis for the classification. The error of such an erroneous typing was impressed on me when a patient with mild hypertension and severe papilledema was grouped as Grade IV and accordingly operated upon with disastrous consequences. Only at autopsy was he discovered to have had pseudotumor cerebri and nothing that could have been attributed to hypertension.

It may be that no one hard and fast classification for hypertensive changes may be possible. Indeed one group of authors [2] concluded that the best classification 'is that based on the separate eye ground features themselves, classified on a two-point scale – present or absent.' Yet for statistical purposes we are pressurized into a digital format. The coding which I found most useful in a large series being screened for possible anti-hypertensive surgery was based on the tendency for differential involvement of the different arteries:

Grade I: Few localized constrictions and possibly minimal diffuse narrowing of the nasal arteries with no involvement of the temporal arteries.

Grade II: Diffuse narrowing of the nasal arteries in addition to localized constriction in the inferior temporal artery with little or no involvement of the superior temporal artery.

Grade III: Diffuse and localized constriction in all retinal arteries but not extreme and usually unaccompanied by conspicuous ensheathing of the arterial walls.

Grade IV: Extreme narrowing of all arteries with, usually, ensheathing of one or more branches.

In the foregoing, hemorrhagic and other changes were noted and taken into consideration for prognostic purposes but were not used as a basis for classification. Age was also taken into account with the tacit assumption that the classification based on narrowing had progressively less validity as the patient was older and the vessels were more 'sclerotic'.

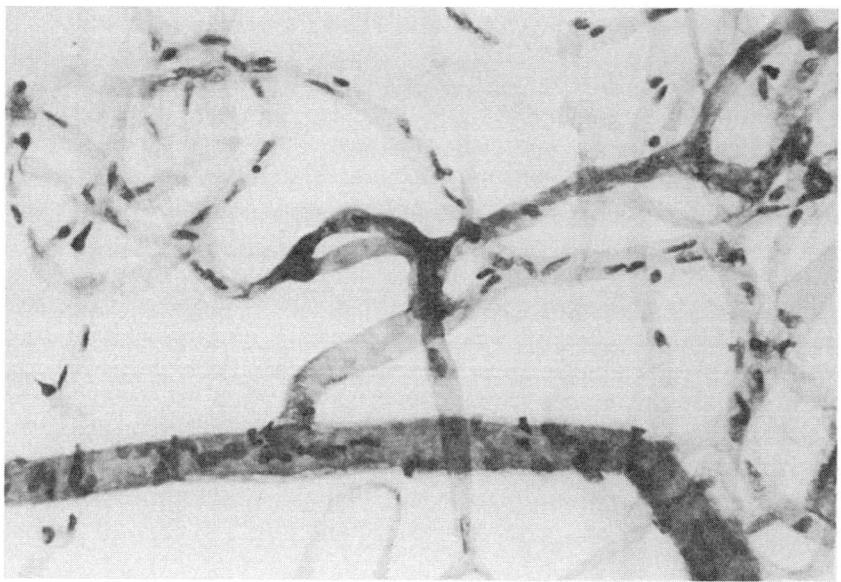

Figure 5. Trypsin digest of the retinal vessels from a patient with hypertension. Note-worthy are the focal increase in stain (PAS) and narrowing of some capillaries. Although the endothelial and mural cells are present in most of the capillaries a few of the capillaries are completely devoid of cells. PAS stain; obj. 25; oc. 10. (Photo from Arch Ophth 65:708–716, 1961.)

PATHOLOGY

Cross-sectional microscopy of eyes with hypertensive retinopathy reveal little more than the expected secondary changes. Narrowing of the arteries, the clinical hallmark of hypertensive retinopathy, is conspicuous only in severe cases. Barring retinal vascular accidents the abnormalities are entirely non-specific. Free blood may be present in all layers of the retina but tend to be especialy massive in the inner layers. What appeared to be cotton-wool spots clinically turn out to be focal swellings of the nerve fibers pathologically. Because they contain aggregates simulating cells they are known microscopically as cytoid bodies; actually they represent debris from focal obstructions of axoplasmic flow. The yellow dots and coalesced masses seen clinically correspond to serum transudate and serum-derived lipid in the deep layers of the retina. Where detached, the retina is separated from the pigment epithelium by serum.

In contrast to the meager information provided by cross-sectional microscopy the changes revealed in trypsin digest preparations are more definite [6]. This method of preparation consists of digesting formalin-fixed whole retinas with trypsin until all neurogial structures are released. The resultant vascular tree is stained by the hematoxylin–periodic acid Schiff method and mounted on a glass slide for microscopy. Preparations from hypertensive patients show a relative acellularity and increased basement membrane staining of the precapillary arteriole as it leaves the parent trunk. This is the minimal manifestation. With further hypertensive retinopathy focal occlusion of the capillaries and loss of capillary endothelium will be added to the precapillary changes. Whether these abnormalities represent a widespread capillaropathy or are peculiar to the retina has yet to be established.

RETINAL VASCULAR ACCIDENTS

Hypertensive patients are at risk of developing vascular accidents in their fundi. It is appropriate, therefore, to comment briefly on the various types of accidents. Most accidents are due either to occlusion of the retinal vessels or of the anterior orbital arteries (posterior ciliary arteries) which supply the

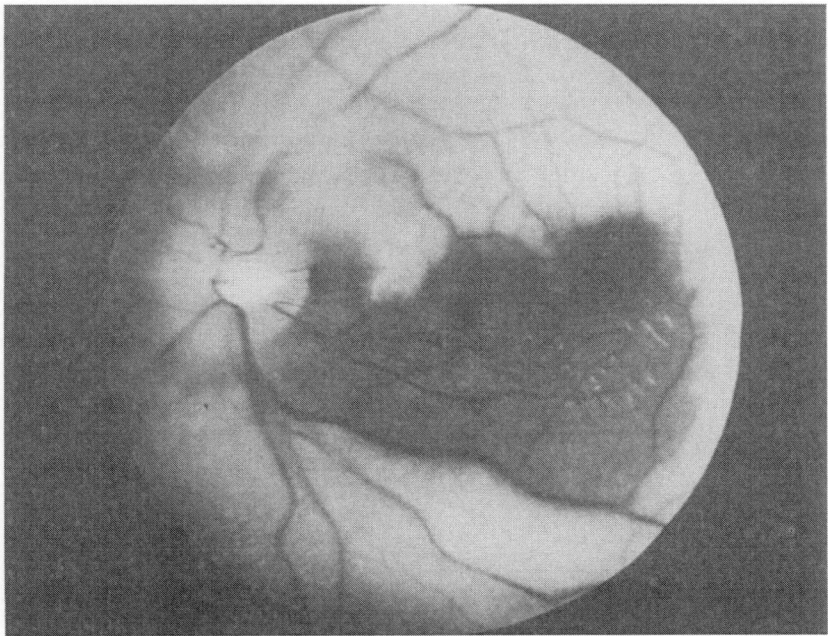

Figure 6. Fresh occlusion of central retinal artery with sharply demarcated sparing of region corresponding to distribution of cilioretinal supply. The dense opacity is due to cloudy swelling of the ganglion cells.

nerve head. The former includes occlusion of the retinal arteries or of the retinal veins or of their branches.

Occlusion of the central retinal artery. This results in a sudden, usually painless, blindness. At times it is preceded by transient black-outs, but once it occurs it is usually permanent. Within a few hours the central area becomes white excepting the most foveal area where the pristine choroidal reflex is preserved as a cherry-red spot. The opacification is due to cloudy swelling of the ganglion cells (Figure 6) and disappears after two to three weeks as the ganglion cells die. The disc then takes on the pallor of optic atrophy.

Branch occlusion shows a similar but segmental opacity of the retina with abrupt borders and corresponding visual field defect. In neither the central nor the branch occlusion are there more than an occasional hemorrhage or transudative features that occur with other types of vascular retinopathy.

The site of occlusion in the central retinal artery is often hidden in the nerve substance so that the clinician is handicapped in ascertaining the cause of the occlusion. With branch occlusion the site of the obstruction is usually at the origin of the branch. Such cases presumably result from thickening of the wall.

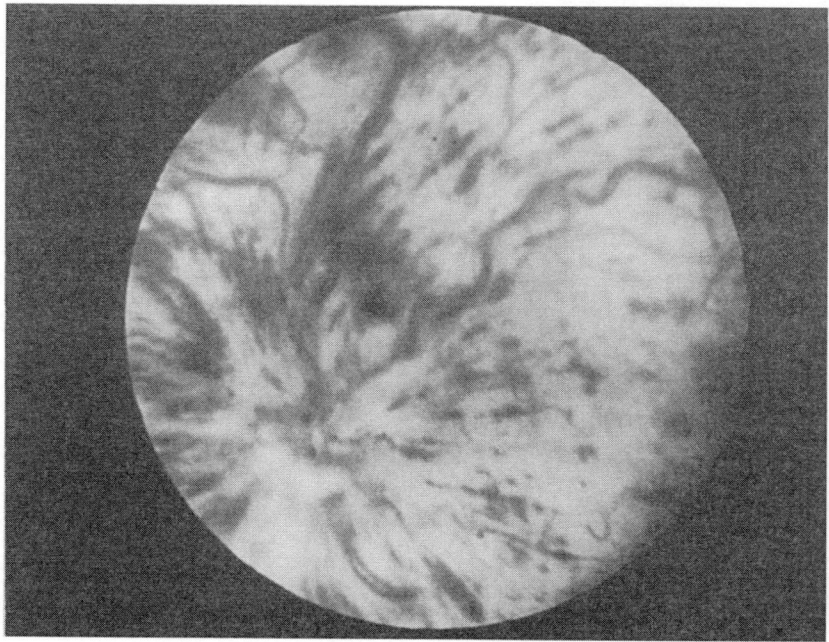

Figure 7. Occlusion of the central retinal vein. The engorged and tortuous veins, together with the arteries and optic disc, are largely hidden by the extensive hemorrhages. These are flame-shaped following the normal distribution of nerve fibers.

On the other hand, most retinal artery occlusions are embolic in origin. Calcific emboli of cardiac or carotid origin lodge preferably at the entrance site of the vessel into the eye, the lamina cribosa, where the fibrous restraint impedes the distensible molding of the vessel. Emboli here are not visible but fragments of the calcific emboli break off and pass onto the disc or into the retina where they become visible as chalk-white intravascular inclusions. The other common embolus is lipid which derives from an ulcerated carotid atheroma. In contrast to the calcific particles these lipid emboli are yellowish, and often multiple, extending into many retinal branches. Cholesterol crystals are a subvariety that are recognizible by their highly reflectile appearance; they are called Hollenhorst plaques [7].

Myxomatous emboli are so rare that most are unrecognized. Yet of all the types this one is perhaps most important, since early identification of the cause and removal of the cardiac myxoma may be life saving.

Local treatment of occlusive arterial disease by anticoagulants, paracentesis, inhalation of CO_2-O_2, or ocular massage is of equivocal benefit. As in the case of myxomatous emboli, therapy should be directed to elimination of the extraocular cause with the hope of preventing further ocular or neurologic deterioration.

Occlusion of the central retinal vein. This is a relatively common vascular accident in the eye. The subjective impairment may be a blur, a severe visual loss or some degree inbetween. Complete blindness is most exceptional unless the retinal artery is also obstructed. The typical ophthalmoscopic appearance in a fresh case is that of massive hemorrhage ('the squashed tomato fundus') which hides all retinal details and obscures the disc margins (Figure 7). The veins emerging over the hemorrhage are grotesquely distended and tortuous. Less degrees of occlusion show correspondingly few hemorrhages and less venous stasis. The site of occlusion of the central retinal vein is at the lamina cribosa where the artery and vein are closely confined in a common and indistensible sheath. The presumption is that the pressure of a rigid artery induces the stasis in the vein and consequent thrombosis. At risk are patients with hypertension, diabetes, multiple myeloma or hyperthrombocythemia and patients with the increased intraocular pressure of glaucoma. With recanalization and establishment of peripapillary anastomosis with the choroid the hemorrhages gradually absorb and considerable recovery of vision may result. However, in a substantial perecentage of the cases a particularly painful form of glaucoma develops in a matter of weeks or months and destroys all useful function.

Branch vein occlusion shows a similar fundus appearance in a sector of the fundus. The obstructive site is at an arteriovenous crossing. Bypass anastomosis ultimately restores the circulation, and the hemorrhagic glaucoma that occurs with central vein occlusion does not follow branch occlusion.

418

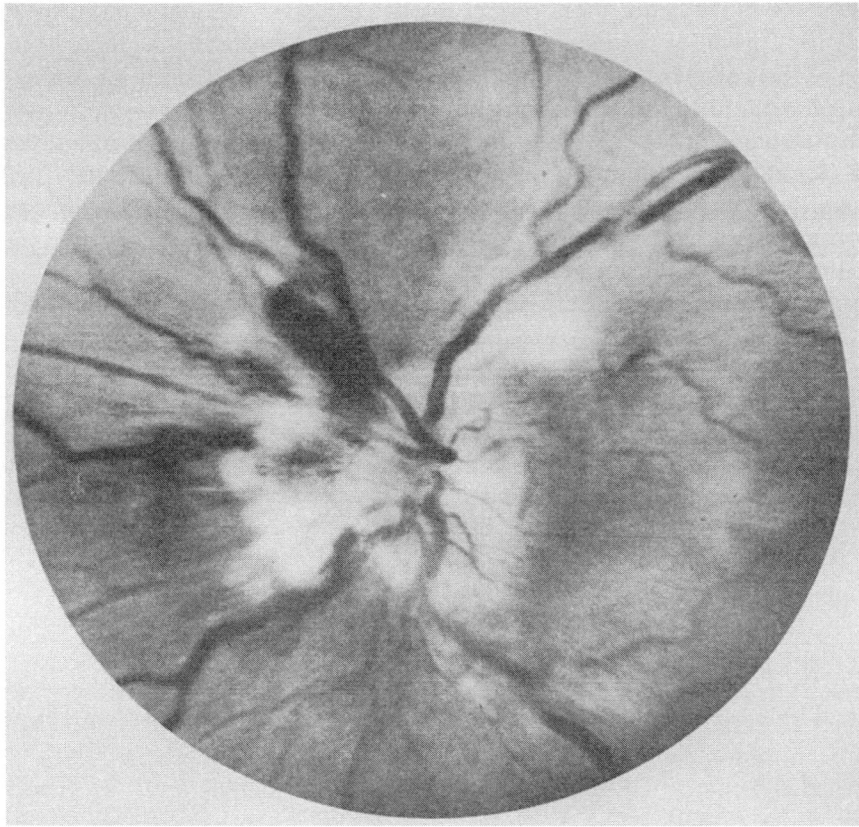

Figure 8. Ischemic optic neuropathy. Characteristic is swelling of the disc with peripapillary hemorrhagic and cotton-wool spots. The appearance may simulate papilledema but is distinguished by the severe visual loss.

Optic nerve ischemia. This is another ocular vascular accident to which hypertensive patients are predisposed. This ischemia results from reduced flow in the posterior ciliary arteries which normally supply the optic nerve. It is generally attributed to arteriosclerosis, but the anatomic evidence for this is yet to be established. The onset is precipitous blindness, complete or partial, occurring spontaneously or after an episode of blood loss. The fundus shows initially a swelling of the disc and a few peripapillary hemorrhages (Figure 8). This is later replaced by optic atrophy and variable field defects. In approximately half the patients the other eye becomes similarly involved in a matter of months and then presents with papilledema in one eye and optic atrophy in the other.

REFERENCES

1. Keith NM, Wagner HP, Barber MW: Some different types of essential hypertension. Their course and prognosis. Amer J Med Sci 197:332–343, 1939.
2. Svärdsudd K, Wedel H, Aurell E, Tibblin G: Hypertensive eye ground changes. Prevalence relation to blood pressure and prognostic importance. The study of men born in 1913. Acta Med Scand 204:159–67, 1978.
3. Breslin DJ, Gifford RW, Fairbairn JF Kearns TP: Prognostic importance of ophthalmoscopic findings in essential hypertension. J Amer Med Assoc 195:335–338, 1966.
4. Pickering GW: High blood pressure. New York: Grune & Stratton, 1955.
5. Kagan A, Aurell E, Dobree J, Hara K, McKendrick C, Michaelson I, Shaper G, Sandaresan T, Tibblin G: A note on signs in the fundus oculi and arterial hypertension: conventional assessment and significance. Bull WHo 34:955–960, 1966.
6. Kuwabara T, Cogan DG: Studies of retinal vascular patterns. Pt I normal architecture. Arch Ophthalmol 64:904–911, 1960.
7. Hollenhorst RW: Significance of bright plaques in the retinal arterioles. Trans Am Ophthalmol Soc 59:252–273, 1961.

27. INFLUENCE OF HYPERTENSION ON THE HEART

R. C. TARAZI

A. GENERAL CONSIDERATIONS

Hypertension is one of the commonest causes of left ventricular hypertrophy and of congestive heart failure, at least amongst the adult population in westernized nations [1, 2]. This strong association between elevated arterial pressure and heart disease has commonly been explained as a simple sequence of cardiac overload leading to myocardial hypertrophy and eventual failure. However, the spectrum of cardiac involvement by the hypertensive process is much wider than a pump response to an increased afterload [3] (Table 1).

Most studies of hypertensive heart disease in the past were based on associations between systemic pressure levels and evidence of cardiac enlargement [4]. Conclusions were, therefore, tentative at best either because of the poor reliability of the signs of ventricular hypertrophy or because of the frequency (in post-mortem series) of coronary atherosclerosis. It was difficult under these conditions to define the role of coronary arterial disease or of other causes of myocardial insults in the development of 'hyperten-

Table 1. Cardiac involvement by hypertension

1. Pressure overload
   a. Direct effect on heart
   b. Indirect effect; increased risk of coronary atherosclerosis
2. Complication of causal disease
   a. Fluid retention as in renal disease
   b. Myocarditis as in renal disease, pheochromocytoma
   c. Pericarditis as in autoimmune diseases, uremia
3. Secondary antihypertensive therapy
   a. Fluid retention (most drugs except for- propranolol and diuretics)
   b. Interference with adrenergic support
   c. Pulmonary hypertension (hyperkinetic or congestive)
4. Postulated neural or humoral effects in some type
   a. Angiotensin myocarditis
   b. Excessive cardioadrenergic drive

From Tarazi et al. [3] (Reproduced with permission).

Amery, A. (ed.) Hypertensive Cardiovascular Disease: Pathophysiology and Treatment
© *1982, Martinus Nijhoff Publishers. The Hague / Boston / London*
ISBN-13: 978-94-009-7478-4

sive' heart disease. The advent of coronary arteriography has since demon-strated that ventricular hypertrophy can develop in hypertensive patients in the absence of coronary disease. More recently, echocardiography has re-vealed a complex picture of myocardial alterations in hypertension; not only can left ventricular hypertrophy be seen very early in the disease [5], but it also appears to respond unexpectedly and rapidly to changes in blood pressure [6].

There is currently a marked renewal of interest in defining the role of the heart in hypertension and particularly in assessing more precisely the car-diac impact of increased arterial pressure. In this process, many notions may have to be modified; thus, although hypertension is commonly defined in terms of diastolic pressure levels, the high diastolic pressure bears only an indirect relationship to cardiac load since the heart's work is defined by the systolic pressure it has to generate. Until recently studies of the heart in hypertension were all too often restricted to determinations of cardiac out-put. There was some delay in the application of more precise indices of cardiac performance to hypertension, in great part because of the inadvisa-bility of left ventricular catheterization in essentially asymptomatic patients. The advent of non-invasive reliable techniques has, therefore, led to a much-needed reassessment of the cardiac impact of hypertension. The effect of increased afterload on cardiac performance has been studied extensively, but in other diseases on experimental models the results obtained did not necessarily apply to the conditions of human hypertension. One of the main reasons for this limitation is the influence of time on ventricular adaptation to the increased load. Both the rate of development of hypertension and its chronicity may influence cardiac responses, so that the situation in essential hypertension is not strictly similar to that produced experimentally by aortic banding.

There are other reasons for the difficulties in extrapolating to hyperten-sion results from aortic stenosis or from studies utilizing aortic constriction. What is often overlooked is the role of the arterial tree in influencing cardiac performance; the aorta and large vessels are involved in accommodating to changes in stroke volume or speed of ejection [7, 8]. Experiments with aor-tic banding prevent or restrict this adaptive role of the large vessels. Coro-nary blood flow is driven by a high head of pressure in hypertension by a relatively low pressure in aortic stenosis. These factors and others can con-siderably influence cardiac responses to increased afterload.

B. PATHOPHYSIOLOGICAL CONSIDERATIONS

1. Arterial pressure and afterload

The diastolic or the mean arterial pressure levels are commonly used as indices of the severity of hypertension, but the pressure load imposed on the heart in hypertension is not adequately defined by either of them. The cardiac impact of hypertension is to a large degree dependent on the increased resistance to left ventricular ejection; that resistance is determined by the instantaneous relationship of pressure and flow during systole ('aortic impedance') [9]. Expressed in a slightly simplified form, outflow impedance includes, amongst other components, a compliant and a resistive component. The former is the sum of those forces opposing a change in the volume of the arterial bed, the latter opposes the run-off of blood from the arterial tree (the total peripheral resistance). It is obvious that neither the diastolic nor mean arterial pressure nor the total peripheral resistance accurately reflect the resistance to ejection from the left ventricle and hence the full extent of the increased work of the heart in hypertension. A closer approximation is given by the systolic blood pressure, which is the pressure that the heart has to develop for effective ejection. A correct measure of 'afterload' (the load that the myocardium begins to bear after beginning its contraction) is given by calculations of aortic impedance [9]. Since this is difficult to obtain in man, an approximation could be derived by adapting the classical resistance formula (R = P/F) to systolic events. Mean resistance to ejection can be calculated as the ration of mean systolic pressure to sytolic flow [10].

The cardiac load in hypertension can also be estimated from the stress that the increased pressure imposes on the ventricular wall. Wall stress is determined by the intraventricular pressure (P), the size and shape of the left ventricle and the thickness of its wall and can be expressed [11]:

$$\sigma = \frac{Pr}{w},\qquad(1)$$

in which r is radium and w is wall thickness. For the left ventricle, meridional wall stress (σ_m) can be approximated from the following calculation described by Grossman et al. [12]:

$$\sigma_m = \frac{P \times EDD}{h\left(1 + \dfrac{h}{EDD}\right)},\qquad(2)$$

where EDD is the internal ventricular diameter measured at end-diastole, and h is the left ventricular (LV) posterior wall thickness. Left ventricular dimensions can be obtained from adequate echocardiographic tracings while systolic pressure reading are approximated from the usual auscultatory arterial pressure measurement [13]. Thus, LV stress can be evaluated by non-invasive methods and its alterations monitored during the evolution of hypertension and its response to treatment. The level of LV wall stress influences cardiac performance markedly; the higher the wall stress the smaller the stroke volume, the lower the ejection fraction and the slower the velocity of ejection.

It is obvious from (1) that wall stress at any given pressure is determined by the ratio of wall thickness to cavity radius or (by extension) to the ratio of LV mass to LV volume [14]. These considerations have important practical implications with respect to not only the evaluation of cardiac conditions in hypertensive patients, but also the effects of antihypertensive therapy on left ventricular mass and function.

2. Ventricular hypertrophy

The development of left ventricular hypertrophy (LVH) is a landmark in the clinical evolution of hypertension (see below). The increased wall thickness reduces wall stress; whether hypertrophy improves or impairs cardiac performance is a hotly debated subject [15]. In this context, two aspects need to be taken into account. One is the effect of hypertrophy on the heart viewed as a muscle, and the other its effect on cardiac performance as a pump. Although obviously closely allied, the two are not synonymous.

One of the clearest conclusions that has emerged from recent studies is that all types of cardiac hypertrophy are *not* similar either in myocardial composition or in functional consequences [16]. Even within the same type of hypertrophy (that resulting from increased pressure load), differences can be found depending on, amongst other factors, the rapidity with which the load is imposed, on the mechanism of rise in pressure and on associated disease. Thus, conclusions from the enormous literature covering other clinical or experimental models cannot be extrapolated without verification to hypertension. Hypertension itself is not a homogenous disease either and hence it is not surprising that the reported alterations in cardiac performance in hypertensive states have covered a wide spectrum from increased to decreased function. The experience of many has been that the ventricular hypertrophy of increased pressure load is associated with diminished contractility. Hearts from hypertensive animals were found unable to eject the same stroke volume as normal hearts at equivalent levels of LV end-diastolic pressure [17]. Consonant with these observations were those of Lund-Johansen [18] who reported the restricted ability of even young hypertensive subjects (from 17 to 20 years old) to increase stroke volume with exercise. These findings have been related to diminished myocardial function or even 'incipient cardiac insufficiency'. However, an alternative explanation is possible. The hypertensive myocardium contains excess hydroxyproline [1]; a diminished ability to increase stroke volume may well result from increased collagen reducing ventricular compliance [3, 17].

424

Table 2. Characterization of left ventricular hypertrophy in hypertension

A. Based on distribution:
   a. Concentric
   b. Asymmetric septal hypertrophy
B. Based on wall stress:
   a. Appropriate: wall stress normalized
   b. Inappropriate: high h/r or LVM/LVV ratio
   c. Inadequate: high stress (low h/r or LVM/LVV)

h/r: wall thickness to radius
LVM/LVV: left ventricular mass to left ventricular volume

In addition to any intrinsic effect of hypertrophy on myocardial contractility, its net effect on pump performance will also be influenced by the way in which it alters ventricular geometry [12, 20]. Ventricular hypertrophy could be defined as *appropriate* if it normalizes wall stress by counterbalancing the increase in wall tension. On this basis, a new classification of hypertrophy has emerged based on the ratio of wall thickness to chamber radius or on the ratio of left ventricular mass to left ventricular volume (Table 2). The full functional implications of these different types still need to be elucidated. Early results in man indicate that inadequate hypertrophy (low mass–volume ratio or thickness–radius ratio) is associated with high ventricular stress, diminished ejection fraction and, possibly, reduced coronary reserve [14].

Another important influence on cardiac performance, particularly in man, is the level of *adrenergic support* available. The heart's ability to sustain an increased pressure load is remarkably dependent on the level of sympathetic activity [21]. The development of LVH in hypertensive animals seems to be associated with a reduced inotropic responsiveness to isoproterenol [22] and possibly with diminished numbers of beta-adrenergic receptors [23]. Saragoca and Tarazi [24] have recently suggested that a subtle shift occurs in experimental hypertensive LVH from dependence on adrenergic support to meet additional work loads to greater reliance on the Frank-Sterling mechanism. In man, the level of cardioadrenergic drive varies widely amongst patients [25, 26], as does the net cardiac effect of sympatholytic or beta-blocking therapy.

3. Coronary blood flow in hypertension

Clinicians have long suspected that myocardial perfusion might be impaired in hypertension. Initial studies, however, showed rather consistently that coronary blood flow per unit mass of myocardium was within normal. Only more recently has the problem been examined in more detail, particularly as regards response of coronary vessels to vasodilator stimuli and the distribution of flow between the endocardium and epicardium [27].

Most studies have indeed confirmed that coronary flow in pressure-LVH was usually normal at rest (in proportion to myocardial mass). However, in response to vasodilator stimuli there was often, albeit not always, found a reduced capacity for coronary vasodilation [28–30]. Apparently, a greater portion of that capacity must have been used to maintain an adequate myocardial perfusion at rest, leaving a reduced coronary vascular reserve. The extent of that reduction differed widely amongst various studies but this is not surprising given the large number of factors that can influence coronary vasodilation. These include the relation of coronary perfusion pressure to degree of LVH and the extent of structural changes in the coronary vessels. In cases with reduced coronary reserve, the coronary flow might not be able to meet the additional demands imposed by increased cardiac work. Under these conditions, the subendocardial region would be at particular risk of ischemic injury [28].

Antihypertensive therapy can influence coronary blood flow in many ways. Fears that therapeutic lowering of a raised blood pressure would lead to coronary insufficiency or to myocardial infarction have *not,* in our experience, been substantiated. On the contrary, reduction of the pressure load and, therefore, of the excessive myocardial oxygen requirements, will help relieve coronary insufficiency and reduce anginal episodes. It is important, however, to avoid in cardiac or in older patients the reflex tachycardia and hyperkinetic circulation that occur with some vasodilators, such as hydralazine diazoxide or minoxidil. In addition to these early pharmacologic effects, one must also consider the long-term consequences of antihypertensive therapy on cardiac hypertrophy and on the coronary vessels.

Wicker and Tarazi found that in rats with renovascular hypertension, reversal of LVH led to restoration of coronary vascular reserve if the latter had been reduced by the hypertrophy. Of particular importance in that respect is the relation between arterial pressure and myocardial mass. Parallel changes in both do not greatly alter coronary blood flow per gram ventricular weight, but reduction of blood pressure without reversal of hypertrophy was associated with a significant reduction in coronary flow response to maximal vasodilation. It is obvious that much remains to be elucidated regarding the coronary effects of prolonged antihypertensive therapy. The situation becomes even more complex if, in addition to the effects of hypertension and of cardiac hypertrophy, are added those of coronary atherosclerosis. Interference with the vasodilating capacity of coronary vessels may aggravate the effects of a coronary stenosis or obstruction.

C. CLINICAL ASPECTS

Cardiac involvement in hypertension is *not* restricted to a ventricular hypertrophy in parallel with the degree of blood pressure elevation. Careful clinical examination will yield important diagnostic data due to the many conditions listed in Table 1, such as the distended neck veins of fluid overload or the bounding arterial pulses and hyperactive apical impulse of hyperkinetic circulation. Subtle signs of cardiac involvement may be revealed by careful palpation of the apex and auscultation for atrial and ventricular diastolic gallop. Technical advances tend sometimes to obscure the wealth of information available from clinical examination; thus, a sustained cardiac apical impulse is a sensitive and quite accurate sign of concentric LVH, certainly more so than a chest X-ray. An accurate history of orthopnea or exertional dyspnea may be the only symptoms of beginning cardiac decompensation that could culminate in acute pulmonary edema or congestive heart failure [31].

1. *Left ventricular hypertrophy in hypertension*

All observers agree on the serious turn of events when signs of LVH appear in the course of hypertension [2, 32]. Even before decompensation occurs, cardiac output is reduced both at rest [33] and during exercise [18] in patients with definite evidence of LVH. By the time the cardiothoracic ratio exceed 50%, LV end-diastolic pressure is usually elevated, although the patient can still be asymptomatic [33]. Sokolow and Perloff [32] have shown in subgroups of hypertensive patients classified by degree of ECG abnormality, that the presence of an increased cardiac transverse diameter was associated with a higher mortality rate. One cannot therefore, await the development of such time-honored and evident signs of cardiac enlargement.

The electrocardiogram is a more sensitive toll than the chest X-ray to detect the concentric LVH of hypertension. The voltage criteria of McPhie (sum of tallest precordial R and S>45 mm, with or without associated 'strain pattern') are quite useful because of their relatively high sensitivity without excessive 'false positives'. A still earlier sign of cardiac involvement is ECG evidence of left atrial enlargement which may be found in the absence of EKG signs of LVH [34]. An abnormal P wave thus can constitute the sole sign of cardiac involvement in some hypertensive patients. This may be associated in many patients with a more accentuated atrial wave in the apex cardiogram (high a/H ratio) [35]. At the bedside, the forcible atrial contraction is reflected in an audible fourth sound with the patient at rest and supine [34]. These signs do not indicate atrial involvement anteceding ventricular hypertrophy, but reflect that atrial overload secondary to diminished compliance of the 'hypertrophying' left ventricle. In fact, there is growing evidence that infringement on the diastolic function of the left ventricle may well constitute one of the earliest signs of cardiac involvement by hypertension. Fouad et al. [36] described a reduced rate of left ventricular filling in hypertensive patients in whom cardiac output, ejection fraction and velocity of ejection were still normal. These early signs, be they hemodynamic or electrocardiographic, are particularly important for two reasons: they may be detected before unequivocal signs of LVH are evident and they may help evaluate the functional impact of slight increases in LV wall thickness.

Determination of LV mass and wall thickness are now available from *echocardiography,* a relative newcomer but a most valuable tool in the evaluation of hypertensive patients. It can reveal very early thickening of the ventricular walls and increases in LV mass when both the EKG and chest X-rays are normal; at the same time, it allows the recognition of coincident valvular heart disease or ischemic myocardial damage. Many studies have reported that echocardiographic estimates of left ventricular function and mass compared favorably with angiographic findings, but many are the pitfalls of quantitative determinations. The sensitivity and limitations of the method require more precise definition before one places too much reliance on the 'security' of numbers offered by a computer print-out. The more complete view of the cardiac chambers obtained from 2-D echocardiography has been very helpful, but exact measurements by this technique are time-consuming and need improved resolution of details.

Early observations by Dunn et al. [37] have confirmed our initial observations regarding the importance of atrial signs in the diagnosis of LVH. Different centers, particularly from Europe, have reported a sizeable incidence of asymmetric septal hypertrophy (ASH), particularly in early hypertension [38, 39]. It has even been suggested that the earliest changes with either the development of LV hypertrophy or its reversal occur in the septal wall [39]. This, however, needs confirmation; although the prevalence of ASH was estimated to be as high as 20–25% by some, other investigators encountered it rarely among their hypertensive patients. Discrepancies among reported series may be related to the stage of hypertension, prevalence of therapy in the group investigated and difficulties in precise delineation of septal thickness. More studies are needed to define the role of hypertension in ASH and the relationship, if any, between hypertensive heart disease and hypertrophic cardiomyopathy.

Echocardiography has also been particularly valuable in determining the performance of the hypertensive hypertrophied heart. The simultaneous noninvasive determination of both left ventricular wall thickness and cavity diameter allows an estimate of wall stress. This proved very helpful in outlining more precisely the impact of different types of hypertrophy on ven-

428

tricular performance. Guazzi et al. [40] contrasted the increased rate of circumferential fiber shortening (Vcf) in patients with concentric ventricular
hypertrophy (increased wall thickness but normal or reduced LV internal
diameter) with the reduced Vcf and impaired performance in patients whose
left ventricular hypertrophy was associated with left ventricular enlargement. The level of ventricular performance amongst their hypertensive
patients was inversely related to the degree of LV stress (Figure 1a and 1b).
These observations are in basic agreement with the studies of Strauer [14],
Gaasch [20], and others, in pointing out the importance of the type of ventricular hypertrophy on the cardiac manifestations of hypertension.

Important as these biophysical considerations are, they are not the only
determinants of cardiac function in hypertensive patients. Alterations in
myocardial contractility, in cardioadrenergic drive and it is not always easy
to define the relative roles they play. Careful individual evaluation will help
select the appropriate approach to therapy. In that evaluation, the relation
between arterial pressure levels and cardiac status deserves particular consideration.

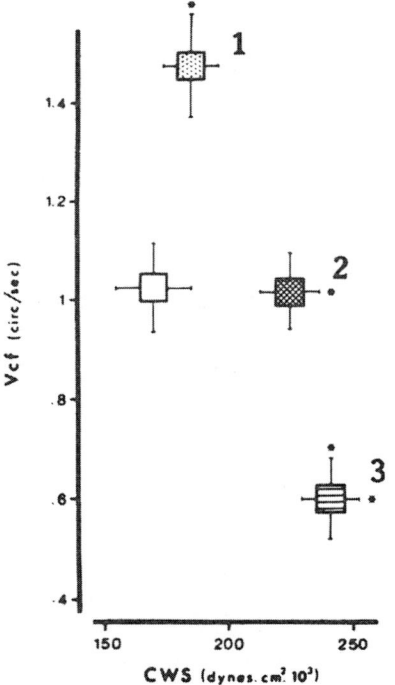

Figure 1a. Circumferential fiber shortening (Vcf) is clearly inversely related to
the circumferential wall stress (CWS) in
three groups of hypertensive patients. 1)
nomal-sized hearts; 2) left ventricular
concentric hypertrophy; and 3) left ventricular hypertrophy and dilation. (Reproduced with permission from [40], Am
J Cardiol 44:1007, 1979.)

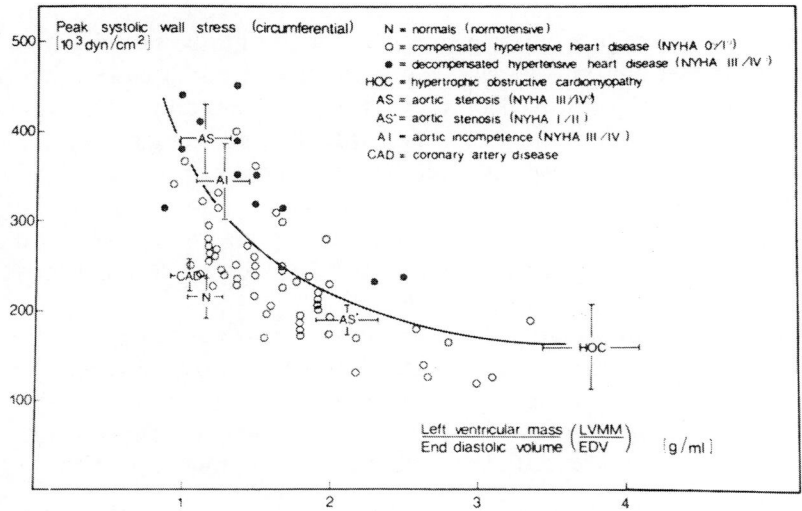

Figure 1b. The same observations illustrated in Figure 1a were also shown by invasive studies of Strauer [14] (Reproduced with permission from Am J Cardiol 44:1007–1012, 1979.)

2. Relationship between blood pressure levels and cardiac hypertrophy in hypertension

Left ventricular hypertrophy with or without dilation is considered a characteristic autopsy finding in hypertension [4]. It is important to point out that the degree of hypertrophy is more closely related to systolic than to diastolic pressure levels. The results of the Framingham studies [1, 2] have clearly indicated that closer attention must be given to systolic pressure levels than is usually done in planning antihypertensive therapy and evaluating response to treatment.

Even with those qualifications, the quantitative relationship between arterial pressure levels and cardiac hypertrophy, albeit significant, is not close. Normal hearts can be seen at autopsy despite severe and prolonged hypertension. On the other hand, enlarged hearts can be found in patients with modest pressure elevation [41, 42]. Definite cardiac hypertrophy is being increasingly recognized in young children and adolescents with borderline hypertension [5], while Sen and associates [43] reported increased ventricular weight in spontaneously hypertensive rats before the development of significant or sustained hypertension.

These exceptions from the expected parallelism between rise in arterial pressure and increase in cardiac weight could be caused by many factors [44]. In man, the complicating effect of coronary arterial disease may play an important role in determining the cardiac response. Indeed, it was thought at one time that hypertension *per se* might not be a sufficient cause for heart disease, but only an aggravating factor in other diseases. This concept has since been disproved in man, as it was in experimental hypertension [3]. Raab [45] had initially suggested that adrenergic disturbances should be considered factors modulating the increase in cardiac size with hypertension. Recent experimental studies with antihypertensive therapy appear to support this hypothesis: good blood pressure control could not *per se* reverse ventricular hypertrophy if the drugs used led to concomitant increase of cardio-adrenergic drive [46].

In summary, a dissociation between blood pressure level and degree of cardiac hypertrophy has so often been documented that, besides pressure, other factors must be playing a significant role in hypertensive heart disease. Their identification is important not only for academic reasons but also because they may influence therapeutic plans attempting reversal of hypertrophy.

3. The cardiac effects of antihypertensive therapy

There is no doubt regarding the life saving value of antihypertensive therapy. Introduction of the first effective drugs led to rapid decline in the cardiac complications and mortality from hypertension [31]. The indications and choice of therapy are discussed elsewhere in this book. However, it seemed important to include here a short review of two items relating specifically to the heart.

a) Secondary cardiac effects of antihypertensive drugs
There are occasions when certain antihypertensive drugs impose an undue strain on the heart or impair its performance through a variety of mechanisms. These include fluid retention withdrawal or blocking of adrenergic support to the myocardium and excessive cardiac stimulation.

i) Fluid retention. Fluid retention and hypervolemia secondary to antihypertensive therapy were first recognized with the introduction of ganglion-blocking drugs. They were subsequently demonstrated to occur with practically all antihypertensive agents except diuretics and beta-blockers [47]. In some instances, the retention may be such as to simulate or even actually precipitate cardiac failure [48].

ii) Interference with adrenergic support to the heart. Adrenergic stimulation is one of the main mechanisms that help the heart to cope with excess demands. Withdrawal or blockade of that support may, under certain conditions, lead to cardiac failure, as was shown both experimentally [49] and in some patients with cardiac disease [50]. Despite the widespread use of sympatholytics and more recently of beta-adrenergic blockers, cardiac decompensation occurred only rarely as a complication of this form of therapy [51]. This is probably because of the simultaneous reduction of cardiac load (blood pressure control), whereas in patients with valvular or coronary heart disease, sympathetic inhibition does not alter the underlying heart problem. Still, cardiac decompensation can occur with these drugs in some hypertensive subjects as reported by Guazzi et al. [52]. Tests of cardiac performance before and after propranolol may help identify patients at special risk of this complication [53]. A minimally invasive approach (Swan-Ganz balloon catheter introduced percutaneously) can be used to determine the effect of increased arterial pressure on the pulmonary wedge pressure. A load–response curve can then be obtained by recording the left ventricular filling pressure response to graded static exercise. Repeating this measurement before and after beta-adrenergic blocker gives an index of the importance of sympathetic contribution to the cardiac response to stress. Demonstration in a patient of marked dependence on adrenergic support might be an indication of caution in using sympatholytics or beta-blockers.

iii) Pulmonary hypertension and vasodilator therapy. Vasodilators can lead to reflex tachycardia, cardiac stimulation and fluid retention. The reflex increase in heart rate and cardiac output may simply inconvenience the patient and interfere with adherence to therapy or, more seriously, it may

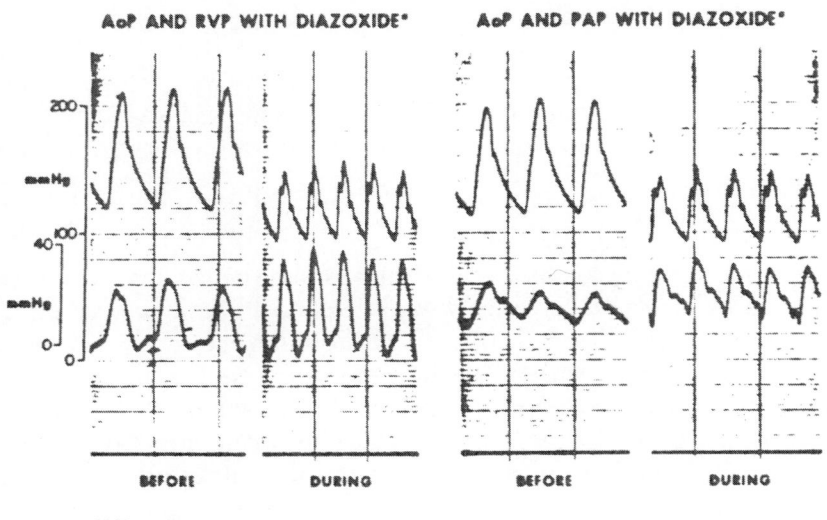

Figure 2. Increased pulmonary artery and right ventricular pressure despite reduction of aortic pressure following diazoxide (300 mg I.V.). The pressure tracings at the right side of the heart obviously indicate a hyperkinetic circulation. (Reproduced with permission from [54] in: Hypertension: Determinants, Complications, and Intervention onesti G, Klimt CR, eds. New York: Grune & Stratton, 1979.)

precipitate chest pain and coronary insufficiency in those with coronary artery disease. Another complication is fluid retention which has been described with hydralazine, minoxidil, and diazoxide [47]; in fact, the fluid retention with minoxidil has been, in our experience, of a higher magnitude than witnessed with any other antihypertensive drug. Significant hemodynamic consequences can result from the combination of volume overload with marked cardiac stimulation.

Less well known, perhaps, than these complications is the effect of vasodilators on the pulmonary circulation [3]. Intravenous injection of diazoxide leads to a slight but significant rise in pulmonary artery pressure even while aortic pressure is declining [54] (Figure 2) and similar findings were seen with parenteral hydralazine and with minoxidil. Vasodilators do not all have the same hemodynamic effects. Drugs with a venodilator action in addition to arteriolar dilatation will produce less of a hyperkinetic circulation and overload of the pulmonary circuit than vasodilator drugs with little or not effects on systemic veins. Some degree of pulmonary hypertension during oral minoxidil therapy was found in about half the patients investigated [3]; the rise in pulmonary artery pressure (PAP) varied from modest to very high. This pulmonary hypertension is not always produced by the same mechanism. Two hemodynamic patterns have been recognized: one is a hyperkinetic pulmonary hypertension similar to that seen with hydralazine or diazoxide, and the other is a congestive pulmonary hypertension associated with more marked increases in pulmonary wedge pressure and expansion of total blood volume; cardiac output decreased as PAP increased. Treatment of the two types differed: the first was usually responsive to adjustment of propranolol therapy, whereas the second indicated the need for more adequate volume depletion and possibly for reduction of minoxidil.

b) Reversal of cardiac hypertrophy
Studies made as early as 1943 and 1954 had shown that removal of the cause of an experimental hypertension was associated with reversal of cardiac hypertrophy [55]. There remained the question, however, of whether medical control of hypertension (as opposed to cure) could lead to the same result. Clinical studies reporting diminished cardiac silhouette or reduction of ECG precordial voltage are very difficult to evaluate precisely. In 1974, Sen et al. were the first to report reversal of cardiac hypertrophy following medical therapy in spontaneously hypertensive rats [19, 43].

The first observation to emerge from these studies was the difference among antihypertensive drugs as regards their ability to reverse hypertrophy. Although methyldopa, hydralazine, and minoxidil were all able to control blood pressure equally, reversal of ventricular hypertrophy occurred only with methyldopa (Figure 3). With hydralazine, ventricular weight

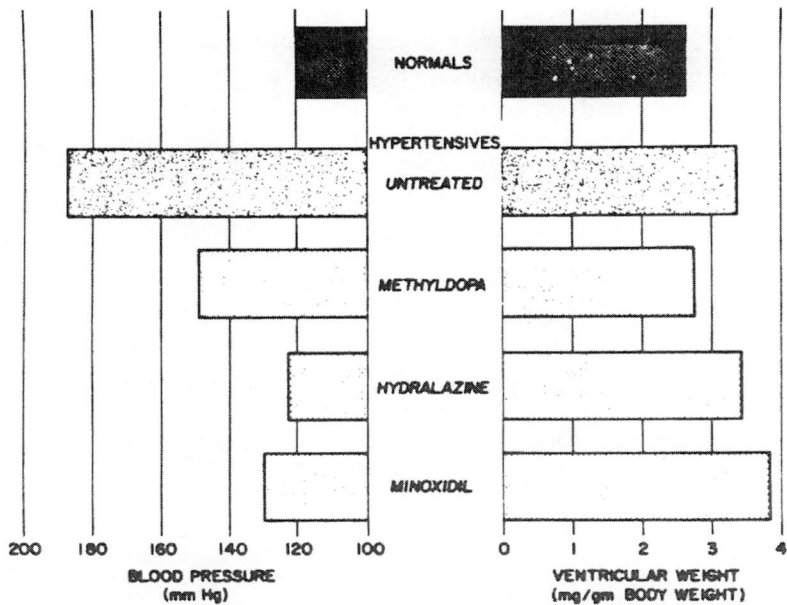

Figure 3. While these three antihypertensive drugs lowered blood pressure to similar levels in spontaneously hypertensive rats, effects on ventricular weight were quite different, as the graph shows. The implication is that reversal of hypertrophy does not depend solely on control of hypertension (From Tarazi RC: The heart in hypertension: its load and its role. Hosp Prac 10:31, 1975, with permission).

remained unchanged and minoxidil actually increased cardiac hypertrophy despite excellent blood pressure control. Reasons for the difference between drugs may be hemodynamic, humoral, or neurogenic [3, 43]. The hyperkinetic circulation of vasodilator therapy may increase cardiac work so as to annul the effects of pressure reduction. On the other hand, a strong argument has been made for a special role of adrenergic factors modulating the hypertrophic response to blood pressure variations [46]. Although these are as yet only speculative interpretations, they carry very important practical implications. Echocardiographic observations in patients have shown that reversal of left ventricular hypertrophy could occur rather rapidly with antihypertensive therapy, and that it did not happen equally with all antihypertensive drugs [6, 56]. Sympatholytics appeared to have a greater effect in reducing left ventricular mass than others. Obviously, a lot more needs to be learned regarding this aspect of antihypertensive therapy, as well as regarding the functional effect of a reduction in myocardial mass. The latter is particularly important in view of the fact that regression of ventricular hypertrophy may be associated with an increased concentration of myocardial hydroxyproline [19].

434

It is probably too early, nor would it be wise, to draw clinical conclusions at this stage. The clinical situation is usually more complex than the monotherapy utilized in many animal experiments. However, the field is advancing rather rapidly and echocardiography has allowed significant observations in hypertensive patients. These new avenues for thought and clinical research may well influence our approach to hypertensive patients in the not too distant future.

REFERENCES *

1. Kannel WB, Castelli WP, McNamara PM, McKee PA, Feinleib m: Role of blood pressure in the development of congestive heart failure. The Framingham Study. N Engl J Med 287:781, 1972.
2. Kannel WB, Gordon T, Offutt D: Left ventricular hypertrophy by electrocardiogram: prevalence, incidence, and mortality in the Frmingham Study. Ann Int Med 71:89, 1969.
3. Tarazi RC, Ferrario CM, Dustan HP: The heart in hypertension. In: Hypertension: Physiopathology and Treatment, p. 738. Genest J, Koiw E, Kuchel O, eds. New York: McGraw-Hill, 1976.
4. Friedberg CK: The heart in hypertension and renal disease. In: Diseases of the Heart, Philadelphia: W. B. Saunders, 1966.
5. Laird WP, Fixler DE: Left ventricular hypertrophy in adolescents with elevated blood pressure: Assessment by chest roentgenography, electrocardiography and echocardiogram. Pediatrics 67:255–259, 1981.
6. Fouad FM, Nakashima Y, Tarazi RC, Salcedo E: Reversal of left ventricular hypertrophy with methyldopa. Am J Cardiol (in press).
7. Cohn JN: Blood pressure and cardiac performance. Am J Med 55:351, 1973.
8. Nichols WW, Pepine CJ, Geiser EA, Conti CR: Vascular load defined by the aortic input impedance spectrum. Fed Proc 39(2):196, 1980.
9. Milnor WR: Arterial impedance as ventricular afterload. Circ Res 36:565, 1975.
10. Tarazi RC, Magrini F, Dustan HP: The role of aortic distensibility in hypertension. In: Recent Advances in Hypertension, p. 133. Milliez P, Safar M, eds. Reims: Boehringer Ingelheim, 1975.
11. Katz AN: Physiology of the Heart, p. 250. New York: Raven Press, 1977.
12. Grossman W, Jones D, McLaurin LP: Wall stress and patterns of hypertrophy in the human left ventricle. J Clin Inves 56:56, 1975.
13. Wilson JR, Teichek N, Hirshfeld J: Noninvasive assessment of load reduction in patients with asymptomatic aortic regurgitation. Am J Med 68:664, 1980.
14. Strauer BE: Ventricular function and coronary hemodynamics in hypertensive heart disease. Am J Cardiol 44:999, 1979.
15. Ross J Jr, Sobel BE: Regulation of cardiac contraction. Ann Rev Physiol 34:47, 1972.
16. Skelton CL, Sonnenblick EH: Heterogeneity of contractile function in cardiac hypertrophy. Circ Res (Suppl 2) 34, 35:83, 1974.
17. Averill DB, Ferrario CM, Tarazi RC, Sen S, Bajbus R: Cardiac performance in rats with renal hypertension. Circ Res 38:280, 1976.
18. Lund-Johansen P: Hemodynamic pattern in essential hypertension at rest and during muscular exercise. Acta Med Scand (Suppl 1) 181:482, 1967.

* This list of references is kept to a minimum.

19. Sen S, Tarazi RC, Bumpus FM: Biochemical changes associated with development and reversal of cardiac hypertrophy in spontaneously hypertensive rats. Cardiovasc Res 10:254, 1976.
20. Gaasch WJ: Left ventricular radius to wall thickness ratio. Am J Cardiol 43:1189, 1979.
21. Bugge-Asperheim B, Kiili F: Cardiac response to increased aortic pressure. Scand J Clin Lab Invest 24:345, 1969.
22. Saragoca M, Tarazi RC: Impaired cardiac contractile response to isoproterenol in the spontaneously hypertensve rat. Hypertension 3:380, 1981.
23. Woodcock EA, Funder JW, Johnston CI: Decreased cardiac β-adrenergic receptors in deoxycorticosterone-salt and renal hypertensive rats. Circ Res 45:560, 1979.
24. Saragoca M, Tarazi RC: Left ventricular hypertrophy in rats with renovascular hypertension: Alterations in cardiac function and adrenergic response. Hypertension 3 (Suppl II): II-171, 1981.
25. Julius S, Esler M: Autonomic nervous cardiovascular regulation in borderline hypertension. Am J Cardiol 36:685, 1975.
26. Ibrahim MM, Tarazi RC, Dustan HP, Bravo EL: Cardioadrenergic factor in essential hypertension. Am Heart J 88:724, 1974.
27. Marcus ML, Mueller TM, Gascho JA, Kerber RE: Effects of cardiac hypertrophy secondary to hypertension on the coronary circulation. Am J Cardiol 44: 1023, 1979.
28. Mueller TM, Marcus ML, Kerber RE, Young JA, Barnes RW, Abboud FM: Effect of renal hypertension and left ventricular hypertrophy on the coronary circulation in dogs. Circ Res 42(4):543, 1978.
29. Bache RJ, Vrobel TR: Effects of exercise on blood flow in the hypertrophied heart. Am J Cardiol 44:1029, 1979.
30. Wicker P, Tarazi RC: Coronary blood flow in renovascular hypertension: Changes during development and reversal of left ventricular hypertrophy. Eur Heart J (in press).
31. Pickering G: High Blood Pressure, pp. 351–355. New York: Grune & Stratton, 1968.
32. Sokolow M, Perloff D: The prognosis of essential hypertension treated conservatively. Circulation 23:697, 1961.
33. Rodriguera E, Narang R, Ahmed S, Fiore JJ, Levinson GE: The significance of cardiomegaly by x-ray in hypertensive heart disease. Circulation 45, 46 (Suppl II):104, 1972 (Abstract).
34. Tarazi RC, Miller A, Frohlich ED, Dustan HP: Electrocardiographic changes reflecting left atrial abnormality in hypertension. Circulation 34:818, 1966.
35. Gibson TC, Madry R, Grossman W, McLaurin LP, Craige E: The A-wave of the apexcardiogram and left ventricular diastolic stiffness. Circulation 49:441, 1974.
36. Fouad FM, Tarazi Rc, Gallagher JH, MacIntyre WJ, Cook SA: Abnormal left ventricular relaxation in hypertensive patients. Clin Sci 59:411s, 1980.
37. Dunn FG, Chandraratna PN, Basta LT, Frohlich ED: Pathophysiological assessment of hypertensive heart disease by echocardiography (ECHO). Am J Cardiol 39:189, 1977.
38. Safar ME, Lehner JP, Vincent MI, Plainfosse MT, Simo ACh: Echocardiographic dimensions in borderline and sustained hypertension. Am J Cardiol 44:930, 1979.
39. Richardson pj, Monaghan M: The role of echocardiography in the assessment of left ventricular hypertrophy in patients with hypertension. In: The Therapeutics of Hypertensions. The Royal Society of Medicine INternational Congress and Symposium Series No. 26, pp. 213–223. Royal Soc of Med (Lond), Academic Press (Lond), Grune & Stratton (New York), 1980.
40. Guazzi M, Fiorentini C, Olivari MT, Polese A: Cardiac load and function in hypertension. Am J Cardiol 44:1007, 1979.
41. Ehrström: Enlargement of the heart in hypertension. Acta Med Scand 103 (Suppl 206):86, 1946.

42. Grant RP: Aspects of cardiac hypertrophy. Am Heart J 46:154, 1953.
43. Sen S, Tarazi RC, Khairallah PA, Bumpus Fm: Cardiac Hypertrophy in spontaneously hypertensive rats. Circ Res 35:775, 1974.
44. Frohlich ED, Tarazi RC: Is arterial pressure the sole factor responsible for hypertensive cardiac hypertrophy? Am J Cardiol 44:459, 1979.
45. Raab W: Hormonal and nueorgenic cardiovascular disorders. Baltimore: Williams & Wilkins, 1953.
46. Tarazi RC, Sen S: Catecholamines and cardiac hypertrophy. In: Catecholamines and the Heart. Royal Society of Medicine International Congress and Symposium Series No. 8, p. 47. Mezey KC, Caldwell ADS, eds. Royal Society of Med (Lond), Academic Press (Lond), Grune & Stratton (New York), 1979.
47. Tarazi RC, Dustan HP, Bravo EL: The importance of plasma volume in the treatment of hypertension. In: Beta-Blockers: Present Status and Future Prospects, p. 102. Schweizer W, ed. Bern: Hans Huber, 1975.
48. Smith AJ: Clinical features of fluid retention complicating treatment with guanethidine. Circulation 31:485, 1965.
49. Vogel JHK, Chidsey CA: Cardiac adrenergic activity in experimental heart failure assessed with beta-receptor blockade. Am J Cardiol 24:198, 1969.
50. Chidsey CA, Braunwald AE, Monow AGL: Catecholamine excretion and cardiac stores of nerepinephrine in congestive heart failure. Am J Med 39:442, 1965.
51. Tarazi RC, Dustan HP, Bravo EL: Haemodynamic effects of propranolol in hypertesnion: a review. Postgrad Med J 52 (Suppl 4):92, 1976.
52. Guazzi M, Magrini F, Fiorentini C, Polese A: Role of the sympathetic nervous system in supporting cardiac function in essential arterial hypertension. Br Heart J 35:55, 1973.
53. alicandri C, Fouad FM, Tarasi RC, Bravo EL: Cardiac performance in hypertension. Circulation 55, 56 (SUPPL III):28, 1977.
54. Tarazi RC: Effects of hypertension on the heart: pathophysiology and clinical implications. In: Hypertension: Determinants, Complications, and Interventions, pp. 211–224. Onesti G, Klimt CR, eds. New York: Grune & Stratton, 1979.
55. Hall O, Hall CE, Ogden E: Cardiac hypertrophy in experimental hypertension and its regression following reestablishment of normal blood pressure. Am J Physiol 174:175, 1953.
56. Devereux RB, Savage DD, Sachs I, Laragh JH: Effect of blood pressure control on left ventricular hypertrophy and function in hypertension. Circulation 62 (Suppl II):II-36, 1980 (Abstract).

28. INFLUENCE OF HYPERTENSION ON THE KIDNEY

HERMAN VILLARREAL

Shortly after the introduction of the sphygmomanometer to measure arterial blood pressure, investigators began to center their attention on the kidney as the responsible organ for essential arterial hypertension [1]. However, debate soon ensued between pathologists and physiologists as to its role in the genesis of the hypertensive process. Pathologists believed the kidney to be the culprit, while physiologists considered it as the victim [2].

Years have passed and still we do not know the etiology of essential arterial hypertension, but we have learned that it is a multifactorial process and that the kidney can be the culprit as well as the victim. This chapter will deal with the kidney as the victim.

Arterial hypertension produces both functional and structural changes in the kidney. Functionally, renal hemodynamics and sodium and water excretion are altered. The structural changes observed are found mainly in the blood vessels.

1. FUNCTIONAL CHANGES PRODUCED IN THE KIDNEY BY ARTERIAL HYPERTENSION

1.1. The effect of arterial hypertension on renal hemodynamics

Established essential arterial hypertension affects renal hemodynamics from the outset. The earliest detectable change is a reduction in renal blood flow (RBF)*, which is thought to result from an increase in the tone of the efferent arterioles [4].

Glomerular filtration rate (GFR) however remains within normal limits despite the significantly diminished renal plasma flow (RPF) (Table 1). This is explained by the fact that intraglomerular pressure is raised due to eleva-

---

* The sodium para-aminohippurate method [3] by which effective renal plasma flow is measured is used for calculating RBF, according to the following formula: RBF = (Effective renal plasma flow)/(1 − hematocrit).

Amery, A. (ed.) Hypertensive Cardiovascular Disease: Pathophysiology and Treatment
© *1982, Martinus Nijhoff Publishers. The Hague / Boston / London*
ISBN-13: 978-94-009-7478-4

Table 1. Mean values of renal hemodynamics in normotensive and hypertensive subjects

	Normotensive subjects [1]	Hypertensive patients [2]
Glomerular filtration rate	124 ml/min	117 ml/min
Renal plasma flow	646 ml/min	484 ml/min
Filtration fraction	19 %	24 %
Maximal tabular excretory capacity [3]	48 mg/min	37 mg/min

[1] Mean values for males and females.

[2] Mean values from 30 patients in the early stage of essential hypertension as judged by the normal values of glomerular filtration rate (100 ml/min or higher).

[3] Values obtained with the diodrast method (Tm_D).

Modified from Goldring W, Chasis H: Hypertension and hypertensive disease. The Commonwealth Fund, 1944.

tion of the arterial blood pressure and also to the increased efferent arteriolar resistance.

Since RPF is diminished and no changes are observed in GFR, the filtration fraction (FF) or percentage of RPF that is filtered is thus increased.

In the early stage of the hypertensive process RPF may regress to normal when a pyrogenic reaction is produced [4]. This indicates that the constriction of the efferent arteriole is functional in nature. When RPF returns to normal, FF also returns to normal since GFR remains unchanged.

In the advanced stage of the hypertensive process RPF decreases further and the alteration now becomes irreversible. At this point an organic lesion is responsible for the change, since arteriolosclerosis of the afferent arterioles and hyalinization of the glomeruli have appeared. These vascular changes reduce the GFR slowly and gradually during the advanced stage of essential hypertension.

Maximal tubular excretory capacity (Tm_{PAH}) is low at the early stage of essential hypertension, decreasing progressively and irreversibly as the pathological process advances. This may be a metabolic process related to the reduction of RPF. However, Tm_{PAH} remains diminished even when RPF returns to normal values under the administration of pyrogenic substances [4].

Maximal tubular reabsorptive capacity (Tm_G) is normal at the early stage of essential hypertension and decreases significantly together with GFR when the hypertensive process is more advanced. Therefore, there is a clearcut difference between tubular capacity to reabsorb glucose and to excrete para-aminohippurate (PAH) at the early stage of essential hypertension. The diminished Tm_{PAH} is characteristic of the hypertensive process and appears prior to glomerular hyalinization, while Tm_G depends upon how far the glomerular lesion has advanced.

1.2. Renal handling of sodium in essential arterial hypertension

It has long been known that the kidney of the hypertensive patient handles sodium differently from that of the normotensive subject [5-10]. The former responds with premature and exaggerated natriuresis to a sodium load in comparison to the latter.

The reason for this response is unclear. Some investigators [11] have considered that increased intrarenal venous pressure may be responsible for this phenomenon. They found that the administration of a hypertonic saline solution produces a significant reduction in afferent and efferent arteriolar resistance which, in turn, favors the increase in intrarenal venous pressure. According to these investigators, when reduction of pre- and postglomerular arteriolar resistance take place, the high arterial pressure passes on to the peritubular capillaries raising intrarenal venous pressure thereby giving rise to exaggerated natriuresis.

Seeking additional support for this hypothesis the same investigators studied the effects of acetylcholine on renal arteriolar resistances, intrarenal venous pressure, and sodium excretion in normotensive subjects. For this purpose they administered the substance in the renal artery of one kidney using the other as a control. They found reduced renal arteriolar resistance, increased intrarenal venous pressure, exaggerated natriuresis in the ipsilateral kidney, and no response in the contralateral one. Furthermore, with intravenous adrenalin administration, renal arteriolar resistance increased, intrarenal venous pressure decreased, GFR was unchanged, and antinatriuresis was observed.

However, in recent studies [12] on exaggerated natriuresis produced by a sodium load in the hypertensive patient the same effect on afferent and efferent arterioles as described above was found but with no change in the intrarenal venous pressure. Therefore, these studies do not support the hypothesis that peritubular capillary physical factors participate in exaggerated natriuresis.

Furthermore, a significant increase in GFR, RPF and FF was found after a sodium load as well as a marked rise in the sodium excretion fraction. This led to the conclusion that both glomerular and tubular factors, particularly the latter, participate in exaggerated sodium excretion. The site in the nephron of altered sodium transport has been located in the ascending loop of Henle [13].

It is evident that the precise mechanisms responsible for exaggerated natriuresis in the hypertensive patient have not yet been elucidated. Intrarenal physical factors have been thought to be responsible for this, but it remains to be determined whether or not other factors, probably of an intra- or extrarenal hormonal character including the so-called natriuretic hormone, play a role in this phenomenon.

1.3. Differences in function between the kidneys in essential hypertension

In studying renal hemodynamics and sodium excretion separately in the two kidneys of essential hypertensive patients [14], it has been found that there are significant differences between them which are not observed in normotensive subjects [15]. In a study on the effect of chlorothiazide in relation to these differences [16] it was found that the discrepancies in renal hemodynamics between the two kidneys tended to disappear under the effect of the drug, while the disparities in sodium excretion remained unchanged being 90% before and 80% after the administration of chlorothiazide (Table 2).

From these findings it may be concluded that essential hypertension effectuates a difference in renal hemodynamics and sodium excretion between one kidney and the other. This discrepancy is functional in nature, and, with respect to sodium excretion, may have a pathogenetic significance, because of its high frequency and persistancy.

1.4. Angiotensin and renal transport of sodium in hypertension

The administration of angiotensin has been found to bring about a decrease in sodium excretion in normotensive subjects and an increase in sodium excretion in hypertensive patients [17, 18]. However, this natriuretic response is not observed in all hypertensive subjects since it appears to be related to the level of the mean arterial blood pressure [19]. In a study of the

Table 2. Sodium excretion in separate kidneys before and after intravenous administration of chlorothiazide in 10 patients with essential arterial hypertension

| Patient | Urinary excretion of sodium (μEq/min) | | | | | |
| | Control | | | Chlorothiazide | | |
	Right	Left	% diff.	Right	Left	% diff.
L.B.	19	26	31	179	225	23
S.M.	34	52	42	164	252	42
C.G.	21	33	44	252	405	45
A.G.	38	37	2	160	217	30
S.P.	25	19	27	222	190	15
J.C.	13	11	18	130	113	14
I.S.	90	112	22	337	411	20
V.G.	44	89	68	216	379	54
M.A.	39	30	26	284	221	25
A.V.	19	16	17	188	229	19

Modified from Villarreal et al. [16]. Significant differences (>15%) were found in 9 patients before and 8 patients after the administration of chlorothiazide.

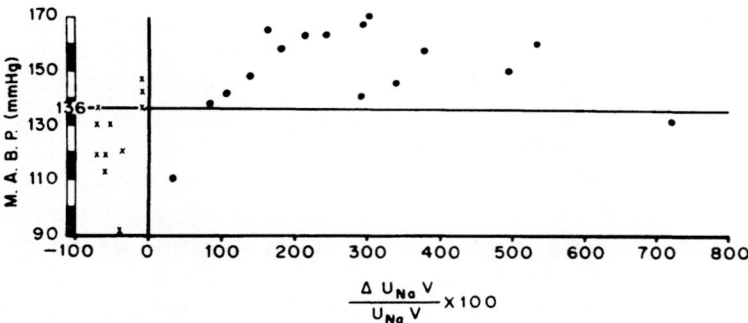

Figure 1. Angiotensin produced a drop in sodium excretion in all but two patients in whom mean arterial blood pressure was 136 mmHg or less and an increase in all but two patients in whom mean arterial blood pressure was above 136 mmHg. (Reproduced by permission of Circulation 35:889–894, 1967.)

early stage of essential hypertension [19], it was observed that when angiotensin was administered, natriuresis occurred in patients whose control mean arterial blood pressure was above 136 mm Hg, while antinatriuresis was found in those whose control blood pressure was below that figure (Figure 1).

Table 3. Effect of angiotensin on sodium excretion and renal hemodynamics in patients with essential hypertension with control mean arterial blood pressure higher and lower than 136 mmHg

	MABP>136 mm Hg			MABP<136 mm Hg		
	Control	Angio-tensin	p	Control	Angio-tensin	p
Mean arterial blood pressure (mmHg)	150	180	<0.001	125	157	<0.001
Sodium excretion (μEq/min)	256	957	<0.001	224	149	<0.01
Glomerular filtration rate (ml/min)	96	106	N.S.	110	99	N.S.
Renal plasma flow (ml/min)	368	298	<0.01	396	288	<0.01
Urine flow (ml/min)	4.90	9.07	<0.01	4.56	1.85	<0.05
Excretion fraction of sodium (%)	1.96	6.74	<0.001	1.51	1.26	<0.05
Excretion fraction of water (%)	4.93	8.74	<0.01	4.16	2.21	<0.05

Modified from Villarreal et al. [19]. Mean values from a group of 16 patients with control mean arterial blood pressure higher than 136 mmHg and 11 patients with control mean arterial blood pressure lower than 136 mmHg.

In hypertensive patients with a mean arterial blood pressure greater than 136 mm Hg, the GFR remained unchanged and RPF was reduced, but the urinary volume, sodium excretion fraction, and water excretion fraction increased significantly (Table 3). The fact that GFR did not change while sodium and water excretion fractions were raised indicates that the natriuresis observed in this group points to a tubular phenomenon. In the group whose control mean arterial blood pressure was below 136 mm Hg, GFR also remained unchanged while RPF, urinary volume, sodium excretion fraction and water excretion fraction decreased significantly. The antinatriuresis found in association with unchanged GFR and decreased sodium and water excretion fractions is a tubular phenomenon as well, although in the opposite direction.

It seems unlikely that the difference in renal handling of sodium in these two groups of patients is due to differences in peritubular physical factors,

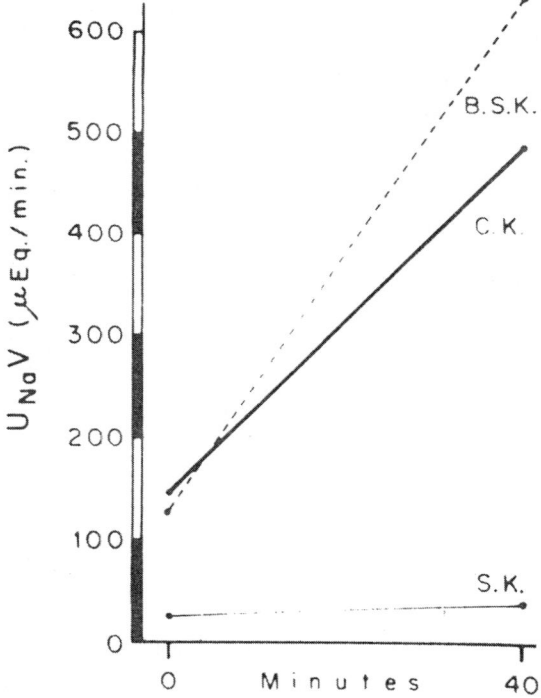

Figure 2. Effect of angiotensin on urinary sodium excretion in 9 patients with unilateral renal artery stenosis and in 2 patients with bilateral renal artery stenosis. There is no increment in the unilateral stenotic kidney (S.K.), whereas the increment was significant in the contralateral kidney (C.K.) and even greater in the bilateral stenotic kidneys (B.S.K.). (Reproduced by permission of Am J Cardiology 19:793–796, 1967.)

since the administration of angiotensin raised the mean arterial blood pressure and renal resistance in both groups.

It appears that the degree of natriuresis produced by angiotensin is proportional to the mean arterial blood pressure transmitted to the kidney. For this reason, the effect of angiotensin was studied in patients with renovascular hypertension [20] in whom there is a difference between the arterial blood pressure in the kidney with stenosis and the contralateral one. Natriuresis was detected in the contralateral kidney and no change was observed in sodium excretion on the ipsilateral one. However, in bilateral stenosis, instead of the expected decrease in natriuresis, a considerable increase in sodium excretion in the two kidneys was found (Figure 2).

The fact that the mean arterial blood pressure was low distal to the arterial stenosis could explain the lack of a natriuretic response by the unilateral stenotic kidney to angiotensin. However, in the bilateral stenotic kidneys distal arterial blood pressure in both kidneys was also low, but nevertheless sodium excretion was markedly increased. This seems to indicate that some unknown factors related to the natriuretic response in renovascular hypertension are present in addition to arterial blood pressure.

It is possible that the natriuretic response obtained with the administration of angiotensin in both essential and renovascular hypertension may be produced by the liberation of prostaglandins from the renal medulla which, on being redistributed by the intrarenal blood flow, are mobilized to the cortex to produce cortical vasodilation and natriuresis [21]. However, this hypothesis is not applicable to the antinatriuresis produced by angiotensin in hypertensive patients in whom the mean arterial blood pressure was below 136 mm Hg.

2. STRUCTURAL CHANGES PRODUCED IN THE KIDNEY BY HYPERTENSION

Three types of vascular lesions are produced by arterial hypertension: atherosclerosis, arteriolosclerosis, and arteriolonecrosis. Atherosclerosis appears mainly in the aorta and large vessels, arteriolosclerosis in the small-caliber arteries and arterioles, and arteriolonecrosis only in the arterioles. Therefore, arteriolosclerosis and arteriolonecrosis are the most important vascular changes found in the hypertensive kidney.

2.1. Arteriolosclerosis

Arteriolosclerosis, a vascular lesion frequently associated with the late stage of essential arterial hypertension, occurs in two forms: hyperplastic arteriolosclerosis and hyaline arteriolosclerosis [22, 23]. These constitute the pa-

444

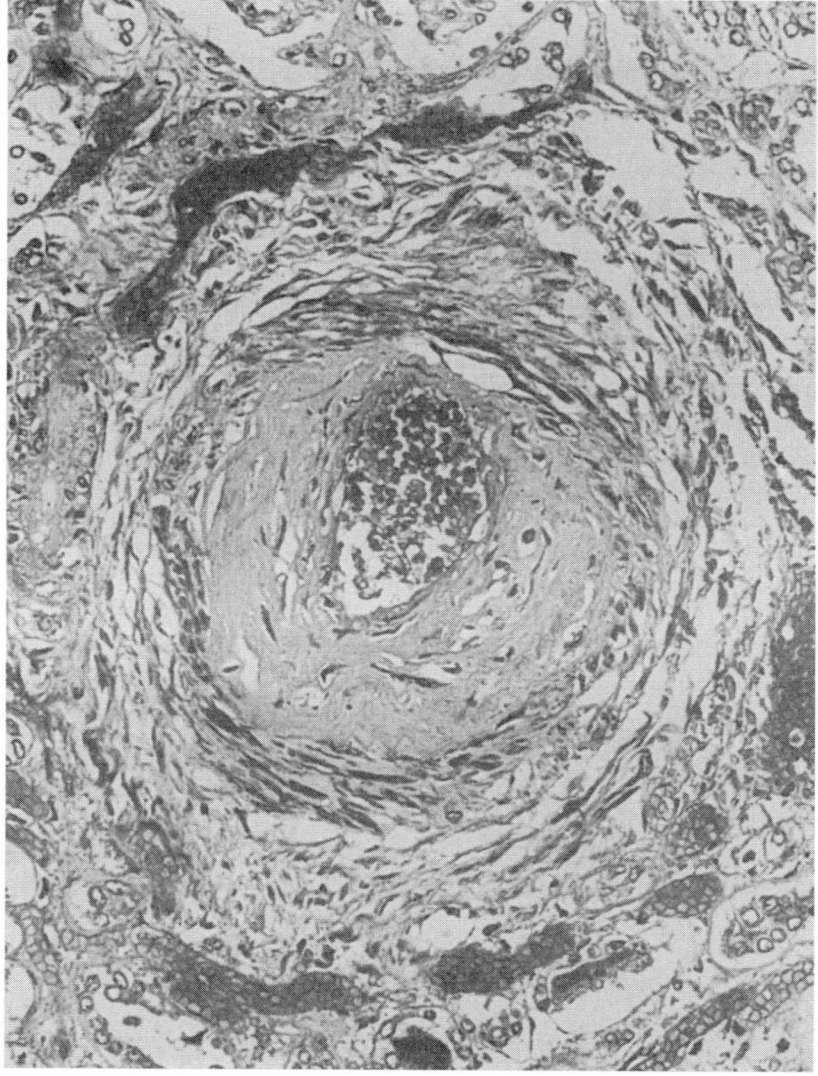

Figure 3. Benign nephrosclerosis. Interlobular artery of the kidney with considerable luminal obliteration due to marked intimal sclerosis. There is also medial fibrosis. (H and E. Original magnification X300. Courtesy of L. Salinas-Madrigal.)

thological vascular substrate of the so-called benign nephrosclerosis (Figures 3 and 4).

In experimental studies [24], it has been observed that alterations in hyperplastic arteriolosclerosis are produced by the migration of smooth muscle cells from the media to the intima, separating the endothelium from

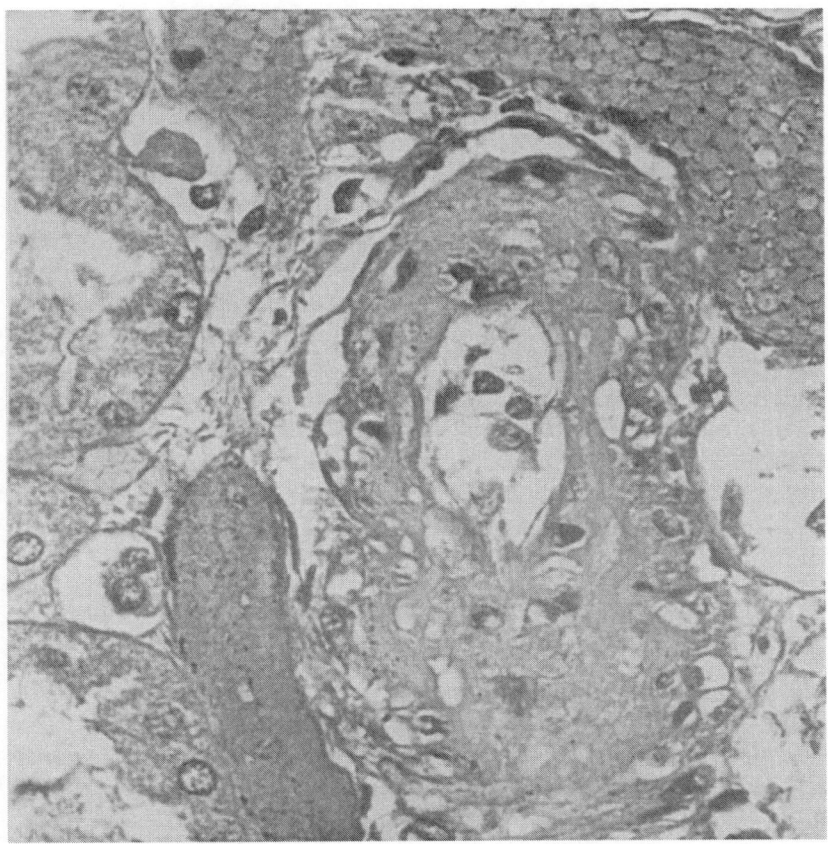

Figure 4. Benign Hypertension. Arteriole of the kidney showing intimal and medial sclerosis with fibrous replacement of the media and luminal narrowing. (H and E. Original magnification X750. Courtesy of L. Salinas-Madrigal).)

the elastic laminae. These cells apparently cross the fenestrae of the elastica to deposit themselves in the intima. Lesions are also present in the endothelium of the arterioles. This has been demonstrated by the finding that colloidal carbon injected intravenously in hypertensive animals appears in the media of the arterioles after a few days. Hyperplasia of the muscular layer and reduplication of the elastica are also observed.

All these changes produce a twofold effect upon the arteriole, wall thickening of the blood vessel and reduction of its lumen. This increased wall–lumen ratio signifies an increment in peripheral vascular resistances and, consequently, further elevation of arterial blood pressure [25].

In contrast to the hyperplastic form hyaline arteriolosclerosis is a focal process. Apparently, the endothelium is damaged by the increased intra-arteriolar pressure and as a result plasma proteins pass through the intima and the elastica to be deposited in the media. The smooth-muscle cells of this layer disappear, giving way to acidophilic deposits of acellular material. Here also, the intravenous administration of colloidal carbon makes it possible to follow the migration, step by step, of plasma proteins in the arteriolar wall.

Although the basic mechanisms by which arteriolosclerosis is produced are not fully understood, there is no doubt that these vascular lesions are directly related to the degree of high blood pressure [24].

2.2. Arteriolonecrosis

Necrotizing arteriolitis, or fibrinoid arteriolar necrosis, is a destructive focal lesion of the arterioles characteristics of malignant hypertension. Exaggerated elevation of arterial blood pressure produces areas of spasm in the arterioles, followed by dilatation. It is at the site of the dilatation where the initial lesion is found, consisting of a rupture of the endothelial layer of the vessel or, rather, in the separation of the endothelial cells [24]. This separation allows the plasma to pass through and invade the intima and media, displacing or destroying the smooth-muscle cells. Deposition at this site resembles that of hyaline arteriolosclerosis. Fibrin is deposited together with the plasma proteins, its organization being the histological characteristic of fibrinoid necrosis (Figure 5). Subsequently, when the lesion heals its histological aspect resembles that of hyperplastic arteriolosclerosis. Plasma proteins are able to pass through the media to come into contact with the basement membrane of the vessel and produce lesions in the adventitia, thus causing periarteritis.

Although the mechanisms producing fibrinoid necrosis are not fully understood, it is generally accepted that sustained, very high arterial blood pressure must be present to produce this condition. Other pathogenetic mechanisms have also been incriminated, such as toxic [26], immunological [27], and humoral [28] factors.

Several investigators are of the opinion that elevated arterial blood pressure is responsible for the vascular damage [29–33]. It is considered that arterioles respond by constriction as the pressure rises until it reaches a critical level of autoregulation. When further elevation of pressure goes beyond this critical point, the arterioles dilate and break.

Those who support this hypothesis explain the vascular lesion by applying Frank's modification of Laplace's law, expressed in the following formula: $T = P \cdot r/w$. According to this law, when the arteriole dilates the radius of the vessel (r) increases and the thickeness of the wall (w) decreases. When this is multiplied by the high arterial pressure (P), a greater increment of the tension on the vessel wall (T) is produced giving rise to the vascular

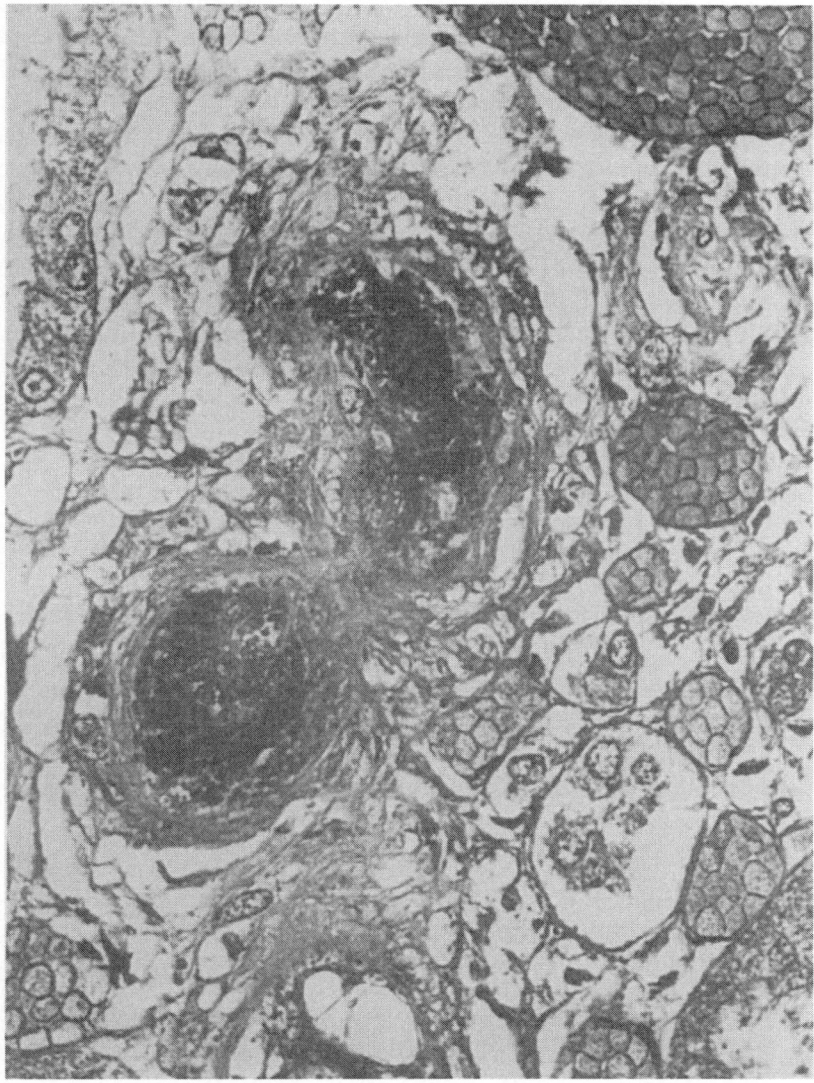

Figure 5. Malignant hypertension. Arteriole of the kidney showing total narrowing due to sclerosis and superimposed 'fibrinoid necrosis' typical of malignant hypertension. (Masson's trichrome. Original magnification X750. Courtesy of L. Salinas-Madrigal).

lesions [24]. However, it is a well-known fact that there are patients with very high arterial blood pressure sustained for a long period who do not have necrotizing arteriolitis [28]. It is important to note in this respect that adaptive changes of the arteriolar walls are observed in arterial hypertension and that they protect them against the effect of hypertension [34].

Various investigators contend that, in addition to high blood pressure, severe arteriolar vasoconstriction produced by vasoactive substances must be present for these lesions to appear [28]. Hence, it has been asserted that the renin–angiotensin system participates in some form in the production of fibrinoid necrosis. This hypothesis is based on the concept that when arterial pressure rises and rapidly reaches a critical level, natriuresis is produced which is responsible for hypovolemia that stimulates the plasma renin activity, producing an even greater increment in the blood pressure and initiating a vicious circle [35]. The hypovolemia is also responsible for hemoconcentration and this, plus the vasoconstriction produced by the angiotensin and the high blood pressure, apparently is the cause of the vascular damage [36]. However, there are experimental models of arterial hypertension, such as that produced in the rat by the administration of deoxycorticosterone in which plasma renin activity is not increased, even though necrotizing arteriolitis is present [37]. The explanation for this is that other vasoactive substances, like catecholamines and vasopressin, may be responsible for the marked vasoconstriction [28].

Apparently, hypovolemia in malignant hypertension is caused not only by natriuresis and diuresis but also by translocation of the fluids of the intravascular space to the interstitial space [38]. The depletion of intravascular volume favors the liberation of vasoconstrictive substances such as vasopressin and catecholamines.

As is evident, the hypothesis of high arterial blood pressure as being the sole factor responsible for the vascular lesion is tenable only if other factors capable of producing vascular damage can be excluded.

REFERENCES

1. Goldblatt H: The Renal Origin of Hypertension. Springfield: Charles C. Thomas, 1948.
2. Smith HW, Goldring WM, Chasis H: Role of the kidney in the genesis of hypertension. Bull NY Acad Med 19:449, 1943.
3. Smith HW, Finkelstein N, Aliminosa L, Crawford B, Graber M: The renal clearances of substituted hippuric acid derivatives and other aromatic acids in dog and man. J Clin Invest 24:388–404, 1945.
4. Goldring W, Chasis H: Hypertension and hypertensive disease. The Commonwealth Fund, 1944.
5. Green DM, Wedell HG, Wald MH, Learned BS: The relation of water and sodium excretion to blood pressure in human subjects. Circulation 6:919–924, 1952.
6. Birchal R, Tuthill SW, Jacobs WS, Trautman WJ Jr, Findley T: Renal excretion of water, sodium and chloride. Comparison of the responses of hypertensive patients with those of normal subjects, patients with specific adrenal or pituitary defects and a normal subject primed with various hormones. Circulation 7:258–267, 1953.
7. Thompson JH, Silva TF, Kinsey D, Smithwick RH: The effect of acute salt loads on the urinary sodium output of normotensive and hypertensive patients before and after surgery. Circulation 10:912–919, 1954.

449

8. Hoobler SW, Weller JM, Cottier PT: Studies on water and electrolyte excretion in essential hypertension. Circulation 14:955, 1956. (Abstract).
9. Brodsky WA, Granbarth HN: Excretion of water and electrolytes in patients with essential hypertension. J Lab Clin Med 41:43–55, 1953.
10. Farnsworth EB: Renal absorption of chlorides and phosphate in normal subjects and in patients with essential arterial hypertension. J Clin Invest 25:897–905, 1946.
11. Lowenstein J, Beranbaum ER, Chasis H, Baldwin DS: Intrarenal pressure and exaggerated natriuresis in essential hypertension. Clin Sci 38:359–374, 1970.
12. Willassen Y, Ofstad J: Renal sodium excretion and the peritubular capillary physical factors in essential hypertension. Hypertension 2:771–779, 1980.
13. Buckalew VM Jr, Puschett JB, Kintzel JB, Goldberg M: Mechanism of exaggerated natriuresis in hypertensive man. Impair sodium transport in the loop of Henle. J Clin Invest 48:1007–1016, 1969.
14. Baldwin DS, Hulet WH, Biggs AW, Gombos EA, Chasis H: Renal function in the separate kidneys of man – II. Hemodynamics and excretion of solute and water in essential hypertension. J Clin Invest 39:395–404, 1960.
15. Hulet WH, Baldwin DS, Biggs AW, Gombos EA, Chasis H: Renal function in the separate kidneys of man – I. Hemodynamics and excretion of solute and water in normal subjects. J Clin Invest 39:389–394, 1960.
16. Villarreal H, Larrondo F, Exaire JE, Revollo A: The effect of chlorothiazide on separate kidney function in essential hypertension. Br Heart J 26:325–329, 1964.
17. Peart WS, Brown JI: The effects of angiotensin (hypertensin or angiotonin) on urine flow and the electrolyte excretion in hypertensive patients. Lancet 1:28–29, 1961.
18. Brown JJ, Peart WS: The effect of angiotensin on urine flow and electrolyte excretion in hypertensive patients. Clin Sci 22:1–17, 1962.
19. Villarreal H, Arcila H, Diaz J, Sierra P: Effect of angiotensin on the renal transport of sodium in essential hypertension. Circulation 35:889–894, 1967.
20. Villarreal H, Arcila H, Diaz J, Sierra P: Effect of angiotensin on renal transport of sodium in renovascular hypertension. Am J Cardiol 19:793–796, 1967.
21. Lee JB: Prostaglandins, neutral lipids, renal intersticial cells, and hypertension. In: Hypertension, Physiopathology and Treatment, pp. 373–393. Genest J, Koiw E, Kuchel E, eds. New York: McGraw-Hill, 1977.
22. Spiro D, Lattes RG, Wiener J: The cellular pathology of experimental hypertension – I. Hyperplastic arteriolosclerosis. Am J Pathol 47:19–49, 1965.
23. Wiener J, Spiro D, Lattes RG: The cellular pathology of experimental hypertension – II. Arteriolar hyalinosis and fibrinoid change. Am J Pathol 47:457–485, 1965.
24. Goldby FS: The pathology of hypertension. In: The Hypertensive Patient, pp. 266–292. Marshall AJ, Barrit DW, eds. Tunbridge Wells: Pitman Medical, 1980.
25. Folkow J: The haemodynamic consequences of adaptive structural changes of the resistance vessels in hypertension. Clin Sci Mol Med 41:1–12, 1971.
26. Muirhead EE, Turner LB, Grollman A: Hypertensive cardiovascular disease. Arch Pathol 51:575–592, 1951.
27. Paronetto F: Immunocytochemical observations on the vascular necrosis and renal glomerular lesions of malignant nephrosclerosis. Am J Pathol 46:901–915, 1965.
28. Möhring J: High arterial pressure versus humoral factors in the pathogenesis of the vascular lesions of malignant hypertension. The case of humoral factors as well as pressure. Clin Sci Mol Med 52:113–117, 1977.
29. Byrom FB: The pathogenesis of hypertensive encephalopathy and its relation to the malignant phase of hypertension. Lancet 2:201–211, 1954.
30. Garner A, Ashton N, Tripathi R, Kohner EM, Bulpitt CJ, Dollery CT: Pathogenesis of hypertensive retinopathy. Br J Ophthalmol 59:3–44, 1975.

31. Heptinstall RH: Malignant hypertension: a study of fifty-one cases. J Pathol Bact 65:423–439, 1953.
32. Pickering G: High blood pressure. Edinburgh: Churchill-Livingstone, 1968.
33. Beilin LJ, Goldby FS: High arterial pressure versus humoral factors in the pathogenesis of the vascular lesions of malignant hypertension. The case for pressure alone. Clin Sci Mol Med 52:111–113, 1977.
34. Byrom FB: Angiotensin and renal vascular damage. Br J Exp Pathol 45:7–12, 1964.
35. Möhring J: Pathogenesis of malignant hypertension: experimental evidence from the renal hypertensive rat. Clin Nephrol 5:167–174, 1975.
36. Brown JJ, Fraser R, Lever AF, Robertson JIS: Hypertension: a review of selected topics. Abstracts of World Medicine 45:549–559, 1971.
37. Goldby FS: The arteriolar lesions of steroid hypertension in the rat. Clin Sci Mol Med 51 (Suppl 3):31s-32s, 1976.
38. Byrom FB: The hypertensive vascular crisis. An experimental study. London: William Heinemann Medical, 1969.

29. INFLUENCE OF HYPERTENSION ON MORTALITY

BERNARD E. KREGER and WILLIAM B. KANNEL

Hypertension kills – less precipitously and less surely than potassium cyanide, but just as definitely. It does not fit the lay person's idea of a disease, since it so rarely evokes recognizable symptoms prior to its culmination in a cardiovascular catastrophe. Yet, hypertension comprises a readily obtained measurement of a physical finding which has come to be acknowledged as a significant indicator of risk of mortality.

Framingham Heart Study data and data from other studies show that risk of morbidity and mortality increases continuously with blood pressure and that there is no well-demarcated line beyond which something called 'hypertension' begins and behind which all are safe. Analyses of mortality risk have been approached from considering blood pressure as a continuous variable, using any of several components: systolic, diastolic, pulse pressure, or mean arterial pressure. Which pressure is used matters little, since there are strong correlations among all blood pressure parameters. Another approach uses arbitrarily established categories of blood pressure levels, such that measurements of <140 mm Hg systolic and <90 mm Hg diastolic are called normotensive, ≥160 mm Hg systolic and/or ≥95 mm Hg diastolic are called definitely hypertensive, and readings inbetween, are classified as borderline or mild. Such categorization has pragmatic utility and simplifies analysis but has stirred needless and illogical controversy about boundary lines.

Although cardiovascular mortality is most relevant in relation to hypertension, death from all causes is also pertinent. Table 1 presents figures from 20-year follow-up data from Framingham. Average annual death rates are related to the blood pressure recorded at each biennial examination. The mortality rate rises with age for both men and women, whatever the blood pressure status, but the rate for people with definite hypertension is about double that of normotensives at each age level. The rate for women in all categories of blood pressure is about half that for men. When these same data are examined considering blood pressure as a continuous variable, the association between increasing blood pressure level and greater mortality is also evident [1]. Even when several risk variables are considered simultaneously in multivariate analysis – including serum cholesterol level, age,

Amery, A. (ed.) Hypertensive Cardiovascular Disease: Pathophysiology and Treatment
© *1982, Martinus Nijhoff Publishers. The Hague / Boston / London*
ISBN-13: 978-94-009-7478-4

452

Table 1. Mortality according to hypertension status – Framingham Study, 20 year follow-up

	Person years	Events	Rate* per 1000	Person years	Events	Rate per 1000	Person years	Events	Rate per 1000	Age-adjusted rate*
	Men aged 45–54			Men aged 55–64			Men aged 65–74			Men 45–74
None	7934	55	6.9	5380	79	14.7	1866	44	23.6	12.1
Borderline	4520	31	6.9	3918	61	15.6	1828	69	37.7	16.7
Definite	2602	40	15.4	2624	75	28.6	1104	47	42.6	23.0
	Women aged 45–54			Women aged 55–64			Women aged 65–74			Women 45–74
None	10746	43	4.0	5904	41	6.9	1586	23	14.5	7.1
Borderline	5292	27	5.1	5524	45	8.1	2758	49	17.8	8.9
Definite	2742	23	6.4	4232	43	10.2	2472	61	24.7	11.1

	Regression coefficient		T-value	
Age	Men	Women	Men	Women
45–54	0.385	0.361	3.47	2.76
55–64	0.344	0.194	4.00	1.75
65–74	0.315	0.269	3.00	2.40
45–74, univariate	0.402	0.421	7.16	6.38
45–74, bivariate	0.334	0.226	5.84	3.24
45–74, multivariate	0.154	0.102	3.15	1.39

* Average annual mortality.

Table 2. Cardiovascular mortality according to hypertension status – Framingham Study, 20 year follow-up

	Person years	Events	Rate* per 1000	Person years	Events	Rate per 1000	Person years	Events	Rate per 1000	Age-adjusted rate*
	Men aged 45–54			Men aged 55–64			Men aged 65–74			Men 45–74
None	7934	20	2.5	5380	45	8.4	1866	18	9.6	5.8
Borderline	4520	17	3.8	3918	41	10.5	1828	37	20.2	9.5
Definite	2602	24	9.2	2624	54	20.6	1104	27	24.5	15.5
	Women aged 45–54			Women aged 55–64			Women aged 65–74			Women 45–74
None	10746	10	0.9	5904	13	2.2	1586	6	3.8	2.3
Borderline	5292	6	1.1	5524	25	4.5	2758	27	9.8	4.1
Definite	2742	11	4.0	4232	24	5.7	2472	46	18.6	7.4

Age	Regression coefficient		T-value	
	Men	Women	Men	Women
45–54	0.662	0.741	4.19	3.15
55–64	0.469	0.449	4.43	2.77
65–74	0.460	0.751	3.17	4.31
45–74, univariate	0.567	0.824	7.62	8.15
45–74, bivariate	0.504	0.587	6.66	5.53
45–74, multivariate	0.261	0.335	3.18	3.18

* Average annual mortality.

453

cigarette smoking, glucose intolerance, left ventricular hypertrophy by electrocardiogram – the mortality risk of hypertension persists and is proportional to be blood pressure level [2]. Even within the borderline and normal range, there is a distinct gradient of risk. It is *blood pressure* that kills, not 'hypertension.'

Table 2 presents similar data regarding death attributed to cardiovascular disease. This group of diagnoses includes myocardial infarction, congestive heart failure, cardiac arrhythmia, aortic and other major vessel dissection, thrombotic and embolic stroke, ruptured aneurysm, and sudden death. Here again, the mortality rate rises with blood pressure level and age, for both men and women, and the age-adjusted rate for women is about half that for men. As expected, the association is more pronounced than for overall mortality, with a threefold excess risk. An even more certain association between elevated blood pressure and mortality from cardiovascular disease is evident than for death from all causes.

Comparison of rates for cardiovascular disease death versus death from all causes shows two things (Table 3). First, high blood pressure increases one's likelihood of having a death, at any age, attributable to cardiovascular disease. Second, though death rates for hypertensive women are lower overall, cardiovascular disease accounts for just as great a portion of their deaths as for men in that blood pressure category.

Among the cardiovascular diseases in hypertensives, coronary heart disease is responsible for a large portion of the mortality. Coronary heart disease mortality shows the same trends in relation to blood pressure as for cardiovascular mortality in general: increasing mortality rate with an increasing blood pressure, even with multivariate analysis. Definite hypertensives have about three times the coronary death rate of normotensives; women have less than half the men's death rate. Although the rate rises with age, in any blood pressure category, at any age and in either sex, hypertensive persons suffer an excess coronary heart disease mortality. About half the coronary heart disease deaths in all subcategories of hypertension are sudden deaths, a picture no different from that for normontensives.

Because of the preponderance of men among coronary heart disease victims, most of the available data about the interrelations between blood

Table 3. Cardiovascular disease as a portion of total death rate*

	Men	Women
Normotension	0.48	0.32
Borderline hypertension	0.57	0.46
Definite hypertension	0.67	0.67

* Ratio of age-adjusted cardiovascular disease death rate to age-adjusted total death rate.

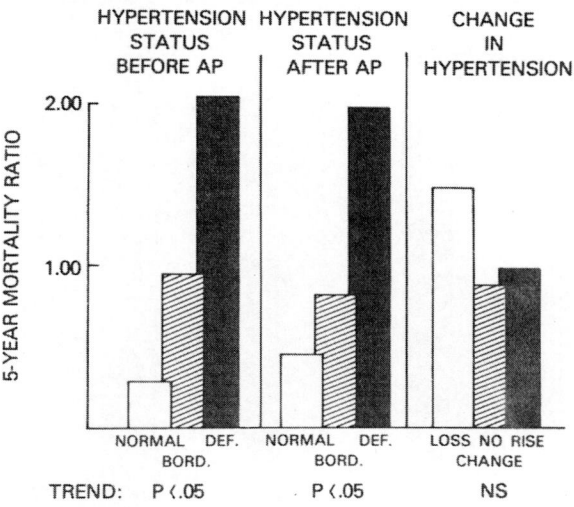

Figure 1.

pressure and coronary heart disease relates to men. Analysis of the relation of blood pressure to mortality after the onset of coronary heart disease is complicated, since the event itself may affect blood pressure. In angina pectoris, blood pressure both before and after the event shows a clear-cut influence on mortality (Figure 1), with elevation posing a definite risk. Little change in blood pressure occurs with the onset of angina pectoris, and such change as is seen seems to have little effect on five-year survival.

For men having their first myocardial infarction, antecedent hypertension is a burden associated with three times the five-year mortality risk of normotensives (Figure 2). Many of these deaths occur at the time of the event or within a month thereafter, and studies have linked hypertension with adverse outcome. Those who survive beyond a month after an acute myocardial infarction comprise a more complex group. On the average, their systolic blood pressure drops 10 mm Hg (7 mm Hg if those receiving antihypertensive medications are omitted). No matter what the antecedent systolic blood pressure level or whether it had been treated, the greater the fall in blood pressure after recovery from infarction, the greater the observed mortality rate over the next few years. A hypertensive who loses his hypertension following infarction has double the risk of dying as compared to one who shows no change in blood pressure status. An interesting, small subgroup is those who sustained a 'silent' or unrecognized myocardial infarction. These men, all of whom had no sudden death or peri-infarction morbidity, are noted to have but a 2 mm fall in systolic blood pressure asso-

MORTALITY FOLLOWING RECOGNIZED MYOCARDIAL INFARCTION

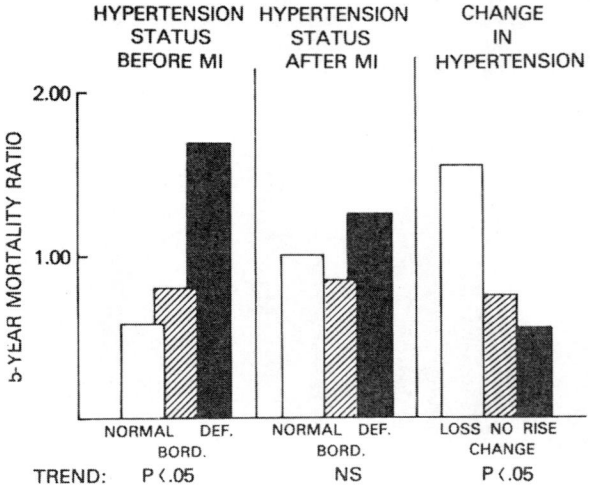

TREND: NORMAL DEF.   NORMAL DEF.   LOSS NO RISE
         BORD.   BORD.   CHANGE
         P < .05   NS   P < .05

Figure 2.

ciated with their infarctions. This assortment of interactions between blood pressure and myocardial infarction results in a lack of demonstrable relation between the postinfarction blood pressure status and mortality rate. It is only in conjunction with preinfarction blood pressure status that the real impact of blood pressure becomes manifest (Figure 2).

CAUSES OF DEATH ACCORDING TO BLOOD PRESSURE STATUS

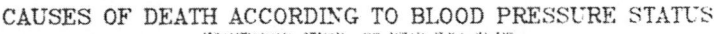

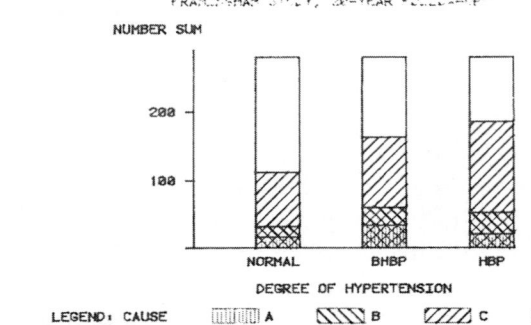

BHBP=BORDERLINE HYPERTENSION
HBP=DEFINITE HYPERTENSION

A=SUDDEN DEATH
B=ALL CORONARY HEART DISEASE
C=ALL CARDIOVASCULAR DISEASES
D=ALL NON-CARDIOVASCULAR DISEASES

Figure 3.

The relation between several causes of death for the three categories of blood pressure – normotension, borderline hypertension, definite hypertension – can be seen in Figure 3. The 867 deaths which occurred in the first twenty years of the Framingham Heart Study are divided almost equally among the blood pressure categories. Thus, two-thirds of the deaths come from less than one-fifth of the total population at risk. Cardiovascular disease accounts for most of the deaths in both mild and definite hypertension categories, with coronary heart disease deaths and the subcategory, sudden death, increasing about proportionally with overall cardiovascular disease. It is of interest that the proportions of deaths attributable to cardiovascular disease in general and coronary heart disease in particular are almost equal for both hypertensive subgroups, emphasizing the impact of even mild hypertension.

Does one particular component of the blood pressure determine the lethality? It used to be taught that diastolic pressure was the key measurement. Long-term studies reveal that this is not the case. An elevation in either diastolic or systolic blood pressure is a hazardous finding. Table 4 illustrates the relationship between death from various causes and systolic versus diastolic blood pressure. Two important facts emerge. First, the regression coefficients are highly significant for all causes of death, in both men and women, and for both systolic and diastolic blood pressure, with but a single exception owing to a small number of events. Equally noteworthy, the coefficient for systolic blood pressure exceeds that for diastolic blood pressure in every instance. Indeed, if anything is to be claimed for the importance of a particular pressure measurement, it appears that the systolic pressure has the greater influence on mortality. This may not be a true,

Table 4. Regression of mortality on systolic versus diastolic blood pressure in men and women 45–74, Framingham Study, 20-year follow-up

		Standardized regression coefficient		T-value	
		Men	Women	Men	Women
Death, all	Systolic BP	0.278	0.266	6.84	5.55
	Diastolic BP	0.185	0.171	4.27	3.39
Death, CVD*	Systolic BP	0.367	0.486	7.19	7.74
	Diastolic BP	0.245	0.300	4.38	4.34
Death, CHD*	Systolic BP	0.408	0.538	4.94	4.69
	Diastolic BP	0.342	0.409	3.79	3.26
Sudden death	Systolic BP	0.322	0.442	2.77	2.37
	Diastolic BP	0.298	0.373	2.43	1.82

* CVD = Cardiovascular disease; CHD = Coronary heart disease.

physiologic difference, since systolic pressures are more accurately determined and span a wider range of values than diastolic pressures.

Another long-held bias has been that a patient whose blood pressure varies widely among repeated readings at a single encounter – including readings ranging from normotensive to well up in hypertensive levels for systolic, diastolic, or both – is in little jeopardy. This suspicion cannot be documented. Not only is an association between the degree of variation in a person's readings on one occasion compared to another occasion two or even twenty years distant lacking, but there is also no demonstrable net effect of any degree of 'lability' of readings on morbidity or mortality [3]. Therefore, it is not safe to rely on the 'basal' or lowest pressure recorded on a patient in judging the need for treatment.

In the days before anti-hypertensive medication became available, the clinical syndrome of malignant or accelerated hypertension was a dreaded and not rare occurrence, causing death from a combination of encephalopathy and renal failure. Today, and indeed for more than two decades, such deaths occur uncommonly and, at least in Framingham, have not been noted as the cause of death since the introduction of effective, potent anti-hypertensive agents.

Now that a wide array of medications is available for the treatment of hypertension, attention has turned to the exact indications for such treatment. Each kind of medication has the potential for causing adverse effects, both symptomatic and chemical, and the question has been raised whether treatment benefits exceed the cost, inconvenience, side effects, and risks. The recently completed Hypertension Detection and Follow-up Program (HDFP) of the National Heart, Lung, and Blood Institute addressed this question in the general population in the United States [4, 5]. It built on the information obtained in prior studies by the Veterans Administration and the United States Public Health Service Hospitals Cooperative Study Group, both of which had limitations imposed by selection of patients [6–8]. In sum, these large studies indicate that the excessive mortality rate among hypertensives can be reduced significantly by treatment; that this reduction occurs not only for those whose blood pressure is far up in the definite range but also for borderline hypertensives. The HDFP also showed that blacks' and women's mortality rates fall, as well as those for white men, and that close attention to ensuring compliance and giving comprehensive care yields the best results, in terms of lowering both the blood pressure and mortality rates.

Certainly then, lower blood pressure is both achievable and efficacious. Still, there remains the practical problem of deciding, for the individual patient, whether to treat. Definite hypertensives offer no dilema: they require blood pressure control. It is the large group of borderline or mild hypertensives who represent the biggest challenge. A rational approach should recognize that this group is not homogeneous. Both their excessive mortality rate and their hypertension itself result from a combination of factors. Thus, the person with an average blood pressure of 146/94, whose serum cholesterol is low to normal, who smokes no cigarettes, who exercises a bit and imbibes alcohol no more than moderately, and who has no impairment of glucose tolerance or electrocardiographic abnormalities, can be observed relatively safely every six months without the administration of antihypertensive medication and without much risk of morbidity. Hygienic measures such as weight control and salt restriction may well succeed in controlling the blood pressure elevation. Though he belongs to the category 'borderline hypertensive', it is not he, but his alter ego with the same blood pressure but a poor cardiovascular risk profile who is subject to the excessive mortality for the group and who should have his pressure treated if he cannot be successfully managed by hygienic means.

Because hypertension plays an important role in the development of cardiovascular disease in the elderly, several observations about their situation are in order. Some clinicians question the wisdom of vigorous treatment in the elderly. Some even consider the rise in pressure with age as an inevitable, normal, physiologic process needed to compensate for progressive arterial sclerosis.

Age trends in blood pressure in the elderly indicate a disproportionate rise in systolic blood pressure consistent with a decrease in arterial capacitance and loss of elasticity with advancing age. Because of this, the prevalence of isolated systolic pressure elevations increases with age so that, over the age of 65, 30% of women and 18% of men have systolic pressures exceeding 160 mm Hg, with diastolic pressures below 95 mm Hg [9].

It is not just for the young that hypertension doubles the risk of death and triples the risk of cardiovascular mortality (Tables 1 and 2). The risk ratio is

Table 5. Risk of cardiovascular mortality according to age in hypertensives. Framingham Study, 20-year follow-up

Age	Incidence per 1000 person years		Risk ratio		Regression coefficient		Attributable risk [2]	
	Men	Women	Men	Women	Men	Women	Men	Women
45–45	9.2	4.0	3.7	4.4	0.662	0.741	6.7	3.1
55–64	20.6	5.7	2.5	2.6	0.469	0.449	11.2	3.5
65–74	24.5	18.6	2.6	4.9	0.460	0.751	14.9	14.8
45–75	15.5	7.4	2.7	3.2	0.501	0.587	9.7	5.1

[1] Risk ratio: ratio of rate in hypertensives to rate in normotensives.

[2] Attributable risk: rate in hypertensives minus rate in normotensives.

Table 6. Two-year morbidity and mortality associated with isolated systolic hypertension. Framingham Study 20-year follow-up [1]

	Rate per 1000 person years		Risk ratio [2]	
	Men	Women	Men	Women
Overall mortality	56	29	2.0	2.0
Cardiovascular mortality	30	24	1.8	4.7
Cardiovascular morbidity	114	50	3.6	3.8

[1] Persons aged 55–74, excluding those having diastolic BP = 95 mmHg at any time over 20 year period.

[2] Risk ratio: ratio of rates in those with isolated systolic hypertension to rates in normotensives.

especially significant in the elderly, in whom cardiovascular disease incidence is substantially greater than in the young. Although the risk over a lifetime is greater in the young hypertensive, the short-term risk of death and disability in the elderly hypertensive is formidable.

Contrary to other cardiovascular risk factors, there is no indication of a diminishing impact of hypertension with advancing age, whether judged from absolute, relative, or attributable risks (Table 5).

As in the young hypertensive, the risk of every major cardiovascular sequela of hypertension is increased in the elderly, with the greatest impact for stroke and least for occlusive peripheral arterial disease. In absolute terms, coronary heart disease is still the commonest sequela and cause of death in the hypertensive elderly as in the young [9].

Contrary to clinical folklore, there is little evidence that elderly women tolerate hypertension any better than men. Relative and attributable risks are actually *greater* in women over the age of 65, and for stroke and cardiac failure absolute risks are no smaller than for men.

In the elderly as well as the young the risk of cardiovascular mortality is no more closely linked to the systolic blood pressure than the diastolic component. Even isolated systolic hypertension in the elderly is far from innocuous, being associated with a two- to fivefold excess of cardiovascular deaths (Table 6). The impact of this type of hypertension is at least equal in the two sexes. Isolated systolic hypertension is not an innocent sign of sclerotic vessels which are producing cardiovascular mortality. Studies at Framingham indicate that systolic hypertension directly contributes to cardiovascular mortality, taking the degree of arterial ridigity into account [9].

Attention to lability of the pressure or to the level of the diastolic component was found to add little to prediction of cardiovascular mortality in relation to blood pressure in the elderly as well as the young hypertensive. It

Table 7. Risk of death and cardiovascular disease according to ECG-LVH [1], persons aged 65–74, Framingham Study, 20-year follow-up

ECG-LVH	Five-year incidence (%)					
	CVD morbidity		CVD mortality		Total mortality	
	Men	Women	Men	Women	Men	Women
None	13.9	10.6	6.4	4.1	14.2	7.9
Possible	27.3	23.0	20.6	15.4	29.4	20.6
Definite	45.0	43.7	40.6	29.9	53.4	36.2
Risk ratio [2]	3.8	4.6	6.3	7.3	3.8	4.6
T-value	8.3	9.2	14.5	11.5	12.7	9.8

[1] ECG-LVH: Left ventricular hypertrophy by electrocardiogram.
[2] Risk ratio: Ratio of rate in those with any ECG-LVH to rate in those with none.

would seem pointless to use the usual level of pressure in the elderly as a normal standard, since a given degree of hypertension carries the same relative risk and a higher absolute risk in the elderly compared to the young.

It is not prudent to await evidence of target organ involvement before instituting treatment in the elderly. One third of cardiovascular catastrophes in the elderly occur before evidence of organ involvement, such as X-ray enlargement of the heart, ECG abnormalities, or albuminuria appears on biennial examination. The first evidence of organ involvement is all too often a lethal coronary attack or a fatal or disabling stroke.

Once ECG evidence of left ventricular hypertrophy appears, the need for antihypertensive treatment becomes urgent. Within five years of its appearance, more than half the men and more than a third of the women will die (Table 7). This is a conservative estimate of the impact, since some of the subjects in the Framingham Study on which the estimated are based received antihypertensive treatment. Cardiovascular mortality rates increase more than sixfold when ECG-LVH appears.

There is no justification for neglect of hypertension in the elderly, and systolic hypertension in particular appears to have been sorely neglected (Table 8). The fact that hypertension in the elderly is common and predominantly systolic does not make it an innocuous condition. There is no reason why arterial vascular damage should derive more from diastolic than from systolic pressure, nor is there evidence that it does.

The benefits and risks of treatment of hypertension in the elderly need further study, and controlled trials are required to determine more clearly the indications, contraindications, best drugs, side effects, benefits, and hazards of treatment in this group. Because of the high morbidity and mortality associated with any type of hypertension in the elderly, its control is a

462

Table 8. Prevalence of antihypertensive drug treatment
At ≥200 mmHg systolic blood pressure*

Age	Percent being treated	
	Men	Women
35–44	40	43
45–54	28	53
55–64	37	40
65–74	21	32

* Framingham Study examinations 1–10.

preventive challenge we must accept. When employed prudently, antihypertensive treatment in the elderly should greatly improve the quality as well as the length of life.

It is evident from the available data that hypertension imposes a substantial risk of mortality. As more information from intervention studies appears, attention can be focused on the effects of controlling blood pressure. The impact of such control will likely be expressed in reduced rates of death from various cardiovascular diseases and, therefore, increased life expectancy. However, the availability of treatment will have little impact unless such treatment is appropriately prescribed and is accepted by hypertensive patients and their physicians. As with cigarette smoking and the non-use of seat belts and helmets, compliance constitutes the greatest challenge in effective management of hypertension. Although it may take decades to accomplish the deed, hypertension kills. This excess mortality should no longer be accepted as an inevitable consequence of aging or genetic make-up.

ACKNOWLEDGEMENTS

Supported in part by contracts numbers NIH-NO1-HV-92922 and NIH-NO1-HV-52971.

REFERENCES

1. Shurtloff D: Some characteristics related to the incidence of cardiovascular disease and Death. Framingham Study: 18-year follow-up. In: An Epidemiological Investigation of Cardiovascular Disease, Section 30. Kannel WB, Gordon T, eds. US Government Printing Office, 1974.

2. Kannel WB, Dawber TR: Hypertension as an ingredient of a cardiovascular risk profile. Br J Hosp Med 2:508, 1974.
3. Kannel WB, Sorlie P, Gordon T: Labile hypertension: a faulty concept? Circulation 61:1183–1187, 1980.
4. Hypertension Detection and Follow-up Program Cooperative Group: Five-Year Findings of the Hypertension Detection and Follow-up Program – I. Reduction in mortality of persons with high blood pressure, including mild hypertension. JAMA 242:2562–2571, 1979.
5. Hypertension Detection and Follow-up Program Cooperative Group: Five-Year Findings of the Hypertension Detection and Follow-up Program – II. Mortality by race, sex and age. JAMA 242:2572–2577, 1979.
6. Veterans Administration Cooperative Study Group on Antihypertensive Agents: Effects of Treatment on Morbidity in Hypertension – I. Results in patients with diastolic blood pressure averaging 115 through 129 mmHg. JAMA 202:1028–1034, 1967.
7. Veterans Administration Cooperative Study Group on Antihypertensive Agents: Effect of Treatment on Morbidity in Hypertension – II. Results in patients with diastolic blood pressure averaging 90 through 114 mmHg. JAMA 213:1143–1152, 1970.
8. United States Public Health Service Hospitals Cooperative Study Group (WF Smith): Treatment of Mild Hypertension: results of a ten-year intervention trial. Circ Res 40 (Suppl 1):98–105, 1977.
9. Kannel WB, Dawber TR, Mc Gee DL: Perspectives on systolic hypertension: the Framingham Study. Circulation:61:1179–1182, 1980.

30. MALIGNANT HYPERTENSION

PRISCILLA KINCAID-SMITH

1. INTRODUCTION

Prior to the advent of effective antihypertensive drugs, the name malignant hypertension was very appropriate for that form of severe hypertension which is associated with papilloedema. Most untreated patients with malignant hypertension died within a few weeks of showing [1] fulminating renal failure.

In 1914 Volhard and Fahr [2] gave a remarkably complete account of the clinical and pathological features of malignant hypertension in their description of 'Die Kombinationsform' or 'Maligne Form der Hypertonie'. They also linked the malignant phase with 'Retinitis Albuminurica'. Keith, Wagener and Barker further elaborated on the ominous prognostic significance of retinal haemorrhages, exudates and papilloedema [3].

2. MALIGNANT HYPERTENSION AND BENIGN HYPERTENSION

We still understand little about the factors which govern the onset of malignant hypertension. There is a striking contrast between an asymptomatic patient with severe but stable 'benign' hypertension, and the weakness and wasting and fulminating uraemia which come on so abruptly in the malignant phase. This transition may occur without any substantial rise in the blood pressure [4]. Indeed, 24-h blood pressure recordings have shown that the extreme ranges of arterial pressure in individual patients with malignant hypertension are quite similar in those with benign hypertension [5].

The lesions in the interlobular arteries of the kidney are the hallmark of malignant hypertension and the cause of the rapidly progressive uraemia. Severe narrowing or occlusion of interlobular arteries and non-function of ischaemic renal parenchyma distal to these arteries, are found at autopsy in uraemic patients.

In benign hypertension in contrast, the kidneys may be normal in size and appearance, and interlobular arteries may show no narrowing even after many years of well-documented very high blood pressure [4].

Amery, A. (ed.) Hypertensive Cardiovascular Disease: Pathophysiology and Treatment
© *1982, Martinus Nijhoff Publishers. The Hague / Boston / London*
ISBN-13: 978-94-009-7478-4

3. MECHANISMS IN MALIGNANT HYPERTENSION

3.1. The central role of vascular lesions

Acute vascular lesions in arteries and arterioles in the kidney and other organs, can explain all the specific clinical manifestations of malignant hypertension. To understand the underlying pathophysiology of malignant hypertension, we have to understand how these lesions develop in arteries and arterioles.

There has been a considerable growth in our knowledge about factors which may contribute to the rapid narrowing of interlobular arteries in the kidney by proliferation of cells in the intima. In 1946 Duguid [6] suggested that thrombus formation may play a part in atherogenesis. It has been proposed that similar mechanisms in the microvasculature could cause the cellular myointimal proliferation which characterises the lesions of malignant hypertension [7, 8]. Endothelial damage followed by platelet aggregation, fibrin deposition and ultimately migration of myointimal cells and their proliferation within the intima, are the steps that lead to progressive narrowing in malignant hypertension [4]. The factors which initiate this intravascular thrombosis by causing endothelial damage are less clearly defined than is the chain of events that follows endothelial damage.

3.2. Initiating factors in malignant hypertension

While there is a strong body of opinion that the height of the blood pressure alone can explain the damage to endothelial cells in malignant hypertension, the same extreme range of blood pressure in benign and malignant hypertension [5] leaves room for doubt about this.

The series of experiments published by Möhring and his co-workers [9–12] throw some light on the factors initiating vascular lesions of malignant hypertension. Möhring and his group studied the two-kidney model of experimental hypertension and the model of deoxycorticosterone hypertension in the rat. In both models, their studies suggested that humoral factors rather than the height of the blood pressure alone, govern the development of the vascular lesions of malignant hypertension.

In the two-kidney model, at the time of onset of malignant hypertension, rats lost weight due to sudden sodium and water loss, and developed very high renin levels and these factors precipitated the onset of vascular lesions of malignant hypertension and a microangiopathic haemolytic anaemia. Remission of both the vascular lesions and the anaemia occurred when the salt and water deficit was corrected by drinking saline. This resolution occurred in the face of blood pressure levels which were maintained as high as they had been during the development of malignant hypertension. Remission was accompanied by a fall in angiotensin II levels and the haematological and vascular lesions of malignant hypertension did not recur, while access to saline was continued. When saline was withdrawn, hyponatraemia and volume depletion rapidly recurred, angiotensin II levels rose and the features of malignant hypertension recurred without significant alteration in the blood pressure level. In this series of experiments the plasma angiotensin II concentrations seemed to be a more important factor governing the onset of malignant hypertension than the blood pressure level. Our own studies in the rat demonstrated a significant correlation between plasma renin activity and vascular lesions in the kidney, but no correlation between the level of the blood pressure and vascular lesions. This was in the aortic ligation two-kidney model with saline loading [13].

In the deoxycorticosterone model, plasma arginine vasopressin levels are very high, and Möhring's observations suggested that this vasoactive substance played an important role in the development of vascular lesions [11, 12].

Even assuming that a certain critical level of blood pressure and certain critical levels of circulating vasoactive substances such as angiotension and vasopressin are necessary for the onset of malignant hypertension, some other precipitating factor on factors are likely to contribute. Not all patients with very high levels of blood pressure and high angiotensin II levels develop malignant hypertension.

The chain of events which led to malignant hypertension in Möhring's experiments was initiated by a sudden loss of salt and water. Many rats develop blood pressure levels of 180–190 mm Hg, but only those which showed this sudden loss of salt and water develop malignant hypertension. The salt and water diuresis led to hypovolaemia and considerable elevation in angiotensin II levels. These changes preceded the development of malignant hypertension defined in terms of onset of vascular lesions and microangiopathic haemolytic anaemia.

In seeking an explanation for the sodium and water diuresis, it has been suggested that this may have been a pressure naturesis [4]. The response to vasoactive substances is enhanced in hypertension [14–16] and the efferent arterioles in the kidney show an increased vasoconstrictor response to both norepinephrine and angiotensin II [17, 18]. In hypertension the lumen of the afferent arteriole is increased in size, whereas the lumen of the efferent arteriole remains unchanged. This difference in lumen size together with increased vascular response in efferent arterioles, could cause a pressure diuresis at certain critical level of circulating vasoactive substances. The pressure diuresis could initiate the chain of events described by Möhring and thus establish the so-called vicious circle of malignant hypertension postulated by Wilson and Byrom in 1939 [19].

4. CAUSES OF SECONDARY MALIGNANT HYPERTENSION

4.1. *Underlying renal disease*

About half the patients who show malignant hypertension have underlying renal disease [1]. Chronic atrophic pyelonephritis (reflux nephropathy) and glomerulonephritis, are by far the commonest associated renal lesions accounting for 80% of associated renal disease in patients with malignant hypertension.

Renal artery stenosis and other renal conditions such as polycystic kidney and polyarteritis, are relatively infrequent in comparison with reflux nephropathy and glomerulonephritis.

The mechanisms which lead to the development of malignant hypertension in patients with renal disease, are not well-defined except in the case of renal artery stenosis which has been clearly established an angiotensin dependent form of hypertension.

There is some evidence, discussed in detail elsewhere, that the renin-angiotensin system may also be involved in reflux nephropathy [4, 20]. In glomerulonephritis, arteriolar and arterial lesions, which resemble those of hypertension, are present in the kidney before hypertension develops [21]. By causing ischaemia of the related nephrons these lesions could also lead to increased renin secretion.

Malignant hypertension is also a relatively frequent complication in analgesic nephropathy and sodium depletion may be a prominent clinical finding accompanying malignant hypertension in such patients [22, 23].

4.2. *Other causes of malignant hypertension*

Oral contraceptives may cause malignant hypertension [24, 25] which may be reversed when the oral contraceptive drug is withdrawn. The renin-angiotensin system is probably involved in this form of hypertension because there is a marked increase in renin substrate in patients taking oral contraceptives.

4.2.1. *Tumours and hyperactivity of the adrenal gland*
Phaeochromocytoma, aldosterone secreting adenomas and Cushing's syndrome have all been described as rare causes of malignant hypertension.

4.2.2. *Renin secreting tumours*
Although these tumours are extremely rare, they are characteristically associated with severe hypertension which may be malignant.

4.2.3. Pregnancy

Malignant hypertension may occur as a complication of pre-eclampsia. The first description of what is now known as post-partum renal failure was published by Counihan and Doniach in 1954 [26] under the title 'Malignant Hypertension Supervening Rapidly on Pre-eclampsia'. The two patients they described and one additional case were included in a study in 1958 [1], all of whom showed unusually florid vascular lesions with prominent fibrin deposition.

While some authors believe that the post-partum renal failure syndrome occurs most frequently in patients who do not develop pre-eclampsia [27], we have most frequently seen this syndrome in association with pre-eclampsia [28, 29].

Fulminating malignant hypertension may also occur as a complication of pregnancy in patients with underlying renal disease [29, 30].

5. CLINICAL FEATURES OF MALIGNANT HYPERTENSION

While some of the clinical features of hypertension are similar to those of benign hypertension, others are distinctive and restricted to malignant hypertension.

5.1. Distinctive clinical features

5.1.1. Visual impairment

Seventy % of patients with malignant hypertension complain of visual disturbances. Blurring of vision is the most frequent complaint [1]. With progression of untreated malignant hypertension, blindness develops as a complication of papilloedema. Sudden temporary or permanent blindness has also been described [1, 31–33].

5.1.2. Weight loss

Weight loss occurs at the onset of malignant hypertension in 75% of patients. This probably reflects loss of salt and water, similar to that which has been well documented by Möhring [10] as an acute event precipitating malignant hypertension in rats.

In some patients, particularly those who suddenly develop malignant hypertension due to renal artery occlusion [34] or analgesic nephropathy [35], extreme sodium depletion may develop with daily loss of as much as 500 mEq of sodium in the urine.

5.1.3. Anaemia

A microangiopathic haemolytic anaemia is a common feature in malignant hypertension [36]. Patients with an underlying renal cause for malignant hypertension tend to have a lower haemoglobin level (mean 9.3 g), than those with no underlying renal disease (mean 11.3 g) [1]. The anaemia in those with underlying renal disease probably reflects chronic impairment of renal function but a microangiopathic haemolytic anaemia may be superimposed on the anaemia resulting from reduced erythropoctin production.

5.1.4. Uraemia

Uraemia is a prominent clinical feature in malignant hypertension and runs a fulminating course to death or end stage renal disease. It is important to emphasize that the vascular lesions of benign hypertension do not cause uraemia. If a patient with benign hypertension becomes uraemic, underlying renal disease is the cause. The only exception to this rule is the group of patients with retinal haemorrhages and exudates, but no papilloedema. These patients may occasionally develop the classical vascular lesions of malignant hypertension before they develop papilloedema and this will result in impaired renal function. Patients with retinal haemorrhages and exudates are recognized to form a separate prognostic group and are not usually included as 'benign' hypertension.

5.2. Other symptoms

5.2.1. Headache

Headache is a common symptom in hypertension. Severe, often incapacitating headache is one of the most frequent symptoms in malignant hypertension and worsening headaches in patients with severe hypertension often herald the onset of the malignant phase. Over 80% of patients with malignant hypertension complain of headache [1].

5.2.2. Cardiac failure

Paroxysmal nocturnal dyspnoea, or left ventricular failure, is frequent in uraemic patients with malignant hypertension. It may also occur quite early in the course of malignant hypertension where there is an abrupt and extreme blood pressure rise.

5.2.3. Neurological manifestations

These were observed in almost half the patients with malignant hypertension before treatment was available. Transient ischaemic attacks were frequent and cerebral thrombosis and hypertensive encephalopathy were also common [37]. Isolated lower motor neuron lesions particularly affecting the

7th nerve, and transient cortical blindness, are among the less frequent neurological manifestations.

6.   TREATMENT OF MALIGNANT HYPERTENSION

6.1. Treatment of underlying causes

Because of the need to commence treatment at once in malignant hypertension, the frequency of underlying disease may be forgotten. More than half the cases will show an underlying cause, and in a few cases reversal of the hypertension is possible by treating the underlying disease. The most widely recognized examples of this are those where removal of a tumour or correction of a renal artery stenosis results in significant lowering of the blood pressure. It is less frequently recognized that malignant hypertension may be reversed in other conditions. In analgesic nephropathy correction of the sodium and water deficit may be followed by a long-term remission of malignant hypertension provided analgesic abuse ceases [35].

Although this is only practical in a few cases, it is important to establish a diagnosis in all patients with an underlying cause, because the disease which is causing the hypertension may warrant treatment in its own right. At least two thirds of children who develop malignant hypertension have underlying reflux nephropathy [38]. In a young child, correct management of the reflux and superimposed infection can prevent further renal scarring and progression to renal failure.

Glomerulonephritis is the most frequent underlying lesion in adults and the value of treatment for both acute and chronic forms of glomerulonephritis is becoming more firmly established as a result of controlled trials [39–42]. The prognosis is also different in patients with different forms of underlying renal disease, and even if treatment is not available it is important to establish the prognosis.

6.2. Treatment of the microangiopathy

The vascular lesions of malignant hypertension are identical to those seen in other forms of thrombotic microangiopathy. The sequence of events which leads to narrowing of renal arteries and arterioles is the same as that in thrombotic microangiopathy, viz. platelet and fibrin deposition and subsequent 'organization' by proliferation of myointimal cells [4].

In experimental vascular lesions similar to those seen in malignant hypertension, certain antithrombotic and anticoagulant agents have been shown to reduce or inhibit the myointimal proliferation which is the factor leading to arterial occlusion and uraemia in malignant hypertension. Anti-platelet serum [43], dipyridamole [44] and heparin [45, 46] have all been shown to reduce or inhibit myointimal proliferation.

In patients with malignant hypertension, arrest of the myointimal proliferation and 'healing' of the vascular lesions is rapidly brought about by lowering the blood pressure [47].

Where renal function is severely impaired, it may gradually improve following reduction of blood pressure levels [47–49]. However, renal function frequently deteriorates in spite of adequate blood pressure control [47]. Malignant hypertension remains an unacceptably frequent cause of end stage renal failure requiring dialysis [50].

Attempts have been made to reverse the vascular lesions in the kidney using heparin and dipyridamole [51], but the risks of bleeding are high unless the blood pressure is rigidly controlled.

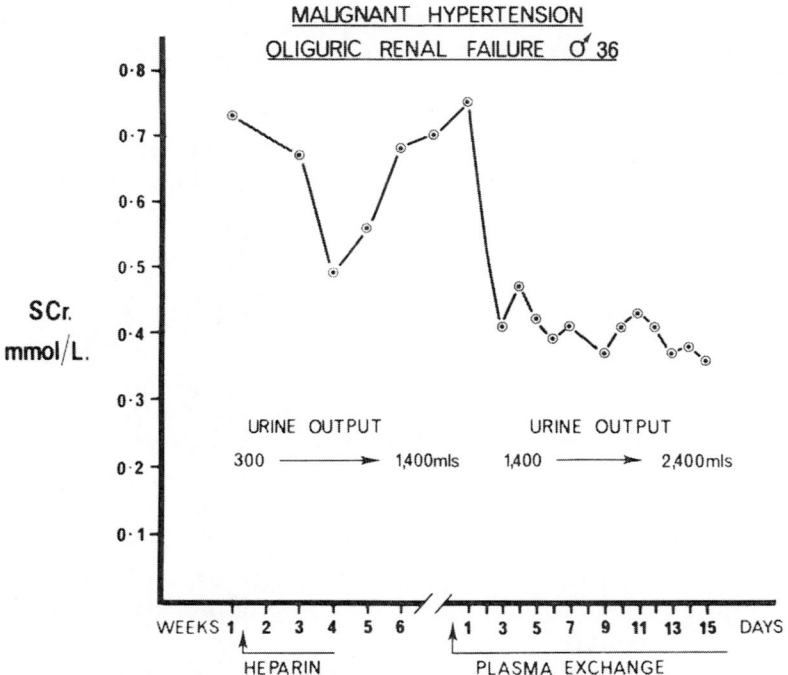

Figure 1. Course of a man aged 36 who presented with apparent end stage renal failure due to malignant essential hypertension. Urine output rose and serum creatinine fell during a period of intravenous heparin, but serum creatinine rose again when heparin was stopped. Serum creatinine fell promptly when plasma exchange was commenced and is still gradually falling 6 weeks later.

Plasma exchange not only lowers the blood pressure in severe hypertension [52], but because it lowers fibrinogen levels, it could also prevent progression and may even reverse early vascular lesions in malignant hypertension. The use of plasma exchange in a few cases has been promising and associated with improvement in renal function in patients showing apparent end stage renal failure due to malignant vessel changes (Figure 1).

6.3. Sodium and malignant hypertension

The rice diet introduced by Kempner in 1944 [53] undoubtedly reversed malignant hypertension in some patients. Compliance was a serious problem, however, and the diet had to be abandoned because of hyponatraemia in about a third of patients [54]. Even without a rice diet, weight loss, due to sodium depletion, occurs in malignant hypertension in man, and sodium depletion may become very severe in some cases [34, 35]. It may be difficult to keep up adequate sodium replacement to maintain renal function in such patients [34, 35]. In addition, Möhring's studies [9–12] clearly demonstrate the importance of salt depletion in the development of malignant hypertension in the rat.

It seems unwise to restrict the sodium intake in patients with malignant hypertension. Indeed, administration of sodium may be necessary to maintain renal function and it may also improve blood pressure control [35, 51, 55].

6.4 Lowering the blood pressure with drugs in malignant hypertension

6.4.1. Hypertensive emergencies in malignant hypertension
Immediate lowering of the blood pressure using parenteral drugs is only necessary in a minority of cases. Hypertensive encephalopathy, acute left ventricular failure, and retinal lesions causing blindness are complications which warrant immediate lowering of the blood pressure. The danger of fits in a pregnant patient with severe hypertension also warrants immediate parenteral antihypertensive medicatoin. Marked paroxysmal rises in blood pressure in any circumstances should probably be treated by immediate lowering of the pressure.

There is a wide choice of agents which will lower the blood pressure (Table 1). Intravenous diazoxide is one of the most reliable agent, but is now usually used in repeated doses of 75 mg rather than a large dose of 300–600 mg. All the drugs have some side-effects and attention has recently been drawn to the potential danger of sudden reduction of the blood pressure [56].

Table 1. Parenteral agents used to lower blood pressure immediately

Drug	Route	Dose
Diazoxide	a) Bolus intravenous injection b) repeated injections	150–300 mg 75–150 mg
Clonidine	Intravenous injection over 10 min	300 µg
Labetolol [1]	Intravenous injection over 5 min	100 mg
Sodium nitroprusside	Intravenous infusion	50–100 mg/l
Hydrallazine	Intravenous infusion	100 mg/l
Phentolamine [2]	Intravenous infusion	200–400 mg/l

[1] Labetolol has been found unsatisfactory in patients already receiving antihypertensive medication [56, 57].
[2] Specifically in patients with sudden catecholamine release.

Intravenous clonidine is a reliable agent for lowering the blood pressure, but because the pressure falls more gradually than following diazoxide [57], it is probably less likely to cause the complications attributed to sudden blood pressure reduction [32, 33, 56].

Labetalol may be effective in patients who have not already received some treatment, but is disappointing in those who have had previous treatment [57, 58].

6.4.2. Oral antihypertensive drugs
Although only complicated cases dealt with in section 6.4.1. require immediate lowering of the blood pressure using parenteral agents, malignant hypertension should be regarded as a medical emergency. Admission to hospital is mandatory and, unless the blood pressure can be brought under adequate control within a few hours, treatment with parenteral agents detailed in section 6.4.1. is justified. Most patients can be treated using conventional drugs, but in those who prove resistant, two drugs, which have a powerful vasodilator effect, have a special place.

Diazoxide and Minoxidil. Diazoxide, a powerful vasodilator, has proved very valuable in the control of severe resistant hypertension [59–61]. Minoxidil, another powerful vasodilator, introduced at about the same time as oral diazoxide [62], is another useful drug in severe refractory hypertension [63, 64].

Both oral diazoxide and minoxidil need to be used in combination with frusemide or another powerful diuretic to control oedema. Diazoxide is diabetogenic and often needs to be combined with an oral hypoglycaemic agent. Mioxidil produces hirsutism which makes it unacceptable to most women. Tachycardia is far more pronounced in patients taking minoxidil than in those taking diazoxide, and minoxidil must invariably be combined with a beta-adrenergic blocking agent to control this tachycardia.

In spite of these side-effects, any referral clinic dealing with patients with severe refractory hypertension will need to use these drugs in some resistant cases.

Prazosin. This drug, which causes vasodilatation, has been used to reduce the blood pressure acutely in patients with severe and malignant hypertension [65].

Conventional antihypertensive medication in treating malignant hypertension. Combination therapy is almost always necessary to achieve adequate control of the blood pressure in malignant hypertension.

Thiazides, introduced over 20 years ago, potentiate the action of all anti-hypertensive drugs. The introduction of thiazides greatly facilitated control of the blood pressure in patients with malignant hypertension [61], And a thiazide diuretic should be included in any drug combintion used to control malignant hypertension.

The two combinations most frequently used in the control of severe hypertension at the present time are either a combination of a thiazide and alpha-methyl dopa or a combination of a thiazide and a beta-adrenergic blocking agent, and a drug causing peripheral vasodilatation, such as prazosin or hydrallazine.

With either dose regimen, a standard dose of thiazide is combined with progressive increase in doses of other drugs until control is achieved. For example, the starting doses would be 0.5 g of chlorothiazide combined with 40 mg of propranolol (or equivalent other beta-adrenergic blocking agent) and 1 mg of prazosin (or 25 mg of hydrallazine). If within two hours, the blood pressure control remains unsatisfactory, doses of propranolol (or equivalent) and prazosin or hydrallazine, can be doubled with further increase after another two hours until maximum doses are reached. Using alpha-methyl dopa, the dose can be progressively increased every two hours to a maximum of a 1 g dose.

Either regimen will achieve blood pressure control in a few hours in almost all patients but parenteral drugs are indicated in those in whom pressure is not adequately controlled,

Other drugs such as labetalol or clonidine can be effective in malignant hypertension in standard doses in combination with a thiazide diuretic.

Captopril. Among newer antihypertensive agents, Captopril, the oral angio-tensin converting enzyme inhibitor, deserves special mention as a drug used in the treatment of severe and malignant hypertension [66]. Although not universally effective in patients with malignant hypertension, very impressive results have been reported in some patients.

Captopril may reverse not only the malignant hypertension, but also the hyponatraemic-hypertensive syndrome of angiotensin-dependent hypertension [67]. Certain forms of malignant hypertension such as scleroderma crises, which have proved resistant to conventional treatment, have responded well to Captopril [68].

REFERENCES

1. Kincaid-Smith P, McMichael J, Murphy EA: The clinical course and pathology of hypertension with papilloedema (malignant hypertension) Q J Med 105 (New Series 27):117–153, 1958.
2. Volhard F, Fahr KT: Die Brightsche Nierenkranheit. Berlin: Springer-Verlag, 1914.
3. Keith NM, Wagener HP, Barker NW: Some different types of essential hypertension: their course and prognosis. Am J Med Sci 197:332–342, 1939.
4. Kincaid-Smith P: Malignant hypertension: Mechanisms and management. Pharmacol Ther 9:245–269, 1980.
5. Bevan AT, Honour AJ, Stott FH: Direct arterial pressure recording in unrestricted man. Clin Sci 36:329–344, 1969.
6. Duguid JB: Thrombosis as a factor in the pathogenesis of coronary atherosclerosis. J Pathol Bact 58:207–212, 1946.
7. Kincaid-Smith P: Histological diagnosis of rejection of renal homografts in man. Lancet 2:849–852, 1967.
8. Penington DG, Kincaid-Smith P: Anaemia in renal failure. Br Med Bull 27:136–141, 1971.
9. Möhring J, Dauda G, Haack D, Hofbauer KG, Homsy E, Naumann HJ, Orth H, Gross F: Malignant phase of renal hypertension in rats. Eur J Clin Invest 2:297, 1972. (Abstract).
10. Möhring J, Petri M, Szokol M, Haack D, Möhring B: Effects of saline drinking on malignant course of renal hypertension in rats. Am J Physiol 230:849–857, 1976.
11. Möhring J, Möhring B, Petri M, Haack D: Vasopressor role of ADH in the pathogenesis of malignant DOC hypertension. Am J Physiol 232:F260–F269, 1977.
12. Möhring J, Möhring B, Petri M, Haack D: Plasma vasopressin concentrations and effects of vasopressin antiserum on blood pressure in rats with malignant two-Kidney goldblatt hypertension. Circulation Res 42:17–22, 1978.
13. Chusilp S, Hua ASP, Kincaid-Smith P: Accelerated hypertension in the rat; relation between renin, renal vascular lesions, salt intake and blood pressure. Clin Sci mol Med 51:69S–71S, 1976.
14. Doyle AE, Fraser JRE: Vascular reactivity in hypertension. Proc of Council for high Blood Pressure Research. Circ Res 9:755, 1961.
15. Folkow B, Hallbäck M, Lundgren Y, Weiss L: Background of increase of flow resistance and vascular reactivity in spontaneously hypertensive rats. Acta Physiol Scand 80:93–106, 1970.
16. Folkow B, Hallbäck M, Lundgren Y, Weiss L: Renal vascular resistance in spontaneously hypertensive rats. Acta physiol Scand 83:96–105, 1971.
17. Click RL, Joyner WL, Gilmore JP: Reactivity of glomerular afferent and efferent arterioles in renal hypertension. Kidney Int 15:109–115, 1979.

476

18. Click RL, Gilmore JP, Joyner WL: Differential response of hamster cheek pouch microvessels to vasoactive stimuli during the early development of hypertension. Circ Res 44:512–516, 1979.

19. Wilson C, Byrom FB: Renal changes in malignant hypertension. Lancet 1:136–139, 1939.

20. Kincaid-Smith P: Vascular obstruction in chronic pyelonephritic kidneys and its relation to hypertension. Lancet 2:1263–1269, 1955.

21. Kincaid-Smith P: The Kidney – A Clinico-Pathological Study, p. 193. Oxford: Blackwell Scientific, 1975.

22. Dawborn JK, Fairley KF, Kincaid-Smith P, King WE: The association of peptic ulceration, chronic renal disease and analgesic abuse. Q J Med 35:69–83, 1966.

23. Kincaid-Smith P: Analgesic nephropathy: a common form of renal disease in Australia. Med J Aust 2:1131–1135, 1969.

24. Harris PWR: Malignant hypertension associated with oral contraceptives. Lancet 2:466–467, 1969.

25. Bock KD, Bohle A: Peracture primary malignant nephrosclerosis with irreversible renal failure and malignant hypertension after taking oral contraceptives. Dtsch Med Wochenschr 98:757–761, 1973.

26. Counihan TB, Doniach I: Malignant hypertension supervening rapidly on pre-eclampsia. J Obstet Gynaecol Br Emp 61:449–453, 1954.

27. Robson JS, Martin AM, Ruckley A, McDonald MK: Irreversible post-partum renal failure. A new syndrome. Q J Med 37: 423–435, 1968.

28. Kincaid-Smith P: The similarity of lesions and underlying mechanism in pre-eclamptic toxaemia and post-partum renal failure. Studies in the acute stage and during follow-up. In: Glomerulonephritis: Morphology,Natural History and Treatment, pp. 1013–1025. Kincaid-Smith P, Mathew TH, Becker EL, eds. New York: John Wiley, 1973.

29. Kincaid-Smith P, Fairley KF. The Changing Spectrum of Acute Renal Failure in Pregnancy and the Post-partum period. Proc. of 8th Symp. Nephrology, Hannover. Contrib Nephrol 25 (24), 1981 (in press).

30. Kincaid-Smith P: The Kidney – A Clinico-Pathological Study, p. 239. Oxford: Blackwell Scientific, 1975.

31. Kincaid-Smith P, Whitworth JA: Danderous antihypertensive treatment. Br Med J 2:737, 1979.

32. Cove DH, Seddon M, Fletcher RF, Dukes DC: Blindness after treatment for malignant hypertension. Br Med J 2:245–246, 1979.

33. Hulse JA, Taylor DSI, Dillon MJ: Blindness and paraplegia in severe childhood Hypertension. Lancet 2:553–556, 1979.

34. Barraclough MA: Sodium and water depletion with acute malignant hypertension. Am J Med 40:265–272, 1966.

35. Nanra RS, Stuart-Taylor J, De Leon AH, White KH: Analgesic nephropathy: etiology, clinical syndrome and clinicopathologic correlation in Australia. Kidney Int 13:72–78, 1978.

36. Brain MC, Dacie JV, Hourihane O'BD: Microangiopathic haemolytic anaemia: the possible role of vascular lesions in pathogenesis. Br J Haematol 8:358–374, 1962.

37. Clarke E, Murphy EA: Neurological manifestations of malignant hypertension. Br Med J 2:1319–1326, 1956.

38. Still JL, Cottom D: Severe hypertension in childhood. Arch Dis Child 42:34–39, 1967.

39. Kincaid-Smith P: The treatment of glomerulonephritis. Aust NZJ Med 10:340–345, 1980.

40. Glassock RJ: The Treatment of Idiopathic Membranous Nephropathy in Adults. In: VIIth Int Congr Nephrol Proc, pp.425–428. Barcelo R, Bergeron M, Carriere S, Dirks J, Drummond R, Guttmann G, Lemieux J, Mongeau J, Seely J, eds. New York: S. Karger, 1978.

41. Mathew TH: Australian Trials on Glomerulonephritis. In: VIIth Int Congr Nephrol Proc, pp. 429–436. Barcelo R, Bergeron M, Carriere S, Dirks J, Drummond R, Guttmann G, Lemieux J, Mongeau J, Seely J, eds. New York: S. Karger, 1978.
42. Tiller DJ: Australian glomerulonephritis trial: membranous glomerulonephritis, mesangio-capillary glomerulonephritis. Aust NZJ Med 1981 (in press).
43. Moore S, Friedman RJ, Singal DP, Gauldie J, Blajchman MA, Roberts RS: Inhibition of injury–induced thromboatherosclerotic lesions by anti-platelet serum in rabbits. Thromb Haemostas 35:70–81, 1976.
44. Harker LA, Ross R, Slichter SJ, Scott CR: Homocystine-induced arteriosclerosis. The role of endothelial cell injury and platelet response in its genesis. J Clin Invest 58:731–741, 1976.
45. Pilcher DB, Barker WF: Retardation of experimental atherosclerosis of heparin and dextran. Am J Surg 120:270–274, 1970.
46. Clowes AW, Karnowsky MJ: Suppression by heparin of smooth muscle cell proliferation in injured arteries. Nature 265:625–626, 1977.
47. Harington M, Kincaid-Smith P, McMichael J: Results of treatment in malignant hypertension. A seven-year experience in 94 cases. Br Med J 2:969–980, 1959.
48. Kincaid-Smith P: The Effects of Antihypertensive Treatment on the Kidney. In: Systemic Effects of Antihypertensive Agents, pp. 21–39. Sambhi MP, ed. New York: Stratton Medical, 1976.
49. Woods JW, Blythe WB, Huffines WD: Management of malignant hypertension complicated by renal insufficiency. A follow-up study. N Engl J Med 291:10–14, 1974.
50. Disney aps, Correll RL: Report of the Australian and New Zealand Combined Dialysis and Transplant Registry. Med J Aust 1:117–122, 1981.
51. Kincaid-Smith P: The management of severe hypertension. Am J Cardiol 32:575–581, 1973.
52. Whitworth JA, d'Apice AJF, Kincaid-Smith P, Shulkes AA, Skinner SL: Antihypertensive effects of plasma exchange. Lancet 1:1205, 1978.
53. Kempner W: Treatment of kidney disease and hypertensive vascular disease with rice diet. NC Med J 5:125, 1944.
54. Newborg JC, Kempner W: Analysis of 177 cases of hypertensive vascular disease with papilloedema: 126 patients treated with rice diet. Am J Med 19:33–47, 1955.
55. Baer L, Parra-Carrillo JZ, Radichevich I, Williams GS: Detection of renovascular hypertension with angiotensin II blockade. Ann Intern Med 86:257–260, 1977.
56. Editorial: Dangerous antihypertensive treatment. Br Med J 2:228–229, 1979.
57. Yeung CK, Thomas gw, Whitworth JA, Kincaid-Smith P: Comparison of labetalol, clonidine and diazoxide intravenously administered in severe hypertension. Med J Aust 2:499–500, 1979.
58. Rosei EA, Brown JJ, Fraser R, Level AF, Morton JJ, Robertson JIS, Trust PM: Labetatol (AH 5158). A competitive alpha- and beta-receptor blocking drug in the management of hypertension. Aust NZ J Med 6:83–88, 1976.
59. Pohl JEF, Thurston H: Use of diazoxide in hypertension with renal failure. Br Med J 4:142–145, 1971.
60. Kincaid-Smith P: The treatment of resistant hypertension. Drugs 11:78–86, 1976.
61. Kincaid-Smith P, Fang P, Laver C: A new look at the treatment of severe hypertension. Clin Sci Mol Med 45:75S–87S, 1973.
62. Chidsey CA: Clinical and pharmacokinetic studies of minoxidil, a new antihypertensive agent. Clin Sci 45: S171–S173, 1973.
63. Limas CJ, Freis ED: Minoxidil in severe hypertension with renal failure. Effects of its addition to conventional antihypertensive drugs. Am J Cardiol 31:355–361, 1973.
64. Pettinger WA, Michell HC: Minoxidil – an alternative to nephrectomy for refractory hypertension. N Engl J Med 289:167–171, 1973.

478

65. Hayes JM: Rapid control of serious high blood pressure with single large oral doses of Prazosin. Med J Aust 1:31–32, 1980.
66. Case DB, Atlas SA, Laragh JH, Sealey JE, Sullivan PA, McKinstry DN: Clinical experience with blockade of the renin–angiotensin–aldosterone system by an oral converting enzyme inhibitor (SQ 14 225, Captopril) in hypertensive patients. Prog Cardiovasc Dis 21:195–206, 1978.
67. Sullivan JM, Ginsburg BA, Ratts TE, Johnston JG, Barton BR, Kraus DH, McKinstry DN, Muirhead EE: Hemodynamic and antihypertensive effects of Captopril, an orally active angiotensin converting enzyme inhibitor. Hypertension 1:397–401, 1979.
68. Lopez-Overero JA, Saal SD, D'Angelo WA, Cheigh JS, Stenzel KH, Laragh JH: Reversal of vascular and renal crises of scleroderma by oral angiotensin-converting-enzyme blockade. N Engl J Med 300:1417–1419, 1979.

31. DEFINITION AND CLASSIFICATION OF HYPERTENSION

Toma Strasser

Commonplace notions do not necessarily have simple definitions; rather the opposite may hold true. Arterial hypertension is a typical case of an often-used medical concept which is more difficult to define than might be assumed at first thought; yet it is imperative to define it well, just *because* the term is so frequently used.

SEMANTICS

First of all a few semantic clarifications are needed. The term 'hypertension' is applied both to the finding of 'high' (i.e. higher than normal) values of systolic and/or diastolic arterial blood pressure (hypertension as a sign) and to morbid conditions characterized by such findings (hypertensive diseases). The two meanings of the term do not necessarily overlap since blood pressure may transitorily be in the hypertensive range without the existence of hypertensive disease, and hypertensive patients may have low blood pressure values, e.g. when in shock or under drug treatment. It is of no avail to replace, with Pickering, the term 'hypertension' by 'high blood pressure', for the ambiguity persists. For the finding of hypertension as a sign we suggest, therefore, to use the term 'blood pressure in the hypertensive range', whenever such usage does not entail an overly clumsy wording.

Another clarification is needed as regards the meaning of hypertension as a morbid condition. In practice, all too often the definition of hypertension as a disease is equated with 'hypertensive disease calling for treatment'. Therapeutic considerations do not automatically follow from the definition of hypertension, unless therapeutic guidelines had been incorporated into the definition. This is often *not* the case, however, definitely not with the World Health Organization definitions to which we shall be referring in particular.

The meaning of the term 'elevated', 'high', or 'hyper-'tension itself presents the major difficulty in defining the concept. Ever since the Pickering–Platt controversy as to whether 'normal' and 'high' blood pressure values

Amery, A. (ed.) Hypertensive Cardiovascular Disease: Pathophysiology and Treatment
© 1982, Martinus Nijhoff Publishers. The Hague / Boston / London
ISBN-13: 978-94-009-7478-4

are discrete categories has been solved on a demographic basis, it is accepted that blood pressure is a graded, quantitative characteristic with a continuous distribution in any population; and yet, mainly in clinical medicine, juxtaposition of 'hypertensive' and 'normotensive' ranges is a practical necessity. We are thus viewing the same phenomenon both as one continuous and two discrete categories, depending on whether the epidemiological or clinical standpoint prevails at a given moment. One way of coping with this paradox is to carefully consider a suitable compromise such as the international definitions quoted in the next section.

THE INTERNATIONAL DEFINITIONS OF HYPERTENSION

'Persistent elevation of the systemic arterial blood pressure' is the definition of the Council for International Organizations of Medical Science (CIOMS) and the International Society and Federation of Cardiology (ISFC), with an added quantitative clause that:

> ... although no sharp dividing line between normal and elevated pressure exists, for practical purposes it is usual to consider repeated sphygmomanometric measurement of over 160 systolic and 95 diastolic as indicative of hypertension. [1]

The definition of the World Health Organization stresses that:

> Any definition of hypertension is based on the arbitrary choice of a threshold value from a continuous distribution of pressure readings. [2]

Nevertheless,

> Hypertension in adults is defined as a systolic pressure equal to or greater than 160 mm Hg (21.3 kPa) and/or diastolic (fifth phase) equal to or greater than 95 mm Hg (12.7 kPa).
> Normal adult blood pressure is arbitrarily defined as a systolic pressure equal to or below 140 mm Hg (18.7 kPa), together with a diastolic (5th Korotkoff phase) equal to or below 90 mm Hg (12.0 kPa).
> The term 'borderline hypertension' is used to denote blood pressure values between the normal and hypertensive ranges as described above. [2]

Mention should be made, however, of certain differences among the above definitions and those promulgated by some other prestigious medical and scientific bodies. Thus, according to the Criteria Committee of the New York Heart Association:

... persistent arterial blood pressures above 140/90 mm Hg in persons under the age of 50 and above 150/100 mm Hg over the age of 50 indicate the presence of hypertension. [3]

On the other hand, according to the 1980 Report of the US Joint National Committee on Detection, Evaluation and Treatment of High Blood Pressure:

The diagnosis of hypertension is confirmed when the average of multiple blood pressure measurements made on at least two subsequent visits is 90 mm Hg or higher. [4]

Obviously, the definition of hypertension is not set once forever. It may change in time, be subject to various considerations, to newly acquired knowledge and to changes in medical attitudes. The 1980 US definition may have been influenced by the recent findings of the Hypertension Detection and Follow-Up Study (HDFP) [5]. As with some other variables, e.g. body weight or serum cholesterol levels, the concept of the biological norm or optimum may be changing. For instance, since in certain primitive populations blood pressure does not increase with age [6], it is still to be elucidated whether the age-related increase, considered to be 'normal' because it is such a common feature, is indeed not a deviation from the biological norm – without entering, at this point, into speculations as to the meaning of the latter. Another example is the downward shift of the clinical concept of the hypertensive range in the elderly during the past decades.

AN INTERCALATION: UNITS FOR EXPRESSING BLOOD PRESSURE

As seen from the WHO definition, blood pressure may be expressed in millimetres of mercury or in kilopascals, the pascal being the pressure unit of the universally adopted Système international d'Unités (SI) [7]. In the discussions that led to setting the policy of WHO in this matter it was agreed that 'while the Système international d'Unités should be adopted by the scientific community, the replacement of the millimetre of mercury by the SI unit, the kilopascal would be premature; rather, both units should be used side by side for a period of time' [2]. Some governmental, scientific and other medical bodies such as the American Heart Association [8], the Canadian Health Protection Branch, Health and Welfare [9], the European Leagues against Hypertension [10], and the International Society of Hypertension [11] considered that introducing the kPa would lead to unnecessary confusion and that the mm Hg should not be replaced by the new SI unit. For these reasons, mm Hg has been retained in the present text.

HOW SHOULD BLOOD PRESSURE BE MEASURED?

Because of the great fluctuations in the individual person, the way *how* the blood pressure values were derived are, in practice, even more important than the issue whether the (anyway arbitrary) limits of the hypertensive range are put 5 mm Hg higher or lower. The WHO Expert Committee on Arterial Hypertension [2] recommended that blood pressure readings be taken under conditions described in detail, observing specifications for the use of the sphygmomanometer and the subject's state, as quoted below.

Blood pressure measurements with a mercury sphygmomanometer should be made by an observer who has been suitably instructed and shown to have normal hearing. The instrument should be kept in good working order. There must be no dust in the rubber tubes linking the inflation bulb with the mercury reservoir and no foreign matter in the space above the mercury column; the deflation valve must be in good working order; and the cuff itself must be in good condition. The standard cuff is 12.5 cm wide and sufficiently long to surround at least two-thirds of the upper arm. Cuffs of different widths are required for blood pressure measurement in children and in obese adults. The following widths have been recommended by the American Heart Association:

under 1 year	2.5 cm
1–4 years	5 or 6 cm
4–8 years	8 or 9 cm
average adults	12.5 cm
obese adults	14 cm

These measurements are a rough guide only; the important point is that the inner bag must be wide enough to cover two-thirds of the length of the circumference of the upper arm, while leaving the antecubital fossa free. For instance, when measuring the blood pressure of obese adults, cuffs 40 cm long are needed. If a choice must be made between a cuff which is too small and one which is too large, the larger one should be chosen. There have been reports that the use of the 2.5 cm cuff on infants produces spuriously high pressures.

The manometer itself should be placed on a horizontal surface. The subject will usually be in the sitting position and it is important that the arm should not be constricted in any way (for example, by clothing). The cuff is adjusted firmly, and the examiner locates the brachial pulse in the antecubital fossa and places a stethoscope over the artery. The cuff is then inflated rapidly to 20–30 mm Hg (3–4 kPa) above the pressure at which the radial pulse disappears to palpation. The cuff is then gradually deflated at a constant rate of 2–3 mm Hg per second (0.25–0.40 kPa per second). The mercury column is watched continuously and carefully. Systolic pressure is taken as the pressure at which the ear distinguishes the first arterial sound. The point at which the last arterial sound disappears (Korotkoff phase 5) is usually taken as the diastolic pressure.

Measurement of arterial pressure with the patient in the sitting position is most practicable for screening purposes. Measurement of arterial pressure with the patient in the lying position and again after he has been standing for 1–5 minutes gives useful information in the clinical examination of the hypertensive patient, particularly when under treatment.

It is valuable also to record the heart rate at the same time as the blood pressure measurement; this is particularly important during treatment with certain drugs (e.g. vasodilators, adrenergic inhibitors and beta-adrenoceptor blockers).

In the presence of cardiac arrhythmias (e.g. atrial fibrillation), repeated measurements are needed in order to obtain a satisfactory approximation to the average systolic and diastolic pressures.

With children, it is important to obtain the confidence of the subject and to ensure that the circumstances of blood pressure measurement are quiet. The Korotkoff phase 4 sound gives the best indication of diastolic pressure in children, because the arterial sound may persist until the cuff pressure has fallen to zero. In pregnant women the Korotkoff phase 4 sound is also used for the indication of diastolic pressure.

There should be no severe exertion, eating, smoking, or exposure to cold immediately preceding the measurement. Considerably lower values may be obtained if the subject is rested or sedated, or following several days in a hospital ware. Nevertheless, for practical clinical and epidemiological purposes, casual pressures have been shown to be reproducible, to give a good indication of the risk of complications, and to demonstrate the effectiveness of treatment.

The number of blood pressure readings are at least as important as the conditions of measurement – an often neglected point. The WHO Expert Committee [2] recommends that 'at least three blood pressure readings be taken on at least two different occasions... except in emergencies', but does not state how the repeated readings should be processed. The US Joint Committee stipulates that:

The diagnosis of hypertension is confirmed when the average of multiple of blood pressure measurements made on at least two subsequent visits is 90 mm or higher. [4]

In practice, however, average (mean) values of multiple readings may not always be used. Some physicians may conclude that a patient is hypertensive if one out of two readings is in the hypertensive range or, on the contrary, may exclude hypertension if one of the readings is in the normotensive range. Sometimes in special studies rather special definitions are applied. Thus, in the Oslo Study on Mild Hypertension the limit of hypertension was defined as:

... the mean of the two highest of three registered systolic blood pressures $\geqslant 150$ mm Hg, and the third not lower than 135 mm Hg. When SBP $\geqslant 150$ mm Hg, there was no lower limit for DBP. When SBP was below 150 mm Hg, however, the two highest of the three diastolic values should not be less that 95 mm Hg and the lowest not lower than 90 mm Hg. [12]

Other studies are based on different, though not necessarily more translucent definitions. The issue would be of minor importance, if the results of such therapeutic trials were not generalized and the conclusions applied to cases of hypertension with different definitions. However, it is still better to give some definition than none at all. As pointed out by Lehane et al. [13], even in prestigious journals two thirds of the publications on hypertension do not carry important information of this type at all.

The impact of blood pressure variations (both those of a biological nature and those due to observer variability) on the validity of the diagnostic con-

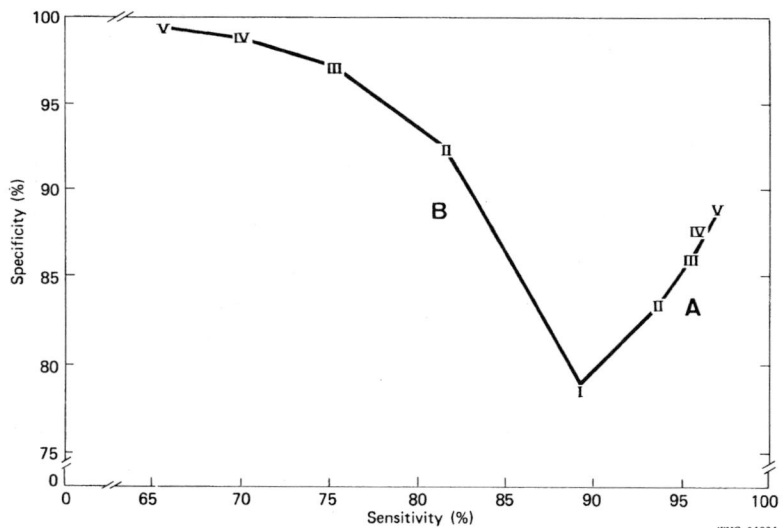

SENSITIVITY AND SPECIFICITY OF CRITERIA FOR HYPERTENSION

Figure 1. Sensitivity and specificity of criteria for hypertension. I, II, III, IV, V: first, second, third, fourth and fifth sessions of measuring blood pressure. Two readings at each session. A) Arithmetic mean of *all* measurements above cutpoint. B) Mean of two measurements at each session above limit.

clusion must never be disregarded. It is mandatory for any definition of hypertension to take into account this variability by exactly defining both the number of measurements and the way of computing the key values which underlie the diagnostic conclusion.

Figure 1 gives an example. The diagnostic decision in favour of 'hypertension' may be reached when the arithmetic mean of *all* double measurements on repeated occasions was above the cut-point (line A). Alternatively, the diagnostic criterion may require that the mean of two measurements be above the limit at *each* of the repeated sessions of double measurements (line B). In the first case, with an increasing number of sessions, the sensitivity of the diagnostic criterion increases (i.e. the likelihood of not missing 'true' hypertensives), together with some increase in specificity. In the second case, the diagnostic specificity (i.e. the likelihood of not including 'false' cases) increases rapidly with the number of repeated sessions, but this happens at the expense of the sensitivity of the diagnosis: by being more specific, more cases will be missed. With inverted signs the same will apply to the decision of considering people to be normotensive [14]. The choice between method A and method B depends on whether high sensitivity or high specificity is aimed at; the important point is, however, to report *how* the key value had been arrived at.

CHILDREN AND ADOLESCENTS, AND THE DEFINITION OF HYPERTENSION

All that has been said above on the definition of hypertension applies to adults. 'What constitutes normal blood pressure in children and adolescents? A child's blood pressure can be readily measured, but what are sound criteria for evaluating it as truly elevated? There are no firm answers to these questions, but there is information that can be used for guidelines'. [15]

While the (arbitrary) definitions of hypertension are derived from longstanding clinical and epidemiological experience with the relationship between adult blood pressure levels and frank disease, no such experience has been gained with children: there is a need for long-term prospective observations of this kind. Many cross-sectional and some longitudinal findings on blood pressure distributions in children are available, however, showing that blood pressure grows with the child's age and that individuals, as time passes, tend to remain at a relatively constant place in the distribution of hypertension for their age – a phenomenon called 'tracking'. Thus, if a child is repeatedly found to have relatively high blood pressures (as compared with his or her peers) it may be justified to extrapolate to a probably similar future position at adult age. However, pending more research, this type of reasoning is conjectural.

486

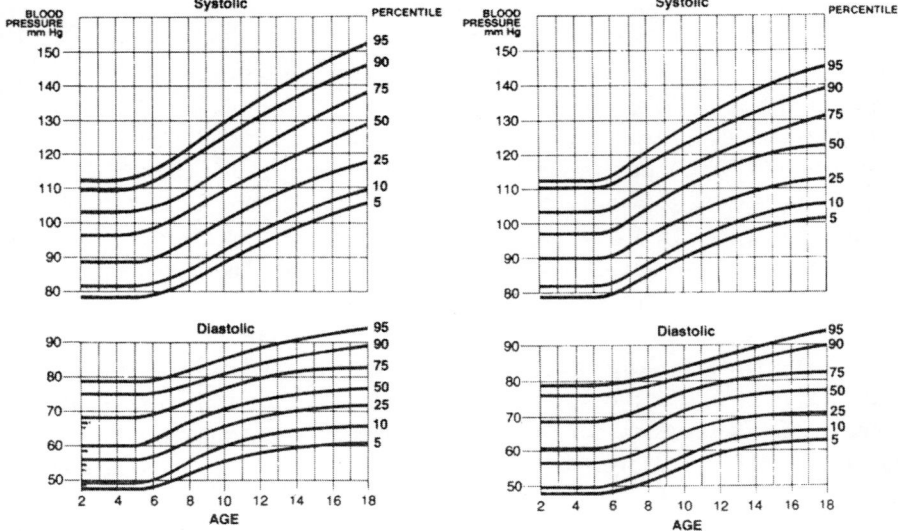

Figure 2. Percentiles of blood pressure measurement (right arm, seated) in boys and in girls. From [15]; with permission of the American Academy of Pediatrics, Evanston, IL, U.S.A.

Information on distributions related to age, sex, height and weight is available from a considerable number of studies reviewed recently [16, 17]. Figure 2 presents the much-quoted nomogram of the National Heart, Lung and Blood Institute [15] and Figure 3 a nomogram by André et al. [18], where blood pressure is presented as a function of height. (According to the latter author, blood pressure in children correlates somewhat better with height than with age.) Sexual maturation has been shown to influence blood pressure in girls greatly [19]; therefore the blood pressure values of adolescent girls should be considered in the light of sexual maturity and body height and weight rather than of age only.

Despite the many unknown factors regarding the definition of hypertension in childhood and adolescence, clinical juvenile hypertension *is* of course a paediatric reality, due almost exclusively to detectable causes. What is unknown at present is the possible continuity between blood pressure levels early in life and adult blood pressure elevations. This is of great relevance to the understanding of the genesis and, potentially, the primary prevention of essential (primary) hypertension, and calls for intensive research. It also refers to the 'precise levels of blood pressure at which hypertension can be defined for children' [2]. It is to be hoped, however, that such 'precise' levels will not be promulgated at all (by definition they cannot be but arbitrary), but that the concept of hypertension will remain a quantitative, probabilistic category as far as blood pressure in childhood and adolescence is concerned.

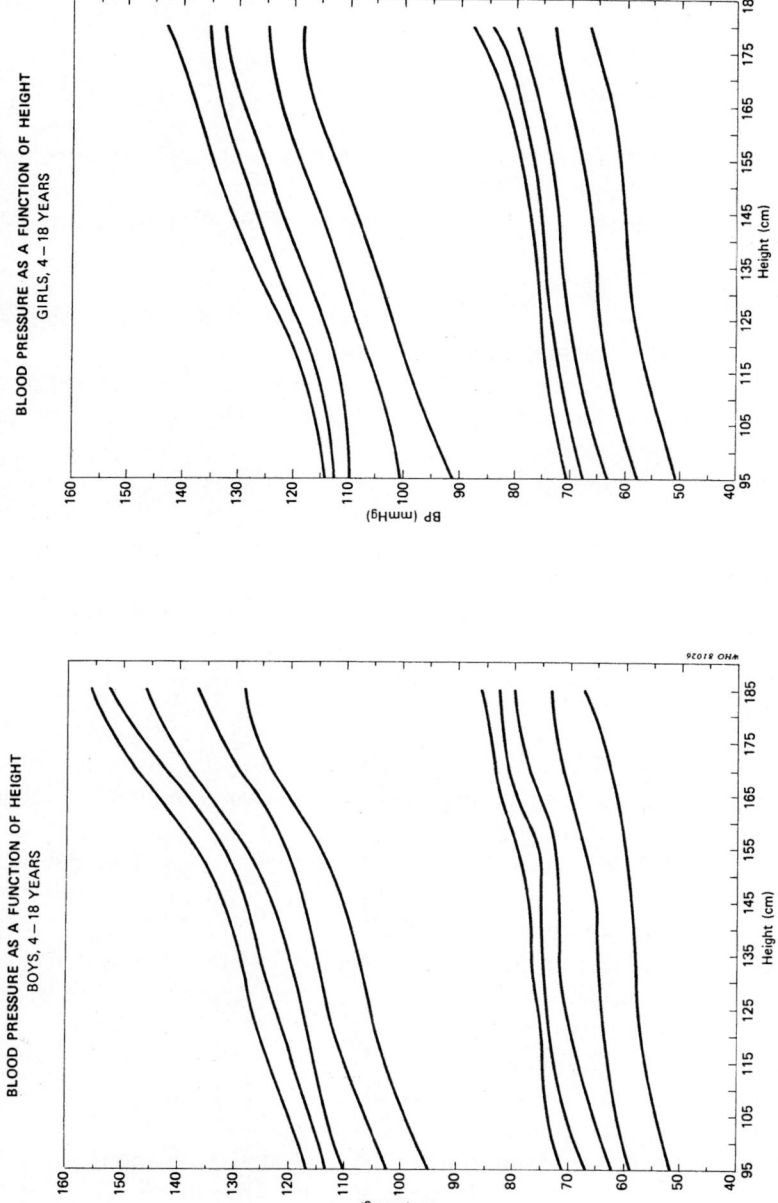

Figure 3. Percentiles of blood pressure measurement by body height; in boys (left); in girls (right). From [18]; with permission of La Nouvelle Presse Médicale, Masson S.A., Paris, France.

CLASSIFICATION OF HYPERTENSION

Patients with hypertensive disease are usually classified according to both the severity of the condition and its causes.

a) Classification by causes

Essential or primary hypertension '... is defined as high blood pressure without evident organic cause.' [2]

'Secondary hypertension is defined as hypertension with an identifiable cause.' [12]

The possible, identifiable causes fall into four groups:

1) Iatrogenic hypertension, due to the administration of drugs (e.g. corticosteroids or ACTH), or oral contraceptives
2) Organic diseases or malformations such as, renal diseases: unilateral or bilateral, surgically untreatable or treatable, parenchymal or non-parenchymal, congenital or acquired, etc.;
   Coarctation of the aorta;
   Endocrine diseases, such as endrino-cortical diseases or diseases of the medulla (phaeochromocytoma).
3) Hypertensive disease of pregnancy
4) Chronic ingestion of certain substances such as liquorice or lead.

b) Classification by severity

Malignant (or accelerated), *severe, moderate* or *mild* hypertension are colloquial labels, descriptive designations often used and based on clinical judgement rather than on accepted definitions.

In certain studies and trials, nevertheless, the term 'mild hypertension' has been used for precisely defined blood pressure levels; these definitions tended to be specific for each study [20].

A simplified stratification by diastolic blood pressure levels is described by the US Joint National Committee on Detection, Evaluation and Treatment of High Blood Pressure [4]:

1) Stratum I (mild): 90–104 mm Hg
2) Stratum II (moderate): 105–114 mm Hg
3) Stratum III (severe): greater than 115 mm Hg.

The most widely accepted and most often-quoted classification, however, is that of WHO [21], dividing hypertension into *three stages* according to the natural history of its evolution in the individual. Thus:

Stage I hypertension is defined as blood pressure in the hypertensive range without any signs of organ changes.

Stage II hypertension is characterized by signs of left ventricular hypertrophy found on physical examination or chest X-ray, electrocardiogram or echocardiogram *.

Stage III hypertension is diagnosed when symptoms and signs have appeared as a result of damage to various organs from hypertensive disease, including heart failure (hypertensive heart disease), cerebrovascular disease, severe eye ground changes, renal failure, arterial aneurysm or occlusion, and coronary heart disease.

In some cases reasoning on pathogenesis may be difficult. Hypertension may have led to organ damage (e.g. renal insufficiency), but hypertension may equally have appeared as its consequence (renal hypertension). At any rate, coexistence of the two conditions suffices for classifying such a patient as having stage III hypertension.

c) Statistical classification

For statistical purposes, the World Health Organization classifies hypertension, within the context of the all-embracing International Classification of Diseases (ICD), in an entirely pragmatic way. ICD results from a long line of decennial revisions of the original Classification of Causes of Death by Jacques Bertillon, adopted by the International Statistical Institute in 1899. This classification must meet several requirements. While keeping abreast with the development of new notions in medicine, it should preserve the continuity of statistics in time. It should also be practical and simple without becoming trivial.

The Ninth Revision of ICD, adopted by the 29th World Health Assembly and in vigour since 1976 [22] classifies arterial hypertension as follows:

Hypertensive disease	ICD Code
Essential hypertension	401
Hypertensive heart disease	402
Hypertensive renal disease	403
Hypertensive heart and renal disease	404
Secondary hypertension	405
Hypertension complicating pregnancy, childbirth and the puerperium	642

Hypertension with clinical involvement of the central nervous system is classified as Cerebrovascular Disease with ICD codes 430–438. The asso-

---

* In 1978, the presence of generalized or focal narrowing of the retinal artery or proteinuria and/or slight elevation of plasma creatine concentrations were added as alternative criteria for stage II hypertension [2].

ciation of coronary heart disease with hypertension is classified as Ischaemic Heart Disease with ICD codes 410–414.

The category 'secondary hypertension' may not be used for mortality purposes; instead, the underlying disease should be stated in the first place.

CONCLUSION

The concept of hypertension has two faces: the qualitative and quantitative aspect, reconcilable only by a pragmatic compromise. The resulting arbitrary but practical definition of hypertension (BP≥160 and/or 95) is reinforced by describing the severity of the condition or defining its stage (WHO stages I–III). It is mandatory to adhere to the accepted blood pressure measurement methods and to specify the calculation of the key (diagnostic) blood pressure value, if a valid standardized definition of hypertension is aimed at. Blood pressure values in childhood and adolescence should be stated in absolute values rather than in terms of 'hypertension' or 'normotension': the (percentile) position of the individual within the age–sex specific distribution is crucial.

The definition of hypertension leads only conditionally to therapeutic considerations. Especially at the lower end of the hypertensive scale, and in the borderline range, the blood pressure value is only one of a whole set of elements to be considered in the decision on treatment. The old clinical adage is still valid: blood pressure levels and the diagnosis of hypertension should be considered in relation to the fact that the patient is a complex and indivisible entity.

REFERENCES

1. CIOMS: Provisional International Nomenclature for Cardiovascular Diseases. Btesh S, ed. Geneva, 1972.
2. Arterial Hypertension. WHO Tech Rep Ser 628, 1978.
3. New York Heart Association Criteria Committee: Nomenclature and Criteria for Diagnosis of Diseases of the Heart and Great Vessels, 7th edn. Boston: Little, Brown & Co, 1973.
4. Report of the Joint National Committee on Detection, Evaluation, and Treatment of High Blood Pressure. National Institutes of Health, Bethesda, Md, 1980.
5. Hypertension Detection and Follow-up Program Cooperative Group: Five-Year Findings of the Hypertension Detection and Follow-up Program – 1. Reduction in Mortality of Persons with High Blood Pressure, Including Mild Hypertension. JAMA, 242:2562–2577, 1979.
6. Epstein FH, Eckoff RD: The epidemiology of high blood pressure – geographic distributions and etiological factors; In: The Epidemiology of Hypertension; Stamler J, Stamler R, Pullman TN, eds. pp. 155–166, New York: Grune & Stratton, 1967.
7. The SI for the Medical Professions. WHO, 1977.

8. American Heart Association Committee Report: Recommendations for human blood pressure determination by sphygmomanometers. Circulation 62:1146A–1155A.
9. Health Protection Branch, Health and Welfare, Canada: Information Letter 583, 15 September 1980.
10. Maintenance of mm Hg as Unit for Measuring Blood Pressure. European Leagues against Hypertension, Newsletter 1:3, 1981.
11. International Society of Hypertension: Resolution on Retaining the Millimeter of Mercury. Meeting of 25 February 1976, Sydney, Australia.
12. Helgeland A: Treatment of mild hypertension: a five year controlled drug trial – the Oslo Study. Am J Med 69:725–732, 1980.
13. Lehane A et al.: Reporting of blood pressure data in medical journals. Br Med J 281:1603–1604, 1980.
14. Strasser T, Dowd E: unpublished results.
15. Report of the Task Force on Blood Pressure Control in Children. Pediatrics 59 (Suppl):803, 1977.
16. Szklo M: Epidemiologic patterns of blood pressure in children. Epidemiol Rev 1:143–169, 1979.
17. Leumann EP: Blood Pressure and hypertension in childhood and adolescence. In: Advances in Internal Medicine & Pediatrics. Frick P, von Harnack G-A, Martini GA, Prader A, Schoen R, Wolff HP, eds. Berlin: Springer-Verlag, 1979.
18. André JL et al.: Pression artérielle chez l'enfant – valeurs rapportées à la taille. Nouv Presse Med 9:1958–1959, 1980.
19. Török E et al.: International collaborative study on juvenile hypertension – I. Study procedures and screening. WHO Bull 59:295–304, 1981.
20. Reader R: Therapeutic trials in mild hypertension ongoing throughout the world. In: Mild Hypertension: To Treat or Not to Treat, vol. 34. Mitchell H Jr, McFate Smith W, eds. Annals of the New York Academy of Sciences, 1978.
21. Arterial Hypertension and Ischaemic Heart Disease – Preventive Aspects. WHO Tech Rep Ser 231, 1962.
22. International Classification of Diseases, Vol 1, 1975 (Revision). WHO, 1977.

V. SECONDARY HYPERTENSION

32. HYPERTENSION SECONDARY TO COARCTATION

Frederick B. Parker Jr., Gunnar H. Anderson Jr. and David H. P. Streeten

Although aortic coarctation has been well known to pathologists for 100 years [1], the hypertension usually associated with coarctation has been appreciated only more recently. In 1912 Gossage [2] suggested that hypertension was essential in patients with coarctation to 'overcome the difficulty of getting blood through the narrow arterial channels.' By 1933 Lewis [3] was able to state in a review of a large number of cases of aortic coarctation that hypertension was present in the upper arms of all patients and that any patient with hypertension must be considered as possibly having coarctation. After reviewing 170 cases of coarctation, King [4] agreed that hypertension was usually present. Furthermore, it is the uncontrolled hypertension which leads to the demise of untreated patients with coarctation, whose average survival is 35 years [5]. Subarachnoid hemorrhage, acute aortic dissection and left heart failure account for the majority of the deaths, and all are directly related to the associated hypertension. It appears obvious that proper therapy of coarctation must be directed towards the relief of the hypertension.

DEFINITION AND DIAGNOSIS OF AORTIC COARCTATION

Aortic coarctation is a constriction of the aorta, opposite the junction with the ligamentum arteriosum (juxta- or postductal type) or in the isthmus proximal to this junction (preductal type). It rarely occurs in the abdominal aorta where some feel it may be an acquired lesion. Usually, systolic blood pressure in the right arm is higher than in age-matched normal subjects [6], and is at least 20 or 30 mm Hg higher than concomitantly measured systolic pressure in the legs. Hypertension is present in 80–85% of patients with coarctation [7]. Inequality of pressures in the two arms may result from origin of the left or right subclavian artery at or below the coarctation. Blood pressure in the legs may be unmeasurable by auscultation, or may be low, normal or high, depending upon the tightness of the aortic stenosis and the extent of development of a collateral circulation; but it is almost always >20 mm Hg lower than in the right arm. Pulse pressure is narrower in the

Amery, A. (ed.) Hypertensive Cardiovascular Disease: Pathophysiology and Treatment
© *1982, Martinus Nijhoff Publishers. The Hague / Boston / London*
ISBN-13: 978-94-009-7478-4

legs than in the arms. Characteristically, femoral arterial pulsations are impalpable or weak, but may be delayed only in comparison with the radial pulse.

Aortic coarctation is often associated with other congenital cardiovascular anomalies, such as patent ductus arteriosus, bicuspid aortic valve, ventricular septal defects, transposition of the great vessels and single ventricle. Clearly, the associated anomalies might have at least as great an effect on the blood pressure as the coarctation itself. We shall confine this discussion to the mechanism and treatment of aortic coarctation uncomplicated by other congenital abnormalities.

MECHANISMS OF THE HYPERTENSION OF COARCTATION

The pathogenesis of hypertension in patients with coarctation has been widely discussed. The evidence for and against the two predominant theories, involving purely mechanical factors on the one hand and renal factors (probably excessive renin release) on the other, will be presented. More recently, the pathogenesis of the paradoxical hypertension which often occurs shortly after surgical correction of coarctation has been studied, and the possible roles of excessive catecholamine release and/or excessive renin release in this form of hypertension will be discussed.

Mechanical factors

In 1931, Blumgart et al. [8] suggested that hypertension in coarctation resulted from resistance to the flow of blood by the stenosis of the aorta and by the collateral vessels. This view was supported by Bing et al. [9] on the basis of their analysis of physiological data from 23 patients, from which they concluded that there was no generalized increase of vascular resistance. However, Steele [10] showed by intra-arterial pressure measurements that diastolic pressures were elevated in the femoral as well as in the radial arteries in 2 out of 3 patients with coarctation, showing that arteriolar tone was increased both below and above the coarctation. Gupta and Wiggers [11] confirmed the frequent existence of diastolic hypertension in the femoral arteries of dogs with aortic coarctation, but considered that this was not necessarily evidence of vasoconstriction in branches of the lower aorta.

There are strong reasons for doubting that simple mechanical obstruction to blood flow is the cause of hypertension in coarctation of the aorta. Scott and his collaborators [12] have studied the B.P. responses to experimental aortic obstruction induced in dogs by transsecting the aorta, closing the proximal end with sutures and anastomosing the much narrower subclavian artery to the distal end of the transsected aorta. This procedure was found to reduce the cross-sectional area of the aortic isthmus by 79 % (mean). Direct intra-arterial blood pressure measurements in 13 dogs revealed a steadily progressive rise in systolic pressure to a stable maximal value of 160–195 (mean 181.5) mm Hg in the carotid artery and 120–175 (mean 134.2) mm Hg in the femoral artery at 5–7 weeks after surgery, (see Scott [12], Table 1), values typical of coarctation. Of great importance, however, was their observation that the blood pressure in these dogs was normal at 72 h after creation of the coarctation, being 120–146 (mean 131.1) mm Hg in the carotid artery and 75–106 (mean 81.8) mm Hg in the femoral artery (except for one dog which was very excited at the time of B.P. measurements and had a systolic value of 180 in the carotid and 120 mm Hg in the femoral artery). With the exception of this one dog, systolic blood pressure remained below 150 mm Hg until at least the ninth day after induction of the aortic constriction. In a subsequent publication, Scott et al. [13] recorded a transient rise in systolic B.P. in the carotid artery for 1–6 h after completion of the surgery, followed by a return to preoperative levels for several days, as had previously been shown to occur by Erlanger and Gasser [14]. Thereafter, blood pressure showed a gradually progressive rise to obviously hypertensive values from the end of the first week to highest values between 5 and 12 weeks. Similarly, 5 dogs subjected to acute ligation of the aortic isthmus were found to manifest carotid arterial hypertension for only $\frac{1}{2}$–2 h after the operation, with return to or below preoperative pressures thereafter [13]. These immediate increases in carotid blood pressures after aortic occlusion confirmed the findings of de Jager [15], Page [16] and Gupta and Wiggers [11], and the transience of these acute changes was reported also by Page [16] and Erlanger and Gasser [14]. However, if the continuing hypertension of coarctation were mechanical in origin, it should not disappear completely for several days and then show a gradual return. One might postulate that the disappearance of the hypertension was secondary to collateral formation, but, if the whole mechanism were purely mechanical, the blood pressure should not again increase subsequently. Thus, although aortic obstruction can cause an immediate, transient, apparently mechanically induced rise in carotid blood pressure, it seems unlikely that the chronic hypertension of coarctation could be the result of a purely mechanical increase in arterial resistance.

Role of the kidney

The classical studies of Goldblatt et al. [17] showed conclusively that moderate degrees of experimental constriction of the renal arteries in dogs resulted in persistent hypertension. Among the various modifications of renal arterial constriction which Goldblatt and his colleagues subsequently studied, one was aortic constriction immediately above the origin of both renal arteries [18]. This form of abdominal aortic coarctation was invariably followed by hypertension, whereas constriction of the aorta below the level of the renal arteries caused no elevation of blood pressure. These observations have stimulated an endless series of subsequent experiments including several related directly to the pathogenesis of hypertension in coarctation. First Rytand [19] showed that in rats partial occlusion of the aorta between the origins of the renal arteries resulted in cardiac hypertrophy which could be prevented by excision of the ischemic kidney. Then, in a series of imaginative experiments, Scott and his colleagues [12] showed that aortic coarctation at the level of the origin of the left subclavian artery caused hypertension in dogs, which could be consistently overcome by transplanting one of the kidneys into the neck and excising the other. Transplantation of the kidney to the groin where it continued to be poorly supplied with blood failed to alleviate the hypertension [12, 13] except when the kidney was subsequently re-transplanted to the normally vascularized cervical area [13]. These experimental observations were confirmed by Svane and Jensen [20], and with slightly different procedures, by Ferguson et al. [21] and Sealy [22] who transferred the source of renal blood to the unobstructed cervical vessels rather than transplanting the kidney itself to the neck. Meacham et al. [23], too, were able to reverse the hypertension induced by aortic coarctation, not by transplanting the ischemic kidney to the neck but by revascularizing it with an aorto-aortic bypass of the coarcted region. Thus, all of these observations strongly implied that the hypertension of experimental aortic coarctation was related to ischemia of the kidneys and could be overcome reproducibly by restoring normal blood flow to the kidneys in spite of continued aortic obstruction. In all cases, the purely mechanical effects of the persistent coarctation failed to cause hypertension as long as renal ischemia was obviated.

MECHANISM OF RENAL ISCHEMIC EFFECT ON COARCTATIONAL HYPERTENSION

Scott et al. [13] tried to show that the ischemic kidneys of dogs with aortic coarctation produced an excess of a blood-borne pressor substance, viz. pherentasin. They succeeded in inducing hypertension in a dog given an infusion of blood taken from the renal vein of a donor animal which had been made hypertensive by the induction of aortic coarctation. The possibility that excessive renin release was the renal mechanism of coarctational hypertension was suggested by the observations of Svane and Jensen [20].

These authors found that the granulation index of the juxtaglomerular apparatus was significantly increased (suggesting excessive renin production) in the kidneys of dogs with aortic coarctation and that the granulation index reverted to normal when such kidneys were transplanted to the neck, with consequent correction of the hypertension.

Many investigators have measured plasma renin activity (PRA) in the peripheral blood of dogs and human patients with coarctation, with variable results. In dogs with experimental coarctation Bagby [24] found that PRA was elevated and associated with reduced renal plasma flow and glomerular filtration rate when studied at 2 years and during strict sodium deprivation. Subsequently, Bagby et al. [25] reported that at 1–12 months after the induction of aortic coarctation and without sodium deprivation, dogs had normal levels of peripheral PRA associated with expansion of the extracellular fluid volume (by 4.1%), plasma volume (by 4.1%) and total blood volume (by 5.1%). Thus, the PRA/volume relationship was abnormal, with PRA levels being inappropriately 'normal' in the presence of hypervolemia.

Other authors who have reported peripheral PRA measurements in dogs with coarctation of the aorta have found elevated levels [23], raised (but not significantly raised) levels [21] and elevated values at 4–21 days thereafter falling to normal [26]. In rabbits coarctation has been found to cause no change in PRA during the first 4 days and a fall to subnormal levels after 6 months [27].

PRA measurements in human patients with coarctation are summarized in Table I. It is evident from the Table that PRA was normal in virtually all patients with coarctation when the measurements were obtained without stimulation by sodium loss and/or orthostasis [28–30, 33, 34, 38]. On the other hand, when the patients were pretreated with a restricted sodium intake and/or diuretic therapy, and/or after standing for 2 h, PRA was elevated above normal limits in many of the patients studied by Fallo et al. [35], Alpert [36], Van Way [34], Ribeiro and Krakoff [37], and Parker et al. [39]. In this respect, the PRA measurements in patients with coarctation are very similar to measurements made in patients with renal arterial stenosis whose hypertension is subsequently shown to be corrected by surgical bypass of the obstructed renal arterial segment(s). In the latter patients, too, peripheral PRA levels are very often 'normal' when measured on a regular sodium diet and without orthostasis [40–44] but are far more frequently excessive after natriuresis and maintenance of the upright posture [45–48]. Even with such stimulation, however, peripheral PRA levels are elevated above the normal range in an average of only 70% of renovascular hypertensive patients [49]. Among reported series of patients with hypertension and renal arterial stenosis, in whom subsequent surgical correction of the stenosis 'cured' the hypertension, peripheral PRA was elevated in the following percentages of patients: 69% [50], 35% [51], 67% [52], 72% [53],

Table 1. Frequency of elevated plasma renin activity and positive saralasin tests in patients with aortic coarctation

Author (reference)	Na intake (mEq/day)	PRA method	Elevated plasma renin activity		+ Furosemide	Saralasin test positive
			Recumbent	Upright		
Strong et al. [28]	ad lib	Bio	2/12			
Brown et al. [29]	ad lib	Bio	0/4			
Amsterdam et al. [30]	ad lib	Bio	1/16			1/1
Sealy et al. [22]	ad lib	Bio	2/5			
Scott et al. [31]	ad lib	RIA	1/1			
Rocchini et al. [32]	ad lib	RIA	1/7			
Werning et al. [33]	110	Bio	1/10	1/10		
Van Way et al. [34]	100	RIA	0/4	3/4		
Fallo et al. [35]	120 or 2 mEq/Kg	RIA		15/37		
Alpert et al. [36]	ad lib	RIA	NS			
	10	RIA	NS			
	ad lib	RIA			$p<0.01$	
Ribeiro et al. [37]	ad lib	RIA		2/2		2/2
Markiewicz et al. [38]	80-110	Bio	0/11		2/11	
Parker et al. [39]	10	RIA			8/8	6/8

RIA = radioimmunoassay of angiotensin I; Bio = Bioassay; NS = not significant. In each case the number of patients with elevated PRA is shown as the numerator, and the total number of patients studied as the denominator.

498

67% [54], 55% [55], 70% [56], 66% [57], 63% [58], 61% [59], 68% [60], giving a mean of 63.0% for all groups. Expansion of the plasma and extracellular fluid volumes has been reported in human patients with aortic coarctation, by Alpert et al. [36].

SARALASIN RESPONSES

When the angiotensin II antagonist, saralasin (1-sar-8-ala-angiotensin II) was infused intravenously into patients with coarctation, blood pressure fell by >10/8 mm Hg in the first 2 patients studied by Ribeiro and Krakoff [37], in 1 of 4 patients studied by Scott et al. [31], and in 6 of 8 patients investigated by Parker et al. [39]. This evidence that a highly specific antagonist of angiotensin II lowered the B.P. in most patients with coarctation revealed the existence of a strong, perhaps exclusively angiotensinogenic component of their hypertension. In this respect, too, these patients with aortic coarctation were very similar to the human counterpart of Goldblatt hypertension, the hypertension of renal arterial stenosis [61–63].

It seems likely, therefore, that in most patients with aortic coarctation, the hypertension is angiotensinogenic in type. As in renovascular hypertensive patients, patients with coarctation probably have some degree of sodium overload resulting from secondary hyperaldosteronism, as the data of Bagby [25] in dogs, and Alpert et al. [36] in man would suggest. The sodium and water retention brought about in this way would be expected to contribute to the hypertension and to inhibit further renin release, thus lowering the PRA towards or into the normal range in many such patients when studied on unrestricted diets and in recumbency. The postulated role of the renin–angiotensin–aldosterone system in the hypertension of aortic coarctation is illustrated in Figure 1.

Role of the sympathetic nervous system

Several investigators have explored the possibility that excessive activity of the sympathetic nervous system might contribute to the pathogenesis of the hypertension of aortic coarctation. Measurements of urinary catecholamine excretion have been uniformly normal [22, 64, 65]. The possible role of the sympathetic nervous system in raising the peripheral vascular resistance of the hind limb in rats with coarctation of the aorta has been studied by Overbeck [66]. He found that vascular resistance in the hind limb was increased, and that part of the increase resulted from sympathetic activity, since it was greatly reduced by sectioning the nerves to the hind limb. In addition, 'chemical sympathectomy' with guanethidine prevented much of

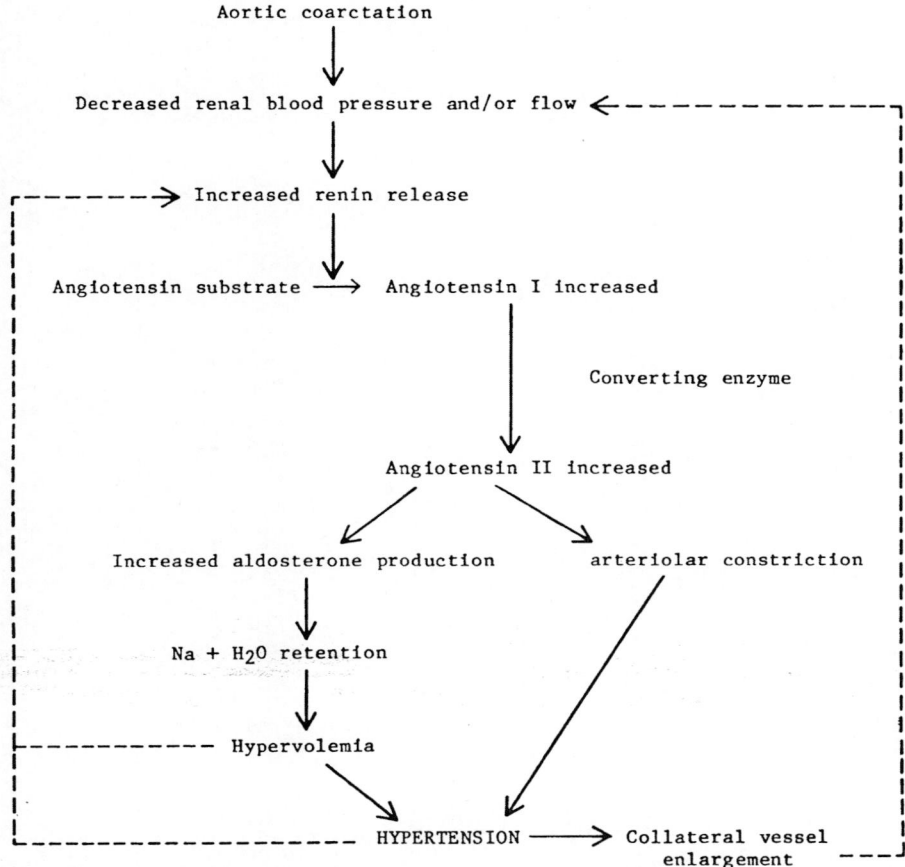

Figure 1. Schematic representation of the pathogenesis of systemic hypertension in aortic coarctation. Stimulatory influences are depicted with solid lines, inhibitory influences with dotted lines.

the hypertension in these rats with aortic coarctation. In another study, however, Prager et al. [67] reported low levels of plasma norepinephrine in puppies with coarctation at 1 year. Since beta-adrenergic stimulation is an important mechanism of increasing renin release, it is quite possible that sympathetic activity in the renal nerves may play a part in the excessive renin release which appears to be present in patients with coarctation of the aorta, without necessarily being reflected by a rise in plasma or urinary catecholamines.

TREATMENT OF COARCTATION

Surgical correction provides definitive therapy for coarctation. It was first performed by Crafoord and Nylin [68] in 1944 and shortly thereafter by

500

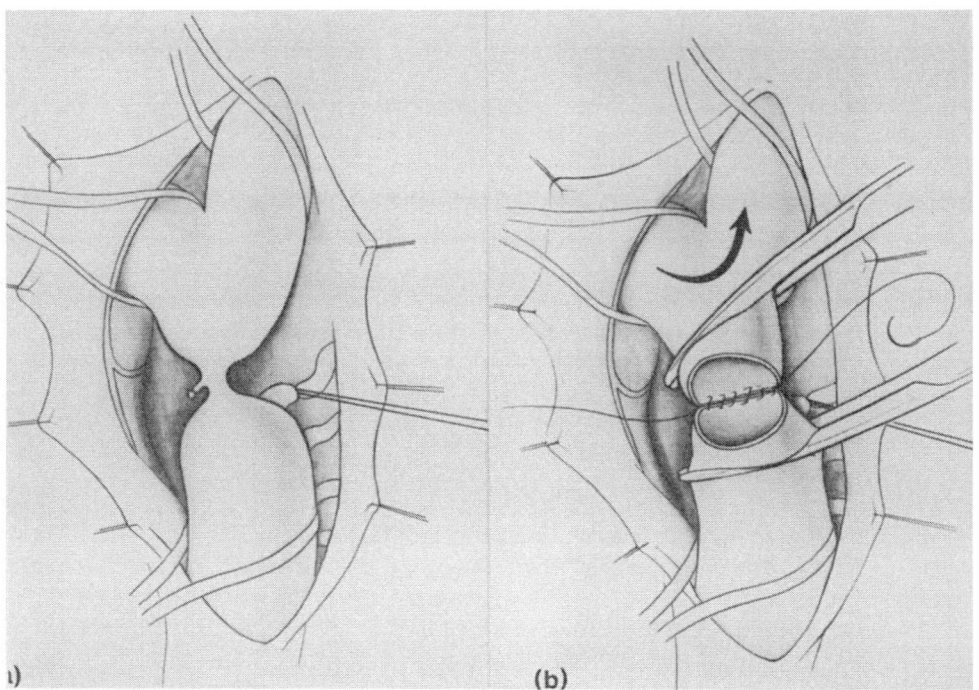

Figure 2. The surgical excision of the aortic coarctation (a) and the end-to-end anastomosis of the ends of the aorta (b) are shown.

Gross [69] in 1945. Although there was significant mortality in the early years of the operation, coarctation repair now enjoys one of the lowest mortalities of the major cardiovascular procedures. The standard surgical correction has been primary excision of the coarcted aortic segment and end-to-end anastomosis (Figure 2). The highest surgical mortality occurs in infants, usually because of some associated congenital cardiac anomaly.

Patients restored to the normotensive state by coarctectomy have few of the well-known complications of uncorrected coarctation. However, 25–40% of surgically corrected patients remain hypertensive. The etiology of this hypertension has never been thoroughly examined, although it is generally believed to be secondary to recurrent coarctation in most cases. A long term retrospective analysis by Maron et al. [70] of 248 corrected coarctation patients revealed a high incidence of premature cardiovascular disease which was related to the duration of preoperative hypertension. Over 40% of the patients studied had no change or an increase in blood pressure over the preoperative value. It must be remembered, however, that this series spans a 25-year period. Technical improvements have probably altered these results.

In our own series of surgically corrected coarctation, 50% of patients with recoarctation had blood pressures above the 95th percentile for the stated age. The vast majority of patients with recoarctation and uncorrected hypertension were derived from those repaired before the age of one year. An end-to-end anastomosis in an aorta with a small transverse diameter sets the stage for future narrowing. The scarring process inhibits aortic growth in the region of the anastomosis and recurrence of the coarctation has been a major problem. It is only recently that improved surgical techniques for coarctation repair in the infant have become available. Subclavian flap angioplasty as described by Waldhausen [71] utilizes the proximal portion of the left subclavian artery as an onlay flap across the narrowed segment. Another recent innovation, patch angioplasty, involves placement of an onlay prosthetic patch across the area of coarctation. This appears to relieve the coarctation, but unlike subclavian angioplasty does not provide living tissue for future aortic growth. These methods are expected to decrease the incidence of recoarctation and to reduce the incidence of residual hypertension in this age group. The problem of persistent hypertension in the older child or adult undergoing coarctation repair appears to be related to the duration of hypertension prior to correction. After a certain number of years, it appears that hypertension may become fixed and that repair does not alter its course. This seems particularly true in the adult. Our own feeling is that all patients should be repaired prior to puberty, preferably between seven and ten years of age. In this age group, there should be no great difficulty in obtaining an adequate lumen at operation, which should prevent recoarctation and reduce residual hypertension. Patients operated upon in our institution between seven and ten years of age have only a 7% risk of recurrent coarctation and no evidence of persistent hypertension. In those operated on below one year of age, only 35% are felt to have a good long-term result. In those operated upon between one and six years 60% are felt to have reasonable persistent benefit from the procedure.

The strong evidence that hypertension in aortic coarctation is angiotensin-dependent leads us to suggest that a trial of therapy with Captopril or other inhibitors of angiotensin-converting enzyme would be of great interest and of considerable potential value in the future.

PARADOXICAL POSTOPERATIVE HYPERTENSION

An important clinical event which occurs frequently during the first week after surgical correction of the coarctation is a paradoxical postoperative rise in blood pressure [72]. Typically, there is *early* elevation predominantly of the systolic pressure during the first 24 h after surgery and subsiding before the 36th hour, and/or *delayed* systolic and diastolic hypertension between the third and the fourteenth postoperative day. At these times pressures rise above preoperative levels or considerably above blood pressure levels observed during the first 6 h after surgery, and the finding of a raised popliteal artery pressure indicates that aortic coarctation has been substantially relieved [73]. In some of the patients who experience severe 'delayed' diastolic hypertension, nausea, vomiting, abdominal distension and tenderness may occur [72, 73]. This is occasionally followed by bowel infarction, and laparotomy or autopsy in such patients has revealed the presence of severe arteritis and arteriolitis of the mesenteric vessels [72, 73, 22].

The mechanism of paradoxical postoperative hypertension was initially postulated to be excessive catecholamine release after surgical correction of the coarctation. Apparent support for this view was derived from the observation that urinary excretion of catecholamines increased postoperatively, most strikingly at the time of the paradoxical hypertension [64]. However, such increases in urinary catecholamine excretion have been seen by others in patients after surgical correction of aortic coarctation [22, 65] and were recorded in control subjects after a variety of surgical procedures not associated with coarctation and not characterized by postoperative hypertension [22, 64, 65]. Moreover, Prager et al. [67] have found that adrenal medullary norepinephrine secretion was actually subnormal in beagles with coarctation acutely subjected to intra-aortic pulsatile pressures of 40, 60 and 80 mm Hg in an attempt to duplicate the pressure changes which presumably follow surgical correction of spontaneous coarctation in human patients. Thus, there is no real evidence to support the theory that sudden catecholamine discharge is responsible for the paradoxical hypertension after surgical correction of coarctation in man.

That an acute renin release might induce the paradoxical hypertension syndrome has been suggested by Rocchini et al. [32]. Seven children who manifested delayed paradoxical hypertension after coarctation resection, were found to show a rise in PRA coincidentally with the hypertension, which was not seen in any of the five control subjects who underwent different types of cardiac surgery and experienced no postoperative hypertension. On the other hand, the early episode of systolic hypertension in these patients was associated with marked depression of the cold pressor response, but only slight elevation in PRA. In the patients who experienced the syndrome of abdominal pain postoperatively it was found that PRA levels were highest at the time when this syndrome was present. The temporal correspondence between delayed hypertension and abdominal pain on the one hand and the rise of PRA on the other, led Rocchini et al. [32] to postulate a causal relationship between renin release and the postoperative hypertension and abdominal pain syndrome in these patients.

These observations are supported and extended by those of Parker et al. [39]. Postoperative paradoxical hypertension was associated not only with elevation of the PRA in 4 out of 8 patients but also with a prompt hypotensive response to infusion of the angiotensin II antagonist, saralasin, in these four individuals. Thus, the postoperative hypertension in many of these patients is not only associated with a rise in PRA but is probably caused by this rise in PRA and the consequent increase in plasma angiotensin II levels which presumably results.

SUMMARY

The hypertension of aortic coarctation is not likely to result from mechanical obstruction per se, since experimental aortic stenosis causes transient hypertension followed by normotension and then a gradually progressive rise in blood pressure despite continued aortic obstruction. Evidence that coarctational hypertension is angiotensinogenic includes observations which show (a) that transplantation of one kidney to the neck or restoration of normal vascularization to the kidney corrects the hypertension; (b) that the granulation index of the juxtaglomerular apparatus of the kidneys is increased in coarctation, but restored to normal by transplanting the kidney to the neck; (c) that, as in renovascular hypertension, peripheral plasma renin activity is usually increased above that of normal control subjects after natriuresis and standing for 2–4 h; (d) that, as in renovascular hypertension, the hypertension of patients with coarctation is usually reversed by the angiotensin antagonist, saralasin.

Surgical correction of aortic coarctation by excision of the stenosed area and end-to-end anastomosis, preferably between the ages of seven and ten years, is the treatment of choice, but the potential usefulness of treatment with Captopril or other angiotensin converting enzyme inhibitors should be explored.

ACKNOWLEDGEMENTS

Supported by a grant (HL 19428) from the National Heart, Lung and Blood Institute and a General Clinical Research Center Grant (RR 229) from the Division of Research Facilities and Resources, U.S. Public Health Service.

REFERENCES

1. Cohnheim J: Lectures on General Pathology. A Handbook for Practitioners and Students. Section I. The Pathology of the Circulation, p. 98. McKee AB, transl. London: New Sydenham Society, 1889.

504

2. Gossage AM: Case of coarctation of the aorta. Proc R Soc Med 6 (Clin Sect):1–5, 1912/1913.
3. Lewis T: Material relating to coarctation of the aorta of the adult type. Heart 16:205–261, 1933.
4. King JT: The blood pressure in stenosis at the isthmus (coarctation) of the aorta; case reports. Ann Intern Med 10:1802–1827, 1937.
5. Reifenstein GH, Levine SA, Gross RE: Coarctation of the aorta. Am Heart J 33:146–168, 1947.
6. Blumenthal S: Standards for children's blood pressure. Pediatrics 59 (Suppl):802–803, 1977.
7. Liberthson RR, Pennington DG, Jacobs ML, Daggett WM: Coarctation of the aorta: review of 234 patients and clarification of management problems. Am J Cardiol 43:835–840, 1979.
8. Blumgart HL, Lawrence JS, Ernstene AC: The dynamics of the circulation in coarctation (stenosis of the isthmus) of the aorta of the adult type. Relation to essential hypertension. Arch Int Med 47:806–823, 1931.
9. Bing RJ, Handelsman JC, Campbell JA, Griswold HE, Blalock A: The surgical treatment and the physiopathology of coarctation of the aorta. Ann Surg 128:803–824, 1948.
10. Steele JM: Evidence for general distribution of peripheral resistance in coarctation of the aorta: report of three cases. J Clin Invest 20:473–480, 1941.
11. Gupta TC, Wiggers CJ: Basic hemodynamic changes produced by aortic coarctation of different degrees. Circulation 3:17–31, 1951.
12. Scott HW, Bahnson HT: Evidence for a renal factor in the hypertension of experimental coarctation of the aorta. Surgery 30:206–217, 1951.
13. Scott HW, Collins HA, Langa AM, Olsen NS: Additional observations concerning the physiology of the hypertension associated with experimental coarctation of the aorta. Surgery 36:445–459, 1954.
14. Erlanger J, Gasser HS: Studies in secondary traumatic shock – II. Shock due to mechanical limitation of blood flow. Am J Physiol 49:151–173, 1919.
15. de Jager S: Experiments and considerations on haemodynamics. J Physiol 7:130–215, 1886.
16. Page IH: The effect of chronic constriction of the aorta on arterial blood pressure in dogs: an attempt to produce coarctation of the aorta. Am Heart J 19:218–232, 1940.
17. Goldblatt H, Lynch J, Hanzal RF, Summerville WW: Studies on experimental hypertension – I. The production of persistent elevation of systolic blood pressure by means of renal ischemia. J Exp Med 59:347–379, 1934.
18. Goldblatt H, Kahn JR, Hanzal RF: Studies on experimental hypertension – IX. The effect on blood pressure of the constriction of the abdominal aorta above and below the site of origin of both main renal arteries. J Exp Med 69:649–660, 1939.
19. Rytand DA: The renal factor in arterial hypertension with coarctation of the aorta. J Clin Invest 17:391–399, 1938.
20. Svane H, Jensen OM: Structure of the juxtaglomerular apparatus in kidneys situated centrally and peripherally to an experimental coarctation of the aorta in dogs. Acta Pathol Microbiol Scand 70:501–511, 1967.
21. Ferguson JC, Barrie WW, Schenk WG: Hypertension of aortic coarctation: the role of renal and other factors. Ann Surg 185:423–428, 1977.
22. Sealy WC: Coarctation of the aorta and hypertension. Ann Thorac Surg 3:15–28, 1967.
23. Meacham PW, Dean RH, Lawson JW, Petracek MR, Burnham SJ, Hollifield JW, Burney P, Scott HW: Study of the renal pressure system in experimental coarctation of the abdominal aorta. Am Surg 43:771–777, 1977.
24. Bagby SP, McDonald WJ, Strong DW, Porter GA, Bennett WM, Bonchek LI: Abnormali-

ties of renal perfusion and the renal pressor system in dogs with chronic aortic coarctation. Cir Res 37:615–620, 1975.

25. Bagby SP, Mass RD, Gray DK: Abnormality of the renin/body-fluid-volume relationship in serially studied inbred dogs with neonatally-induced coarctation hypertension. Hypertension 2:631–642, 1980.
26. Yagi S, Kramsch DM, Madoff IM, Hollander W: Plasma renin activity in hypertension associated with coarctation of the aorta. Am J Physiol 215(3):605–610, 1968.
27. Fujii J, Murata K, Yamaguchi H, Kuramachi M, Seki A, Ikeda M: Pathogenesis of hypertension in rabbits with coarctation of the abdominal aorta. Tohoku J Exp Med 99:115–119, 1969.
28. Strong WB, Botti RE, Silbert DR, Liebman J: Peripheral and renal vein plasma renin activity in coarctation of the aorta. Pediatrics 45:254–259, 1970.
29. Brown JJ, Davies DL, Lever AF, Robertson JIS: Plasma renin concentration in human hypertension – II. Renin in relation to aetiology. Br Med J 20:1215–1219, 1965.
30. Amsterdam EA, Albers WH, Christlieb AR, Morgan CL, Nadas AS, Hickler RB: Plasma renin activity in children with coarctation of the aorta. Am J Cardiol 23:396–399, 1969.
31. Scott HM, Dean RH, Boerth R, Sawyers JL, Meacham P, Fisher RD: Coarctation of the abdominal aorta. Pathophysiologic and therapeutic considerations. Ann Surg 189:746–757, 1979.
32. Rocchini AP, Rosenthal A, Barger AC, Castaneda AR, Nadas AS: Pathogenesis of paradoxical hypertension after coarctation resection. Circulation 54:382–387, 1976.
33. Werning C, Schönbeck M, Weidmann P, Baumann K, Gysling E, Wirz P, Siegenthaler W: Plasma renin activity in patients with coarctation of the aorta. A comment on the pathogenesis of prestenotic hypertension. Circulation 40:731–737, 1969.
34. Van Way CW 3rd, Michelakis AM, Anderson WJ, Manlove A, Oates JA: Studies of Plasma renin activity in coarctation of the aorta. Ann Surg 183:229–238, 1976.
35. Fallo F, Armanini D, Maragno I, Mantero F: Plasma renin activity in coarctation of the aorta before and after surgical correction. Br Heart J 40:1415–1418, 1978.
36. Alpert BS, Bain HH, Balfe JW, Kidd BSL, Olley PM: Role of the renin–angiotensin–aldosterone system in hypertensive children with coarctation of the aorta. Am J Cardiol 43:828–834, 1979.
37. Ribeiro AB, Krakoff LR: Angiotensin blockade in coarctation of the aorta. N Engl J Med 295:148–150, 1976.
38. Markiewicz A, Wojczuk D, Kokot F, Cicha A: Plasma renin activity in coarctation of aorta before and after surgery. Br Heart J 37:721–725, 1975.
39. Parker FB, Farrell B, Streeten DHP, Blackman MS, Sondheimer HM, Anderson GH Jr: Hypertensive mechanisms in coarctation of the aorta. J Thorac Cardiovasc Surg 80:568–573, 1980.
40. Brown JJ, Davies DL, Lever AF, Robertson JIS: Renin and angiotensin. A survey of some aspects. Postgrad Med J 42:153–176, 1966.
41. Laragh JH, Sealey JE, Sommers S: Patterns of adrenal secretion and urinary excretion of aldosterone and plasma renin activity in normal and hypertensive subjects. Circ Res 18:158–174, 1966.
42. Veyrat R, deChamplain J, Boucher R, Genest J: Measurement of human arterial renin activity in some physiological and pathological states. Can Med Ass J 90:215–220, 1964.
43. Creditor MC, Loschky UK: Plasma renin activity in hypertension. Am J Med 43:371–382, 1967.
44. Brown JJ, Davies DL, Lever AF, Robertson JIS: Plasma renin concentration in human hypertension – II. Renin in relation to aetiology. Br M J 2:1215–1219, 1965.
45. Cohen EL, Rovner DR, Conn JW: Postural augmentation of plasma renin activity; importance in diagnosis of renovascular hypertension. J Am Med Ass 197:973–978, 1966.

46. Streeten DHP, Schletter FE, Clift GV, Stevenson CT, Dalakos TG: Studies of the renin–angiotensin–aldosterone system in patients with hypertension and in normal subjects. Am J Med 46:844–861, 1969.
47. Hunt JC, Strong CG: Renovascular hypertension. Mechanisms, natural history and treatment. Am J Cardiol 32:562–572, 1973.
48. Nielsen J, Nerstrom B, Jacobsen JG: The postural plasma renin response in renovascular hypertension. Acta Med Scand 189:213–220, 1971.
49. Streeten DHP, Anderson GH Jr, Sunderlin FS Jr, Mallov JS, Springer J: Identifying Renin Participation in Hypertension. In: Frontiers in Hypertension Research. Laragh JH, ed. New York: Springer, 1981, pp. 204–207.
50. Gunnells JC, McGuffin WL, Johnsrude I, Robinson RR: Peipheral and renal venous plasma renin activity in hypertension. Ann Intern Med 71:555–575, 1969.
51. Hussain RA, Gifford RW, Stewart BH, Meaney TF, McCormick LJ, Vidt DG, Humphrey DC: Differential renal venous renin activity in diagnosis of renovascular hypertension. Am J Cardiol 32:707–715, 1973.
52. Tucker RM, Strong CG, Brennan LA, Sheps SG, Brown RD, Weinshilboum RM: Renovascular hypertension. Relationship of surgical curability to renin-angiotensin activity. Mayo Clin Proc 53:373–377, 1978.
53. Vaughan ED, Bühler FR, Laragh JH, Sealey JE, Baer L, Bard RH: Renovascular hypertension: renin measurements to indicate hypersecretion and contralateral suppression, estimate renal plasma flow, and score for surgical curability. Am J Med 55:402–414, 1973.
54. Stockigt JR, Collins RD, Noakes CA, Schambelan M, Biglieri EG: Renal-vein renin in various forms of renal hypertension. Lancet 1:1194–1198, 1972.
55. Bianchi G, Campolo L, Vegeto A, Pietra V, Piazza U: The value of plasma renin concentration per se, and in relation to plasma and extracellular fluid volume in diagnosis and prognosis of human renovascular hypertension. Clin Sci 39:559–576, 1970.
56. Marks LS, Maxwell MH, Kaufman JJ: Renin, Sodium and vasodepressor response to saralasin in renovascular and essential hypertension. Ann Intern Med 87:176–182, 1977.
57. Grim CE, Luft FC, Weinberger MH, Grim CM: Sensitivity and specificity of screening tests for renal vascular hypertension. Ann Intern Med 91:617–622, 1979.
58. Poutasse EF, Gonzalez-Serva L, Wendelken JR, Franz JP: Saralasin tests as a diagnostic and prognostic aid in renovascular hypertensive patients subjected to renal operation. J Urol 123:306–310, 1980.
59. Kaufman JJ: Editorial comment. J Urol 123:310, 1980.
60. Streeten DHP, Anderson GH Jr: Outpatient experience with saralasin. Kidney Int 15:S44–52, 1979.
61. Brunner HR, Gavras H, Laragh JH, Keenan R: Angiotensin II blockade in man by sar^1-ala^8-angiotensin II for understanding and treatment of high blood pressure. Lancet 2:1045–1048, 1973.
62. Streeten DHP, Anderson GH Jr, Freiberg JM, Dalakos TG: Use of an angiotensin II antagonist (saralasin) in the recognition of 'angiotensinogenic' hypertension. N Engl J Med 292:657–662, 1975.
63. Baer L, Parra-Carrillo JZ, Radichevich I, Williams GS: Detection of renovascular hypertension with angiotensin II blockade. Ann Intern Med 86:257–260, 1977.
64. Verska JJ, DeQuattro V, Woolley MM: Coarctation of the aorta. The abdominal pain syndrome and paradoxical hypertension. J Thorac Cardiovasc Surg 58:746–753, 1969.
65. Srouji MN, Trusler GA: Paradoxical hypertension and the abdominal pain syndrome following resection of coarctation of the aorta. Can Med Ass J 92:412–416, 1965.
66. Overbeck HW: Pressure-independent increases in vascular resistance in hypertension: role of sympathoadrenergic influences. Hypertension 2:780–786, 1980.
67. Prager RL, Dunn J, Harness J, Seaton J, Harrison T, Behrendt DM: The adrenergic

response to pulsatile abdominal blood flow in laboratory animals with chronic coarctation of the thoracic aorta. Surgery 85:695–701, 1979.

68. Crafoord C, Nylin G: Congenital coarctation of the aorta and its surgical treatment. J Thorac Surg 14:347–361, 1945.
69. Gross RE: Surgical correction for coarctation of the aorta. Surgery 18:673–678, 1945.
70. Maron BJ, Humphries JO, Rowe RD: Prognosis of surgically corrected coarctation of the aorta. A 20-year postoperative appraisal. Circulation 47:119–126, 1973.
71. Waldhausen JA, Nahrwold DL: Repair of coarctation of the aorta with a subclavian flap. J Thorac Cardiovasc Surg 51:532–538, 1966.
72. Sealy WC: Indications for surgical treatment of coarctation of the aorta. Surg Gynecol Obstet 97:301–306, 1953.
73. Sealy WC, Harris JS, Young WG Jr, Callaway HA: Paradoxical hypertension following resection of coarctation of aorta. Surgery 42:135–147, 1957.

33. HYPERTENSION SECONDARY TO RENAL PARENCHYMAL DISEASE

James Gibb Johnson and James C. Hunt

Disease of the renal parenchyma is the most common cause of secondary hypertension. In studies of hypertensive populations, some form of kidney disease other than renal artery stenosis is found in approximately 5–10% of patients [1–3]. Not only is there a relatively high frequency of kidney disease among hypertensives, but also the elevated blood pressure tends to occur earlier and become more severe in patients with parenchymal disease [4]. In addition, the hypertensive state accelerates the deterioration of renal function in these patients [5].

The earliest recognition of the association between hypertension and renal parenchymal disease is generally attributed to Richard Bright. In this classic observations at Guy's Hospital in London between 1820 and 1836, he noticed the striking association of contracted kidneys, albuminous urine, and hypertrophy of the heart [6]. He speculated that the kidneys were responsible, that they chemically altered the blood, causing a resistance to the outflow from the heart. Althgouh blood pressure was not measured clinically at that time, the introduction of blood pressure measurement into clinical medicine quickly confirmed Bright's observations.

As we have learned more about the natural histories of the various renal diseases and have become more sophisticated in classifying them, we have gained insights into the interaction of kidney disease and hypertension. Although our understanding is far from complete, basic and clinical investigations have yielded clues regarding the pathogenesis. In addition, we are learning about the effect of the hypertensive state on the deterioration of renal function in some renal diseases. We are also making headway in the application of more rational treatment goals and methods.

OCCURRENCE AND SEVERITY OF HYPERTENSION IN VARIOUS RENAL DISEASES

The expression of hypertension is quite variable among patients with renal disease. Although there is a striking association of hypertension in some, it is almost non-existent in others. In some, hypertension occurs early in the

Amery, A. (ed.) Hypertensive Cardiovascular Disease: Pathophysiology and Treatment
© 1982, Martinus Nijhoff Publishers. The Hague / Boston / London
ISBN-13: 978-94-009-7478-4

course of renal functional impairment, whereas in others it is delayed until end stage, and even then may appear only with the accumulation of excess sodium and water. Similarly, the hypertension is usually mild at the outset, becoming more severe as the disease progresses; but in some the blood pressure elevation may be severe from the beginning.

Examples of those diseases with a relatively high frequency and severity of hypertension are shown in Table 1. Severe hypertension is seen in renin producing tumors of the kidney cortex [7–11], bringing them to medical attention. Likewise scleroderma kidney disease, renal infarcts, and segmental renal hypoplasia often are associated with severe and malignant hypertension [12–14]. Acute and chronic glomerulonephritis are associated with high frequency, but the severity of the hypertension is quite variable and often related to the degree of sodium retention [15].

Table 2 shows examples of diseases with either mild or non-existent hypertension until renal failure is superimposed. Minimal change nephropathy and focal glomerulopathy with benign hematuria are derangements of the glomeruli which fall into this category [16, 17]. Oligonephronia, meduallry cystic-nephronophthisis complex and many of the acute tubulointerstitial diseases also have little hypertension without renal failure [18–20]. Furthermore, at end stage, hypertension is frequently absent in the diseases

Table 1. Renal diseases with high occurrence and severity of hypertension

I.   Renal infarction
     Emboli involving the small renal arteries
     Post-traumatic renal infarction

II. Diseases involving the interlobular arteries
     Polyarteritis nodosa of the kidney
     Scleroderma kidney disease

III. Glomerular diseases with prominent small artery involvement
     Acute glomerulonephritis due to SLE and other systemic vasculitides
     Diabetic glomerulosclerosis
     Hemolytic-uremic syndrome and its varients
     Rapidly progressive glomerulonephritis

IV. Diffuse lesions of the glomerular capillaries
     Acute post-infectious glomerulonephritis
     Chronic glomerulonephritis

V.   Renin producing tumors of the kidney
     Juxtaglomerular cell tumor
     Renin producing hamartomas
     Renin producing Wilms' tumor

VI. Renal hypoplasia
     Segmental hypoplasia (ask-upmark kidney)

Table 2. Renal diseases with low occurrence of hypertension

I.	Reduced nephron population without scarring Bilateral renal hypoplasia with oligonephronia Simple renal hypoplasia
II.	Tubulointerstitial diseases Acute tubulointerstitial nephritis Balkan nephritis Medullary cyctic-nephronophthisis complex Medullary sponge kidney
III.	Glomerular diseases Focal glomerulopathy with benign hematuria Minimal change disease

primarily affecting the tubulointerstitial structures, providing a valuable diagnostic clue to the type of the underlying disease.

The diseases listed in Table 3 on the other hand, are sometimes reported to be associated with severe hypertension; however, the occurrence and severity of hypertension in these diseases is at times found to be low.

Although the primary glomerular diseases presenting as nephrotic syndrome do not usually manifest hypertension unless renal failure supervenes, idiopathic membranous glomerulonephritis and focal glomerulosclerosis patients sometimes are found to have prominent hypertension unrelated to corticosteroid therapy or renal insufficiency [21–23]. Also hypertension may persist despite a remission of the other clinical manifestations of membranous glomerulonphritis [15]. Most patients with the idiopathic nephrotic syndrome, however, are normotensive until moderate or advanced renal insufficiency develops [24, 25].

Analgesic nephropathy is a disease which has been reported to have both a high and a low occurrence of hypertension [26]. In Australia hypertension

Table 3. Renal diseases with variable occurrence and severity of hypertension

I.	Glomerular diseases with prominent proteinuria Focal glomerulosclerosis with hyalinosis Membranous nephropathy
II.	Tubulinointerstitial diseases Analgesic nephropathy Bilateral chronic pyelonephritis Unilateral chronic pyelonephritis Unilateral obstructive uropathy
III.	Cystic kidney disease Adult polycystic disease Childhood polycystic disease Multicystic kidney disease

appears to be common among patients with this disease, and in Europe the frequency of hypertension is relatively low. This curious geographic difference has been attributed to differences in the extent of papillary necrosis and to be differences in the analgesic compounds used in the two areas [26].

The relationship between hypertension and the diseases caused by bacterial infection of the kidney has been a subject of much investigation and confusion. Acute pyelonephritis rarely causes hypertension unless it is associated with either papillary necrosis, acute renal failure and overload, or obstructive uropathy. Chronic pyelonephritis is complicated by hypertension in a high percentage of cases [26]. This association seems to be related to the presence of parenchymal scarring [27]. Vesicoureteral reflux with scarring has been demonstrated to be strongly associated with hypertension in some children [28, 29]. Unilateral atrophic pyelonephritis as a cause of hypertension has been a subject of much debate. The early reports of surgical cures of hypertension were in patients whose contracted kidneys were supposedly scarred from pyelonephritis [30, 31], and this entity was felt to be the most frequent cause of surgically correctable hypertension. Since the early reports, however, it has become apparent that the histopathologic picture in such patients is mimicked by ischemic atrophy from either renal artery stenosis or segmental renal hypoplasia [32–34]. As arteriography was not yet in clinical use, and the pathologic criteria did not distinguish adequately the cause of atrophy, many of these early patients were likely to have renal artery stenosis or segmental hypoplasia [35]. Still there are a few cases of surgical cure of hypertension in well-documented pyelonephritis; however, they are mostly seen in children in whom vesicoureteral reflux has been demonstrated to be the cause of scarring [36]. Experimental attempts to cause hypertension by unilateral pyelonephritis have been successful primarily when vesicoureteral reflux has been introduced by a variety of methods [37].

Some patients with polycystic kidney disease have elevated blood pressure with little impairment of glomerular filtration rate long before other symptoms appear. Others may manifest normal blood pressures with far-advanced renal insufficiency [38]. However, this is an exception to the usual expectation that most patients with polycystic renal disease develop hypertension as renal function becomes impaired, and the blood pressure elevation becomes more severe with progression of the disease.

RELATIONSHIP OF HISTOPATHOLOGIC AND FUNCTIONAL
ALTERATIONS WITH HYPERTENSION

The renal anatomical and functional alterations which are commonly found in the diseases with prominent hypertension are different from those found in the diseases without hypertension. These differences provide important clues to the pathogenesis of the hypertensive rate in renal diseases. It is important to note, however, that some diseases a predominance of factors which are either not present in others or, at least, not present to the same degree. Thus it appears that the hypertensive state may be influenced more by one set of factors in one group of diseases and different factors in other diseases.

Careful study of patients with renin secreting tumors of the renal cortex affords us a view of an experiment of nature in which an excess of renin is clearly the initiating and sustaining factor. A hypertensive state occurs which is severe and frequently develops a malignant phase [7, 9, 39]. Secondary aldosteronism occurs, although hypertension persists when adrenalectomy is performed or aldosteronism is opposed with spironolactone [7, 8, 40], indicating that aldosterone excess is not essential to the maintenance of the hypertensive state. The blood volume is diminished in some patients when aldosteronism is eliminated; and hypotension has been reported upon removal of the tumor [8], a phenomenon also seen in patients with pheochromocytoma. Since angiotensin has a powerful venoconstrictor action, the low blood volume seen in these renin-secreting tumor patients is likely secondary to the effect of angiotensin on capacitance vessels. In addition to the peripheral effects of angiotensin, the intrarenal circulation is affected in a manner which is likely to contribute to the maintenance of hypertension. Both anatomic arterial stenosing lesions and reversible vasoconstriction within the kidney occur. The secondary vascular lesions include the gamut from hyaline arteriolar change to angiosclerosis of the interlobular arteries [7, 8]. The intrarenal functional and anatomic narrowing act to diminish renal blood flow more than glomerular filtration, thus causing a tendency for enhancement of sodium reabsorption by the kidney. This increase in filtration fraction has been demonstrated in one case which was also studied with an inhibitor of angiotensin [40]. The administration of angiotensin inhibitor was attended by a further drop in renal blood flow and rise in filtration fraction. Thus it appears that even in a syndrome of almost pure renin excess causing vasoconstriction, there are also abnormalities in the renal circulation which alter the glomerular tubular balance for sodium, an abnormality which has been felt by some to be very important in the pathogenesis of hypertension of many varieties [41].

Ischemia-producing vascular lesions are seen in many of the hypertensive renal diseases. In polyarteritis the inflammatory lesions narrow and obstruct arteries of various sizes, particularly by the interlobular and arcuate arteries [42]. Scleroderma kidney disease is characterized by marked narrowing of the interlobular arteries with ischemia of the glomeruli [43, 44]. In embolic and thrombotic infarctions, arteries of varying size are partially or completely occluded causing ischemia along with the infarction.

In each of the diseases listed in Table 1 a common denominator is vascular narrowing with ischemia of the supplied tissue, except in the types of acute glomerulonephritis without system vasculitis. In these glomerular diseases the dominant lesion is obstruction to blood flow through the glomeruli with interference with the normal filtration of sodium and water, and it is with sodium and water retention that the connection with hypertension is felt to exist.

It is useful to contrast the renal hypoplasia of the kidney. Simple hypoplasia and bilateral oligonephronia have few or no vascular lesions, and hypertension occurs only when the ability to excrete sodium is impaired [18]. Segmental hypoplasia, on the other hand, has areas of atrophic scarring within the kidney associated with marked vascular narrowing and ischemia and is often characterized by severe hypertension [18, 45].

The focal glomerulonephritides likewise have an interesting correlation between vascular lesions and hypertension. Patients with focal glomerular lesions and no system manifestations have few vascular lesions and are normotensive. However, patients with systemic diseases whose renal lesions are characterized by focal inflammation or scarring within the glomeruli frequently have vascular lesions and hypertension [23, 17].

Patients with medullary cystic-nephronophthisis complex and some other forms of chronic tubulointerstitial disease comprise another interesting group. They often waste sodium and have *low* blood pressure on a normal sodium diet [19], and the histopathologic renal lesions primarily affect the tubular structures rather than the vessels or the glomeruli.

Thus it appears that those patients who have a tendency to develop severe hypertension before the appearance of renal failure have histopathologic lesions characterized by vascular narrowing and ischemia on the one hand or glomerular obstruction, scarring or obliteration on the other. Patients who tolerate early and moderate insufficiency without hypertension have neither of the above abnormalities to any major degree, and patients with a tendency to develop hypotension are likely to have lesions which interfere with tubular function and are particularly prone to sodium wasting.

HEMODYNAMIC AND FLUID VOLUME CHARACTERISTICS OF RENAL HYPERTENSION

We are also learning about the nature of renal hypertension from examining hemodynamic and fluid volume alterations in the various disease states. Clues regarding both pathogenesis and information are helpful in designing therapeutic regimens are obtained.

Acute Glomerulonephritis

The hemodynamic and fluid volume pattern seen with acute glomerulon-ephritis and acute renal failure represent one end of the spectrum of patterns. The severely affected patients have oliguria and sodium retention leading to a congested circulation [46–48], with increases in the extracellular and plasma volumes [49]. The cardiac output is elevated in most patients when measured at the height of the circulatory congestion [46, 47]. Peripheral resistance has been found either to be increased or 'inappropriately normal' in the face of an elevated cardiac output [46, 47]. In some older patients cardiac output is normal while peripheral resistance is elevated. This raises the possibility that patients with acute glomerulonephritis may enter a phase in which the blood pressure is maintained by a high peripheral resistance with normal cardiac output [49]. Patients exhibiting this pattern have also been shown to have either an elevated plasma renin activity or an inappropriately normal level of renin activity for the degree of sodium and water excess [49]. It is likely that inappropriately normal renin levels in such patients contribute to an inappropriately normal or elevated peripheral resistance.

Chronic Nephritis

In hypertensive patients with chronic glomerulonephritis or pyelonephritis, the hemodynamic pattern is not so sharply defined. There is, however, evidence that many non-uremic patients have an elevated cardiac index initially which reverts to normal as hypertension becomes more severe [50]. Despite this tendency to an increase in systemic flow, renal blood flow is reduced by the renal disease [51]. Diminished venous distensibility has also been found in the early stage in such patients [52]. Thus in chronic nephritis small increases in angiotensin may be contributing to the elevated output by reducing the capacity of the vascular bed, inordinately enhancing return to the heart for the level of blood volume. Under such circumstances even a 'normal' blood volume is inappropriately high. Other studies have also indicated inappropriately high blood volumes in patients with chronic renal parenchymal disease and hypertension [53].

Plasma renin and angiotensin measurements in patients with chronic glomerulonephritis and chronic pyelonephritis have mostly been within the normal range [54, 55]. Angiotensin blockade has not lowered the blood pressure [54]. On the other hand, studies of sodium loading in such patients have shown that the plasma renin activity remains inappropriately normal for the level of sodium and water expansion [56], again raising the possibility that the hypertensive state may be sustained in these patients by the interaction of the pressor angiotensin with an inappropriately elevated volume. There is also evidence that inappropriately elevated suppressor doses of angiotensin may contribute to hypertension by central stimulation of sympathetic outflow and venous constriction [57, 58].

End Stage Renal Disease

The hemodynamic characteristics of end stage renal hypertensive patients have been well defined. In non-nephrectomized dialysis patients two general patterns are present. The majority of end stage patients develops a largely volume-dependent type of hypertension as the glomerular filtration rate (GFR) becomes nil, although renin plays a role causing generalized vasoconstriction [59]. This pattern occurs regardless of the underlying disease. Excess dietary ingestion of sodium and water or inadequate removal with dialysis results in the worsening of the hypertension. The blood pressure correlates directly with blood volume and exchangeable sodium, as well as with plasma renin activity [60]. Both cardiac output and total peripheral resistance are elevated [61] even when patients are at a clinically dry weight, although it appears that anemia accounts for the elevated cardiac output [62]. Following bilateral nephrectomy, blood pressure and peripheral resistance fall to normal, and cardiac output is unchanged unless the anemia is corrected, in which case the cardiac output reverts to normal [62].

A minority of hypertensive patients on dialysis have a more severe type of hypertension which cannot be controlled with dialysis, restriction of sodium and water, and sympatholytics [63]. These patients frequently develop a malignant phase of hypertension and have elevated renin levels [64] and excessive thirst. The thirst is felt to be secondary to renin stimulation of the thirst center [65]. In these patients bilateral nephrectomy promptly corrects the hypertension and thirst [64, 65], although current antihypertensive regimens using storng vasodilators and angiotensin opposing drugs also have controlled the syndrome [66]. In these patients the peripheral resistance is often so high that cardiac output is found to be low despite anemia. Nephrectomy or successful medical management is associated with a fall of the pressure and peripheral resistance and a rise in the cardiac output.

In the minority of patients for whom nephrectomy is desired, a new pattern occurs in the anephric state. The patients whose hypertension was severe prior to nephrectomy develop greater pressure elevations with sodium loading than do those patients whose pressures were normal [67]. Thus one group can be said to be 'salt sensitive' and one 'salt resistant' in the sense that sodium loading in the anephric state tends to raise the pressure in one group more sharply than in the other [22]. Hence it appears that even following the removal of renal factors, humans have a variability in their blood pressure sensitivity to sodium loading.

PATHOGENESIS OF RENAL HYPERTENSION

Obviously, with the variation in structural, functional and hemodynamic derangements, it is apparent that renal hypertension is not a homogeneous entity. A number of derangements have been incriminated as possible pathogenetic factors in the various disease states. It is probable that the degree of participation of any individual abnormality and the pattern of interaction of the involved factors vary from one disease to another and from one patient to another. It is important to keep in mind that the maintenance of an elevated blood pressure usually requires the interaction of two or more factors, as the normal control mechanisms tend to compensate for single factor variations, such as an excess of only vasoconstriction or volume.

Two factors which clearly seem to be involved in the pathogenesis in many patients have been discerned. Much evidence for glomerulotubular imbalance of sodium [68], and the excess stimulation of the renin–angiotensin system exists in various types of renal disease, although the interaction of these two factors does not wholly account for the hypertensive problem seen in all renal parenchymal diseases.

Some diseases appear to have a mechanism similar to that seen in stenosis of the main renal artery. Diseases such as renal scleroderma, segmental hypoplasia with prominent vascular involvement and surgically correctable unilateral atrophic pyelonephritis from vesicoureteral reflux fall into this category. It is possible that patients with non-uremic chronic glomerular and interstitial disease with prominent vascular involvement and surgically correctable unilateral atrophic pyelonephritis from vesicoureteral reflux fall into this category. It is possible that patients with non-uremic chronic glomerular and interstitial disease with prominent vascular involvement also have a similar pthogenetic sequence. In these patients the two important factors seem to be stimulation of the renin–angiotensin system and glomerulotubular imbalance for sodium.

The reduced vascular bed and ischemia seen in these diseases leads to sodium reabsorption from altered regional hemodynamics within the kidney. Firstly, reduced renal perfusion is known to be followed by a relatively greater efferent than afferent arteriolar constriction as an autoregulatory response to maintain glomerular filtration, thus increasing the filtration fraction [69]. Post-glomerular capillary hydrostatic pressure falls under this circumstance while the oncotic pressure is increased. Both these factors enhance tubular sodium reabsorption relative to filtration [70, 71], causing a transient expansion of blood volume until a pressure rise overcomes the increased vascular resistance and restores glomerulotubular balance, albeit at higher pressure [68]. In addition stimulation of the renin system causes enhanced sodium reabsorption through an aldosterone mechanism. Thus both sodium retention and the stimulation of the renin–angiotensin system interact in causing hypertension in this general category of prominent vascular lesions.

In some patients little evidence exists to incriminate the renin–angiotensin system, and sodium-volume factors predominate. Anephric hypertensive patients have this type of hypertension. Hypertension seen in the early phase of acute post-infectious glomerulonephritis also appears to be largely secondary to sodium and water retention. Hypertension associated with acute renal failure and sodium and water overload is another example.

Other factors are likely to play a role in the pathogenesis of hypertension. It is possible that renal pressor systems other than the renin–angiotensin system exist [72, 73]. Studies in uremic hypertensive patients show that even when PRA is normal, a dramatic drop in peripheral vascular resistance may occur with nephrectomy implying that removal of the kidneys rids the patient of yet another renal pressor factor [5].

Finally, there is evidence that indicates that a renal vasodepressor system may exist which helps modulate the blood pressure, opposing the kidneys' prohypertensive factors by elaborating antihypertensive factor(s). Vasodepressor lipids which appear to be released from renal interstitial cells have been shown to modify hypertension in several experimental models [74]. The effect of renal scarring, reduced medullary blood flow, enhanced sodium reabsorption or excess renin release within the kidney on such a system in man is at present unknown. Transplants of renal medulla to locations in the body outside the constraints of the renal circulation modify various forms of experimental hypertension, including renoprival and renovascular hypertension in the dog and rabbit [75].

Measurements of urinary kallikrein, a renal enzyme which catalyzes the production of the vasodilating and natriuretic kinins and thus serves as a marker of the renal kinin system activity, have shown that patients with renal parenchymal disease and hypertension excrete smaller than normal amounts [76]. A deficiency of this renal vasodilating system may influence the development of hypertension by decreasing renal sodium and water excretion via a diminution in renal perfusion [77]. It is as yet unclear what role, if any, is played by abnormalities of this system in the pathogenesis of renal hypertension.

CLINICAL ASPECTS

Effect of Hypertension on Renal Function

There is a growing body of evidence to confirm a long-held clinical view that elevated blood pressure has a particularly adverse effect on renal func-

518

tion in patients with various forms of renal parenchymal disease. In scleroderma kidney disease a phase occurs with elevated pressure generating still higher pressures and a deterioration of renal function [44]. Stimulation of excess renin by ischemia is important in this process [44]. Typical scleroderma lesions of the interlobular arteries and afferent arterioles cause a positive feedback wherein the lesions become so ischemia-producing that the pressure spirals upward while the renal lesions progress, stimulating further renin release and rendering the kidney more bloodless and thus more functionless. Control of the pressure in these patients used to require nephrectomy [44, 78]. However, recent vigorous attempts to control pressure using beta-blocking or other renin suppressing drugs along with vasodilators and sodium removal have been successful in controlling pressure and halting the progression of renal insufficiency in a few cases. In some there has been a marked improvement in the renal functional impairment [79, 80]. Although this is the most dramatic example of the importance of blood pressure control in preserving renal function in patients with renal disease, the principle applies to other types of hypertensive renal parenchymal diseases as well. In diabetic glomerulosclerosis a correlation exists between glomerular nodular lesions and blood pressure elevation [81]. Treatment of hypertension in patients with diabetic renal disease has been shown to reduce proteinuria and to cause a slow decline of renal function [82]. In patients with polycystic kidney disease control of hypertension has also been associated with prolonged renal survival. It is felt that the same effect is seen clinically in many renal diseases including the chronically rejecting transplanted kidney, chronic pyelonephritis, and chronic glomerulonephritis. Marked improvement of uremia and renal insufficiency associated with the malignant transformation of essential hypertension has been seen following blood pressure control in a few isolated instances [83, 84]. With the recent introduction of the potent vasodilator, minoxidil, which has allowed more strict blood pressure control in drug resistant hypertensive patients, this phenomenon has become more common [85].

Detection of Renal Parenchymal Disease

In the diagnostic evaluation of the hypertensive patient, underlying parenchymal disease will be apparent in most of those in whom it is present. Rarely will patients with chronic glomerular disease, chronic pyelonephritis, or one of the systemic vasculitides present with hypertension as the only apparent clinical feature. There are, however, many patients with chronic nephritis, and other renal diseases whose underlying problem is relatively cryptic. Special care should therefore be taken during the initial evaluation and on subsequent early follow-up visits to detect these patients, as the early detection may be important in preserving renal function and designing an appropriate antihypertensive regimen.

Inquiry regarding previous nephritic and nephrotic episodes should be included in the evaluation. Periods of weight gain or edema should be sought. A history of flank pain, discoloration of the urine, dysuria and frequency, and unexplained chills and fever may offer clues. Particular attention should be paid to a history of polyuria and nocturia, for this is often the first signal of renal insufficiency as the renal concentrating ability becomes impaired.

Evaluation of the optic fundus not only is important as an indication of target organ damage, but also detection of microaneurysms may uncover diabetes and lead to finding diabetic glomerulosclerosis in a previously unsuspected diabetic. The examination of the integument and musculoskeletal system may provide clues to underlying hereditary renal diseases. Adenoma sebaceum and other lesions of tuberous sclerosis may signal renal hamartomas. Partial lipodystrophy may be associated with membranoproliferative glomerulonephritis. Hypotropic nails with small or absent patellas constitute a syndrome with chronic glomerulonephritis or renal dysplasia. Polycystic kidney disease may be associated with skeletal abnormalities. Examination of the abdomen may discover the nephromegaly of polycystic disease or hydronephrosis.

The urinalysis is the most valuable diagnostic test for underlying renal disease. For this reason, measures should be taken to insure that the maximum benefit is obtained from a complete urinalysis. The specimen should be a freshly voided concentrated one. A second voided morning specimen after overnight dehydration and while still fasting is strongly preferred. The presence of moderate or severe proteinuria should alert one to parenchymal disease. Hematuria and red cell casts suggest glomerular disease, and other sediment changes are likely to point to the kidney.

The serum creatinine serves as a useful guide to underlying renal insufficiency, although it should be kept in mind that significant impairment of function may exist with only modest increase of the creatinine, particularly in the elderly patient. Hypokalemia indicates secondary aldosteronism more often than primary, and many severe hypertensives with a variety of diseases will present with modest hypokalemia, even prior to diuretic therapy. This is especially true of the patient with a very high sodium intake.

The existence of hypertension in the young, especially if severe, should alert one to possible underlying renal disease as this group in particular has a high occurrence of secondary hypertension. In the follow-up period patients who exhibit drug resistant hypertension or who escape control despite dietary sodium restriction should be re-evaluated for possible underlying renal or renovascular disease.

Principles of Medical Management

Patients whose disease is characterized by vasculopathy and ischemia and intense vasoconstriction are managed differently from those whose problem is acute sodium and fluid overload due to glomerulopathy. Likewise patients with severe hypertension, those with renal insufficiency, and those with congested circulation are managed differently from the mild patients, the ones with normal GFR, and the ones with renal parenchymal disease begins with an assessment which taken into account the underlying disease process, the severity of the hypertension, the degree of renal insufficiency, and a clinical assessment of sodium and volume status including an evaluation of dietary sodium intake.

Following pretreatment diagnostic evaluation which should include quantitation of renal function, a number of general features should be considered in establishing and maintaining an appropriate medical antihypertensive regimen.

The aim of therapy is to maintain the pressure within the normal range, not only to protect the cerebral and cardiac circulation, but also to prevent or slow the deterioration of renal function. Although rises in the serum creatinine may occur in some patients upon normalization of the blood pressure, in the majority of patients the rise is of only a few days and is followed by a restoration of the renal blood flow and GFR to the pretreatment levels. One must be aware, however, that an occasional patient with very fixed resistance, such as is seen in some older atherosclerotic patients, will manifest a true deterioration in renal function if the blood pressure is reduced to normal and kept there. Also precipitous drops in pressure with parenteral agents have been accompanied by the development of acute renal failure. Therefore, except for emergencies, one should use oral agents and avoid a *precipitous* drop in pressure to normal or hypotensive levels which will not maintain adequate renal perfusion. In restoring the blood pressure to absolute normal levels persistence rather than haste should be the watchword.

Sodium restriction and control of the sodium-volume status is the keystone to therapy in most patients with renal hypertension. However, special considerations exist. Renal patients not only have a tendency to develop sodium retention, they frequently lose the ability to conserve sodium as renal insufficiency becomes severe. This relative sodium wasting upon severe sodium restriction is seen more commonly in the patients with less vascular disease and more interstitial disease (including polycystic disease), but is highly variable among patients with the same disease process. Therefore, those patients with advanced renal insufficiency and hypertension need careful monitoring while receiving severe sodium restriction and diuretics so that pre-renal azotemia and hypovolemia with frank or postural hypotension can be avoided.

In renal hypertensive patients with near-normal glomerular function, the thiazide diuretics can be used; however, these should be avoided in favor of the loop diuretics when the GFR falls below approximately 30–40% of normal. Spironolactone and other potassium sparing diuretics have potential dire consequences by causing life-threatening hyperkalemia when used in renal insufficiency and should be avoided when the GFR is less than 50% of normal. In addition, diabetic and interstitial nephritis patients may have hyporeninemia and a tendency to develop hyperkalemia. These patients in particular should not be given potassium-sparing diuretics.

As renal insufficiency progresses, adjustemnts must be made in dosages of drugs which are primarily eliminated by the kidney. Modification of the dosage of those antihypertensive medications including methyldopa and clonidine may be indicated. Nevertheless, we have found methyldopa in association with careful control of dietary sodium (monitored by 24 h urine sodium output) to be an effective agent for the management of many hypertensives with parenchymal renal disease.

The use of sodium restriction alone is successful in many of the early patients with mild hypertension and with mild to moderate reduction of GFR. As the process progresses, however, the addition of diuretics, beta-adrenergic blockers or drugs which have sympatholytic effects, and drugs which have a vasodilating action are added in a stepwise fashion. The combination of sodium restriction (75–100 mEq/24 h), loop diuretics, beta-adrenergic blockade and a vasodilator is often useful in the severely hypertensive patient with moderate or advanced renal insufficiency.

In the end stage dialysis patients, the use of a proper dietary management including strict compliance of sodium and water restriction coupled with the administration of beta-adrenergic blockade or converting enzyme inhibition (experimental) and vasodilation has obviated the need for nephrectomy to control hypertension in many patients. In some instances patients who otherwise would have been subjected to nephrectomy because of a malignant phase have had sufficient return of blood flow to the kidneys by prolonged blood pressure control that they gain enough renal function to escape dialysis, and a rare patient has demonstrated marked improvement [85].

SUMMARY

Hypertension in patients with renal parenchymal disease occurs in association with a combination of factors which alter the kidneys' role in the normal regulation of blood pressure and fluid volume homeostasis. Clues regarding the pathogenesis of renal hypertension are obtained from observations of these pathological and functional associations. Although management of these patients in general parallels the management of essential hypertension, knowledge of the altered hemodynamics and other structural and functional derangements aids in tailoring therapy.

522

REFERENCES

1. Earle DP: Hypertensionin parenchymal renal disease. Prog cardiovas Dis 8:195–209, 1965.
2. Gifford RW Jr: Evaluation of the hypertensive patient. Milbank Mem Fund Q 47:170, 1969.
3. Bech K, Hilden T: The frequency of secondary hypertension. Acta med Scand 197 (1-2):65–69, 1975.
4. Paul O: Epidamiology of hypertension. In: Hypertension, Genest J, Kiow E, Kuchal O, eds. New York: McGraw-Hill, 1977.
5. Tuttle E: Hypertension Complicating Renal Disease. In: Hypertension Update: Mechanisms, Epidemiology, Evaluation, Management, pp. 76–84. Bloomfield, NJ: Health Learning Systems, 1980.
6. Bright P: Cases and observations, illustrative of renal diseases accompanied with the secretion of albuminous urine. Guy Hosp. Rep 1:338–379, 1836.
7. Robertson PW, Klidgian A, Harding LK, Walters G: Hypertension due to a renin secreting renal tumor. Am J Med 43n(6):963–976, 1967.
8. Valdes G, Lopez JM, Martinez Pk, Rosenberg H, Barriga P, Rodriquez JA, Otipka N: Renin secreting tumor. Hypertension 2:714–718, 1980.
9. Orjavik OS, Aas M, Fauchild P, Hovig T, Oystese B, Brodwall EK, Flatmark A: Renin-secreting renal tumor with severe hypertension. Acta Med Scand 197:329–335, 1975.
10. Mimran A, Leckie BJ, Fourcade JC, Baldet P, Navratil H, Barjon P: Blood pressure, renin angiotensin system and urinary kallikrein in a case of juxtaglomerular cell tumor. Am J. Med 65:527–536, 1978.
11. Brown JJ, Fraser R, Lever AF, Morton JJ, Robertson JIS, Tree M: Hypertension and secondary hyperaldosteronism associated with renin-secreting renal juxtaglomerular cell tumor. Lancet 2:1228-1232, 1973.
12. LeRoy EC, Fleischmann RM: The management of renal scleroderma: experience with dialysis, nephrectomy and transplantation. Am J Med 64:974–978, 1978.
13. Ben-Asher S: Hypertension caused by renal infarction. Ann. Intern Med 23:433–436, 1945.
14. Sobel JD, Hampel N, Kursbaum A, Adler O, Gellei B: Hypertension due to Ask-Upmark Kidney. Br J Urol 49:447–480, 1977.
15. Brod J: Acute diffuse glomerulonephritis. Am J Med 7(9):317–335, 1949.
16. Cameron JS, Turner DR, Ogg CS, Sharpstone P, Brown DB: The nephrotic syndrome in adults with 'minimal change' glomerular lesions. Q J Med 43(171:461–488, 1974.
17. Ferris TF: Focal glomerulonephritis. In: Nephrology, pp. 310–313. Stein Jay H, ed. New York: Grune and Stratton, 1980.
18. Royer P: Renal Hypoplasia. In: Nephrology, pp. 1059–1069. Hamburger WB, ed. Philadelphia: Saunders, 1968.
19. Gardner KD Jr: Juvenile Nephronophthisis and Renal Medullary Cystic Disease: An Analytic Review. In: Cystic Diseases of the Kidney, pp. 173–185. Gerdner KD Jr, ed. New York: John Wiley, 1976.
20. Ooi BS, Wellington J, First MR: Mancilla R, Pollack VE: Acute interstitial nephritis: a clinical and pathologic study based on renal biopsies. Am J Med 59:614–629, 1975.
21. Noel LH, Zanetti M, Droz D, Barbanel C: Long-term prognosis of idiopathic membranous glomerulonephritis. A study of 116 untreated patients. Am J Med 66:82–90, 1979.
22. Mandel AK, Chrysant K, Nordquist JA, Kraikitpanitch S, Xoung DT, Lindeman RD: Focal glomerular sclerosis. South Med. J. 69:997–1004, 1976.
23. Kincaid-Smith P: Hypertension and the Kidney. In: The Kidney: a clinico-pathologic study, pp. 205–221. Oxford: Blackwell Scientific, 1975.

24. Pollak VE, Rosen E, Pirani CL, Muehrcke RC, Kark RM: Natural history of lipoid nephrosis and of membranous glomerulonephritis. Ann Intern Med 69:1171–1196, 1968.
25. Schreiner GE: Nephrotic Syndrome. In: Diseases of the Kidney, pp. 503–636. Strauss MR, welt LC, eds Boston: Little, Brown & Co, 1971.
26. Kincaid-Smith P: Parenchymatous Diseases of the Kidney and Hypertension. In: Hypertension. Genest J, Kiow E, Kuchel O, eds. pp. 794–815. New York: McGraw-Hill, 1977.
27. Kincaid-Smith P: Pyelonephritis, Chronic Interstitial Nephritis and Obstructive Uropathy. In: Nephrology, pp. 553–582. Hamburger J, Corsnier J, Grunfield J, eds. New York: Wiley-Flammarion, 1979.
28. Holland NH, Kotchen T, Bhathena D: Hypertension in children with chronic pyelonephritis. Kedney Int. (Suppl):S243–S251, 1975.
29. Stecker JF, Read BP BP, Poutasse EF: Pediatric hypertension as a delayed sequela of reflux-induced chronic pyelonephritis. J Urol 118:644–646, 1977.
30. Butler NW: Chronic pyelonephritis and arterial hypertension. J Clin Invest 16:889–897, 1937.
31. Barker NW, Waters W: Hypertension associated with unilateral chronic atrophic pyelonephritis: treatment by nephrectomy. Proc. Staff Meet Mayo Clinic 13:118–121, 1938.
32. Pfau A, Rosenmann E: Unilateral chronic pyelonephritis and hypertension: coincidental or causal relationship? Am J Med 65(3):499–506, 1978.
33. Heptinstall RN: The Limitations of the Pathologic Diagnosis of Chronic Pyelonephritis. In: Renal Disease, pp. 350–381. Black DAR, ed. Oxford: Blackwell Scientific, 1967.
34. Haycock GB: Hypertension associated with unilateral renal disease in childhood. Acta Pediatr. Scand 64:299–304, 1975.
35. Gifford RW, McCormack LJ, Poutasse EF: The atrophic kidney, its role in hypertension. Mayo Clin Proc 40:834–852, 1965.
36. Poutasse EF, Stecker JF, Ladaga LE, Sperber EE: Malignant hypertension in children secondary to chronic pyelonephritis: laboratory and radiologic indications for partial or total nephrectomy. J Urol 119:264–267, 1978.
37. Tsuchida S, Yamaguchi O, Arai S, Fukuchi S: Hypertension and plasma renin activity in experimentally induced chronic pyelonephritis. Nephron 17:215–223, 1976.
38. Nash DA: Hypertension in polycystic kidney disease with renal failure. Arch Intern Med 137:1571–1575, 1977.
39. Eddy RL, Sanchez SA: Renin-secreting neoplasms and hypertension with hypokalemia. Ann Intern Med 75:725–729, 1971.
40. Conn JW, Cohen EL, Lucas CP, McDonald WJ, Major GH, Blough WM, Eveland WC, Bookstein JJ, Lapides J: Primary reninism. Arch Intern Med 130:682–696, 1972.
41. Guyton AC, Coleman TG: Quantitative analysis of the pathophysiology of hypertension. Circ Res (Suppl 1):1–15, 1969.
42. Kincaid-Smith P: Polyarteritis Nodosa and Other Forms of Arteritis. In: The Kidney: A Clinico-Pathologic Study, pp. 295–301. Oxford: Blackwell Scientific, 1975.
43. Moore HC, Sheehan HL: The kidney of scleroderma. Lancet 1: 68–70, 1952.
44. Cannon PJ, Hassar M, Case DB, Casarella WJ, Sommers SC, Le Roy EC: The relationship of hypertension and renal failure in scleroderma to structural and functional abnormalities of the renal cortical circulation. Medicine 53:1–46, 1974.
45. Fay R, Winer R, Cohen A, Brosman SA, Bennett C: Segmental renal hypoplasia and hypertension. J Urol 113(4):561–564, 1975.
46. Eichna LW, Farber SJ, Berger AR, Rader B, Smith WW, Albert RE: Non-cardiac circulatory congestion simulating congestive heart failure. Trans Assoc Am Physicians 67:72–85, 1954.
47. DeFazio V, Christensen RC, Regan TJ, Baer LJ, Morita Y, Hellems HK: Circulatory changes in acute glomerulonephritis. Circulation 201(2):190–200, 1959.

524

48. Agrest A, Finkielman S: Hemodynamics in acute renal failure, pathogenesis of hyperkinetic circulation. Am J Cardiol 19(2):213–220, 1967.
49. Birkenhager WH, Schalekamp MA, Schalekamp-Kuyken MP, Kolsters C, Drauss XH: Interrelations between arterial pressure, fluid-volumes and plasma-renin concentration in the course of acute glomerulonephritis. Lancet 1:1086–1087, 1970.
50. Brod J: Chronic renal parenchymal disease and hypertension. Kidney Int 8 (Suppl):S235–S242, 1975.
51. Brod J, Hejl Z, Ulrych M, Fend V, Jorka J: Hemodynamický podklad renální hypertense. Csl Fysiol 10:228, 1961.
52. Brod J: Hypertension and renal parenchymal disease: mechanisms and management. Cardiovasc. Clin 9(1):137–164, 1978.
53. Dustan HP, Iarazi RC, Bravo EL, Dout RA: Plasma and extracellualr fluid volumes in hypertension. Circ Res 32 (Suppl 1):73–83, 1973.
54. Brod J: Hypertension and Renal Parenchymal Diseaseb: mechanisms and Management. In: Hypertension: Mechanisms, Diagnosis and Treatment, pp. 137–164. Onest G, Brest AN, eds. Philadelphia: F.A. Davis, 1978.
55. Brownn JJ, Davies DL, Lever AF et al.: Plasma renin concentration in human hypertension – II. Renin in relation to aetology. Br Med J II(5472):1215–1262, 1965.
56. Warren DJ, Ferris TF: Renin secretion in renal hypertension. Lancet 1:159–162, 1970.
57. Severs WB: Cardiovascular effects of angiotensin II medicated by the central nervous system. In: Regulation of Blood Pressure by the Central Nervous System, the Fourth Hahemann International Symposium on Hypertension, p. 203. Onesti G, Fernandes M, Kim KE, eds. New York, 1975.
58. Cachovan M, Brod J, Bahlmann J et al.: The effect of intravenous angiotensin of the peripheral circulation with particular reference to its bearing onthe general hemodynamics, p. 96. 4th Meeting of International Society for Hypertension, Sidney, 1976.
59. Schalekamp MA, Beevers DG, Briggs JD et al.: Hypertension in Chronic renal Failure: an Abnormal relation between Sodium and the Renin–angiotensin System. In: Hypertension Manual, Laragh J, ed. New York: Yorke Medical/Dun-Donnelly, 1977.
60. Dathan JR, Goodwin FJ: The relationship between body fluid compartment volumes, renin and blood pressure in chronic renal failure. Clin Sci 43:2P, 1972.
61. Kim K, Onesti G, Schwartz AB, Clinitz JL, Swartz C: Hemodynamics of hypertension in chronic end-stage renal disease. Circulation 46:456–464, 1972.
62. Neff MS, Kim DE, Persoff M, Onesti G, Swartz C: Hemodymanics of uremic anemia. Circulation 43:876–883, 1971.
63. Vertes V, Cangiano JL, German LB, Gould A: Hypertension in end-stage renal disease. N Eng J Med 280:978–981, 1969.
64. Lazarus JM, Hampers CL, Bennett AH, Vandam LD: Urgent bilateral nephrectomy for severe hypertension. Ann Intern Med 66:733–739, 1972.
65. Rogers PW, Kurtzman NA: Renal failure, uncontrollable thirst and hyperreninemia: cessation of thirst with bilateral nephrectomy. JAMA 225:1236–1238, 1973.
66. Hull AR, Long DL, Prati RC, Pettinger WA, Parker TF: The control of hypertension in patients undergoing regular maintenance hemodialysis. Kidney Int (Suppl 2):184–187, 1975.
67. Onesti G, Kim KE, Fernandes M, Neff MS, Greco JA, del Guercia ET, Flynn JJ, Swartz C: Hypertension of Parenchymal Disease: Hemodynamic Patterns and Mechanisms. In: Proceedings of the Sixth International Congress of Nephrology, pp.284–303. Giovanettei S, Bonomini V, D'Amico G, eds. Florence/Basel, 1976.
68. Guyton AC, Hall JE, Balfe JW, Lohneier TE, Jackson TE, Norman RA: Pathophysiological Renal Mechanisms that Cause hypertension, Hypotension and Uremia. In: Proceedings, VII International Congress of Nephrology, Montreal, S. Karger, Basel, 1978.

69. Stamey TA: Functional Changes in the Nonoccluded Kidney after Nephrectomy for Unilateral Renal Artery Occlusive Disease. In: Renovascular Hypertension, pp. 110–134. Baltimore: Williams & Wilkins, 1963.
70. Earley LE, Martino JA, Fridler RM: Factors affecting sodium reabsorption by proximal tubule as determined during blockade of distal tubule sodium reabsorption. J Clin Invest 45:1668–1684, 1966.
71. Lewy JE, Windhager EE: Peritubular control of proximal tubular sodium reabsorption in the rat kidney. Am J Physiol 214:943–954, 1968.
72. Grollman A, Williams, JR, Harrison TR: The preparation of renal extracts capable of reducing blood pressure of animals with experimental hypertension. J Biol Chem 134:115, 1940.
73. Skeggs LT, Kahn JR, Levine M, Dorer FE, Lentz KE: Chronic one kidney hypertension in rabbits – III Renopressin, a new hypertensive substance. Cir Res 40:143, 1977.
74. Muirhead EE: Antihypertensive function of the kidney. Hypertension 2:444–464, 1980.
75. Muirhead EE, Rightsel WA, Leach BE, Byers LW, Pitcock JA, Brooks B: Reversal of hypertension by transplants and lipid extracts of cultured renomedullary interstitial cells. Lab Invest 36:162–172, 1977.
76. Mitas JA, Levy SB, Holle R, Frigon RP, Stone RA: Urinary kallidrein activity in the hypertension of renal parenchymal disease. N Eng J Med 299:162–165, 1978.
77. Warren SE, O'Connor DT: Does a renal vasodilator system mediate racial differences in essential hypertension? Am J Med 69:425–429, 1980.
78. Shapiro CB, Lerner NE, Ackad AS: Malignant hypertension and uremia in scleroderma; efficacy of nephrectomy and hemodialysis. Clin Nephrol 8:321–323, 1977.
79. Mitnick PD, Feig PU: Control of hypertension and reversal of renal failure in scleroderma. N Eng J Med 299:871–872, 1978.
80. Wasner C, Cooke CR, Fries JF: Successful medical treatment of scleroderma renal crisis. N Eng. J Med 299:873–875, 1978.
81. Kuhlmann H, Mehnert H: Zur des blutdrucks durch eine nephropathie bei diabetikern. Klin. Wochenschr 47:276, 1969.
82. Morgensen CE: Progression of nephropathy in long-term diabetics with proteinuria and effect of initial anti-hypertensive treatment. Scand. J Clin Lab Invest 36:384–388, 1976.
83. Woods JW, Blythe WB: Management of malignant hypertension complicated by renal insufficiency. N Eng J Med 277:57–61, 1967.
84. Mamdani BH, Lim VS, Mahurkar SD, Katz AI, Dunea G: Recovery from prolonged renal failure in patients with accelerated hypertension. N Eng J Med 291:1343–1344, 1974.
85. Mitchell HC, Graham RM, Pettinger WA: Renal function during long-term treatment of hypertension with minoxidil: comparison of benign and malignant hypertension. Ann Intern Med 93:676–681, 1980.

34. HYPERTENSION SECONDARY TO RENOVASCULAR DISEASE

Morton H. Maxwell

Arterial hypertension caused by occlusive lesions of the renal arterial vasculature is the most common cause of potentially curable hypertension. Nevertheless, neither reliable guidelines for the choice of appropriate diagnostic tests nor precise criteria for the selection of patients for corrective surgery have been established. In this chapter, I shall review the current status of diagnosis and therapy, emphasizing such recent developments as the use of angiotensin-inhibitors as diagnostic tools, and in ascertaining their potential use as therapeutic agents in long-term treatment, and preliminary comparison of percutaneous transluminal angioplasty versus traditional operative techniques in renal artery vascularization. Because of editorial restrictions as to chapter length, bibliographic citations will be selective.

DIAGNOSIS OF RENOVASCULAR HYPERTENSION

Since renal artery stenosis may be present in the absence of hypertension, a distinction must be made between *renovascular disease* and *renovascular hypertension*. Renovascular disease is defined as the presence of stenotic lesions of a main or segmental renal artery demonstrable by arteriography or at the time of surgery. Renovascular hypertension is defined as arterial hypertension which responds favorably, i.e., cured or benefited, to operative treatment of renovascular disease. Renovascular hypertension is thus a retrospective diagnosis; our task is to make it a prospective diagnosis.

The Cooperative Study of Renovascular Hypertension, with 14 participating institutions, had the advantage of a large (2442 patients) prospective study with rigid protocol requirements and central interpretation of all data, permitting valid statistical conclusions and the elimination of individual bias. Furthermore, there has been no substantial contradiction of the results of this study by subsequent publications. I shall, therefore, briefly review the results of the Cooperative Study [1].

Amery, A. (ed.) Hypertensive Cardiovascular Disease: Pathophysiology and Treatment
© *1982, Martinus Nijhoff Publishers. The Hague / Boston / London*
ISBN-13: 978-94-009-7478-4

Clinical characteristics [2]

The first question asked was: Do patients with renovascular hypertension have clinical characteristics which differentiate them from patients with essential hypertension? For this purpose, 339 patients with unequivocal essential hypertension (normal renal arteriograms) were compared with 175 patients with renovascular disease who were cured by corrective operation and were, therefore, considered to be unequivocal cases of renovascular hypertension.

A number of significant differences were related to age, sex, race and diastolic blood pressure, and were no longer significant when 131 patients in each group were individually paired to eliminate these variables. In the matched series, patients with renovascular hypertension were found to have a shorter duration of hypertension, more frequent onset of hypertension after the age of 50 years, less hypertension in the family, more severe retinopathy, more abdominal or flank bruits, higher blood urea nitrogen (BUN) and serum carbon dioxide content, lower serum potassium concentration and greater frequency of urinary casts and proteinuria than patients with essential hypertension. Although the presence of an abdominal or flank bruit was six to eight times as frequent in renovascular as in essential hypertension, its diagnostic value is limited by the greater frequency of essential hypertension in the hypertensive population.

Renovascular hypertension is not homogeneous, but rather must be divided according to the two major lesions responsible for renal artery stenosis. Patients with renal arterial *atherosclerosis* were older (mean age 50 years), had a higher systolic blood pressure and more frequent arterial disease in areas outside of the kidney, and were more likely to develop target organ damage than patients with essential hypertension. Patients with renal arterial *fibromuscular hyperplasia* were younger (mean age 35 years), predominately female, more likely to have no family history of hypertension and less prone to develop cardiomegaly.

The differences in clinical characteristics between patients with renovascular hypertension and those with essential hypertension were quantitative rather than qualitative. Truly distinctive features of renovascular hypertension, suggested by a number of investigators, were not found. Thus renovascular hypertension may occur in either sex at any age, and may range in severity from mild to very severe. It would appear, however, that renovascular hypertension is far less frequent in black than in white persons.

Intravenous urogram [3]

The rapid sequence intravenous urogram has been widely applied as a screening procedure for renovascular hypertension, since some of the mea-

Table 1. Comparison of rapid sequence urogram and radioisotope renogram in essential hypertension and unilateral renovascular disease

Diagnosis	n	Positive urogram (%)	Positive renogram (%)
Essential hypertension	1,051	11.4	24.6
Renovascular disease			
<50%*	170	22.3	43.5
50–80%	148	64.0	68.9
>80%	133	82.8	77.4
100%	50	95.7	94.0
Total (50–100%)	331	78.2	76.1

* Percent estimated stenosis.

sured parameters reflect the renal hemodynamic and functional changes which occur distal to renal artery stenosis. The urogram and the radioisotope renogram (see below) have the further advantage of widespread availability as safe and relatively inexpensive outpatient procedures.

Major urographic features considered were: disparity in renal length, calyceal appearance time and concentration on late films. The incidence of a positive urogram (at least one major feature abnormal) in renovascular disease as compared with essential hypertension can be seen in Table 1. The single most prevalent urographic abnormality in renovascular disease was delayed pyelocalyceal appearance time. With increasing severity of the stenosis as judged on the arteriograms, the frequency of all major urographic abnormalities, single or in combination, increased. In essential hypertension, 11% of patients had a falsely positive urogram; few patients had more than one abnormality.

The rapid sequence urogram was thus relatively effective in distinguishing patients with renovascular disease from those with essential hypertension. Within renovascular disease, however, there was no significant difference in the incidence of urographic abnormalities, either singly or in combination, between the groups with favorable and unfavorable responses to operation. Eighty-three percent of those responding favorably to surgery had positive urograms compared with eighty-one percent of those who failed to respond.

Elimination of the criterion of disparity of contrast medium concentration on the late films, a subjective feature, eliminated many false-positive urograms and made the urogram more discriminative.

Radioisotope renogram [4]

The speed, safety and simplicity of the ^{131}I-Hippuran renogram as a screening test are advantageous, but its interpretation and reliability are still challenged.

Analyses of the renograms by the usual simple visual technique as either 'normal' or 'abnormal', i.e., negative or positive, in the patient population is seen in Table 1. If greater than 50% stenosis as judged by arteriography can be considered to represent 'significant' renal artery stenosis, then the sensitivity of the renogram is comparable to that of the rapid sequence urogram, i.e., 76.1 versus 78.2 positive tests, respectively. There is, however, a significantly greater proportion of renograms judged to be abnormal in patients with lesser degrees of stenoses as well as in essential hypertension (false-positive tests). For this reasons, the usual visual renogram is less discriminatory than the urogram in stratifying patients with hypertension. A

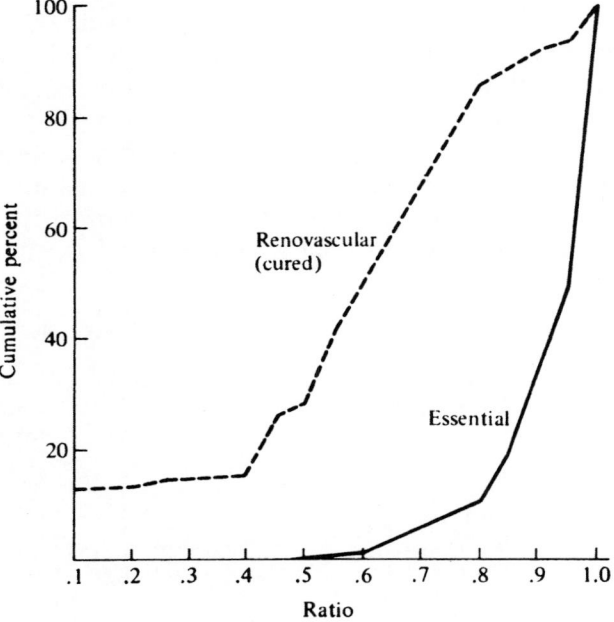

Figure 1. Cumulative percentage of radioisotope renogram ratios in patients with essential hypertension and patients with renovascular hypertension. The ratio (R value) represents an index of functional asymmetry between the two kidneys (see text). It can be seen that there is good discrimination between the two types of hypertension. A ratio of 0.8, for example, would include only 10% of the essential hypertension group and 90% of the renovascular hypertension group.

530

positive renogram is of no value in distinguishig between renovascular disease and renovascular hypertension. The renogram was positive in 76.4% of those with a favorable surgical response, and in 82.9% of surgical failures.

In an effort to improve the renogram, a computer technique is being used to compare the ratios of several parameters of the curves suggested in the literature. An index of functional asymmetry (R value) was obtained by comparing a ratio of two ratios of radioactivity: the ratio at the time of first kidney peak divided by the ratio at the time of one-half its maximum value (T $\frac{1}{2}$ Max). In comparing 152 curves from patients with essential hypertension with 164 curves from patients with renovascular hypertension, the R value proved to be remarkably discriminative (Figure 1). This technique is now being utilized for reanalysis of all study patients.

Decision as to further tests (arteriography, renal vein renins) [1]

Generally, the suspicion of renovascular disease is made on the basis of clinical characteristics, the intravenous urogram and the radioisotope renogram. This decision is compounded by the fact that even if a given test of abnormality is clearly more frequent in renovascular than in essential hypertension, it still may fail to discriminate significantly between these two populations because of the much greater prevalence of essential hypertension. For example, even if abdominal bruits were ten times more frequent in renovascular disease than in essential hypertension, if the prevalence of

Table 2. Percentile distribution of abnormal features in essential hypertension and in patients with over 50% renal artery stenosis*

Prevalence in total population	Abnormalities	Essential hypertension (N = 605)	Renovascular hypertension (N = 445)
57.5	None	98.4	1.6
6.3	B	91.8	8.2
20.1	R	94.6	5.4
3.0	B, R	65.2	34.8
4.1	I	91.2	8.8
1.2	B, I	60.1	39.9
4.8	R, I	43.0	57.0
3.0	B, R, I	5.0	95.0
100.0			

B: abdominal bruit; R: renogram; I: intravenous urogram.
* Table is adjusted for a prevalence ratio of essential hypertension 90% and renovascular hypertension 10%.

renovascular disease is 10% of the total hypertensive population, then a hypertensive patient discovered to have an abdominal bruit has an equal chance of having either disorder.

Utilizing the three most discriminating features in the patient work-up (abdominal bruit, intravenous urogram, radioisotope renogram), there are eight mutually exclusive combinations, ranging from all three normal to all three abnormal (Table 2). Weighting the table for a prevalence ratio of essential hypertension to renovascular disease of 90% to 10%, then any particular cluster of abnormalities results in an a posteriori specific chance of detecting renovascular disease by arteriography. For example, if all three features are normal, a situation which constitutes 57.5% of the total hypertensive population only 1.6% of all arteriograms done will demonstrate renal artery stenosis of over 50%. Conversely, if all three features are abnormal (3% of the total population), then 95% of the arteriograms will be abnormal.

Analyzing each of the three features individually, regardless of the other two, then the chance of renovascular disease is as follows: abdominal bruit, 36%; positive renogram, 25%; positive urogram, 49%.

Maximal discrimination will be achieved if arteriography is performed when two or more of the three features are abnormal, or when there is simply a positive 'quantitative' renogram (Figure 1). Utilizing this stopping rule, then arteriography will be performed on 9.7% of the total hypertensive population; 7.6 of the arteriograms (79.5%) will demonstrate significant renal artery stenosis, and 2.1 arteriograms per 100 patients will be performed in subjects who have essential hypertension [1].

Arteriography [5]

As expected, interpretation of the renal arteriogram was generally predictive of the etiology and locations of renal artery lesions, as confirmed at surgery and by tissue examination. In addition, the degree of renal artery stenosis as judged by arteriograms correlated well with functional asymmetry in the urogram, renogram and individual kidney function studies. Atherosclerotic lesions were more frequent in males, on the left side, and in the proximal portion of the renal artery, whereas fibromuscular hyperplasia showed a striking predilection for females and for the mid and distal portions of the right renal artery. Both types of lesions were bilateral in approximately 25% of the cases. The arteriogram had only limited value in predicting the response to surgery, and there was no relationship between surgical response and the presence of collateral circulation or poststenotic dilations.

532

Individual kidney function tests [1]

Individual kidney function studies were often of value in establishing an ischemic pattern, but they were of limited use in predicting operative cure or failure, i.e., in diagnosing renovascular hypertension. They are not without risk (acute renal failure, kidney infection) and should probably be used only in special situations, such as the need to determine the contribution to overall renal function of a stenotic kidney prior to possible nephrectomy.

In summary, the Cooperative Study of Renovascular Hypertension demonstrated that there is no combination of clinical characteristics which distinguish patients with renovascular hypertension from those with essential hypertension; although elderly patients with widespread atherosclerosis and a late onset or acceleration of hypertension are suspect for atherosclerotic renovascular disease, and young or middle-aged hypertensive women with an abdominal bruit should be investigated for fibromuscular dysplasia. The Cooperative Study was generally limited to adults, but others have emphasized the relatively high incidence and curability of renovascular disease in hypertensive children [6–8]. The rapid sequence urogram and the radioisotope renogram are usually abnormal in patients with significant renal artery stenosis but because the prevalence of renovascular hypertension is probably less than 5% of the total hypertensive population [1], the overall misclassification with these tests is in the neighborhood of 25%. The usual decision matrix for the diagnosis of renovascular hypertension is illustrated in Figure 2. This type of patient work-up has been criticized for not being cost-effective [9].

Contribution of the Renin–Angiotensin System to Renovascular Hypertension

Renin determinations were not included in the protocol of the Cooperative Study, and the use of angiotensin-inhibitors is relatively recent. Are the tests of the renin–angiotensin system more specific for the diagnosis of renovascular hypertension? As is the case in *chronic* experimental two-kidney one-clip renovascular hypertension [10], in human renovascular hypertension peripheral renin activity (PRA) levels often may be within so-called normal limits [11]. This apparent dilemma led to the theory that although renovascular hypertension is initiated by increased renin secretion, a different mechanism is involved in its chronic phase [12]. Rapid lowering of blood pressure following nephrectomy or a corrective vascular operation in unilateral renal artery stenosis, however, indicates that it is *renal-mediated,* even in its chronic form. In chronic 2-kidney Goldblatt hypertension in the dog, we demonstrated significantly increased renal renin secretion from the ste-

DECISION-TREE FOR DIAGNOSIS OF RENOVASCULAR
HYPERTENSION

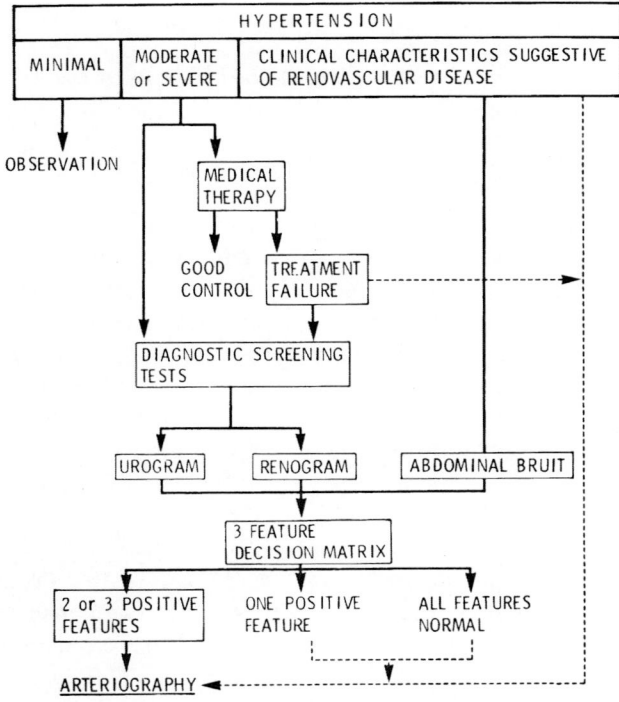

Figure 2. Usual decision-tree for diagnosis of renovascular hypertension.

notic kidney despite normal PRA and concluded that the high blood pressure is maintained because of increased vascular responsiveness to renin and angiotensin [13].

The failure of angiotensin antagonists to cause significant reductions in blood pressure after the first few weeks of experimental 2-kidney renal hypertension suggested that the renin–angiotensin system does not have a significant pressor role in the chronic phase [14]. However, in animals which are resistant in the sodium replete state, angiotensin antagonists may significantly lower blood pressure following sodium depletion [15], apparently unmasking a renin-dependence of the hypertension. Also, prolonged infusions of saralasin (8 substituted A-11 analogue) [16] or single doses of captopril (converting enzyme inhibitor) [17] lower blood pressure in the chronic phase, although there are conflicting results [18]. These results in animals combined with the successful use of angiotensin antagonists in diagnosis and treatment lead to the conclusion that chronic human renovascular hypertension is largely renin-mediated [19, 20]. Therefore, clinical tests of the renin–angiotensin system should be useful in diagnosing this disorder.

PRA, Renal Vein Renins and Angiotensin Antagonists in the Diagnosis of Renovascular Hypertension

Plasma renin activity (PRA)

There is general agreement that PRA is of little value in stratifying patients with renovascular hypertension from those with essential hypertension because of considerable overlap in values [21]. When a PRA is inappropriately high in a patient with hypertension, however, more extensive investigation for renovascular disease or parenchymal renal disease is indicated. Diuretic-induced salt depletion generally causes a greater rise in PRA in renovascular than in essential hypertension, and the further increase of PRA after saralasin administration clearly differentiates the two groups (see below) [22].

Renal Vein Renin Ratios (RVRR)

In patients with essential hypertension, a RVRR of 2.0 or higher falls beyond the 95% confidence limit and therefore may be considered abnormal [23]. Of 57 patients with proved renovascular hypertension (benefited by corrective surgery), 53% had RVRR of less than 2.0 [24]. Renal vein renin ratios thus represent a continuum in both populations, with no arbitrary value lower than 2.0 being statistically discriminative. All 34 patients with clearly lateralizing renin data by the usual criteria of ipsilateral hypersecretion and contralateral suppression (RVRR of 1.5 or higher and contralateral/caval ratio of 1.3 or lower) benefited by operation; and none of the 9 patients with renovascular disease who did not benefit from operation (presumed renovascular disease, but not renovascular hypertension) fulfilled these renin criteria. However, 23 additional patients without renin lateralization also benefited from operation. No previously proposed scheme or mathematical formulas for renin data analysis detected more than 75% of those with proved renovascular hypertension [24]. These results were confirmed by a critical review of the literature [25] and more recent publications [21].

Therefore, an abnormal RVRR is 95% predictive of curability, but a normal ratio may be found in the presence of correctible renovascular hypertension [27]. Since not all patients were studied during conditions of renin stimulation, it is possible that changes in test conditions (sodium depletion, diazoxide [28], captopril [29]) might increase the percentage with renin lateralization in patients with renovascular hypertension.

Angiotensin Antagonists [19]

The majority of studies of renovascular hypertension have used saralasin (Sar^1-Ala^8-angiotensin II). This angiotensin analogue competes with and displaces angiotensin II from its receptor sites, including the peripheral vasculature [30]. A vasodepressor response to the administration of saralasin presumably indicates renin-mediated hypertension, including renovascular hypertension. In 1973 Donker and Leenen reported a vasodepressor response to saralasin infusion in two subjects with renovascular hypertension [31]. In 1975 Streeten et al. reported on the use of saralasin infusion as a screening procedure for renin-mediated hypertension [32]. In the same year, our investigative group described the saralasin bolus test (rapid intravenous injection) [32].

We subsequently extended our observations and reported that the saralasin bolus test was positive (blood pressure lowering effect) in 95% of patients with renovascular hypertension and was more sensitive and specific than RVRR; a positive response in essential hypertension was limited to patients with high PRA levels. The test was most discriminative when performed under conditions of mild sodium depletion [34]. Similar results have been reported by others [20, 35–38]. In a large prospective study, Hollenberg et al. found a significant vasodepressor response to saralasin in 86.1% of patients with renovascular hypertension, with a false-positive rate in essential hypertension of 9.5% [20]. Others have had less favorable results [39], and in one large series the rapid sequence intravenous urogram was more discriminative than the saralasin test [21].

These combined data suggest that a vasodepressor response to an angiotensin inhibitor is a reliable way to diagnose renin-mediated, largely renovascular, hypertension, and further suggests that chronic renovascular hypertension is renin-mediated.

More recently, we showed that PRA increases disproportionately in renovascular hypertension after the combined stimuli of mild sodium depletion and a saralasin bolus [22]. The post-saralasin PRA is more sensitive than the fall in blood pressure and results in fewer misclassifications. This was subsequently confirmed by others [40], and a similar hyperresponse of PRA in patients with renovascular hypertension was shown to occur after an oral captopril test [41].

Figure 3, which may be contrasted with Figure 2, shows a potential decision matrix in screening patients for renovascular hypertension [19, 20]. Hypertensive patients would receive a diuretic for at least one week. If the blood pressure normalizes and there are no clinical indications of renovascular disease (abdominal bruit, inappropriate age of onset), no further tests are required. In clinically suspect patients and in those with an inadequate blood pressure response, the diuretic will have served to prepare the patient for the test. Test results would be judged by blood pressure and PRA

536

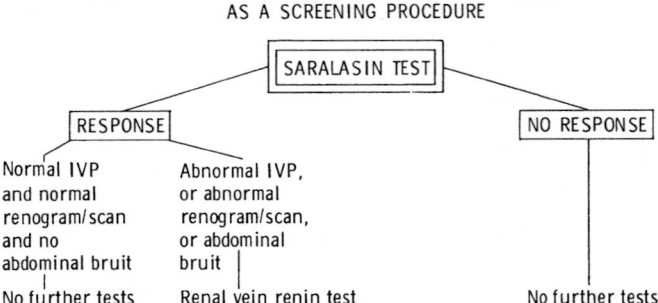

FLOW DIAGRAM FOR THE IDENTIFICATION OF PATIENTS WITH
RENOVASCULAR HYPERTENSION BASED ON THE SARALASIN TEST
AS A SCREENING PROCEDURE

Figure 3. Decision-tree for diagnosis of renovascular hypertension based on the saralasin test as an initial screening procedure. Patients whose hypertension responded to a one-week trial of a diuretic drug would be classified as probable essential hypertensive and would not have a saralasin test.

responses. Only those with a positive test response would undergo further testing. This sequence would be cost-effective and avoid unnecessary invasive procedures.

THERAPY OF RENOVASCULAR HYPERTENSION

Renovascular hypertension is considered a potentially 'curable' from of high blood pressure insofar as the elevated blood pressure often decreases to normal limits following nephrectomy or corrective revascularization. Therefore, operative treatment has been the preferred therapy, with drug treatment reserved for certain subgroups of patients. Very recently, data have appeared on the short term results of percutaneous transluminal angioplasty.

Results of Operative Treatment

In the Cooperative Study of Renovascular Hypertension, the blood pressure response to operative treatment in 502 patients was: cured in 51%, improved in 15%, and failed in 34% [42]. Patients with unilateral fibromuscular disease had a favorable response (79.8%) more frequently than the patients with unilateral atherosclerosis (63.4%) (Table 3). In bilateral steno-

537

sis a favorable operative result occured in 56%. The percentage of patients who were benefited by reconstructive surgery was approximately the same as those who were benefited by nephrectomy, i.e., 72.1 and 69.3% respectively.

Follow-up arteriography showed an unexpectedly high rate of thrombosis of the reconstructed artery in patients who failed to respond to surgery. In addition, 26 patients (23 surgical failures) who had no prior evidence of functional disparity between the kidneys by any of the diagnostic tests underwent surgery. After excluding 41 patients with known anatomically unsuccessful arterial resconstructions (thrombosis) or no prior evidence of functional disparity, the overall benefited rate in unilateral stenosis increased from 69.3 to 78.7% (numbers in parentheses in Table 3). Furthermore, when technical failures were excluded, then reconstructive surgery had a significant higher benefited rate than nephrectomy (86.5 versus 72.1%, respectively) [42]. Reconstructive surgery has the further advantage of preservation of renal mass. When thrombosis or restenosis of an initial arterial reconstruction occurred, the results of secondary nephrectomy were not significantly different from results of initial nephrectomy.

In defining 'cure' of hypertension, a postoperative blood pressure of less than 90 mm Hg was demanded. The apparent higher success rate in fibromuscular hyperplasia than in atherosclerosis was found to be age- and sex-related, i.e., the patients with atherosclerosis were 15 years older than those with fibromuscular hyperplasia and consisted largely of males. Adjusting the postoperative blood pressures by age and sex eliminated any difference in operative results between atherosclerosis and fibromuscular hyperplasia; the results of reconstructive surgery were confirmed to be significantly better than nephrectomy [1].

Subsequent data from large operative series have generally reported somewhat better results than those from the Cooperative Study [43–52],

Table 3. Favorable response to surgery related to type of procedure and type of renal artery lesion

Procedure	Renal artery lesion		Total
	AS (%)	FM (%)	
Nephrectomy	62.1 (65.6)	77.8 (78.7)	69.3 (72.1)
Reconstruction	64.4 (83.3)	82.4 (90.9)	72.1 (86.5)
Total	63.4 (74.4)	79.8 (83.8)	
Overall	69.3	(78.7)	

AS: Atherosclerosis; FM: Fibromuscular hyperplasia.
Numbers in parentheses included only best-defined surgical candidates.

538

with benefited rates generally around 90-95%. This difference may be largely attributable to improvements in operative techniques which have increased the frequency of technically successful revascularization. Cures (normal blood pressure) are highest in unilateral fibromuscular dysplasia and lowest in bilateral atherosclerosis [45, 47, 53], although overall benefited rate (cured and improved) may be equal in both disorders [53]. Adjustment of postoperative blood pressures by age and sex, as was done in the Cooperative Study [1] (see above), might eliminate any difference in operative results between fibromuscular dysplasia and atherosclerosis in these reports. Improvement of renal function in the affected kidney [43] and regression of target organ damage [48] occurred following revascularization. A 55% cure rate of hypertension was reported in patients with total renal artery occlusion prior to surgery [43].

Operative Mortality

In the Cooperative Study, the overall operative mortality was 5.9% [54]. The primary causes of death were largely uremia, extensive hemorrhage or myocardial infarction. The operative mortality was 9.3% in patients with atherosclerotic disease versus 3.4% with fibromuscular hyperplasia. Operative mortality was associated with the presence of coronary artery disease, renal function impairment and left ventricular hypertrophy. It was unacceptably high in patients undergoing complicated and prolonged bilateral procedures. In more recent reports the operative mortality has generally been lower than in the Cooperative Study, ranging from 0% [46, 49, 50, 53] to 5% [47].

CONCLUSIONS

From the data, the following conclusions would appear to be warranted: a) corrective surgery is seldom indicated without evidence of functional renal disparity by appropriate diagnostic tests; b) when technically feasible, renal arterial reconstruction should be the preferential procedure for the initial operation; c) follow-up arteriography should be performed when blood pressure remains elevated following reconstructive surgery, and secondary nephrectomy considered for technical failures; d) antihypertensive drug therapy may be the treatment of choice in elderly patients with long-standing hypertension and evidence of coronary artery disease.

Renovascular hypertension in children and in kidney transplantation

Renovascular disease is not uncommon as the cause of hypertension in children, with generally favorable results from surgery [6] especially utilizing the techniques of ex vivo and autotransplantation [7, 8]. Renal artery stenosis is usually suspected because of an abnormal intravenous urogram [6].

Following kidney transplantation, stenosis of the renal artery supplying the graft occurs in approximately 10–15% of patients [55, 56], usually heralded by severe hypertension occurring within a few months after transplantation [57]. These stenoses may be corrected surgically or by angioplasty (see below).

Results of percutaneous transluminal angioplasty (PTA)

The development of a double lumen balloon catheter by Gruntzig [58] has been followed by reports of the successful use of PTA in occlusive lesions of peripheral, coronary and renal arteries. The potential advantages of PTA as compared to operative treatment of renal artery stenosis are decreased morbidity and mortality and greater cost-effectiveness.

When dilatation of a stenosed renal artery is technically feasible by the PTA technique, there is always an acute reduction of systemic blood pressure [59–63], a marked decrease in renal vein renin from the stenotic kidney as well as a reduction in PRA [59, 64]. There are few long term follow-up studies, however, so that the precise indications for PTA cannot yet be delineated.

Successful initial dilatation appears to be possible over 90% of the cases [60, 63, 65], the main reason for technical failure being stenosis so severe that the guide wire or the balloon catheter cannot be inserted. There have been no patient deaths reported, and the immediate morbidity appears to be about 5% [66]. The most common complications associated with PTA appear to be acute renal failure, severe groin hematomas and renal artery dissection [63, 67]. PTA may be attempted in patients who are poor operative risks. In this regard, PTA has resulted in decreased blood pressure and some improvement in renal function (6-month follow-up) in azotemic patients with bilateral artery stenosis or a single functioning kidney [66].

As noted above, the mortality associated with the usual operative revascularization is much higher in elderly patients with atherosclerotic renal artery stenosis and evidence of coronary and/or peripheral atherosclerosis than in the younger females with fibromuscular dysplasia. Therefore, it was initially hoped that the safer procedure of PTA could replace surgery in the former group of patients. Unfortunately, several investigators have noted frequent and early restenoses of atherosclerotic renal artery stenosis follow-

540

ing PTA [60, 62, 67, 68]. Successful redilatation by PTA, however, has been repeated in some patients up to four times [67, 68].

PTA has been used successfully (6-month follow-up) in patients with postrenal transplantation renal artery stenosis [69].

In summary, the short- and intermediate-term results (up to 1 year) of PTA in patients with fibromuscular lesions of the renal artery appear to be equivalent to those following conventional vascular reconstructive surgery. In patients with atherosclerotic renal artery stenosis, PTA is safer than operation and may be attempted in patients who are prohibitive operative risks. Restenosis of atherosclerotic lesions may occur within one year in approximately 50 % of patients, although repetitive PTAs are possible. A more precise assessment of the role of PTA in the treatment of renal artery stenosis must await long-term follow-up studies.

Treatment of renovascular hypertension with antihypertensive drugs

There have been no published prospective, randomized trials of medical versus operative therapy of renovascular hypertension. Furthermore, available reports vary widely with regard to selection of patients, definition of renovascular hypertension, types of medications used and length of follow-up.

Two of the earliest reports indicated that standard antihypertensive drugs were effective in lowering the blood pressure of *some* patients with renovascular hypertension [70, 71], presenting an alternative mode of therapy for patients who were poor operative risks or who had inoperable renal arterial lesions. The largest comparative study showed much better long-term results in operated patients [72]. During a 7-year follow-up period almost 40 % of the medically treated patients died, mainly of vascular complications, compared to only 16 % of the surgically treated patients. Of the surviving patients, blood pressure was significantly lower in the operative group. Other reasons for favoring operative treatment, at least in patients at lower surgical risk (young individuals with normal renal function and lack of diffuse vascular disease), are the possibility of cure of the hypertension and prevention of renal damage due to progressive occlusion of the renal artery [73].

The better results of medical therapy in more recent reports have been attributed to the use of newer antihypertensive drugs, particularly beta-blockers and captopril [74]. In a non-randomized study of 28 patients, after 24 months of follow-up there was no significant difference in blood pressure between the surgically and medically treated groups; the types of medications used were not specified [75]. In a retrospective study of 114 cases of renovascular hypertension followed from 18 months to 9 years, good blood pressure control was obtained in 45% of operative patients versus 63% of medically treated patients, most of whom received beta-blockers [76]. Guedon et al. [77], on the other hand, found that the effects of beta-blocker therapy were variable.

The results of therapy with the oral converting enzyme inhibitor, captopril, usually in combination with a diuretic, have been outstanding. Captopril alone controlled the hypertension in 7 patients with renovascular hypertension treated for 6 weeks [78], and in 7 patients treated for 4 weeks [79]. Captopril alone, or more often in combination with a diuretic agent, significantly decreased blood pressure in 8 patients followed from 1 to 7 months [80]; in 4 patients followed from 3 days to 12 months [81], and in 12 patients with severe hypertension followed for a mean period of 4.9 months [82].

Although the mean plasma renin activity was generally higher in patients with renovascular than with essential hypertension, in none of these studies did the intermediate- or long-term blood pressure lowering effect of capto-

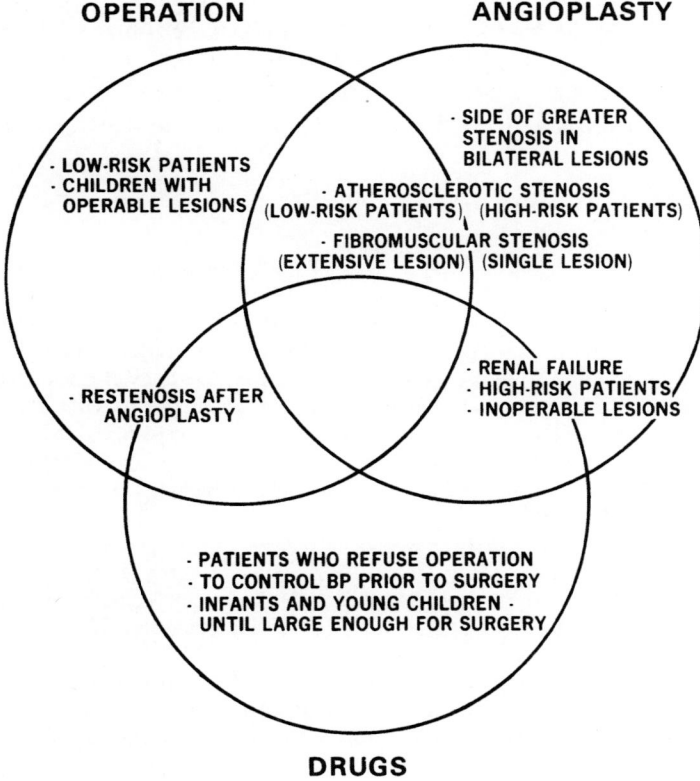

Figure 4. Proposed decision matrix for choice of therapy.

542

pril correlate with pretreated angiotensin II or plasma renin activity. In one report [80] the *acute* reduction in blood pressure following captopril was related to control PRA. There is no evidence that tolerance to the effects of captopril develop during prolonged therapy. These effects include decreased systolic and diastolic blood pressures; unaltered cardiac output and extra-cellular fluid, and reduced total peripheral resistance [79]; reduced plasma angiotensin II and aldosterone with converse increases in plasma renin and blood angiotensin I [78]; unaltered plasma norepinephrine and epineph-rine [79, 83]. Untoward side effects of captopril occur in about 15% of treated patients, and consist of a skin rashes, an impairment of taste, pro-teinuria, and leucopenia or agranulocytosis [83].

The development of percutaneous transluminal angioplasty and oral con-verting enzyme inhibitors has presented variable alternatives to operative therapy in renovascular hypertension. Their precise roles must await reports of long-term results on a larger number of patients (Figure 4). At the present time corrective surgery may be the treatment of choice in low risk patients with operable fibromuscular dysplasia and in children with renovascular hypertension. PAT may be tried in patients at high surgical risk and in renal artery lesions judged to be inoperable as judged by renal arteriography. Medical therapy with captopril may also be tried in high surgical risk patients or inoperable lesions; in infants and very young children whose arteries are still too small for operative repair; and in restenoses following operation or PAT.

REFERENCES

1. Maxwell MH, Varady PD: Cooperative Study of renovascular hypertension. In: Contribu-tions to Nephrology. Berlyne GM, Giovannetti S, eds. Basel: Karger S, 1976.
2. Simon N, Franklin SA, Bleifer KH, Maxwell MH: Cooperative study of renovascular hyper-tension. Clinical characteristics of renovascular hypertension. JAMA 220:1209, 1972.
3. Bookstein JJ, Abrams HL, Buenger RE, Lecky J, Franklin SS, Reiss MD, Bleifer KH, Klatte EC, Varady PD, Maxwell MH: Cooperative study of renovascular hypertension. Radiologic aspects of renovescular hypertension. 2. The role of urography in unilateral renovascular disease, JAMA 220:1225, 1972.
4. Maxwell MH: Cooperative study of renovascular hypertension: current status. Kid Intern (Suppl) 8:s153, 1975.
5. Bookstein JJ, Abrams HL, Buenger RE, Reiss MD, Lecky JW, Franklin, SS, Bleifer KH, Varady PD, Maxwell MH: Cooperative study of renovascular hypertension. 3. Appraisal of arteriography. JAMA 221:368, 1972.
6. Broyer J, Lenoir G, Guesry P, Levy-Bentolia D, Gubler MC: Arterial hypertension caused by anomaly of the renal artery or its branches in children. Arch Mal Coeur 72:35, 1979.
7. Kyriakides GK, Najarian JS: Renovascular hypertension in childhood: successful treatment by renal autotransplantation. Surgery 85:611, 1979.
8. Menezes de Go'es G, Arap S, D'Enes FT: Renovascular hypertension in children. Urol Int 35:206, 1980.

9. McNeil BJ, Varady PD, Burrows BA, Adelstein SJ: Measures of clinical efficacy, N Eng J Med 293:216, 1975.
10. Page IH, McCubbin JA, eds.: In: Renal Hypertension. Chicago: Year Book Medical, 1968.
11. Kaplan NM: Clinical Hypertension, 2nd edn. Baltimore: Williams & Wilkins, 1978.
12. Koletsky S, Rivera-Velez JM, Marsh DJ, Pritchard WH: Relation of renal arterial pressure to activity of the renin–angiotensin system in renal hypertension. Proc Soc Exp Biol Med 118:96, 1965.
13. Lupu AN, Maxwell MH, Kaufman JJ: Mechanisms of hypertension during the chronic phase of one-clip, two-kidney model in the dog. Circ Res (Suppl 1) 40:1–57, 1977.
14. Thurston H, Swales JD: Comparison of angiotensin II antagonist and antiserum infusion with nephrectomy in the two-kidney Goldblatt hypertensive rat. Circ Res 35:325, 1974.
15. Gavras H, Brunner HR, Thurston H, Laragh JH: Reciprocation of renin dependency with sodium volume dependency in renal hypertension. Science 188:1316, 1975.
16. Riegger AJG, Millar JA, Lever AF, Morton JJ, Slack B: Correction of renal hypertension in the rat by prolonged infusion of angiotensin inhibitors. Lancet 2:1317, 1977.
17. Thurston H, Bing RF, Marks ES, Swales JD: Response of chronic renovascular hypertension to surgical correction or prolonged blockade of the renin–angiotensin system by two inhibitors in the rat. Clin Sci 58:15, 1980.
18. Fernandez M, Fiorentini R, Onesti G, Bellini G, Gould AB, Hessan H, Kim KE, Swartz C: Effect of administration of Sar^1-Ala^8-angiotensin II during the development and maintenance of renal hypertension in the rat. Clin Sci 54:633, 1978.
19. Maxwell MH: Use of Angiotensin Antagonists in Experimental and Human Renovascular Hypertension. In: Advances in Nephrology, Year Book Medical Publishers, Inc., Chicago, London, 8:297, 1979.
20. Hollenberg NK, Williams GH, Adams DF, Moore T, Brown C, Borucki LJ, Leung F, Bavli S, Solomon HS, Passan D, Dluhy R: Response to saralasin and angiotensin's role in essential and renal hypertension. Medicine 58:115, 1979.
21. Grim CE, Luft FC, Weinberger MH, Grim CM: Sensitivity and specificity of screening tests for renal vascular hypertension. Ann Intern Med 91:617, 1979.
22. Maxwell MH, Varady P, Zawada ET, Burkhalter JF, Waks U, Marks L: Maximal discrimination of renovascular from essential hypertension by the saralasin test. Clin Sci 55:297s, 1978.
23. Maxwell MH, Marks LS, Varady PD, Lupu AN, Kaufman JJ: Renal vein renin in essential hypertension. J Lab Clin Med 86:901, 1975.
24. Maxwell MH, Marks LS, Lupu AN, Cahill PJ, Franklin SS, Kaufman JJ: Predictive value of renin determinations in renal artery stenosis. JAMA 238:2617, 1977.
25. Marks LS, Maxwell MH: Renal vein renin. Value and limitations in the prediction of operative results. Urol Clin North Am 2:311, 1975.
26. Poutasse EF, Gonzales-Serva L, Wendelken JR, Franz JP: Saralasin test as a diagnostic and prognostic aid in renovascular hypertensive patients subjected to renal operation. J Urol 123:306, 1980.
27. Marks LS, Maxwell MH, Varady PD, Lupu AN, Kaufman JJ: Renovascular hypertension: Does the renal vein renin ratio predict operative results? J Urol 115:365, 1976.
28. Armanini D, Fallo F, Opocher G, Scaroni C, Boscaro M, Mantero F: Diazoxide-induced acute stimulation of plasma renin activity in renal veins for diagnosis and prognosis in hypertensive patients. G Ital Cardiol 9:1351, 1979.
29. Re R, Novelline R, Escourrou MT, Athanasoulis C, Burton J, Haber E: Inhibition of angiotensin-converting enzyme for diagnosis of renal-artery stenosis. N Eng J Med 298:582, 1978.
30. Pals DT, Masucci FD, Sipos F, Denning GS, Jr: A specific competitive antagonist of the vascular action of angiotensin II. Cir Res 29:664, 1971.

31. Donker AJM, Leenen FHH: Infusion of angiotensin II analogue with unilateral renovascular hypertension. Lancet 2:1535, 1974.
32. Streeten DHP, Anderson GH, Freiberg JM, Dalakos TG: Use of an angiotensin II antagonist (Saralasin) in the recognition of 'angiotensinogenic' Hypertension. N Eng J Med 292:657, 1975.
33. Marks LS, Maxwell MH, Kaufman JJ: Saralasin bolus test. Rapid procedure for renin mediated hypertension. Lancet 2:784, 1975.
34. Marks LS, Maxwell MH, Kaufman JJ: Renin, sodium, and vascular response to saralasin in renovascular and essential hypertension. Ann Intern Med 87:176, 1977.
35. Wilson HM, Wilson JP, Slaton PE, Foster JH, Liddle GW, Hollifield JW: Saralasin infusion in the recognition of renovascular hypertension. Ann Intern Med 87:36, 1977.
36. Baer L, Parra-Carrillo JZ, Radichevich J, Williams GA: Detection of renovascular hypertension with angiotensin II blockade. Ann Intern Med 86:257, 1977.
37. Bönner G, Helber A, Meure KA, Hummerich W, Wambach G, Kaufman W: The saralasin test in the diagnosis of hypertension. Dtsch Med Wochenschr 104:432, 1979.
38. Buda JA, Baer L, Arora SP, Parra-Carrillo JZ, Radichevich I: Evaluation of surgical response in renovascular hypertension using angiotensin II blockade. Surgery 84:664, 1978.
39. Krakoff LR, Ribeiro AB, Gorkin JU, Felton KR: Saralasin infusion in screening patients for renovascular hypertension. Am J Cardiol 45:609, 1980.
40. Case DB, Atlas SA, Laragh JH: Reactive hyper-reninaemia to angiotensin blockade identifies renovascular hypertension. Clin Sci 57:313s, 1979.
41. Imai Y, Abe K, Otsuka Y, Sakurai Y, Yoshinaga K: A screening test for renovascular hypertension by means of orally active angiotensin I converting enzyme inhibitor, captopril (SQ 14225). Tohoku J Exp Med 131:311, 1980.
42. Foster JH, Maxwell MH, Franklin SA, Bleifer KH, Trippel OH, Julian OC, DeCamp PT, Varady PT: Renovascular occlusive disease, results of operative treatment. JAMA 231:1043, 1975.
43. Polterauer P, Dean RH, Hollifield JW: Surgical treatment of renovascular hypertension: results of operation in 400 patients with renal artery stenosis. Wien Klin Wochenschr 92:433, 1980.
44. Pinkerton JA Jr, Crouch TT, Sharma JN: Surgical treatment of renovascular hypertension. Am J Surg 138:759, 1979.
45. Vetter W, Vetter H, Tenschert W, Kuhlmann U, Studer A, Glänzer K, Pouliadis G, Largiader F, Furrer J, Siegenthaler W: Renovascular hypertension. Prognostic value of renal venous renin determinations. Klin Wochenschr 57:863, 1979.
46. Starr DS, Lawrie GM, Morris GC Jr: Surgical treatment of renovascular hypertension. Long-term follow-up of 216 patients up to 20 years. Arch Surg 115:494, 1980.
47. Lankford NS, Donohue JP, Grim CE, Weinberger MH: Results of surgical treatment of renovascular hypertension. J Urol 122:439, 1979.
48. McNair A, Neilsen MD, Gammelgaard PA, Giese J, Ibsen H, Kappelgaard AM, Lund JO, Mathiesen F, Munck O, Tonnesen KH: A follow-up study of hypertensive patients after operative treatment of unilateral renovascular or renal disease. Acta Med Scand 205:569, 1979.
49. Stoney RJ, Silane M, Salvatierra O, Jr: Ex vivo renal artery reconstruction. Arch Surg 113:1272, 1978.
50. Nordhus O, Ekeström S, Liljeqvist L, Tidgren B: Renal artery reconstruction in renovascular hypertension. Scand J Thorac Cardiovasc Surg 12:111, 1978.
51. Stefanini P, Benedetti-Valentini F Jr, Fiorani P: Selection for surgery and long-term results in renovascular hypertension. Int Surg 63:73, 1978.
52. Bergentz SE, Ericsson BF, Husberg B: Technique and complications in the surgical treatment of renovascular hypertension. Acta Chir Scand 145:143, 1979.

545

53. Dean RH, Lawson JD, Hollifield JW, Shack RB, Polterauer P, Rhamy RK: Revascularization of the poorly functioning kidney. Surgery 85:44, 1979.
54. Franklin SS, Young JD Jr, Maxwell MH, Foster JH, Palmer JM, Cerny J, Varady PD: Cooperative study of renovascular hypertension. Operative mordidity and mortality in renovascular disease. JAMA 231:1148, 1975.
55. Lacombe M: Artery stenosis in renal transplantation. Acta Chir Belg 79:1, 1980.
56. Woo KT, Yeung CK, D'Apice AJ, Kincaid-Smith P: Transplant renal artery stenosis. Aust NZ J Surg 49:613, 1979.
57. Klarskov P, Brendstrup L, Krarup T, Jorgensen HE, Egeblad M, Palbol, J: Renovascular hypertension after kidney transplantation. Scand J Urol Nephrol 13:291, 1979.
58. Gruntzig A, Kumpe DA: Technique of percutaneous transluminal angioplasty with the Gruntzig balloon catheter. AJR 132:547, 1979.
59. Millan VG, Mast WE, Madias NE: Non-surgical treatment of severe hypertension due to renal-artery intimal fibroplasia by percutantaneous transluminal angioplasty. N Eng J Med 300:1371, 1979.
60. Tegtmeyer CJ, Dyer R, Teates CD, Ayers CR, Carey RM, Wellons HA Jr, Stanton LW: Percutaneous transluminal dilatation of the renal arteries: techniques and results. Radiology 135:589, 1980.
61. Lux E, Seybold D, Gross-Vorholt R, Zeitler E, Gessler U: Percutaneous transluminal catheter dilatation of kidney artery stenoses in patients with renovascular hypertension. Fortschr Med 17:563, 1980.
62. Kulmann U, Vetter W, Furrer J, Lütolf U, Siegenthaler W, Grüntzig A: Renovascular hypertension: treatment by percutaneous transluminal dilatation. Ann Intern Med 92:1, 1980.
63. Schwarten DE, Yune HY, Klatte EC, Grim CE, Weinberger MH: Clinical experience with percutaneous transluminal angioplasty (PTA) of stenotic renal arteries. Radiology 135:601, 1980.
64. Laragh JH, Sealey JE, Vaughan ED Jr, Pickering TG, Case DB, Sos TA, Sniderman KW: Renal venous renin secretory patterns before and after percutaneous transluminal angioplasty, p. 31. Proc 8th Int Congr Nephrol Athens, 1981.
65. Geyskes GG, Puylaert CB, Oei HY, Boomsma JH: Intraluminal dilatation of renal artery stenosis. Clin Sci (Suppl 5) 57:441s, 1979.
66. Schwarten DE: Transluminal angioplasty of renal artery stenosis: 70 Experiences. AJR 135:969, 1980.
67. Grim CE, Luft FC, Yune HY, Klatte EC, Weinberger MH: Balloon dilatation of renal artery stenosis causing hypertension: Contrasting cure rate by lesion type, p. 1154. Proc 8th Int Congr Nephrol Athens, 1981.
68. Barbaric Z, Kaufman JJ, Maxwell MH: Unpublished data.
69. Sniderman KW, Sos TA, Sprayregen S, Saddekni S, Cheigh JS, Tapia L, Tellis V, Veith FJ: Percutaneous transluminal angioplasty in renal transplant arterial stenosis for relief of hypertension. Radiology 135:23, 1980.
70. Dustan HP, Page IH, Poutasse EF, Wilson L: An evaluation of treatment of hypertension associated with occlusive renal arterial disease. Circulation 27:1018, 1963.
71. Pinedo HM, Degraeff J, Struyvenberg A: Prognosis in arteriosclerotic renovascular hypertension. Clin Sci (Suppl 2) 45:309s, 1973.
72. Hunt JC, Strong CG: Renovascular hypertension: mechanisms, natural history and treatment. Am J Cardiol 32:562, 1973.
73. Meaney TF, Dustan HP, McCormack LJ: Natural history of renal arterial disease. Radiology 91:881, 1968.
74. Brunner HR, Gavras H: Medical Therapy of Renovascular Hypertension. Proc 8th Int Congr Nephrol Athens, 1981.

75. Whelton PK, Harris AP, Russell RP, Walsh PC, Williams GM, Harrington DP, Walker WG: Renovascular hypertension: comparison of medical and surgical therapy. Clin Sci 57:445s, 1979.
76. Zech P, Pozet N: Hypertension renovasculaire: Variations du pronostic selon le traitement
77. médical ou chirurgical. Nouv Presse Med 8:495, 1979.
77. Guedon J, Lucsko M, Cuche JL, Chaignon M: Renovascular hypertension and beta blockers. Theoretical and practical implications. Arch Mal Coeur 72:9, 1979.
78. Atkinson AB, Brown JJ, Fraser R, Leckie B, Lever AF, Morton JJ, Robertson JIS: Captopril in hypertension with renal artery stenosis and in intractable hypertension; acute and chronic changes in circulating concentrations of renin, angiotensins I and II and aldosterone, and in body composition. Clin Sci 57:139s, 1979.
79. de Bruyn JHB, Man in 't Veld AJ, Wenting GJ, Boomsma F, Derkx FHM, Schalekamp MADH: Cardiovascular effects of captopril monotherapy in low-renin versus high-renin hypertension. In: Recent Advances in Hypertension Therapy: Captopril. Brunner HR, Gross F, eds. p. 41. Amsterdam: Excerpta Medica, 1981.
80. Brunner HR, Gavras H, Waeber B, Kershaw GR, Turini GA, Vukovich RA, McKinstry DN, Gavras I: Oral angiotensin-converting enzyme inhibitor in long-term treatment of hypertensive patients. Ann Intern Med 90:19, 1979.
81. Sullivan JM, Ginsburg BA, Ratts TE, Johnson JG, Barton BR, Kraus DH, McKinstry DN, Muirhead EE: Hemodynamic and antihypertensive effects of captopril, an orally active angiotensin converting enzyme inhibitor. Hypertension 1:397, 1979.
82. Studer A, Luscher T, Greminger P, Siegenthaler W, Vetter W: Captopril in therapy-resistant essential and renovascular hypertension. In: Recent Advances in Hypertension Therapy: Captopril, p. 31. Brunner HR, Gross F, eds. Amsterdam: Excerpta Medica, 1981.
83. Biollaz J, Brunner DB, Gavras H, Brunner HR: An overview of clinical experience with captopril. In: Recent Advances in Hypertension Therapy: Captopril, p. 15. Brunner HR, Gross F, eds. Amsterdam: Excerpta Medica, 1981.

35. HYPERTENSION SECONDARY TO ADRENAL CORTICAL DISEASE

WŁODZIMIERZ JANUSZEWICZ and JOLANTA CHODAKOWSKA

PRIMARY ALDOSTERONISM

The term primary aldosteronism refers to those patients with arterial hypertension in whom elevation of blood pressure results from selective oversecretion of aldosterone, this single hormonal abnormality underlying the clinical syndrome, defined first by Conn in 1955 [1].

In about 85% of cases hypersecretion of aldosterone is caused by adrenal cortical adenoma, while in the remaining cases it is associated with diffuse cortical hyperplasia.

The adenomas (aldosteronomas) found in clinically recognised cases are usually small, solitary tumours, measuring less than 3 cm in diameter. When multiple, which occurs in about 10% of cases, in most instances they are confined to one adrenal.

Selective oversecretion of aldosterone by an adrenal cancer seems extremely rare, but cases of cortical carcinoma with predominant features of aldosteronism have been described [2].

Diffuse hyperplasia of the micronodular or macronodular type affects both adrenals, although one of the glands may sometimes be more hypertrophied than the other.

Most statistics estimate the incidence of primary aldosteronism at 1–2% of all hypertensive patients, a smaller proportion than the 20% suggested by Conn, but, in view of the prevalence of hypertension in modern communities, a large number of potentially curable cases.

Pathophysiology

Fairly convincing evidence, coming from clinical studies and corroborated by experimental data, suggests that sodium conservation is the first consequence of aldosterone excess. The ensuing increase of intravascular volume and, possibly, the deposition of sodium in the arterioral wall, seem responsible for the development of arterial hypertension, which sets in early in the course of the disease. Sodium retention is not a continuous process. At a certain stage a new sodium balance becomes re-established by a mechanism

Amery, A. (ed.) Hypertensive Cardiovascular Disease: Pathophysiology and Treatment
© *1982, Martinus Nijhoff Publishers. The Hague / Boston / London*
ISBN-13: 978-94-009-7478-4

548

known as 'escape phenomenon'. This mechanism, probably involving dopamine, causes diminution of sodium reabsorption at the proximal tubule [3]. However, the effects of increased amounts of aldosterone continue at the target sites, with the resulting loss of potassium mainly via the distal tubule of the kidney and the alimentary tract. Continuous potassium loss depletes body stores with all the ensuing consequences. The initial increase of intravascular volume and, possibly, altered tubular sodium load at the macula densa, associated with the 'escape phenomenon', cause inhibition of renin release from the juxtaglomerular cells [4].

Thus the most characteristic early humoral abnormality present in patients with primary aldosteronism consists of excessive aldosterone secretion with suppressed secretion of renin, a feature distinctly separating them from hypertensive patients with secondary, renin-dependent aldosteronism, such as that associated with malignant hypertension, renal artery stenosis, reninoma or certain diseases of the kidney.

Aldosterone secretion in primary aldosteronism is autonomous in regard to the regulatory effect of the suppressed renin–angiotensin system. However, it is not clear to what extent it is independent of other regulatory mechanisms. Some facts suggest that ACTH and potassium may stimulate secretion of aldosterone in patients with adenoma but not in those with hyperplasia [5, 6]. On the other hand, the latter cases have been shown to respond with increased aldosterone excretion to subtle increments of the still subnormal plasma renin activity [6].

Clinical picture

Although affecting patients of all ages, the disease is most often recognised in the third or fourth decade of life, about twice as often in women as in men.

The clinical picture of primary aldosteronism is related directly to the abnormal secretion of aldosterone and potassium depletion, while its severity and the array of symptoms may vary depending probably on the natural history of the disease, with clinically asymptomatic cases at the earliest stage, and the full-blown syndromes, like that of the classical Conn's description, following marked prolonged aldosterone excess [4, 7].

Arterial hypertension is the constant feature. It is usually mild or moderate, but severe elevation of blood pressure and advanced vascular complications are also encountered, malignant hypertension being no exception [8].

Headaches are a common and early symptom and are probably related to hypervolaemia [4, 8]. Most of the other typical signs and symptoms of primary aldosteronism are the result of potassium deficiency and hypokalaemia. Of these, the most frequent include muscular weakness, polyuria, particularly marked at night, and polydipsia. The patient's history may also include paraesthesia, periodic paralysis, and tetany [4].

Physical examination will reveal signs related to hypertensive complications, such as left ventricular hypertrophy and fundoscopic changes, which are usually moderate. Although suggestive findings such as positive Chvostek's and Trousseau's signs and diminished tendon reflexes may be present in advanced cases, pysical examination is often non-contributory to the diagnosis.

Laboratory findings

Hypokalaemia is the most important abnormality found by routine laboratory examinations included in the diagnostic work-up of patients suspected on clinical grounds as well as in the usual screening procedure for hypertensive patients. The low plasma level of potassium is associated with abnormally high urinary excretion of this ion, exceeding 30 mmol/24 h with normal intake.

Obviously, recent administration of diuretics must be excluded. It should be kept in mind that in some patients, especially those harbouring small adenomas, and at an early stage of the disease, the plasma potassium level may be normal. In some of them, repeated examinations of the blood will reveal intermittent hypokalaemia [4, 7].

Alkalosis is usually present, especially in hypokalaemic patients, and is reflected by elevated plasma bicarbonate. While hypernatraemia is consistent with aldosterone excess, plasma sodium concentration is often normal.

The concentrating and acidifying ability of the kidney is diminished; therefore, the urine is usually alkaline or neutral and its specific gravity is low and unresponsive to fluid restriction or administration of Pitressin.

Abnormal glucose tolerance of the diabetic type may be demonstrated in some patients. The electrocardiogram may show features of hypokalaemia.

The urinary excretion of 17-hydroxysteroids and 17-ketosteroids is normal.

Diagnosis

The final diagnosis of primary aldosteronism requires demonstration of excessive secretion of aldosterone with supressed renin secretion, unresponsive to physiological stimuli.

Since the increased secretion of aldosterone is paralleled by augmented urinary excretion of the hormone, examination of the 24-h urine aliquot obtained in basal conditions is usually sufficient for the diagnosis of aldosteronism, but repeated examinations of the urine are sometimes necessary.

Plasma renin activity is measured in basal conditions of normal sodium intake in the recumbent body position and then again following stimulation, which may be achieved by upright posture, ambulation, sodium depletion, or combinations of these stimuli.

When in a patient without other signs of adrenal cortical hyperfunction urinary excretion of aldosterone is increased and plasma renin activity subnormal and unresponsive to stimulation, the diagnosis of primary aldosteronism is established.

Adenoma versus hyperplasia

Once the diagnosis has been made, it is crucial to define the nature and location of the adrenal lesion which will determine the therapeutic approach.

Differential etiological diagnosis on the basis of the standard biochemical and hormonal studies is insufficient, although it has been pointed out that patients with hyperplasia tend to demonstrate less profound abnormalities than those with adenoma. In some centres multifunctional analysis of the humoral profile has been fairly successful in preoperative prediction of the nature of the adrenal pathology [9]. However, one would not expect this procedure to be sensitive enough in early cases of adenoma, especially those of the normokalaemic type. On the other hand, dynamic hormonal studies seem more discriminative. The diagnosis of bilateral hyperplasia may be suggested or supported upon finding an increase of plasma aldosterone level following 4-h upright posture. This response does not occur in patients with adenoma in whom plasma aldosterone under these conditions usually remains unchanged or indeed falls [5, 10].

Older radiological methods, such as intravenous pyelography, nephrotomography, retroperitoneal tomography, and arteriography are of little help in delineating the small adenomas with their poor vasculature.

Of the newer invasive methods, adrenal phlebography and bilateral adrenal vein catheterisation with determination of aldosterone levels in the adrenal venous effluents has proved to be of great diagnostic value. In expert hands, adrenal phlebography yields 70–85% of correctly diagnosed cases of adrenal cortical adenoma, the accuracy of the method being limited by the size of the tumour. In general, adenomas smaller than 7 mm in diameter are below the resolving power of phlebography [11, 12].

551

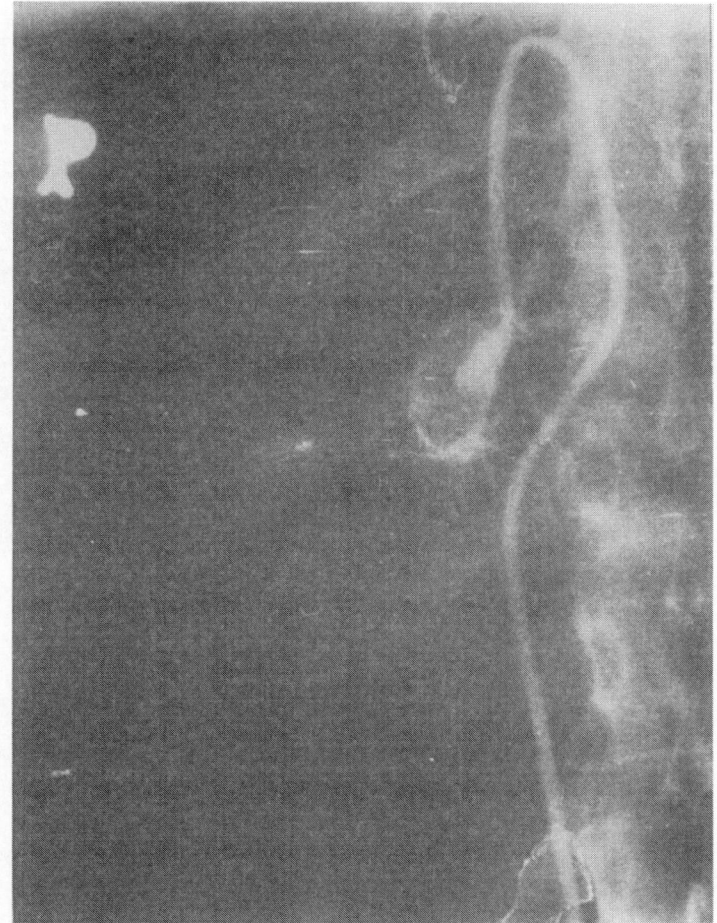

Figure 1. Phlebography of the right adrenal gland demonstrating an adenoma in a patient with primary aldosteronism.

Adrenal vein blood sampling is usually performed at the time of phlebography. Joint evaluation of the results of these two procedures, if both technically correct, increases the diagnostic accuracy to almost 100% [13]. Determination of aldosterone level in the adrenal venous blood is helpful in the diagnosis of even very small unilateral adenomas, not discernible by phlebography. Suppression of the renin-dependent aldosterone secretion from the normal adrenal, which occurs in patients with adenoma, exaggerates the difference in aldosterone concentration in the venous effluents of the two glands.

552

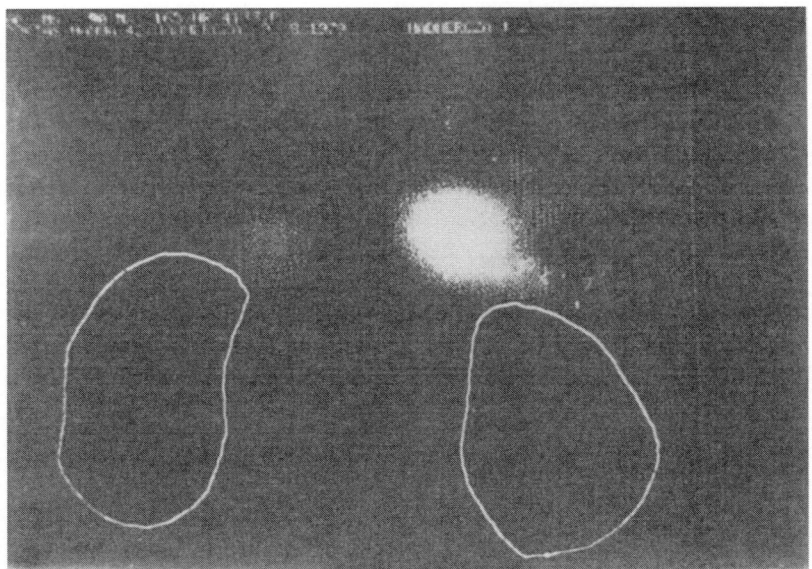

Figure 2. Standard adrenal scintiscan in a patient with primary aldosteronism, demonstrating a right-sided adenoma. Postero-anterior projection.

These two invasive methods employing catheterisation of the adrenal veins are not free of technical difficulties, concerned especially with introduction of the catheter into the right adrenal vein. The rate of complications of phlebography, reported from leading centres, reaches 5%, of which perforation of the adrenal vein with extravasation of the dye and haemorrhage to the adrenal are the most important ones.

Recent years have witnessed successful introduction of non-invasive methods very useful in the diagnosis of adrenal abnormality underlying the syndrome of primary aldosteronism, namely adrenal scintiscanning and computerised tomography of the adrenals.

Scintiscanning of the adrenal glands is performed with the use of cholesterol salts labelled with radioisotopes of iodine or selene which accumulate in rapidly metabolizing adrenal tissue such as functioning adenoma or the hyperplastic gland, while their uptake by the normal tissue is slower and smaller [14]. This difference in the uptake of radio-cholesterol can be further increased by administration of dexamethasone which suppresses the activity of the normal adrenal cortex, but not that of adenoma [4, 5]. Administration of dexamehtasone for three to six days will also suppress the uptake of the isotope by the hyperplastic adrenals: therefore, the comparison of the standard scan with the suppression scan may contribute to the diagnosis of adrenal cortical hyperplasia. The reported rate of correct diag-

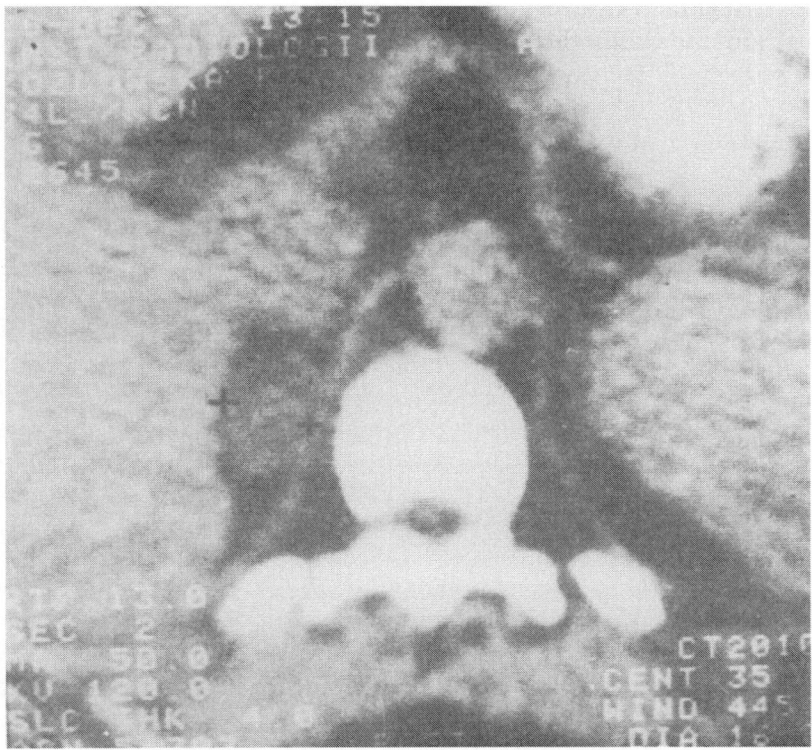

Figure 3. Computerised tomography scan made in the case illustrated in Figure 1. Crosses denote a tumour of the right adrenal gland.

nosis of adenoma offered by adrenal scintiscanning varies from 70–80% with standard scanning, and from 80–94% with suppression scanning, the latter procedure increasing the probability of demonstration of very small active aldosteronomas [16, 17].

Computerised tomography of the adrenals represents the most recent addition to the array of diagnostic methods for visualisation of adrenal adenoma. In our own series it has proved capable of discerning surgically confirmed aldosterone-producing adenoma as small as 8 mm. Although requiring costly equipment, it has the great advantage of being free from any risk for the patient, who can be examined on an out-patient basis [17, 18].

Investigation of the patient by these two non-invasive methods, adrenal scintiscanning with dexamethasone suppression and computerised tomography, may be sufficient to demonstrate and localise the adrenal adenoma in most patients.

Positive recognition of bilateral hyperplasia is more difficult, although the use of the full range of methods described above may provide a fairly con-

554

vincing diagnosis. However, since these patients are not usually referred to the surgeon, the confirmation of the diagnosis will be lacking.

Treatment

In the past, surgical treatment was offered to all patients with primary aldosteronism. The experience accumulated over the subsequent period has shown that in patients with bilateral hyperplasia treated by subtotal adrenalectomy, the late effects are not encouraging. Since these patients usually respond to medical treatment with spironolactones it is now considered unjustified to subject them to the consequences of total removal of the adrenal tissue. Chronic administration of spironolactone (Aldactone), 200–400 mg daily, is usually sufficient to normalise the biochemical abnormalities and the blood pressure. This goal may be also achieved by amiloride (Midamor), 10–20 mg daily. Larger doses of the drugs may be required in an occasional case.

In patients with proven aldosterone-producing adenoma, surgical removal of the tumour is the therapeutic method of choice. The modern diagnostic procedures provide preoperative localisation of the tumour which enables the surgeon to apply the relatively sparing unilateral lumbar approach. Prior

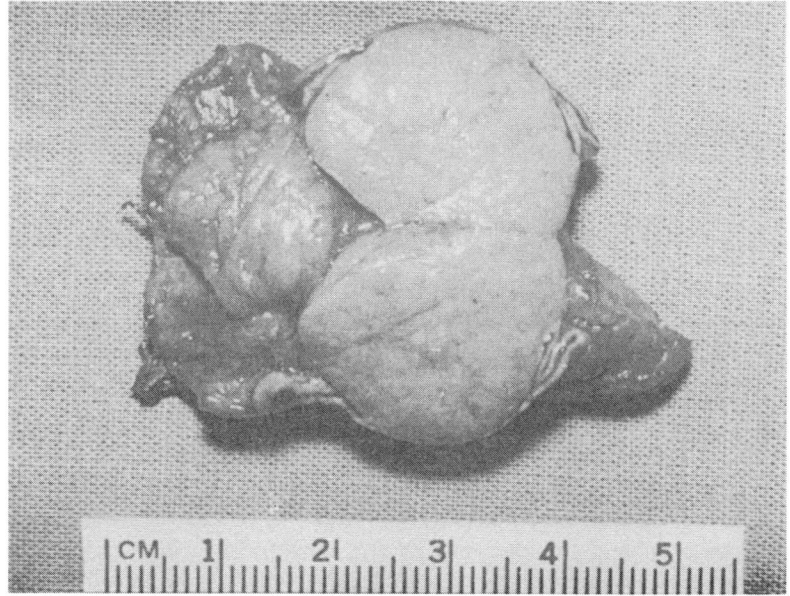

Figure 4. An aldosterone-producing adenoma of the adrenal gland, removed at surgery.

to surgery, the patient's potassium stores should be repleted to minimise the hazard of complications, particularly that of arrhythmia, at the time of operation and in the postoperative period. For this purpose, spironolactone or amiloride and potassium chloride are administered over two to six weeks.

Successful removal of the aldosterone-producing adenoma reverts the humoral abnormalities. Immediately after operation, urinary excretion of aldosterone falls transiently to subnormal levels before it becomes normal. Lack of this response indicates that another adenoma has been missed or suggests bilateral hyperplasia.

In most surgically treated cases of adenoma, a lasting normalisation of blood pressure is achieved. Hypertension may persist in patients with advanced secondary renal vascular lesions; however, it is usually responsive to conventional hypotensive therapy including the diuretic agents. Successful surgery for aldosterone-producing adenoma does not preclude later development of essential hypertension.

Glucocorticoid – remediable aldosteronism

Mention should be made of a rare form of primary aldosteronism, which can be corrected by administration of glucocorticoids. The disease, characterised by familial occurrence, has been recognised in children and in adults. Bilateral adrenal cortical hyperplasia could be demonstrated in a few cases.

CUSHING'S SYNDROME

Cushing's syndrome is a rare cause of secondary hypertension and accounts for less than 0.2% of all cases of hypertension. It represents the clinical consequence of overproduction of glucocorticoids, mainly that of cortisol, by the adrenal cortex.

In about 75–85% of cases the syndrome is caused by bilateral cortical hyperplasia secondary to excessive secretion of ACTH. Oversecretion of ACTH is due to pituitary adenoma or microadenoma, albeit hypothalamic mechanisms seem implicated in some cases. The pituitary-dependent syndrome, habitually termed Cushing's disease, is characterised by elevated plasma ACTH level. Less frequently the ACTH-dependent Cushing's syndrome is associated with ectopic secretion of ACTH by extra-pituitary malignant tumours, classically by oat cel carcinoma of the lung. The remaining 15–30% of cases of Cushing's syndrome are caused by adrenal cortical tumours, usually unilateral benign adenomas, adrenal cancer being found in about $\frac{1}{4}$ of tumour cases. These patients are characterised by low plasma ACTH levels.

Pathophysiology

Arterial hypertension is present in about 80% of all cases of Cushing's syndrome, regardless of etiology, and represents a frequent clinical symptom, only obesity occurring more frequently. However, the syndrome caused by ectopic secretion of ACTH is characterised by lower incidence of high blood pressure. Probably in these cases the rapid development of other clinical symptoms precedes the slower onset of hypertension. It should be pointed out that arterial hypertension develops in about 20% of patients with iatrogenic Cushing's syndrome caused by chronic administration of natural glucocorticoids or their synthetic derivatives. In all likelihood, the occurrence of hypertension in this situation depends on the dosage of the hormones and the duration of treatment.

The mechanisms of hypertension in Cushing's syndrome are not completely understood. Although the action of physiologic amounts of glucocorticoids on sodium metabolism is relatively weak, it is presumed that their excess leads to sodium retention and hypervolaemia with resultant elevation of blood pressure. The renin–angiotensin–aldosterone system also seems to be involved. It has been shown that exogenous cortisol increases the synthesis of renin substrate, and patients with Cushing's syndrome indeed may have elevated plasma renin substrate levels [19]. Moreover, in some of them infusion of the angiotensin antagonist Saralasin causes reduction of elevated blood pressure [20]. However, in most instances plasma renin activity and urinary aldosterone excretion are normal. Increased arteriorial sensitivity to pressor substances caused by excess of cortisol represents yet another postulated hypertensive mechanism [21]. Finally, in some cases increased viscosity of the blood related to polycythaemia may contribute to the elevation of arterial pressure.

For discussion of pathophysiology of other manifestations of Cushing's syndrome, the reader is referred to textbooks of endocrinology.

Clinical picture

Cushing's syndrome is usually recognised in the third and fourth decade of life, about four times as frequently in women as in men. In typical cases the diagnosis may be obvious already at the bedside or in the office, if the patient presents with hypertension in connection with characteristic features such as central obesity, plethoric face, hirsutism, muscular weakness, dysmenorrhoea in woman and impotence in man, acne, skin bruises, psychic depression and backache [22]. The clinical impression is less suggestive in patients in whom the disease is superimposed on simple obesity lacking the characteristic central distribution of the adipose tissue; they are frequently erroneously regarded as having essential hypertension.

Symptomatology is often atypical in Cushing's syndrome associated with ectopic secretion of ACTH and may be misleading, especially if other manifestations of the underlying malignancy are not apparent. Hypertension in Cushing's syndrome is usually mild or moderate, but hypertensive complications may contribute to the clinical picture and the malignant phase may develop, particularly in neglected cases.

Laboratory findings

Patients with Cushing's syndrome are usually screened out from the hypertensive population on the basis of the clinical picture alone. However, usual screening laboratory procedures may be helpful in cases of atypical clinical presentation.

The suggestive routine laboratory findings include hypokalaemic alkalosis, blood and urine glucose values indicative of overt or chemical diabetes and polycythaemia. Routine chest film or intravenous pyelography may incidentally reveal signs of osteroporosis, while very infrequently they would suggest the presence of an adrenal or bronchogenic tumour.

Diagnosis

In order to establish the diagnosis suspected on clinical grounds, oversecretion of cortisol must be ascertained by chemical methods. In most cases urinary excretion of 17-hydroxysteroids is augmented, but demonstration of excessive excretion of urine-free cortisol has greater screening value as it discriminates between Cushing's syndrome and simple obesity. Augmented urinary excretion of 17-ketosteroids is a less constant finding, but it may be very marked in cases of adrenal cancer.

Standard determination of blood cortisol level has limited diagnostic usefulness due to significant variability occurring both in patients with Cushing's syndrome and in healthy people. However, the blood assays are very valuable when combined with exogenous steroid suppression.

The single-dose overnight dexamethasone suppression test is considered the most sensitive screening procedure for Cushing's syndrome [23–25]. The patient is given 1 mg of dexamethasone by mouth at 11.0 p.m. and the cortisol level is determined in the blood sample obtained at 8.0 a.m. the following morning. In contrast to patients with Cushing's syndrome, in healthy persons the blood cortisol at 8.0 a.m. should be below 138 nmol/l, although some authors suggest 193–280 nmol/l as the discriminating value.

The low-dose dexamethasone suppression test provides confirmation of the diagnosis of Cushing's syndrome in most cases. This test requires administration of 0.5 mg of dexamethasone every 6 h for two consecutive days which, on the second day, should cause significant reduction of urinary corticosteroid excretion in healthy people, while significant suppression does not occur in patients with Cushing's syndrome [26].

Etiological diagnosis

When the diagnosis of hypercortisolism has been confirmed, it is necessary to recognise the etiology of Cushing's syndrome since treatment depends on the nature of the underlying pathological process. Subsequent measures will be directed at anatomical localisation of the suspected tumour, providing the confirmation of the diagnosis on the one hand, and guiding the surgeon on the other.

Etiological diagnosis employs tests based on hormonal assays with various suppression procedures. The most useful of these are the high-dose dexamethasone suppression test, the metyrapone test and determination of plasma ACTH level [23–26].

The high-dose dexamethasone test demonstrates suppression of urinary steroid excretion occurring in patients with pituitary-dependent Cushing's disease and absent in those with adrenal tumour. The patient is given 2 mg of dexamethasone every 6 h for two days. On the second day urinary excretion of 17-hydroxysteroids or 17-ketogenic steroids in the ACTH-dependent cases should fall by 40% or more of the baseline value. Lack of this response indicates adrenal tumour.

The metyrapone test is based on the inhibition of cortisol synthesis at an early stage, caused by metyrapone. Compensatory increase of ACTH secretion occurs in normal subjects and in patients with pituitary-dependent Cushing's disease, but not in patients with adrenal tumour who do not demonstrate the corresponding increase in urinary 17-hydroxysteroids. Thus, following 6 oral doses of metyrapone, 750 mg every 4 h, urinary excretion of 17-hydroxysteroids falls in patients with Cushing's syndrome due to adrenal tumour, while in patients with pituitary-dependent disease it increases significantly as compared with the baseline.

Determination of plasma ACTH level has become particularly useful with the introduction of very sensitive radioimmunoassays. In patients with Cushing's syndrome associated with adrenal tumours plasma ACTH levels are low or undetectable. In contrast, patients with ACTH-dependent disease, either of pituitary origin or due to ectopic ACTH secretion, exhibit elevated to normal blood levels of this hormone. In the rare instances when it is difficult to distinguish between these two causes of ACTH oversecretion, it may be helpful to resort to determinations of ACTH levels in the blood samples obtained by selective catheterisation of pituitary venous drainage and other veins draining the regions suspected of harbouring the malignancy which ectopically secretes ACTH [27].

Anatomic localisation of the lesion underlying the Cushing's syndrome depends largely on various radiologic techniques. Large pituitary tumours may be detected by tomography of the sella turcica, while nephrotomography, intravenous pyelography and retroperitoneal tomography are sometimes useful in demonstrating large adrenal masses. However, in the majority of cases of Cushing's syndrome these conventional methods fail to disclose the small adrenal tumour and the still smaller pituitary adenoma.

The anatomic diagnosis of the adrenal disease may be obtained by one of the newer radiologic methods, viz. selective adrenal arteriography and particularly adrenal phlebography. This latter procedure can be coupled with determination of cortisol levels in the adrenal venous effluent. However, the results of the cortisol assays in the adrenal blood should be interpreted with

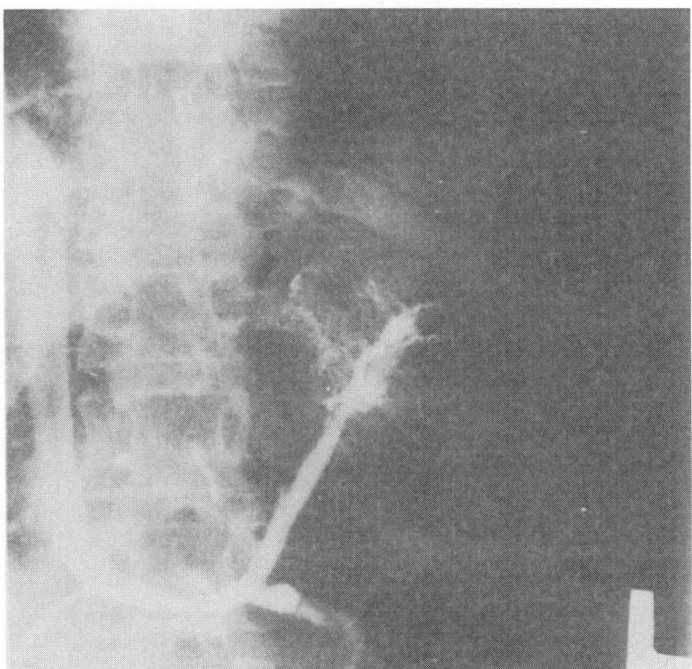

Figure 5. Phlebography of the left adrenal gland demonstrating an adenoma in a patient with Cushing's syndrome.

560

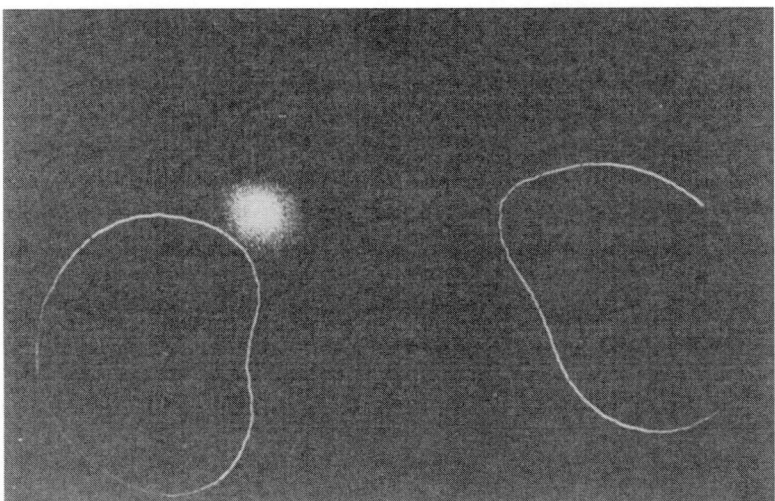

Figure 6. Adrenal scintiscan in the same patient as in Figure 5 demonstrating a left-sided adenoma. Postero-anterior projection.

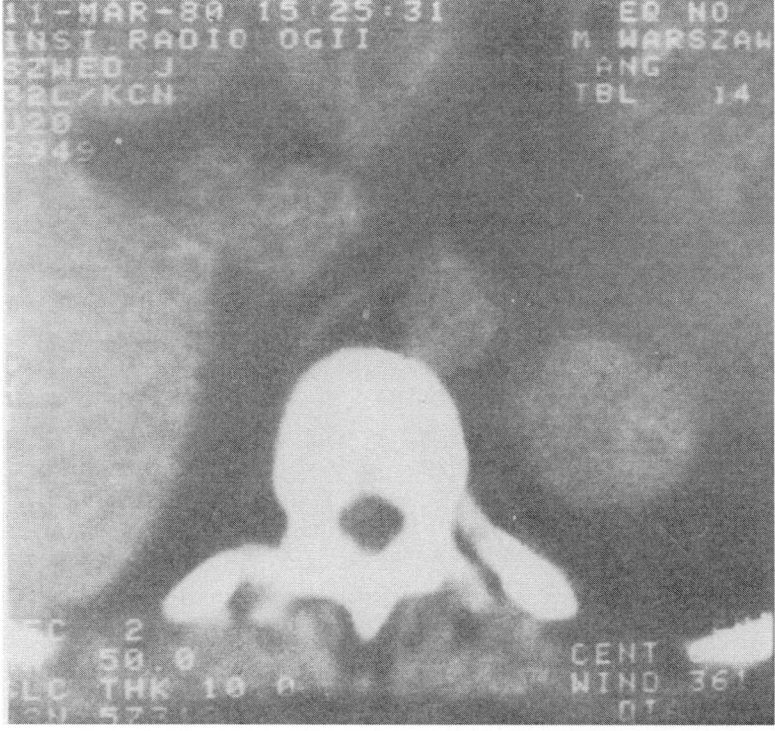

Figure 7. Computerised tomography scan made in the case illustrated in Figure 5. Crosses indicate a tumour of the left adrenal.

caution because significant fluctuations of cortisol secretion occur both in patients with Cushing's syndrome and in normal subjects.

The growing experience with the use of adrenal scintiscanning and abdominal computerised tomography indicates that these two reliable non-invasive methods are sufficient for identification of the adrenal lesion in the vast majority of cases, while cranial computerised tomography may disclose the larger pituitary adenoma [18, 24–25]. However, the prevailing minute pituitary lesion remains undetectable by any visualisation technique short of surgical exploration.

Management

Surgical excision is the therapeutic method of choice in patients with the adrenal tumour. Substitution treatment with corticosteroids may be required postoperatively until the suppressed function of the remaining adrenal is fully restored.

In the past, most patients with pituitary-dependent Cushing's syndrome were treated by bilateral adrenalectomy. At present, in view of the progress of techniques of hypophyseal surgery, total adrenalectomy can be avoided. The transphenoidal approach permits selective excision of pituitary adenoma without the ablation of the entire gland [28]. Since the presence of an adenoma undetected by other means can often be ascertained by the surgeon, attempts at hypophyseal surgery are recommended in all cases properly selected by the hormonal studies.

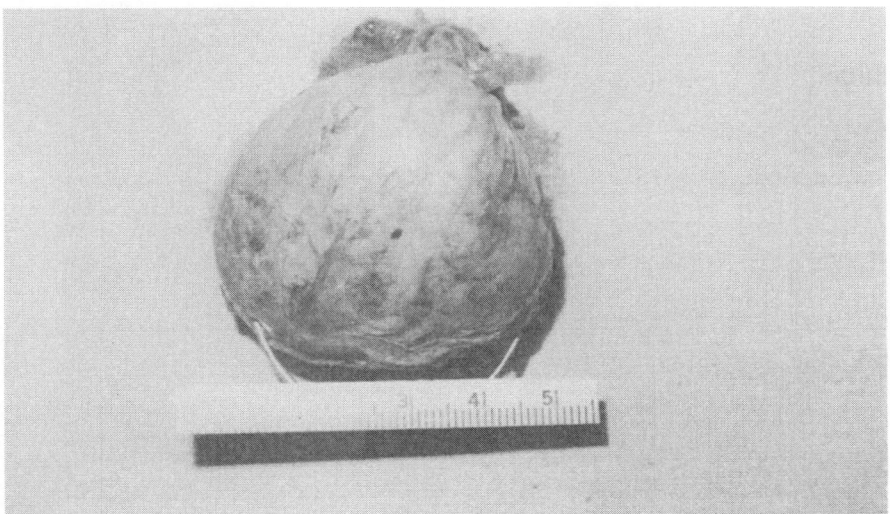

Figure 8. An adenoma removed at surgery in the case illustrated in Figures 5–7.

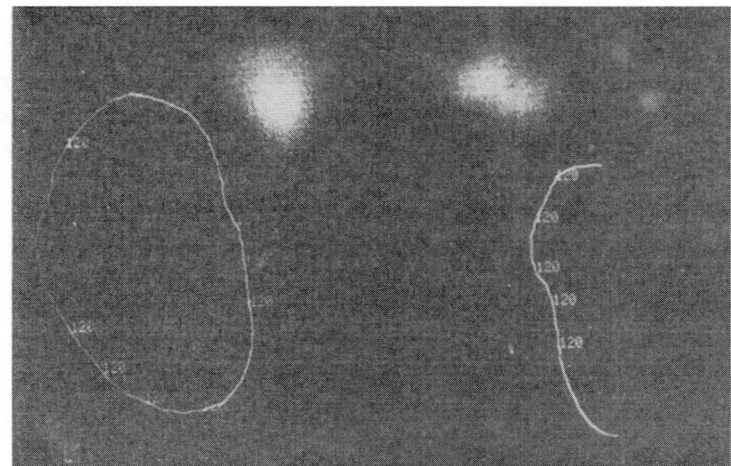

Figure 9. Adrenal scintiscan in a patient with Cushing's syndrome due to bilateral cortical hyperplasia.

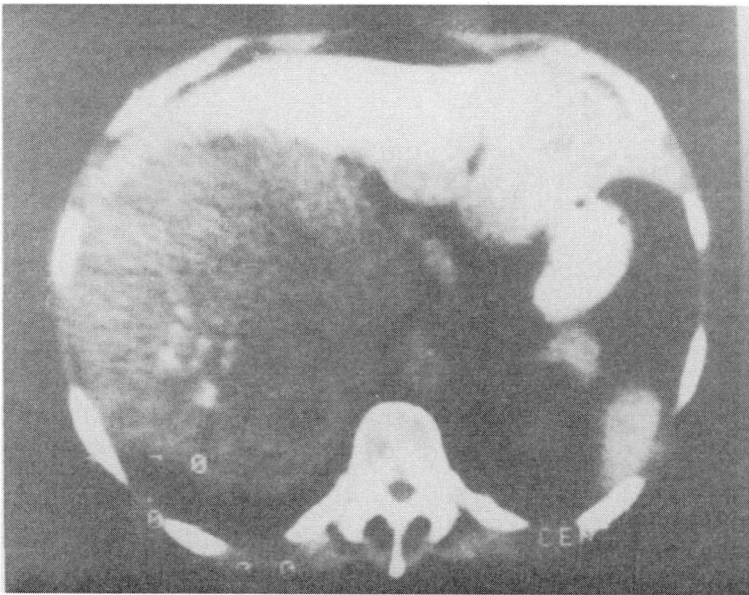

Figure 10. Computerised tomography scan made in a patient with Cushing's syndrome, demonstrating a very large tumour of the right adrenal. Surgery confirmed the diagnosis of cancer.

Various forms of pituitary radiation have been used in the past for treatment of Cushing's disease. Of these, cobalt irradiation has been the most successful method, particularly in the young patient with mild clinical picture [29].

Pharmacological treatment has limited application in Cushing's syndrome, although patients with advanced adrenal carcinoma may benefit from steroid-inhibiting agents like aminoglutethimide (Elipten) or mitotane (op'- DDD, Lysodren). A serotonin antagonist cyproheptadine (Periactin, Peritol) has been used with some success in milder cases of pituitary-dependent disease [30].

Surgical treatment brings about normalisation of blood pressure in the majority of cases of Cushing's syndrome. However, in some patients with advanced, long-standing hypertension, the blood pressure may remain elevated in spite of the regression of other clinical symptoms. These patients require hypotensive drug therapy according to usual principles.

HYPERTENSION DUE TO ENZYMATIC DEFECTS OF ADRENAL STEROID SYNTHESIS

Hypertension may be associated with certain forms of congenital adrenal hyperplasia characterised by enzymatic blocks of steroid synthesis, caused by deficiency of 11-hydroxylase or 17-hydroxylase [31–33].

The deficiency of 11 beta-hydroxylase is responsible for inhibition of synthesis of cortisol, corticosterone and aldosterone. The resultant compensatory ACTH oversecretion provokes excessive production of desoxycorticosterone, desoxycortisol and adrenal androgens. The clinical syndrome of hypertension and virilism becomes usually manifest in early childhood.

Deficiency of 17 alpha-hydroxylase blocks the synthesis of cortisol as well as that of adrenal androgens and estrogens. The compensatory increase in ACTH secretion leads to excessive synthesis of desoxycorticosterone and corticosterone. The disease is usually recognised at the age of puberty when hypogonadism becomes apparent.

Both these enzymatic blocks are characterised by volume-dependent hypertension due to excess of desoxycorticosterone, suppressed plasma renin activity, diminished urinary aldosterone excretion and hypokalaemic alkalosis. Administration of glucocorticoids leads to normalisation of blood pressure and reverts the biochemical abnormalities.

ACKNOWLEDGEMENTS

The authors gratefully acknowledge the generous help of Tadeusz Feltynowski with the preparation of the illustrations.

564

REFERENCES

1. Conn JW: Primary aldosteronism: a new clinical syndrome: J Lab Clin Med 45:6–17, 1955.
2. Filipecki S, Feltynowski T, Popławska W, Łapińska K, Kruś S, Wocial B, Januszewicz W: Carcinoma of the adrenal cortex with hyperaldosteronism. J Clin Endocrinol Metab 35:225–229, 1972.
3. Kuchel O, Buu NT, Hamet P, Nowaczyński W, Genest J: Free and conjugated dopamine in pheochromocytoma, primary aldosteronism and essential hypertension. Hypertension 1:267–273, 1979.
4. Conn JW: Primary hyperaldosteronism. In: Hypertension, Physiopathology and Treatment, p. 768. Genest J, Koiw E, Kuchel O, eds. New York: McGraw-Hill, 1977.
5. Ganguly A, Melada GA, Luetscher JA, Dowdy AJ: Control of plasma aldosterone in primary aldosteronism: distinction between adenoma and hyperplasia. J Clin Endocrinol Metab 37:765–775, 1973.
6. Vetter H, Vetter W: Regulation of aldosterone secretion in primary aldosteronism. Horm Metab Res 7:417–424, 1975.
7. Kaplan NM: Clinical Hypertension. New York: Medcom Press, 1973.
8. Chodakowska J, Januszewicz W, Wocial B, Ignatowska-Świtalska H, Feltynowski T, Skórka B: Primary hypertaldosteronism – some clinical aspects. Kard Pol 19:463–476, 1976.
9. Ferris JB, Beevers DG, Brown JJ, Fraser R, Lever AF, Padfield PL, Robertson JIS: Low Renin ('primary') hyperaldosteronism. Differential diagnosis and distinction of subgroups within the syndrome. Am Heart J 95:641–658, 1978.
10. Ignatowska-Świtalska H, Feltynowski T, Wocial B: Blood aldosterone changes caused by upright posture in patients with primary aldosteronism. Pol Arch Med Wewn 62:495–503, 1979.
11. Cerny JC, Nesbit RM, Conn JW, Bookstein JJ, Rovner DR, Cohen EL, Lucas CP, Warshawsky A, Southwell T: Preoperative tumour localization by adrenal venography in patients with primary aldosteronism: a comparison with operative findings. J Urol 103:521–528, 1970.
12. Yune HY, Klatte EC, Grim CE, Weinberger MH, Donohue JP, Yum MN, Wellman HN: Radiology in primary aldosteronism. Am J Roentgenol 127:761–767, 1976.
13. Weinberger MH, Grim CE, Hollifield JW, Kem DC, Ganguly A, Kramer NJ, Yune HY, Wellman H, Donohue JP: Primary aldosteronism. Diagnosis localization and treatment. Ann Intern Med 90:386–395, 1979.
14. Conn JW, Morita R, Cohen EL, Beierwaltes WH, McDonald WJ, Herwig KR: Primary aldosteronism. Photoscanning of tumors after administration of ^{131}I-19-Iodocholesterol. Arch Intern Med 129:417–425, 1971.
15. Seabold JE, Cohen EL, Beierwaltes WH, Hinerman DL, Nishiyama RH, Bookstein JJ, Ice RD, Balachandrans S: Adrenal imaging with ^{131}I-19-Iodocholesterol in the diagnostic evaluation of patients with aldosteronism. J Clin Endocrinol Metab 42:41–51, 1976.
16. Conn JW, Cohen EL, Herwig KR: The dexamethasone-modified adrenal scintiscan in hyporeninemic aldosteronism/tumor versus hyperplasia. A comparison with adrenal venography and adrenal venous aldosterone. J Lab Clin Med 88:841–856, 1976.
17. Feltynowski T, Pacho R, Jakubowski W, Chodakowska J, Januszewicz W: Value of computer tomography and scintigraphy in preoperative recognition of adenoma in patients with primary aldosteronism. In: Secondary forms of Hypertension: Current Diagnosis and Management. Proceedings of the Second International Symposium of Nephrology at Montecatini, 1980, pp. 243–250, Blaufox MD, Bianchi C, eds. New York: Grune & Stratton, 1981.
18. Ganguly A, Pratt JH, Yune HY, Grim CE, Weinberger MH: Detection of adrenal tumors by

computerized tomographic scan in endocrine hypertension. Arch Intern Med 139:389–390, 1979.
19. Krakoff L, Nicolis G, Amsel B: Pathogenesis of hypertension in Cushing's syndrome. Am J Med 58:217–220, 1975.
20. Dalakos TE, Elias AN, Anderson GH Jr, Streeten DHP, Schroeder ET: Evidence for an angiotensinogenic mechanism of the hypertension of Cushing's syndrome. J Clin Endocrinol Metab 46:114–118, 1978.
21. Mendlowitz M, Gitlow S, Noftchi N: Work of digital vasoconstriction produced by infused norepinephrine in Cushing's syndrome. J Appl Physiol 13:252–256, 1958.
22. Ross EJ, Marshall-Jones P, Friedman M: Cushing's syndrome diagnostic criteria. Q J Med 35:149–192, 1966.
23. Nugent CA, Nichols T, Tyler FH: Diagnosis of Cushing's syndrome. Single dose dexamethasone suppression test. Arch Intern Med 116:172–176, 1965.
24. Gold EM: The Cushing syndromes: changing views of diagnosis and treatment. Ann Intern Med 90:829–844, 1979.
25. Crapo L: Cushing's syndrome: a review of diagnostic tests. Metabolism 28:955–977, 1979.
26. Liddle GW: Tests of pituitary-adrenal suppressibility in the diagnosis of Cushing's syndrome. J Clin Endocrin Metab 20:1539–1560, 1960.
27. Corrigan DF, Schaaf M, Whaley RA, Czerwiński CL, Earll JM: Selective venous sampling to differentiate ectopic ACTH secretion from pituitary Cushing's syndrome. N Engl J Med 296:861–862, 1977.
28. Wilson CB, Dempsey LC: Transsphenoidal microsurgical removal of 250 pituitary adenomas. J Neurosurg 48:13–22, 1978.
29. Jennings AS, Liddle GW, Orth DN: Results of treating childhood Cushing's disease with pituitary irradiation: N Engl J Med 297:957–962, 1977.
30. Krieger DT, Amorosa L, Linick F: Cyproheptadine-induced remission of Cushing's disease: N Engl J Med 293:893–896, 1975.
31. Bongiovanni AM, Root AW: The adrenogenital syndrome. N Engl J Med 268:1283–1289, 1963.
32. New MI, Seaman MP: Secretion rates of cortisol and aldosterone precursors in various forms of congenital adrenal hyperplasia. J Clin Endocrinol Metab 30:361–371, 1970.
33. Biglieri EG, Herron MA, Brust N: 17-hydroxylation deficiency in man. J Clin Invest 45:1946–1954, 1966.

36. HYPERTENSION SECONDARY TO PHEOCHROMOCYTOMA

WILLIAM M. MANGER and RAY W. GIFFORD JR.

The clinical expressions of pheochromocytoma are often dramatic and explosive, and are so variable that it has rightly earned the title of the 'great mimic' [1]. One cannot determine histologically whether a pheochromocytoma is benign or malignant. Although only 10% of these neoplasms are pathologically malignant, as evidenced by metastasis or invasion of adjacent tissue, lethal complications from the effects of excessive circulating catecholamines (epinephrine and norepinephrine) almost invariably result if the disease is not appropriately treated. All patients with manifestations even remotely suggestive of pheochromocytoma must be screened for this disease.

The incidence of pheochromocytoma is unknown, but at least 0.1% of the population with persistent diastolic hypertension has this tumor. In calculating the prevalence of pheochromocytoma it should be remembered that about 50% of pheochromocytoma patients have only paroxysmal hypertension.

Pheochromocytomas may occur at any age, but the greatest frequency is seen in the fourth and fifth decades with a slight predilection for women; in children, approximately two thirds of these tumors occur in boys [2].

Pheochromocytoma arises from chromaffin cells of the sympathoadrenal system. Major sites of occurrence are the adrenal medulla, where it is located 90% of the time, the paraganglia cells of the sympathetic nervous system, and the organ of Zuckerkandl. It may also arise in the chest (<2%) and neck (<0.1%). Multiple and extra-adrenal tumors are far more common in children (35% of cases) than in adults (8% of cases). Familial pheochromocytomas almost invariably arise from the adrenal medulla and are bilateral in 70% of cases, or more.

Most pheochromocytomas secrete both norepinephrine and epinephrine, but norepinephrine is usually the predominant amine. Some tumors secrete only norepinephrine and, rarely, only epinephrine may be secreted. Very rarely, dopamine, dopa, or serotonin are secreted by these tumors [3].

Amery, A. (ed.) Hypertensive Cardiovascular Disease: Pathophysiology and Treatment
© *1982, Martinus Nijhoff Publishers. The Hague / Boston / London*
ISBN-13: 978-94-009-7478-4

1. CLINICAL PRESENTATION

Manifestations encountered in patients with pheochromocytoma are so numerous that they have been described as kaleidoscopic; about 80 manifestations have been reported [4]. Often symptoms arise in a dramatic, explosive fashion when the tumor suddenly releases catecholamines into the circulation. Rarely, sudden death may occur with the initial attack in a patient who has been asymptomatic, or patients may show manifestation of one of the complications of these tumors. About 50 % of patients with persistent hypertension experience a sudden onset of symptoms, usually associated with episodic increases in hypertension; in patients with persistent hypertension symptoms are generally less pronounced than in patients with only paroxysmal hypertension. Very rarely, a patient with either paroxysmal or sustained hypertension may remain relatively asymptomatic [5].

Episodes may occur only once every few months or as often as 25 times daily and persist for from less than a minute to as long as one week. Paroxysms may also occur daily at the same time, but they usually occur quite irregularly. About 75 % of patients with pheochromocytoma experience one or more attacks weekly, and the remainder have one or more daily [6]. Attacks invariably subside more slowly than they start. They may be elicited by any of the following factors: massage or steady pressure for a minute or two in the area of the tumor; lying in a particular position; postural changes, especially involving flexion and bending of the body; exercise; anxiety; having the blood pressure taken; eating, ingestion of certain food or alcoholic beverages that contain tyramine, (e.g., cheese, beer and wine) or of fruit juice rich in synephrine; hyperventilation; increased intra-abdominal pressure; parturition; the Valsalva maneuver; tight clothing; laughing; pressure on the carotid sinuses; certain odors; micturition; bladder distention; straining at stool; smoking a cigarette; shaving; gargling; sneezing; sexual intercourse; trauma; pain; changes in body temperature; intramuscular or subcutaneous administration of certain drugs such as histamine, glucagon, epinephrine, tyramine, tetraethylammonium, methacholine, succinylcholine chloride (Anectine), nicotine, adrenocorticotropic hormone (ACTH), phenothiazines, or saralasin and other angiotensin II analogs; intubation, anesthesia, or operative manipulation.

1.1. *Symptoms*

Symptoms of pheochromocytoma are due either to pharmacologic effects of excessive circulating catecholamines or to complications of hypertension. Table 1 cites the symptoms, of which the three most commonly experienced are headache, generalized sweating, and palpitations.

568

Additional manifestations due to complications, or coexisting diseases or syndromes are also listed in Table 1. Headaches are almost always paroxysmal in character, frequently throbbing and bilateral, and usually very severe during a paroxysm of hypertension. Abrupt in onset, they subside as the

Table 1. Symptoms reported by patients [a] with pheochromocytoma associated with paroxysmal or persistent hypertension

Symptoms due to excessive catecholamines or hypertension	Paroxysmal (37 patients)	Persistent (39 patients)
Headaches (severe)	92 [b]	72 [b]
Excessive sweating (generalized)	65	69
Palpitations ± tachycardia	73	51
Anxiety or nervousness (± fear of impending death, panic)	60	28
Tremulouness	51	26
Pain in chest. abdomen (usually epigastric). lumbar regions, lower abdomen, or groin	48	28
Nausea ± vomiting	43	26
Weakness, fatigue, prostration	38	15
Weight loss (severe)	14	15
Dyspnea	11	18
Warmth ± heat intolerance	13	15
Visual disturbances	3	21
Dizziness or faintness	11	3
Constipation	0	13
Paresthesia or pain in arms	11	0
Bradycardia (noted by patient)	8	3
Grand mal	5	3

Miscellaneous (A large number of miscellaneous symtoms have been reported. Especially noteworthy are painless hematuria, frequency, nocturia, and tenesmus in pheochromocytoma of the urinary bladder).

Manifestations due to complications

Congestive heart failure ± cardiomyopathy
  Myocardial infarction
  Cerebrovascular accident
  Ischemic enterocolitis ± megacolon
  Azotemia
  Dissecting aneurysm
  Encephalopathy
  Shock
  Hemorrhagic necrosis in a pheochromocytoma

[a] Total of 76 patients; almost all adults.
[b] Approximate percentage.
From: Manger WM, Gifford RW Jr: Cardiovasc. Med. 3: 292, 1978.

Table 1 (Continued).

Manifestations due to coexisting diseases or syndromes

  Cholelithiasis

  Medullary thyroid carcinoma $\pm$ effects of secretions of serotonin, calcitonin, prostaglandin, or ACTH-like substance

  Hyperparathyroidism

  Mucocutaneous neuromas with characteristic facies

  Thickened corneal nerves (seen only with slit lamp)

  Marfanoid habitus

  Alimentary tract ganglioneuromatosis

  Neurofibromatosis and its complications

  Cushing's syndrome (rare)

  von Hippel-Lindau disease (rare)

  Virilism, Addison's disease, acromegaly (extremely rare)

Symptoms caused by encroachment on adjacent structures or by invasion and pressure effects of metastases

blood pressure returns toward normal; frequently they are accompanied by nausea and vomiting. Often they are occipital or frontal, or both, in location, but at times are generalized and characterized by an intense sensation of pressure, occasionally including a throbbing in the temporal regions. Some patients are awakened by severe headache in the early morning. Although headache may be severe in patients with sustained hypertension, sometimes it is mild to moderate and indistinguishable from tension headache and that experienced in patients with essential hypertension.

About two thirds of our patients have had excessive perspiration, sometimes 'drenching' in nature, that was generalized but more so in the upper body and not confined to one area. The most profuse sweating appears during paroxysmal attacks of hypertension, but it may appear as the crisis recedes.

Palpitations, the third most common symptom, are usually accompanied by tachycardia, although reflex bradycardia may be elicited by the increased blood pressure. Patients frequently complain of 'pounding' in the chest.

1.2. Signs

The clinical signs of pheochromocytoma encountered in 76 patients are cited in Table 2. In 138 patients with pheochromocytoma seen at the Mayo

Table 2. Signs observed in patients* with pheochromocytoma

Blood pressure changes

± Hypertension ± wide fluctuations (rarely, paroxysmal hypotension or hypertension alternating with hypotension)

Hypertension induced by physical maneuver such as exercise, postural change, or palpation and massage of flank or mass elsewhere

Orthostatic hypotension ± postural tachycardia.

Paradoxic BP response to certain antihypertensive drugs and marked pressor response with induction of anesthesia

Other signs of catecholamine excess

Hyperhidrosis

Tachycardia or reflex bradycardia; very forceful heartbeat; arrhythmia

Pallor of face and upper part of body (rarely flushing)

Anxious, frightened, troubled appearance

Hypertensive retinopathy

Dilated pupils (very rarely exophthalmos, lacrimation, scleral pallor or injection; pupils may not react to light)

Leanness or underweight

Tremor (± shaking)

Raynaud's phenomenon or livedo reticularis (occasionally puffy, red. cyanotic hands in children); skin of extremities wet, cold, clammy, pale; gooseflesh; occasionally, cyanotic nail beds

Fever

Mass lesion

Palpable tumor in abdomen (rare), neck pheochromocytoma or chemodectoma, thyroid carcinoma, or thyroid swelling (very rare and only during hypertensive paroxysm)

Signs caused by encroachment on adjacent structures or by invasion and pressure effects of metastases

Manifestations rolated to complications or coexisting diseases or syndromes (see table 1)

---

* Total of 76 patients, almost all adults.

From: Manger WM, Gifford RW Jr: Cardiovas. Med. 3: 293, 1978.

Clinic, 91% had hypertension; in 42%, hypertension was paroxysmal, whereas in 49% it was sustained [7]. A small percentage of pheochromocytomas may cause manifestations without hypertension. Some tumors cause no signs or symptoms, either because they are nonfunctioning or because they release only relatively small amounts of catecholamines into the circulation; these tumors may be found accidentally by X-ray examination, at operation, or at autopsy [8–10].

The type of hypertension tends to be consistent in members of a family afflicted with pheochromocytoma, i.e., all family members harboring the tumor will have sustained hypertension or all will have paroxysmal hypertension [5]. A few patients have hypotensive episodes, sometimes alternating with hypertension. During a paroxysm of hypertension the blood pressure may on rare occasions be unobtainable with a sphygmomanometer because of severe peripheral vasoconstriction.

Orthostatic hypotension in a hypertensive patient not being treated with antihypertensive medication suggests pheochromocytoma. Some have claimed that orthostatic hypotension occurs in 70% of patients with sustained hypertension caused by this tumor [11, 12].

A paradoxic blood pressure response to certain antihypertensive drugs, such as ganglionic blocking agents and guanethidine, and a marked pressor response frequently observed during induction with almost any anesthetic agent should also suggest pheochromocytoma [2].

Although pallor of the face and upper part of the body has been observed in 60% of patients having paroxysmal hypertension and in 28% of those with sustained hypertension, flushing of the face may rarely be observed alone or following the pallor [2].

Retinopathy, of Group 3 or 4 classification [13], was found in about half of our patients with persistent hypertension due to pheochromocytoma, but was indistinguishable ophthalmologically from that seen in primary hypertension. Retinopathy was not observed in patients with paroxysmal hypertension [2].

1.3. Atypical manifestations

When pheochromocytoma occurs in childhood or in pregnancy, or if the tumor arises in the urinary bladder, atypical manifestations are frequently evident.

It is important to measure the blood pressure routinely in children, since over 90% of those with pheochromocytoma have sustained hypertension. Visual complaints, nausea, vomiting, and weight loss occur more frequently in children than in adults. A puffy, red, cyanotic appearance of hands, is occasionally seen in children, but not in adults [2].

Pregnancy complicated by pheochromocytoma may be confused with toxemia of pregnancy, preeclampsia, or a ruptured uterus, when the patient goes into shock during or immediately after labor [14]. Attacks may be aggravated by pregnancy in some patients, whereas in others attacks may subside during pregnancy.

Pheochromocytomas of the urinary bladder frequently cause paroxysmal attacks which occur during or shortly after micturition or with distention of the bladder; 65% of patients have painless hematuria [15].

2. PATHOLOGIC ENTITIES SOMETIMES ASSOCIATED WITH PHEOCHROMOCYTOMA

Conditions occurring in patients with pheochromocytoma more frequently than in the general population should be kept in mind.

Familial pheochromocytoma in association with multiple endocrine neoplasms or hyperplasia of the thyroid and parathyroid was originally designated MEN (multiple endocrine neoplasia) type 2 [5]. Development of neoplasms in other endocrine glands, or the presence of multiple endocrine neoplasia in relatives establishes the diagnosis. The coexistence of pheochromocytoma, medullary thyroid carcinoma, mucosal neuromas, thickened corneal nerves, alimentary tract ganglioneuromatosis, and frequently a marfanoid habitus constitutes still another familial entity: MEN type 3 [16], also designated type 2B or 2b [17-20].

Hyperparathyroidism occurs in about 50% of patients with MEN type 2, whereas it is rare in MEN type 3 [16]. The increased incidence of cholelithiasis (up to 30%) in patients with pheochromocytoma remains unexplained [2].

Association of neurocutaneous lesions with pheochromocytoma is best explained by the fact that these lesions are of neuroectodermal origin. Neurofibromatosis (von Recklinghausen's disease) with or without café-au-lait spots, occurs in 5% of patients with pheochromocytoma; the incidence of pheochromocytoma in neurofibromatosis is less than 1% [21]. Vascular anomalies (coarctation, renal artery stenosis, or renal artery aneurysm) sometimes occur with neurofibromatosis and may cause hypertension [2]. Rarely, pheochromocytoma occurs in association with von Hippel-Lindau disease (cerebellar hemangioblastoma and retinal angioma) or acromegaly.

3. DIFFERENTIAL DIAGNOSIS

In the differential diagnosis of pheochromocytoma (discussed in detail elsewhere [2]) the clinician may have to consider the disease entities listed in Table 3. Preoperative diagnosis must be confirmed by demonstrating significant elevations of catecholamines or their metabolites in the urine or plasma. A careful history and physical examination can be of great value in deciding which patients with sustained or paroxysmal hypertension to screen for pheochromocytoma since approximately 95% are symptomatic. All symptomatic patients with sustained or paroxysmal hypertension should be screened unless the cause of their hypertension is known. Asymptomatic patients with hypertension of unknown cause should be screened if they have diseases known occasionally to occur with pheochromocytoma or abnormal laboratory findings that may be caused by increased circulating catecholamines.

Conditions that may be accompanied by hypertension and an increased urinary excretion of catecholamines or their metabolites, have been asterisked in Table 3. Clinical manifestations suggesting pheochromocytoma in a person having access to vasopressor drugs, should suggest the remote pos-

Table 3. Differential diagnosis of pheochromocytoma

All hypertensive states (sustained and paroxysmal)
Anxiety, tension states, psychoneurosis, psychosis
Hyperthyroidism
Paroxysmal tachycardia
Hyperdynamic beta-adrenergic circulatory state
Menopause
Vasodilating headache (migraine and cluster headaches)
Coronary insufficiency syndrome
Acute hypertensive encephalopathy
Diabetes mellitus
Renal parenchymal or renal arterial disease with hypertension
Focal arterial insufficiency of the brain
Intracranial lesions ($\pm \uparrow$ intracranial pressure)*
Autonomic hyperreflexia*
Diencephalic seizure and syndrome
Toxemia of pregnancy (or eclampsia with convulsions*)
Hypertensive crises associated with monoamine oxidase inhibitors
Carcinoid*
Hypoglycemia*
Mastocytosis
Familial dysautonomia
Acrodynia*
Neuroblastoma* ganglioneuroblastoma* ganglioneuroma*
Acute infectious disease
Rare causes of paroxysmal hypertension (acute porphyria, acute lead poisoning, clonidine withdrawal, tetanus, Guillain-Barré syndrome, factitious, etc.)*
Fortuitous circumstances simulating pheochromocytoma such as coarctation of the abdominal aorta, renal cyst, and adrenocortical adenoma with hypertension

* Conditions reported to cause occasional increased excretion of catecholamines or their metabolites or both.
From: Manger WM, Gifford RW Jr: Cardiovac. Med. 3: 294, 1978.

sibility of factitious production of symptoms, i.e., pseudopheochromocytoma [22].

Finally, the extreme importance of recognizing hemorrhagic necrosis in a pheochromocytoma cannot be overstated. This condition may present as an acute abdomen or a cardiovascular catastrophe, and without prompt treatment and extirpation of the tumor, the patient will almost certainly die.

4. DIAGNOSIS

Guidelines for screening patients for pheochromocytoma are given in Table 4.

574

Table 4. Indications for screening patients for pheochromocytoma

---

Hypertensives (sustained or paroxysmal) with:
  symptoms (see Table 1)
  group 3 or 4 retinopathy of unknown cause
  weight loss
  hyperglycemia
  hypermetabolism without hyperthyroidism

Persons with marked hyperlability of blood pressure

Recurrent attacks of symptoms (see Table 1) and signs (see Table 2), even if hypertension not
  demonstrated

Severe pressor response during:
  anesthesia induction
  surgery
  angiography
  parturition
  antihypertensive therapy

Unexplained circulatory shock
  during anesthesia
  during pregnancy, delivery, or in puerperium
  during operation or postoperatively
  following administration of phenothiazine drugs

Family history of pheochromocytoma, especially if hypertensive (also screen siblings and children)

Hypertensives with diseases sometimes associated with pheochromocytoma (see Table 1)

Apparent toxemia of pregnancy with hyperlabile blood pressure or severe hypertension

Transient abnormal electrocardiogram during hypertensive episodes

X-ray evidence of suprarenal mass

4.1. Pheochromocytoma 'pearls'

Table 5 cites several facts that are worth emphasizing. The two types of multiple endocrine neoplasia that are associated with familial pheochromocytoma have been grouped separately according to their pathologic features and manifestations. Also, four conditions that occur more frequently than in the general population begin with the letter 'C' and are grouped together as a memory aid.

4.2. Laboratory and EKG findings

The following laboratory abnormalities may be helpful clues in diagnosing pheochromocytoma: hyperglycemia, impaired glucose tolerance, glycosuria,

Table 5. Pheochromocytoma fact sheet

The 5 H's	*MEN-type 3 sextet* [b]
hypertension	medullary thyroid carcinoma
headache	bilateral familial
hyperhidrosis	pheochromocytoma (frequent)
hypermetabolism	mucosal neuromas
hyperglycemia	thickened corneal nerves
	marfanoid habitus
95% of patients will have one or more	alimentary tract
of the following:	ganglioneuromatosis
headache	(very rarely, hyperparathyroidism)
hyperhidrosis	
palpitation	*The 4 C's*
	cholelithiasis
Rough rule of 10	Cushing's syndrome (rare)
10% familial	cutaneous lesions
10% bilateral (adrenal) [a]	cerebellar hemangioblastoma (rare)
10% malignant	
10% multiple	*Pheochromocytoma*
(other than bilateral adrenal) [a]	*manifestations*
10% extra-adrenal [a]	*may appear*
10% occur in children	*during pregnancy.*
MEN-type 2 triad	
medullary thyroid carcinoma	
bilateral familial	
pheochromocytoma (frequent)	
hyperparathyroidism (~50%)	

[a] Adults and children combined.
[b] MEN = multiple endocrine neoplasia.
From Manger WM Gifford RW Jr: Cardiovasc. Med. 3: 298, 1978.

hypermetabolism, and increased free fatty acids. Rarely, polycythemia, transitory leukocytosis or hyperreninemia may occur. Furthermore, when a patient with pheochromocytoma has a coexisting disease or complication (see Table 1), other abnormal laboratory findings may be reported.

A wide variety of abnormal EKG findings have been reported in patients with pheochromocytoma. They are nonspecific, but appearance of EKG changes during paroxysmal hypertension and their reversibility with subsidence of the paroxysm suggests pheochromocytoma, especially in the absence of another cause [2].

4.3. Pharmacologic tests

Rarely is there need for performing a phentolamine test; however, when a patient presents in a hypertensive crisis or with sustained malignant hypertension the blood pressure response to intravenous phentolamine may be of value in the differential diagnosis. False-positive phentolamine test results may be obtained in some patients with malignant hypertension [2].

Occasionally, glucagon or histamine provocative tests, when combined with chemical quantitation of urine or plasma catecholamines or their metabolites, can prove indispensable in the diagnosis of a paroxysmally secreting pheochromocytoma. Adequate precautions to counteract hypertensive crises, arrhythmias, or hypotension must be observed in performing provocative tests. Our experience and that at the Mayo Clinic have indicated that provocative tests are safe if performed correctly and with proper precautions [2]. Provocative tests should be performed or supervised by one thoroughly familiar with the procedure and preferably in a hospital setting.

4.4. Biochemical tests

A conditio sine qua non for preoperative diagnosis of pheochromocytoma is demonstration of elevated catecholamines or their metabolites in urine or elevated plasma catecholamines. Exploratory surgery without chemical confirmation or radiologic evidence of a tumor is indefensible.

Patients with pheochromocytoma who have sustained hypertension due to excessive circulating catecholamines will invariably have elevated plasma and urinary catecholamines or metabolites. Rarely, some patients have normal concentrations of catecholamines and their metabolites when the blood pressure is normal. When evaluating these patients, it is imperative that plasma or urine be obtained during a hypertensive period, either occurring spontaneously or induced by a provocative agent, since occasionally a preoperative diagnosis can be made only through this approach.

Measurement of total metanephrines (metanephrine plus normetanephrine) in a 24-h urine specimen has proved to be the most reliable method of detecting pheochromocytoma. More than 95% of patients have elevated excretion of total metanephrines; furthermore, quantitation of total metaphrines is comparatively easy, and fewer drugs interfere with its assay than with assays of urinary catecholamines or VMA (vanilmandelic acid). Substances that can interfere with quantitation of urinary catecholamines or their metabolites are listed in Table 6, which also cites the upper limit of normal concentrations in adults. It is essential that drugs significantly altering urinary assays be avoided for at least one week before urine specimens are collected. We are unaware of any patients with pheochromocytoma in whom drug therapy lowered the excretion rate of the catecholamines or their metabolites to a normal range. Severe renal insufficiency may possibly result in markedly impaired excretion of catecholamines and their metabolites.

Table 6. Effects of drugs and interfering substances on concentrations of urinary catecholamines and their metabolites [a]

Catecholamine or metabolite	Upper limit of normal range (adult) (mg per 24 h)	Effects of drugs and interfering substances
Catecholamines		↑ catecholamines [b], ↑ drugs containing catecholamines; ↑ isoproteranol [c]; ↑ L-dopa; ↑ methyldopa; ↑ tetracyclines [c]; ↑ erythromycin [c]; ↑ chlorpromazine [c]; ↑ other fluorescent substances [c] (for example, quinine, quinidine, bile in urine); ? ↑ rapid clonidine withdrawal [d]; ↑ ethanol; ↓ fenfluramine (large doses) [e]
Epinephrine	0.02	
Norepinephrine	0.08	
Total	0.10	
Dopamine	0.20	
Metanephrines		↑ catecholamines; ↑ drugs containing catecholamines; ↑ MAO inhibitors [f]; ? ↑ rapid clonidine withdrawal; ↑ ethanol; ↑ diatrizoate meglumine and diatrizoate sodium (Renovist, Renografin); ↓ fenfluramine (large doses)
Metanephrine	0.4	
Normetanephrine	0.9	
Total	1.3	
VMA	6.5	↑ catecholamines (minimal increase); ↑ drugs containing catecholamines (minimal increase); ↑ L-dopa; ↑ nalidixic acid [c]; ? ↑ rapid clonidine withdrawal; ↓ clofibrate; ↓ disulfiram; ↓ ethanol; ↓ MAO inhibitors; ↓ fenfluramine (large doses)

[a]   As determined by most reliable assays.
[b]   ↑ = Increases apparent value.
[c]   Probably spurious influence.
[d]   ? = Uncertain if significant increase can occur.
[e]   ↓ = Decreases apparent value.
[f]   Monoamine oxidase.
From Manger WM and Gifford RW Jr: Cardiovasc. Med. 3: 303, 1978.

Conditions other than pheochromocytoma that may be accompanied by significantly increased or decreased excretion of catecholamines and their metabolites are listed elsewhere [2]. Patients requested to collect 24-h urine specimens for assay should be instructed to avoid severe stress (e.g., strenuous physical activity or exposure to extreme cold) during the collection period, since stress may result in significantly elevated levels of the substances assayed.

The finding that a significant fraction of urinary catecholamines is epinephrine or its metabolite metanephrine, or that plasma epinephrine is elevated, strongly suggests that the pheochromocytoma is located in the adrenal area. Rarely, tumors secreting significant amounts of epinephrine have occurred in extra-adrenal sites [2].

578

4.5. Preoperiative location of pheochromocytoma

In addition to demonstrating increased concentrations of epinephrine or metanephrine in urine or plasma, suggesting an intra-adrenal tumor, radiography and central venous blood sampling for catecholamine assay can be of great value in locating the site of pheochromocytoma.

Nephrotomography was successful in locating 67 % of abdominal pheochromocytoma [7]. Angiography (i.e., aortography, selective arteriography, and adrenal phlebography) is exceptionally valuable for locating pheochromocytomas; it has the advantage of demonstrating vascular abnormalities in many intra-adrenal and extra-adrenal tumors. Aortography will almost always demonstrate adrenal pheochromocytomas that are large and well vascularized. However, sometimes only selective arteriography or adrenal

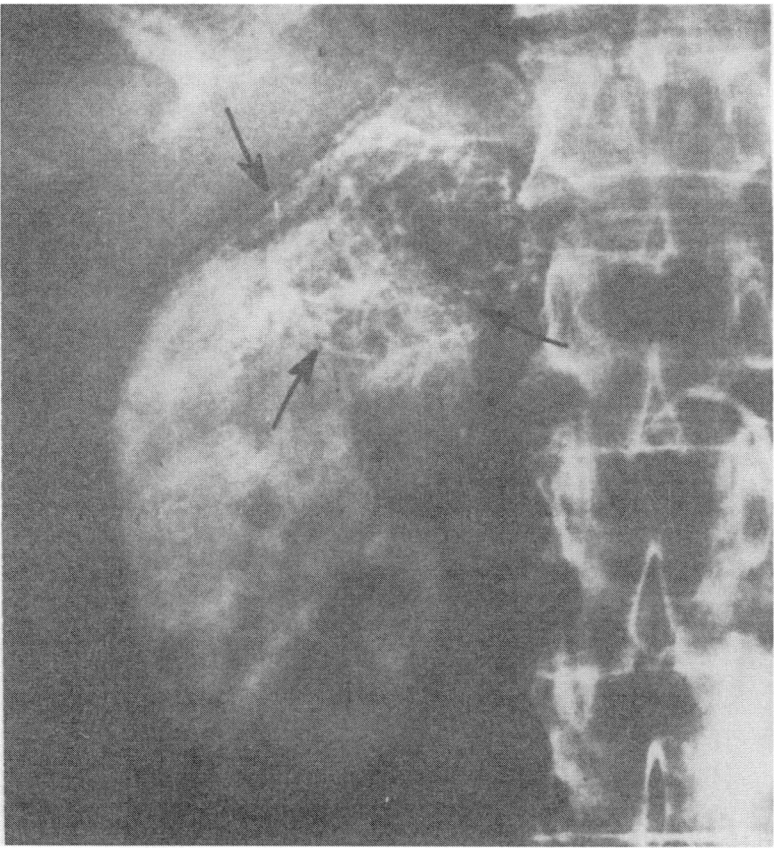

Figure 1. Demonstration of a pheochromocytoma in the right adrenal gland by angiography. Courtesy of Dr. Thomas Meaney, Cleveland Clinic Foundation.

phlebography will demonstrate the tumor. Computerized axial tomography appears as reliable as angiography in detecting adrenal and extra-adrenal pheochromocytomas [23] (Figure 1 and 2). Angiography and computerized axial tomography can be of great value in locating tumors in the thorax and neck. Oblique chest X-ray films should be obtained routinely when the diagnosis of pheochromocytoma is considered, since these tumors usually are located near the spine.

Controversy exists as to whether alpha-adrenergic blockade should be induced in all patients suspected of harboring a pheochromocytoma prior to angiography, to avoid hypertensive crises that may be precipitated by injection of contrast media. In most instances patients should be blocked during angiographic studies. However, a prior negative exploratory laparotomy is an indication for avoiding adrenergic blockade, since a hypertensive response during selective arteriography can be an important aid in confirming the diagnosis and in locating the tumor. Appropriate precautions must be taken to treat hypertensive crises, arrhythmias, or hypotension if angiography is performed in the unblocked patient.

When feasible, vena caval catheterization and central venous blood sampling for catecholamine assay, followed by adrenal phlebography, should be performed when pheochromocytoma has not been located by other radiographic procedures. Central venous sampling can be particularly helpful when tumors are very small, multiple, or metastatic; it usually permits exclusion of cervical or intrathroacic pheochromocytoma. Although we have not found it necessary to induce alpha-adrenergic blockade prior to catheterization for blood sampling, precautions recommended for angiography in unblocked patients should be observed.

5. TREATMENT

5.1. Preoperative evaluation and management

Expertise and teamwork are essential to successful management of pheochromocytoma. Preoperatively, one must exclude other conditions that may cause increased excretion of catecholamines and their metabolites. If there is evidence suggesting familial pheochromocytoma, it is mandatory to determine if medullary thyroid carcinoma or hyperparathyroidism is present.

Occurrence of Cushing's syndrome in patients with pheochromocytoma requires preoperative evaluation, but ACTH infusion tests, if indicated, should be performed with extreme caution because of the risk of severe hypertensive crises [5]. Since malignant pheochromocytomas may metastasize, metastatic lesions should be identified whenever possible.

Angiographic studies can provide the surgeon with a vascular 'road map'

580

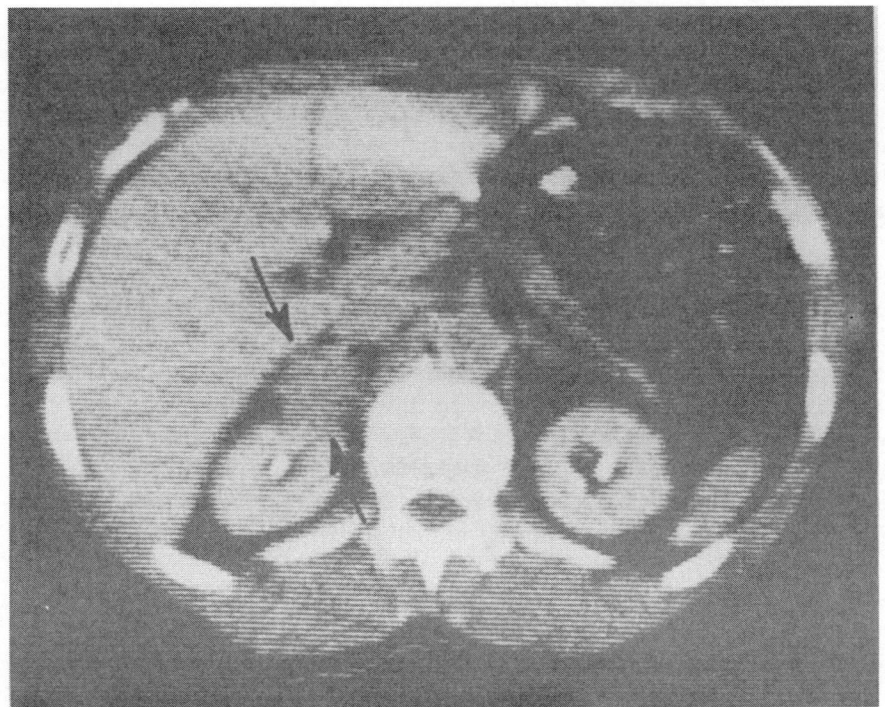

Figure 2. Demonstration of pheochromocytoma in the right adrenal gland by computerized axial tomography. Courtesy of Dr. Thomas Meaney, Cleveland Clinic Foundation.

that may aid in removal of the tumor. If there is indication of pheochromocytoma in the urinary bladder, cystoscopy should be carried out under alpha-adrenergic blockade.

Any diagnostic procedure, including abdominal palpation, that entails even a minor degree of trauma or stress should be performed with caution and with drugs available to treat hypertensive crises, arrhythmias, or hypotension.

Occasionally, patients with pheochromocytoma may present with acute or malignant hypertension or with acute abdominal or cardiovascular complications requiring immediate medical and surgical therapy. In managing an acute hypertensive crisis, either before or during surgery or induced by angiography or a provocative test, we usually use bolus injections of phentolamine, giving 5 mg at a time but leaving the needle and syringe in place so that if there is no response within a minute or two another 5 mg can be given and repeated until the crisis is brought under control. Since the effect of phentolamine is transient, it may be necessary, especially during spontaneous crises and during operation, to control blood pressure by infusing phentolamine or sodium nitroprusside (usually 100 mg of either drug mixed with 500 ml of 5% dextrose in water) at a rate adequate to keep blood pressure at a relatively normal range. In the presence of impaired renal function or with prolonged infusion of nitroprusside, the thiocyanate level in the blood should be monitored, since concentrations >10 mg/dl may cause toxic psychosis.

Preoperative and intraoperative management remains controversial. Advocates of preoperative alpha-adrenergic blockade continued to the time of operation argue that blockade prevents severe preoperative clinical manifestations, reverses the hypovolemia that frequently exists, and promotes smooth induction of anesthesia and a relatively stable blood pressure during operation. Those who oppose alpha-adrenergic blockade up to the time of operation feel that if blockade is complete, the surgeon will not have the advantage of utilizing increases in blood pressure as a guide to tumor location or of immediately recognizing, by persistence of hypertension, that another tumor may be present. Although preoperative use of alpha-adrenergic drugs in moderate dosage is indicated if sustained hypertension or paroxysmal attacks are very severe or if the patient is precariously ill, we feel that complete blockade is contraindicated, especially when the location of the tumor is uncertain or when the likelihood of encountering multiple tumors is anticipated. To induce alpha-adrenergic blockade we recommend starting with 10 mg of phenoxybenzamine twice daily and increasing the dosage with gradual increments, usually to 20–40 mg two or three times a day, until an optimal dosage is obtained as judged by blood pressure control.

Prazosin hydrochloride selectively blocks postsynaptic alpha receptors and has been shown to be effective in controlling hypertension due to pheochromocytoma [24]. Patients with pheochromocytoma are frequently unusually sensitive to prazosin and we recommend starting with 1 mg, which may control the hypertension for 8–12 h. Severe pheochromocytic hypertension often can be controlled with 1 or 2 mg of prazosin two or three times daily. Prazosin can be used for preoperative alpha-adrenergic blockade and probably will become the drug of choice if further experience indicates that it produces fewer side effects and is as effective as phenoxybenzamine.

Preoperative beta-adrenergic blockade with propranolol is indicated in the presence of presistent tachycardia or arrhythmias that appear hazardous or if angina pectoris occurs, provided there are no contraindications to its use. *Propranolol should never be given to a patient with pheochromocytoma without first creating alpha-adrenergic blockade,* since beta-blockade, even in the presence of alpha-blockade, may significantly elevate blood pressure.

582

To induce beta-blockade, 10 mg of propranolol is given twice daily and increased by 10 mg increments every day or two, usually to 40 mg two or three times daily, until the tachycardia and/or arrhythmia is controlled. The intravenous administration of a bolus of propranolol (0.5 mg in 15–30 sec) or lidocaine (50–100 mg) may be required to correct significant arrhythmias [2].

Labetalol, a drug with both alpha- and beta-adrenergic blocking action, was reported effective when given orally or intravenously in controlling blood pressure and clinical manifestations in some patients with pheochromocytoma [25].

In expert hands operative mortality (0–3.3%), does not appear to have been influenced by preoperative alpha- and beta-adrenergic blockade.

Certain drugs (e.g., morphine and phenothiazines) should be avoided since they may precipitate hypertensive crises or hypotension. If bilateral adrenalectomy is anticipated, appropriate steroid replacement therapy should be instituted before operation [2].

5.2. Operative and postoperative management and follow-up

Careful monitoring of arterial pressure, EKG, and central venous pressure is crucial to successful intraoperative management. Intubation must be performed with appropriate premedication. Enflurane or halothane appear to be suitable anesthetic agents [2].

Prompt control of hypertensive crises and arrhythmias during operation is critical; appropriate use of phentolamine, sodium nitroprusside, propranolol, lidocaine, and volume expanders has been discussed in detail elsewhere [2]. Of paramount importance in preventing postoperative hypotension is preoperative and intraoperative correction of blood volume deficits; vasopressor agents are rarely indicated.

The anterior transperitoneal approach is mandatory when operating for an intra-abdominal pheochromocytoma, since these tumors may be multiple and extra-adrenal. Surgical strategy varies but we believe the desirable strategy is immediate ligation of tumor vasculature followed by extirpation and thorough exploration for residual tumors [2]. Because of the high incidence of coexisting cholelithiasis, the gallbladder should be examined during exploration.

Pheochromocytomas of the neck and chest require specialized surgical techniques, but preoperative, intraoperative, and postoperative management is similar to that described for intra-abdominal tumors. Management of the pregnant patient depends somewhat on the duration of pregnancy when a diagnosis of pheochromocytoma is made. In early pregnancy, extirpation of the tumor has been recommended, whereas in the later months of pregnancy, patients may be treated with adrenergic blocking agents as indicated until close to term [26]. We consider it adviseable to remove a pheochromocytoma as soon as it is discovered, regardless of the duration of pregnancy. If pregnancy is carried to term, we recommend cesarean section with tumor extirpation without allowing the patient to undergo the stress of vaginal delivery [2].

Monitoring and close observation should be continued postoperatively until the patient's condition is stable. Bleeding at operative sites may well be the cause of postoperative hypotension. Postoperative hypertension may result from fluid overload, pain, residual pheochromocytoma, or inadvertant ligation of a renal artery. Severe hypoglycemia, sometimes causing central nervous system manifestations with coma, has been reported in several patients within two hours postoperatively. It is a transient phenomenon, perhaps due to increased insulin release and should be treated with infusion of dextrose in water [27, 28].

The five-year survival rate of patients with benign tumors is 96%, whereas it drops to 44% for patients with malignant pheochromocytomas [7]. Approximately 75% of patients are normotensive following surgical removal, while the remainder show sustained hypertension without evidence of residual tumor. The cause of this sustained hypertension remains uncertain.

5.3. Chronic medical management

If a pheochromocytoma has metastasized or cannot be totally resected, one must remove as much of the tumor as possible to reduce functioning tissue to a minimum. Radiotherapy and chemotherapy have usually been relatively ineffective. By blocking peripheral effects of catecholamines, chronic medical treatment with phenoxybenzamine has proved very successful in controlling blood pressure and manifestations of excessive circulating catecholamines. Alpha-methyl-L-tyrosine (Demser) has been used effectively to decrease synthesis of catecholamines in patients with pheochromocytoma. As it can occasionally cause serious side effects (crystalluria, extrapyramidal effects, sedation, psychic disturbances, diarrhea), Demser should be used cautiously.

ACKNOWLEDGEMENTS

The valuable and very expert assistance of Mildred Hulse and Margaret Forsyth is gratefully acknowledged.

584

REFERENCES

1. Decourcy JL, Decourcy CB: Pheochromocytomas and the General Practitioner. Cincinnati: Barclay Newman, 1952.
2. Manger WM, Gifford RW Jr: Pheochromocytoma. New York: Springer-Verlag, 1977.
3. Winkler H, Smith AD: Pheochromocytomas and other catecholamine-producing tumors. In: Catecholamines, p. 900. Blaschko H, Muscholl E, eds. New York: Springer-Verlag, 1972.
4. Hermann H, Mornex R: Human Tumours Secreting Catecholamines: Clinical and Physiopathological Study. Oxford: Pergamon, 1964.
5. Steiner Al, Goodman AD, Powers SR: Study of a kindred with pheochromocytoma, medullary thyroid carcinoma, hyperparathyroidism and Cushing's disease: multiple endocrine neoplasia type 2. Medicine 37:371, 1968.
6. Thomas JE, Rooke ED, Kvale WF. The neurologist's experience with pheochromocytoma. A review of 100 cases. J Am Med Assoc. 197:754, 1966.
7. Remine WH, Chong GC, van Heerden JA, Sheps SG, Harrison EG Jr: Current management of pheochromocytoma, Ann Surg 179:740, 1974.
8. Minno AM, Bennett WA, Kvale WF: Pheochromocytoma; a study of 15 cases diagnosed at autopsy. N Engl J Med 251:959, 1954.
9. Aranow H Jr: Pheochromocytoma. In: Monographs in Medicine, p. 179. Bean WE, ed. Series 1. Baltimore: Williams & Wilkins, 1952.
10. Taubman I, Pearson OH, Anton AH: An asymptomatic catecholamine-secreting pheochromocytoma. Am J Med 57:953, 1974.
11. Sjoerdsma A: Sympatho-adrenal system: Pheochromocytoma. In: Cecil Loeb Textbook of Medicine. Beeson PB, McDermott W, eds. 13th edn, p. 1832. Philadelphia: W. B. Saunders, 1971.
12. Engelman K, Zelis R, Waldmann T, Mason DT, Sjoerdsma Am: Mechanism of orthostatic hypertension in pheochromocytoma. Circulation (suppl 6) 38:72, 1968.
13. Keith NM, Wagener HP, Barker NW: Some different types of essential hypertension: their course and prognosis. Am J Med Sci 197:332, 1939.
14. Hume DM: Pheochromocytoma in the adult and in the child. Am J Surg 99:458, 1960.
15. Leestma JE, Price EB Jr. Paraganglioma of the urinary bladder. Cancer 28:1063, 1971.
16. Khairi MR, Dexter RN, Burzynski NJ, Johnston CC Jr: Mucosal neuroma, pheochromocytoma and medullary thyroid carcinoma: Multiple endocrine neoplasia type 3. Medicine 54:89, 1975.
17. Carney JA, Go VL, Sizemore GW, Hayles AB: Alimentary-tract ganglioneuromatosis. A major component of the syndrome of multiple neoplasia, type 2b. N Engl J Med 295:1287, 1976.
18. Carney JA, Sizemore GW, Lovestedt SA. Mucosal ganglioneuromatosis, medullary thyroid carcinoma, and pheochromocytoma: Multiple endocrine neoplasia, Type 2b. Oral Surg 41:739, 1976.
19. Chong GC, Beahrs OH, Sizemore GW, Woolner LH: Medullary carcinoma of the thyroid gland. Cancer 35:695, 1975.
20. Robertson DM, Sizemore GW, Gordon H. Thickened corneal nerves as a manifestation of multiple endocrine neoplasia. Trans Am Acad Ophthalmol Otolaryngol 79:772, 1975.
21. Brasfield RD, Das Gupta TK: Von Recklinghausen's disease: a clinicopathological study. Ann Surg 175:86, 1972.
22. DeQuattro V, Chan S: Raised plasma-catecholamines in some patients with primary hypertension. Lancet 1:806, 1972.
23. Stewart BH, Bravo EL, Haaga J, Meaney TF, Tarazi R: Localization of pheochromocytoma by computed tomography. N Engl J Med 299:460, 1978.

585

24. Wallace JM, Gill DP: Prazosin in the diagnosis and treatment of pheochromocytoma. J Am Med Assoc 240:2752, 1978.
25. Rosei EA, Brown JJ, Lever AF. Treatment of phaeochromocytoma and of clonidine withdrawal hypertension with labetalol. Br J Clin Pharmacol 3 (suppl 3):809, 1976.
26. El-Minawi MF, Paulino E, Cuesta M, Ceballos J: Pheochromocytoma masquerading as pre-eclamptic toxemia. Am J Obstet Gynecol 109:389, 1971.
27. Allen CT, Imrie D: Hypoglycemia as a complication of removal of a pheochromocytoma. Can Med Assoc J 116:363, 1977.
28. Wilkins GE, Schmidt N, Doll WA. Hypoglycemia following excision of pheochromocytoma. Can Med Assoc J 116:367, 1977.

37. HYPERTENSION SECONDARY TO THYROID DYSFUNCTION

HERBERT G. LANGFORD

Numerous papers have suggested that decreased thyroid function would ameliorate or slow the development of experimental hypertension. In addition, a number of papers have documented decrease in one parameter or another of thyroid function in various types of experimental hypertension. The clinical literature has suggested that hypothyroidism may be associated with hypertension which certainly would not be anticipated from the animal studies. There is relatively little about any causal role of hyperthyroidism in the development of diastolic hypertension in humans. This article will first review the clinical literature on hypothyroidism and hyperthyroidism and then discuss the experimental literature.

HYPOTHYROIDISM

Hypothyroidism has been listed as a cause of hypertension since a report of W. O. Thompson in 1931 [1]. The recent paper of Endo et al. casts doubt on the basic observation [2]. Endo determined blood pressure in 1601 female subjects and documented the usual progressive increase in blood pressure with age, and therefore the progressive increase in the percentage of the population that could be classified as hypertensive. Thyroid function was determined in 73 apparently normal women, spanning the same age ranges. All of these women were euthyroid, and their blood pressure followed exactly the pattern found in the largest survey. Next, the blood pressure was ascertained in three groups of hypothyroid patients, separated according to the severity of their hypothyroidism. Slightly hypothyroid patients were those whose T_4 levels were slightly elevated at the lower limits of normal and basal TSH (20 ± 2.2 mμ/ml). There were 38 patients in this group, and their blood pressure was indistinguishable from the normal control patients. Patients defined as having moderate hypothyroidism (T_4 3.1 ± 0.1 mg/100 ml) also had normal blood pressures. There were 17 in this group.

A deviation from normal appeared only in those diagnosed as having severe hypothyroidism. These patients were said to have typical symptoms

Amery, A. (ed.) Hypertensive Cardiovascular Disease: Pathophysiology and Treatment
© *1982, Martinus Nijhoff Publishers. The Hague / Boston / London*
ISBN-13: 978-94-009-7478-4

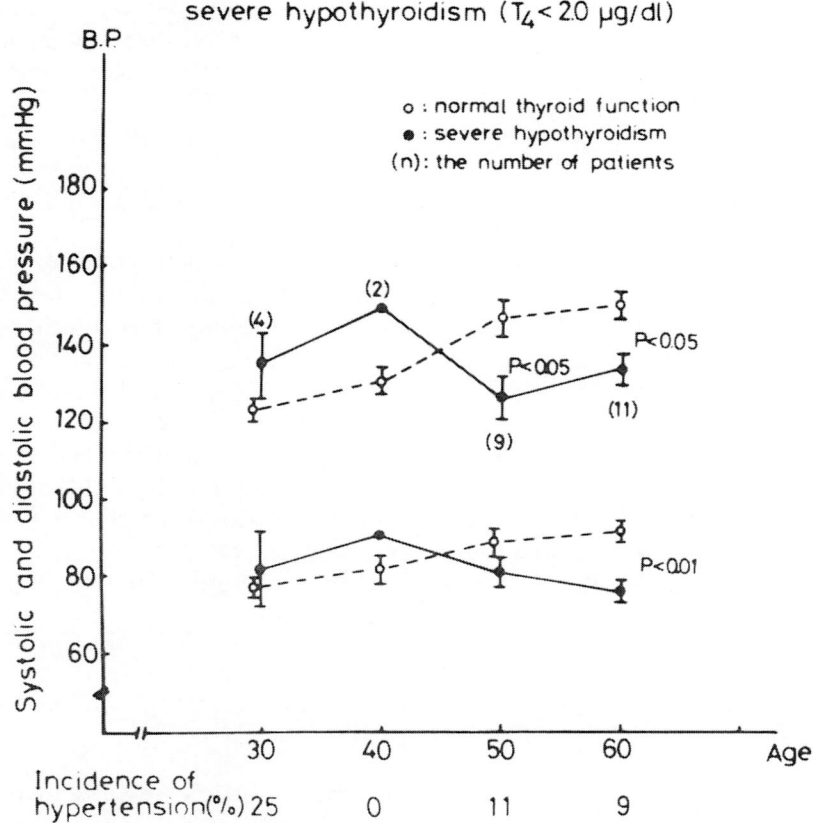

Figure 1. Mean systolic (above) and diastolic (below) blood pressures and incidence of hypertension in severe hypothyroid patients. for comparison, blood pressure in known euthyroid subjects (dotted line) was indicated. Circles and vertical lines indicate mean ± SE. (From Endo et al., [2].)

of hypothyroidism. Their T_4 value averaged 1.2 ± 0.1 mg/100 ml, and their basal TSH was 163.6 ± 6.4 mμ/ml. Figure 1 taken from Endo's paper shows that systolic blood pressure was significantly lower in the 50- and 60-year-old group, and diastolic blood pressure was significantly lower in the 60-year-old group *in the hypothyroid patients.*

There is one possible flaw in this otherwise excellent report. The circumstances of measuring blood pressure of the hypothyroid patients may have been different from the circumstances surrounding the control patients. It seems unlikely that this difference would be enough to create 'hypertension' in the hypothyroid patients, when the only difference demonstrated by Endo was significantly lower blood pressure in the severely hypothyroid patients. In addition, this finding of lowered blood pressure accompanying severe hypothyroidism is more in keeping with the reduction in blood pressure by hypothyroidism produced in spontaneously hypertensive rats and in rats with hypertension produced by renal encapsulation. If there is an effect of hypothyroidism on blood pressure, it seems to lower it.

HYPERTHYROIDISM AND HYPERTENSION

The frequency of elevated diastolic blood pressure in hyperthyroidism does not seem to have been studied. Elevated systolic pressures are very frequent as would be anticipated from the increased cardiac output found in hyperthyroidism. Boone and Langford [3] documented that the production of euthyroidism by either radioiodine therapy or propylthiouracil produced a significant drop in systolic blood pressure. The mean systolic blood pressure of thyrotoxic patients treated with propylthiouracil was 153 mm Hg before therapy and 129 mm Hg after therapy, $p = 0.01$. A 4 mm drop of diastolic blood pressure noted in this group was not statistically significant. Patients treated with radioiodine had a drop of systolic pressure from 151 mm Hg to 134 mm Hg. In other words, hyperthyroidism is a cause of systolic hypertension which remits after successful therapy.

ANOMALIES OF THYROID FUNCTION IN EXPERIMENTAL FORMS OF HYPERTENSION

Renal encapsulation hypertension in the rat is associated with thyroid enlargement, increased excretion of a dose of radioiodine, and decreased thyroidal uptake of radioiodine [4]. The decrease in thyroidal radioiodine uptake was significantly negatively correlated with the attained systolic blood pressure. These studies do not seem to have been repeated since methods became available to measure the level of circulating thyroxine. The changes in radioiodine homeostasis are those that would be anticipated from the action of a goitrogen. There are no reports of similar findings in human hypertension. Hypertension due to a perirenal constricting membrane is extremely rare, but the compression of renal parenchyma found in polycystic kidney disease might replicate the abnormality found in renal encapsulation hypertension. It would be of interest to see if similar changes in thyroid physiology occur in conjunction with polycystic kidneys.

Serum levels of thyroxine and triiodothyronine are suppressed in rats with the Okomoto variety of spontaneous hypertension, and TSH is elevated [5]. Thyroidal radioiodine uptake is increased.

The pattern of thyroid dysfunction is quite different from that seen in renal encapsulation hypertension, and apparently is an independent genetic abnormality. Therapy with thyroxine does not affect the hypertension.

EFFECT OF CHANGE OF THYROID FUNCTION ON EXPERIMENTAL HYPERTENSION

Removal of the thyroid and parathyroid glands of rats markedly decreased hypertension produced by desoxycorticosterone and saline. Blood pressure was apparently measured by a method that reflects only systolic pressure. Cardiac hypertrophy was effectively prevented by the operation, suggesting that the reported decrease in occurrence of hypertension was not an artifact produced by a lower systolic pressure with a maintained diastolic pressure [6]. Replacement of thyroxine alone restored hypertension, suggesting that hypocalcemia was not the cause of the lowered blood pressure. Induced hypothyroidism in the dog did not lower blood pressure, and treatment of post-desoxycorticosterone hypertension with propylthiouracil produced a temporary fall in blood pressure with later return of blood pressure to the initial hypertensive levels in one or two weeks [7].

THYROID FUNCTION AND THE SYMPATHETIC NERVOUS SYSTEM

Clinical hyperthyroidism simulates a state of increased sympathetic function; clinical hypothyroidism simulates a state of decreased thyroid feeding and experimental hypothyroidism is associated with a marked increase in cardiac norepinephrine turnover and biosynthesis. Moreover, plasma norepinephrine is low or normal in hyperthyroid patients and significantly increased in patients with hypothyroidism [8]. Therefore, changes in sympathetic nervous function cannot explain the effects of changes in thyroid function on the development of experimental hypertension.

SUMMARY

Clinical hyperthyroidism is associated with systolic hypertension without any systematic demonstrated effect on diastolic blood pressure. Severe hypothyroidism probably lowers blood pressure in humans. The development of experimental mineralocorticoid hypertension is slowed by hypothyroidism and accelerated by hyperthyroidism. Changes in sympathetic function probably cannot explain the effect of level of thyroid function on the development of hypertension.

ACKNOWLEDGEMENTS

Supported in part by grants NIH-DRR-MO1-RR00626 and NHLBI-1-R01-HL24369.

590

REFERENCES

1. Thompson WO, Dickie LFN, Morris HE, Hilkevitch BH: The high incidence of hypertension in toxic goiter and in mycedema. Endocrinology 15:265–272, 1931.
2. Endo T, Komiya I, Tsukui T, Yamada T, Izumiyama T, Nagata H, Kono S, Kamata K: Re-evaluation of a high possible incidence of hypertension in hypothyroid patients. Am Heart J 98:684–688, 1979.
3. Boone G, Langford HG: Effect of propylthiouracil and ^{13}I on blood pressures of thyrotoxic patients: A retrospective study. S Afr Med J 60:24–25, 1967.
4. Fregly MJ: Modification of thyroid activity during development of experimental renal hypertension in rats. Texas Reports in Biology and Medicine. 29:63–73, 1971.
5. Koizuma Y, Aizawa T, Tawata M, Yamata T, Yamori Y, Okomoto K: Effect of normalization of hypometabolic state on blood pressure in spontaneously hypertensive rats and in patients with essential hypertension. J Am Gen Soc XXIV:454–457, 1976.
6. Salgado E, Green DM: Mechanisms of desoxycorticosterone action XII. Influence of the thyroid. Am J Physiol. 188:519–523, 1957.
7. Green DM, Saunders FJ, Wahlgreen N, Craig RL: Self-sustaining, post-DCA hypertensive cardiovascular disease. AM J Physiol. 170:94, 1952.
8. Landsberg L: Catecholamines and the sympathoadrenal system. In: The Thyroid 5th edn., pp. 791–800. Werner SC, Ingbar SH, eds. New York: Harper & Row, 1978.

38. PARATHYROID FUNCTION AND HYPERTENSION

HERBERT G. LANGFORD and J.C. NAINBY-LUXMOORE

The relationship between parathyroid function and blood pressure is complex. At least four questions must be considered: (1) Are patients with hyperparathyroidism more likely to be hypertensive? (2) If they are hypertensive, is it due to renal damage produced by the disease? (3) Could hypertension affect calcium homeostasis in any manner? (4) How does antihypertensive therapy affect serum calcium, parathyroid function, and urinary calcium excretion? The profound effect that renal failure has on calcium metabolism and renal function must be kept in mind, but will not be discussed at length in this article.

HYPERPARATHYROIDISM AND HYPERTENSION

Two recent reports have compared the mean blood pressure of individuals with hyperparathyroidism and without. Christensson, Hellstrom, and Wengle found that in individuals with hyperparathyroidism blood pressure was 19/9 mm Hg higher than those without hyperparathyroidism [1]. Their data, which was derived from a community screening program, was similar to the results found by Nainby-Luxmoore and Langford et al. in a case-comparison study in hospital [2]. A difference of 12/8 mm Hg was found. The latter investigators found a relative risk of hypertension in the hyperparathyroid patients of 1.7 which was very close to the relative risk of 1.98 which Heath, Hodgson, and Kennedy found, although they used a different definition of hypertension [3]. Nainby-Luxmoore found that the difference in blood pressure persisted even when those with elevated creatinine were removed from the computation or when the elevated creatinine was partialled out by statistical maneuvers. The difference in blood pressure between cases and controls disappeared after surgical correction of the parathyroid abnormality. The authors concluded that the effect of hyperparathyroidism was to shift the blood pressure distribution curve 10 mm Hg to the right and that it was reasonable to expect that successful parathyroid surgery would lower blood pressure on the average by that much. In other words, hyperparathyroidism produces modest blood pressure elevation. Renal damage is not obligatory

Amery, A. (ed.) Hypertensive Cardiovascular Disease: Pathophysiology and Treatment
© *1982, Martinus Nijhoff Publishers. The Hague / Boston / London*
ISBN-13: 978-94-009-7478-4

for hypertension to occur, and the blood pressure elevation may be reversible.

Hypertension associated with hyperparathyroidism seems to be a direct consequence of the stimulating effect of the increased ionized calcium on the arterial and arteriolar vasculature. Sympathetic blockade does not reduce the effect. The direct effect of calcium infusion into the kidney is an increase of sodium excretion, and the direct effect of calcium chloride infusion into the kidney is a decrease of renin secretion. Both of these effects, if quantitatively important, should serve to decrease the hypertensive consequences of elevated serum calcium. The evidence that elevated parathyroid hormone is not the cause of the hypertension is indirect. There is no immediate effect of parathyroid hormone injection on blood pressure. States of calcium depletion which are associated with increased parathyroid hormone levels are not classically associated with hypertension. Calcium elevation from nonparathyroid hormone causes, such as Vitamin D overdosage or malignancy, is associated with hypertension [4].

EFFECT OF HYPERTENSION ON CALCIUM HOMEOSTASIS

McCarron has demonstrated that moderately severe essential hypertension is characterized by slight elevation of the parathyroid hormone level, increased calcium excretion after standardization for sodium excretion, and slightly lower phosphorous [5]. In other words, there appears to be a calcium leak associated with hypertension and compensatory hyperparathyroidism. As the blood pressure goes higher, the leak is more intense. Apparently, this is not due to renal damage in the usual sense because the creatinine levels were actually slightly lower in the hypertensive patients than in the normotensive controls. McCarron postulates that the distal tubule is the site of the abnormality in calcium handling and that the hypertensive patient may be more prone to thiazide-produced hypercalcemia than a normotensive subject. He also implies that the increased prevalence of 'primary' hyperparathyroidism in hypertension is a *consequence* of the calcium leak, presumably with later development of parathyroid autonomy.

EFFECT OF ANTIHYPERTENSIVE THERAPY ON CALCIUM

The administration of thiazide diuretic institutes a complex series of changes which may simulate or unmask hyperparathyroidism. The majority of serum calcium is protein-bound calcium. Therefore, diuretic-produced hemoconcentration directly increases the total serum calcium because protein concentration is increased. In addition, calcium excretion in the urine

DIASTOLIC B.P.

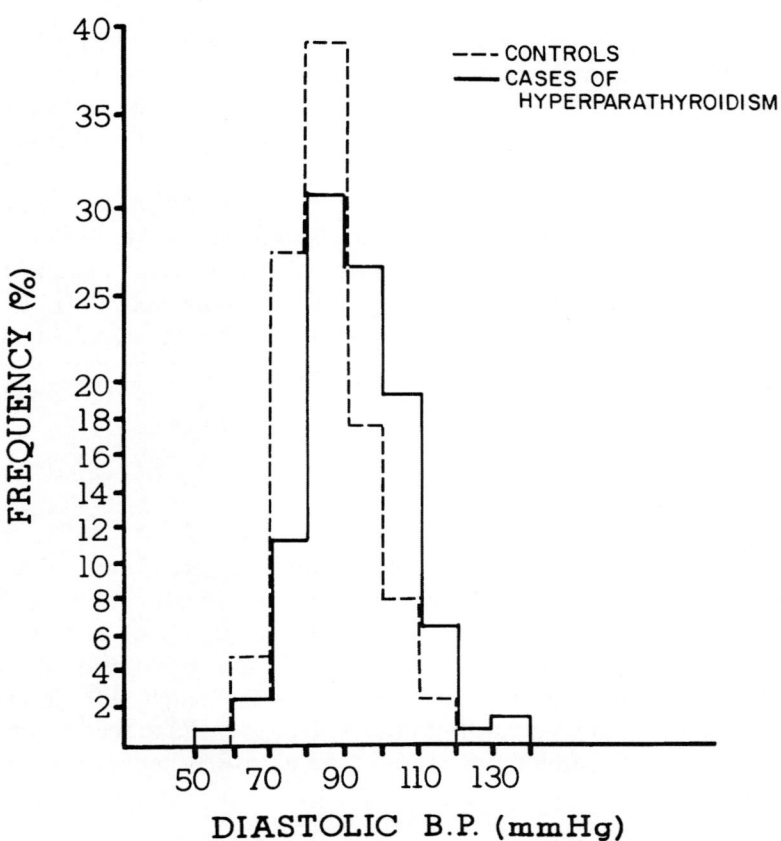

Figure 1. Diastolic pressures of cases and controls. Distribution of 5th phase diastolic blood pressures on admission to hospital of cases of hyperparathyroidism and controls. The blood pressure distribution of the cases is shifted to the right.

falls. This is probably due to the joint action of two mechanisms. The sodium depletion produced by thiazide diuretics increases bulk absorption in the proximal tubule where the majority of filtered calcium is reabsorbed. In addition, thiazide diuretics directly increase the distal reabsorption of calcium. The consequence of the decreased excretion of calcium means that hypercalcemia must surely result, unless there is some change in other aspects of calcium dynamics. It is attractive to think that parathyroid hormone secretion will normally decrease and, as a final result, the gut absorption of calcium will decrease. If this postulated change occurs, it is likely

594

that the compensation is less than perfect. Curb, Langford et al. noted recently that therapy with diazide diuretics was associated with a decrease in serum alkaline phosphatase in post-menopausal women [6]. There is now considerable evidence that these women are in negative calcium balance normally. Therefore, it is quite possible that the positive calcium balance produced by thiazide diuretics causes increased bone mass and therefore less elevation of serum alkaline phosphatase. This hypothesis must remain conjectural at the moment.

The modest elevation of 0.2-0.3 mg/percent serum calcium seen regularly when thiazide diuretics are started usually subsides towards normal with continued therapy. However, some patients will have persistent and increasing calcium elevations. As hyperparathyroidism is more frequent in hypertensive patients than in the rest of the population, these patients must be carefully evaluated and referred for surgery if they are felt to have the disease.

HYPOPARATHYROIDISM

As hyperparathyroidism is associated with modest hypertension, and as elevated serum calcium causes vasoconstriction, one might anticipate that hypoparathyroidism with its associated hypocalcemia would be associated with hypotension. Abrupt decrease in serum calcium by infusion of compounds which complex calcium is known to be associated with decreased myocardial contractility and at times shock. However, there seems to be no systematic study of the blood pressure of the untreated patient with hypoparathyroidism.

ACKNOWLEDGEMENTS

Supported in part by grants NIH-DRR-M01-R00626 and NHLBI-1-R01-HL24369.

REFERENCES

1. Christensson T, Hellstrom J, Wengle B: Blood pressure in subjects with hypercalcemia and primary hyperparathyroidism detected in a health screening programme. Eur J Clin Invest 7:109–113, 1977.
2. Nainby-Luxmoore JC, Langford HG, Nelson NC, Watson RL, Barnes T: A case-comparison study of hypertension and hypertarathyroidism. Clin Res 28:333A, 1980.
3. Heath H, Hodgson SF, Kennedy MD: Primary hyperparathyroidism. N Eng J Med 302:189–193, 1980.

4. Earll JM, Kurtzman NA, Moser RH: Hypercalcemia and hypertension. Ann Intern Med 64:378–381, 1966.
5. McCarron DA, Pingree PA, Rubin RJ, Gauches SM, Molitch M, Krutzik S: Enhanced parathyroid function in essential hypertension: A homeostatic response to a urinary calcium leak. Hypertension 2:162–169, 1980.
6. Curb D, Langford HG, Harrist R, Molteni A, Mastbaum L, Tyroler H, williams W: Effect of age and thiazide diuretics on alkaline phosphatase. Hypertension Detection and Follow-Up Program. Clin Res, 1981 (in press).

39. HYPERTENSION IN PREGNANCY

E. Malcolm Symonds

HYPERTENSION IN PREGNANCY

The most dramatic manifestation of hypertension in pregnancy is the development of eclampsia, the premonitory signs and clinical manifestations of which have been documented in the medical literature since the time of Hippocrates [1]. However, eclampsia represents a very small and extreme section of hypertension in pregnancy and by far the commonest situation is the development of mild hypertension, with or without the presence of proteinuria, in the third trimester of pregnancy. In its severe forms, hypertension in pregnancy is associated with a significant risk to maternal and foetal life. In its mildest form, arising in late pregnancy for the first time, hypertension appears to be associated with no significant maternal hazard and improved foetal growth and survival [2, 3].

Classification

Numerous attempts have been made to classify hypertension in pregnancy and none of them are entirely satisfactory because most claim a precision in diagnosis that is not justifiable. For example, the Committee on Terminology of the American Committee on Maternal Welfare have classified hypertension in pregnancy as:
A) the disease peculiar to pregnancy
  1) Pre-eclampsia
  2) Eclampsia
B) diseases independent of pregnancy
C) pre-eclampsia or eclampsia superimposed upon chronic hypertension
D) transient hypertension
E) unclassified hypertensive disorders.
Pre-eclampsia has been defined as development of hypertension during pregnancy associated with either oedema or proteinuria. In fact, the grouping of oedema with proteinuria is spurious as oedema is so common in pregnancy that it has virtually no measurable significance whereas the appearance of proteinuria has the gravest prognostic signifcance for both mother and child.

Amery, A. (ed.) Hypertensive Cardiovascular Disease: Pathophysiology and Treatment
© *1982, Martinus Nijhoff Publishers. The Hague / Boston / London*
ISBN-13: 978-94-009-7478-4

The inclusion of a classification of transient hypertension in this context is meaningless as all hypertension associated with pregnancy is transient. There is no proven temporal line that allows a sub-classification of this type. In addition, the term pre-eclampsia is gradually being abandoned and being replaced by pregnancy-induced hypertension.

Thus, the common form of hypertension in pregnancy arises during pregnancy in a previously normotensive woman, and is known as pregnancy-induced hypertension or gestational hypertension. This group should simply be divided into those women who develop hypertension alone and those who also develop proteinuria with or without fits.

The only other group is those patients where the hypertension predates and is complicated by pregnancy and where the condition may be further worsened by the superimposition of pregnancy-induced hypertension and proteinuria.

The term hypertension in this context is defined as the occurrence of a sustained systolic pressure of 140 mm Hg or more and a sustained diastolic pressure of 90 mm Hg or more. A rise of 30 mm Hg or more in systolic pressure and 15 mm Hg or more in diastolic pressure is also considered significant on the basis that a lower starting pressure leads to greater significance to a relative rise in blood pressure. In practice, the differences in maternal or foetal mortality in pressures below 140/90 is insignificant and it is therefore preferable to adhere to a definition of hypertension based on the occurrence of a blood pressure of 140/90 on two or more occasions within 6 h. Page and Christianson [4] have suggested that mean arterial pressure should be used but this has not received general recognition. It would have much to commend it and would have the advantage of simplicity without loss of risk definition.

Incidence

It is about impossible to present a cohesive statement on the incidence of pregnancy-induced hypertension. The condition shows a markedly variable incidence in relation to race and geography, but has also shown remarkable changes in relation to time. Figures published over two decades ago are almost certainly no longer relevant. Furthermore, comparisons are often extremely difficult as diagnostic criteria often vary with different studies. MacGillivray [5] reviewed incidence figures in the United Kingdom in 1961 and reported an incidence of proteinuric hypertensive disease varying from 2.9% in London to 4.1% in Scotland. At the Nottingham City Hospital, figures over the last five years show an incidence of 12-17% for hypertension alone and 3-8% of these women develop proteinuric hypertension [2] so that by far the commonest problem is the management of mild forms of hypertension with or without oedema but without proteinuria.

598

Pathogenesis

No single factor can adequately explain the mechanism for the development of hypertension during pregnancy, but it seems likely that a series of factors may act as a triggering mechanism. The two central features that characterise pregnancy-induced hypertension are arteriolar vasospasm and disseminated intravascular coagulation and the acute pathological manifestations in the kidney and uteroplacental bed are a direct consequence of these changes. There is considerable debate as to whether the vasospasm precedes the coagulation changes or whether the primary mechanism is initiated through intravascular fibrin deposition. Page [6] has suggested that a circle of events occurs whereby vasospasm in the uterine vasculature results in the release of trophoblastic material into the maternal circulation. This material is rich in thromboplastins which precipitate intravascular coagulation and hence the changes in renal function and in the retention of sodium and water with increasing vascular sensitivity to angiotensin II and worsening of the vasospasm. Page also suggests that a variety of external factors may tend to accelerate this process. The aetiology of the vasospasm is therefore central to the mechanism of pregnancy-induced hypertension and further consideration will be given to this phenomenon. A modification of the sequence of events suggested by Page is shown in Figure 1.

Arteriolar vasospasm

There is considerable evidence to suggest that there is a humoral factor responsible for the vascular changes in pregnancy-induced hypertension.

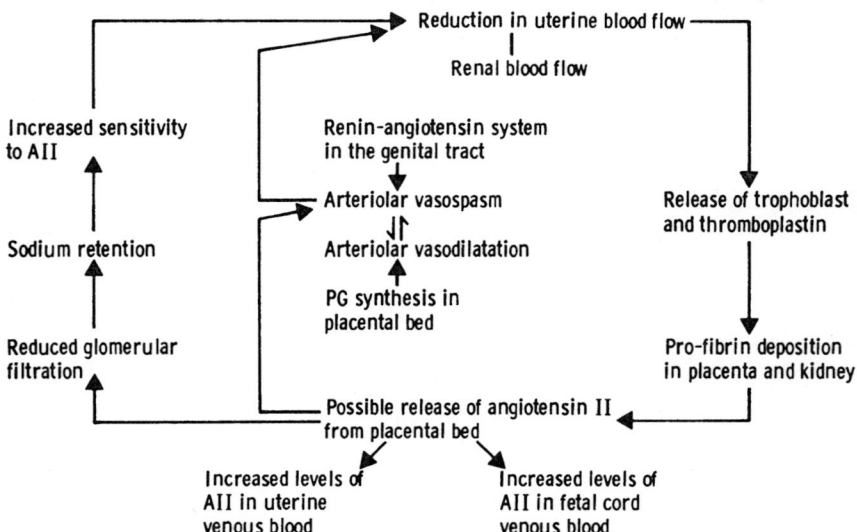

Figure 1. Modification of the 'inner vicious circle' of events described by Page [6].

Various pressor peptides have been investigated and vascular responses have been shown to vary markedly. Zuspan, Nelson and Ahlquist [7] demonstrated an increased sensitivity to epinephrine in pre-eclamptic women and Talledo, Chesley and Zuspan [8] demonstrated similar changes with infusions of norepinephrine but did not show any differences in response between normal pregnant and non-pregnant females. Chesley and Valenti [9] also demonstrated enhanced responses to vasopressin in women with pregnancy-induced hypertension.

THE RENIN-ANGIOTENSIN SYSTEM

The renin–angiotensin system has been of particular interest in this respect, partly as a result of the changes that occur in vascular sensitivity in pregnancy and partly because renin is produced both in the kidney and in the genital tract. Talledo et al. [10] showed that vascular response to angiotensin II was markedly impaired in normal pregnancy. Gant et al. [11] have shown not only that sensitivity increases in women who develop pre-eclampsia, but also that the increased sensitivity predates the actual onset of hypertension.

Plasma renin activity and plasma renin concentration show a marked increase in normal pregnancy [12–15] and a high percentage of renin (70 %) [16] in early pregnancy is in the inactive or acid-activated form. Nearly all published data have shown that plasma renin activity and plasma renin concentration are suppressed in women with pregnancy induced hypertension [17–19]. However, there is evidence of a positive correlation between blood pressure and angiotensin II [20], and similarly high levels have been demonstrated in cord venous blood of infants born to mothers with pregnancy-induced hypertension. Any theory that seeks to explain the role of the renin–angiotensin system in pregnancy hypertension must take into account the mechanism by which vascular sensitivity is altered, and recently it has been suggested that prostaglandins may play an important role in mediating these effects [22]. O'Brien et al. [23] have shown in pregnant rabbits that infusion in PGE_2 produces a marked reduction in sensitivity to infused angiotensin II. Furthermore, dietary deprivation of essential fatty acids [24] has been shown to induce a state of hypersensitivity. There is evidence to suggest that infused angiotensin II stimulates the release of PGE_2 in the uteroplacental bed, thus stimulating local vasodilatation and that this effect can be blocked by the infusion of saralasine [25]. Thus, the inability of the placenta to produce local vasodilator prostaglandins would result in vasoconstriction and elevated blood pressure. Similar changes would almost certainly show a similar pathogenesis in the kidney.

Coagulation changes

In 1893, Schmorl [26] first recorded the presence of thrombosis in the small blood vessels of women dying from eclampsia. This phenomenon was extensively investigated in the 1950s by MacKay [27] and since then a great deal of research has been directed towards further understanding the condition. Chesley [28] has pointed out that signs of consumptive coagulopathy are not likely to be detected in mild cases of pre-eclampsia because the factors consumed will be replaced at a comparable rate and equilibrium will be re-established.

In general terms, significant changes in clotting factors have not been identified and measurement of fibrinogen levels in eclampsia [29] have not shown any consistent or significant reduction. However, decreased platelet counts are an important feature of the disease and have been identified by many authorities. There is also evidence of increased fibrinolysis as demonstrated by the presence of fibrin degradation products. However, many women with severe pre-eclampsia [30] fail to show any evidence of abnormal levels of FDPs. It should be emphasised that not all pathologists believe that capillary thrombosis is an important feature of eclampsia and Sheehan and Lynch [31] found renal fibrin thrombi to be rare in fatal cases of eclampsia. Fibrin deposition in the placenta occurs in normal pregnancy, and this process appears to be exaggerated in pre-eclampsia [32] with intervillous thromboses and increased deposits on the villi.

It has been suggested that the process of disseminated intravascular coagulation may be initiated by the release of trophoblastic tissue rich in thromboplastin from the uteroplacental bed into the general circulation [33]. It is also possible that thromboplastin may arise from platelets as in the Schwartzman reaction [34] and this hypothesis is supported to some degree by the evidence of thrombocytopenia in severe pre-eclampsia.

Immunologic factors

Normal pregnancy constitutes an allogeneic graft and it is perhaps not surprising that the possibility of antigen–antibody reaction as the cause of placental damage, and hence preeclampsia, has been under consideration for the last eighty years. Nevertheless, the situation still remains uncertain. Chesley [35] has suggested that major potential antigenic differences may occur between ABO and Rh blood group antigens, HLA antigens and tissue antigens of the placenta. With the exception of severe rhesus iso-immunisation, there is no evidence to support any relationship between blood groups and pregnancy hypertension. Carrette et al. [36] demonstrated anti-HLA antibodies with increased frequency in women with pre-eclampsia, although the findings in other studies have been variable [37].

Conflicting studies have been published on complement and levels of IgG and IgM, some workers demonstrating reduced levels in eclampsia [38] whilst others have found no difference [39]. Similar discrepancies have emerged in studies on complement in the kidney. Studies on renal biopsy material obtained from women with severe pre-eclampsia have shown evidence of IgG and IgM in the glomeruli [40] with occasional complement, although Spargo and his co-workers [41] found only occasional evidence of these globulins and complement in patients with classical features of glomerular capillary endotheliosis.

Pathology

It is not possible to describe all the pathological changes in a review of this size. Nevertheless, some general points need discussion because they relate in general to the relevance and nature of therapy. It must be remembered that with the possible exception of the placenta, nearly all the morphological characteristics described in the literature relate to the severe form of the disease. Where it is possible to obtain tissue in cases other than autopsy material, there is little evidence of histological change. This particularly applies to the kidney where the characteristic lesions only appear where there has been clinical evidence ofproteinuria.

Cerebral haemorrhage is now the commonest cause of death in severe pre-eclampsia and eclampsia. The brain does not exhibit any evidence of oedema and the findings may vary from those of small cortical petechiae to massive haemorrhage in the basal ganglia and pons with occasional intraventricular extension.

The characteristic features in the kidney include swelling of the glomerular tuft, swelling of the endothelial/mesangial cells, the appearance of electron-dense material under the basement membrane of the glomerular capillary, and vacuolation of epithelial cells. Renal failure may occur from either cortical or tubular necrosis in the advanced stages of the disease.

The common hepatic lesions are the presence of periportal haemorrhage and infarction which probably results from intense arteriolar spasm.

It must be emphasised that all these lesions represent one end of the spectrum, and are not relevant to the common problem of mild pregnancy-induced hypertension.

Management

In the absence of any clear understanding of the cause of pregnancy-induced hypertension, a logical approach to therapy remains difficult.

602

Chesley [42] has reviewed the incredible range of lethal forms of treatment that have been inflicted on women with eclampsia ranging from renal decapsulation to post-partum curettage and oophorectomy.

Certain basic guide-lines can be proposed which are based on the known pathology of the particular form of hypertension. In general terms, there are three major divisions in relation to therapy:

1) the management of mild hypertension arising during pregnancy and uncomplicated by proteinuria
2) the management of severe hypertension and proteinuria occasionally progressing to eclampsia
3) the management of pregnancy complicating pre-existent forms of hypertension and sometimes additionally complicated by superadded pregnancy-induced hypertension.

The management of mild pregnancy-induced hypertension

The commonest problem facing obstetricians in Western European countries is the management of mild hypertension arising in late pregnancy sometimes accompanied by oedema but rarely by proteinuria. The problem has considerable importance as it represents the commonest reason for hospital admission to antenatal wards. The management still practised is based on the observations of Hamlin [43] that eclampsia could be prevented by the strict enforcement of a policy of early hospital admission for mild hypertension. Such a policy has advantages as it enables careful scrutiny of maternal blood pressure and proteinuria. It also enables careful monitoring of foetal welfare with the use of serial placental function tests, serial ultra-

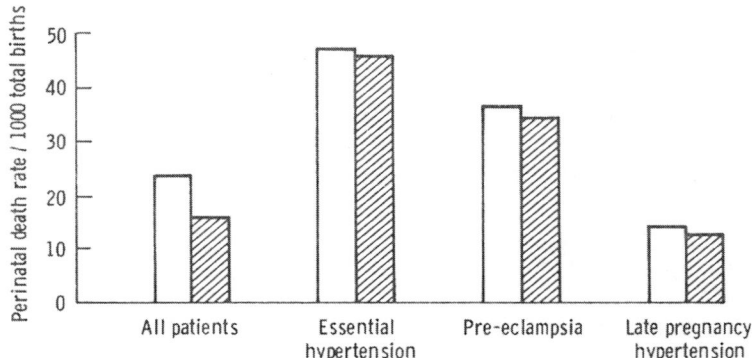

Figure 2. Perinatal death rates in different forms of hypertension in pregnancy. Open lines represent uncorrected perinatal death rates. Hatched lines represent corrected perinatal death rates. From Clinch J, J Ir Med Assoc 73:348, 1980.

sonograms and non-stressed cardiotocography. Appropriately timed intervention and induction of labour completes the cycle of management.

Nevertheless, it is appropriate at this time to begin to question the current dogma surrounding this type of management. It is both socially disruptive and associated with the potential hazards of prolonged immobilisation. It may also lead to unnecessary induction of labour when the patience of the mother and the obstetrician wear thin. Recent publications on the mild form of pregnancy-induced hypertension [3] (Figure 2) suggest not only that perinatal mortality rates are not elevated, but also that the rate is significantly reduced below overall hospital rates. These figures represent a biased population as they apply to a group where gestational age has been selected in favour of foetal survival. The question arises as to whether the current programme produces the excellent results associated with mild hypertension or whether mild hypertension carries positive benefits to the foetus.

A recent randomised study of home management [44] based on self-assessment of proteinuria has suggested that comparable results can be obtained at home as compared with hospital management provided admission was arranged with the appearance of proteinuria or severe hypertension. Current studies in Nottingham with self-assessment of blood pressure suggest that, on the condition that additional supervision is provided in the home, it may be possible to maintain a high degree of safety with home management, but careful scrutiny of this approach will be necessary if serious sequelae are to be avoided. The development of proteinuria and hyperuricaemia herald a significant change in prognosis for both mother and foetus and in the presence of worsening hypertension, constitutes an indication for induction of labour.

Sedatives and tranquillisers

For many years barbiturates were employed for sedation of mothers admitted to hospital with hypertension. The justification for this therapy was always dubious and it probably served only to reduce the patient's mobility. These drugs have no specific effect in lowering blood pressure and, at best, are weak anticonvulsants. The most widely used tranquilliser used in the United Kingdom is diazepam [45] and this drug is administered principally for its anticonvulsant action as it has no direct effect on blood pressure. Yet, it must be remembered that this drug also has significant effects on the foetus. Both diazepam and its metabolite desmethyldiazepam are metabolically active and cross the placental barrier. Accumulation of these compounds in the foetus results in hypotonia and hypothermia. Provided one is aware of these problems, there appears to be no long-term hazard for the infant. However, unless there is evidence of hyperreflexia or imminent evidence of fitting, it is doubtful that diazepam has any useful role in mild pregnancy-induced hypertension.

Diuretics

Hypertension as a result of pregnancy is uncommon in that it is character-ised in its severe form by hypovolaemia. There seems little doubt that the reduction in glomerular filtration results in a reduced sodium clearance but this does not result in an expansion of plasma volume. On this basis, the use of thiazide diuretics seems unlikely to provide any great benefit and may further reduce plasma volume. In addition, there is no conclusive evidence that increased sensitivity to angiotensin II is mediated by increased sodium content in the maternal arteriolar walls. Campbell and MacGillivray [46] have shown that prolonged use of diuretics is associated with lower birth weight infants. Furthermore, there is no convincing evidence that prophy-lactic use of diuretics reduced the incidence of the development of hyper-tension and proteinuria.

The main role of diuretics in pregnancy lies in the management of essen-tial hypertension and the relief of symptomatic oedema.

Antihypertensive drugs

As previously mentioned, the results of conservative management of preg-nancy-induced hypertension are generally satisfactory. Thus, to prove a spe-cific benefit of antihypertensive therapy, it will be necessary to prove that any benefits to the mother or foetus will outweigh any deterimental effects that may result from the drug. A wide range of drugs have been used in pregnancy and many have been abandoned because of serious side-effects on the foetus. Methyldopa is the drug most widely used in pregnancy at the present time. Studies by Redman et al. [47] have demonstrated a reduction in mid-trimester abortion and perinatal loss in women treated for mild pregnancy-induced hypertension with methyldopa. The drug does not ap-pear to reduce the incidence of subsequent proteinuria. The drug has signif-icant maternal side-effects and for this reason is sometimes rejected by the mother.

β-adrenergic blockers

The use of β-blockers in pregnancy has been approached with considerable caution in view of early observations [48] that propranolol might interfere with the ability of the foetal heart to adapt its rate to hypoxic stress. Retrospective studies of the use of propanolol [49] in pregnancy certainly suggested an adverse outcome for the foetus, although subjects being compared on differing therapies were also suffering from different forms of hypertension. A historical non-concurrent study on 25 women with essential hypertension [50] did show evidence of a marked improvement in perinatal outcome in these women after their blood pressures were controlled with propranolol. However, this is a different question from whether these drugs are beneficial in the management of pregnancy-induced hypertension. Gallery et al. [51] randomly allocated 53 women, the majority of whom had developed hypertension during the course of pregnancy, to treatment with either oxprenolol or methyldopa. There were no still births in either group and 2 neonatal deaths in the methyldopa group. However, the interesting finding in this study was the significantly higher birth weight in the oxprenolol group. There was no significant difference in gestational ages at birth. It has been suggested that these differences may be due to an expansion of plasma volume in the oxprenolol-treated group with a consequent improvement in uteroplacental perfusion.

A further study [52] using a combination of propranolol and hydralazine has also been reported in essential hypertension in pregnancy with apparent beneficial effects to the foetus. More recently, a randomised study comparing the combined α- and β-blocker, labetalol, has shown a favourable outcome in the labetalol group [53], and this study included only patients with pregnancy-induced hypertension. Thus, at the present time, the evidence available points to certain advantages to using β-blockers in hypertension in pregnancy with the one possible exception of hypertension secondary to underlying primary renal disease.

The management of severe hypertension proteinuria in pregnancy

The management of severe pre-eclampsia and eclampsia presents a medical emergency which necessitates prompt and efficient treatment if maternal and foetal deaths are to be avoided. The three essential guide-lines in management are:
1) control the convulsions
2) control the blood pressure
3) deliver the patient.

Control of convulsions

For many years, magnesium sulphate has been extensively used for the treatment of eclampsia and the recent reports from Pritchard [54] from a large series of eclamptics have shown excellent results for both mother and foetus. The drug regime recommended by Pritchard includes an initial intra-venous injection of 4 g of magnesium sulphate followed by an intramuscular injection of 10 g with 4-hourly injections of 5 g according to the state of consciousness on the serum levels of magnesium. The exact mechanism of action remains uncertain, although recent studies [55] on the effect of mag-nesium ions on thrombus formation in vivo suggest that at least part of its action may be due to the ability of extracellular Mg^{2+} to reduce platelet aggregation.

Magnesium sulphate is not used extensively in the United Kingdom and convulsions are usually controlled with diazepam given by intravenous and intramuscular injection [45]. The use of chlormethiazole by intravenous infusion is advocated by some authors [56], but the administration of the drug requires careful supervision and strict attention to maintenance of the patient's airway.

Control of blood pressure

The emergency control of a hypertensive crisis is best achieved with the intravenous infusion of hydrallazine. Any drug used to lower blood pressure should not jeopardise uterine blood flow and on this basis, there is animal evidence [57] to show that, whereas drugs such as diazoxide will lower blood pressure at the expense of reducing uterine blood flow, hydralazine lowers blood pressure but tends to increase uterine blood flow at the same time. Acute control of blood pressure can also be achieved with the intravenous administration of labetalol [53] although the control is often short-lived as a rebound hypertension tends to follow the initial period of control.

Anticoagulant therapy

In view of the changes that occur in the haematological system, it has been suggested that the use of heparin in severe pre-eclampsia may arrest the process of intravascular coagulation and thrombocytopenia. In fact, none of the studies performed with heparin [58, 59] have shown any evidence of improvement in the condition even when the haematological changes have been corrected and it would seem that magnesium sulphate is much safer in this situation.

The management of essential hypertension in pregnancy

There is general agreement that the control of blood pressure from early in pregnancy is an important ingredient of management and of minimising perinatal losses. Studies with methyldopa [60, 61] have shown that perinatal survival is enhanced by early and adequate control of blood pressure and, as previously mentioned, similar benefits appear to result from the use of propanolol [50] either alone or in combination with hydralazine [52]. Control may be enhanced where a diuretic is used in this situation, although Chesley [62] suggests that the antihypertensive drug should be changed to methyldopa or hydralazine and diuretics discontinued.

There is significantly greater risk that women with essential hypertension in pregnancy will develop superadded pre-eclampsia and this carries an increased risk for the foetus. There is no evidence to suggest that pregnancy has any significant effect on the long-term prognosis of essential hypertension.

Chronic renal disease and hypertension

The association of chronic glomeronephritis and pregnancy does not appear to carry a significantly worse prognosis for the foetus except where the condition is complicated by hypertension [63]. Under these circumstances the perinatal loss is as high as 45% and the outlook is generally poor even with antihypertensive therapy. As previously suggested, this is one situation where β-blockers may be contra-indicated, although, as the complication is reasonably rare, no randomised study has been performed in this situation. Chronic interstitial nephritis is often associated with severe hypertension and foetal prognosis is once again largely determined by the level of the blood pressure. The results reported by Felding [64] suggest that perinatal loss is not significantly increased above the normal pregnancy levels where the pregnancy is uncomplicated by hypertension and, although there is insufficient information available to assess the effect of blood pressure control in this situation, it seems reasonable to assume that adequate control will result in improved prognosis for the foetus.

Renal involvement in lupus erythmatosis carries a poor prognosis for the foetus but is not commonly associated with hypertension [65], and in this case the hypertension does not appear to be a major determinant in prognosis.

CONCLUSIONS

Hypertension arising during pregnancy is the commonest antenatal complication facing clinicians at the present time.

Mild forms of hypertension uncomplicated by proteinuria appear to carry a beneficial prognosis for the foetus but this situation alters dramatically with the development of proteinuria.

608

The pathogenesis of the condition results from a complex series of changes which are interrelated and which are dependent on the balance between vasopressor and vasodilator effects associated with the regulation of blood pressure.

Active drug therapy appears to significantly improve perinatal outcome in chronic hypertensive disease and there is evidence to suggest that similar beneficial effects will result from the use of antihypertensive drugs in hypertension arising during pregnancy.

REFERENCES

1. The Medical Works of Hippocrates. Translated by Adams F, p. 715. London: The Sydenham Society, 1849.
2. Symonds EM: Hypertension in pregnancy. In: Recent Advances in Obstetrics and Gynaecology, p. 167. Stallworthy j, Bourne G, eds. Edinburgh: Churchill Livingstone, 1979.
3. Clinch J: Late pregnancy hypertension – a harmless condition. J Ir Med Assoc 73:348, 1980.
4. Page EW, Christianson R: The impact of mean arterial pressure in the middle trimester upon the outcome of pregnancy. Am J Obstet Gynecol 125:740–745, 1976.
5. MacGillivray I: Pre-eclampsia in Great Britain and Ireland. Pathol Microbiol 24:504, 1981.
6. Page EW: On the pathogenesis of pre-eclampsia and eclampsia. J Obstet Gynaecol Br Commonw 79:863–894, 1972.
7. Zuspan FP, Nelson GH, Ahelquist RP: Epinephrine infusions in normal and toxemic pregnancy – I. Nonesterified fatty acids and cardiovascular alterations. Am J Obstet Gynecol 90:88–96, 1964.
8. Talledo OE, Chesley LC, Zuspan FP: Renin–angiotensin system in normal and toxemic pregnancies – III. Differential sensitivity to angiotensin II and norepinephrine in toxemia of pregnancy. Am J Obstet Gynecol 100:218–221, 1968.
9. Chesley LC, Valenti C: The evaluation of tests to differentiate pre-eclampsia from hypertensive disease. Am J Obstet Gynecol 75:1165–1173, 1958.
10. Talledo OE: Renin–angiotensin system in normal and toxemic pregnancies – I. Angiotensin infusion test. Am J Obstet Gynecol 96:141–143, 1966.
11. Gant NF, Daly GL, Chand S, Whalley PJ, MacDonald PC: A study of angiotensin II pressor response throughout primigravid pregnancy. J Clin Invest 52:2682–2689, 1973.
12. Weir RJ, Brown JJ, Fraser R et al.: Relationship between plasma renin, renin-substrate, angiotensin II, aldosterone and electrolytes in normal pregnancy. J Clin Endocrinal Metab 40:108, 1975.
13. Skinner SL, Lumbers ER, Symonds EM: Analysis of changes in the renin–angiotensin system during pregnancy. Clin Sci 42:479, 1972.
14. Gordon RD, Symonds EM, Wilmshurst EG, Pawsey CGK: Plasma renin activity, plasma angiotensin and plasma and urinary electrolytes in normal and toxaemic pregnancy including a prospective study. Clin Sci Mol Med 45:115, 1973.
15. Lammintausta R, Erkkola R: Renin–angiotensin aldosterone system and sodium in normal pregnancy. A Longitudinal study. Acta Obstet Gynecol Scand 56:221, 1977.
16. Skinner SL, Cran EJ, Gibson R et al.: Angiotensins I and II, active and inactive renin, renin substrate, renin activity and angiotensinase in human liquor amnii and plasma. Am J Obstet Gynecol 121:626, 1975.
17. Symonds EM, Andersen GJ: The effect of bed rest on plasma renin in hypertensive disease of pregnancy. J Obstet Gynaecol Br Commonw 81:676, 1974.

18. Weir RJ, Brown JJ, Fraser R et al.: Plasma renin, renin-substrate, angiotensin II and aldosterone in hypertensive disease of pregnancy. Lancet 1:291, 1973.

19. Kokot F, Cekanski A: Plasma renin activity in peripheral and uterine vein blood in pregnant and non-pregnant women. J Obstet gynaecol Br Commonw 79:72, 1972.

20. Symonds EM, Broughton Pipkin F, Craven DJ: Changes in the renin–angiotensin system in primigravidae with hypertensive disease of pregnancy. Br J Obstet Gynaecol 82:643, 1975.

21. Broughton Pipkin F, Symonds EM: Angiotensin II and the placenta in normal pregnancy and pregnancy complicated by hypertension. J Physiol 256:121, 1975.

22. Speroff L, Dorfman GS: Prostaglandins and pregnancy hypertension. Clin Obstet Gynaecol 4:635. London: Saunders, 1977.

23. O'Brien PMS, Filshie GM, Broughton Pipkin F: The effect of Prostaglandin E2 on the cardiovascular response to angiotensin II in pregnant rabbits. Prostaglandins 113:171, 1977.

24. O'Brien PMS, Broughton Pipkin F: The effects of deprivation of prostaglandin precursors on vascular sensitivity to angiotensin II and on the kidney in the pregnant rabbit. Br J Pharmacol 65:29, 1979.

25. Speroff L: An autoregulatory role for prostaglandins in placental hemodynamics. Their possible influence on blood pressure in pregnancy. J Reprod Med 15:181, 1975.

26. Schmorl G: Pathologisch-anatomische Untersuchungen über Puerperal-Eklampsie. Leipzig: Vogel, 1893.

27. McKay DG, Merrill SJ, Weiner AE, Hertig AT, Reid DE: The pathologic anatomy of eclampsia, bilateral renal cortical necrosis, pituitary necrosis and other acute fatal complications of pregnancy, and its possible relation to the generalised Schwartzman phenomenon. Am J Obstet Gynecol 66:507, 1953.

28. Chesley LC: In: Hypertensive Disorders in Pregnancy, p. 105. New York: Appleton-Century-Crofts, 1978.

29. Pritchard JA, Cunningham FG, Mason RA: Coagulation changes in eclampsia: their frequency and pathogenesis. Am J Obstet Gynecol 124:855, 1976.

30. Hyde E, Joyce D, Gurewich V, Flute PT, Barrera S: Intravascular coagulation during pregnancy and the puerperium. J Obstet Gynaecol Br Commonw 80:1059, 1973.

31. Sheehan HL, Lynch JB: In: Pathology of Toxaemia of Pregnancy. London: Churchill Livingstone, 1973.

32. McKay DG: Clinical significance of the pathology of toxaemia of pregnancy. Circulation 30 (Suppl 2):66–75, 1964.

33. Jaameri KEU, Koivuniemi AP, Carpen EO: Occurence of trophoblasts in the blood of toxaemic patients. Gynaecologia 160:315, 1965.

34. McKay DG, Goldenberg V, Kaunitz H, Csavossy I: Experimental eclampsia: an electron microscope study and review. Arch Pathol 84:1557, 1967,

35. Chesley LC: In: Hypertensive disorders in Pregnancy, p. 467. New York: Appleton-Century-Crofts, 1978.

36. Carretti N, Chiaramonte P, Pasini C, Zanetti M, Fagiolo U: Association of anti-HL-A antibodies with toxemia in pregnancy. In: First International Symposium on Immunology in Obstetrics and Gynaecology, Amsterdam, p. 221. Centaro A, Carretti N, eds. Amsterdam: Excerpta Medica, 1974.

37. Scott JR, Beer AE, Stastny P: Immunogenetic factors in pre-eclampsia and eclampsia. Erythrocyte, histocompatibility and Y-dependent antigens. JAMA 235:402, 1976.

38. Yang SL, Kleinman AM, Wei PJ: Immunologic aspects of term pregnancy toxemia: study of immunoglobulins and complement. Am J Obstet Gynecol 122:727, 1975.

39. Burdash NM, Blake JM Jr, Hester LI Jr: Immunoglobulin levels and liver function tests in normal and toxemic pregnancies. Am J Obstet Gynecol 116:827, 1973.

40. Petrucco OM, Thomson NM, Lawrence JR, Weldon MW: Immunofluorescent studies in renal biopsies in pre-eclampsia. Br Med J 473, 1974.
41. Spargo BH, Lichtig C, Luger AM, Katz AI, Lindheimer MD: The renal lesion in pre-eclampsia: examination by light and electron and immunofluorescence microscopy. In: Hypertension in Pregnancy, p. 129. Lindheimer MD, Katz AI, Zuspan FP, eds. New York: J. Willey & Sons, 1976.
42. Chesley LC: In: Hypertensive Disorders in Pregnancy, p. 309. New York: Appleton-Century-Crofts, 1978.
43. Hamlin RHJ: The prevention of eclampsia and pre-eclampsia. Lancet 1:64, 1952.
44. Matthews DD: A randomized controlled trial of bed rest and sedation on normal activity and non-sedation in the management of non-albuminuric hypertension in late pregnancy. Brit J Obstet Gynaecol 84:108, 1977.
45. Chamberlain GVP, Lewis PJ, De Swiet M, Bulfitt CJ: How obstetricians manage hypertension in pregnancy. Brit Med J 1:626, 1978.
46. Campbell DM, MacGillivray I: The effect of a low calorie diet or a thiazide diuretic on the incidence of pre-eclampsia and on low birth weight. Br J Obstet Gynaecol 82:572, 1975.
47. Redman CWG, Beilin LJ, Bonnar J: Fetal outcome in trial of antihypertensive treatment in pregnancy. Lancet 2:753, 1976.
48. Rudolph AN, Heyman MA: Foetal and Neonatal Physiology. Rudolph AN, Heyman MA, eds. Cambridge: Cambridge University Press, 1973.
49. Lieberman BA, Stirrat GM, Cohen SL, Beard RW, Pinker GD, Selsey E: The possible adverse effects of propanalol on the foetus in pregnancies complicated by severe hypertension. Br J Obstet Gynaecol 85:678, 1978.
50. Eliahou HE, Silverberg DS, Reisin E, Romem J, Mashiachi S, Serr DM: Propanalol for the treatment of hypertension in pregnancy. Br J Obstet Gynaecol 85:431, 1978.
51. Gallery EDM, Saunders DM, Hungor SN, Gyory AZ: Randomised comparison of methyl dopa and oxprenolol for the treatment of hypertension in pregnancy. Br Med J 1:1591, 1979.
52. Bott-Kanner G, Schweitzner A, Reisner SH, Joel-Cohen SJ, Rosenfeld JB: Propanolol and hydrallazine in the management of essential hypertension in pregnancy. Br J Obstet Gynaecol 87:110, 1980.
53. Lamming GD, Broughton Pipkin F, Symonds EM: Comparison of the alpha and beta blocking drug labetalol and methyl dopa in the treatment of moderate and severe pregnancy-induced hypertension. Clin Exp Hypertension 2:865, 1980.
54. Pritchard ja: Standardised treatment of 154 consecutive cases of eclampsia. Am J Obstet Gynecol 123:543, 1975.
55. Adams JH, Mitchell JRA: The effect of agents which modify platelet behaviour and of magnesium ions on thrombus formation in vivo. Thromb Haemostas 42:603, 1979.
56. Duffus GM, Tunstall ME, Condie RG, MacGillivray I: Chlormethiazole in the prevention of eclampsia and the reduction of perinatal mortality. J Obstet Gynaecol Br Commonw 76:645, 1969.
57. Brinkman CR, Assali NS: Uteroplacental hemodynamic response to antihypertensive drugs in hypertensive pregnant sheep. In: Hypertension in Pregnancy. p. 363. Lindheimer MD, Katz AI, Zuspan FP, eds. New York: J Wiley & Sons, 1976.
58. Bonnar J: Coagulation disorders. J Clin Path 29 (Suppl 10): 35, 1976.
59. Howie PW, Prentice CRM, McNicol GP: Failure of heparin therapy to affect the clinical course of severe pre-eclampsia. Br J Obstet Gynaecol 82:711, 1975.
60. Kincaid-Smith P, Bullen M, Mills J: Prolonged use of methyl dopa in severe hypertension in pregnancy. Br Med J 1:274, 1966.
61. Leather HM, Humphreys DM, Baker P, Chadd MA: A controlled trial of hypertensive agents in hypertension in pregnancy. Lancet 2:488, 1968.

62. Chesley LC. In: Hypertensive Disorders in pregnancy, p. 482. New York: Appleton-Century-Crofts, 1978.
63. Ferris TF: Renal disease. In: Medical Complications during Pregnancy, p. 20. Burrow GN, Ferris TF, eds. Philadelphia: Saunders, 1975.
64. Felding C: Obstetric aspects in women with histories of renal disease. Acta Obstet Gynecol Scand 48 (Suppl 2):1, 1969.
65. Budman DR, Steinberg Ad: Hypertension and renal disease in systemic lupus erythematosis. Arch Intern Med 136:1003, 1976.

40. HYPERTENSION SECONDARY TO CONTRACEPTIVE AGENTS

R. J. WEIR

Agents used to prevent conception are generally of five main types:
1) mechanical barriers, e.g. sheaths and cervical diaphragms.
2) intra-uterine devices; these may be inert plastic, or contain a metal such as copper, or be impregnated with a hormone such as progesterone.
3) spermicidal creams, jelly or paste.
4) oral hormonal steroids; in combinations or as single hormones.
5) intra-muscular long acting hormonal steroids.

There is no evidence that mechanical barrier methods, spermicides or IUDs influence blood pressure in any way, and these methods will not be discussed further.

TYPES OF ORAL AND I-M CONTRACEPTIVE AGENTS

1. Combined oestrogen – progestagen oral contraceptives

The mechanism of action of the combined oestrogen-progestagen pill is mainly one of suppression of ovulation, with effects also on endometrium cervical mucus and ovary. They are taken for the first 21 days of each menstrual cycle, and have the highest contraceptive effect of any agent, with a failure rate of about 0.1 per 100 women years. Two oestrogens are used, either ethinyloestradiol or its 3-methyl-ether, mestranol. The progestagens used are derived from 19-nortestosterone (norethynodrel, norethisterone, ethynodiol diacetate, lynoestrenol, norgestrel) or from 17-α-hydroxyprogesterone (medroxyprogesterone acetate, megestrol acetate, chlormadinone acetate). The derivatives of nortestosterone may be metabolised to a small extent to oestrogenic compounds.

Initially, these combined preparations contained 100 μg oestrogen and 1–4 mg progestagen. Following reports of a relationship between the dose of oestrogen and the incidence of thrombo-embolic disorders [1], the oestrogen content was reduced to 50 μg and now many preparations contain 20, 30 or 35 μg. Although some combinations continue to have up to 4 mg norethisterone acetate, others now have smaller doses of progestagen, e.g. 150 μg

Amery, A. (ed.) Hypertensive Cardiovascular Disease: Pathophysiology and Treatment
© 1982, Martinus Nijhoff Publishers. The Hague / Boston / London
ISBN-13: 978-94-009-7478-4

levonorgestrel. A recent development has been the administration of small dose combination tablets containing ethinyloestradiol 30 µg and levonorgestrel 50 µg in the first 6 days of the menstrual cycle, increasing to 40 µg and 75 µg respectively for 5 days, then 30 µg ethinyloestradiol and 125 µg levonorgestrel for the next 10 days.

2. Progestagen only oral contraceptives

These are rather less effective contraceptive agents than the combined preparations, with a failure rate of about 0.5–3.1 per 100 women years, depending upon the dose and type of progestagen used. They are also more likely to cause menstrual disturbances with irregular bleeding or amenorrhoea. Preparations in current use in the U.K. contain norethisterone 350 µg, ethynodiol diacetate 500 µg, levonorgestrel 30 µg and norgestrel 75 µg.

3. Intramuscular injection of progestagen

The intramuscular injection of depot medroxy-progesterone acetate and norethisterone oenanthate at intervals of 3 or 6 months has a similar incidence of failure and menstrual irregularity as the oral progestagens. The long-acting effect is a disadvantage if side-effects occur and there is a continuing controversy about a possible relationship with breast cancer.

BLOOD PRESSURE CHANGES INDUCED BY CONTRACEPTIVE STEROIDS

Studies of blood pressure changes associated with oral contraceptives are based mainly on the 50–100 µg oestrogen combinations, although some information has been reported recently in women taking low dose oestrogen and progestagen only pills.

The first case report of hypertension induced by an oestrogen-progestagen oral contraceptive was published in 1962 [2], and was followed by a number of other reports in the U.S.A. [3–5]. In 1969 a retrospective study in the U.K. showed a small increase in blood pressure after three years [6].

In 1969 a prospective study was started in Glasgow in which the changes in blood pressure in a group of women taking oral contraceptives were compared with those found in a control group of women using cervical diaphragms or IUDs [7]. Blood pressure was measured under standardised conditions by a doctor who had no knowledge of the contraceptive technique being used, and the London School of Hygiene sphygmomanometer was used to reduce observer bias. Five brands of oral contraceptives were taken with oestrogen contents of 50–100 μg and progestagen contents of 1.0–4.0 mg. Blood pressure was less than 140/90 mm Hg in every case before oral contraceptives were started. In the 15 women who took oral contraceptives for five years, the mean systolic blood pressure had risen significantly after one year (p<0.05), and after five years the mean increase was 12.3 mm Hg (p<0.01). Mean diastolic pressure showed a significant rise after two years (p<0.05) and had increased by 8.8 mm Hg after five years

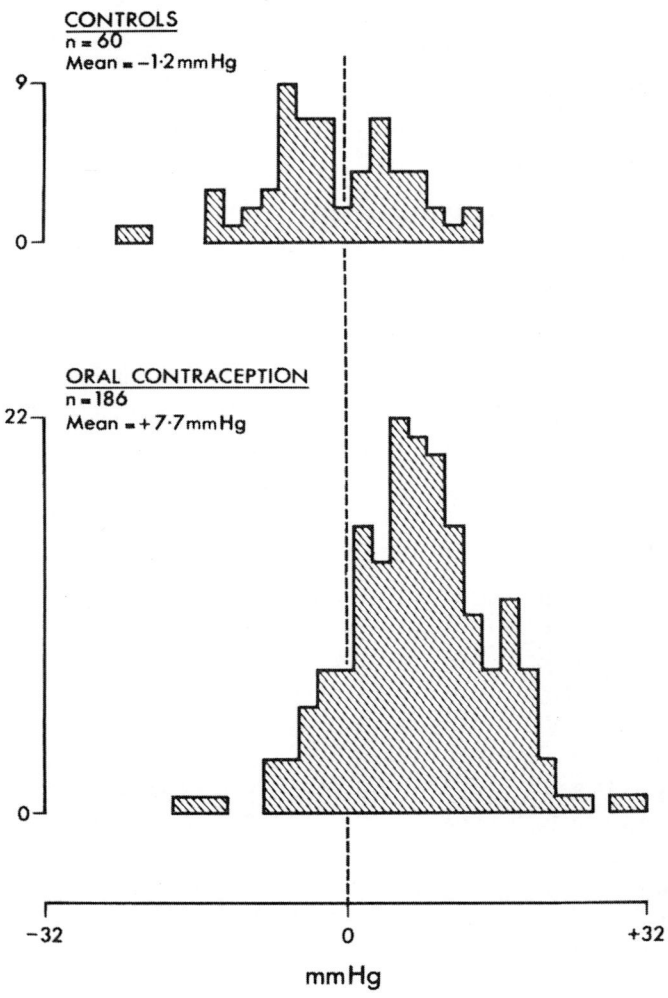

Figure 1. Changes in systolic bloodpressure after two years in women taking oestrogen-progestagen oral contraceptives and in controls.

(p<0.01). No significant change had occurred in either the systolic or diastolic pressure after five years in a control group of 10 women. Of 186 women who had taken oral contraceptives for two years, systolic pressure had risen in 164 cases (p<0.01) and diastolic pressure in 150 cases (p<0.05). Sixty women in the control group showed no significant change (Figure 1).

The results of this survey suggest that the increase in blood pressure induced by combined oestrogen-progestagen oral contraceptives generally occurs within the first two years of their administration. However, in some women the blood pressure may continue to rise progressively for at least five years.

The effect of lower dose oestrogen-progestagen oral contraceptives on blood pressure is less well defined. A cross-sectional population study in London showed the blood pressure to be higher in women taking 30 µg oestrogen containing pills than in those taking 50 µg oestrogen combinations [8]. However, in a prospective study of 58 normotensive women, combined oral contraceptives containing 30 µg ethinyl oestradiol plus 150 µg levonorgestrel showed no significant effect on blood pressure after three years, compared with a significant rise of blood pressure in women taking a 50 µg oestrogen combination for the same time [9].

In 1978, a prospective controlled study was set up in Glasgow to compare the effects on blood pressure of oral contraceptives containing 30 µg ethinyl oestradiol plus 150 µg levonorgestrel, with a control group using barrier methods or IUDs. Preliminary data after nine months follow-up are shown in Table 1. During this time blood pressure had risen significantly (p<0.01) by a mean of 8.0 mm Hg in 20 women taking the low dose oestrogen oral contraceptives, compared with no significant change in the control group. However, there is a marked difference in age between these groups which

Table 1. Effect on blood pressure after 9 months in women taking oral contraceptives containing ethinyloestradiol 30 µg plus levonorgestrel 150 µg, or norethisterone 350 µg or norgestrel 75 µg

	No. at 9 months	Mean age	Mean ± SE Systolic BP		Mean ± SE Diastolic BP	
			0	9	0	9
Controls	20	32	109±3	105±4	72±2	67±2
Ethinyl Oestradiol 30 µg + Levonorgestrel 150 µg	20	22	103±3	111±3	68±2	69±2
Norethisterone 350 µg	8	33	117±5	112±4	79±4	75±5
Norgestrel 75 µg	8	29	119±5	116±5	78±4	69±5

may explain the lower initial pressures of the low dose oestrogen group and further analysis of larger numbers at one and two years' follow-up will be required before definite conclusions can be made.

The same prospective controlled study has included two groups of women taking progestagen alone, either norethisterone 350 µg or norgestrel 75 µg. As shown in Table 1, preliminary analysis after nine months has shown no significant change in blood pressure in these two groups. This is in agreement with other studies of progestagens used alone [10-12].

INCIDENCE OF HYPERTENSION INDUCED BY ORAL CONTRACEPTIVES

In the standardised, controlled prospective Glasgow study described in the previous section [7], two women had increases in systolic pressure to over 160 mm Hg and diastolic pressure to over 90 mm Hg, i.e. about 1 % of the group studied. Other workers studying other populations and using varying criteria for the diagnosis of hypertension, have reported an incidence of hypertension between 1 % and 15 % of oral contraceptive users [13-16].

In a large U.K. non-standardised multi-centre study by the Royal College of General Practitioners [17], 23 000 pill users were compared with a control group of non-users. The incidence of hypertension diagnosed after five years was 2.6 times higher in the users versus the non-users and appeared to increase with the duration of oral contraceptive use and the age of the taker. Similar data were obtained in the U.S.A. [18] when 13 358 women were studied for three years, with an incidence of hypertension in the users five times greater than non-users.

FACTORS PREDISPOSING TO ORAL CONTRACEPTIVE INDUCED HYPERTENSION

There is some evidence that women who have high blood pressure when taking combined oestrogen-progestagen oral contraceptives are those who would be likely to develop hypertension spontaneously, i.e. those who are older and heavier and have a family history of hypertension and cardiovascular disease [11, 14, 15, 17]. Women with pre-existing hypertension do not appear to be more susceptible [19], but the evidence for susceptibility in those with previous pregnancy-induced hypertension is conflicting [11, 14, 20, 21].

There is no evidence to suggest that the rise in blood pressure is associated with a concurrent gain in weight, fluid retention, cigarette smoking or social class [7]. Data from a recent study, however, suggests that hypertension is less likely to occur in black women taking oral contraceptives, no significant change in mean blood pressure being found in a group of 2000 black women followed for up to two years [22].

THE ROLE OF THE OESTROGEN AND PROGESTAGEN COMPONENTS IN THE RISE OF BLOOD PRESSURE

In the large study conducted by the Royal College of General Practitioners [17] the incidence of hypertension appeared to be related to the dose of progestagen but not to the dose of oestrogen. However, this was a non-standardised study in which the participating doctors were asked to report the diagnosis of hypertension based on their own individual criteria and the data must therefore be interpreted with some reservations. In the standardised, controlled, prospective Glasgow study [7], no relationship was demonstrated between the rise in blood pressure and the type or dose of progestagen used. In a more recent study comparing different doses of norethisterone acetate (1.0, 2.5, 3.0 and 4.0 mg) combined with 50 µg ethinyloestradiol, no relationship was found with the incidence of hypertension [23]. Also, there is no evidence to date that progestagens given alone will affect blood pressure in previously normotensive women [10–12, 24].

An increase in systolic blood pressure has been demonstrated during intravenous infusion of oestrogens [25], and administration of oral oestrogens, especially ethinyl oestradiol in doses equivalent to those in the combined contraceptive pill, caused significant increases in blood pressure [11]. However, the use of smaller doses of oestrogen did not cause a significant change in blood pressure [26]. It seems likely, therefore, that it is the oestrogen component which is the main culprit, but perhaps there is a synergistic action with the associated progestagen.

PATHOGENESIS OF HYPERTENSION INDUCED BY ORAL CONTRACEPTIVES

A number of mechanisms for the rise in blood pressure have been examined:

1. *Renin and angiotensin.* Oestrogens increase the hepatic synthesis of renin-substrate [27] and it is not surprising that plasma renin-substrate levels are raised in women taking oestrogen-progestagen contraceptives [4, 28–34]. Plasma renin activity is also increased in these women [4, 5, 28, 31, 32, 34, 35]. Plasma renin concentration, however, is normal or low [28, 30, 31, 33, 34, 36]. Plasma angiotensin II concentrations have been reported to be raised [31] or normal [36]. Plasma pro-renin levels remain unchanged [35].

As the changes in the renin–angiotensin system were at first demonstrated

618

in women with hypertension while taking oral contraceptives, it was thought that these changes might have induced the rise in blood pressure. It was suggested that the normal or reduced plasma renin concentration might be due to a feedback mechanism associated with the raised plasma renin substrate concentration and augmented plasma renin activity, and that impairment of this suppression of renin might result in an increase in blood pressure in some women. It has since been found that women with hypertension induced by oral contraceptives have plasma renin concentrations similar to or lower than women with normal blood pressure while taking the pill. Plasma renin substrate concentrations, plasma renin activity and plasma angiotensin II concentrations are the same in both groups [37].

There is, therefore, no evidence that the raised blood pressure is due to increased circulating levels of angiotensin II, nor is there evidence that the levels of angiotensin II are inappropriately high in relation to concurrent sodium balance [37]. A study of two women showed no change in sensitivity to infused angiotensin II while taking and after withdrawal of oral contraceptives [38]. One study has shown that the administration of the competitive angiotensin II inhibitor, saralasin to a small number of hypertensive women taking oral contraceptives resulted in a fall in blood pressure in the women whose pressure subsequently returned to normal when the pill was stopped, but no change in those whose pressure remained high when off the pill [39]. However, no significant fall in blood pressure was found in another similar study [40]. The role of angiotensin, therefore, remains uncertain.

2. *Aldosterone, cortisol, DOC.* Increased aldosterone secretion and excretion rates in some women given oestrogen-progestagen contraceptives, and increased plasma protein binding of aldosterone, have been described [4, 5, 32, 41]. Plasma concentrations of aldosterone may be increased [34] or normal [30, 37]. Plasma cortisol levels show a consistent rise mainly due to increased protein binding but an increase in free cortisol may also occur [30, 41, 42]. Plasma DOC levels also rise [37]. These changes in plasma concentrations of aldosterone, cortisol and DOC are not related to changes in blood pressure [37] and there is no evidence to incriminate these hormones in the development of hypertension in women taking oral contraceptives. In fact, a case has been described of oral contraceptive induced hypertension occurring in a women after adrenalectomy and hypophysectomy [43].

3. *Sodium and fluid retention.* It is generally thought that most women gain weight while taking oestrogen-progestagen oral contraceptives and Walters and Lim [44] found a significant increase after three months. The Glasgow prospective controlled study showed a significant mean increase of 2.4 kg (p<0.05) in the oral contraceptive takers but there was no correlation with the changes in blood pressure [7].

One study has shown that ethinyl oestradiol and the synthetic progestagens ethynodiol diacetate, norethisterone and chloromadinone increased total exchangeable sodium when given alone to 10 normal subjects for three weeks [45]. However, in another study [37] no significant difference in total exchangeable sodium or potassium was found in 5 women assessed while taking and three months after stopping oestrogen-progestagen combinations; total body water measured in 3 women also showed no consistent change. When measured in 11 women, no correlation was found between blood pressure and total exchangeable sodium [37].

4. *Plasma volume and cardiac output.* In 1970, Walters and Lim described an increase in body weight, plasma volume, stroke volume, and cardiac output in a group of normotensive women who had taken oestrogen-progestagen oral contraceptives for three months [44]. This was associated with a small increase in systolic blood pressure. It seemed possible, therefore, that the hypertension induced in some women might be related to a greater increase in plasma volume and cardiac output. However, another study [46] showed no significant change in plasma volume, stroke volume or cardiac output in 10 women before and three months after stopping oestrogen-pro-

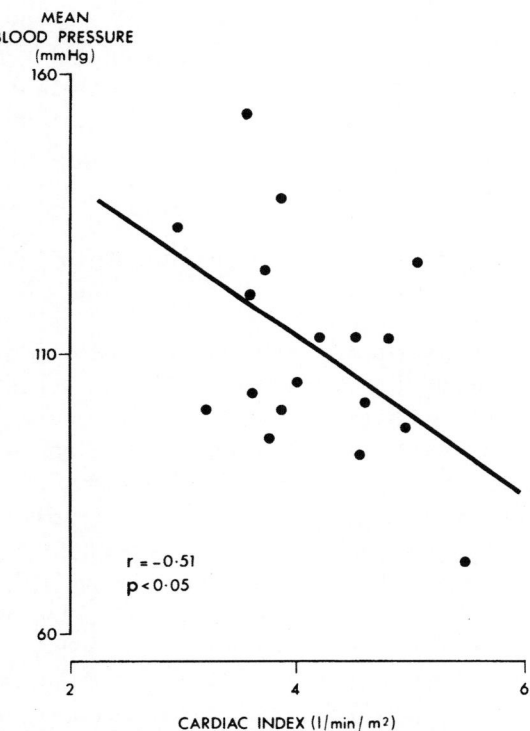

Figure 2. Relationship between mean blood pressure and cardiac index in 18 women taking oestrogen-progestagen oral contraceptives.

gestagen pills. The same report described a negative correlation between blood pressure and plasma volume, stroke volume and cardiac output in 18 women who had taken oral contraceptives for up to ten years, with a significant positive correlation to calculated total peripheral resistance (Figure 2). Women with established oral contraceptive-induced hypertension do not have a high output state and appear to have the same cardiovascular changes as patients with essential hypertension.

5. *Catecholamines and sympathetic nervous activity.* Rockson and colleagues [48] found higher plasma levels of dopamine β-hydroxylase in women taking oral contraceptives. This suggests an increase in sympathetic nervous activity but the mechanism by which this occurs and its relevance remains to be assessed.

6. *Renal changes.* Hollenberg and colleagues [48] found that in most women taking oestrogen-progestagen oral contraceptives there was a reduction of 25 % in mean renal blood flow. An arteriographic study [49] showed narrowing of the peripheral renal vessels in 5 hypertensive women taking oestrogen-progestagen oral contraceptives; 3 of these women also had mild vascular changes on renal biopsy. Whether these changes are a cause or effect of the hypertension is uncertain.

In summary, the combined oestrogen-progestagen oral contraceptive may induce certain biochemical, hormonal, haemodynamic and vascular changes. Some of these appear to be related to the oestrogen component. To date, none of these changes has been shown to be causally related to the rise in blood pressure and the mechanism for this remains to be elucidated.

COMPLICATIONS OF ORAL CONTRACEPTIVE-INDUCED HYPERTENSION

The increases in blood pressure as found in the Glasgow prospective survey of normotensive women [7] were not accompanied by clinical complications and would not generally be regarded as clinically important. Nevertheless, mortality and morbidity statistics from the Framingham Study and Insurance Company data suggest that a relatively small increase in blood pressure within the range found in these pill taking women carries a distinct risk. These steroids are now being taken by large numbers of women throughout the world and the number of women using them in the U.K. alone is over 3 million. If about 1 % of these women develop clinical hypertension, a very significant number of women will be at greater risk. Most of these women have levels of diastolic pressure between 100 and 120 mm Hg. More severe hypertension is uncommon [13] and malignant (accelerated) phase hypertension is rare and usually associated with renal failure [50, 51].

There is now evidence of an increased incidence of cardiovascular mortality in young women who have taken combined oestrogen (50–100 µg) and progestagen (1–4 mg) oral contraceptives [52]. The risks are five times greater in such women, and 10 times greater if the pill has been taken for five years or more. Major complications are more likely to occur if the women is over the age of 35 and if she smokes cigarettes. Beral [53] has shown a statistical correlation between the rising use of oral contraceptives and the increasing incidence of cardiovascular mortality in women aged 15–44 in twenty-one countries.

Thrombo-embolic disorders are well-documented complications of oral contraceptive use [1] and are likely to play a major role in the development of cardiovascular disease. Raised blood pressure is also an important risk factor, especially for cerebro-vascular disease. The Collaborative Group for the Study of Stroke in Young Women [54] implicated oestrogen-progestagen oral contraceptives in a significant number of cases and this has been confirmed by the Royal College of General Practitioners Study [52] and the Oxford/FPA study [55]. An increased risk of subarachnoid haemorrhage has been reported [52, 56] but a case control study in England and Wales in 1976 showed no significant increase in deaths from this condition [57]. Vertebral artery occlusion appears to be more common in these women [50].

In 1974, Oliver reported a 52% use of oral contraceptives in women with myocardial infarction, a greater proportion than expected and these women showed the same prevalence of risk factors as non-users [59]. He concluded that oral contraceptives only increased the risk of myocardial infarction in the presence of one or more of the major risk factors such as smoking, hypertension, diabetes and hyperlipidaemia. Confirmation of increased risk of myocardial infarction, even in the absence of other risk factors, was published by Mann and his colleagues in 1975 and 1976 [60, 61] and the proportion is about 2:1, increasing to 19:1 in women who smoke 25 cigarettes or more daily. This has been confirmed by some workers [62] but not by others [63].

In addition to their effect on coagulation factors, oestrogens have been shown to affect carbohydrate and lipid metabolism [64, 65]. These effects are less marked on the 30 µg than the 50 µg oestrogen combinations and do not seem to occur with progestagens alone [8]. However, they do seem to be related to the dose of progestagen taken with the combined pill and a positive association has been found between the dose of norethisterone acetate and deaths from stroke and ischaemic heart disease [23].

MANAGEMENT OF HYPERTENSION INDUCED BY ORAL CONTRACEPTIVES

When a women taking oral contraceptives is found to have a raised blood pressure, this should be checked on at least one other occasion to confirm a sustained hypertension. Not uncommonly the blood pressure may be high at one clinic visit, perhaps due to anxiety about a cervical smear test, or to other factors, and is normal at subsequent visits. If it is found to be consistently high, a full history and physical examination should be carried out, with particular attention to blood pressure recordings before starting the pill and evidence of complications of raised blood pressure, such as left ventricular enlargement and optic fundal changes. If thought necessary, renal or adrenal causes for the hypertension should be excluded by further radiological and biochemical assessment, bearing in mind the biochemical alterations induced by oral contraceptives which have been discussed earlier.

The rise in blood pressure is reversible in most women when the pill is stopped. In the Glasgow prospective survey of normotensive women [7], 32 women who had taken oral contraceptives for up to three years stopped the pill and three months later the blood pressure had returned to pre-treatment levels in all cases. In another study [66] of 26 women with established hypertension induced by oral contraceptives, 24 showed a fall in blood pressure to pre-treatment normotensive levels after stopping the pill, some taking up to one year before normotensive pressures were reached and

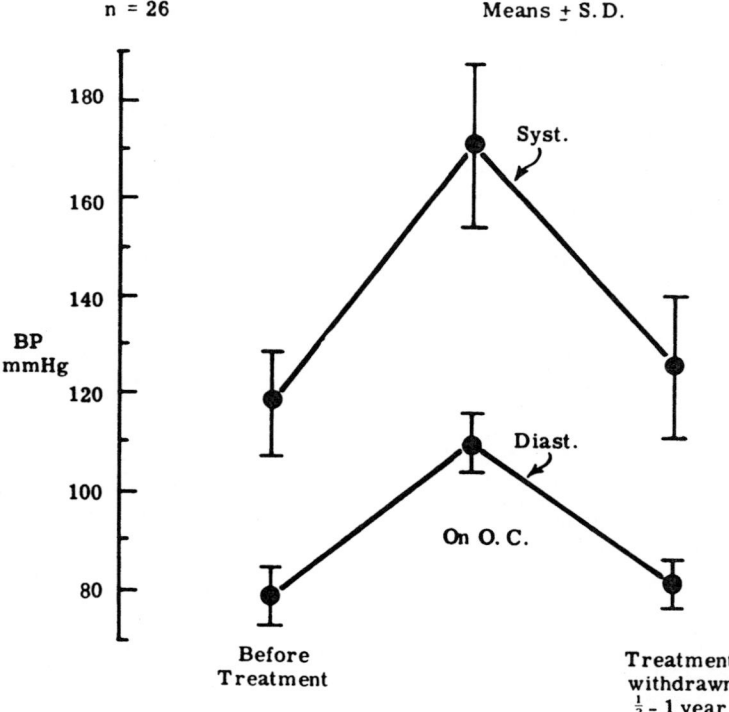

Figure 3. Change in blood pressure after withdrawal of oral contraceptives in 26 women with hypertension induced by oestrogen-Progestagen oral contraceptives.

maintained (Figure 3). In 2 of these 26 women, the blood pressure remained mildly raised and it is possible that these women had essential hypertension unmasked by oral contraceptives. Among 14 women whose blood pressure had returned to normal after the pill was stopped, Woods and colleagues [67] found 7 who developed hypertension within the next six years.

Preferably, then, the oral contraceptives should be stopped and alternative methods of contraception advised, such as occlusive methods. IUDs, sterilisation or vasectomy. These other methods, however, may be inappropriate, unacceptable or associated with troublesome side-effects, in which case a lower dose oral contraceptive may be prescribed (Table 2).

Table 2. Summary of management of hypertension in women taking oral contraceptives

---

1. Check BP on at least two occasions to establish persistently high BP

2. If BP persistently high:
   a) Change to low dose (30 μg) oestrogen-progestagen or progestagen-only preparation; continue to monitor BP;
   b) If BP stays high, stop oral contraceptive.
   Or

3. Stop oral contraceptive; recommend alternative contraceptive measure.
   a) Continue to monitor BP;
   b) If BP stays high 6 months after stopping oral contraceptive, investigate for renal or adrenal cause of hypertension.
   c) If BP is still high one year after stopping oral contraceptive, treat with hypotensive drug.

4. If severe or accelerated (malignant) phase hypertension, stop oral contraceptive and treat with hypotensive drugs urgently.

5. If BP continues to be raised and it is considered necessary to continue the oral contraceptive, treat with hypotensive drug (e.g. β-blocker and/or thiazide diuretic); monitor BP regularly.

What is the effect of changing from a high to a low dose oestrogen-progestagen combination?

In a study of 8 women with hypertension induced by combinations containing 50 μg oestrogen and 1–4 mg progestagen, these were replaced by 'low dose' combinations containing 30 μg ethinyl oestradiol plus 150 or 250 μg levonorgestrel [68]. After one year the mean blood pressure had dropped from 170/109 to 156/95 ($p < 0.05$). In a further 6 women in whom the 50 μg combination had been withdrawn six months previously because of hypertension, the mean blood pressure rose from 137/80 to 155/95 ($p < 0.05$) six months after starting the low dose combination; when this was stopped, the pressure fell again to 134/82 ($p < 0.05$) six months later.

What is the effect of changing from a high dose oestrogen-progestagen combination to a progestagen alone?

In 10 women with hypertension induced by combinations containing 50 μg oestrogen and 1–4 mg progestagen, the mean blood pressure fell from 174/112 to 136/90 (p<0.05), one year after changing to 350 μg norethisterone alone [68]. In 6 women in whom the 50 μg oestrogen combination had been withdrawn six months previously because of hypertension, the mean pressure rose from 132/83 to 144/95 (p<0.05) six months after starting norethisterone 350 μg alone; when this was withdrawn, the pressure fell again to 132/86 (p<0.05) six months later.

On present evidence, if a woman has hypertension induced by a 50 μg oestrogen-progestagen combination, it is likely that her blood pressure will fall significantly when the pill is changed to a lower dose combination, and more so if changed to a progestagen alone. The risks of cardiovascular and cerebrovascular complications should be reduced, but the blood pressure may not return entirely to pre-treatment levels. It is important, therefore, to check the pressure regularly at three- or four-monthly intervals, and if it does not return to normal after one year, then the oral contraceptive should be stopped in most cases (Table 2).

Can the oral contraceptive be continued and the blood pressure controlled by hypotensive drugs?

Occasional situations occur where alternative contraceptive measures are contra-indicated, impractical or unacceptable. If in such a case the woman needs contraception for medical, psychological or social reasons then it is justified to continue with the oral contraceptive, while at the same time a hypotensive drug is administered. A β-adrenocepter blocker and/or a thiazide diuretic will control the blood pressure in most cases, but occasionally the addition of another hypotensive agent may be required.

What is the management of severe and malignant (accelerated) phase hypertension induced by oral contraceptives?

Malignant phase hypertension is a medical emergency and urgent hypotensive treatment is mandatory as discussed in the chapter by Sannerstedt. The oral contraceptive should of course, be stopped. As the hypertensive effects of the oral contraceptive diminish over weeks or even months, it should be possible to gradually decrease the dose of the hypotensive drugs. Some women may eventually show normal blood pressure levels without treatment. Others may need to continue hypotensive treatment indefinitely; it is not clear whether such women have had a predisposition to hypertension which may have been unmasked by the pill, or whether the pill has induced permanent renal and/or vascular changes.

Will the blood pressure be affected in future pregnancies?

As stated earlier, there is conflicting evidence as to whether women who have had pregnancy-induced hypertension are more likely to develop raised blood pressure while taking oral contraceptives. To date, it has not been shown that women with oral contraceptive-induced hypertension are more likely to develop hypertension in future pregnancies. There is, therefore, no need to advise against future pregnancies on this account but it seems sensible to monitor the blood pressure particularly carefully during such pregnancies.

REFERENCES

1. Inman WHW, Vessey MP, Westerhold B, Engelund A: Thrombo-embolic disease and the steroid content of oral contraceptives. A report to the Committee on Safety of Drugs. Br Med J 2:203–209, 1970.
2. Brownrigg GM: Toxaemia in hormone-induced pseudo-pregnancy. Can Med Ass J 87:408–409, 1962.
3. Woods JW: Oral contraceptives and hypertension. Lancet 2:653–654, 1967.
4. Laragh JH, Sealey JE, Ledingham JGG, Newton MA: Oral contraceptives. Renin, aldosterone, and high blood pressure. J Am Med Ass 201:918–922, 1967.
5. Weinberger MH, Collins RD, Dowdy AJ, Nokes GW, Leutscher JA: Hypertension induced by oral contraceptives containing oestrogen and gestagen. Ann. Intern Med 71:891, 1969.
6. Loudon NB, Burton JL: Oral contraceptives and blood pressure. Lancet 2:217, 1969.
7. Weir RJ, Briggs E, Mack A, Naismith L, Taylor L, Wilson E: Blood pressure in women taking oral contraceptives. Br Med J 1:533–535, 1974.
8. Meade TW, Haines AP, North WRS, Chakrabarti R, Howarth DJ, Stirling Y: Haemostatic, lipid, and blood pressure profiles of women on oral contraceptives containing 50 µg or 30 µg oestrogen. Lancet 2:948–951, 1977.
9. Briggs M, Briggs M: Oestrogen content of oral contraceptives. Lancet 2: 1233, 1977.
10. Mackay EV, Khoo SH, Adam R: Contraception with a six-monthly injection of progestogen – I. Effects on blood pressure, body weight and uterine bleeding pattern, side effects, efficacy and acceptability. Aust NZJ Obstet Gynaec 11:148–155, 1971.
11. Spellacy WN, Birk SA: The effect of intra-Uterine devices, oral contraceptives, and progestagens on blood pressure. Am J Obstet Gynec 112:912–919, 1972.
12. Hawkins DF, Benster B: A comparative study of three low dose progestagens, chlormadinone acetate, megestrol acetate and norethisterone, as oral contraceptives. Br J Obstet Gynaec 84:708–713, 1977.
13. Wallace MR: Oral contraceptives and severe hypertension. Aust NZ J Med 1:49–52, 1971.
14. Clezy TM, Foy BM, Hodge RL, Lumbers ER: Oral contraceptives and hypertension. An epidemiological survey. Br Heart J 34:1238–1243, 1972.
15. Fisch IR, Freedman SH, Myatt AV: Oral contraceptives, Pregnancy and blood pressure. J Am Med Ass 222:1507–1510, 1972.
16. Stern MP, Brown BW, Haskell WL, Farquhar JW, Wehrle CL, Wood PDS: Cardiovascular risk and use of oestrogens or oestrogen-progestagen combinations. Stanford Three Community Study. J Am Med Ass 235:811–815, 1976.
17. Royal College of General Practitioners: Oral contraceptives and health. London, 1974.
18. Fisch IR, Frank J: Oral contraceptives and blood pressure. J Am Med Ass. 237:2499–2503, 1977.
19. Spellacy WN, Birk SA: Fert Ster 25:467, 1974.
20. Smith RW: Hypertension and oral contraceptives. Am J Obstet Gynec 113:482–487, 1972.

626

21. Pritchard JA, Pritchard SA: Blood pressure response to oestrogen-progestin oral contraceptives after pregnancy-induced hypertension. Am J Obstet Gynec 129:733–739, 1977.
22. Blumenstein BA, Douglas MB, Hall WD: Blood pressure changes and oral contraceptives use: a study of 2676 black women in the South-eastern United States. Am J Epidemiol 112:539–552, 1980.
23. Meade TW, Greenberg G, Thompson SG: Progestagens and cardiovascular reactions associated with oral contraceptives and a comparison of the safety of 50- and 30-μg oestrogen preparations. Br Med J 1:1157–1161, 1980.
24. Weir RJ, Wilson E, Cruikshank J: A prospective controlled study of blood pressure changes in women taking low dose oestrogen and progestagen only oral contraceptives. (To be published.)
25. Lim YL, Lumbers ER, Walters WAW, Whelan RF: Effect of oestrogens on the human circulation. J Obstet Gynaec Br Comwlth 77:349–355, 1970.
26. Gow J, Macgillivray I: Metabolic, hormonal and vascular changes after synthetic oestrogen therapy in oophorectomised women. Br Med J 2:73–77, 1971.
27. Helmer OM, Judson WE: Influence of high renin substrate levels on renin–angiotensin system in pregnancy. Am J Obstet Gynec 99:9–17, 1967.
28. Skinner SL, Lumbers ER, Symonds EM: Alteration by oral contraceptives of normal menstrual changes in plasma renin activity, concentration and and substrate. Clin Sci 36:67–76, 1969.
29. Saruta T, Saade GA, Kaplan NM: A possible mechanism for hypertension induced by oral contraceptives. Arch Intern Med 126:621–626, 1970.
30. Weir RJ, Tree M, Fraser R: The effect of oral contraceptives on blood pressure and on plasma renin, renin-substrate and corticosteroids. J Clin Pathol 23 (Suppl 3):49–54, 1970.
31. Cain MD, Walters WA, Catt KJ: Effects of oral contraceptive therapy on the renin–angiotensin system. J Clin Endocrinol Metab 33:671–676, 1971.
32. Crane MG, Harris JJ, Winsor W: Hypertension, oral contraceptive agents and conjugated oestrogens. Ann Intern Med 74:13–21, 1971.
33. Kotchen TA, Kotchen JM, Guthrie CP, Cottrill CM: Plasma rennin activity, reactivity, concentration and substrate following hypertension during pregnancy. Effect of oral contraceptive agents. Hypertension 1:355–361, 1979.
34. Beckerhoff R, Vetter W, Armbruster J, Luetscher JA, Siegenthaler W: Plasma aldosterone during oral contraceptive therapy. Lancet 1:1218–1220, 1973.
35. Hedlin AM, Loh AY, Osmond DH: Fibrinolysis, renin activity, and prorenin in normal women: effects of exercise and oral contraceptive medication. J Clin Endocrinol Metab 49:663–671, 1979.
36. Weir RJ, Tree M, McElwee G: Changes in blood pressure and in plasma renin, renin substrate and angiotensin II concentrations in women taking contraceptive steroids. Proc 4th Int Congr Endocrinol, Washington, 1972. Excerpt Med Int Congr Series 273:1019, 1974.
37. Weir RJ, Davies DL, Fraser R, Morton JJ, Tree M, Wilson A: Contraceptive steroids and hypertension. J Steroid Biochem 6:961–964, 1975.
38. Weir RJ, Tree M, Fraser R, Chinn RH, Davies DL, Düsterdieck GO, Robertson JIS, Horne CHW, Mallinson AC: The effect of combined oestrogen-progestagen oral contraceptives and of their separate components on plasma levels ofrenin, renin-substrate, angiotensin and aldosterone and on blood pressure. Proc 3rd Int Congr Hormonal Steroids, Hamburg, Excerpt Med Int Congr Series 219:929–937, 1971.
39. Streeten DHP, Anderson G, Dalakos TG: Angiotensin Blockade; its clinical significance. Am J Med 60:817–824, 1976.
40. Broughton-Pipkin F, Hunter JC, Oats J, Symonds M: Hypertension and oral contraceptives. Br Med J 2:278, 1978.
41. Layne DS, Meyer CJ, Vaishwanar PS, Pincus G: The secretion and metabolism of cortisol

and aldosterone in normal and in steroid-treated women. J Clin Endocrinol Metab 22:107–118, 1962.

42. Burke CW: Biologically active cortisol in plasma of oestrogen treated and normal subjects. Br Med J 2:798–800, 1969.

43. Lindheimer MD, Landau RL, Oparil S: Oral contraceptive-induced hypertension after adrenalectomy and hypophysectomy. Arch Intern Med 136:1029–1031.

44. Walters WAW, Lim YL: Haemodynamic changes in women taking oral contraceptives. J Obstet Gynaec Br Cmwlth. 77:1007–1012, 1970.

45. Crane MG, Harris JJ: Effect of oestrogens and gestagens on exchangeable sodium. In: Oral contraceptives and High Blood Pressure. Fregly MJ, Fregly MS, eds. Gainsville FL: The Dolphin Press, 1974.

46. Weir RJ, Moseley H, Kennedy JA: The relationship of plasma volume and cardiac output to raised blood pressure induced by steroid contraceptives. Abstract, 8th World Congr Cardiol, Tokyo, 1978.

47. Rockson SG, Stone RA, Gunwells JC, Schanberg SM, Kirschner M, Robinson RR: Plasma dopamine-β-hydroxylase activity in oral contraceptive hypertension. Circulation 51:916–923, 1975.

48. Hollenberg NK, Williams GF, Burger B, Chenitz W, Hoosmand I, Adams DF: Renal blood flow and its response to angiotensin II. An interaction between oral contraceptive agents, sodium intake, and the renin–angiotensin system in healthy young women. Circ Res 38:35–40, 1976.

49. Boyd WN, Burden RP, Aber GM: Intrarenal vascular changes in patients receiving oestrogen-containing compounds. A clinical, histological and angiographic study. Q J Med 175:415–431, 1975.

50. Harris RWR: Malignant hypertension associated with oral contraceptives. Lancet 2:466, 1969.

51. Dunn FG, Jones JV, Fife R: Malignant hypertension associated with the use of oral contraceptives. Br Heart J 37:336–338, 1975.

52. Royal College of General Practitioners' Oral contraception study. Mortality among oral-contraceptive users. Lancet 2:727–731, 1977.

53. Beral V: Cardiovascular disease mortality trends and oral contraceptive use in Young women. Lancet 2:1047–1052, 1976.

54. Collaborative Group For The Study of Stroke in Young Women. Oral contraceptives and increased risk of cerebral ischaemia or thrombosis. N Engl J Med 288:871–878, 1973.

55. Vessey MP, McPherson K, Johnson B: Mortality among women participating in the Oxford/Family Planning Association Contraceptive Study. Lancet 2:731–733, 1977.

56. Petitti DB, Wingerd J: Use of oral contraceptives, cigarette smoking, and risk of subarachnoid haemorrhage. Lancet 2:234–236, 1978.

57. Inman WHW: Oral contraceptives and fatal subarachnoid haemorrhage. Br Med J 2:1468–1470, 1979.

58. Ask-Upmark E, Bickerstaff ER: Vertebral artery occlusion and oral contraceptives. Br Med J 1:487–488, 1976.

59. Oliver MF: Ischaemic heart disease in young women. Br Med J 4:253–259, 1974.

60. Mann JI, Vessey MP, Thorogood M, Doll R: Myocardial infarction in young women with special reference to oral contraceptive practice. Br Med J 2:241–245, 1975.

61. Mann JI, Inman WHW: Oral contraceptive use in older women and fatal myocardial infarction. Br Med J 2:445–447, 1976.

62. Shapiro S, Slone D, Rosenberg L, Kaufman DW, Stolley PD, Miettinen OS: Oral contraceptive use in relation to myocardial infarction. Lancet 1:743–747, 1979.

63. Rosenberg L, Armstrong B, Jick J: Myocardial infarction and oestrogen therapy in post-menopausal women. N Engl J med 294:1256–1259, 1976.

64. Wallace RB, Hoover J, Barrett-Connor E: Altered Plasma lipid and lipoprotein levels associated with oral contraceptives and oestrogen use. Lancet 2:111-114, 1979.

65. Wynn V, Godsland I, Niththyananthan R: Comparison of effects of different combined oral contraceptive formulations on carbohydrate and lipid metabolism. Lancet 1:1045-1049, 1979.

66. Brown JJ, Cumming AMM, Lever AF, Robertson JIS, Weir RJ: Hypertension and coronary heart disease in young women. In: Coronary Heart Disease in Young Women, pp. 162-172. Oliver MF, ed. Edinburgh: Churchill Livingston, 1978.

67. Woods JW, Algray WA, Stier FM: Oral contraceptives and hypertension. Circ 46 (Suppl 2):82, 1972.

68. Weir RJ: Reduced hypertensive risks of low dose contraceptive steroids. In: Prophylactic Approaches to Hypertensive Diseases. Perspectives in Cardiovascular Research, Vol 4, pp. 15-20. Yamori Y, Lovenberg W, Freis ED, eds. New York: Raven Press, 1979.

VI. EXAMINATION OF THE HYPERTENSIVE PATIENT

41. CLINICAL EXAMINATION OF THE HYPERTENSIVE PATIENT INCLUDING BLOOD PRESSURE MEASUREMENT

DESMOND FITZGERALD, EOIN O'BRIEN and KEVIN O'MALLEY

1. INTRODUCTION

Until quite recently there has been a tendency to perform detailed investigatios on all patients with hypertension. Despite a 20% prevalence of this condition, rising to 50% in the elderly [1], only a quarter of hypertensive subjects are on treatment [2]. As public awareness of the dangers of hypertension grows and screening programs are initiated, the numbers attending for assessment will increase. The incidence of secondary hypertension in such a screened population is small, about 2% [3] compared with 5–10% of a referred population [4], and as most of the newly diagnosed patients will have mild hypertension, the incidence of end-organ damage will also be less. Faced with a poor yield from these investigations and a rising population of people identified as hypertensive, detailed laboratory evaluation is therefore no longer feasible nor indeed indicated. We are now more dependent on clinical evaluation as a means of identifying patients who have secondary hypertension and end-organ damage. Only where clinical assessment suggests an underlying cause, or the patient is young with severe or progressive hypertension, should the patient be referred for detailed investigations. Otherwise, routine urinalysis, serum electrolytes and an electrocardiogram are adequate.

Hypertension can only be diagnosed by a sphygmomanometer. The technique gives an indirect assessment of the intra-arterial pressure and the results must be interpreted in the light of the many factors which affect this method. Further, the technique records blood pressure at one particular point in time. Blood pressure varies greatly and so attempts are being made to assess blood pressure behaviour by various methods, including home recording by the patient [5] and ambulatory measurement using automatic blood pressure recorders [6]. While these techniques make us less dependent on single measurements, in general the diagnosis and management of hypertension is based on a few measurements with the conventional sphygmomanometer. We must ensure, therefore, that our technique is accurate and that we avoid the many pitfalls which can affect the results of indirect blood pressure measurement. With increasing accuracy fewer people will be mislabelled as hypertensive and those with mild hypertension will be offered the benefits shown to result from treatment [7].

Amery, A. (ed.) Hypertensive Cardiovascular Disease: Pathophysiology and Treatment
© *1982, Martinus Nijhoff Publishers. The Hague / Boston / London*
ISBN-13: 978-94-009-7478-4

In this chapter we shall discuss the clinical evaluation of the hypertensive patient with emphasis on identifying possible secondary hypertension and end-organ effects of high blood pressure. We shall also describe in some detail the pitfalls in indirect blood pressure measurement and how they may be avoided.

2. HISTORY

2.1. Symptoms

Elevated blood pressure does not cause symptoms per se unless extremely high or complications are present. There have been descriptions of a characteristic headache, occipital in position, worse in the morning and relieved by rising. However, the incidence of headache is the same in normotensive and hypertensive people [8]. Further, headaches are more common in patients who know they have high blood pressure than in those who are not aware of it [9]. Despite this, the incidence of sustained hypertension among patients with headache in one study was 40% higher than in a normal population [8]. Raised intracranial pressure with stretching of pain sensitive structures is the most likely cause of the headache of malignant hypertension, which is generally worse in the morning and may be associated with vomiting. An association has been described between hypertension and migraine. Migraine sufferers have diastolic blood pressures which are, on average, 10 mm Hg higher than in the normal population [10]. Other symptoms which occur more commonly in hypertensive subjects are breathlessness and tinnitus. Epistaxis is frequently considered a symptom of hypertension, and although in one study there was a higher incidence of hypertension when no local cause was found for the epistaxis than when a nasal lesion was detected [11], it is more probable that epistaxis is a chance occurrence which brings the high blood pressure to the attention of the doctor. The frequent finding of epistaxis and hypertension in the same patient is due to the fact that both conditions are common. Many symptoms of hypertension result from end-organ damage. Angina, dyspnoea, intermittent claudication and cerebrovascular symptoms all indicate the presence of end-organ disease. Urinary symptoms are rare and, in patients with little other evidence of end-organ involvement, suggest primary renal or urinary tract disease.

2.2. Causative factors

A positive family history of raised blood pressure occurs more commonly in essential than secondary hypertension, though in some secondary causes, such as multiple endocrine adenoma syndromes and polycystic renal disease, it can nearly always be elicited. A positive family history emphasises the importance of the disease to the patient and may encourage him to persuade family members to attend for screening.

Though there is still some doubt regarding the effectiveness of salt restriction in hypertension, recent evidence suggests that sodium restriction combined with increased potassium intake reduces blood pressure in mild hypertensives [12]. Patients with a high salt intake should therefore be advised to limit its use. A rough estimate of salt intake may be made by grading the patient according to whether he adds salt to his food, adds it only after tasting the food or adds it routinely to all food. A history of prescribed and non-prescribed medications that elevated blood pressure, such as steroids, sympathomimetics, carbonoxalone or other liquorice derivatives, and analgesics, which may damage the kidney, should be determined. Oral contraceptives are probably the most common cause of secondary hypertension [13]. The blood pressure rises in most women taking oestrogen preparations, in 4% of cases to hypertensive levels [14]. Other risk factors, such as smoking, alcohol intake and a history of diabetes should be noted. Patients should be questioned regarding symptoms which may give clues to other secondary causes of hypertension. Intermittent symptoms of sweating, palpitation and nervousness suggest a phaechromocytoma, though anxious patients and those with the hyperkinetic heart syndrome may have have similar complaints [15]. Weakness may result from hypokalaemia secondary to Conn's syndrome.

3.   CLINICAL EXAMINATION

3.1. *General examination*

The general appearance of the hypertensive patient may suggest a possible cause or aggravating factor. There may be features indicating a poor life style such as obesity and nicotine staining of the fingers. Evidence of diabetes, such as glycosuria, fundal changes and peripheral vascular disease may be present. Xanthelesma and xanthomata suggest hyperlipidaemia. Cushing's syndrome, chronic renal failure and polycythaemia are usually self-evident. Skin lesions, such as neuromas and pigmented patches suggest neurofibromatosis which is occasionally associated with phaeochromocytoma and hypertension due to renal artery compression [4]. Ischaemic leg ulcers due to dermal end-artery occlusion are an uncommon complication of severe hypertension which resolves with treatment [16]. Sweating, tremor and nervousness may be due to anxiety or may indicate an underlying phaeochromocytoma.

Evidence of vascular disease suggested by bruits in large arteries, tortuous vessels, absent or reduced peripheral pulses and aneurysm of the abdominal aorta should be sought. A careful neurological examination may detect occult neurological signs due to a previous minor cerebrovascular accident.

Secondary causes of hypertension are detected in the majority of cases by careful physical examination and urinalysis [13]. Coarctation of the aorta is suggested by an ejection murmur at the left sternal border radiating under the left clavicle, in association with a delayed and reduced femoral pulse. Confirmatory signs include a palpable arterial pulsation and bruit over the medial scapular border. Abdominal examination may detect enlargement of one or both kidneys due to polycystic disease, hypernephroma or hydronephrosis. Dipstick urinalysis is in our view an important part of the physical examination. Routine culture and microscopy is not indicated unless the urinalysis is abnormal.

3.2. Cardiovascular assessment

3.2.2.1. The pulse
Examination of the pulse in hypertensive patients is generally unhelpful. Earlier writers emphasised the increased tension of the pulse in patients with strokes prior to there being any method of blood pressure measurement [17]. Palpation of the radial artery as a means of detecting arterial wall disease has often been stressed though it bears no relationship with pathological findings [18]. Atrial fibrillation and ectopic activity may be detected. Their occurence probably reflects underlying ischaemic heart disease.

3.2.2. Taking the blood pressure
This forms the most important aspect of the evaluation of the hypertensive patient and is discussed in greater detail later. In general, an inflatable rubber bladder of suitable size enclosed in a cloth cuff is wrapped around the upper arm so that its lower edge lies above the antecubital fossa with the tubing facing upwards. The bladder is inflated rapidly to a pressure 30 mm Hg above the point of disappearance of the radial pulse. During slow deflation, at a rate not exceeding 2–3 mm Hg per pulse, the examiner auscultates over the brachial artery below the cuff edge. The appearance of the first Korotkoff sound corresponds to the systolic pressure, while both the point of muffling and disappearance (phases IV and V) should be recorded as the diastolic pressure. The time of day, the position of the patient, whether lying, standing or sitting, and whether or not the patient appears anxious or distressed are all factors which should be recorded. For example, the blood pressure might be recorded as 142/94/90 (lying, relaxed) [19].

3.2.3. The apex

A heaving apex beat is the most common sign of left ventricular hypertrophy. Mechanical methods of assessing the cardiac impulse have shown that in normal subjects the outward movement of the apex is short and does not extend into the latter one third of systole. In hypertensive patients with left ventricular hypertrophy, the outward deflection is prolonged, sometimes beyond the second sound. This is referred to as a heaving apex and is best appreciated by simultaneous auscultation and palpation of the apex beat with the patient supine [20]. The area occupied by the cardiac impulse may also be increased beyond the normal one rib space. The least sensitive sign of left ventricular hypertrophy is displacement of the apex relative to the midclavicular line. Factors which interfere with the proper assessment of the apex include obesity and emphysema. A cardiac aneurysm produces a prolonged and enlarged cardiac impulse. Although usually distinguishable by its position, above and medial to the apex beat, it may occupy the ventricular apex.

3.2.4. Auscultation

Much emphasis has been placed on the loudness of the second heart sound in hypertension. This may reflect a period when blood pressure measurement was of doubtful accuracy and a loud second sound was used as an aid to diagnosis [21]. Although quoted as being present in as many as 70% of hypertensive patients [23], there is no evidence that this sign gives any information as to the state of the heart or the patients prognosis. The origin of the second sound has been variously attributed to vibrations in a column of blood or myocardium after valve closure, sudden tension in a flaccid membrane and apposition of valve cusps. Part of the sound is due to closure of the pulmonary valve and opening of the atrioventricular valves [24]. More recently, in the laboratory study of porcine and human valves mounted in a transparent medium, the second heart sound has been shown to be the result of diastolic vibration of the valve cusps. The amplitude of the sound produced depends on the amplitude of the valve motion which is directly related to the rate of change of pressure across the aortic valve [25]. This in turn depends on the aortic diastolic pressure and the rate of diastolic isovolumic relaxation of the left ventricle. Therefore, in a hypertensive patient with a normal left ventricle, the rate of change of pressure across the valve in early diastole is high, producing a loud second heart sound. However, in heart failure where the rate of isovolumic relaxation is poor and there is a fall in the rate of pressure change across the valve, the amplitude of the second sound becomes diminished [26]. Rarely, paradoxical splitting of the second sound may occur in which the aortic component of the second sound is delayed maximally during expiration. It is more common when hypertension is complicated by left bundle branch block.

Another common auscultatory finding in hypertension is a presystolic or fourth heart sound, present in 50 % of cases [23]. It correlates well with electrocardiographic P-wave abnormalities and is probably due to decreased left ventricular compliance. It may also be due to underlying myocardial ischaemia and is frequently first head after beta blockade. A protodiastolic or third heart sound is heard in 30 % of hypertensives, frequently in association with other signs of left ventricular failure or accelerated hypertension.

Systolic murmurs are common in hypertensive patients, present in up to 70 % of cases [23]. They are usually ejection type murmurs best heard at the apex or base of the heart. Amyl nitrate inhalation increases their intensity though aortic valvular lesions are rarely found at post mortem. In contrast, the regurgitant murmurs of mitral incompetence are rare in hypertensive patients and are usually due to organic disease. Apical mid-diastolic murmurs are occasionally heard and must be distinguished from a presystolic or pèrotodiastolic sound. They are most commonly due to organic mitral stenosis, a condition associated with an increased incidence of hypertension. Rarely they occur in the absence of organic disease and are probably the result of increased flow across the mitral valve. Finally, functional aortic regurgitant murmurs may occur in patiens with severe hypertension [23, 27].

3.2.5. Renovascular hypertension

The presence of a renal artery bruit is the only sign of discriminatory value between renovascular hypertension and essential hypertension. In the Co-operative Study on Renovascular Hypertension, 12 % of patients with renal artery stenosis and 1 % of patients with essential hypertension had an abdominal bruit [28]. However, in other studies abdominal bruits were found in 88 % of cases due to renal artery dysplasia and 36 % of cases due to atherosclerosis [29]. Further, they have been detected in 18 % of normal subjects [30]. Careful auscultation is as successful in the detection of abdominal bruits as phonarteriography [31]. The patient should be examined in a quiet room without undue compression of the abdominal wall by the stethoscope. Renal artery bruits are best heard above the umbilicus on or lateral to the midline. Occasionally, the murmur is heard well up into the epigastrium. It frequently radiates to one or other side, and this might help to lateralise the lesion, though it can be misleading. Higher pitched murmurs and those with a diastolic component are more significant, the latter predicting a successful surgical outcome in patients with renal artery dysplasia [32]. By far the commonest cause of abdominal bruit is coeliac artery stenosis. Other causes include stenosis of mesenteric, splenic and hepatic arteries, collateral vessels around complete vascular occlusions, aortic aneurysm and vascular tumours. A history of worsening hypertension in a young person with an abdominal bruit suggests renovascular hypertension secondary to renal artery dysplasia. In older subjects, atherosclerosis is a more common cause and there is frequently widespread vascular disease [4].

3.2.6. Fundoscopy

Fundoscopic vascular changes indicate that there is end-organ damage elsewhere [33] and are of prognostic significance in treated and untreated patients. Moreover, their resolution with treatment offers objective evidence of adequate control. Three disorders are manifested in the fundal changes of the hypertensive; hypertensive neuroretinopathy, arteriosclerosis and atherosclerosis [34]. Hypertensive neuroretinopathy presents as generalised arteriolar narrowing with later focal narrowing (grades I and II). This is difficult to assess as generalised narrowing is common, occuring in 33% of normotensive men aged 40–60 years [35] and attempts to derive an index of arteriolar narrowing have failed to distinguish normal and hypertensive subjects. Focal narrowing may also occur in the absence of hypertension. It has been postulated that narrowing of arterioles is an autoregulatory response to increased pressure. This compensatory mechanism may fail resulting in endothelial damage and arteriolar occlusion presenting as flame shaped haemorrhages and cotton wool exudates (grade III). At higher pressures, ischaemia of the optic nerve head results in papilloedema due to interruption of axoplasmic flow (grade IV). Grades III and IV hypertensive retinopathy occur in malignant hypertension.

Arteriosclerotic changes result in an increased light reflex from the arteriolar wall and venular compression by crossing arterioles. Though considered to reflect the duration rather than the degree of hypertension, the relationship of arteriosclerotic changes to hypertensive disease is unknown. An abnormal light reflex occurs in 30% of middle aged normotensive men [35] and venular compression may also be seen in the absence of hypertension. Further, these changes may resolve on treatment of hypertension casting doubt on their proposed underlying pathological cause.

Atherosclerotic changes of the central retinal artery may present as ischaemic neuropathy of the optic nerve and central retinal artery thrombosis. Retinal vein occlusion may occur due to an atherosclertoic plaque eroding into the vein from an adjacent artery as both lie within a single sheath [36]. In patients with transient ischaemic attacks embolic material may be seen at arteriolar bifurcations [34].

Resolution of vascular changes usually occurs with treatment. Haemorrhages and exudates may resolve over 2–10 weeks, the latter becoming granular and later hard and waxy in appearance before complete resolution. Papilloedema may take some months to resolve.

636

4. BLOOD PRESSURE MEASUREMENT

4.1. Equipment

Indirect blood pressure measurement is a valuable clinical technique frequently taken for granted. Students and nurses are poorly trained, equipment is badly maintained and attention to detail is often lacking. Further, failure to standardise the technique and changing recommendations from authoriative bodies have created confusion. These factors tend to make blood pressure measurement more inaccurate than need be.

The two devices most frequently used in blood pressure measurement are the mercury-in-glass and aneroid sphygmomanometers. Both anaeroid and mercury manometers are accurate but the mercury manometer retains its accuracy longer and is easier to maintain [37]. Mercury may be lost from the reservoir of the mercury device so that the meniscus lies below zero with no pressure applied to the cuff. Dirty tubing and oxidised mercury may obscure the meniscus. A blocked air vent at the top of the mercury column may cause sluggish movement of the mercury during inflation and deflation and result in overestimation of blood pressure [38]. Calibration of each new device must be corrected for the fall of mercury in the reservoir as the mercury column rises so that the scale indicates the differences between the levels of mercury in the tube and in the reservoir. This error is small, 1 % or less, if the diameter of the reservoir is over ten times the diameter of the tube [39].

An anaeroid manometer utilises a metal bellows which elongates when pressure is applied. A gear sector transmits the movement to an indicator needle. In some devices there is a stop at the zero position of the scale so that zero drift cannot be detected. The device should be tested regularly throughout the entire pressure range against a mercury-in-glass manometer by connecting both devices to a single cuff using a T-tube connector. In one study, 32% of all hospital anaeroid sphygmomanometers deviated from the limits laid down by the American National Bureau of Standards (± 3 mm Hg) [40]. Such deviations are less frequent where there is a policy of regular servicing. Anaeroid manometers are more convenient to use but must be calibrated against a mercury standard every six months and returned to the manufacturers for servicing if inaccurate. Moreover, errors, and their causes, are less easily identified and corrected than with mercury sphygmomanometers.

Both devices are subject to leaks due to worn valve washers, old tubing or ruptured bladders. These can be detected by inflating a cuff to 250 mm Hg. With the valve closed, the leak rate should not exceed 2 mm Hg in 10 s after the system has been allowed to equilibrate [37]. By clamping the circuit in sections, the site of the leak will be identified. Difficulty in inflating the cuff may be due to a blocked air vent within the valve apparatus. This is easily removed and cleaned.

4.2. Blood pressure measurement

An adult sized cuff should be placed snugly round the patients arm above the antecubital fossa. Ideally the bladder should completely encircle the arm and if it does not the bladder centre must be over the brachial artery [41]Ç. A loosely applied cuff acts as a narrow cuff and gives a falsely high measurement [42]. Inflation should be rapid to 30 mm Hg above the point of disappearance of the pulse. Slow inflation causes congestion of the arm resulting in attenuation of Korotkoff sounds and false elevation of the diastolic blood pressure [43]. Deflation should not exceed 3 mm Hg per pulse if underestimation of systolic blood pressure and overestimation of diastolic blood pressure are to be avoided. Tilting of the mercury column causes underestimation of blood pressure. The pressure should be read to the nearest 2 mm Hg from the top of the mercury meniscus which should be at eye level to avoid parallax error.

The patient should be in a resting position with the arm supported by the observer to prevent the elevation in blood pressure due to the isometric exercise of maintaining posture [44]. The arm should be at heart level to avoid the affect of hydrostatic pressure. In most subjects, the intra-arterial pressure is equal in both arms [43]. There may, however, be a difference of 10 mm Hg between arms when simultaneous indirect recordings are compared; this difference occurs more frequently when the pressures in the two arms are recorded sequentially because of the additional effect of physiological variation. Therefore, though a difference in pressure recordings between arms occurs in patients with widespread atherosclerosis, dissecting aortic aneurysm and coarctation of the aorta, it commonly occurs in patients with no vascular lesion. The pressure should be recorded in both arms initially and the higher measurement accepted as the true pressure. The arm with the highest pressure should be used for future measurement. In general, the pressure is highest in the right arm.

The frequency range of Korotkoff sounds in 40–120 cycles per second with maximum amplitude centred about 100 cycles/s. Upon muffling (Phase IV), the higher frequencies are attenuated and the maximum amplitude then centres about 60 cycles/s [46]. The diaphragm of the stethoscope is usually made of stiff linen bakelite designed to attenuate lower frequencies. The open chest piece, or bell, however, has a lower natural frequency and is four times more sensitive to low frequency sounds. The acoustic range of Korotkoff sounds is therefore better suited to the bell of the stethescope. However, it is usually easier for nurses and trained technical staff to use the diaphragm and stethescopes used by nurses may not have a bell attachment. A single tubed stethescope avoids extraneous noise caused by two tubes rubbing against each other and, by reducing the volume of the device increases the efficiency of sound transmission to the ear. The stethescope head should be placed as near as possible to the point of compression of the artery, below the lower edge of the cuff.

4.3. Korotkoff sounds

In his thesis on indirect blood pressure measurement, Korotkoff described three phases in the arterial sounds heard during cuff deflation [47]. The appearance of the first sound corresponded to systolic pressure. This was followed by a louder murmur and finally disappearance of the sound which correspoded to the diastolic pressure. In the subsequent decade, five phases of Korotkoff sounds were described.

Phase I   – First appearance of a clear tapping sound.
Phase II – Period during which a swishing quality is heard.
Phase III – Period during which sounds become crisper.
Phase IV – Period of abrupt muffling of the sounds.
Phase V   – Disappearance of sound.

Another phenomenon that may occur during cuff deflation is the auscultatory gap when the sounds disappear temporarily, reappearing at a lower pressure. If auscultation is not continued beyond this gap, a falsely high diastolic pressure will be recorded.

No one hypothesis for the production of Korotkoff sounds has found general acceptance. Theories have included a sudden localised change in the shape of the compressed artery, a water–hammer affect of the wave front striking a stationary column of blood below the cuff, fluid turbulence and resonance of air within the cuff. Studies using a Doppler technique [46] to differentiate arterial wall movement and fluid turbulence suggest that the Korotkoff sounds consist of a higher frequency component due to sudden arterial wall movement, and a lower frequency component due to fluid disturbance. At the point of muffling, the higher frequency component disappears. This point corresponds with the period in which the artery first remains open throughout the cardiac cycle, though the relationship is not consistent. Theoretically, therefore, this would appear to be the most logical end-point for diastole because in order for the artery to remain open throughout the cardiac cycle, cuff occlusive pressure must be lower than diastolic pressure. According to the analysis of Anliker [48], the production of Korotkoff sounds results from dynamic instability of the vessel wall induced by the cuff pressure. At this point oscillations induced in the arterial wall by the wave front are amplified and are detected as Korotkoff sounds. The limits of cuff pressure which induce dynamic instability correspond to the systolic and diastolic auscultatory pressures. Outside these limits, above the systolic or below the diastolic pressure, no sounds are heard.

4.4. Diastolic dilemma

It is not surprising, therefore, that as the origin of the Korotkoff sounds is not satisfactorily explained, their relationship to intra-arterial pressure has been studied in detail. Many of these studies are not comparable because of differences in technique. Some authors have compared direct and indirect recordings from the same artery. However, it seems probable that an indwelling catheter would alter sound production from an artery. In many earlier studies, the transducer-catheter systems for intra-arterial pressure measurements were of doubtful accuracy and in some the frequency–amplitude characteristics were not given. This varies greatly depending on length and bore of tubing, transducer type and volume of transducer chamber [49]. In some studies, the direct radial pressure in one limb has been compared with indirect recordings from the opposite brachial artery. The systolic pressure in the radial artery, however, is about 6 mm Hg higher than in the brachial artery and there may be a difference in indirect pressure recordings between arms.

The sphygmomanometers used as standard for comparison with intra-arterial recordings have varied between studies and this may alter results. The London School of Hygiene Sphygmomanometer [50] has been used in two studies which favoured phase IV Korotkoff sounds as the diastolic end-point [51, 52]. We have found that this device tends to underestimate blood pressure for two reasons. Firstly, a calibration error in the device leads to an underrecording of 4 mm Hg at higher pressures- Secondly, there is a difference in decision end-points between this device and the standard method of blood pressure measurement. During deflation of the London School of Hygiene Sphygmomanometer, three mercury columns hidden from the observers view monitor cuff pressure. The fall of mercury in each column may be halted independently so that separate recordings for systolic and diastolic phase IV and V pressure are made. In order to ensure that the systolic end-point has been reached, the second Korotkoff sound must be taken as the systolic end-point. Similarly, the diastolic end-point is some variable pressure below the last sound, that point where a sound would be expected but fails to occur. Further, the London School of Hygiene Sphygmomanometer has been shown to give lower recordings of indirect blood pressure than other methods, including the standard mercury device [51, 53]. This may explain why in these two studies indirect blood pressure measurement with the London School of Hygiene Sphygmomanometer was lower than direct intra-arterial measurement.

In general, most authors have found that phase V corresponds more closely with the intra-arterial diastolic pressure. The American Heart Association has variously recommended phase V [54] and phase IV [55] as the diastolic end-point, whereas the World Health Organisation recommends that both phase IV and phase V be recorded. There is greater agreement between observers using the silent rather than the muffled end-point, a matter of great importance in training observers. We recommend that phase V be taken as the diastolic pressure. To avoid confusion, however, we support the suggestion that the fourth and fifth phases should always be noted. In patients with a high velocity of blood flow, Korotkoff sounds may be heard right down to zero pressure. In such cases the fourth phase should be taken as the diastolic end-point.

Many factors influence the difference between the indirect and direct pressure recordings. The mercury or anaeroid sphygmomanometer measures cuff pressure and it is assumed that this reflects intra-arterial pressure. In general, however, the indirect method tends to underestimate the intra-arterial systolic pressure and the fifth phase diastolic end-point tends to have a variable relationship to intra-arterial diastolic pressure. The relationship between indirect and direct blood pressure recording depends on the elasticity, wall thickness and radius of the artery under compression [56]. It might be expected, therefore, that in elderly subjects the pressure required to collapse the artery would be increased. This would lead to an overestimation of the true intra-arterial pressure by the indirect method in the elderly, a phenomenon referred to as 'pseudohypertension' [57].

4.5. Bladder size

Another potential source of error is the bladder size. If the inflatable bladder within the cuff is not matched for arm circumference indirect measurements become unreliable. The zone of effective pressure exerted by the bladder narrows in deeper tissues so that in an obese subjects the pressure within a standard bladder (12 cm × 23 cm) may not be fully exerted on the artery. Therefore, in order to compress an adequate length of brachial artery the bladder must be inflated to pressures higher than in non-obese subjects. Another possible explanation is that in obese subjects the bladder balloons into the soft tissues and therefore acts as an exceptionally narrow bladder [41]. Ideally the cuff bladder width should be 40% of the arm circumference [58]. Bladder width, however, is less critical if a bladder of sufficient length to completely encircle the arm is used and indirect recordings with such a bladder correlate best with intra-arterial recordings [37]. We recommend that for adults the bladder should be at least 35 cm long and 12 cm wide. If the bladder fails to encircle the arm, the centre of the bladder, often marked on the cuff, must be placed directly over the artery to be compressed.

4.6. Variability of indirect blood pressure measurement

Repeated indirect blood pressure recordings have demonstrated that casual recording may bear little relationship to the patients overall blood pressure behaviour. Raftery [59] has shown the considerable variation in blood pressure over 24 h with direct intra-arterial pressure measurements. This may also be demonstrated using non-invasive technique for ambulatory blood pressure recording (Figure 1). These devices are providing useful especially in patients with borderline hypertension and in those in whom blood pres-

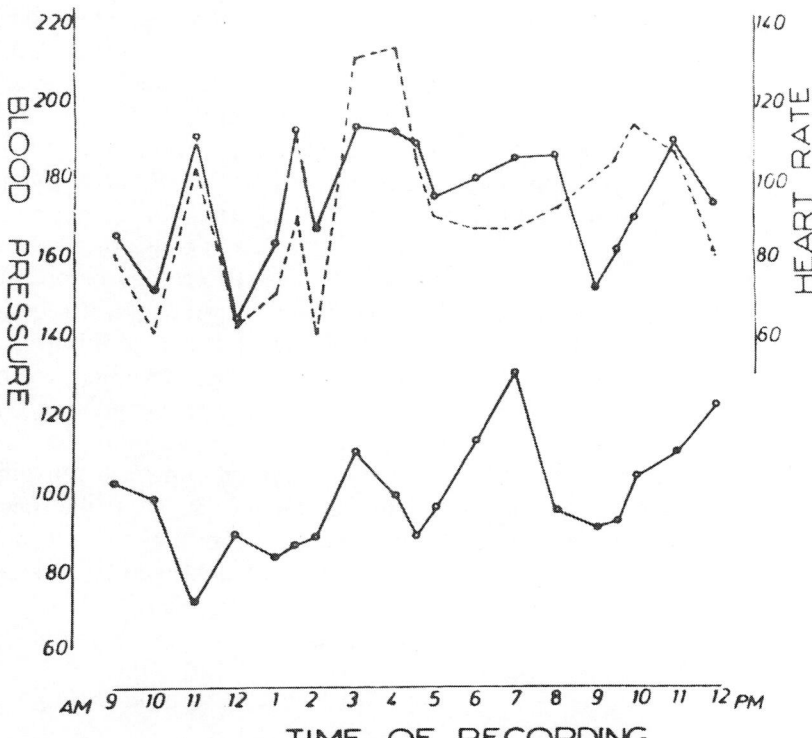

Figure 1. Ambulatory systolic and diastolic blood pressure (—) and heart rate (— — —) recordings over a sixteen-hour period (Remler M2,000 semiautomatic portable blood pressure recorder).

sure control is difficult. Blood pressure behaviour may also be assessed by home recording of blood pressure by the patient or a relative. This is a simple technique, requiring only a small amount of training and inexpensive equipment [5]. The initial recording of blood pressure tends to be higher especially in the clinical environment presumably due to anxiety. Over 50% of patients found to have high blood pressure at their first visit are normotensive on subsequent examination [2]. Further, repeated measurements on a single occasion may be highly variable, the first recording tending to be highest [60] with a gradual fall to basal levels after four recordings at ten-minute intervals. In practice, the average of three recordings, two at the start and one at the end of the examination, is considered adequate [61]. These should be repeated at one other visit before a decision is made on diagnosis or management. However, in cases of severe or accelerated hypertension, treatment may have to be started earlier.

Observer error accounts for some of the variation in blood pressure recordings and is high for medical staff [62]. This is partly due to a difference between observers which reflects inadequate training and the continueing difference in diastolic decision end-points. Nurses and doctors should be trained in blood pressure measurement using either a film or, more simply, a binaural stethescope so that teacher and trainee are auscultating the same sounds [63]. A further component of observer variability is observer bias. This describes an unconscious tendency of raising or lowering a patient's blood pressure. For example, there might be observer bias in over-reading blood pressure so that a patient is included in a drug trial. Similarly, we may under-record blood pressure in a young healthy man and so not label him hypertensive. Digit preference describes the tendency to record blood pressures with figures ending in 0 or 5, such as 80 and 95. Adequate discussion during training makes the observer aware of such bias and minimises its affect. Special instruments have been designed to overcome this problem especially during research. The London School of Hygiene reduces both observer bias and digit preference but has disadvantages already referred to and is expensive and cumbersome. The Hawkesley random-zero sphygmomanometer is a mercury-in-glass sphygmomanometer which has the special feature of obscuring the zero point for each recording until after the systolic and diastolic end-points have been read. The results must then be corrected for the zero point which varies between 0 and 60 mm Hg [64]. It has the advantage of being not much larger than the standard mercury sphygmomanometer and is reasonably priced.

4.7. Blood pressure measurement in special situations

Blood pressure determination in children and infants is difficult because of the effect of anxiety, restlessness and crying, and in addition, it is more difficult to auscultate the Korotkoff sounds. Further, blood pressure is labile and it is especially important to rely on repeated measurements for diagnosis. Proper cuff bladder size is essential for recording accurate pressure readings. Too large a cuff underestimates and too small a cuff overestimates blood pressure. In general, the cuff bladder should be wide enough to cover two-thirds of the upper arm and long enough to fully encircle it [65]. Cuff bladder widths range from 2.5 cm for infants to 9.5 cm for older children. Muffling of sound is recommended as the best index of diastolic pressure [66]. In 50% of children, only one diastolic auscultatory criterion occurs in that there is no discernable muffling before disappearance of the sounds. In neonates, poor sound production may exclude accurate recordings by auscultation and other techniques may be necessary. The Arteriosonde is a device which detects arterial wall movement by an ultrasonic method. It has been shown to give accurate results when compared with both other indirect methods and intra-arterial recordings [67]. Another device, the Infrasonde 3000, detects the low frequency sounds produced by the fluttering of the arterial wall when the pulse wave passes into the collapsed segment. Although outside the acoustic range of the human, this device reproduces these frequencies into an audiosigual. Despite its accuracy in recording systolic pressures, this device is inaccurate for diastolic recordings [67]. Other methods used in children include the flush method, which gives an estimate of the mean pressure [68], and oscillometry [69].

In cardiac dysrhythmias, such as atrial fibrillation, stroke volume, and therefore the blood pressure, varies depending on the preceeding pulse interval. The point of onset and disappearance of the Korotkoff sounds vary so that the average of three recordings should be taken [37].

In clinical shock, brachial artery pulsations may be greatly diminished and the blood pressure is difficult to estimate though central pressure may be well maintained. Ultrasonic detection of arterial wall movement (Arteriosonde) or of blood flow (Accoson) and intra-arterial recordings are more accurate in this condition.

The blood pressure should be recorded in the thigh when coarctation of the aorta is suspected. A cuff containing a bladder 18 cm wide and long enough to fully encircle the thigh should be used. The cuff is wrapped around the thigh and the patient lays prone. The pressure is recorded by auscultating over the popliteal artery. Simultaneous intra-arterial femoral and brachial pressures are equal and the tendency to record higher formal systolic pressures by the indirect method reflects inadequate cuff size.

SUMMARY

With a rising population of patients identified as hypertensive through screening programmes, the importance of clinical as opposed to laboratory investigations is becoming increasingly apparent. A clinical evaluation exploring the areas of secondary causes and end-organ disease combined with an evaluation of blood pressure behaviour will accurately diagnose hypertension in the majority of patients. Further, most cases of secondary hypertension will be identified and the number of laboratory investigations reduced. The inaccuracies of indirect blood pressure measurement are magnified by poor technique, inadequate training of staff, improperly maintained equipment and the continuing debate regarding which phase of the Korotkoff sounds should be taken as the diastolic end point. However, with attention to detail, this technique is accurate except in infancy, marked hypotension and possibly the elderly hypertensive.

REFERENCES

1. O'Malley K, O'Brien E: Management of hypertension in the elderly. N Eng J Med 302 (25):1397–1401, 1980.
2. Carey RM, Reid RA, Ayers RC, Lynch SS, McLain WL, Vaughan DE: The Charlottesville Blood Pressure Survey. Value of repeated blood pressure measurements. JAMA 236 (7):847–851, 1976.
3. Berglund G, Anderson O, Wilhelmson L: Prevalence of primary and secondary hypertension: studies in a random population study. Br Med J 2:554–556, 1976.
4. Kaplan NM, Lieberman E: Clinical hypertension. 2nd edn. Baltimore: William & Wilkins, 1978.
5. Laher MS, O'Boyle CP, Quinn C, O'Brien ET, O'Malley K: The training of relatives for home recording of blood pressure. Ir Med J. (In press.)
6. Sokolow M, Perloff D, Cowan R: Contribution of ambulatory blood pressure to the assessment of patients with mild to moderate elevation of blood pressure. Cardiovasc Rev Rep 1 (4):295–303. 1980.
7. Management Committee: The Australian therapeutic trial in mild hypertension. Lancet 1:1261–1267. 1980.
8. Moser M, Wish H, Freidman AP: Headache and hypertension. JAMA 180 (4):301–306, 1962.
9. Stewart IMG: Headache and hypertension. Lancet 1:1262–1266, 1953.
10. Walker CH: Migraine and it's relationship to hypertension. Br Med J 2:1430–1433, 1959.
11. Mitchell JRA: Nose-bleeding and high blood pressure. Br Med J 1:25–27, 1959.
12. Parfrey PS, Vandenburg MJ, Wright P, Holly JMP, Goodwin FJ, Evan SJW, Ledingham JM: Blood pressure and hormonal changes following alteration in dietary sodium and potassium in mild essential hypertension. Lancet 1:59–64, 1981.
13. Ferguson RK: Cost and yield of hypertensive evaluation. Ann Intern Med 82:761–765, 1975.
14. Editorial: Hypertension and oral contraceptives. Br Med J 1:1570–1571, 1978.
15. Ibrahim MM, Tarazi RC, Dustan HP, Bravo EL, Gifford RW: Hyperkinetic heart in severe hypertension: a separate clinical haemodynamic entity. Am J Cardiol 35:667–674, 1975.
16. Wooling KR: Hypertensive-ischaemic ulcer. An atypical ischaemic necrosis of the skin. JAMA 157 (3):196–201, 1964.
17. Herrison J: The sphygmomanometer, an instrument which renders the action of the arteries

apparent to the eye. London: Longman Blundell ES (transf), 1835.

18. Martyn CN, Carroll RJM, Frier BM, McClement M, French EB: Why palpate the radial artery. Lancet 1:89–90, 1981.
19. O'Brien ET, O'Malley K: ABC of blood pressure measurement. Technique. Br Med J 2:982–984, 1979.
20. Conn RD, Cole JS: The cardiac impulse. Clinical and angiographic correlations. Ann Intern Med 75:185–191, 1971.
21. Janeway TC: A clinical study of hypertensive cardiovascular disease. Arch Intern Med 12:755–797, 1913.
22. O'Brien ET, O'Malley K: ABC of blood pressure measurement. The patient. Br Med J 2:920, 1979.
23. Barlow J, Kincaid-Smith P: The auscultatory findings in hypertension. Br Heart J 21:505–514, 1959.
24. Luisada AA, Lia CK, Aravanis C: On the mechanism of production of the heart sounds. Am Heart J 55:383–399, 1958.
25. Stein PD, Sabbah HN: Origin of the second heart sound: clinical relevance of new observations. Am J Cardiol 41:108–110, 1978.
26. Stein PD, Sabbah HN, Khaja F, Anbe DT: Exploration of the cause of the low intensity aortic component of the second sound in nonhypotensive patients with poor left ventricular performance. Circulation 57:590–593, 1978.
27. Evans W: Hypertonia or uneventful high blood pressure. Lancet 2: 52–59, 1957.
28. Simon N, Franklin, Franlkin SS, Bleifer KH, Maxwell MH: Clinical characteristics of renovascular hypertension. JAMA 220:1209–1218, 1972.
29. McLoughlin M, Colapinto RF, Hobbs BB: Abdominal bruits. Clinical and angiographic correlation. Jama 231:1238–1242, 1975.
30. Rivin A: Abdominal vascular sounds. JAMA 221:688–690, 1972.
31. Zoneraich S, Zoneraich O: Value of auscultation and phonoarteriography in detecting atherosclerotic involvement of the abdominal aorta and its branches. Am Heart J 83:620–629, 1972.
32. Eipper DF, Gifford RW, Stewart BH, Alfidi RJ, McCormack LF, Vidt DG: Abdominal bruits in renovascular hypertension. Am J Cardiol. 37:48-52, 1976.
33. Keith NM, Wagener HP, Barker NW: Some different types of essential hypertension: their course and prognosis. Am J Med Sci 197:332–343, 1939.
34. Hedges TR: The retina and hypertension. Postgrad Med 45:120–128, 1969.
35. Van Buchem FSP, v.d. Heuvel-Aghina JWM Th, v.d. Heuvel JEA: Hypertension and changes of the fundus oculi. Acta Med Scand 176:539–546, 1964.
36. Editorial: Postural response of intra-occular pressure in vascular disease. Lancet 1:314, 1981.
37. O'Brien ET, O'Malley K: ABC of blood pressure measurement. The sphygmomanometer. Br Med J 2:851–853.
38. Shaw A: Sphygmomanometers: errors due to blocked vents. Br Med J 1:789–790, 1979.
39. Malindzak GS, Rapela CE, Green HD: Static method for simultaneous calibration of several pressure transducer systems. Med Res Eng 3:39–42, 1968.
40. Perlman LV, Chiang BC, Keller J, Blackburn H: Accuracy of sphygmomanometers in habitual practice. Arch Intern Med 125:1000–1003, 1970.
41. King GE: Errors in clinical measurement of blood pressure in obesity. Clin Sci 32:223–237, 1967.
42. Nuessle WF: The importance of a tight blood pressure cuff. Am Heart J 53(6):905–907, 1956.
43. Ragan C, Bordley J: Measurements of blood pressure. Bull Johns Hopkins Hosp 69:526, 1941.

44. Viol GW, Goebel M, Lorenz GJ, Ing TS: Seating as a variable in clinical blood pressure measurement. Am Heart J 98(6):813–814, 1979.
45. Harrison EG, Roth GM, Hines EA: Bilateral indirect and direct arterial pressures. Circulation 22:419–436, 1960.
46. McCutcheon EP, Rushmer RF: Korotkoff sounds: an experimental critique. Circulation 20:149–161, 1967.
47. Korotkoff MS: On the subject of methods of measuring blood pressure. Bull Imp Milit Med Acad St. Petersburg 11:365–367, 1905.
48. Anliker M, Raman KR: Korotkoff sounds at diastole – a phenomenon of dynamic instability of fluid filled shells. Int J Solids Structures 2:467, 1966.
49. Cronvich JA, Burch GE: Frequency characteristics of some pressure transducer systems. Am Heart J 77:792–797, 1969.
50. Rose GA, Holland WW, Crowley EA: A sphygmomanometer for epidemiologists. Lancet 1:296–300, 1964.
51. Ulrych M, Burianova B, Hornych A, Mydlik M, Dousa T, Hejl Z. Comparisons of direct and indirect methods of measurement of arterial blood pressure in man. Cor Vasa 8:77–88, 1966.
52. Halland WW, Humerfelt S: Measurement of blood pressure. Comparison of intra-arterial and cuff valves. Br Med J 2:1241–1243, 1964.
53. Hunyor SN, Flynn JM, Cochineas C: Comparison of performance of various sphygmomanometers with intra-arterial blood pressure readings. Br Med J 2:159–162, 1978.
54. Bordley J, Connor CAR, Hamilton WF, Kerr WJ, Wiggers CJ: Recommendations for human blood pressure determinations by sphygmomanometers. Circulation 4:503–509, 1951.
55. Kirkendall WM, Burton AC, Epstein FH, Freis ED: Recommendations for human blood pressure determination by sphygmomanometers. Circulation 36:980–988, 1967.
56. Sacks AH: Indirect blood pressure measurements: a matter of interpretation. Angiology 30:683–695, 1979.
57. Spence JD, Sibbald WJ, Cape RD: Direct, indirect and mean blood pressures in hypertensive patients: the problem of cuff artefact due to arterial wall siffness, and a partial solution. Clin Invest Med 2:165–173, 1980.
58. Geddes LA, Tivey R: The importance of cuff width in measurement of blood pressure indirectly. Cardiovasc Res Cent Bull 14:69b–79, 1976.
59. Raftery EB: The methodology of blood pressure recording. Br J Clin Pharmac 6:193–201, 1978.
60. Armitage P, Rose GA: The variability of measurements of casual blood pressure. 1. A laboratory study. Clin Sci 30: 325–335, 1966.
61. Souchek J, Stamler J, Dyer AR, Paul O, Lepper MH: The value of two or three versus a single reading of blood pressure at a first visit. J Chron Dis 32:197–210, 1979.
62. Rose G: Standardisation of observers in blood pressure measurement. Lancet 1:673–674, 1965.
63. O'Brien ET, O'Malley K: ABC of blood pressure measurement. The Observer. Br Med J 2:775–776, 1979.
64. Wright BM, Dore CF: A random-zero sphygmomanometer. Lancet 1:337–338, 1970.
65. American Task Force on blood pressure control in children. Pediatrics 59 (Suppl 1):797–820, 1977.
66. Moss AJ, Adams FH: Index of indirect estimation of diastolic blood pressure. Am J Dis Child 106:364–367, 1963.
67. Savage JM, Dillon MJ, Taylor JFN: Clinical evaluation and comparison of the Infrasonde and Arteriosonde, and mercury sphygmomanometer in measurement of blood pressure in children. Arch Dis Child 54:184–189, 1979.

68. O'Brien ET, O'Malley K: ABC of blood pressure measurement. Infancy and childhood. Br Med J 2:1048–1049, 1979.
69. Ashworth AM, Neligan GA, Rogers JE: Sphygmomanometer for the newborn. Br Med J 1:801–804, 1959.

42. LABORATORY EXAMINATION OF THE HYPERTENSIVE PATIENT

Mohinder P. Sambhi

LABORATORY EXAMINATION OF THE HYPERTENSIVE PATIENT

Laboratory examination of a patient with hypertension ought not to be viewed as an entity separate from the total work-up, but rather as an integral part of it, including the clinical and the radiological examinations. This subdivision is made here in the interest of descriptive clarity and emphasis, albeit at the unavoidable expense of some repetition as well as diversity of opinion and approach.

The objectives and the scope of the laboratory work

It may be appropriate to discuss the laboratory investigation in the context of the major objectives of the work-up of a patient with hypertension.

(A) The first objective would perhaps be to confirm the diagnosis (or the label) of hypertension. This objective today is largely, indeed exclusively, achieved through clinical examination, discussed in the preceding chapter. At the time of this writing, no definitive marker test is proven or established as diagnostic of primary essential hypertension. Current research on possible genetic markers, consisting of a fundamental or characteristic fault in the membranous transport of cation is being actively pursued [1]. The existence of genetic markers, if confirmed in the future, may provide the basis of a simple in vitro test (studying the cation flux across the red blood cells of a hypertensive patient) as an important diagnostic aid even in the prehypertensive stage.

(B) Another important objective of the investigations in a hypertensive patient is to identify or to exclude the known causes of the 'curable' types of secondary hypertension. This benefit should theoretically be extended to every new patient with hypertension, and also to patients who may experience unexplained exacerbation in the course of the disease. In practice, the cost effectiveness of the extensive work-up needs to be balanced against the benefits and risks that accrue for the patient.

The secondary types of hypertension have been discussed in detail earlier

Amery, A. (ed.) Hypertensive Cardiovascular Disease: Pathophysiology and Treatment
© *1982, Martinus Nijhoff Publishers. The Hague / Boston / London*
ISBN-13: 978-94-009-7478-4

in this volume. The description of the definitive diagnostic procedures need not be repeated here. In this chapter we shall limit ourselves to a discussion of screening procedures required for routine exclusion of secondary hypertension in the work-up of every newly discovered hypertension patient. The question of how extensive this screening work-up for secondary hypertension should be for every patient continues to be a matter of debate. Arguments for and against a thorough and extensive work-up for secondary hypertension can be advanced depending upon whether the investigations are performed in an academic institution or in the private office of a physician, and upon whether the expense of the investigation is borne by the patient himself, an insurance company, or a socialized system supporting medical care. There is a good deal of room for differences of opinion regarding what is commensurate with 'good' medical practice. It should be recognized that the objective of ruling out a secondary cause for hypertension, if considered worthwhile, should not be relegated to chance by arbitrarily limiting the investigation to a predetermined recipe or a battery of tests for all patients. Investigations need to be individualized for each patient just as much as the treatment. Limitations of routine screening tests, even with a high degree of reliability and accuracy, can be illustrated by the following example. Assuming that the prevalence of renovascular hypertension is 2.5% in the hypertensive population at large, a screening test with the impressive record of 97.5% positive identification for renovascular hypertension, if performed routinely on every patient with hypertension, will result in a 50% rate of false negative results.

(C) If the diagnosis of primary hypertension appears to be likely, the next objective of the modern clinician is to attempt to classify the patient in a subset of essential hypertension, with the hope that the process will aid in planning long-term management and the selection of specific pharmacotherapeutic agents. There is a general consensus regarding this objective as far as it is achievable on clinical grounds, e.g., classification as borderline hypertension, systolic hypertension, complicated hypertension, etc. There is intense controversy, on the other hand, on whether laboratory investigation leading to the classification of low, normal, or high renin hypertension (or a similar profiling of patients based on plasma catecholamine levels) is essential, desirable, helpful, or useless in the therapeutic management of a hypertensive patient. This question will be briefly discussed later on.

(D) Another major objective of a hypertensive work-up is to assess the degree of existing hypertensive cardiovascular disease or vascular damage in the target organs caused by hypertension. In the central nervous system and the retina, this assessment is at present made clinically. In contrast, the estimation of the extent of renal damage is almost entirely dependent upon laboratory examination and will be discussed below. The assessment of cardiac hypertrophy and function is predominantly in the realm of clinical and radiological examinations, although recent work indicates that the low pressure receptors in the area of the heart and the great veins have a significant role in the control of renin secretion [2]. Preliminary evidence is available to suggest that regulation of plasma renin is abnormal in the hypertensive patient with cardiac involvement [3].

(E) The next major objective of hypertensive work-up almost entirely in the realm of laboratory investigation, is to identify associated diseases, overt or subclinical metabolic, endocrine, or other systemic abnormalities that may influence the course and the natural history of essential hypertension. The frequently occurring and well-known examples are diabetes, gout, and atherosclerosis; rare instances include familial hypercholesterolemia or hyperlipoproteinemia, collagen diseases, and porphyruria.

It must be reiterated that the objectives listed above are not applicable uniformly to all patients. Accordingly, the 'optimal' work-up should be tailored to the needs of the individual patient taking into account age and sex, as well as the magnitude of the index of clinical suspicion or the available circumstantial evidence for or against the existence of secondary hypertension, target organ damage, and other associated disorders.

The discussion of the labortory examination will therefore be approached as applicable to a newly discovered ptient with hypertension, presumably essential.

LABORTORY EXAMINATIONS

All measurements should ideally be made while the patient is off all medications and on normal habitual dietary intake. Laboratory investigation of a new patient should begin with simple screening for health survey, such as a complete hemogram, routine blood and urine chemistries, and urinalysis (including a urine culture in the female). Many of these tests are now available as a package.

Urinalysis and 24-hour urinary electrolyte determinations

Chemical and microscopic examination of a freshly voided midstream morning specimen of urine should be made. In uncomplicated essential hypertension, urinalysis is normal. A careful examination may in other cases provide many useful clues.

(A) A normal capacity of urine to acidify itself and achieve a pH value close to 5.0 can rather conclusively exclude primary aldosteronism as the basis of hypertension. Alkaline urine is a feature of Conn's syndrome, and no exception has been reported in the world literature.

(B) Discovery of a low urinary osmalarity or specific gravity should be reconfirmed and taken as an indication for further investigations for possible underlying renal disease. Traces of protein or sugar if discovered should be quantitated in 12- or 24-hour urine samples to be meaningful.

(C) Microscopic examinations of urine should also be conducted on a 12-(overnight) or 24-hour urinary collection. Quantitative counts of red blood cells, white blood cells, and casts can provide an index of suspicion regarding pre-existing chronic parenchymal disease. In the female, urine culture and even asymptomatic bacteriuria should be quantitated by microscopic methods.

(D) Whenever feasible, 24-hour urinary electrolytes, total creatinine, and urinary volume should be measured. Under uncontrolled but stable conditions of dietary intake, urinary sodium and potassium provide a measure of habitual dietary consumption of sodium and potassium, an information of fundamental importance in planning the therapeutic range of dietary manipulation. On a normal intake of salt and without diuretic administration, a urinary loss greater than 60 mEq/l is probably excessive for most patients, and justifies further screening tests to exclude aldosteronism, such as the behavior of serum potassium and a measurement of urinary aldosterone.

Twenty-four hour urinary excretion of catecholamines and the two major metabolites is commonly used as a routine test in screening for pheochromocytoma. As a single screening test, determination of total metanephrines is considered reliable, with a lower incidence of false negative results. Methylglucamine contained in several X-ray opaque dyes may, however, interfere with metanephrine measurements for three to four days following the radiographic procedures. Measurements of vanillymandelic acid (VMA) and free catecholamines in the 24-hour urinary sample are used as supplemental procedures.

Total urinary creatinine serves as a rough guide to the adequacy of complete urine collection, and allows a gross estimation of endogenous creatinine clearance and of sodium creatinine ratio in the urine. These derived parameters are subject to inherent and wide variations and lack precision as indices of glomerular filtration rate and the filtered fraction of sodium. Despite these limitations they have the virtue of simplicity and of being byproducts of the 24-hour urine collection.

Hemogram

In addition to being a reflection of general health, a hemogram serves to exclude anemia or polycythemia, which in hypertensives may accompany renal disease or rare neuroendocrine disorders. Red cell morphology may be abnormal in certain cases of accelerated hypertension.

Serum Chemistries

These measurements are important not only as diagnostic indicators but also as baseline controls for future reference during therapeutic interventions.

Serum creatinine is considered superior to blood urea nitrogen as an indicator of renal function or for derivation of glomerular filtration rate. It should be recognized, however, that elevation of serum creatinine is a late and crude indicator of renal insufficiency, requiring almost two thirds of the renal parenchyma to be nonfunctional.

Serum sodium is usually normal. Under appropriate conditions, it may reflect mineralcorticoid or vasopressin excess. Serum potassium should be carefully measured under conditions of normal diet and off medications. A consistently normal serum potassium virtually rules out the presence of a primary aldosteronism. In borderline cases, an administered sodium load may expose the tendency towards hypokalemia. Rarely, a potassium-losing kidney or excessive ingestion of liquorice may be the underlying cause of hypokalemia. Mild to moderate elevations of serum potassium are observed in hyporeninemic hypoaldosteronism.

Serum calcium and phosphorus measurements are indicated to exclude primary hyperparathyroidism, an entity considerably more common among patients with hypertension than in the general normotensive population.

A routine measurement of plasma cortisol, thyroid hormones, and liver function tests is generally included in a complete laboratory survey.

Estimation of carbohydrate tolerance, serum uric acid, serum cholesterol and triglycerides

The association of atherosclerosis and hypertension and the potentiating influence of each on the other is well known. During the asymptomatic stage mild hypertension has a meager incidence of so-called pressure-dependent complications. Potentiation of atherosclerotic complications, including ischemic heart disease, is the major risk associated with mild hypertension.

The risk is further enhanced in the subset population with manifestations of mild to moderate carbohydrate intolerance, hyperuricemia, and hyperlipidemia. Several antihypertensive medications induce metabolic abnormalities in certain patients during long-term therapy [4]. The significance of induced abnormalities, however, is not entirely clear. These considerations, discussed fully elsewhere in this volume, dictate that a careful assessment of these risk factors is prudent in every patient with hypertension. The presence of these metabolic abnormalities may be important in the decision of when to start treatment of mild hypertension, how aggressively to treat hypertension in a given patient, and what drugs to employ preferentially for the management of the individual patient.

As many as 20% of untreated patients with hypertension may have elevated serum uric acid. Serum uric acid and fasting and two-hour postprandial plasma glucose should be measured routinely. In case of manifest carbohydrate intolerance, a glucose tolerance test should be performed. Serum cholesterol and fasting serum triglycerides should be measured routinely. In patients showing elevated values, particularly in association with mild elevations of plasma glucose and uric acid, lipoprotein electrophoresis should be employed as an aid in the classification of hyperlipidemia.

The value of plasma renin and catecholamine profiling on the management of a patient with hypertension

Renin sodium profiling
Measurements of plasma renin and catecholamines are valuable tools for the diagnosis of the renal and adrenal causes of secondary types of hypertension. The diagnostic use of plasma renin activity in primary aldosteronism, of bilateral renal venous renin measurements in renal hypertension, and of plasma catecholamines for pheochromocytoma have been fully discussed under the respective titles. The controversial aspects of low renin hypertension as an entity have also been treated in a separate chapter. However, one of the most controversial topics in the area of routine laboratory work-up of a new patient with essential hypertension continues to be the question of whether renin measurements are of significant and fundamental value in planning the therapeutic management. It is beyond the scope of the present discussion to review all aspects of the arguments in this issue. A brief summary is presented.

In a series of publications since 1972, Laragh and coworkers have been articulating an attractive thesis suggesting that the maintenance of hypertension may be usefully viewed as the dual interaction of volume and vasoconstriction, depending upon the sodium and renin components. The hypertensive population can be profiled into low, normal, and high categories in comparison with the curvilinear relationship of a 24-hour urinary sodium and plasma renin activity measurements in normal subjects. Based on retrospective analysis, these investigators found a striking lack of morbid events and complications of hypertension in patients classified as low renin vs. normal and high renin. Plasma renin was therefore viewed as an important determinant of vascular damage secondary to hypertension, and the measurement of plasma renin was proposed as a reliable predictor of future hypertensive complications. Accordingly, antihypertensive drugs lowering plasma renin were considered desirable, those elevating renin for prolonged periods as potentially harmful and less efficacious. It was recommended that the selection of antihypertensive drugs suitable to the individual patient should be based upon the renin status of the patient and the renin suppressant or elevating effect of the therapeutic agent [5, 6].

Numerous studies have been addressed to the questions raised above. Although the results of these studies have in some cases been sharply negative, in other cases they have provided partial support to aspects of the Laragh thesis. The following general statements can be made:

(A) Several studies have failed to confirm the suggestion that the low renin patient is significantly protected against hypertensive complications. However, it is generally accepted that elevated plasma renin is either a marker for the existence of hypertensive complications [7], or in borderline hypertension may reflect the level of adrenergic activity at least in some patients [8].

(B) The controversy is unresolved on whether it is possible for investigators to preselect efficacious antihypertensive drugs by studying the renin sodium profiling of a patient prior to the initiation of therapy. It is, however, generally recognized that in the presence of elevated renin, a greater component of the elevated blood pressure is being maintained by the renin–angiotensin system, as can be usually demonstrated by the use of angiotensin blockers.

Nevertheless there are valid arguments in favor of the recommendation that for the practitioner, renin sodium profiling is at present of little help in planning antihypertensive therapy. Some of these arguments are listed below.

(1) Dr. Laragh contends [9] that one of the major reasons why other investigators have failed to confirm the findings of his group is because no one has used precisely the same methodology for renin measurement. To this author's knowledge, this contention has never been challenged through a controlled comparison; not a facile study to undertake, to be sure.

(2) There are many pitfalls and variables in the construction and the use of a renin sodium profile in hypertensive patients as well as in a representative sample of the normotensive population. Each laboratory needs to use its own control data. It is difficult to standardize renin measurements from different laboratories, and these problems are well known and appreciated [10, 11]. Additionally, a single measurement of 24-hour urinary sodium, too difficult, inconvenient, and often unreliable a procedure in a doctor's office or the outpatient clinic to be used as appropriate renin sodium profiling, implies that the subject is in a reasonable sodium balance and that factors other than sodium influencing the level of renin activity are of relatively minor importance. Both of these assumptions may not be correct in a given patient.

(3) If changes in diet, antihypertensive therapy, and factors other than sodium-regulating renin release can influence plasma renin to a sufficient degree, resulting in a change of the patient's classification into low, normal, or high categories over relatively short periods of time, renin profiling as a static concept ceases to offer the promise faithfully to predict the dynamic situation. If deemed useful, frequent and continuous assessment of renin sodium profiling of a patient under well-controlled conditions clearly falls in the realm of a specialized laboratory of hypertension research and not in a clinician's office.

In view of these considerations, routine plasma renin measurements for every patient with essential hypertension represents an unnecessary expense and inconvenience to the patient in whom other appropriate clinical, radiological and laboratory investigations have been made and indicate the initiation of drug treatment. As a research tool, renin sodium profiling of patients with hypertension needs to be evaluated more widely in better controlled studies than hitherto attempted.

Measurements of inactive renin are at this time of research interest only [12]. The biological significance of inactive renin is not yet entirely clear [13].

Plasma catecholamines

Perhaps there is a small group of young patients in the early stages of essential hypertension who have elevated plasma catecholamines, generally associated with elevated plasma renin activity, and who manifest symptoms of a hyperdynamic heart and circulation and of a so-called 'hyperadrenergic' state. Adrenergic beta blocking agents administered to these individuals tend to normalize the symptoms of increased sympathetic activity and are the preferred mode of therapy. Measurements of plasma catecholamines, however, are not essential for the clinical diagnosis of this subgroup.

In patients with essential hypertension, measurements of catecholamines in the basal state do not correlate with the hemodynamic status [14].

SUMMARY

Laboratory examination of a hypertensive patient is an integral part of the total work-up and investigation. The objectives of the work-up are to establish the diagnosis of the type of hypertension, to exclude secondary causes of hypertension, to assess the degree of existing target organ damage, to identify pertinent associated disorders and risk factors, and to aid in the plan-

656

ning of therapeutic management. Carefully conducted routine survey of simple tests on urine and blood, inconjunction with the clinical and radiological survey is usually adequate in achieving these objectives or defining the need for further investigation.

REFERENCES

1. Parker JC: Hypertension and the red cell. (Editorial). N Eng J Med 302:804–805, 1980.
2. James TN, Hapman GR, Urthaler F: Anatomic and physiologic considerations of a cardiogenic hypertensive chemoreflex. Am J Cardiol 44:852–859, 1979.
3. Sambhi MP: Unpublished observations.
4. Antihypertensive drugs, plasma lipids and coronary disease. (Editorial). Lancet ii:19–20,1980.
5. Laragh JH: Vasoconstriction – volume analysis for understanding and treating hypertension: the use of renin and aldosterone profiles. Am J med 55:261–274, 1973.
6. Laragh JH, Sealey JE: Renin-sodium profiling: why, how and when in clinical practice. Cardiovasc Med 2:1053–1078, 1977.
7. Christlieb Ar, Gleason RE, Hickler RB, Lauler DP: Renin: a risk factor for cardiovascular disease? Ann Intern Med 81:7–10, 1974.
8. Esler MD, Julius S, Randall OS et al.: Relation of renin status to neurogenic vascular resistance in borderline hypertension. Am J Cardiol 36:708–715, 1975.
9. Laragh JH: Renin as a predictor of hypertensive complications: Discussion. In: Mild Hypertension: to Treat or Not to Treat. Perry M, Smith J, eds. Ann NY Acad Sci 304:165–174, 1978.
10. Bangham DR, Robertson I, Robertson JIS Robinson CJ, Three M: An international collaborative study of renin assay; establishment of the international reference preparation of human renin. Clin Sci Mol Med 48:135s, 1975.
11. Sambhi MP: Renin substrate reaction. An embarkation premise. Circ Res 41:11S1–4, 1977.
12. Sambhi MP: Hetrogeneity of renin and renin substrate. Amsterdam: Elsevier Scientific, 1981.
13. Lijnen P, Fagard R, Staessen J, Verschueren L, Amery A: Biological significance of active and inactive renin in hypertensive patients. J Endoctinal 85:137–143, 1980.
14. Birkenhager WH, Falke HE: Circulating catecholamines and blood pressure. Utrecht: Bunge, 1978.

43. RADIOLOGICAL EXAMINATION OF THE HYPERTENSIVE PATIENT

A. FOURNIER, J. P. CECILE, M. TONNELIER, R. MAKDASSI, J. F. DE FREMONT, A. REMOND and J. GRUMBACH

Radiology has a preeminent place in the evaluation of an hypertensive patient in order (a) to assess its consequence on the heart and the great vessels and (b) to establish the diagnosis of most secondary hypertensions. Besides the routine chest X-ray, the clinician is offered a great variety of techniques such as excretory urogram, aortography and selective arteriographies, phlebographies, various venous samplings, and non-invasive investigations such as ultrasonography, computed tomography and scientigraphies.

The choice of these techniques depends mainly on the previous basic clinical and biological evaluation upon which the clinician will decide whether or not it is worthwhile for the benefice of the patient to look for secondary forms of hypertension, and in which of the main four directions he should first look for (1) aortic coarctation, (2) renal parenchymal diseases, (3) renovascular diseases, (4) adrenal diseases. Therefore, we shall discuss the radiologic evaluation of an hypertensive patient according to these four main directions, after rapidly reviewing the informations given by the chest X-ray.

I. THE CHEST X-RAY

Chest X-ray gives both prognostic and etiologic information. From a prognostic point of view, it allows the assessment of cardiomegaly, left cardiac failure and aortic atheroma. Left ventricular hypertrophy and dilatation gives a prominent inferior left curvature on the frontal view and a prominent inferior curvature on the left anterior oblique view. Global cardiomegaly is diagnosed on a cardio-thoracic ratio greater than 0.5 in the adult. For valuable comparison of size over the years it was found that the film should be taken with the X-ray source placed at least two meters from the patient and always at maximum inspiration. Pulmonary complications of left cardiac failure may be objectivated by images of pulmonary edema and pleural effusions. Atheroma of the aortic arch is visualized by a prominent left superior curvature, sometimes with calcifications. Etiologic information

Amery, A. (éd.) Hypertensive Cardiovascular Disease: Pathophysiology and Treatment
© *1982, Martinus Nijhoff Publishers. The Hague / Boston / London*
ISBN-13: 978-94-009-7478-4

may be provided by the chest X-ray, since it may give indirect signs of aortic coarctation and show intrathoracic paravertebral localization of a pheochromocytoma (best seen at an oblique view).

II. RADIOLOGICAL EXAMINATION OF A PATIENT WITH SUSPECTED COARCTATION OF THE AORTA

1. In the child and the adult

In the child and the adult, coarctation of the aorta is postductal, i.e. located just after the left subclavicular artery. It represents a surgically curable cause

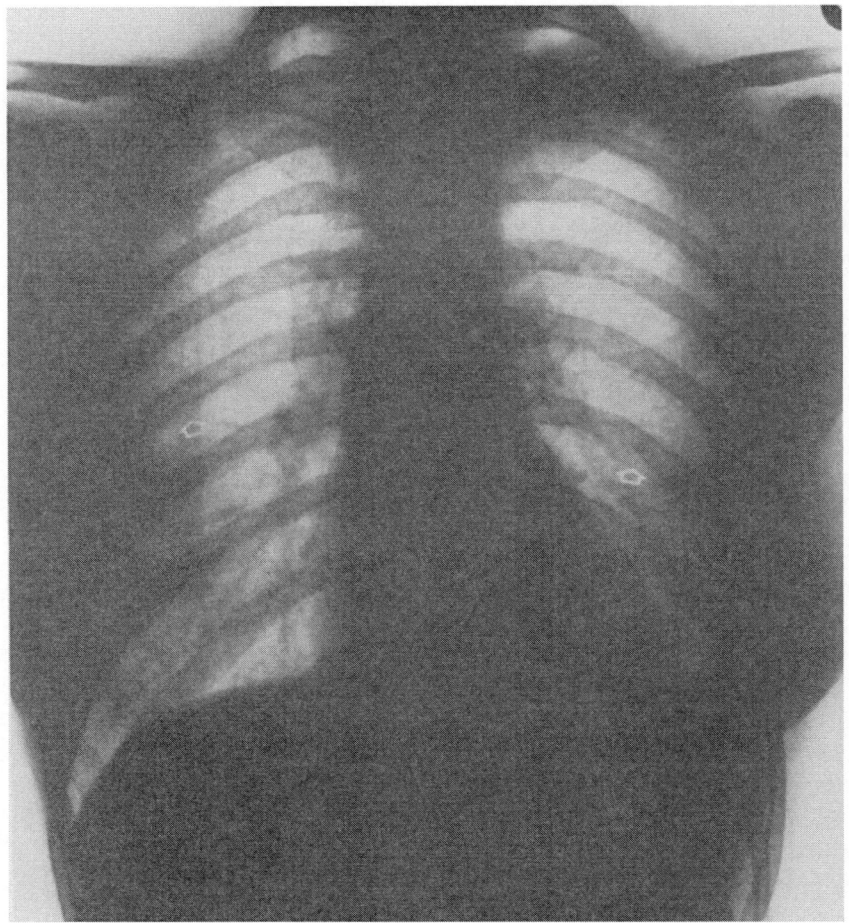

Figure 1a. Standard chest X-ray of a patient with coarctation showing the 'chimney' pattern of the arterial pedicle (no aortic curvature) and notches of the inferior border of the ribs (arrows).

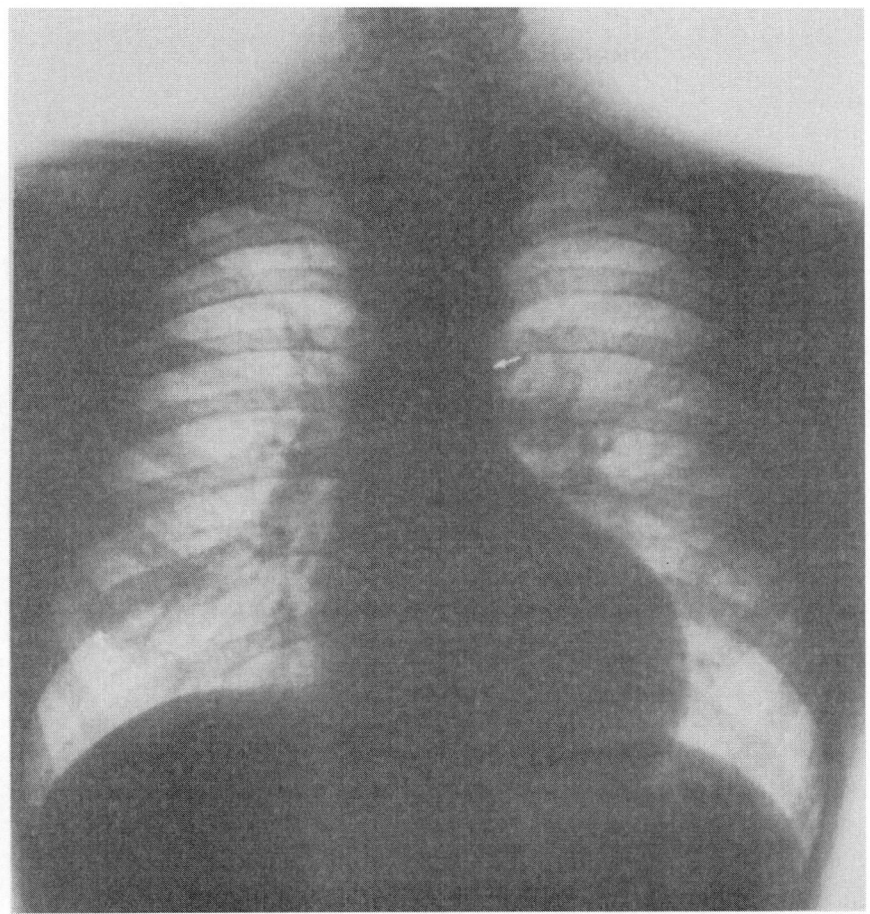

Figure 1b. Standard chest X-ray of a patient with coarctation showing the indentation of the left border of the descending aorta and a big inferior curvature of the heart suggestive of left ventricular hypertrophy.

of hypertension which should always be looked for by the systematic palpation of the femoral pulses and heart auscultation. When the femoral pulses are absent or only decreased, the diagnosis of coarctation is made and has to be confirmed or excluded by radiological means.

1.1. *The standard chest X-ray* may give some indications such as (1) the absence of aortic arch, giving the 'chimney' pattern (Figure 1a), (2) the dilatation of the ascending aorta, (3) the dilatation of the left subclavicular artery giving an opacity of the left apex, (4) the notches of the inferior borders of the upper ribs (3–9th) (Figure 1a), (5) the direct visualization of the stenosis by an indentation of the aortic left border because of the dilated left subclavicular artery and the post stenotic dilatation (Figure 1b).

660

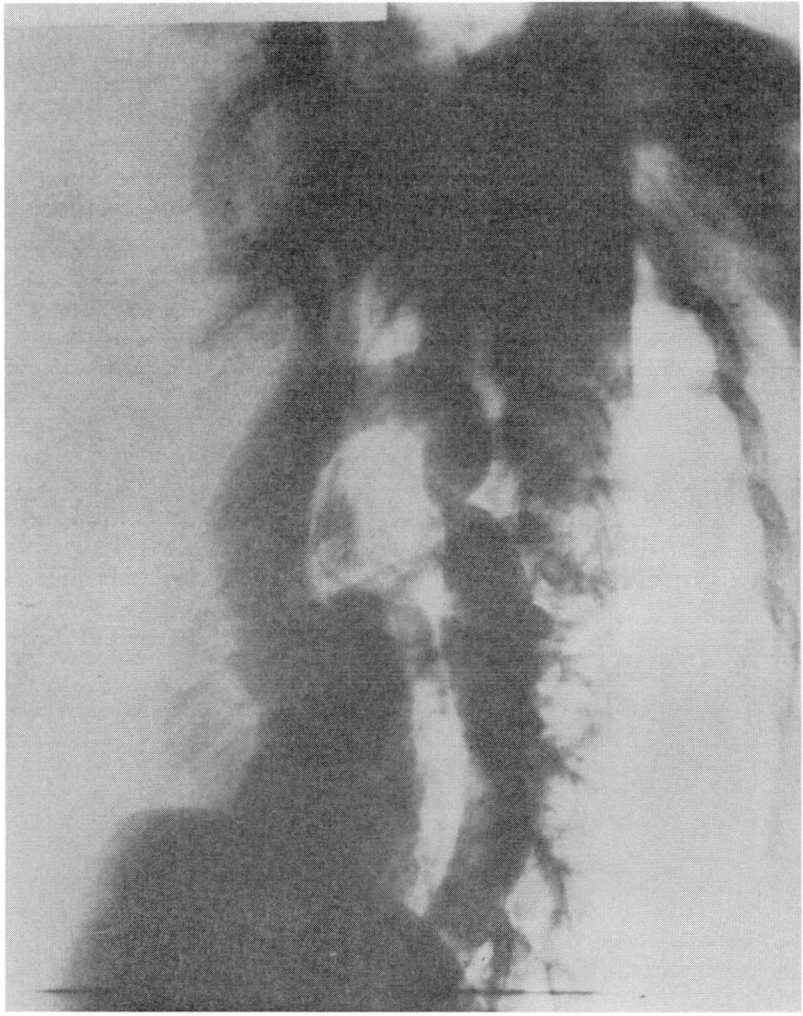

Figure 1c. Intravenous angiocardiography in a patient with coarctation. Left anterior oblique view showing the coarctation.

1.2. *Radiological angiography* establishes the diagnosis using either the intravenous angiocardiography (Figure 1c) or the retrograde arteriography by humeral arteriotomy or puncture of the axillary or of the humeral artery [1]. It is best carried out under two orthogonal incidences and with a rapid film changer or a radiocinema. It is always associated with an hemodynamic study of the right and left hearts. The angiography will define the location of the coarctation (usually isthmic, rarely located before the left carotid), its length, its diameter and its axis. Sometimes, it may show an

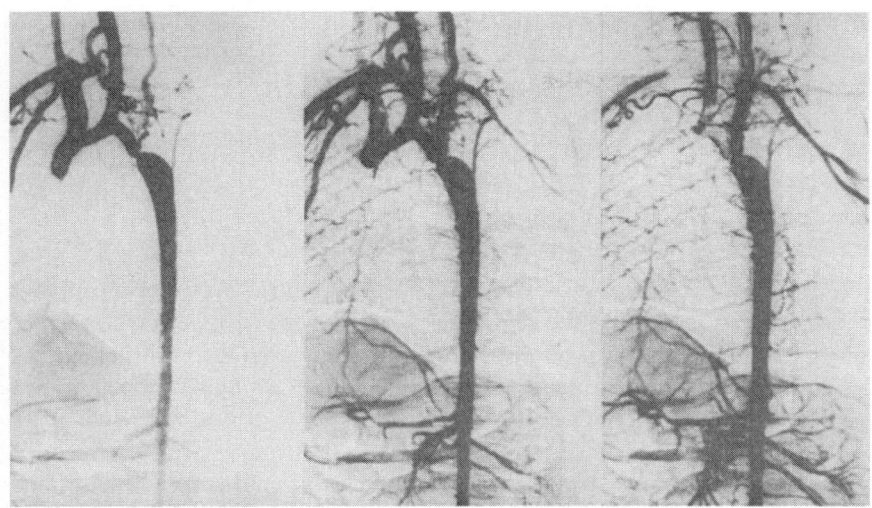

Figure 1d. Infant of 8 weeks (4.2 kg) with coarctation syndrome as evidenced on an aortography by retrograde carotid puncture at three successive periods. The figure at the left shows the hypoplasia of the aortic arch and the coarctation, the two other figures reveal the important collateral circulation and the excellent opacification of the abdominal aorta.

overlapping of the superior and inferior segments. In favor of a tight stenosis, are the delay and persistence in the opacification of the substenotic aorta and the importance of the collateral circulation (dilated internal mammary and intercostal arteries) (Figure 1d).

Associated lesions should always be looked for: aneurysm of the ascending aorta; bicuspidia (25%), aortic insufficiency (15%), aortic stenosis (6,4%), auriculoventricular shunt or arterial duct.

1.3. *The advent of cross-sectional echocardiography* [2] allows to-day a non-invasive diagnosis of coarctation of the aorta. This procedure can show the narrowing of the aorta after the left subclavicular artery and the hyperpulsatility of the ascending aorta. The pictures are satisfactory in 80% of the cases [2]. In 20% of cases, pulmonary emphysema prevents one from obtaining a good picture because the ultrasounds are absorbed. When possible this investigation has to be carried out before invasive angiography.

2. In the new born and the infant

The coarctation is preductal and gives a rapidly progressive cardiac failure. For these small weights (<10 kg), we have developed a technique of aortography by retrograde carotid puncture [3]. The Figure 1d shows that coarctation is often not located at the isthmus but widespread, giving an aortic arch hypoplasia. It is often associated with other cardiac malformations (patient ductus, intraventricular communication, great vessel transposition).

III. RADIOLOGIC EXAMINATION OF A PATIENT WITH POSSIBLE RENAL PARENCHYMAL DISEASE [4, 5]

Glomerulonephritis, chronic pyelonephritis, segmental hypoplasia, polycystic kidneys are the most frequent causes of secondary hypertension. More rarely hydronephrosis, renal cysts, Wilms' tumors, adenocarcinoma and juxtaglomerulo-apparatus tumors may be the cause of hypertension. These causes are usually discovered by a *standard excretory urogram,* which has been easily decided because of the presence of urinary symptoms and/or proteinuria, and/or hematuria, and/or leucocyturia, and/or renal insufficiency. Glomerulonephritis gives no alteration of the excretory urogram when renal function is normal. In acute glomerulonephritis with renal failure, the excretory urogram may be very pale or not even visible, but the nephrograms show that the two kidneys are increased in size. In chronic glomerulonephritis with renal failure, the urogram is very pale or absent and the nephrography shows two small regular kidneys.

Chronic pyelonephritis has a typical urographic aspect with convex calices and cortical scarrings. The lesions may be uni- or bilateral. They cannot be radiologically differentiated from those of the so called 'segmental hypoplasia' about which there is still a controversy whether or not it is only a 'reflux nephropathy'. Evidence of chronic pyelonephritis lesions should yet lead to a *micturition cystography,* when possible at the end of the intravenous pyelography after the pyelogram has disappeared and, if this is not possible, by means of a *retrograd cystography.* When pyelonephritic lesions are strictly unilateral, the question may arise whether or not it would be beneficial for the patient to have a nephrectomy of this kidney in order to cure his hypertension. This is a very controversial question that is beyond the scope of this chapter. Let us only say that the integrity of the contralateral kidney (best assessed on the importance of its compensatory hypertrophy) is a prerequisite for the decision and that excretory urogram and renal arteriography should be carefully reviewed for that purpose [4] (Figure 2).

Polycystic kidneys give a typical excretory urogram with two big kidneys (greater than $3\frac{1}{2}$ vertebrae) with lacunar nephrographies, stretched and distorded pyelograms. Renal tumors (cysts or cancers) are best seen during an intravenous pyelography when a nephrotomography is performed at 15–30 s after the injection of a big bolus of contrast medium. Typically, a benign cyst gives a pale round image with the spike sign, whereas the well-vascularized cancer gives a round image, more dense than the rest of the

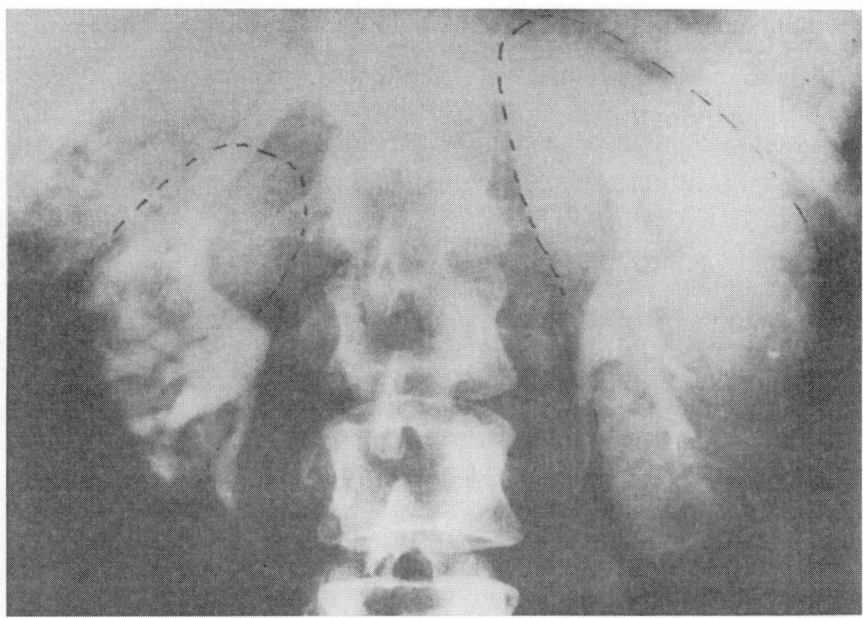

Figure 2. Small pyelonephritic kidney with convex calices and cortical scarrings in the middle and lower part of the right kidney, whereas the left kidney has a compensatory hyperplasia.

parenchyma. On the later films, both tumors may give a compression of the pyelogram. Further evaluation of the tumor syndrom is based, first on ultrasonography or computed tomography and only secondarily on arteriography by the Seldinger technique and/or the puncture of the dubious liquid tumors. The use of the intravenous arteriography for the diagnosis of renovascular disease as described below, has the advantage to give the diagnosis by the first radiological examination, since it shows the hypervascularization of the cancer. Only necrotized cancers will be undiagnosed by this technique and necessitate computed tomography and/or puncture of the liquid tumors.

Renin-producing tumors are exceptional and very difficult to visualize. Most of them are juxtaglomerular apparatus tumors, but a few are in relation with an adenocarcinoma, a Wilms' tumor or even with an extrarenal carcinoma (lung, liver, orbitis). As regards the juxtaglomerular apparatus tumors, the excretory urogram was normal in the 15 cases reported, whereas selective renal arteriography could show an avascular cortical tumoral zone in 10 cases [6]. The diameter ranged from 0.8–4 cm. This investigation was guided by the fact that, in a young patient with severe hypertension, hypokalemia and high plasma renin activity, a global renal arteriography showed no abnormalities of the renal arteries, but the renal vein blood samplings showed evidence of unilateral high renin secretion [6]. Although no experience has been reported with computed tomography, this examination should be performed in this situation, since it can diagnose a tumor of 1.5 cm in diameter.

IV. RADIOLOGIC EXAMINATION OF A PATIENT WITH POSSIBLE RENOVASCULAR DISEASE

Incidence of renovascular disease, i.e. the presence of stenosis or thrombosis of the renal arteries, is quite high in the hypertensive population that has undergone radiological evaluation. In this selected population, McNeil [7] estimated this incidence to be 10%. In our systematic study of 848 hypertensive patients, by intravenous arteriography, this incidence was 7% [8]. This renovascular disease may be the cause of true renovascular hypertension, i.e. a hypertension curable by nephrectomy or revascularization by surgery or transluminal percutaneous angioplasty, in about 1–3% of the investigated population [8]. Furthermore, in all cases, it represents a risk of ischemic destruction of the renal parenchyma. Therefore, the search of a renovascular disease is a major concern for the clinician in the evaluation of any hypertensive patient.

The classical approach for the diagnosis of renovascular disease is to perform a renal arteriography by the Seldinger technique, in patients selected on the basis of the clinical examination and the rapid sequence urography. As a matter of fact, the Seldinger technique is the most accurate way to visualize renal artery disease, but its systematic use in hypertensive patients is not recommended because it would be too expensive for the community and too hazardous for the patient population regarding the low prevalence of renovascular disease [7]. In the American Cooperative Study on Renovascular Hypertension, the mortality rate of the Seldinger technique was 0.1% and severe hemorrhages or thromboses occured in 1.3% of the cases [9]. Therefore, we shall describe the technique and the information given by the rapid sequence urography and the renal arteriography by the Seldinger technique, before presenting our personal diagnostic approach with the intravenous arteriography combined with the excretory urogram.

1. Rapid sequence excretory urography (E.U.) and pyelogram wash-out

1.1. Pathophysiology of the urographic signs of renovascular disease
There are three main urographic signs for renovascular disease: (a) size disparity, (b) delayed caliceal appearance time, (c) increased late pyelogram density, spontaneously evident or unmasked by wash-out.

Figure 3a. Pathophysiological scheme of the functional urographic signs.

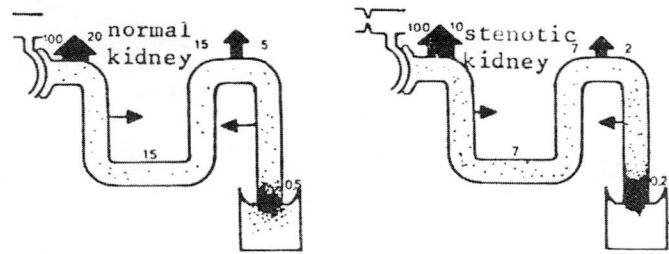

• delayed calciceal appearance time on early films is explained by the decreased delivery of contrast medium secondary to the decrease in GFR;

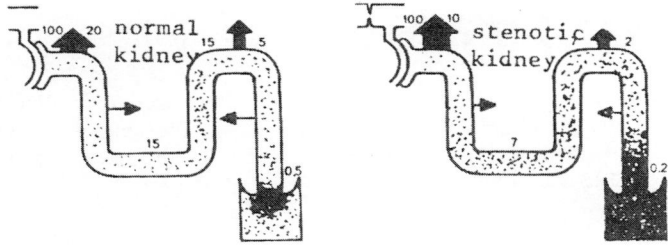

• late pyelogram hyperdensity occurs when the urine with hyperconcentrated contrast medium has filled completely the excretion cavities.

(a) *Size disparity.* Decreased blood flow to one kidney leads to a reduction in size of the kidney involved. This sign can easily be assessed on an excretory urogram. Since the length of the left kidney is usually greater than that of the right one by 0.4 cm, the left kidney is considered smaller than the right one if it is 1 cm smaller, whereas right kidney is considered smaller than the left one if it is 1.5 cm smaller.

(b) *Delayed caliceal appearance time* (Figure 3a). Modern contrast media used for urography are only filtred by the glomerulus and the rate of its delivery to the pyelocaliceal system is only dependent on the GFR of the kidney. Decreased perfusion pressure due to unilateral stenotic lesion will decrease GFR of the ipsilateral kidney and this will lead to a decreased delivery of contrast medium to the pyelocaliceal system. Therefore, during the first minutes after the injection the concentration of iodine in the excretory cavities of the side involved will be lower and these cavities will be visualized with a delay in comparison to the controlateral kidney. As the normal appearance caliceal time is 2 min after the intravenous injection of the contrast medium, early films taken at 2 and 3 min are mandatory to catch this delay, which would be missed if the first film were taken only 5 min later as for a standard E.U. Only exceptionally are films at 1 or 4 min useful for catching this delay [10], so they may be omitted.

666

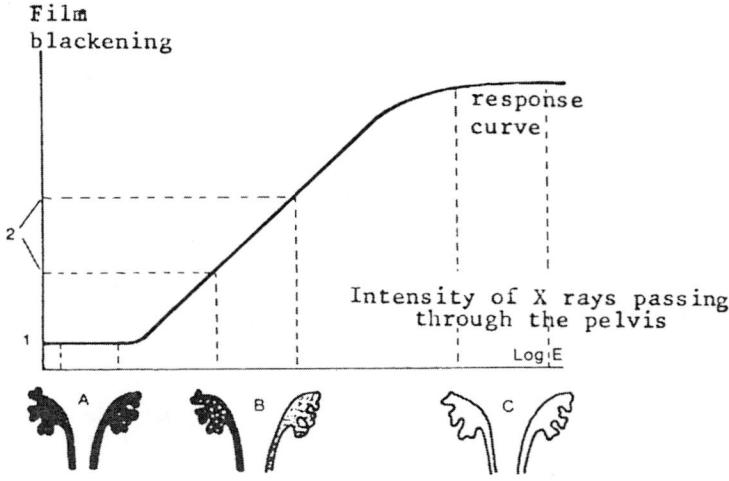

Figure 3b. Scheme showing the relation between the blackening of the film and the intensity of the X-rays falling on the film (cf. text for explanation). Note that, compared to usual IVP, the pyelograms are black when opaque and white when washed-out.

(c) *Increased late pyelogram density and delayed pyelogram wash-out.* It is shown in figure 3a that, although the delivery rate of contrast medium is smaller on the side involved, its concentration in the urine arising from the collecting ducts is greater because of the increase of salt and water fractional tubular reabsorption as evidenced by bilateral ureteral catheterization (Howard test). When the whole pyelocaliceal system has been filled by the urine containing the contrast medium at the same higher concentration as in the collecting duct, the concentration of iodine in the pelvis of the side involved will be higher. This should give a higher radiographic density in comparison to the controlateral kidney. This actually occurs only for a certain range of X-ray intensities for which the film chemical reaction is proportional to the X-ray intensity (situation B on Figure 3b). This does not occur in situation A of Figure 3b, where the same patient (with a right renal artery) has no difference in pyelogram density because, on both sides, the intensity of X-rays is insufficient to provoke a chemical reaction to blacken the film, the concentration of iodine being too great even on the non-stenotic side. To transform situation A into situation B, i.e. to unmask the increased density in relation to the actual difference in iodine concentration, it is necessary to dilute the urine. This is most rapidly done either by infusion of osmotic diuretics like mannitol or urea and more easily by intravenous injection of 40 mg of furosemide [11–13].

When the dilution is very great (situation C), the intensity of X-rays showig on the film is so great that the film blackening is maximum at both sides and both pyelograms are completely 'washed out'. To catch this phenomenon, it is usually necessary to take three small films every 5 min after the start of urea infusion (30 g urea and 10 g mannitol in 250 ml of isotonic saline) and every 2 min after the furosemide injection. The advantage of furosemide wash-out over urea wash-out is its better tolerance, since urea may cause headaches and vomiting in 20% of the cases [12, 13]. It is very important to stress that late pyelogram density (either the spontaneous one or the wash-out unmasked one) is suggestive of renovascular disease only when the following causes of pyelogram density asymmetry have been eliminated:

1. any obstacle to urine flow: the error is easily detected since the pelvis is then not only more dense but also bigger, whereas it is thinner or at least of the same size in case of renovascular disease.
2. a malrotation of the kidney; the pelvis is always seen laterally and appears more dense also on the early films and not only on the late films.
3. a unilateral pyelonephritis with unilateral lower urine concentration will make the uninvolved pyelogram appear more dense.

It should also be pointed out that after an intravenous furosemide injection, it is not possible to accurately detect a vesico-ureteral reflux because of the transient nature of the dilution by furosemide and the persistence of contrast medium filtration so that the upper cavities reappear after the wash-out (situation C is transformed into situation B or A).

(d) *Other urographic signs of renovascular disease.* These are less common and include:

1. asymmetry in nephrographic density, the early nephrography being less dense but the late nephrography being more dense on the stenotic side; the assessment of these variations needs serial films and is very subjective.
2. ureteral notching due to the print of a rich collateral circulation.
3. the decrease in the increase of kidney area induced by urea infusion or furosemide injection; this increase is typically less than 5% on the stenotic side, whereas it ranges from 7–20% on the uninvolved side [14].

The latter sign may be particularly useful to screen bilateral and symmetrical renal artery stenosis which is otherwise overlooked since the other urographic signs are based on asymmetry between both kidneys.

1.2. Value of the rapid sequence urogram and wash-out as a screening test for renovascular disease

The cooperative study of Maxwell and the cost–effectiveness calculations of McNeil have established the rapid sequence urogram as the method of choice for the screening of renovascular hypertension. Our own previous

668

experience [4] fully agrees with this statement, although we found that the pyelogram wash-out, which was not performed in the American Cooperative Study, may enhance the chances to discover curable renovascular hypertension: in a series of 43 cases improved by surgery E.V. was normal in only 1 case when early films and washout were performed, whereas it was normal in 4 cases when only early films were taken and in 9 cases when only the standard films were taken. However, a delayed wash-out is not specific of renovascular disease. A recent survey of the litterature [8] totalizing 2275 hypertensive patients who have had Seldinger arteriography and E.U. with wash-out can be summarized as follows:

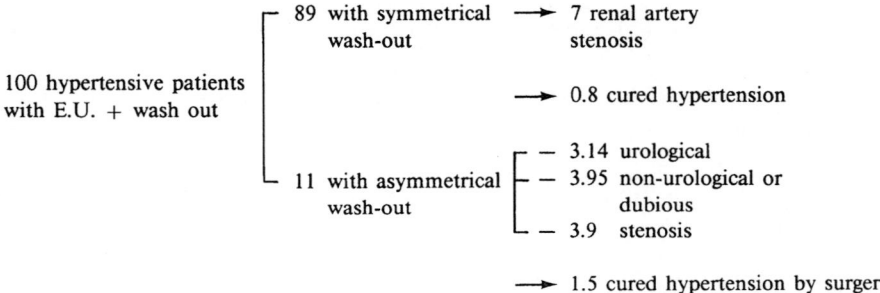

Thus, in only 35% of the cases with positive wash-out, a renal artery stenosis will be found and in only 13% of the cases with a positive wash-out, the hypertension will be cured by surgery. When the urological causes of delayed wash-out are eliminated, the specificity of this sign for the diagnosis of curable renovascular hypertension is a little improved but still poor: $(1.5 \times 100)/(11 - 3.14) = 20\%$. However, a review of the literature has shown that the other screening tests for renovascular hypertension such as the isotopic renogram, the angiotensin test, the measurement of basal or upright peripheral plasma renin activity or the Saralasin test were not better [4, 15]. As regards the Cooperative Study, rapid sequence urogram without wash-out, was positive in 78% patients with renovascular disease and falsely positive in 11% of the patients with essential hypertension.

1.3. Prognostic value of the delayed wash-out

The late pyelogram hyperdensity or the delayed pyelogram wash-out on the side of the stenosis are indirect assessments of the Howard test. The latter evaluates the functional consequence of a renal artery stenosis mainly on the increase in fractional reabsorption of sodium and water, as assessed by its consequence: the increased urinary concentration of substances like creatinine, insulin or contrast medium which are only filtered and not reabsorbed by the tubule. Therefore, it is not surprising that this sign has been shown to accurately predict the correction of hypertension by surgery. In the review of 132 patients with renovascular disease who underwent surgery and who had previously an E.U. with wash-out, the results of surgery on hypertension were correctly predicted in 115 patients (87%), whereas there was surgical failure in spite of positive wash-out in 7 cases (5.5 false-positive) and surgical success in spite of negative wash-out in 10 cases (7.5% false-negative). This prognostic value is comparable to that of the Howard test (74% of good prediction) and that of the ratio of plasma renin activity in the renal veins (75% of good prediction) [4]. The apparent discrepancy between the poor specificity of a positive wash-out as a screening test for renovascular hypertension and its quite good practical prognostic value may be explained by the great selection of the patients who undergo surgery. As regards the prognostic value of the delayed pyelocaliceal appearance time, we agree with Maxwell that it is poor [4].

2. The renal arteriography by the technique of Seldinger

2.1. The technique
Previously, aortography was performed by direct translumbar aortic puncture (Dos Santos technique). Seldinger has proposed to introduce the catheter along a guide previously introduced through a needle punctured into the femoral artery at the Scarpa triangle. The catheter is then placed about 2 cm above the renal artery and the contrast medium is injected. A global aortography with bilateral visualization of the renal arteries is thus performed in supine position. When ostium stenosis is suspected on this first investigation, a second global aortography is performed in oblique position. When the artery lesions are poorly defined because of vascular superposition and especially when distal involvement of the artery branches is suspected, a selective arteriography with a specially curved catheter has to be performed. Otherwise, selective arteriographies are not very useful and may lead to fallacious diagnosis of stenosis because they may provoke arterial spasms at the tip of the cathether introduced into the renal artery.

2.2. Results
The renal arteriography by the Seldinger technique is a highly reliable technique to delineate precisely the renal arterial tree. However, there is no means to evaluate false-negative results since surgery is not performed when the arteriogram is normal. False-positive results are mainly observed in the case of selective arteriography. Renal arteriography establishes the diagnosis of renovascular disease and assesses its location and its extension, precisions that are critical in determining operability. Furthermore, it allows one to determine with a certain probability the histological nature of the stenotic lesion.

Atherosclerotic lesions are found in about two thirds of the cases. They

Figures 3c–3g give various morphological aspects of renal artery stenosis according to their histological nature.

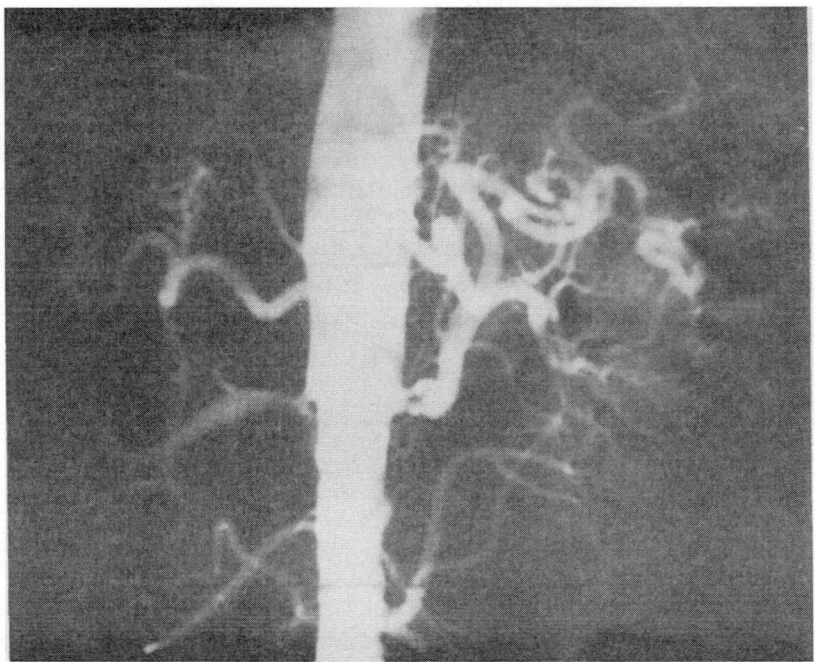

Figure 3c. Proximal bilateral renal artery stenosis due to atherosclerosis. Note atherosclerotic lesions of the aorta.

are preferentially proximal and asymmetrical and often associated with atherosclerotic lesions of other vessels (aorta, coronaries, carotids, iliac arteries). They are often bilateral and complicated with thrombosis and dissection. They are mostly observed in men over 50 years old (Figure 3c), whereas young women are more likely to have stenosis by fibrous dysplasia.

Stenosis by fibrous dysplasia has been variously classified. According to the classification of McCormack and Harrison (Cleveland Clinic and Mayo Clinic), we can distinguish [17]:

1. Stenosis by intimal fibrosis (10% of the fibrous dysplasia) which is generally distal. It progresses frequently to thrombosis and dissection (Figure 3d). It may involve other arteries. It is the lesions seen in the neurofibromatosis of Recklinghausen.

2. Stenosis by medial fibroplasia with microaneurysms (which is too often wrongly called fibromuscular hyperplasia, because muscular hyperplasia is actually lacking) is the most common fibrous stenosis (75%). It is easily recognized by its 'string of beads' pattern due to the presence of a series of fibrous rings interspersed with short segment of aneurysmal dilatation, the diameter of which is equal or greater to the proximal normal artery lumen

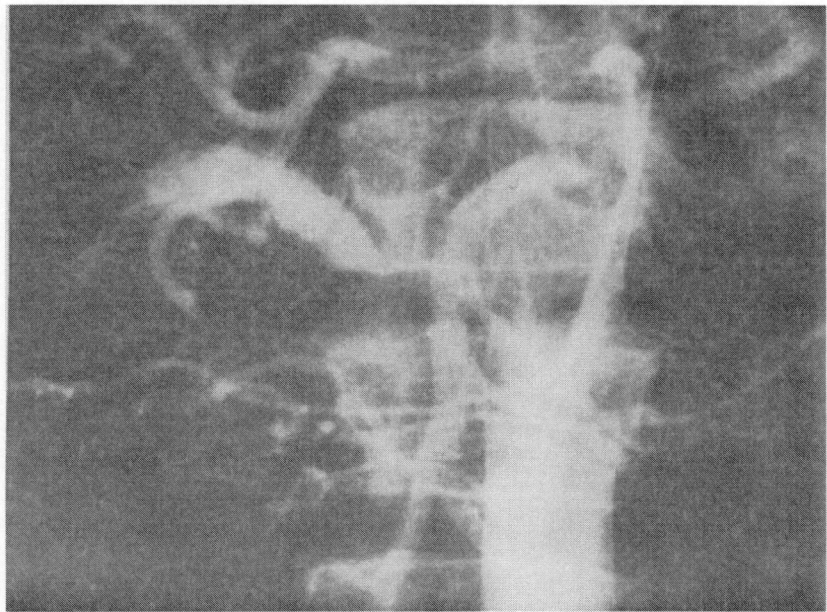

Figure 3d. Dissection of the right renal artery due to intimal fibrosis. On this late film only the dissection canal is opaque because of contrast medium stagnation.

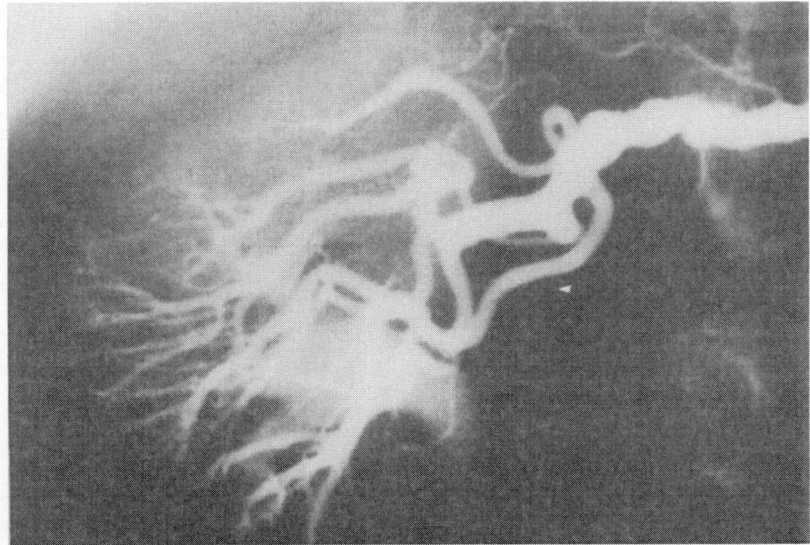

Figure 3e. String of beads pattern of the medial fibroplasia with microaneurysms of a right artery.

672

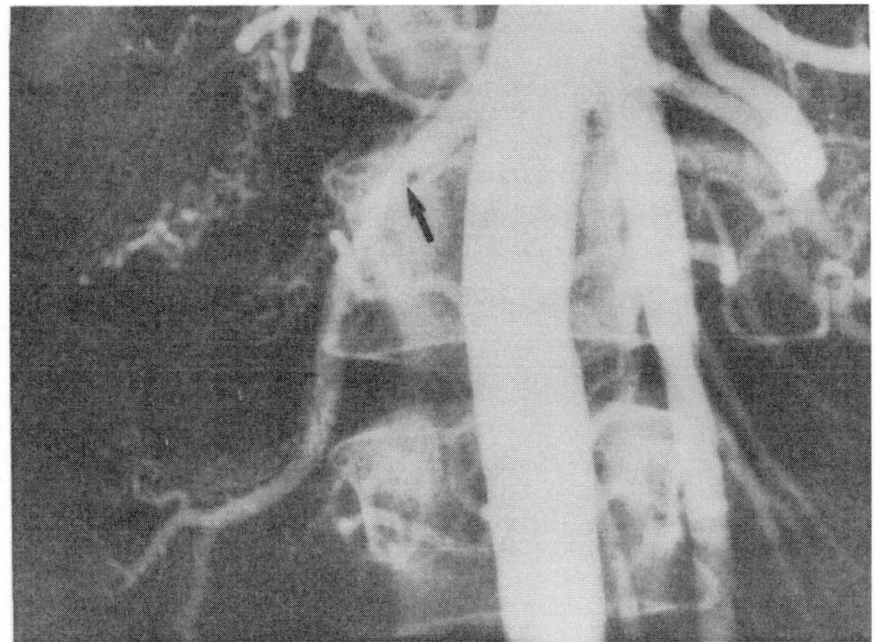

Figure 3f. 'String of beads' pattern of a subadventitial fibroplasia.

(Figure 3e). These lesions are often bilateral and are less likely to progrees to thrombosis [17], although this is not always the case [18].

3. Stenosis by subadventitial or perimedial fibroplasia (12% of the fi-

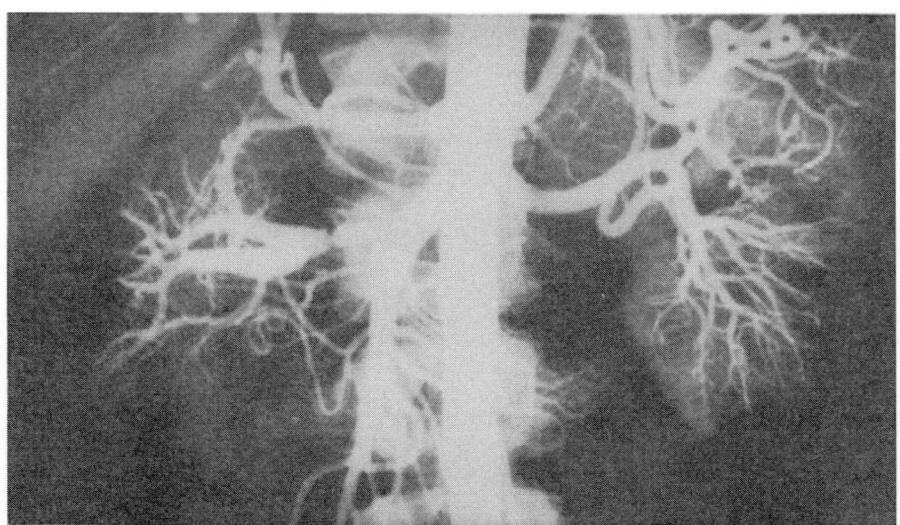

Figure 3g. 'Collar pattern' of a focal subadvential fibroplasia.

brous dysplasia) has two main angiographic aspects: (a) the string of beads pattern which differs from that of the medial fibroplasia by the fact that careful examination shows that the caliber of the normal segment is not exceeded by the beads and by the frequent occurence of extensive collateral circulation (Figure 3f); (b) the collar or diaphragm pattern (Figure 3g). These lesions have a serious prognosis since they frequently progress and are complicated by thrombosis.

2.3. The value of renal arteriography to predict the result of surgery is limited

The degree of stenosis has some importance since Bookstein observed that in atherosclerotic lesion favorable response to surgery is 43% when the reduction in luminal diameter is less than 50% and that it is 68% when the reduction is greater than 50%. In fibrous dysplasia, favorable response is observed in 72% of the stenosis with less than 50% reduction and in 91% of the stenosis with more than 80% reduction. Presence of collateral circulation and of post-stenotic dilatation could not be correlated to surgical results in spite of the fact that the length of the post-stenotic dilatation is proportional to the lumen reduction. The delay of small arteries filling and of nephrography appearance assessed on the global aortography (with the tip of the catheter checked 2 cm above the renal arteries to secure adequate mixing of the contrast medium) has a modest prognostic significance: 68% correct prediction, 18% false-positive and 14% false negative [4].

3. Intravenous arteriography combined with the excretory urogram

3.1. Technique

The idea to visualize the renal arteries by intravenous injection of contrast medium is old: earlier attempts go back to 1939 in the U.S. with Robb and to 1956 in France with Viallet. The technique was then improved by Cecile in France [20], Schockert in Belgium [21] and Ingrish in Germany [23]. The technique of Cecile [20] consists in injecting a bolus of 2–3 ml/kg of a 38% contrast medium (Telebrix®) at a speed of 22 ml/s in young patients and 15 ml/s in older subjects, or in patient with pulmonary hypertension or with beta-blocking drugs, using a 14 Butterfly needle and an automatic injector. Twelve seconds after the end of the injection, a film changer with six films is turned on so as to present a film every 2 s in the young patients and every 3 s in the older ones. The first film which preceedes the opacification of the abdominal aorta is used for substraction. An excretory urogram is then performed with two films at 5 and 15 min after the bolus administration. When a stenosis is visualized, a pyelogram wash-out is performed and three small films are taken at 2-min intervals. When no film changer is available, only one arteriographic film is taken when the opaque bolus, followed on TV screen, reaches the 11th dorsal vertebra, and early films at 2–3 min are also taken to assess the delayed caliceal appearance time. The technique of Ingrish [23] consists of the rapid injection of 1 ml/kg of contrast medium (Telebrix 38®) within 3–5 s, then the determination of the circulation time between injection site at the arms and the aorto-abdominalis using the addition of 0,2 mCi 99 Tc to the contrast medium and next, performing a single tomography with a multileaf cassette with five films, each 1 cm apart.

3.2. Results

The technique of Cecile has been performed in 4155 patients for various reasons; in 848 of them because of hypertension [22]. Renovascular disease was present in 7 % of these cases. As shown on Figures 3h–3k, the contrast is sharper with the Seldinger arteriography but the information provided by the intravenous arteriography is similar. An adequate renal arteriography was obtained in 95 % of the cases, even in obese patients, when six films were taken with a film changer. When only one arteriographic film is taken, Cecile obtains adequate arteriogram in 70 % of a series of 300 cases [8].

Figures 3h–3k concern a 40-year-old man with a fibrous stenosis of the left renal artery causing a severe hypertension resistant to beta-blockers.

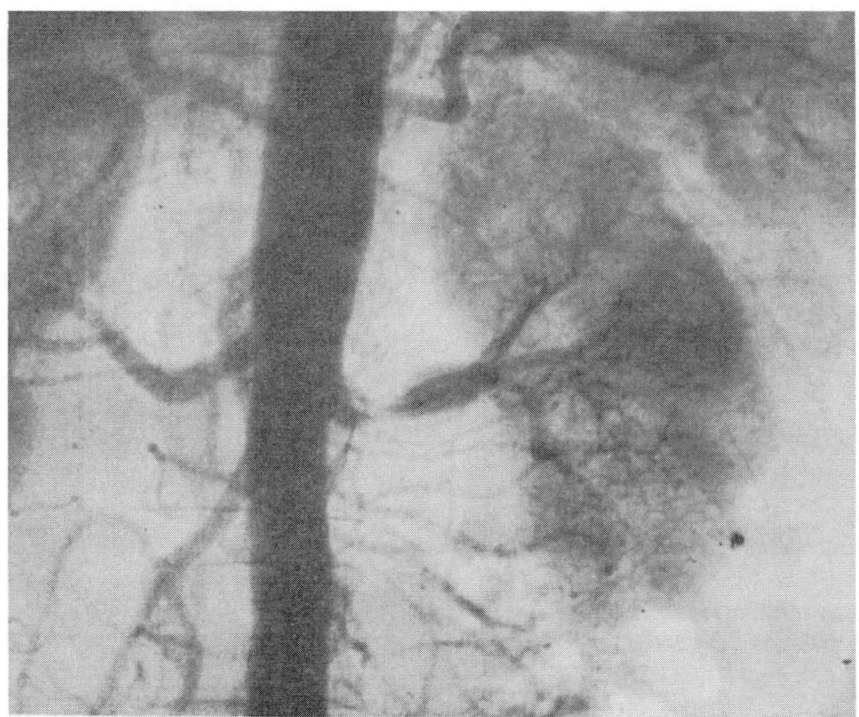

Figure 3h. Intravenous arteriogram showing the severe stenosis.

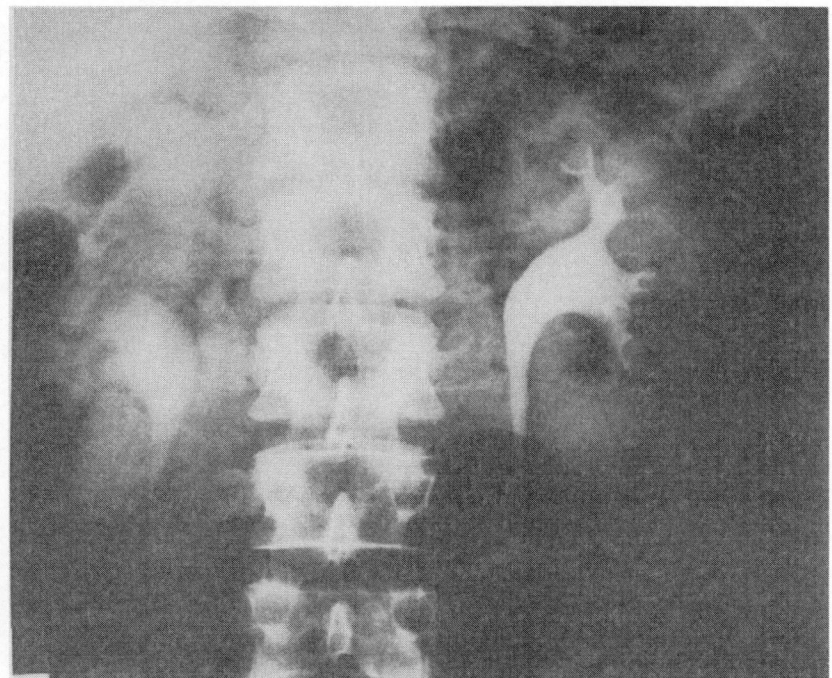

Figure 3i. Pyelogram 5 min after the injection of 40 mg of furosemide: Only the left pyelogram is clearly visible, whereas the right one is washed-out. Plasma renin activity in the renal vain was 3.3. ng/ml/h in the right vein and 24 in the left one. A dilatation with the Gruntzig catheter was performed.

When 5 simultaneous tomographies are taken, Ingrish obtains clearly outlined main renal arteries in 83% of the cases [23]. The tolerance of these techniques is good and they can be performed on outpatients. Headaches and flushes are common (60%) but transitory. They were related to the hypertonicity of the contrast medium, and are less frequent with new nonionic contrast medium. Immunoallergical reactions are less frequent (0.15%) than with classical urography (5%). Increase in serum creatinine was absent, except in patients with diabetes and abnormal renal functions. The irradiation cost is comparable to that of the rapid sequence urogram since both procedures need about the same number of films. Radiation dose has been evaluated at about 255 millirads in women and 95 millirads in men.

4. Digital subtraction angiography

Digital subtraction angiography is a new radiological technology, wich allows intravenous arteriography of good quality. The images are acquired

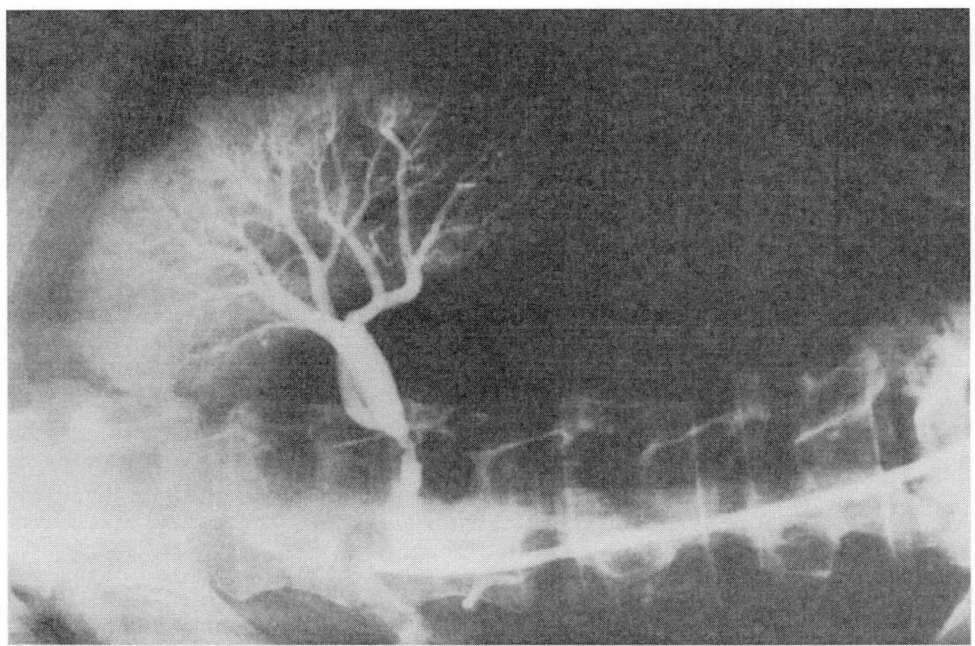

Figure 3j. Selective arteriogram performed by the Seldinger technique just before dilatation.

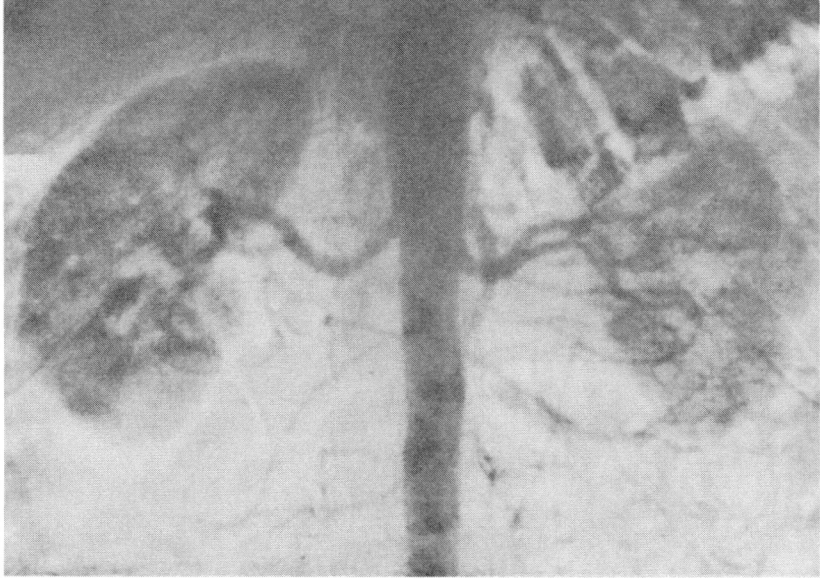

Figure 3k. Intravenous arteriogram performed 6 months later when subject was normo-tensive without drug at 140–80 mmHg.

directly by image intensifier and are then digitized and transmitted to a computer storage complex. Precontrast images are electronically subtracted from images obtained after the contrast medium reaches the renal vasculature.

Because electronic subtraction enhances the contrast, the quantity of contrast medium is smaller than with the Cécile's technique: Hillman et al. (Radiology 1981:139, 277) use 45 ml of 76% meglumine diatrizoate (Renographin 76). These authors inject this contrast medium at a rate of 30 ml/s into an antecubital vein via a 16-Angiocath or via a 7-F pigtail catheter placed into the distal superior vena cava. Exposures are taken at a rate of one per second and continued for 20 s.

The use of a balloon to displace stomach and small bowel may sometimes be necessary to prevent artifacts due to subtraction of moving bowel gas and feces.

Subsequent reviewing of the videotape allows the radiologist to select the best pictures to be printed on small radiographic films. The procedure can easily be repeated to obtain oblique views when necessary. Satisfactory examination was achieved in 92% of the cases.

5. Cost effectiveness comparison of the classical approach and the intravenous arteriography

The cost of investigating 100 hypertensive patients has been evaluated at $ 27,500 with the classical approach and at $ 24,181, i.e. 12% less, with the intravenous arteriography. Since the effectiveness of the intravenous arteriography in discovering renovacular disease is greater, the cost of finding a case of renovascular disease is $ 3626 with this method against $ 4849 with the classical approach, i.e. a difference of 25%. In order to assess its functional significance, the intravenous arteriography combined with a pyelography and a pyelogram wash-out with furosemide appears to us the method of choice for the screening and the diagnosis of renovascular disease, since it is more effective, cheaper and less hazardous than the classical approach [22].

Since a renovascular disease may be associated with a parenchymal disease, combined intravenous arteriography and excretory urogram may be preferred as the first radiological examination in an hypertensive patient with symptoms or biological signs of nephropathy.

6. Indications for the radiological screening of renovascular disease

Whether the classical approach or the intravenous arteriography is used for the screening of renovascular disease, the major problem to solve is how to decide that it is worthwhile doing so. The solution of this problem would need information that is not available such as a controlled prospective comparison of surgical or angioplastic treatment [24] to medical treatment of hypertension with renovascular disease, and a precise evaluation of the future compliance of a given patient to medical therapy. Summarizing an editorial review on this subject [25], we may say that, in selected cases, surgical and possibly angioplastic revascularization are better than medical treatment, because they allow a better control of hypertension and a better protection against renal failure. Therefore, radiological screening is justified when the clinician has first judged that he would like to perform a revascularization procedure in case a stenotic lesion is found, because the hypertension is severe and the patient young. The existence of an abdominal murmur, of an emboligenic cardiopathy, of a lumbar trauma in the anamnesis and of a hypokalemia, will favor radiological screening. Since the advent of percutaneous transluminal angioplasty, presence of renal failure or of other atheromatous complications should no more be a contra-indication for this research. On the contrary, renal failure would be an indication to a rapid visualization of the renal arteries by intravenous arteriography even in older patients, since transluminal angioplasy may improve their renal function in case of a severe stenotic lesion of a functionally unique kidney [24]. However, because of the cost of radiology and because of the low prevalence of renovascular disease, we think radiological screening should be decided in patients over 50 years old without renal insufficiency only when medical treatment is inadequate, and in patients under 50 years only when their untreated diastolic pressure is permanently $\geqslant 115$ mm Hg.

V. RADIOLOGICAL EXAMINATION OF A PATIENT WITH POSSIBLE ADRENAL DISEASES

Three main adrenal diseases may cause hypertension: pheochromocytoma, primary aldosteronism and Cushing syndrom. The diagnosis of these diseases is based on clinical and biological examinations primarily and the radiologic examination comes only secondary, in order to localize a pheochromocytoma, and to precise the histological nature of primary aldosteronism or of the Cushing syndrom. Since the problems are different with each disease, they will be discussed successively.

1. Localization of a pheochromocytoma

Pheochromocytoma is a rare cause of hypertension (<0.5%). However, the superiority of surgical treatment is obvious in most cases [26, 27]. There-

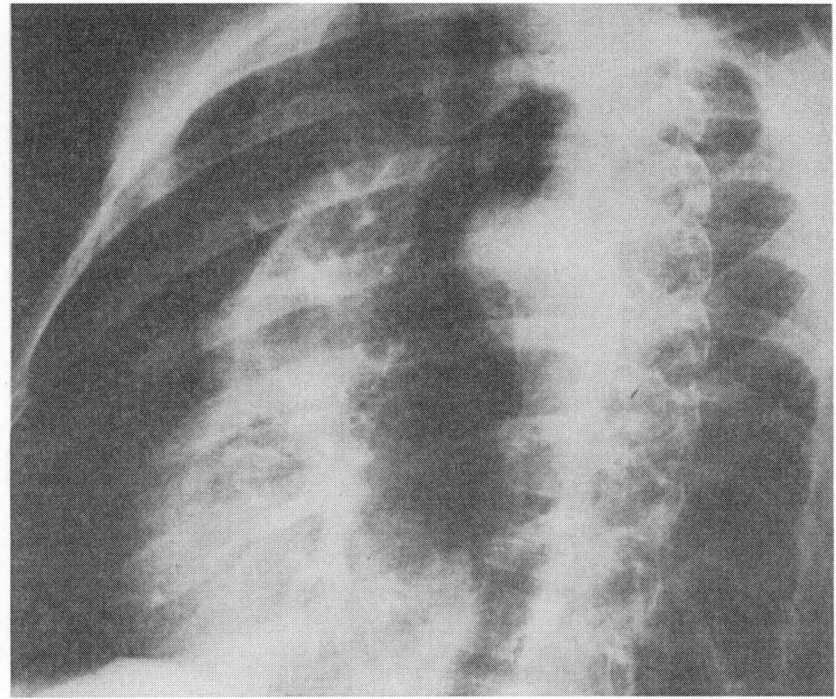

Figure 4a. Lateral anterior oblique view of the chest showing a latero-vertebral thoracic pheochromocytoma.

fore, its diagnosis is systemiatically made before any hypertension with suggestive clinical symptoms (hypertensive crisis, profuse sweating, tachycardia, familial endocrinopathies, diabetes). It is confirmed mainly by biological measurements showing increased catecholamine secretion (increased urinary vanyl mandelic acid or metanephrines, increased plasma catecholamines) and occasionally by pharmacological tests.

Pheochromocytoma may be localized all along the anterior paravertebral region, from the base of the skull to the sacrum. However, about 95% are located in the abdomen and intra-adrenal localization occurs in 90% of the adults but only in 78% of the children. Multiple localizations occur in about 10%. Since most authors agree [26, 27] that proper localization of pheochromocytoma will decrease the hazards of surgery, the radiologist has a preeminent role to play. After the routine chest X-ray with an oblique view, which will be systematically performed to discard a thoracic localization (Figure 4a), he will be faced with the choice of a variety of techniques orientated to abdominal localization. We shall review their information and risks before discussing their choice.

1.1. Excretory urogram with nephrotomography

This exceptionally induces increases in blood pressure (1 out of 54 cases according to Tcherdakoff [27]) and provides valuable information in many cases. E.U. alone can detect pheochromocytoma in only 23% of the cases, but nephrotomography after rapid injection of a big bolus of contrast medium can accurately localize pheochromocytoma in 67% in the series of the Mayo Clinic [26]. Although we do not have any pheochromocytoma in our series of 848 hypertensive patients who had the intravenous arteriography combined with E.U., it can safely be predicted from its value for diagnosing other vascular retroperitoneal tumors and from the usual quality of its nephrographies, that this technique would give adequate localization in 80–90% of the cases. Like the Seldinger arteriography, this technique also has the potential advantage to show multiple abdominal localizations.

With these examinations, pheochromocytoma is either directly visualized as a round vascular tumor of various size, or only indirectly suggested by modifications of the kidneys' positions (kidneys may be lowered and have their oblique longitudinal axis verticalized by a suprarenal mass), by compression of the excretory cavities or even by urographic signs of renovascular hypertension (delayed caliceal appearance time, late pyelogram hyperdensity). Furthermore, E.U. is mandatory before surgery to make sure that there are two normal functioning kidneys as, sometimes, the surgeon has to take out one kidney when the pheochromocytoma cannot be dissected from the kidney (hilar pheochromocytoma, for example). It should be stressed that left adrenal pheochromocytoma should be distinguished from gastric big tuberosity, because it gives a round image persisting on a procubitus film.

1.2. Retroperitoneal pneumography

This procedure combined with E.U. and nephrotomography may increase the chance to visualize pheochromocytoma. In fact, it was widely used before Seldinger arteriography or bolus nephrotomography became widespread. It allowed localization in about 50% of the cases. However, this procedure is unpleasant and dangerous for the patients because it sometimes causes dramatic increases in blood pressure or collapses which have been fatal. Therefore this procedure is now abandoned [26, 27].

1.3. Arteriography

Aortography by the technique of Seldinger, completed by selective arteriographies, has become increasingly popular and accurate as a diagnostic procedure for detecting pheochromocytoma. In a review of 150 cases, Agee [28] reported an accurate detection in 80–85% of the cases. With the experience of 34 patients at the Cleveland Clinic, Zelch [29] states that the angiographic sequence is the key to a safe and accurate study and recommends the following procedure:

1. if localization is suggested by E.U. (or now by sonography or computed tomography) to perform a selective arteriography on the suspected side,
2. to perform a selective right renal arteriogram, because of the higher incidence of pheochromocytoma on the right side, if no previous localization is suggested
3. to perform a left renal arteriogram, if the right selective arteriogram is negative
4. following the above procedure, to perform a high (cathether tip above the coeliac axis) and a low (cathether above the inferior mesenteric artery) aortography.

The above sequence is preferred since injection of contrast medium into the aorta may initiate a hypertensive crisis before tumor localization. Injection into a renal artery not feeding the tumor will not significantly elevate blood pressure. On the contrary, a hypertensive response to selective angiography is considered to be a positive sign to pheochromocytoma. With this technique, he could localize 29 out of the 37 tumors studied by the aortogram. Selective arteriography was critical for four other tumors and adrenal phlebography for remaining the four.

Beside localizing pheochromocytoma, arteriography may show associated true intrinsic renal artery stenosis, renal artery compression by hilar pheo-

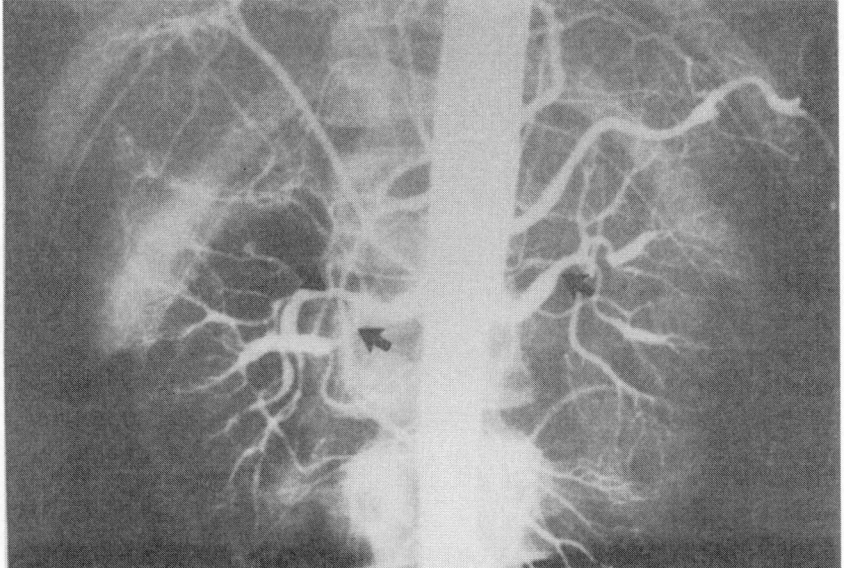

Figure 4b. Vascular phase of an aortography in a patient with a right adrenal pheochromocytoma (surrounded by corbelling vessels above the right kidney). Multiple spasms of the renal and extrarenal arteries are also seen.

682

chromocytoma and sometimes multiple spasms of the renal arteries or of other arteries (Figure 4b). Furthermore, arteriography may sometimes show hypervascularized metastasis of the liver, indicating the malignant nature of the pheochromocytoma.

Although arteriography is the best technique to diagnose multilocal pheochromocytoma, it is not without hazards because of the hypertensive crises it may provoke in about 50 % of the cases. A few fatalities have been reported, namely three in the early times of direct aortography [26], but also with the Seldinger technique (one personal patient who was already in shock state before performing the arteriography). For this reason, arteriography should certainly not be performed in critically ill patients before his condition has improved by a treatment with α- and β-blocking drugs (dibenzyline or phentolamine and beta-blockers, or labetalol which has both α- and β-blocking properties). In the other cases, previous α-blocking therapy is questionable since hypertension crisis will be prevented and one will miss the localization value of these crises. In most of the cases, this additional aid will be of little value since an abdominal tumor will be detected in the majority of the patients. However, when the biological diagnosis is uncertain or when previous radiological, surgical exploration has been negative,

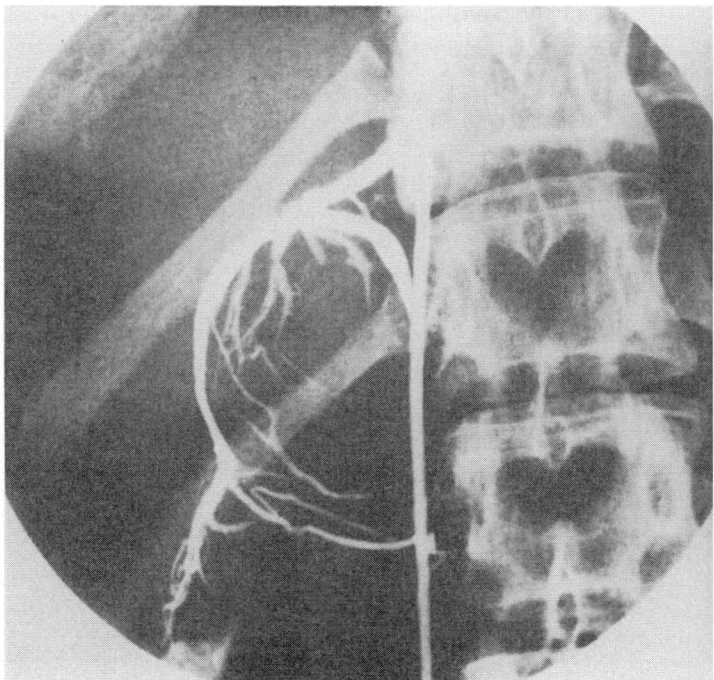

Figure 4c. Adrenal Phlebography showing a right adrenal pheochromocytoma.

arteriography induced hypertension crisis will gain diagnostic significance and therefore alpha-blockade should be avoided in that case. The radiologist and anesthesiologist should then be alert to promptly combat this crisis by pentolamine or sodium nitroprusside intravenous administration under continuous monitoring of blood pressure and ECG.

1.4. Adrenal phlebography

This difficult and hazardous technique is rarely indicated for the localization of pheochromocytoma but may be helpful when bolus nephrotomography, arteriography or comptued tomography have failed. Thus, in the series of 74 pheochromocytoma recorded by one of us (Tonnelier), phlebography was diagnostically useful in only four cases [30] (Figure 4c).

1.5. Ultrasonography

The interest of this non-invasive method is rather limited since conventional technique cannot detect tumor with a diameter smaller than 3 cm and necessitates a great skill from the operator. However, recent advance in sonography technology (gray scale) would allow for defining correctly normal adrenal glands in 85% of the cases and thus diagnose small tumors of 1.5 cm in diameter [31]. In practice, the experience in sonographic diagnosis of pheochromocytoma is limited and not very encouraging, since it shows only five out of eight adrenal pheochromocytoma discovered by surgery missing one tumor of 4 cm and another of 8 cm in diameter [32].

1.6. Computed axial tomography (CT)

This non-invasive procedure is gaining still greater popularity since it allows for a proper delineation of normal adrenal glands in 78% of the cases. Normal shape [33, 34, 38] of the right adrenal is linear ($\int$) in 87%, V-shaped (Λ) in 9%, whereas that of the left is Λ-shaped in 50%, λ-shaped in 32% and triangular (Δ) with concave sides in 8%. Their length is about 2–4 cm, their width 2–2,5 cm and their thickness less than 1 cm (usually 3–4 mm for the linear shape of the right adrenal gland). Therefore, small tumor of more than 0.5 cm at right and 1 cm at left could be detected.

The value of CT in the diagnosis of pheochromocytoma has been established only in small series but with promising results: the location of 10 pheochromocytoma out of 11 patients in the series of Stewart [35], 4 pheochromocytoma out of 4 in series of Ganguly [36] and the 13 pheochromocytoma out of 13 in the 10 patients in the series of Thomas [37]. Thus, for localizing pheochromocytoma, CT appears as accurate as selective angiography, without the hazards of the latter. It can even better detect avascular or necrotized pheochromocytoma. The only disadvantage is that it may be necessary to perform centimetric scans from the base of the skull to the pelvis if no tumor is found in the suprarenal regions. This would not be acceptable as regards the irradiation cost and would also be time-consuming. Only when angiographic studies and central venous samples for catecholamines assays are also negative, should such an investigation be performed.

1.7. Isotopic localization of pheochromocytoma

Adrenal pheochromocytoma may be visualized by compression or displacement of radioactive cortical tissue after administration of ^{131}I-19 iodocholesterol. Experience with this method is limited and not promising (3 abnormal visualization of adrenal cortex in 5 cases of pheochromocytoma) [32]. Administration of a catecholamine precursor such as monoidotyrosine or dopamine labeled with radioactive iodine would allow visualization of pheochromocytoma at any localization. However, experience is limited in this case as well [26, 27].

1.8. Central venous samples for catecholamine assays

It is a time-consuming procedure, necessitating a reliable laboratory to measure plasma catecholamine and giving results often difficult to interprete. It is therefore generally performed when the other procedures have failed and when the secretion of catecholamines has been demonstrated to be made only of norepinephrine, since the presence of epinephrine hypersecretion is associated with adrenal localization in 95 % of the cases. It consists in performing a femoral vein catheterization and blood samples from various vena cava levels: lumbar 4, 2 and 1, T12 and just above and below the entrance into the right atrium. Samples should be taken form both renal veins (L1 for the left and L2 for the right) and when possible from both adrenal veins (the right drains into IVC at T12 and the left drains into the left renal vein). Finally, when there is any suspicion of a chromaffinoma in the neck or the head, samples will be taken from the internal jugular veins. During the whole procedure, it is mandatory to record the timing of blood samples and the variations in blood pressure and heart rate every minute in order to evaluate eventual changes in basal secretion rate of the pheochromocytoma and interprete changes in plasma concentrations appropriately.

1.9. Proposed scheme for localizing a pheochromocytoma

Since non-invasive procedures like computed tomography (and possibly gray scale ultrasonography) are as effective as arteriography in detecting the most common localizations of pheochromocytoma (the upper abdominal region), it is tempting with Stewart [35] to recommend it as the one and only procedure when it shows a tumor. However, this attitude disregards the possibility of ectopic localizations present in 10 % of the cases in the adult and in 22 % of the cases in the children, as well as the necessity to know whether the patient has two normally functioning kidneys, since surgical removal of pheochromocytoma may sometimes lead to nephrectomy. For these reasons, we would rather recommend to perform (with the routine chest X-ray with oblique view) the intravenous arteriography which gives good vascular and parenchymal opacification of the whole abdomen and may disclose associated abnormalities of the other arteries and of the excretory cavities. Computed tomography should be performed in a second stage and when it fails to diagose a pheochromocytoma in the upper abdomen, arteriographies with the Seldinger technique, according to the sequence of Zelch would be recommended. Scanning with CT of the pelvis, thorax and neck and/or adrenal phlebography with central venous samples for catecholamines assays will be the ultimate diagnostic means.

2. Radiologic examination of a patient with primary aldosteronism

Primary aldosteronism is a rare cause of hypertension (<1%). It is readily diagnosed in patients with hypertension because of persistent hypokalemia, elevated plasma or urinary aldosterone and suppressed plasma renin activity. This condition is due in two thirds of the cases to an unilateral adenoma of the adrenal cortex and is then cured in 70–80% of the cases by unilateral adrenalectomy. However, in one third of the cases, this condition is related to a bilateral adrenal hyperplasia [39–42]. Therefore, it is of crucial importance to distinguish between these two subgroups: the one with the true Conn syndrome and the other with the so-called idiopathic hyperaldosteronism, usually managed with medical treatment. This distinction remains a major diagnostic challenge for which radiologic examinations are of prime importance since confirmation of the presence and ultimate localization of an adenoma may be accomplished either by adrenal scintigraphy [43], or by adrenal arteriography and venography with the measurement of aldosterone in adrenal venous blood [30, 40, 45] or, more recently, by computed tomography [42, 47].

2.1. Adrenal scintigraphy

Conn has proposed to use adrenal scintigraphy with ^{131}I-iodocholesterol after administration of lugol to saturate the thyroid and of dexamethasone for 5–6 days in order to suppress the corticol secreting parenchyma [43]. In the case of a unilateral adenoma there is a marked unilateral hyperfixation, whereas in the case of idiopathic hyperplasia, fixation of the isotope is poor and symmetrical. This procedure is non-invasive and can be performed on an outpatient. However, the irradiation cost is not negligible (4 rads for testis, 6 rads for ovaries, 60 rads for the adrenals) and the examination is costly, time-consuming and reserved to highly specialized centers. Furthermore, although the recent series of Leger on 42 cases proposes this procedure of localization as the first one to perform, other authors [41, 42] have not confirmed its diagnostic accuracy. It is explained by the fact that it cannot detect adenoma smaller than 1 cm and that Conn adenoma is usual-

686

ly very small, since in a series of 42 patietns Tonnelier found that it had a mean diameter of 1 cm.

2.2. Adrenal venography
It is certainly the most accurate procedure to detect small adenoma of the adrenal cortex. It is however also the most hazardous one, since adrenal necrosis may ensue. It should therefore be performed by a well-trained and skilled angiographer. Its realization is much more difficult for the right than for the left adrenal vein. Venography should laways be accompanied by blood samplings for measurement of aldosterone. Weinberger [41] advises to measure both aldosterone and cortisol concentrations during ACTH administration so as to reduce the error induced by episodic production of aldosterone as well as by dilution of blood by non-adrenal venous sources. Figure 4d, 4e and 4f show examples of adrenal venographic findings in Conn adenoma and bilateral hyperplasia. In his series of 62 patients with primary aldosteronism, Tonnelier found an adenoma in 70% of the cases and a bilateral hyperplasia in 30%. Phlebography alone was diangostic in

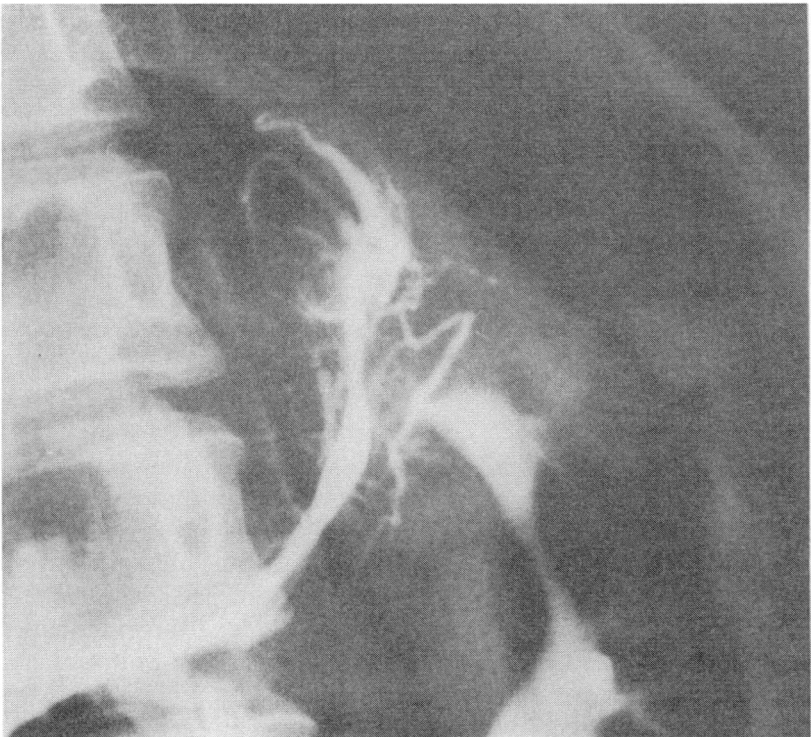

Figure 4d. Typical adenoma of 1.5 cm secreting aldosterone (6500 ng/100 ml of aldosterone onthis side vs. 100 on the other side).

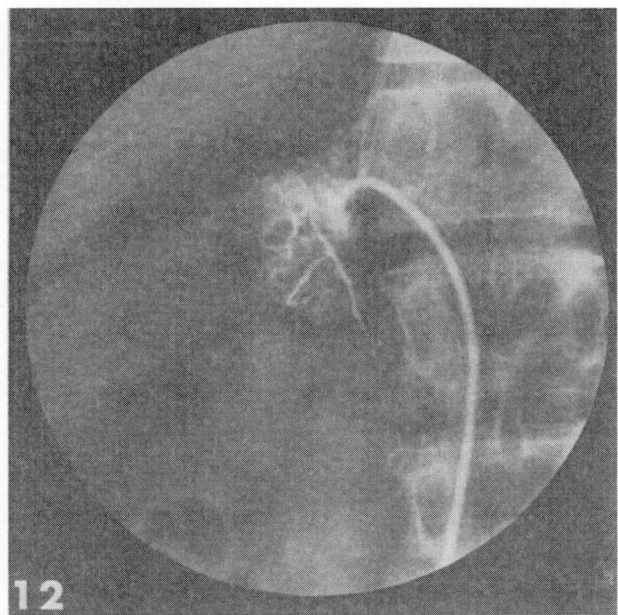

Figure 4e. Small adenoma secreting aldosterone of 0.5 cm in diameter in a right hyperplasia gland (700 ng/100 ml of aldosterone in the venous blood).

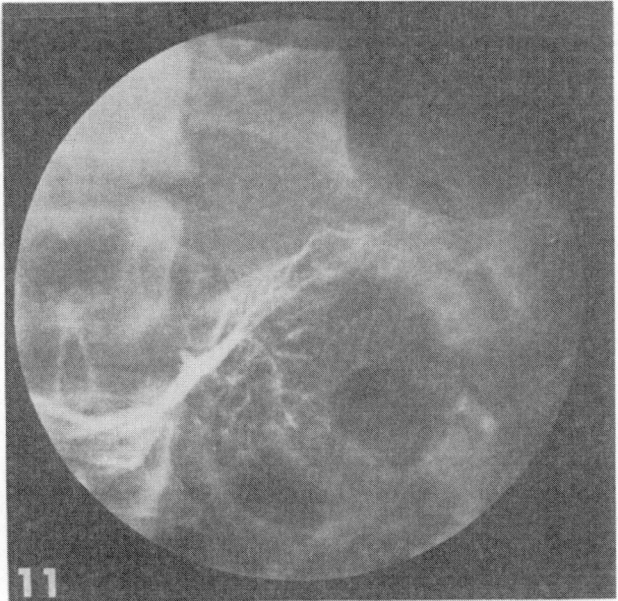

Figure 4f. Nodular hyperplasia of the left adrenal gland.

688

80% of the cases and aldosterone measurement allowed for such a conclusion in the other 20%.

2.3. Computed tomography

Recent advances in computed tomography theoretically enable us to detect an adrenal tumor greater than 0.5 cm for the right and 1 cm for the left side. CT may therefore detect Conn adenoma in most cases. This was confirmed in the series of White. On 22 patients with primary aldosteronism, 12 out of 16 with biological criteria suggestive of adenoma had unilateral adrenal mass that was clearly demonstrated and confirmed by surgery in the 11 cases who underwent surgery. In the remaining 4 patients no definite diagnosis could be made, whereas in the 6 patients with biological criteria suggestive of idiopathic hyperaldosteronism, CT showed either normal or bilateral hyperplasia. Earlier report by Linde was less enthusiastic since CT scan failed to identify 3 adenomas in 9 patients. These adenomas measured 1 cm (Figure 4g).

2.4. Indication of the radiologic procedure

Since they are usually negative, we have not discussed about excretory urography and aortography. Intravenous arteriography and pyelography may be interesting only when surgery is decided to look for eventual coincidental abnormalities of the kidneys. Otherwise, the first examination to propose for diagnosing a Conn adenoma should be computed tomography rather

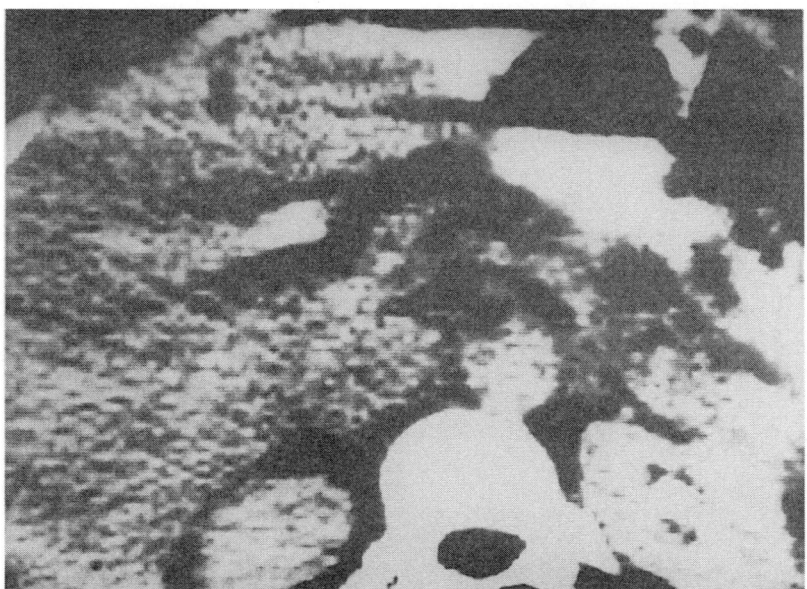

Figure 4g. Conn adenoma of the left adrenal gland (located between the left kidney and the aorta) on a computed tomography (Courtesy of Dr. Masselot of Villejuif).

than idiocholesterol scintigram after dexamethasone, since it exposes the patient to less radiation. The choice between these two possibilities currently depends mainly on local availability. Because of its hazards and the necessity of a skilled angiographer and of a reliable laboratory, adrenal venography with blood samples for aldosterone determination is proposed as the ultimate step.

3. Radiologic examination of an hypertensive patient with Cushing's syndrom

Although hypertension is a frequent complication of Cushing's syndrome, the latter represents a rare cause of hypertension (<0.8%). This syndrome is mostly due to bilateral hyperplasia in relation to ACTH hypersecretion, but may be also due to adrenal cortical adenoma or carcinoma. Since the Liddle suppressive test by high doses of dexamethasone is not always conclusive and since measurement of plasma ACTH is not readily available, radiologic examination has an important place for the etiological diagnosis of this syndrome by showing either bilateral hyperplasia or unilateral tumor.

In a comparative study of ultrasound, ^{131}I-19 iodocholesterol scintigraphy and aortography in defining adrenal lesions in 14 cases of Cushing's syndrome. Kehlet et al. found that scintigraphy was the best diagnostic procedure for detecting the five adenomas, whereas ultrasonography failed to detect one of them and aortography two of them. Since the advent of computed tomography, however, the latter method represents the procedure of choice, since, theoretically at least, it is as sensitive as the scintigraphy, exposes the patient to less radiation and is less time-consuming [48]. Furthermore, it allows for determining the eventual extension of a malignant tumor to the neighborhood structures. Because of its hazards, adrenal venography is contra-indicated in Cushing's syndrome [48].

In conclusion, the anatomical diagnosis of a Cushing's syndrome should be based in the first place on computed tomography or gray scale sonography and in the second place on scintigraphy.

REFERENCES

1. Pinet F, Amiel M, Devic J: Les coarctations de l'aorte. Encycl Med Chir, Paris Radiodiagnostic III, 4.3.11, 32015-D25.
2. Weyman AC, Caldwell RL, Hurwitz RA, Girod DA, Millon JC, Feigenbaum W, Green D: Cross-sectional echocardiography detection of aortic obstruction in coarctation of the aorta. Circulation 57:498, 1978.
3. Remond A, Grumbach Y, Risbourg B, Dieval M, Deramond H: L'aortographie par voie carotidienne rétrograde chez le nouveau-né et le nourrisson. Technique et résultats. A propos de 21 observations. J Radiol 60:175–180, 1979.
4. Fournier A, Vaysse J, Lacombe M: Rein et hypertension artérielle. Paris: Edition Baillères, 1978.

5. Emmet JL, Witten DM: Clinical urography. Philadelphia: Saunders C, 1971.
6. Mimran A: Hypertension artérielle et tumeur rénine secrétantes. In: Hypertension artérielle, pp. 188-197. Tcherdakoff P, ed. Rueil Malmaison: Sandoz, 1980.
7. McNeil BJ, Varady PD, Burrow SB: Measure of clinical éfficacy–cost effectiveness calculations in the diagnosis and treatment of hypertensive renovascular disease. N Engl J med 293:216-221, 1975.
8. Fournier A, Cecile JP, Remond A: Le temps artériel de l'urographie intraveineuse dans l'hypertension artérielle rénovasculaire. Ann Med Intern 131:272-277, 1980.
9. Maxwell MH, Varady PD: Cooperative study of renovascular hypertension: clinical characteristics, diagnostic test and results of surgery. Contr Nephrol 3:1-19, 1976.
10. Plantureux P, Plainfosse MC: Faut-il encore pratiquer une UIV complète systématiquement à toute HTA en 1977? Ann Radiol 20:545-555, 1977.
11. Amplatz K: Two radiographic tests for assessment of renovascular hypertension. A preliminary report Radiology 79:807, 1962.
12. Amiel M, Pinet F, Froment A, Pipard G, Plantier S: Une nouvelle méthode d'étude des hypertensions artérielles rénovasculaires: le wash-out à la furosémide. Lyon Medical 229:453, 1973.
13. Fournier A, Safar M, Benmaiz H, Girard J, Plainfosse MC, Laval-Jeantet m, Bernard J, Milliez P: Urography with urea wash-out in renovascular hypertension. A comparison with split renal function tests and predictive value. Acta Radiol (Diagn) 14:315-325, 1973.
14. Dorph S, Ølgaard A: Variations in renal size in the diagnosis of renovascular hypertension. Br J Radiol 46:187-190, 1973.
15. Grim CE, Luft FC, Weinberger MH, Grim CM: Sensitivity and specificity of screening tests for renovascular hypertensions. Ann Intern Med 91:617-622, 1979.
16. Seldinger SI: Catheter replacement of the needle in percutaneous arteriography. Acta Radiol Dig 39:368-376, 1953.
17. Stewart BH, Dustan HP, Kiser WS, Meaney TF, Straffon RA, McCormack LJ: Correlation of angiography and natural history in evaluation of patients with renovascular hypertension. J Urol 104:231-238, 1970.
18. Sheps SG, Kincaid DW, Hunt JC: Serial, renal function, and angiographic observation in idiopathic fibrosis and fibromuscular stenosis of renal arteries. Am J Cardiol 30:55-60, 1972.
19. Bookstein JJ, Abrams HL, Buenger RE, Reiss MD, Lecky JW, Franklin SS, Varady PD, Maxwell M: Radiologic aspects of renovascular hypertension - III. Appraisal of arteriography. JAMA 221:368-374, 1972.
20. Cecile JP, Fournier A, Lelong M: Phleboarteriography in the diagnosis of abdominal masses in children Clin Radiol 23:340-348, 1972.
21. Schockert J, Bollaert A, Demanet JC: Intérêt de l'aortographie par voie veineuse comme examen systématique chez l'hypertendu. J Urol Nephrol 73:750-753, 1973.
22. Fournier A, Cecile JP, Remond A, de Fremont JF, Makdassi R, Andrejak M, Hardin JM, Grumbach Y: Value of combined intravenous renal arteriography and pyelography in the diagnosis of renovascular hypertension. Clin Sci Mol Med 59:423s-425s, 1980.
23. Ingrish H, Holzgreve H, Frey KW: Visualization of the renal arteries during excretory urography. Clin Sci Mol Med 59:419s-422s, 1980.
24. Schwarten DE, Yune HY, Klatte EC, Grim CE, Weinberger MH: Clinical experience with percutaneous transluminal angioplasty of stenotic renal arteries. Radiology 135:601-604, 1980.
25. Fournier A: Faut-il encore rechercher, quand et comment, une hypertension artérielle rénovasculaire en 1980? Ou les indications du temps artériel de l'urographie intraveineuse. Ann Med Intern 131:261-265, 1980.
26. Manger WM, Gifford RW: Pheochromocytoma, pp. 247-276. New York: Springer-Verlag, 1977.

691

27. Tcherdakoff P, Colliard M, Dumont D: Localisation des phéochromocytomes,pp. 226–231. In: Hypertension artérielle Tcherdakoff P, ed. Rueil Malmaison: Sandoz, 1980.
28. Agee OF, Kaude J, Lepason J: Preoperative localization of pheochromocytoma. Acta Radiolog (Diagn) 14:545–560, 1973.
29. Zelch JV, Meaney TF, Belhobek GH: Radiologic approach to the patient with suspected pheochromocytoma. Radiology 111:279–284, 1974.
30. Ecoiffier J, Tonnelier M: Radiologie des surrénales chez l'adulte. Encycl Med Chir – Radiodiagnostic 345$_{50}$, B$_{20}$ and B$_{30}$ 1–20.
31. Sample WF, Sarti D: Computed tomography and gray scale ultrasonography of the adrenal gland. Am J Roentgen 130:963–966, 1978.
32. Kehlet H, Blichert-Toft M, Hancke S, Pedersen JF, Hasner E: Comparative study of ultrasound, [131]I-19 iodocholesterol scintigraphy and aortography in localising adrenal lesions. Br Med J 2:665–667, 1976.
33. Montagne JP, Kressel HY, Korobkin R, Moss AA: Computed tomography of the normal adrenal glands Am. J Roentgen 130:963–966, 1978.
34. Heithoff KB: Computerized tomography of the adrenals. J Belg Radiol 61:383–398, 1978.
35. Stewart BH, Bravo EL, Haaga J, Heaney TF, Tarazi R: Localization of pheochromocytoma by computed tomography. N Engl J Med 299:460–467, 1978.
36. Gangula A, Henry DP, Yune HY, Pratt JH, Grim CE, Donohve JP, Weinberger MH: Diagnosis and localization of pheochromocytoma. Detection by measurement of urinary norepinephrine excretion during sleep, Plasma norepinephrine concentration and computerized axial tomography (CT scan). Am J Med 67:21, 1979.
37. Thomas JL, Bernardino ME, Samaan NA, Hickey RC: CT of pheochromocytoma. Am J Roentgen 135:477–482, 1980.
38. Elie G, Le Treut A, Dilhuydy MH, Bruneton JN, Calabet A: Tomodensitométrie de la surrénale pathologique tumorale de l'adulte. J Radiol 61:597–601, 1980.
39. Salvador M, Chamontin B, Guittard J: Les hyperminéralocorticismes. In: Hypertension artérielle, pp. 210–219. Tcherdakoff. P, ed. Rueil Malmaison: Sandoz, 1980.
40. Corvol P, Houde M, Benguigui L, Tonnelier M, Menard J, Milliez P: Le diagnostic de l'hyperaldostéronisme primaire. Nouv Presse Med 6:2483–2488, 1977.
41. Weinberger MH, Grim CE, Hollifield JW, Kem DC, Yune HY, Wellmann H, Donohue JP: Primary aldosteronism. Diagnosis, localization and treatment. Ann Intern Med 90:386–395, 1979.
42. White EA, Schambelan M, Rost CR, Biglieri EG, Moss A, Korobkin M: Use of computed tomography in diagnosing the cause of primary aldosteronism. N Engl J Med 303:1503–1507, 1980.
43. Conn JW, Cohen EL, Herwig KR: The dexamethasone modified adrenal scintiscan in hyporenihemic aldosteronism (tumor versus hyperplasia). A comparison with adrenal venography and adrenal venous aldosterone. J Lab Clin Med 88:841–856, 1976.
44. Leger FA, Requeda E, Beach G, Plouin PF, Savoie E: Scintigraphie corticosurrénalienne au [131]I-19 iodocholesterol. Nouv Presse Med 10:395–399, 1981
45. Kahn PC, Kelleher MD, Egdahl RH, Melby JC: Adrenal arteriography and venography in primary aldosteronism. Radiology 101:71–78, 1971.
46. Nicolis GL, Mitty HA, Modlinger RS, Gavrilove JL: Percutaneous adrenal venography. A clinical study of 50 patients. Ann Intern Med 76:899–909, 1972.
47. Linde R, Coulam C, Battino R, Rhamy R, Gerlock J, Hollifield J: Localization of aldosterone producing adenoma by computed tomography. J Clin Endocrin Metab 49:642–645, 1979.
48. De Gennes JL, Chatelain C, Turpin G, Richard F, Cariou G: Exploration actuelle des tumeurs de la corticosurrénale. Séminaires d'Uronephrologie, pp. 40–57. Kuss R, Legrain M, eds. Paris: Masson, 1981.

VII. ANTIHYPERTENSIVE THERAPY

44. NON-DRUG TREATMENT OF HYPERTENSION

HENRY R. BLACK

In the past decade there has been considerable interest in treating hypertension (HBP) with non-pharmacologic methods, both old (sodium (Na$^+$) restriction and weight reduction) and new (behavioral therapy and exercise). Yet, in its 1980 report the Joint National Committee on Detection, Evaluation, and Treatment of High Blood Pressure recommended some forms of non-drug therapy for HBP in some patients with little enthusiasm [1]. They felt that obese hypertensive patients should be encouraged to lose weight; that modest Na$^+$ restriction (85 mEq/day) was a reasonably adjunctive therapy in all patients but that behavioral methods could not yet be considered a substitute for pharmacologic treatment. No recommendations were made about exercise. The rationale for non-pharmacologic treatment of HBP (Na$^+$ restriction, weight reduction, stress reduction, and exercise) is based on experimental and epidemiologic evidence suggesting a role for excess Na$^+$ intake, obesity, and stress in causing HBP in man.

1. SODIUM RESTRICTION

There is ample evidence from antiquity that salt was scarce and very valuable, and only in the past several centuries could most members of acculturated societies count on having adequate Na$^+$ available. Fries suggested, in fact, that the epidemic of essential hypertension in Western society is caused by our recently acquired habit of eating large quantities of salt and that adequate reduction of salt intake by susceptible members of the population will lead to a disappearance of HBP as a problem [2]. The evidence for this hypothesis comes from epidemiologic surveys and extensive animal studies on the role of Na$^+$ intake in the development of HBP in genetically susceptible animals.

Although lowering dietary Na$^+$ has been considered as therapy for HBP since early in the 20th century [3, 4], Kempner's success in reducing BP with a very low Na$^+$ (<5 mEq/day) 'rice-fruit diet' [5] was the major impetus for others to try this approach to treat HBP. The diastolic (D) BP in the majority of patients who could adhere to this diet fell more than 10 mm Hg, while

Amery, A. (ed.) Hypertensive Cardiovascular Disease: Pathophysiology and Treatment
© *1982, Martinus Nijhoff Publishers. The Hague / Boston / London*
ISBN-13: 978-94-009-7478-4

in 13% DBP decreased 30 mm Hg or more. Although many patients lost weight while on the rice-fruit diet, Dole et al. [6] showed that adding back even small amounts of Na^+ caused a rise in BP and they concluded that extreme Na^+ restriction was responsible for the hypotensive effect of the diet.

Grollman et al. had minimal success with a one gram salt diet in six hospitalized patients [7] and when inexpensive oral diuretic therapy became available for treating HBP in the late 1950s, interest waned in using Na^+ restriction.

Because of the known metabolic effects [8] and potential long-term toxicity of diuretic therapy and the failure of non-diuretic drugs consistently to reduce BP when used alone, the use of dietary Na^+ restriction as primary or adjunctive treatment has been re-examined. In a crossover design, Parijs et al. [9] compared the hypotensive effect of modest Na^+ restricted diets (90–100 mEq/day) or usual diets (193 mEq Na^+/day) when diuretic therapy or placebo were used concomitantly. Na^+ restriction alone reduced BP 7.7/4.4 mm Hg, while diuretics alone caused a 16.1/8.1 mm Hg drop. The combination of diet and diuretics was best as BP fell 20.7/10.8 mm Hg. They suggested a drop in salt intake from 10 to 5 g/day would reduce BP by 10/5 mm Hg. Morgan and colleagues studied 132 Australians with mild HBP and randomized them into four groups of 31 patients each [10]. One group received no treatment; one got dietary instruction designed to reduce Na^+ intake to 70–100 mEq/day; a third were given thiazide diuretics and alpha-methyl dopa if needed; and the last diuretics and propranolol. Although more of the patients treated with drugs became normotensive (DBP <90 mm Hg), DBP in $\frac{1}{3}$ of the Na^+ restricted group was less than 90 mm Hg at two years. This good result occurred even though the urinary Na^+ fell only to 157 mEq/day compared to 190 mEq/24 h in all other groups. In an Italian study quoted by Heyden et al., a three gram salt diet was as effective as drugs in reducing BP [11]. The group given drugs dropped from 164/98 mm Hg to 158/91 mm Hg, while the patients treated only with Na^+ restriction went from 160/101 mm Hg to 147/90 mm Hg. In this study, actual Na^+ excretion and degree of weight loss, if any, is not specified.

Hunt and Margie treated more than 3000 patients with combined dietary therapy and pharmacologic agents if needed [12]. Most of the patients who could reduce their urinary Na^+ below 75 mEq/day had DBP fall to below 90 mm Hg; half of those with a DBP above 115 mm Hg who could do so became normotensive. At five years, however, only 40% of all the patients were still on diet therapy alone.

One very important observation was that whatever drug regimen was used, the less Na^+ a patient excreted, and presumably ate, the better the success with any drug regimen. Hunt feels that there is no real reduction in BP until Na^+ excretion is less than 90 mEq/day. Since these were also hypocaloric diets, many patients also lost weight and 70% of the patients who became normotensive had lost 10% of their body weight or more.

Potassium (K^+) depletion may play a significant role in causing HBP and may be as important as Na^+ excess [13]. In 1928, Addison claimed that K^+ salts reduced BP [14] and other early investigators made similar suggestions [15, 16]. Meneely has recently reviewed the data on the role of the low K^+ environment and pointed out that all low Na^+ diets are also high K^+ diets [17]. The Kempner diet contains approximately 75 mEq/K^+ and Hunt's regimen is a 100 mEq/day K^+ diet. To date, no one has systematically studied the effect of K^+ supplementation as treatment for HBP, but in normal man Luft and co-workers showed that maintaining K^+ balance will prevent the rise in BP seen with very high Na^+ intakes (800–1500 mEq Na^+/day) [18].

Conclusion

There is little doubt that Na^+ intake is a key determinant of BP, especially in large quantities in genetically susceptible individuals. Proof is lacking, however, that most patients will be able to restrict adequately their intake in our modern society. Hunt's work, however, has shown that Na^+ restriction may play a very important role in treatment, both alone and as adjunctive therapy with drugs, and it may be worth the effort to get patients to reduce their Na^+ intake. Salt restriction even to very low levels [19] is generally very safe, although Longworth et al. have suggested that BP will rise in some patients when sodium is restricted [20]. While Na^+ restriction has a central but limited role in the non-drug treatment of hypertension, the value of high K^+ diets has not been adequately studied. If K^+ does protect against the rise in BP induced by Na^+ then, perhaps, in patients with normal renal function deliberately high K^+ diets or K^+ supplementation, whether or not patients were being treated with kaluretic agents, would reduce BP.

2. WEIGHT REDUCTION

Considerable disagreement exists as to whether obesity is an important cause of HBP or even of cardiovascular disease. The newly published Build Study of the Society of Actuaries [21] confirmed the finding of the 1959 Build and Blood Pressure Study [22] and showed that significant obesity was correlated with increases in BP and a greater risk of death from cardiovascular disease. Stamler [23] and others [24, 25] agreed that obesity is a major risk factor in cardiovascular disease, but some groups [26, 27] have concluded that obesity does not itself contribute to premature cardiovascular disease except insofar as it causes HBP.

The Framingham Study demonstrated a strong association between obesity and HBP in adults at all ages and in both men and women [28]. For children and adolescents numerous population studies have indicated that there is a strong correlation between obesity and HBP [29–32]. Chiang et al. reviewed the association of obesity and HBP and concluded that, while the mechanism for obesity causing HBP was unclear, there was no question that obesity in a patient with HBP worsened the prognosis and that weight reduction was beneficial for the hypertensive individual [33]. Mann is more cautious and correctly points out the difficulty physicians have in successfully treating this 'relatively incurable disorder' [34].

Reisin and colleagues [35] treated 24 new hypertensive patients with weight reduction only and randomly selected 57 patients from a group of 83 already on drugs to receive dietary treatment in addition. The other 26 patients on pharmacologic agents got no dietary therapy and served as controls. Since Dahl had always claimed that calorie restriction worked because all hypocaloric diets were also low Na^+ diets [36], this group encouraged patients to eat heavily salted foods. All patients who were given dietary treatment (800–1200 calorie diets) lost at least 3 kg (mean loss was 10.5 kg). Thirty-nine of the 81 patients had a reduction of weight to within 10% of ideal weight, while another 37 patients lost more than 5% of initial body weight. Weight did not change in 96% of the untreated groups. BP became normal in 53 of the diet treated group (75% of those were on no drugs) and only 10 of 81 patients in the weight loss group did not show a reduction in BP. The loss of weight and fall in BP were strongly correlated. Twenty-four of the 26 patients on drugs alone had the same or higher BP at the end of the six-month study. Since these patients were encouraged to eat salty foods and had high urinary Na^+ excretions (165–185 mEq/l) when tested at the conclusion of the weight reduction program, Reisin and colleagues felt that the beneficial effects of the diet were due entirely to its hypocaloric effect and not to concomitant Na^+ restriction. Unfortunately, they provide no data on Na^+ excretion soon after calorie restriction began and their weight loss group might have been in significant negative Na^+ balance early in the program. The follow-up period for this study is only six months and the recidivism rate or applicability in a less committed population is unknown. Without these data, the usefulness of weight reduction diets this strict for the general hypertensive population cannot be predicted. In the Chicago Coronary Prevention Program [37], men with mild and borderline HBP were given dietary counseling. The patients lost small amounts of weight (11 pounds) but had a significant reduction in BP (13/9 mm Hg). No mention is made of changes in Na^+ intake or excretion. Early reviews [38] emphasized the difficulty in treating obesity and a recent study by Currey et al. cast serious doubts on even new behavior modification techniques [39].

Conclusion

The association of obesity and HBP is primarily statistical. Many obese subjects are normotensive and many hypertensive patients are not over-weight. Weight reduction can significantly reduce BP in obese hypertensives but problems with adherence to the diet seriously limit this form of therapy. Perhaps the less stringent and combined approaches of Stamler et al. [23] and Hunt [12] may be more generally useful. While Reisin's study has convincingly shown that the beneficial efforts of weight reduction can be separated from those of salt restriction in HBP, some doubt still remains and this issue can only be settled by more careful balance studies.

3. EXERCISE

Physical inactivity, like obesity, has been associated with increased susceptibility to coronary artery disease (CAD) and HBP in many population studies [40–43]. Montoye et al. [44] and Cooper and colleagues [45] have tried to quantitate physical activity and have shown that subjects who are physically active by history or by direct measurments of conditioning, tend to have lower BP even when body fat is accounted for. Scheuer and Tipton, on the other hand, feel that most studies have not demonstrated a significant effect of physical fitness on BP [46].

The value of exercise as therapy for both experimental and clinical HBP is even more controversial. In several different models of HBP in rats, Tipton and colleagues showed that an exercise program of running on a treadmill will delay the onset and magnitude of HBP, but not reduce resting BP to normal in adult hypertensive animals [47]. Training by swimming also reduced BP in experimental HBP [48], but one study found no effect of 16 weeks of running in the same animal model [49]. In man, Boyer and Kasch showed that a modest individualized exercise program of walking and jogging after adequate warm up, reduced BP a mean of 13.5/11.8 mm Hg after six months in the 23 men studied [50]. No drugs were used and BP fell in all patients. Body weight did not change in the majority of the patients and no serious complications occurred. Choquette and Ferguson reduced BP from 136/90 mm Hg to 122/86 mm Hg in groups of 37 borderline hypertensive men with a six-month program of calisthenics, jogging, and volleyball performed once a week for two hours [51]. These subjects were also advised to do 10–15 min of daily calisthenics at home. Wilmore and colleagues achieved similar results with a program of jogging thrice weekly whether done for 12 or 24 min/day [52]. Other studies have not been as successful in lowering BP [53, 54], but it is clear that exercise programs are safe even in the previously sedentary individuals [53], even if elderly [54]. In fact, complications of supervised exercise programs are relatively free of risk even in patients recovering from myocardial infarctions [55, 56]. Gibbons et al. reported only two cardiac events, none fatal, in nearly 3000 unselected adults who ran or walked more than 2 700 000 km in 374 798 person hours [57]. Haskell surveyed cardiac rehabilitation programs in high-risk patients and found that one non-fatal event occurred every 34 673 patient hours and a fatal event every 116 402 patient hours [55].

Conclusion

The specific beneficial effect of exercise therapy in HBP has not been proven. In uncommitted patients, compliance with the program may be only 30–50% [52, 58], and in high-risk individuals the exercise program should be initiated under careful supervision. When properly supervised, however, exercise is safe, should be inexpensive, and offers the additional benefits of weight loss and psychological well-being to the patient.

4. BEHAVIORAL THERAPY

Behavioral treatment for HBP is designed to reduce the excessive stress or the abnormal response to stress that may be a critical factor in the development of HBP and CAD [59–62]. Two basic approaches, relaxation and biofeedback, have been used extensively both separately and together to treat HBP.

Relaxation

Although Jacobson was perhaps the first to utilize relaxation techniques therapeutically [63], Benson pointed out that techniques to induce a state of relaxation have been used for thousands of years usually in a religious context [64]. He feels the central nervous system, probably the hypothalamus, not only controls the well-known response to stress (the fight or flight reaction) but also can elicit an opposite reaction designed to protect against 'overstress'. This reaction is a state of decreased sympathetic activity characterized by a decrease in BP, heart rate, respiratory rate and O_2 consumption, and an increase in skeletal muscle blood flow and alpha waves on electroencephalogram. Benson and colleagues note that regular practitioners of transcendental meditation (TM), an Eastern religious relaxation technique, successfully achieved this hypometabolic state [65] including a lowered BP and so they devised a non-cultic equivalent to TM they called the Relaxation Response (RR). Four maneuvers are necessary to elicit this response: (1) sitting quietly in a comfortable position, (2) closing one's eyes, (3) progressively and deeply relaxing all muscle groups beginning at the feet, and (4) breathing deeply through one's nose and becoming aware of this breathing while repetitively repeating a phrase with each expiration. In TM, the phrase is a mantra given by the instructor and with RR the number 'one' is used. These techniques are designed to help the subject maintain a passive attitude and ignore extraneous thoughts. The initial 'dose' prescribed for the RR was twenty minutes twice a day and, like TM, it can be learned in a few short sessions.

The RR has been studied extensively as a treatment for HBP. Benson initially reported a reduction in BP in 22 untreated patients of 7.0/3.8 mm Hg (146.5/94.6 to 139.5/90.8 mm Hg) [66] and of 10.6/4.9 mm Hg (145.6/91.9 to 135/87 mm Hg) in 14 patients who remained on but did not change their antihypertensive therapy [67]. BP was always measured at a time remote from the exercise. This experiment lasted approximately six months and when subjects stopped practicing relaxation, BP rose to pretreatment levels within four weeks.

Other groups have had similar results with these and related techniques. Blackwell and colleagues reduced BP in six of seven subjects with TM [68] and Stone and DiLeo used Buddist meditation exercises [69] and lowered BP from 141/90 mm Hg to 132/82 mm Hg compared to a control group whose BP was unchanged during the same time period. In this study, plasma dopamine beta-hydroxylase levels (a measure of sympathetic activity) were reduced and the fall correlated with the fall in BP. Datey et al. in India [70] also used yogic exercise ('Shavasan') with a good response in about 50% of the patients. Taylor and colleagues [71] used relaxation techniques with pharmacologic agents and compared the results to drugs and to 'nonspecific' supportive therapy. The group treated with relaxation and drugs had a greater reduction in BP than either drugs or supportive care alone. A reduction of 12.0/6.2 mm Hg was seen with combined treatment compared to 6.8/1.5 mm Hg for drugs and 4/3.5 mm Hg for nonspecific therapy. Pollack et al. [72], on the other hand, reported limited success with TM in a group of 20 patients but they did comment that most of their subjects had an enhanced sense of well-being even if their BP remained at pretreatment levels and 14 of the 20 asked to continue meditation even though it had failed as therapy. Deabler and colleagues [73] compared relaxation techniques and hypnosis in 6 untreated and 9 drug-treated patients. The group given relaxation had a reduction in BP, but the group given hypnosis did better.

Several investigators have combined relaxation with other methods of behavioral therapy. Patel and North [74] in a well-designed crossover trial, divided 34 patients into two groups. Group I was given a modified program of TM and biofeedback of skin resistance. These patients also had a red disc placed on their wristwatches to 'remind' them to relax. Group II was seen as often, but was given no special instructions or reminders. Subjects were then followed biweekly for nearly three months. In the treated group, BP fell 26.1/15.2 mm Hg compared to 8.9/4.2 mm Hg in the controls. After a two-month interval of no therapy, the control group was given the same training as Group I and Group II was merely followed. After three additional months, BP had fallen 28.1/15.0 mm Hg in the patients now given 'active' therapy (Group II). The BP of Group I had risen only slightly during the interval and did not change appreciably during the remainder of the trial (10 month follow-up). Patel has also shown that this combination may reduce the exaggerated BP response to stress seen in hypertensive patients [75]. Shoemaker and Tasto also had good results using relaxation techniques and non-continuous biofeedback of BP [76]. Frankel and colleagues [77] combined biofeedback, both of DBP and frontalis muscle tone with relaxation techniques including autogenic training [78]. They failed to find any BP reduction in their treated group during a 16-week trial. Roberts and Forester taught meditation in a group session [79], while their control group met to discuss 'medical topics of interest'. In this study, the reduction in BP was very small and not different between the groups.

Conclusion

In general, the results of relaxation therapy are disappointing. The reduction in BP is small at best and some side effects of the treatment (failure, insomnia, psychosis) have been reported [64]. The treatment is certainly inexpensive and some patients may be able to reduce their doses of insulin or beta-blockers as the degree of their sympathatic stimulation is reduced. Better designed long-term studies are needed before this therapy can be recommended for most patients as anything more than an adjunct to drugs.

More research is also needed to determine whether it is the increased attention given to patients, the enthusiasm of the therapists or a placebo effect [80] that makes relaxation 'work'. Ayman in 1930 [81] and Goldring et al. [82] in 1956 pointed out the value an enthusiastic therapist can have in lowering BP. As Schwartz et al. have stated, relaxation and other non-pharmacologic treatment for HBP should be analyzed with the same rigor customarily applied to the evaluation of pharmacologic therapy [83]. In any case, whether or not relaxation techniques reliably reduce BP, patients who practice them feel better. In fact, patients may feel so much better that they may neglect their pills and their BP may rise. This ontoward 'side effect' must be watched for and patients must be constantly reminded of the need to continue their drugs even if they are meditating.

Biofeedback

Biofeedback is the second major type of behavioral treatment used to treat HBP. Biofeedback uses modern instrumentation to monitor a physiologic process and to convert that information into some other signal that is easily recognized by the subject. The instrumentation may be complex, such as that used to monitor SBP [84] or be very simple like the temperature-sensitive cuffs that can be wrapped around the finger, measure skin temperature and 'feedback' the actual level to the subject.

It has long been assumed that physiologic processes such as BP that were under the control of the autonomic nervous system could not be voluntarily modified. In the late 1960s work in animals demonstrated that the functions of the autonomic nervous system were amenable to traditional operant conditioning and in 1969 Shapiro and colleagues showed that young male college students could be taught to lower and raise SBP. BP was monitored by means of a microphone placed over the brachial artery and a BP cuff was set to inflate to approximate SBP. The presence of the first Korotokoff sound was picked up by the microphone which then beeped and also connected to a red light which went on simultaneously. The subjects were told that they would be rewarded if they kept the light on and the beeps going (in subject required to raise BP) or if they kept them off (in those who were to lower BP). In this way the process (SBP) was monitored and information on its level was 'fed back' to the subject, who was then rewarded for changing that process in the desired direction. In one training session, small but significant elevations and reductions in SBP were achieved. In 1971, similar techniques were used on hypertensive patients and of the seven patients trained in from 8 to 32 sessions, five had a significant reduction in SBP (16.1–33.8 mm Hg) with a mean fall of 16.5 mm Hg (164.9–148.4 mm Hg) for the group, including the two failures [85]. Kristt and Engel trained five hypertensive patients (three of whom were on pharmacologic therapy) to control their SBP [86]. Home BP was measured both before and after a three-week training period and was reduced 18/8 mm Hg. All patients who were taking antihypertensive drugs were able to reduce their dosages. Blanchard et al. used simple instrumentation in four patients with reductions in SBP of between 9 and 55 mm Hg, but only one patient had even as much as two weeks of follow-up [87]. Elder et al. [88] used DBP biofeedback in groups of four patients with and without 'semi-quantitative' verbal encouragement. The patients given feedback and encouragement had a greater fall in BP than those with biofeedback alone and both groups did better than controls. Goldman and colleagues [89] also showed that trained subjects had a greater reduction in BP than controls, but others [90] were unable to show the superiority of true biofeedback over 'sham' feedback. In this study, irrelevant feedback was given and no differences in BP response were seen.

Biofeedback has also been used to treat other abnormalities both cardio-vascular (rhythm disturbances and hypotension) and non-cardiovascular (Raynaud's syndrome, migraine and tension headaches, functional diarrhea, fecal incontinence, and neuromuscular abnormalities) with mixed but generally encouraging results [91, 92]. For HBP, however, all the studies reported are small, short-term, poorly controlled, if controlled at all, and the responses reported are generally unimpressive. Several authors [91, 92] have suggested that what beneficial results occur from biofeedback may not actually be a result of the technique but rather occur from biofeedback may not actually be a result of the technique but rather of some associated phenomena. Subjects, for example, may use the opportunity as a time to relax, and perhaps, the same hypometabolic state seen with TM or RR can be achieved. Kristt and Engel's study [86], however, showed that when BP went down, muscle tone, respiratory rate, and alpha waves did not, as would be expected if relaxation occurred. Schwartz has also shown that subjects can be taught to lower BP and *raise* heart rate which would not occur with relaxation [93].

The work of Patel and North [74], however, suggest that biofeedback of functions other than BP may be useful. They gave frontalis muscle tone biofeedback and felt this technique was additive to the relaxation exercise used. While BP biofeedback may be difficult to do and of minimal value, feedback of other indices of anxiety and tension might be additive with relaxation.

Biofeedback may help for other reasons as well. It provides the patient with a sense of control over his or her disease and makes the patient an active participant in his or her care. The ability to lower BP successfully by these means may be a positive achievement, but failure to do so may be devastating. Furthermore, the placebo effect of biofeedback or the effect of the enthusiasm of the clinician is unknown. Goldring [82] after all, had excellent results in many patients treating them with an 'electron gun' and a dedicated nurse. Benson's warning [66] that biofeedback may be detrimental to achieving relaxation since the patient had to 'concentrate' on something rather than trying to remain passive, is probably unwarranted.

Conclusion

BP biofeedback is not an important technique in treating HBP. The equipment is too expensive and cumbersome and the effect too small and probably too transient to warrant its widespread application. Perhaps biofeedback of other indices of anxiety such as reduced skin temperature or muscle tension may serve well to monitor a patient's success in achieving the relaxation response.

702

Other behavioral techniques

Shapiro et al. [94] and Frumkin and colleagues [95] have recently reviewed other non-pharmacologic behavioral methods to treat HBP. *Psychotherapy* successfully reduced BP in approximately one-half of the patients treated by Reiser and colleagues [96] but few other studies showing benefit have been done. Shapiro [97] showed that hospitalization, a form of *environmental modification,* can have a dramatic therapeutic effect (average fall of 25.4 mm Hg in mean BP) but most of those patients had extremely elevated baseline BP levels. He and others [80] confirmed the effect of hospitalization in a later study in patients whose initial BP's were lower. Other techniques such as hypnosis and autogenic training [78] are forms of relaxation and probably work by a similar mechanism. Perhaps, *home BP monitoring* could be viewed as another non-pharmacologic approach to treating HBP. Laughlin et al. [98] trained 60 patients to take their own BP twice a day at home. Patients were followed for a month and most patients had a reduction in their home BP within a few days. At the end of the follow-up period, 43% had reductions of 10 mm Hg or more in SBP and/or DBP and in 17 patients the dose of drugs were reduced. Clinic BP readings also fell significantly from 154.8/99.9 to 147.4/94.2 mm Hg.

5. CONCLUSIONS

Non-pharmacologic methods of treating hypertension are certainly safe and inexpensive but the efficacy and applicability of these treatments to general hypertensive population remains to be proven. Modest salt restriction can almost certainly be achieved, especially if we modify the eating habits of our children and younger adults. Avoiding obesity and getting adequate exercise should be recommended for all adults whether or not they have HBP. All of these methods are useful adjuncts to pharmacologic therapy but will not replace drugs for the majority of hypertensive patients. Behavioral methods of reducing BP are still new and untested but our early enthusiasm must be tempered by the fact that the results of the majority of these treatments have been disappointing. I think we must continue to look for ingenious ways to combine non-pharmacologic methods with drugs in order to achieve our goal of controlling HBP and its complications, and to do so with a minimum of risks to the patient.

1. The 1980 Report of the Joint National Committee on Detection, Evaluation, and Treatment of High Blood Pressure. Arch Intern Med 140:1280–1284, 1980.

2. Freis ED: Salt, volume and the prevention of hypertension. Circulation 53:589–595, 1976.
3. Ambard L, Beujard E: Causes l'hypertension arterielle. Arch Gen Med 193:520–533, 1904.
4. Allen FM, Sherrill JW: The treatment of arterial hypertension. J Metab Res 2:429, 1922.
5. Kempner W: Treatment of hypertensive vascular disease with rice diet. Am J Med 4:545–577, 1948.
6. Dole VP, Dahl LK, Cotzias GC, Eder HA, Krebs ME: Dietary treatment of hypertension. Clinical and metabolic studies of patients on the rice-fruit diet. J Clin Invest 29:1189–1206, 1950.
7. Grollman A, Harrison TR, Mason MF, Baxter J, Crampton J, Reichsman F: Sodium restriction in the diet for hypertension. JAMA 129(8):533–537, 1945.
8. Dustan HR, Tarazi RC, Bravo EL: Diuretic and diet treatment of hypertension. Arch Intern Med 133:1007–1013, 1974.
9. Parijs J, Joossens JV, Van der Linden L, Verstreken G, Amery AKPC: Moderate sodium restriction and diuretics in the treatment of hypertension. Am Heart J 85:22–34, 1973.
10. Morgan T, Gillies A, Morgan G, Adam W, Wilson M, Carney S: Hypertension treated by salt restriction. Lancet 1:227–230, 1978.
11. Heyden S, Nelius SJ, Hames CG: Obesity, salt intake, and hypertension. J Cardiovasc Med 11:987–994, 1980.
12. Hunt JC, Margie JD: The influence of diet on hypertension management. Hypertension Update 4:37–47, 1979.
13. Haddy FJ: Mechanism, prevention and therapy of sodium-dependent hypertension. Am J Med 69:746–758, 1980.
14. Addison W: The uses of sodium chloride, potassium chloride, sodium bromide and potassium bromide in cases of arterial hypertension which are amenable to potassium chloride. Can Med Assoc J 18(2):281–285, 1928.
15. McQuarrie I, Thompson WH, Anderson JA: Effects of excessive ingestion of sodium and potassium salts on carbohydrate metabolism and blood pressure in diabetic children. J Nutr 11:77–101, 1936.
16. Priddle WW: Observations on the management of hypertension. Can Med Assoc J 25:5–8, 1931.
17. Meneely GR, Battarbee HD: High sodium–low potassium environment and hypertension. Am J Cardiol 38:768–785, 1976.
18. Luft FC, Ranin LI, Weinberger MH: The role of potassium (K^+) in the responses to extremes of sodium (Na^+) intake in man. Clin Res 26(5):698A, 1978.
19. Oliver WJ, Cohen EL, Neel JV: Blood pressure, sodium intake and sodium relted hormones in the Yanomamo Indians, a 'no-salt' culture. Circulation 52(1):146–152, 1975.
20. Longworth DL, Drayer JIM, Weber MA, Laragh JH: Divergent blood pressure responses during short-term sodium restriction in hypertension. Clin Pharmacol Ther 27:544–546, 1980.
21. Society of Actuaries and Association of Life Insurance Medical Directors of America: Build Study 1979. Recording & Statistical Corp., USA, March 1980.
22. Society of Actuaries: Build and Blood Pressure Study, 1959, Vols 1 and 2, Chicago, 1959.
23. Stamler J: Research related to risk factors. Circulation 60:1575–1586, 1979.
24. Rabkin SW, Mathewson FAL, Hse PH: Relation of body weight to development of ischemic heart disease in a cohort of young North American men after a 26 year observation period: the Manitoba Study. Am J Cardiol 39:452–458, 1977.
25. Messerli FH, Christie B, DeCarvalho JGR, Aristimuno GG, Suarez DH, Dreslinski GR, Frohlich ED: Obesity and essential hypertension: Hemodynamics, intravascular volume, sodium excretion, and plasma renin activity. Arch Intern Med 141:81–85, 1981.

26. Keys A, Aravanis G, Blackburn H, Van Buchen FSP, Buzino R, Djordjevic BS, Fidanza F, Karvonin JM, Menotti A, Pudda V, Taylor HL: Coronary heart disease: Overweight and obesity as risk factors. Ann Intern med 77:15–27, 1972.
27. Weinsier RL, Fuchs RJ, Kay TD, Triebwasser JH, Lancaster MC: Body fat: its relationship to coronary heart disease, blood pressure, lipids and other risk factors measured in a large male population. Am J Med 61:815–824, 1976.
28. Kannel WB, Brand N, Skinner JJ, Dawber TR, McNamara P: The relation of adiposity to blood pressure and development of hypertension. The Framingham Study. Ann Intern Med 67:48–59, 1967.
29. Voors AW, Foster TA, Frerichs RR, Webber LS, Berenson GS: Studies of blood pressures in children, ages 5–14 years, in a total biracial community: the Bogalusa Heart Study. Circulation 54:319–327, 1976.
30. Rames LK, Clarke WR, Conner WE, Reiter MA, Lauer RM: Normal blood pressures and the evaluation of sustained blood pressure elevation in childhood: the Muscatine Study. Pediatrics 61:245–251, 1978.
31. Harlan WR, Cornoni-Huntley J, Leaverton PE: Blood pressure in childhood. The national health examination survey. Hypertension 1:559–565, 1979.
32. Munoz S, Munoz H, Zambrano LF: Blood pressure in a school-age population. Distribution, correlations, and prevalence of elevated values. Mayo Clin Proc 55:623–632, 1980.
33. Chiang BN, Perlman LV, Epstein FH: Overweight and hypertension. A review. Circulation 39:403–421, 1969.
34. Mann GV: The influence of obesity on health. N Engl J Med 291:178–232, 1974.
35. Reisin E, Abel R, Modan M, Silverberg DS, Eliahou HE, Modan B: Effect of weight loss without salt restriction on the reduction of blood pressure in overweight hypertensive patients. N Engl J Med 298:1–6, 1978.
36. Dahl LK, Silver L, Christie RW: Role of salt in the fall of blood pressure accompanying reduction of obesity. N Engl J Med 258:1186–1192, 1958.
37. Stamler J, Farinaro E, Mojonnier LM, Hall Y, Moss D, Stamler R: Prevention and control of hypertension by nutritional-hygienic means. JAMA 243:1819–1823, 1980.
38. Stunkard A, McLaulin-Hume M: The results of the treatment for obesity. Arch Intern Med 103:79–85, 1959.
39. Currey H, Malcolm R, Riddle E, Schachte M: Behavioral treatment of obesity. Limitations and results with the chronically obese. JAMA 237:2829–2831, 1977.
40. Dawber TR: Risk factors in young adults: The lessons from epidemiologic studies of cardiovascular disease: Framingham, Tecumseh, and Evans County. J Am Coll Health Assoc 22:84–95, 1973.
41. Fox S, Skinner J: Physical activity and cardiovascular health. Am J Cardiol 14:731–746, 1964.
42. Morris Jn, Chave SPW, Adam C, Sirey C, Epstein L, Sheehan DJ: Vigorous exercise in leisure-time and the incidence of coronary heart disease. Lancet 1:333–339, 1973.
43. Paffenbarger RS, Hale WE: Work activity and coronary heart mortality. N Engl J Med 292:545–550, 1975.
44. Montoye HJ, Metzner HL, Keller JB, Johnson BC, Epstein FH: Habitual physical activity and blood pressure. Med Sci Sports 4:175–181, 1972.
45. Cooper KH, Pollack ML, Martin RP, White SR, Linnerud AC, Jackson A: Physical fitness levels vs selected coronary risk factors. A cross-sectional study. JAMA 236:166–169, 1976.
46. Scheuer J, Tipton CM: Cardiovascular adaptations to physical training. Ann Rev Physiol 39:221–251, 1977.
47. Tipton CM, Matthes RD, Callahan A, Tcheng TK, Lais LT: The role of chronic exercise on resting blood pressures of normotensive and hypertensive rats. Med Sci Sports 9:168–177, 1977.

48. Evenwel R, Struyker-Boudier H: Effect of physical training on the development of hypertension in the spontaneously hypertensive rat. Pfluegers Arch 381:19–24, 1979.
49. Weiss L: Adaptive cardiovascular changes to physical training in spontaneously hypertensive and normotensive rats. Cardiovasc Res 12:329–333, 1978.
50. Boyer JL, Kasch FW: Exercise therapy in hypertensive men. JAMA 211:1668–1671, 1970.
51. Choquette G, Ferguson RJ: Blood pressure reduction in 'borderline' hypertensives following physical training. Can Med assoc J 108:699–703, 1973.
52. Wilmore JH, Royce J, Girandola RN, Katch FI, Katch VL: Physiological alterations resulting from a 10-week program of jogging. Med Sci Sports 2:7–14, 1970.
53. Frick MH, Konttinen A, Sarajas HSS: Effects of physical training on circulation at rest and during exercise. Am J Cardiol 12:142–147, 1963.
54. Barry AJ, Daly JW, Pruett EDR, Steinmetz JR, Page HF, Birkhead NC, Rodahl K: The effects of physical conditioning on older individuals – I. Work capacity, circulatory-respiratory function, and work electocardiogram. J Gerontol 21:182–191, 1966.
55. Konig K: Changes in physical capacity, heart size and function in patients after myocardial infarction, who underwent a 4- to 6-week physical training program. Cardiology 62:232–246, 1977.
56. Haskell WL: Cardiovascular complications during exercise training of cardiac patients. Circulation 57:920–924, 1978.
57. Gibbons LW, Cooper KH, Meyer BM, Ellison C: The acute cardiac risk of strenuous exercise. JAMA 244:1799–1801, 1980.
58. Reid EL, Morgan RW: Exercise prescription: A clinical trial. Am J Public Health 69:591–595, 1979.
59. Henry JP, Cassel JC: Psychosocial factors in essential hypertension. Recent epidemiologic and animal experimental evidence. Am J Epidemiol 90:171–200, 1969.
60. Buell JC, Eliot RS: The role of emotional stress in the development of heart disease. JAMA 242:365–368, 1979.
61. Jenkins CD: Recent evidence supporting psychologic and social risk factors for coronary disease. N Engl J Med 294:987–994 1nd 1033–1038, 1976.
62. Shekelle RB: Psychosocial factors and high blood pressure. Cardiovasc Med 12:1249 1253, 1979.
63. Jacobson E: Variation of blood pressure with skeletal muscle tension and relaxation. Ann Intern Med 12:1194–1212, 1939.
64. Benson H: Systemic hypertension and the relaxation response. N Engl J Med 296:1152–1156, 1977.
65. Wallace RK, Benson H, Wilson AF: A wakeful hypometabolic physiologic state. Am J Physiol 221:795–799, 1971.
66. Benson H, Rosner BA, Marzetta BR, Klemschuk HP: Decreased blood pressure in borderline hypertensive subjects who practiced meditation. J Chron Dis 27:163–169, 1974.
67. Banson H, Marzetta BR, Rosner BA, Klemschuk HM: Decreased blood pressure in pharmacologically treated hypertensive patients who regularly elicited the relaxation response. Lancet 1:289–291, 1974.
68. Blackwell B, Bloomfield S, Gartside P, Robinson A, Hanenson I, Magenheim H, Nidich S, Zigler R: Transcendental meditation in hypertension. Lancet 1:223–226, 1976.
69. Stone RA, DeLeo J: Psychotherapeutic control of hypertension. N Engl J Med 294:80–84, 1976.
70. Datey KK, Deshmukh SN, Dalvi CP, Vinekar SL: 'Shavasan': A yogic exercise in the management of hypertension. Angiology 20:325–333, 1969.
71. Taylor CB, Farquhar JW, Nelson E, Agras S: Relaxation therapy and high blood pressure, Arch Gen Psychiatry 34:339–342, 1977.

72. Pollack AA, Case DB, Weber MA, Laragh JH: Limitations of transcendental meditation inthe treatment of essential hypertension. Lancet 1:71–73, 1977.
73. Deabler HL, Fidel E, Dillenkoffer RL, Elder ST: The use of relaxation and hypnosis in lowering high blood pressure. Am J Clin Hypn 16:75–83, 1973.
74. Patel C, North WRS: Randomised controlled trial of yoga and biofeedback in management .of hypertension. Lancet 1:93–95, 1975.
75. Patel C: Yoga and biofeedback in the management of 'stress' in hypertensive patients. Clin Sci Mol Med 48:171s–174s, 1975.
76. Shoemaker JE, Tasto DL: The effects of muscle relaxation on blood pressure of essential hypertensives. Behav Res Ther 13:29–43, 1975.
77. Frankel BL, Patel DJ, Horwitz D, Friedewald WT, Gaarder KR: Treatment of hypertension with biofeedback and relaxation techniques. Psychosom Med 40:276–293, 1978.
78. Luthe W: Autogenic Therapy. New York: Grune & Stratton, 1969.
79. Roberts BW, Forester WE: Group relaxation–acute and chronic effects on essential hypertension. Cardiovasc Med 5:575–580, 1979.
80. Moutsos SE, Sapira JD, Scheib ET, Shapiro AP: An analysis of the placebo effect in hospitalized hypertensive patients. Clin Pharmacol Ther 8:676–683, 1967.
81. Ayman D: An evaluation of therapeutic results in essential hypertension – I. The interpretation of symptomatic relief. JAMA 95:246–249, 1930.
82. Goldring W, Chasis H, Schreiner GE, Smith HW: Reassurance in the management of benign hypertensive disease. Circulation 14:260–264, 1956.
83. Schwartz GE, Shapiro AP, Redmond DP, Ferguson DCE, Ragland DR, Weiss SM: Behavioral medicine approaches to hypertension: An integrative analysis of theory and research. J Behav Med 2:311–363, 1979.
84. Shapiro D, Tursky B, Gershon E, Stern M: Effects of feedback and reinforcement on the control of human systolic blood pressure. Science 163:588–590, 1969.
85. Benson H, Shapiro D, Tursky B, Schwartz GE: Decreased systolic blood pressure through operant conditioning techniques in patients with essential hypertension. Science 173:740–742, 1971.
86. Kristt DA, Engel BT: Learned control of blood pressure in patients with high blood pressure. Circulation 15:370–378, 1975.
87. Blanchard EB, Young LD, Haynes MR: Technique innovations. A simple feedback system for the treatment of elevated blood pressure. Behavior Ther 6:241–245, 1975.
88. Elder ST, Ruiz RZ, Deabler HL, Dillenkoffer RL: Instrumental conditioning of diastolic blood pressure in essential hypertensive patients. J Appl Behav Anal 6:377–382, 1973.
89. Goldman H, Kleinman KM, Snow MY, Bidus DR, Korol B: Relationship between essential hypertension and cognitive functioning: Effects of biofeedback. Psychophysiology 12:569–573, 1975.
90. Frankel BL, Patel D, Horwitz D, Friedwald WT, Gaarder KR: Clinical ineffectiveness of a combination of psychophysiologic therapies. Psychosom Med 39:51–52, 1977.
91. Weiss T: Biofeedback training for cardiovascular dysfunctions. Med Clin North Am 61:913–928, 1977.
92. Orne MT: The efficacy of biofeedback therapy. Ann Rev Med 30:489–503, 1979.
93. Schwartz GE: Voluntary control of human cardiovascular integration and differentiation through feedback and reward. Science 175: 90–93, 1972.
94. Shapiro AP, Schwartz GE, Ferguson DCE, Redmond DP, Weiss SM: Behavioral methods in the treatment of hypertension. A review of their clinical status. Ann Intern Med 86:626–636, 1977.
95. Frumkin K, Nathan RJ, Prout MF, Cohen MC: Nonpharmacologic control of essential hypertension in man: A critical review of the experimental literature. Psychosom Med 40:294–320, 1978.

96. Reiser MF, Brust AA, Ferris EB, Shapiro AP, Harrison MB, Ransohoff W: Life situations, emotions, and the course of patients with arterial hypertension. Psychosom Med 13:133–319, 1951.
97. Shapiro AP: Consideration of multiple variables in evaluation of hypotensive drugs. JAMA 160:30–39, 1956.
98. Laughlin KD, Fisher L, Sherrard DJ: Blood pressure reductions during self-recording of home blood pressure. Am Heart J 98:629–634, 1979.

45. DIURETICS AS ANTIHYPERTENSIVE AGENTS

Franz H. Messerli and Edward D. Frohlich

Diuretics are pharmacological agents that contract the extracellular fluid volume by increasing renal sodium and water excretion. Hence, the terms saluresis and natriuresis have been used to describe more precisely their specific action. They are often considered as the first step therapy used for the management of the hypertensive diseases. Three main classes of diuretic agents, each differing in its site of action, are currently available for clinical use: thiazides and similarly acting congeners; high-ceiling or 'loop' diuretics (Table 1); and potassium-sparing agents. Each of these drugs can significantly reduce arterial pressure in over two-thirds of patients with hypertensiion. Moreover, it is possible to manage over 50 % of patients with mild essential hypertension with a diuretic alone and as many as 75 % when therapy is supplemented by a prudent sodium-restricted diet [1]. These compounds are, in general, safe, relatively inexpensive, and produce minimal side effects.

MECHANISMS OF DIURESIS

Proximal convoluted tubule

As much as 70 % of the filtered load of sodium and water is reabsorbed in the proximal tubule. Apparently, this process is related to the glomerular

Table 1. Differences between loop diuretics and thiazides

Loop diuretics		Thiazide congeners
+ + +	natriuresis	+
+	antihypertensive effect	+ +
+	potassium loss	+ +
↑	calcium clearance	↓
↓	urine concentration	—
↓	urine dilution	↓↓
↑ or −	renal blood flow	↓
+ +	effective in renal failure	—

Amery, A. (ed.) Hypertensive Cardiovascular Disease: Pathophysiology and Treatment
© *1982, Martinus Nijhoff Publishers. The Hague / Boston / London*
ISBN-13: 978-94-009-7478-4

filtration rate as well as to the state of expansion or depletion of the extracellular fluid volume compartment [2, 3]. Although volume expansion will reduce proximal tubular sodium reabsorption, and contraction of extracellular fluid volume will increase proximal tubular salt and water reabsorption [2, 4, 5], the precise mechanisms involved are not known completely, but perhaps involve changes in peritubular forces. Thus, chronic volume depletion, such as achieved with long-standing diuretic therapy, will in turn promote adaptive mechanisms that serve to increase salt and water reabsorption, thereby limiting the natriuretic effect. Most of the commonly used diuretics have little effect on the proximal tubule. However, the thiazide diuretics (as well as the 'loop' agents) act as mild carbonic anhydrase inhibitors, and therefore serve to reduce reabsorption of sodium, bicarbonate, chloride, and water at the level of the proximal convoluted tubule. Recently it has been shown that the fractional chloride reabsorption was decreased by chlorothiazide to about the same extent as with the carbonic anhydrase inhibitor *benzolamide* [6]. Since the thiazide diuretics' carbonic anhydrase-inhibiting action and their volume-depleting effect antagonize each other at the proximal tubule, the overall influence in a given patient will depend on the fluid volume state.

Loop of Henle

The ascending limb of the loop of Henle is responsible for the reabsorption of approximately 20 % of the filtered sodium load and the remaining 10 % is absorbed by the distal tubule and collective ducts [7]. These sodium-and-water conservation mechanisms are highly efficient at the loop of Henle, involving a countercurrent system that provides the major means for concentrating the urine. Since the loop diuretics inhibit salt reabsorption in the ascending limb of Henle's loop, they interfere with the medullar countercurrent system, thereby impeding urinary concentration mechanisms. The mechanism whereby the high-ceiling diuretics act (furosemide and ethacrynic acid) involves the inhibition of the active chloride ion transport at the ascending limb of Henle's loop [8, 9]. Thus, by actively inhibiting chloride reabsorption they are also responsible for the concomitant reabsorption of the sodium ion as well as other major cations.

Cortical diluting segment and distal convoluted tubule

Although less than 10 % of the filtered salt and water load is conserved at this level (and by the collecting ducts), it is a key site for active sodium and water transport and conservation. The more proximal area of the distal tubule is impermeable to the passage of water, but it is a potent site for active sodium reabsorption and urinary dilution. At a more distal tubular level (and in the cortical collecting duct) sodium, potassium, and hydrogen ion excretion is controlled by aldosterone-mediated active exchange mechanisms [10, 11]. Other mechanisms influencing active sodium transport at the distal tubular level implicate the interactions of the kinin-kallikrein, aldosterone, and possibly other systems [12].

The thiazide diuretics act between the ascending limb of the loop of Henle and the more distal tubule in the cortical diluting segment [13]. Accordingly, the more proximal urinary concentration mechanisms are not affected by these drugs; however, they commonly impair urinary dilutional ability by decreasing free-water clearance [14]. This mechanism has been exploited therapeutically with some success in patients with renal diabetes insipidus. However, with diuretic-induced impairment of free-water clearance, hyponatremia may be produced, and in susceptible patients this may even lead to water intoxication [15]. Indeed, one patient with psychogenic polydipsia and hyponatremia died after thiazide ingestion [16].

The distal convoluted tubule is still another site of action for the thiazide diuretics where they predominantly inhibit sodium and chloride reabsorption [6]. The effect of the thiazide diuretics and their congeners on distal tubular sodium and chloride reabsorption may be clinically most important and also account for their action in the 'cortical diluting segment' [14]. The potassium-sparing agents, i.e., spironolactone, triamterene, and amiloride, also exert their principal actions at the distal tubular level. These latter compounds decrease urinary potassium and hydrogen ion excretions while increasing fractional sodium excretion by only about 2% [17]. Amiloride and probably triamterene act independently of aldosterone and seem to decrease luminal sodium permeability and reverse negative transtubular electrical potential, resulting in a fall in potassium reabsorption [18]. Part of this mechanism may be mediated by amiloride's direct interaction with the kallikrein system [19]. Amiloride seems to account for a greater natriuresis and antihypertensive effect than triamterene. In contrast to triamterene and amiloride, spironolactone competitively binds with aldosterone receptors in the distal tubule to inhibit aldosterone's action and promote natriuresis and potassium conservation. Its potency as a diuretic and antihypertensive agent is probably intermediate between triamterene and amiloride and is most useful in primary and secondary states with mineralocorticoid excess. Conversely, spironolactone will be ineffective in the absence of aldosterone.

ANTIHYPERTENSIVE ACTIONS

Figure 1 schematizes the antihypertensive actions following diuretic therapy.

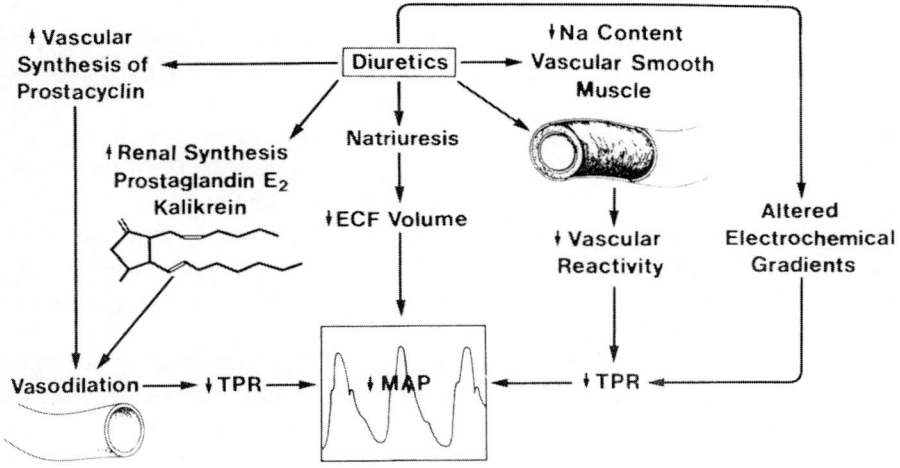

Figure 1. Possible mechanisms by which diuretics lower arterial pressure.

Hemodynamics

By their prompt natriuretic effect, diuretics contract plasma and extracellular fluid volumes [20, 21]. As a result, cardiac output initially falls [22, 23] and this effect can be totally prevented by ureterocaval shunting of urine into the intravascular compartment or by dextran-induced volume expansion [23–26]. Within a brief time, arterial pressure also falls and this pressure reduction is associated with a continued reduction in cardiac output and an unchanged (or even slightly increased) total peripheral resistance [20, 22, 23, 25–29]. At this time the attenuation of the infused pressor stimuli and potentiation of depressor stimuli may be entirely reversed by infusion of salt-free dextran [21, 24]. However, even in the absence of volume contraction or a direct hemodynamic effect, the thiazides will attenuate pressor and accentuate depressor phenomena [30, 31].

With continuing diuretic therapy the reduced plasma volume and cardiac output, observed initially, tends to return to pretreatment levels [20, 27], although even with prolonged diuretic therapy for two years or more some reports have indicated that plasma volume remains contracted and plasma renin activity is increased [29, 32, 33]. Following discontinuation of the diuretic the plasma volume rebounds within one week to greater than pretreatment levels; and this reexpansion of plasma and extracellular fluid volume is associated with a reduction of plasma renin activity to pretreatment levels [33]. In a comparison of patients who responded to thiazide therapy with a significant arterial pressure fall with patients who failed to demonstrate as great a fall in pressure, the significant hypotension was associated with a persistent fall in total peripheral resistance [29, 34]. Hence, the long-term antihypertensive effect of the thiazides (and probably the other diuretics) seems to be mediated hemodynamically by reduced total peripheral resistance.

The question may be raised as to the precise mechanism(s) explaining the reduction in vascular resistance induced by the diuretics in patients with hypertension. The following hypotheses have been reported:

(a) From the earliest studies it was suggested that because of the possibility of excess sodium and water in the blood vessel wall in hypertension [35], diuretics may reduce vascular resistance passively by diminishing this excess sodium and 'waterlogging' effect [36, 37].

(b) The vasoconstrictor and vasodepressor effects of circulating naturally occurring vasoactive agents may be blunted and potentiated, respectively, by diuretic therapy [22, 24]. Indeed, this is most likely since it explains the augmented effect of diuretics when they are used with other antihypertensive drugs.

(c) Responsiveness of the vascular smooth muscle to neural stimuli may be altered [38].

(d) Vascular smooth muscle tone may be reduced by altered transmembrane ionic gradients [39].

(e) More recently, some investigators have suggested an active indirect action whereby the thiazide may stimulate production of naturally occurring vasodilating prostacyclin in vascular walls [40] or the kallikrein system [41].

(f) A direct vasodilating effect of the diuretics on arterioles has been suggested, but these assertions have never been adequately demonstrated. Arguments have been offered concerning a direct vasodilating effect of the thiazides by citing the immediate arteriolar (but not venular) dilation and hypotension induced by the nondiuretic thiazide congener diazoxide [42, 43]. A few studies have shown variable effects on vascular resistance with the loop-acting diuretics [44–46].

It might therefore be concluded that diuretics lower arterial pressure immediately by decreasing plasma and extracellular fluid volumes. This volume contraction is associated with a fall in cardiac output and a rise in plasma renin activity. With time these volumes tend to reexpand, although the extracellular fluid volume seems to remain significantly reduced while elevated plasma renin activity persists. The long-term hypotensive action is associated with a reduced total peripheral resistance that may be explained, in part, by: altered vascular responsiveness to vasoactive agents; possible reversal in vascular 'waterlogging'; active vasodilation mediated either directly or by induced, naturally occurring vasodilators (e.g., prostacyclin); by altered responsiveness to neural stimuli; or by a modified transmembrane ionic gradient of vascular smooth muscle.

To what degree is arterial pressure lowered by diuretics? Recent studies have shown that when used alone the thiazides achieve a decrease in arterial pressure varying from 9/8 to 19/13 mm Hg (average 15/10 mm Hg) [47]. It has been estimated that perhaps over 50% of patients with hypertension may be treated with a diuretic alone and that the addition of a sodium-restricted diet (100 mEq/day or less) will control arterial pressure in upwards of 75% of patients with mild hypertension [1]. It is not known with any great degree of certainty whether this antihypertensive effect differed from one diuretic to another. Several studies have shown that the thiazides are more effective in reducing arterial pressure in a patient with uncomplicated essential hypertension with normal renal function than are the loop diuretics [48–51]. However, the hypotensive action with the thiazides does not follow a linear dose–response relationship. Thus, after taking, e.g.'s 100–150 mg hydrochlororthiazide per day, further dose increases will not reduce pressure any further. In contrast, as long as some renal function persists in a patient with parenchymal renal disease and volume-dependent hypertension, increasing the dose of furosemide will eventually produce some diuresis and an antihypertensive action [52]. The potassium-retaining agents, spironolactone and triamterene, have less antihypertensive effects than the thiazide diuretics [53–57], although a recent multicenter study with amiloride seemed to suggest that this agent may be of equivalent potency with hydrochlorothiazide in patients with mild, uncomplicated essential hypertension [58].

Renal hemodynamics

Renal blood flow and glomerular rate usually are somewhat diminished during treatment with thiazide diuretics [59]. This may be related to the contraction in intravascular volume; however, low doses of furosemide have been shown to increase renal blood flow and glomerular filtration rate [59, 60]. Whether this is a drug-related phenomenon or related to changes in cardiac output is not known. Nevertheless, this effect has been used to increase urine flow (and possibly renal perfusion) in patients with oliguric renal failure with or without hypertension. However, with prolonged diuretic therapy, volume depletion in these patients may override the increased renal blood flow, and renal perfusion and GFR may return to or below pretreatment levels [61]. Moreover, since intravascular volume tends to return to pretreatment levels, this mechanism does not entirely explain the persistent slight reduction in glomerular filtration rate that is associated with prolonged diuretic therapy. The recent studies of Wright and Schnermann indicate that the decrease in GFR may, at least to some extent, be mediated by an intrarenal feedback mechanism by which distal tubular

714

solute load directly influences filtration rate [62, 63]. These decreases in renal blood flow and glomerular filtration rate are associated with mild persistent, but significant, increases in the concentrations in blood urea nitrogen and serum creatinine despite return of plasma volume and cardiac output to pretreatment levels (see also Table 1) [29].

Renin–angiotensin–aldosterone system

All diuretics increase circulating plasma renin activity, plasma angiotensin II, and serum aldosterone levels in patients with or without hypertension. These effects are most likely mediated through several mechanisms: contraction of plasma and extracellular fluid volumes; sympathetic nervous stimulation of the kidney in response to the contracted volume and fall in arterial pressure (renal baroreceptors); reduction in intrarenal perfusion pressure; increased levels of sodium (or chloride) concentration at the macula densa; and probably other effects [64, 65]. An early rise in renin secretion can be observed within five minutes following intravenous furosemide [66]. This rise in plasma renin activity will occur despite ureterovenous anastomosis or other maneuvers to prevent volume contraction, thereby excluding salt and water loss or volume contraction and reduced renal perfusion pressure as the sole mechanism(s) [66–70]. Conceivably, at least

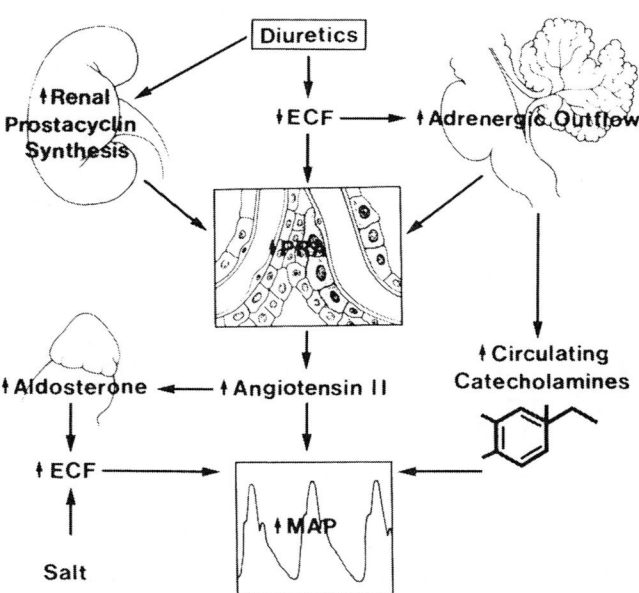

Figure 2. Effects of diuretics on endocrine factors.

one stimulus for renin release is mediated by the number or concentration of sodium and/or chloride ions that reach the cells of the macula densa [71]. This effect may be more pronounced with the loop diuretics and they could deliver a higher distal tubular load than the thiazide congeners [66]. A late renin secretion takes place 1–2 h after the intravenous administration of a diuretic, regardless of its chemical structure [66]. The later rise in renin secretion can also be prevented by beta-adrenergic receptor blockade and ureterovenous anastomosis; beta-blockers and anastomosis cannot prevent the earlier rise [66]. Hence, it appears that the early renin hypersecretion is caused by a direct renal mechanism involving the increased sodium and chloride concentration at the luminal site of the macula densa.

Catecholamines

Lake and collaborators recently have shown that the initial increased vascular resistance that is found with diuretic treatment is associated with increased plasma norepinephrine levels [72]. Even after prolonged treatment plasma norepinephrine levels remain elevated suggesting that the fall in vascular resistance was not achieved solely by a decreased sympathetic nervous activity. Plasma norepinephrine levels were higher in both supine and standing positions after 9 and 47 days of treatment, whereas dopamine β-hydroxylase was not affected. Conceivably, enhanced sympathetic activity counteracts the antihypertensive effect of the diuretics. Hence, this study provides rationale for concurrent use of diuretics with agents that diminish sympathetic outflow or interfere with the effects of circulating catecholamines.

Prostaglandins and kinins

Several observations suggest that renal prostaglandins are partially involved in mediation of the saluretic effect of diuretics. First, concomitant use of an inhibitor of prostaglandin synthetase, indomethacin, attenuates the natriuresis, the increase in plasma renin activity produced by loop diuretics [73–75] and other natriuretic agents [76].

Renal vasodilator kallikrein increases following furosemide [77, 78]. Other studies have indicated that urinary kallikrein excretion may be regulated by mineralocorticoids [78, 79] and that the increased urinary secretion of prostaglandin and kallikrein observed following furosemide may be mediated by the renin–angiotensin–aldosterone system [79, 80]. However, the increase in urinary kallikrein-kinin and prostaglandin E after furosemide has correlated closely with its diuretic and natriuretic effects [78]. This work suggested that the diuretic directly facilitated the renal generation of kallikrein and prostaglandin E. However, since no correlation was found between plasma renin activity and urinary prostaglandin E or kallikrein excretion, the investigators concluded that the renin–angiotensin–aldosterone system did not participate directly in mediating the increased prostaglandin E and kallikrein [78].

A novel diuretic agent (MK 447) has recently been found that seems to stimulate prostaglandin E2 synthesis [81]. This drug lowered arterial pressure in spontaneously hypertensive rats at lower doses than those required for diuresis, and both diuretic and antihypertensive effects were antagonized by indomethacine [81]. These observations suggest that at least some diuretics may induce diuresis and lower arterial pressure by increasing renal synthesis of prostaglandins. Moreover, Webster et al. have shown that bendroflumethizide significantly increased plasma levels of 6-Oxo PGF_2d after 3 days and 10 weeks of treatment [40]. The chemical hydrolysis product of prostacyclin is 6-Oxo PGF_2d, a potent vasodilator that may be produced in vascular smooth muscle. Hence, thiazides may reduce vascular resistance by increasing local prostacyclin synthesis.

OTHER METABOLIC EFFECTS OF DIURETICS

A number of metabolic effects are associated with the natriuretic, hypovolemic and hypotensive responses to diuretic therapy. These include changes in electrolyte concentrations such as hypokalemia, metabolic alkalosis, hyponatremia, and altered carbohydrate, uric acid and lipid metabolism.

Hypokalemia

Distal tubular potassium secretion predominantly depends on the volume and rate of urine flow in the distal tubule [82]. Since most diuretics increase the volume load to the distal tubule, more potassium will be available for exchange with sodium and more will be wasted. In addition, all of the factors that are stimulated to facilitate the release of renin from the juxtaglomerular cells serve to increase the circulating levels of angiotensin II, thereby stimulating the secretion of aldosterone from the adrenal cortex. This state of secondary hyperaldosteronism will promote sodium absorption and potassium secretion by the distal convoluted tubule. Furthermore, this resulting metabolic alkalosis also stimulates distal tubular potassium secretion. The loop diuretics furosemide and ethacrynic acid also inhibit potassium reabsorption at the loop of Henle [83, 84]. Consequently, distal tubular potassium load will be higher and a potassium waste could occur by this mechanism too.

However, this diuretic-induced potassium loss is usually self-limited. Since diuretics lead to a significant extracellular volume contraction, proximal tubular reabsorption of sodium and chloride will increase as the distal tubular flow falls. Further, the induced hypokalemia will, in turn, decrease the aldosterone secretion from the adrenal cortex. Hence, both factors, hypokalemia and volume contraction, will limit the long-term wastage of urinary potassium and permit the establishment of a new level of potassium balance.

From a clinical point of view, it must be borne in mind that during diuretic treatment distal tubular potassium excretion importantly depends on distal tubular sodium load [85]. This relationship has two major clinical considerations: 1) high sodium intake will also serve to reexpand extracellular fluid volume to override the antihypertensive effect of the diuretic. Thus, not only will a low sodium diet augment the antihypertensive effectiveness of the diuretic, but it will also decrease the amount of sodium available at the distal tubular level to minimize potassium wastage. This important physiological consideration is the rationale for educating a patient to follow a sodium-restricted diet during antihypertensive treatment, and in particular with diuretic therapy.

Although serum potassium falls in all patients who are treated with diuretics, the clinical implications of the induced hypokalemia remain unclear. Thus, it has been estimated that between 20 and 50% of patients treated with conventional diuretics will develop hypokalemia as defined by a serum potassium concentration of lower than 3.5 mEq/l [86–90]. The serum potassium concentration starts to fall within a few hours of the first dose of chlorothiazide or furosemide [91, 92] and the maximal fall is said to occur by the end of the first week of treatment [93]; the dose of the diuretic given does not seem to make a marked difference [93]. In other words, it has been reported that whether daily doses of 50, 100 or 200 mg hydrochlorothiazide are given there will be a similar fall in serum potassium concentration during long-term treatment [93]. Thiazide diuretics in general seem to produce a significantly greater loss in potassium than furosemide [93, 94]. Morgan and Davidson compared published data on different diuretics and found that chlorthalidone and hydrochlorothiazide produced a mean fall in serum concentration of 0.62 mEq/100 ml, whereas furosemide and cyclopanthiazide resulted only in a fall of 0.30 and 0.31 mEq, respectively [93].

When evaluating possible effects of potassium loss, it must be remembered that the serum potassium concentration, which accounts for less than 1% of total body potassium, does not usually reflect the total body store of potassium. Moreover, a patient may experience a fall in serum potassium concentration without having significant loss of total body potassium stores. Although most patients with essential hypertension show a fall in serum potassium concentration with diuretic treatment, total body potassium apparently does not change significantly [95, 96]. Wilkinson reported a fall of total body potassium by 3% after one year of bendrofluazide therapy, whereas serum potassium dropped from a mean value of 4.26 to 3.86 mEq (p<0.02) [96].

The question may appropriately be posed as to just what the clinical consequences are of a diuretic-induced hypokalemia. Davidson and Surawicz found that serum potassium levels between 3 and 3.5 mEq/dl did not increase the prevalence of ectopic beats or atrioventricular conduction disturbances [97]. More recently, however, Steiness and Olesen found that patients receiving maintenance digoxin therapy whose serum potassium fell into the range of 3-3.5 mEq/dl did experience cardiac arrhythmias [98]. However, most authorities would agree that serum potassium concentrations that are less than 3.0 mEq/dl may be potentially harmful to the patient, but even at these low levels most patients will not experience any symptoms of hypokalemia. When symptoms do occur they include polyuria, muscle weakness, and possible enhancement of signs of digitalis toxicity. Severe hypokalemia, as produced experimentally, has been associated with renal structural changes (e.g., vacuolization of tubular epithelium, interstitial nephritis) [99]. The cardiac effects have ranged from well-known electrocardiographic changes of rhythm and conduction to myocardial necrosis [100]. Potassium-deficient skeletal muscle may develop rhabdomyolysis during periods of intensive exercise [101], a problem which is of potential importance to joggers and individuals who exercise heavily, as exercise per se may lead to volume depletion, activation of the renin–angiotensin–aldosterone system and subsequent potassium deficiency. Nevertheless, in most instances, diuretic-induced hypokalemia is most often benign, self-limited, and of little practical clinical consequence. To a certain degree, potassium-rich foods together with a low-sodium diet may also help to prevent potassium loss; however, most of these foods are high in calories, which makes them undesirable in patients with hypertension. In our experience, most patients' hypokalemia can be managed primarily by sodium restriction and also with potassium-rich foods.

A useful maneuver to validate problems of electrolyte homeostasis is the determination of 24-h urine excretion of sodium and potassium concentrations. However, if the patient has unexplained consistently low serum potassium levels (with or without diuretic therapy), a review of the entire problem (and reassessment of the initial diagnosis) may be helpful. The patient may have primary aldosteronism, other adrenal cortical hormonal excess, or hyperreninemia from other causes (renal artery stenosis, renin-producing tumor). A common exogenous cause of hypokalemia is laxative abuse or chronic diarrhea and vomiting. There may be a history of ingesting substances that have mineralocorticoid activity, e.g., licorice, anabolic steroids, nonsteroidal anti-inflammatory drugs [102]. Even tobacco chewing has been identified as a cause of pseudomineralocorticoidism [103]. Further, administration of insulin and glucose infusion may provoke hypokalemia. Other diseases with mineralocorticoid excess such as Cushing's, Bartter's or Liddle's syndromes are commonly accompanied by low potassium values.

After having excluded these causes of hypokalemia in the few patients who are potassium-wasters, the deficiency should be corrected. Since a chloride-responsive metabolic alkalosis coexists with diuretic-induced potassium deficiency, the potassium supplements are best prescribed as the chloride salt [104]. Thus, potassium citrate or other salts will not correct the hypochloremic alkalosis, and, a result, the intracellular potassium deficiency. Perhaps the simplest and most inexpensive means for correcting potassium deficiency with supplements is with potassium chloride-containing commercial salt substitutes [105]. They are considerably less expensive and most often better tolerated than commercially available potassium supplements [105]. In the few patients with persistent hypokalemia, a potassium-sparing agent needs to be prescribed in conjunction with the thiazide diuretics without need for other potassium supplements. Liquid potassium chloride is better absorbed and less irritating to the gastrointestinal tract than tablets or slow-release preparations. However, they are unpalatable for most patients and produce nausea and vomiting. This is especially undesirable in clinical situations when cardiovascular stability should be maintained, such as post myocardial infarction or stroke [106]. But when potassium chloride supplements are prescribed with the diuretic, the patient should receive between 40 and 60 mEq of potassium supplements per day in addition to the dietary intake to overcome thiazide-induced hypokalemia [107]. Addition of potassium supplements to diuretic therapy already containing a potassium-sparing agent may be disastrous in a patient with impaired renal function. In any event, it is always important to monitor the serum potassium levels at regular intervals, at least initially, to insure that hyperkalemia does not develop and to see whether the hypokalemia has been corrected.

Metabolic alkalosis

Diuretic-induced potassium depletion accelerates distal tubular excretion of hydrogen ion. An increased excretion of ammonium in the urine is needed to buffer these H-ions. Accordingly, for each equivalent of ammonium secreted into the tubular lumen, one equivalent of bicarbonate will replace the chloride in the extracellular fluid volume. Since the diuretics also lead to an extracellular fluid volume contraction, the rate of reabsorption of sodium bicarbonate will be increased. Chloride and potassium ion depletion together with extracellular volume contraction may augment renal bicarbonate reabsorption, further aggravating metabolic alkalosis [14]. Diuretic-induced metabolic alkalosis is 'chloride responsive'. However, at least partial correction of the potassium (by potassium chloride) deficit or even discontinuation of diuretic treatment is required before metabolic alkalosis will respond.

Hyponatremia

Thiazide diuretics acting at the distal convoluted tubule (cortical diluting segment) commonly interfere with urinary dilution mechanisms [14, 108]. Hence, free water clearance becomes limited and excessive water intake will lead to hyponatremia. Moreover, extracellular fluid volume contraction further stimulates antidiuretic hormone (ADH) release, thereby facilitating free water reabsorption and dilutional hyponatremia [109]. The normal homeostatic mechanisms for sodium conservation are usually adequate to prevent severe diuretic-induced hyponatremia. However, especially in older patients and under conditions of heavy exercise in hot weather with water-drinking, hyponatremia may become clinically significant. This may also be encountered in patients receiving intravenous fluid therapy and with fluid replacement after heavy transpiration with exercise. Although loop diuretics interfere with urinary dilution by blocking chloride and sodium reabsorption, they also may inhibit free water reabsorption and directly interfere with the action of ADH on the collecting duct [110]. Hence, furosemide has been used for acute and long-term correction of hyponatremia in patients with inappropriate secretion of ADH [111, 112].

Calcium Metabolism

Up to 30 % of the filtered calcium load is reabsorbed at the site of sodium and chloride reabsorption in the ascending thick limb of Henle's loop. This process may be similar to the passive sodium reabsorption by active chloride transport, although evidence for an independent active calcium transport system has been found [113, 114]. The high ceiling loop diuretics inhibit sodium and calcium reabsorption to about the same degree and, therefore, seem to increase urinary calcium excretion in parallel to sodium [115]. The thiazide diuretics, on the other hand, decrease calcium clearance by about 50 % [115]. Micropuncture studies have revealed that chlorothiazide produces a dissociation between sodium and calcium reabsorption in the distal tubule; thus, intraluminal sodium concentration increases significantly, but calcium concentration remains unchanged [115]. Middler et al. have suggested that the thiazide diuretics increase the renal effects of parathyroid hormone to retain calcium and that in turn the increased serum calcium levels would suppress the parathyroid glands [116]. Nevertheless, hypercalcemia is not a common clinical problem associated with long-term thiazide therapy in previously normocalcemic patients [117]. It may occur more frequently, however, in those who are taking vitamin D or who have antecedent hyperparathyroidism and prolonged thiazide administration has even been associated with secondary hyperparathyroidism and parathyroid adenomas despite unchanged plasma parathyroid hormone (PTH) levels [118, 119]. The fact that thiazide reduce renal calcium clearance can be used prophylactically in patients with idiopathic hypercalcuria who have a tendency to stone formation. On the other hand, acute increase in calcium clearance after furosemide has been taken advantage of in the management of hypercalcemic states.

Other ions

Recently it has been shown that chlorthalidone and thiazide diuretic increase urinary zinc excretion by about 60% [121–123]. In contrast, during treatment with loop diuretics, urine zinc concentration diminished and the total amount excreted was less than during therapy with thiazides, whereas triamterene seemed to have no significant effect [123]. Although the clinical implication of these findings is unknown, it has to be kept in mind that zinc has been recognized as an essential element for human health. Similarly to hypokalemia, hypomagnesemia has been found during long-term diuretic therapy [124]. Magnesium loss predisposes to potassium loss [125] and if hypomagnesemia is present it seems to be very difficult to correct hypokalemia [126]. Furthermore, aldosterone may increase renal excretion of magnesium. Magnesium deficiency may lead to arrhythmias and other cardiovascular disorders [127] and it has even been suggested that patients with diuretic-induced hypokalemia should receive magnesium together with potassium supplements.

Diuretics have also been found to reduce renal lithium clearance [128]. Accordingly, diuretic therapy may increase the risk of lithium intoxication in lithium-treated patients [129]. Although chlorothiazide has a beneficial effect in the renal diabetes insipidus [108], it seems not to improve the urinary concentration capacity in lithium-treated patients.

Hyperglycemia

After the thiazides were introduced for the treatment of hypertension, several cases were reported of patients developing diabetes mellitus while receiving this therapy [130, 131]. Diabetes mellitus has been observed also in patients receiving furosemide [132]. Surprisingly, no deterioration of glucose tolerance was observed in 137 patients who were treated with an oral diuretic for one year [133]; and insulin and free fatty acid levels also remained unchanged on therapy [133]. However, when 51 of these patients were observed for over six years, a significant deterioration of the glucose tolerance occurred [134]. Speculative mechanisms that could explain the development of carbohydrate intolerance include inhibition of the pancreatic release of insulin from the beta-cells and blockade of peripheral glucose utilization. Such a mechanism seems to account for the effect of diazoxide (orally) in patients with islet cell tumors. It has been suggested that the carbohydrate intolerance may be related to diuretic-induced hypokalemia [135]. However, in the above-mentioned long-term study, no correlation was found between the degree of hypokalemia and hyperglycemia [134]. Even in patients with established hypokalemia, no deterioration of glucose tolerance had taken place. Despite the low prevalence of hyperglycemic complications, it should be borne in mind that thiazide diuretics have been associated with hyperosmolar hyperglycemic nonketotic coma in older patients with maturity-onset diabetes [136]. In general, it has been held, however, that diabetes mellitus does not develop in patients treated with the thiazides (or other diuretic) unless carbohydrate intolerance was present prior to initiating the diuretic.

Hyperuricemia

Mild hyperuricemia may occur in between 20 and 30 % of untreated patients with essential hypertension [137, 138]. We have recently shown that uric acid closely parallels the magnitude of renal vascular resistance and hence may be an indicator of early hypertensive renal disease. Long-term use of thiazides more than doubles the incidence of hyperuricemia. Both thiazides and the loop diuretics decrease renal uric acid clearance by decreasing the tubular secretion of uric acid. This may be related to a fall in the renal blood flow [139], a rise in renal vascular resistance [139], or to intravascular volume depletion [140]. Rarely does hyperuricemia precipitate symptoms of gout requiring treatment. However, most authorities recommend that a uricosuric agent (e.g., probenecid) or an inhibitor of urate synthesis (e.g., allopurinol) be given to those patients whose serum uric acid concentration exceeds 10–11 mg/100 ml. When prescribing probenecid one must consider that it also inhibits the diuretic effect since it prevents reabsorption of the diuretic at the proximal tubule and thus from reaching its site of action.

The clinical significance of prolonged mild hyperuricemia is not known. Clearly, most agree that urate nephropathy has not aggravated hypertension; nor has symptomatic gout been a major problem. Nevertheless, hyperuricemia is a risk factor for coronary heart disease [141]. Moreover, it has been suggested that chronic mild hyperuricemia may lead to low grade hyperuricemic nephropathy and contribute to a deterioration in the renal function in essential hypertension [137]. On the other hand, Beevers et al. have shown that patients who had been receiving thiazides for up to 15 years showed no evidence of urate nephropathy or other diuretic-induced kidney changes [142]. Further, Fessel has recently shown that mild hyperuricemia probably was not of any clinical importance unless uric acid levels exceeded 13 mg per deciliter in men [143]. Also, no appreciable loss of renal function was noted in 112 patients with gout as compared to normouricemic subjects followed for up to 12 years [144]. Despite these reassuring long-term studies, a distinct increase in serum uric acid with diuretic treatment remains somewhat disturbing for most physicians. Hopefully, newer diuretics that are uricosuric and are safe as the thiazides will become available in the near future. This apparently was not the case with ticrynafen [47].

Hyperlipidemia

Ames and Hill have shown that a rise in serum cholesterol and triglycerides of 12 and 36 mg/dl, respectively, was found in patients treated with chlorthalidone which could be accounted for by a distinct increase in about half of their patients from low pretreatment levels [145]. More recently in a joint Veterans Administration/National Heart, Lung, and Blood Institute study of mild hypertension, it was found that chlorthalidone produced an increase in total cholesterol and triglyceride levels of 10 and 9.8 mg/dl, respectively, and of low density lipoprotein cholesterol of 12.6 mg/dl after one year of treatment [146]. Helgeland found a 9% increase in triglycerides, but no change in cholesterol levels [147]. The rise occurred primarily in patients with increased uric acid levels, who had gained weight, or received adrenergic inhibition therapy. In contrast to these reports, the Framingham study did not report increases in serum cholesterol in any of their patients who had been treated for years with diuretics [148]. Grimm et al. have recently shown that the diuretic-induced increase in cholesterol and triglycerides of 8 and 16%, respectively, could be prevented with a fat-controlled diet [149]. The clinical significance of the mild rise in lipids while receiving chlorthalidone is unknown. But based on the prospective Framingham data, a 10 mg/dl rise in cholesterol should lead to a 12% increase in risk of coronary heart disease in a 35-year-old man.

THIAZIDES AND RELATED COMPOUNDS

Although by 1948 diuretics [150] and sodium restriction [151] had been shown to reduce arterial pressure in hypertensive patients, it was not until

10 years later that the feasibility of long-term antihypertensive treatment with chlorothiazide [152, 153] was demonstrated. Subsequently, the chemical structure of this sulfanilamide derivative has been changed to produce more potent or longer-acting derivatives. Chlorthalidone, metalazone, and quinethazone have a different structure, although they retain the sulfamil group and the adjacent halogen. Nevertheless, manipulation of the chemical structure seems to provide little clinical benefit [154]. The compounds with a longer duration of action may produce a somewhat less brisk diuresis. This may be an advantage and possibly could enhance patient adherence. However, no convincing clinical evidence has been provided that the antihypertensive effect of the shorter-acting thiazide is less than that of the longer-acting compounds.

Pharmacokinetics

Thiazide diuretics are well absorbed from the gastrointestinal tract and are predominantly excreted in the urine. Chlorothiazide, the best documented thiazide congener, passes through the placenta and is also known to be easily distributed throughout the extracellular space [155]. In contrast, chlorthalidone is more slowly excreted, probably caused by its binding to red blood cells.

Table 2. Adverse reactions to thiazide diuretics and congeners

I. Metabolic:	Hypokalemia, Hyponatremia, Azotemia, Metabolic alkalosis, Hypercalcemia, Secondary hyperparathyroidism, Hyperglycemia, Hyperlipidemia, Hyperuricemia, Zinc and magnesium depletion.
II. Gastrointestinal:	Anorexia, Gastric irritation, Nausea and vomiting, Cramping, Diarrhea, Constipation, Jaundice (intrahepatic, cholestatic), Pancreatitis, Sialadenitis, Flatulence, Gallstones, Colitis.
II. Central nervous system:	Vertigo, Dizziness, Headache, Xantopsia, Paresthesias, Coma, Insomnia, Blindness, Tinnitus.
IV. Cardiovascular:	Orthostatic hypotension, Tachycardia, Palpitations, Acute pulmonary edema.
V. Hematologic:	Leukopenia, Agranulocytosis, Thrombocytopenia, Aplastic anemia, Hemolytic anemia, Splenomegaly, Lymphadenopathy.
VI. Allergic reactions:	Necrotizing angiitis, Fever, Glomerulonephritis, Interstitial nephritis, Urticaria, Rash, Photosensitivity, Purpura, Anaphylactic reaction, Steven-Johnson Syndrome.
VII. Miscellaneous:	Change in libido, Muscle cramps, Spastic cranial facial syndrome, Rebound hypertension.

Precautions and adverse effects

Apart from the previously mentioned metabolic adverse effects on the serum chemistry, thiazide diuretics may occasionally produce various other adverse reactions (see also Table 2). The most important is pancreatitis [156–158], which has been associated with hyperosmolar nonketotic hyperglycemic coma [136, 159]. Occasionally, thiazide-induced jaundice has been shown to complicate antihypertensive treatment [160]. Paradoxical pulmonary edema [161], pneumonitis [162], and other allergic reactions such as photosensitivity, interstitial nephritis [163], and glomerulonephritis [164], renal vasculitis [165] and exfoliative dermatitis [166] have been reported. Hematologic adverse effects as bone marrow aplasia (one case) [167], purpura thrombocytopenic [168] or nonthrombocytopenic [169], eosinophilia and hemolytic anemia [170] have rarely been found. Among the neurologic effects, spastic cranial facial syndrome, tinnitus, paresthesis, blurring of vision, and even cortical blindness with hyperpyrexia [171] have been observed.

Clinical use

When prescribing thiazide diuretics either alone or in combination with other antihypertensive drugs, a few points should be remembered. Many

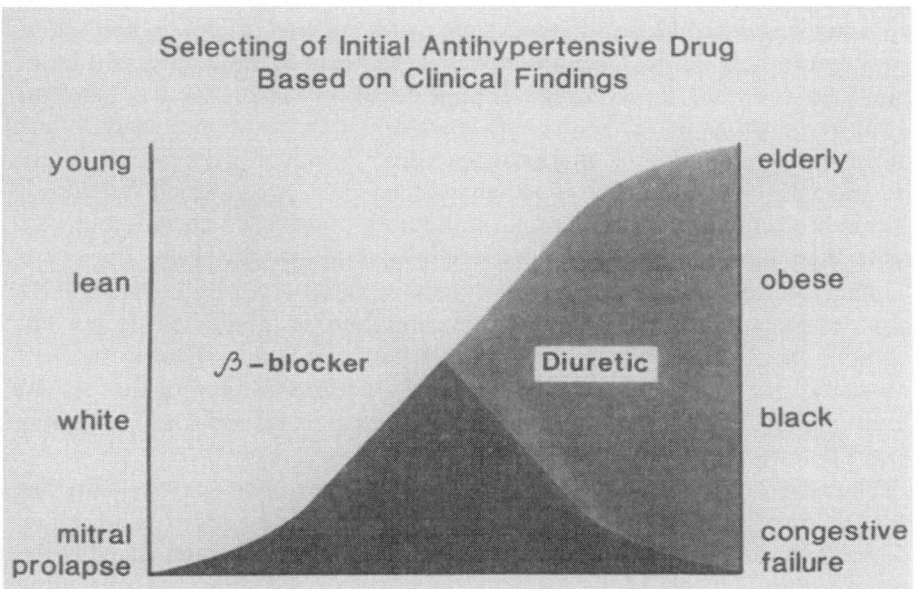

Figure 3. When to use a diuretic versus a β-blocker as a first-step agent.

patients with essential hypertension can be controlled by a thiazide alone, especially with a sodium-restricted diet [1]. We consider a diuretic as the initial drug of choice in elderly patients, in obese subjects, and also in black patients (Figure 3). On the other hand, in young white subjects, especially in those who are lean and have symptoms and signs of an increased adrenergic drive, it is our policy to start with a beta-blocker. As previously discussed, thiazides are more potent antihypertensive drugs than the loop diuretics. Hence, they should be preferred in uncomplicated essential hypertension. However, in contast to loop diuretics, they have a flat dose-response curve with regard to natriuresis so that once an effective dose is reached, little more can be gained from a higher dose. Although a higher dose will not have any additional antihypertensive or diuretic effect, it may increase the prevalence of adverse reactions [172]. The effective dose also depends on the dietary salt intake [173–176]. Patients receiving a low sodium diet will favorably react to a relatively low diuretic dose, i.e., hydrochlorothiazide or chlorothalidone of 25 mg/day. On the other hand, patients with a 'normal' salt intake require a higher dose, and it is a common clinical observation that a high salt intake can completely override the antihypertensive effect of a diuretic. Despite the lack of an antihypertensive effect, potassium loss will be greatly accelerated. As previously mentioned, potassium loss increases with a high salt intake since a higher sodium load is available at the distal tubular level.

When prescribing thiazides as part of combination therapy, we propose not only to lower blood pressure, but also to prevent extracellular fluid volume expansion. Most antiadrenergic drugs such as reserpine, methyldopa, prazosin, clonidine, guanethidine, etc., will lead to water and salt retention after a few days or weeks [117]. Such a volume expansion may manifest itself by weight gain and edema and can override the antihypertensive effect of the antiadrenergic drug and even may precipitate congestive heart failure in susceptible patients [178]. This phenomenon has been termed 'pseudotolerance' to antiadrenergic therapy. It is rarely observed with beta-blockers since they usually do not affect extracellular fluid volume [179]. Pseudotolerance can easily be prevented and treated by diligent use of diuretics. With most antiadrenergic drugs, a simple thiazide diuretic is sufficient to prevent volume expansion. Only with minoxidil fluid retention seems to be very resistant, and loop diuretics are commonly needed to protect the patient from massive fluid retention and from developing edema and congestive heart failure [180].

The question whether the diuretic should be given once or twice daily has not yet been resolved. The antihypertensive effect of even a short-acting drug seems not to depend upon the frequency of administration. Usually the clinical situation and/or the patient's convenience will dictate at what time of the day the drug should be taken.

LOOP DIURETICS

Furosemide, ethacrynic acid, bumethanide, piretanide, and muzolimine are fast-acting and extremely potent diuretics. Because they inhibit sodium and chloride reabsorption in the ascending limb of the loop of Henle, they are even effective in patients who are not responsive to the thiazide diuretics.

Pharmacokinetics

The loop diuretics are easily absorbed from the gastrointestinal tract and circulate in the intravascular space bound to plasma proteins [152]. They are rapidly excreted in the urine by glomerular filtration and secretion in the proximal tubule. A substantial amount of furosemide seems also to be excreted in the feces. Diuresis occurs within a few minutes after intravenous injection. With oral ingestion a diuretic response can be expected within an hour. The diuretic effect peaks after 2–3 h and ends after 6–8 h [152]. In severe renal failure, biliary excretion of the drug may exceed 60% [181].

Table 3. Adverse reactions to loop diuretics

I. Metabolic:	Hypokalemia, Hyponatremia, Hypochloremia, Alkalosis, Hyperglycemia, Hyperuricemia, Hyperlipidemia, Azotemia, Hypophosphalemia, Hypomagnesiemia.
II. Cardiovascular:	Orthostatic hypotension, Tachycardia, Volume depletion, Thromobophlebitis, Non-occlusive mesenteric infarction
III. Central nervous system:	Dizziness, Vertigo, Paresthesias, Headache, Xantopsia, Blurred vision, Tiniitus and hearing loss, Hallucination, Somnolence, Diaphoresis, Sweet taste.
IV. Allergic:	Purpura, Photosensitivity, Rash, Urticaria, Necrotizing angiitis, Erythema multiforme, Pruritus, Interstitial nephritis, Bullous hemorrhagic lesions, Phototoxic blisters, Exfoliative dermatitis.
V. Hematologic:	Anemia, Leukopenia, Agranulocytosis, Thrombocytopenia, Aplastic anemia, Eosinophilia.
VI. Gastrointestinal:	Anorexia, Gastric irritation, Nausea, Vomiting, Cramping, Diarrhea, Constipation, Jaundice (intrahepatic, cholestatic), Pancreatitis, Flatulence.
VII. Miscellaneous:	Ototoxicity, Acute bladder spasm and urine retention, Sudden death, Muscle spasm, Restlessness.

Adverse reactions

The renal effects of loop diuretics (Table 3) include hyponatremic metabolic alkalosis, hypokalemia, hyperuricemia, as well as other disturbances of the blood chemistry such as hyperglycemia and hyperlipidemia and are similar to those of the thiazide diuretics. Occasionally the diuretic response, especially with intravenous application, may be excessive and life-threatening [182]. Patients with hepatic cirrhosis seem to be at higher risk of developing prerenal azotemia and hepatic coma due to the decrease in renal and hepatic blood flow [183]. Sudden death has been observed after intravenous or intramuscular administration [184, 185]. Gastrointestinal side effects with nausea and diarrhea are common. Nonocclusive mesenteric infarction [186], pancreatitis and jaundice [187], and nonketotic hyperosmolar diabetic coma [188] have been reported. Skin reactions are rare and include phototoxic blisters [189], erythema multiforma, and necrotizing vasculitis [190]. Fatal thrombocytopenia [191] and reversible leukopenia and eosinophilia have been occasionally observed. Other allergic reactions such as anaphylaxis and interstitial nephritis have also been reported [192, 193]. Neurologic side effects include hallucinations [194], nonspecific paresthesis, vertigo and somnolence. Hearing loss with or without tinnitus may occur, especially with high doses [195, 196]. Ototoxicity seems most often to be reversible with furosemide but not always with ethacrynic acid [197]. Piretanide has been reported to be somewhat less ototoxic. Paradoxical diuretic-induced edema caused probably by ADH-induced water retention has been observed and should be borne in mind when treating patients with these drugs [198–200].

Clinical use

The loop diuretics have a steep dose–response curve with regard to sodium excretion and a relatively shallow one with regard to the antihypertensive effect. Accordingly, they should be used predominantly in patients whose blood pressure is volume-dependent, (renal parenchymal disease) or who are not or less responsive to thiazide diuretics (renal failure). The principal indications for the use of diuretics in the treatment of hypertension are the following.

1) Patients with renal failure, i.e., a creatinine level higher than 2 mg/dl. Thiazide diuretics may reduce arterial pressure even in anephric patients to some extent. However, most often hypertension is associated with extracellular fluid retention, and the lowering of blood pressure depends on an

effective diuresis. Accordingly, in this clinical setting a high-ceiling compound is preferable over a thiazide diuretic.

2) Hypertensive patients who have edema or congestive heart failure. The natriuretic potency of thiazide congeners may not suffice in patients with congestive heart failure, and the patient may require a loop diuretic.

3) Hypertensive emergencies. When a rapid volume depletion is desirable, the intravenous application of a loop diuretic will achieve a faster diuresis than a thiazide diuretic.

4) In combination with the vasodilators minoxidil and diazoxide. Both minoxidil and diazoxide are potent vasodilators that commonly lead to severe fluid retention and peripheral edema. In our experience, thiazide diuretics are not sufficient to deal with such a volume overload as caused by these two vasodilators, and most often loop diuretics are needed.

Treatment is usually started with 40 mg furosemide or 50 mg ethacrynic acid once or twice a day. In older ptients, especially in the ones with congestive heart failure, a lower initial dose of 20 or 25 mg once or twice a day is indicated. The range of the optimal dosage varies from 40 to 200 mg/day. In hypertensive emergencies as well as hypertension associated with congestive heart failure, the intravenous application of 20 to 100 mg is useful.

POTASSIUM-SPARING DIURETICS

Renal potassium excretion can be influenced by steroids with mineralocorticoid activity or by drugs that act directly on the distal nephron. Spironolactone is a competitive aldosterone antagonist acting only in the presence of aldosterone and probably competing for distal tubule receptor sites since its effect is overriden by increasing aldosterone concentrations [201]. Triamterene and amiloride, on the other hand, act directly on the distal nephron independent of adrenal steroids [19].

Pharmacokinetics

Spironolactone is easily absorbed from the gastrointestinal tract and metabolized to canrenone [202]. The drug and its metabolites are mostly bound to plasma proteins. Canrenone and other metabolites are predominantly excreted by the kidney but a certain percentage has been recovered in the bile [56]. Triamterene is excreted in the urine with a peak in the renal excretion within 2 h after oral intake [203]. The total duration of action is about 24 h. About half of it is bound to protein in the plasma [154]. In the urine most of the drug is present in the form of metabolites. Amiloride is absorbed to about 20–30% of an oral dose from the gastrointestinal tract and its action reaches a peak within 6 hours and usually lasts for about 24 h [154]. The drug is excreted unchanged in the urine.

Adverse effects

The effects of these potassium-sparing agents are listed in Table 4. Spironolactone commonly produces hyperkalemia, hyponatremia, mild acidosis, and an increase in BUN [204]. Nonspecific gastrointestinal complaints are occasionally observed [204]. More disturbing are the effects of the drug on the endocrine system. In men a decrease in libido, gynecomastia, and impo-

Table 4. Potassium-sparing agents

A. Triamterene	
1. Metabolic:	Hyperkalemia, Hyperglycemia, Hyperuricemia, Azotemia, Metabolic acidosis, Hyperuricemia, Kidney stones (Oxalate and Triamterene)
2. Gastrointestinal:	Diarrhea, Nausea, Vomiting
3. Central nervous system:	Dizziness, Weakness, Headache, Agitation, Insomnia
4. Allergic:	Anaphylaxis, Photosensitivity, Rash, Pruritus, Urticaria
5. Other	Hot and cold flushes, Paresthesias, Bitter taste, Dry mouth
B. Amiloride	
1. Metabolic:	Hyperkalemia, Hyponatremia, Azotemia, Hyperchloremia
2. Gastrointestinal:	Diarrhea, Flatulence, Cramps, Gastric upset, Nausea, Vomiting, Anorexia, Gastrointestinal bleeding
3. Allergic:	Skin rash, Pruritus, Hives
4. Nervous System:	Paresthesias, Dizziness, Weakness
5. Other:	Salivary gland inflammation, Constipation, Vertigo, Abnormality of liver function tests, Visual blurring, Mental confusion, Mild proteinuria, Glucosuria
C. Spironolactone	
1. Metabolic:	Hyperkalemia, Azotemia, Metabolic acidosis, Hyponatremia
2. Gastrointestinal:	Nausea, Vomiting, Cramping, Diarrhea, Dry mouth
3. Central nervous system:	Drowsiness, Lethargy, Headache, Mental confusion, Ataxia
4. Endocrine:	Irregular menstruation, Amenorrhea, Postmenopausal bleeding, Hirsutism, Deepening of the voice in the female, Impotence, Decreased libido, Gynecomastia in male
5. Allergic:	Maculopapular or erythematous cutaneous eruptions, Urticaria, Pruritus

tence [205] may be observed, and in women amenorrhea, postmenopausal bleeding, hirsutism, and deepening of the voice may occur [206]. Although androgen-like side effects are usually reversible, they are common and restrict the use of the drug. They seem to be caused by an increased metabolic clearance rate and an accelerated conversion rate of testosterone into estradiol in patients treated with spironolactone [207]. Skin rashes and urticaria are occasionally observed [208].

Similar to spironolactone, triamterene may cause hyperglycemia, hyperuricemia, and an increase in BUN and creatinine [209]. More recently, it has been shown that kidney stones may be related to triameterine therapy [210]. The kidney stones seemed to be composed of triamterene crystals alone or a mixture of calcium oxalate and triamterene [210]. Megaloblastic anemia has been reported especially in patients with alcoholic cirrhosis [211]. Triamterene seems to inhibit dehydrofolate reductase and this effect may have clinical consequences in suspectible patients [212].

Amiloride can also produce hyponatremia and mild proteinuria and glycosuria. Gastrointestinal side effects are nonspecific. Occasional abnormalities of liver enzymes are observed. Skin rashes, pruritus, and paresthesia are rarely associated with amiloride therapy [202].

Clinical Use

The natriuretic properties of potassium-sparing diuretics are, in general, mild and their antihypertensive effect is somewhat smaller than the one seen with thiazide diuretics. However, since thiazide diuretics and high-ceiling diuretics produce a renal potassium loss, the addition of a potassium-sparing compound seems at least theoretically very attractive. Spironolactone is a somewhat more effective antihypertensive agent than triamterene, especially when used in hypermineralocorticoid states. Because of the antagonistic effect on potassium metabolism, various combination preparations of thiazides and potassium sparing compounds have been marketed. These fixed combination drugs may be useful in the few patients who are potassium wasters or in the few with high mineralocorticoid levels. Nevertheless, most patients with uncomplicated essential hypertension can be treated with a thiazide diuretic alone. There is no reason to expose a patient to possible hazards (such as kidney stones or gynecomastia) of a second drug when a thiazide diuretic alone would suffice. The prescription of a fixed-drug combination does not absolve the physician from monitoring potassium levels since both hypokalemia and more often hyperkalemia have been reported under these circumstances [213]. Needless to say, patients treated with potassium-sparing drugs should not receive additional potassium supplements. The tendency to develop hyperkalemia is especially important to remember in patients with progressive renal failure. In early parenchymal kidney disease, a tendency to potassium loss may be present; however, as renal failure progresses, potassium will be retained and life-threatening hyperkalemia may develop.

Spironolactone is an effective diuretic when used in the setting of congestive failure, hepatic cirrhosis, or other edematous states with mineralocorticoid excess [214]. It has been found to be an excellent agent in treating patients with primary aldosteronism because of its competitive antagonism at the mineralocorticoid receptor level [215, 216]. When prescribing spironolactone for the treatment of resistant edema or congestive failure, it should be borne in mind that it takes 2–3 days until a significant diuretic effect will take place. Because of its dose-dependent adverse effects, the dose should be kept as low as possible. In patients with essential hypertension who need a potassium-sparing drug, 50 to at most 100 mg will suffice.

Amiloride's antihypertensive effects seem to be equivalent to the thiazide diuretics, and both amiloride and triamterene serve to protect against the hypokalemic effect of the thiazides. Accordingly, they are most often prescribed for the potassium-sparing action in conjunction with a high-ceiling or a thiazide diuretic. The usual dose of triamterene is 100 mg twice daily. As with all potassium-sparing agents, serum potassium levels should be monitored freqeuntly. Amiloride is given in a dose of 5 to 10 mg a day.

Other Diuretics

Indacrinic Acid. This is an experimental agent that inhibits urate reabsorption in the proximal tubule and sodium chloride reabsorption in the ascending limb of the loop of Henle. Accordingly, it has diuretic and uricosuric effects.

Ticrynafen (tienilic acid). Another uricosuric diuretic that has been recently withdrawn from the market because of its hepatic toxicity.

MK-447 is an experimental compound with natriuretic effects that are similar to those of furosemide. It exerts an antihypertensive effect at doses lower than those required for its diuretic activity. This suggests that its diuresis and antihypertensive properties may be mediated by enhancement of the synthesis of renal or vascular prostaglandins.

Indapamide. Indapamide is said to produce a good antihypertensive effect in low doses with only minimal diuresis. The hypotensive effect has been attributed to a direct smooth muscle relaxation and seems to be independent of the diuretic action. Preliminary clinical studies have shown that indapamide is well tolerated and effective in a dose of 2.5 mg daily. In contrast to thiazide diuretics, it does not affect either serum potassium or uric acid levels. These pharmacologic characteristics may make it a promising antihypertensive agent in the management of essential hypertension.

733

Piretanide is a new high-ceiling diuretic that has been claimed to be less ototoxic and less phosphate-depleting than furosemide.

REFERENCES

1. Hunt JC: Management and treatment of essential hypertension. In: Hypertension: Physiopathology and Treatment, pp. 1068–1084. Genest J, Koiw E, Kuchel O, eds, New York: McGraw-Hill, 1977.
2. Dirks JH, Cirksena WJ, Berliner RW: The effect of saline infusion on sodium reabsorption by the proximal tubule of the dog. J Clin Invest 44:1160–1170, 1965.
3. Dirks JH, Cirksena WJ, Berliner RW: Micropuncture study of the effect of various diuretics on sodium reabsorption by the proximal tubules of the dog. J Clin Invest 45:1875–1885, 1966.
4. Weinman EJ, Kashgarian M, Hayslett JP: Role of peritubular protein concentration in sodium reabsorption. Am J Physiol 221:1521–1528, 1971.
5. Weiner MW, Weinman EJ, Kashgarian M, Hayslett JP: Accelerated reabsorption in the proximal tubule produced by volume depletion. J Clin Invest 50:1379–1385, 1971.
6. Kanau RT Jr, Weller DR, Webb HL: Clarification of the site of action of chlorothiazide in the rat nephron. J Clin Invest 56:401–407, 1975.
7. Hamburger J, Crosnier J, Grunfeld JP, eds: Nephrology. New York: Wiley, 1979.
8. Burg M, Stoner LC, Cardinal J, Green N: Furosemide effect on isolated perfuse tubules. Am J Physiol 225:119–124, 1973.
9. Berg M, Green N: Effect of ethacrynic acid on the thick ascending limb of Henle's loop. Kidney Int 4:301–303, 1973.
10. Hierholzer K, Wiederholt M, Holzgreve H, Giebisch G, Klose RM, Windhager: Micropuncture study of renal transtubular concentration gradients of sodium and potassium in adrenalectomized rats. Pfluegers Arch 285:193–210, 1965.
11. Herholzer K: Intrarenal action of steriod hormones on sodium transport in renal transport and diuretics. In: Renaler Transport and Diuretics, Internationales Symposium, Feldafing, 21–23 Juni 1968, pp. 153–171. Thurau K, Jahrmaker H, eds. New York: Springer Verlag, 1969.
12. Geller RG, Margolius HS, Pisano JJ, Keiser HR: Effects of mineralocorticoids, altered sodium intake, and adrenalectomy on urinary kallikrein in rats. Circ Res 31:857–861, 1972.
13. Goldberg M: The renal physiology of diuretics. In: Handbook of Physiology. Section 8: Renal Physiology, pp. 1003–1031. Orloff J, Berliner RW, eds. Washington D.C., American Physiological Society, 1973.
14. Seely JF, Dirks JH: Site of action of diuretic drugs. Kidney Int 11:1–8, 1977.
15. Kennedy RM, Earley LE: Profound hyponatremia resulting from a thiazide-induced decrease in urinary diluting capacity in a patient with primary polydipsia. N Engl J Med 282:1185–1186, 1970.
16. Raskind M: Psychosis, polydipsia and water intoxification. Arch Gen Psychiatry 30:112–114, 1974.
17. Duarte CG, Chomety F, Giebisch G: Effect of amiloride, ouabain and furosemide on distal tubular function in the rat. Am J Physiol 221:632–639, 1971.
18. Stoner LC, Burg MB, Orloff J: Ion transport in cortical collecting tubule, effect of amiloride. Am J Physiol 227:453–459, 1974.
19. Margolius HS, Chao J: Amiloride inhibits mammalian renal kallikrein and a kallikrein-like enzyme from toad bladder and skin. J Clin Invest 65:1343–1350, 1980.

734

20. Conway J, Lauwers P: Hemodynamic and hypotensive effects of long-term therapy with chlorothiazide. Circulation 21:21–27, 1967.
21. Freis ED, Wanko A, Wilson IM et al.: Chlorothiazide in hypertensive and normotensive patients. Ann NY Acad Sci 71:450–455, 1958.
22. Dustan HP, Cumming GR, Corcoran AC, Page IH: A mechanism of chlorothiazide-enhanced effectiveness of antihypertensive ganglioplegic drugs. Circulation 19:360–365, 1959.
23. Frohlich ED, Schnaper HW, Wilson IM, Freis ED: Hemodynamic alterations in hypertensive patients due to chlorothiazide. N Engl J Med 262:1261–1263, 1960.
24. Freis ED, Wanko AM, Schnaper HW, Frohlich ED: Mechanism of the altered blood pressure responsiveness produced by chlorothiazide. J Clin Invest 39:1277–1281, 1960.
25. Crosley AP Jr, Castillo C, Freeman DJ, White DH Jr, Rowe GG: The acute effects of carbonic anhydrase inhibitors on systemic hemodynamics. J Clin Invest 37:887, 1958.
26. Lohmoller G, Lohmoller R, Pfeffer MA, Pfeffer JM, Frohlich ED: Mechanism of the immediate hemodynamic effects of chlorothiazide. Am Heart J 89:487–492, 1975.
27. Conway J, Palmero H: The vascular effect of the thiazide diuretics. Arch Intern Med 111:203–207, 1963.
28. Aleksandrow D, Wysznacka W, Gajewski J: Studies on the mechanism of hypotensive action of chlorothiazide. N Engl J Med 260:51–55, 1959.
29. De Carvalho JGR, Dunn FG, Frohlich ED: Hemodynamic correlates of prolonged thiazide therapy. Clin Pharmacol Ther 22:875–880, 1977.
30. Gillenwater JY, Scott JB, Frohlich ED: Effects of chlorothiazide upon the response of the renal bed to vasoactive substances. Circ Res 11:283, 1962.
31. Frohlich ED, Thurman AE, Pfeffer MA, Brobmann GF, Jacobson ED: Altered vascular responsiveness: intial hypotensive mechanisms of thiazide diuretics (36639). Proc Soc Exp Biol Med 140:1190–1196, 1972.
32. Leth A: Changes in plasma and extracellular fluid volumes in patients with essential hypertension during long-term treatment with hydrochlorothiazide. Circulation 41:479–485, 1970.
33. Tarazi RC, Dustan HP, Frohlich ED: Long-term thiazide therapy in essential hypertension: evidence for persistent alteration in plasma volume and renin activity. Circulation 41:709–717, 1970.
34. Van Brummelen P, Veld A, Schalekamp MA: Hemodynamics during long-term thiazide treatment in essential hypertension: differences between responders and non-responders. Clin Sci 57:359s–362s, 1979.
35. Tobian L, Binion JT: Tissue cations and water in arterial hypertension. Circulation 5:754–758, 1952.
36. Tobian L: Interrelationship of electolytes, juxtaglomerular cells, and hypertension. Physiol Rev 40:280–312, 1960.
37. Tobian L: Why do thiazide diuretics lower blood pressure in essential hypertension? Ann Rev Pharmacol 7:399–408, 1967.
38. Aoki VS, Brody MJ: The effect of thiazide on the sympathetic nervous system of hypertensive rats. Arch Int Phamacodyn Ther 177:423–434, 1969.
39. Zsoter TT, Hart F, Radde IC: Mechanism of antihypertensive action of prolonged administration of hydrochlorothiazide in rabbit and dog. Circ Res 27:717–725, 1970.
40. Webster JA, Dollery CT: Antihypertensive action of bendroflumethazide: increased prostacyclin production. Clin Pharmacol Ther 28:751–758, 1980.
41. O'Conner DT, Preston RA, Mitas JA et al.: Urinary kallikrein activity and renal vascular resistance. Hypertension 3:139–147, 1981.
42. Bhatia K, Frohlich ED: Hemodynamic comparison of agents useful in hypertensive emergencies. Am Heart J 85:367–373, 1973.

43. Rubin AA, Zitowitz L, Hausler L: Acute circulatory effects of diazoxide and sodium nitrite. J Pharmacol Exp Ther 140:46–51, 1963.
44. Ogilvie RI, Reudy J: Hemodynamic effects of ethacrynic acid in anephric dogs. J Pharmacol Exp Ther 176:389–396, 1971.
45. Ogilvie RI, Schlieper E: Comparative effects of ethacrynic acid, furosemide and diazoxide in the perfused dog hindlimb. Can J Physiol Pharmacol 49:1038–1043, 1971.
46. Dikshit K, Vyden JD, Forrester JS, Swan HJC: Renal and extrarenal hemodynamic effects of furosemide in congestive heart failure after acute mycardial infarction. N Engl J Med 288:1087–1090. 1973.
47. Frohlich ED: Ticrynafen: a new thiazide-like but uricosuric diuretic. N Engl J Med 301:1378–1382, 1979.
48. Anderson J, Gosfrey BE, Godfrey BE, Hill DM, Munro-Faure AD, Sheldon J: A comparison of the effects of hydrochlorothiazide and of frusemide in treatment of hypertensive patients. Q J Med 40:541–560, 1971.
49. Bariso CR, Hanenson IB, Gaffney TE: A comparison of the antihypertensive effects of furosemide and chlorothiazide. Curr Ther Res 12:333–340, 1970.
50. Finnerty FA, Maxwell MH, Lunn J, Moser M: Long-term effects of furosemide and hydrochlorothiazide in patients with essential hypertension: a two-year comparison of efficacy and safety. Angiology 28:125–133, 1977.
51. Araoye M, Freis E et al.: Furosemide compared to hydrochlorothiazide in hypertension. Circulation (Suppl III), 30:55–56, 1977.
52. Muth RG: Diuretic properties of furosemide in renal disease. Ann Intern Med 69:249–261, 1968.
53. Cranston WI, Semmence AM, Richardson DW, Barnett CF: Effect of triamterene on elevated arterial pressure. Am Heart J 70:455–460, 1965.
54. Heath WC, Freis ED: Triamterene with hydrochlorothiazide in the treatment of hypertension. JAMA 186:119, 1963.
55. Patterson JW, Dollery CT, Huston RM: Amiloride hydrochloride in hypertensive patients. Br Med J 1:422, 1968.
56. Crane MG, Harris JJ: Effect of spironolactone in hypertensive patients. Am J Med Sci 260:311, 1970.
57. Drayer JIM, Kloppenborg PWC, Festen J, Van 't Laar A, Benraad TJ: Intrapatient comparison of treatment with chlorthalidone, spironolactone and propranolol in normorenic essential hypertension. Am J Cardiol 36:716–721, 1975.
58. Multicenter Diuretic Cooperative Study Group: Multicenter comparison of amiloride, hydrochlorothiazide, and hydrochlorothiazide plus amiloride in patients with essential hypertension. Arch Intern Med 141:431–434, 1981.
59. Hook JB, Blatt AH, Brody MJ, Williamson HE: Effects of several saluretic-diuretic agents on renal hemodynamics. J Pharmacol Exp Ther 154:667, 1966.
60. Ludens JH, Heitz DC, Brody MJ, Williamson HE: Differential effects of furosemide on renal and limb blood flows in the conscious dog. J Pharmacol Exp Ther 171:300–306, 1970.
61. Dirks JH: Mechanism of action and clinical uses of diuretics. Hosp Prac 9:99–110, 1979.
62. Wright FS: Intrarenal regulation of glomerular filtration rate. N Engl J Med 291:135–141, 1974.
63. Wright FS, Schnermann J: Interference with feedback control of glomerular filtration rate by furosemide, trilocin and cyanide. J Clin Invest 52:1695–1708, 1974.
64. Davis JO: Review: what signals the kidney to release renin? Circ Res 28:301–306, 1971.
65. Kotchen TA, Guthrie GP: Renin-angiotensin-aldosterone and hypertension. Endocrine Reviews 1:78–99, 1980.

66. Imbs JL, Schmidt M, Velly J, Schwartz J: Comparison of the effect of two groups of diuretics on renin secretion in the anaesthetized dog. Clin Sci Mol Med 52:171–182, 1977.
67. Vander AJ, Carlson J: Mechanism of the effects of furosemide on renin secretion in anesthetized dogs. Circ Res 25:145, 1969.
68. Meyer P, Menard J, Papanicolaou N, Alexandre JM, Devaux C, Miller P: Mechanism of renin release following furosemide diuresis in rabbit. Am J Physiol 215:908, 1968.
69. Eide I, Loying E, Langaid O, Løyning E, Langård Ø, Kill F: Influence of ethacrynic acid on intrarenal renal renin release mechanisms. Kidney Int 8:158–165, 1975.
70. Bonvalet JP, Nenard JP: Influence of furosemide and propranolol on glomerular filtration rate and renin secretion in the rat. Pfluegers Arch 346:107, 1974.
71. Tuck ML, Dluhy RG, Williams GW: A specific role for saline or the sodium ion in the regulation of renin and aldosterone secretion. J Clin Invest 53:988, 1974.
72. Lake CR, Zeigler MG, Coleman MD, Kopin IJ: Hydrochlorothiazide-induced sympathetic hyperactivity in hypertensive patients. Clin Pharmacol Ther 26:428–432, 1979.
73. Patak RV, Mookerjee BK, Bentzel CJ, Hysert PE, Babeu M, Lee JB: Antagonism of the effects of furosemide by indomethacin in normal and hypertensive man. Prostaglandins 10:649–659, 1975.
74. Romero JC, Dunlop CL, Strong CG: The effects of indomethacin and other anti-inflammatory drugs on the renin-angiotensin system. J Clin Invest 58:282–290, 1976.
75. Tan SY, Mulrow PJ: Inhibition of the renin-aldosterone response to furosemide by indomethacin. J Clin Endocrinol Metab 45:174–176, 1977.
76. Lopez-Ovejero JA, Weber MA, Drayer JIM, Sealey JE, Laragh JH: Effects of indomethacin alone and during diuretic or adrenoreceptor-blockade therapy on blood pressure and the renin system in essential hypertension. Clin Sci Mol Med 55:203s–205s, 1978.
77. Croxatto HR, Roblero J, Garcio R, Corthorn J, San Marin M: Urinary kallikrein under furosemide and plasma kininogen levels in normal and hypertensive rats. Acta Physiol Lat Am 23:556–558, 1973.
78. Abe K, Seino M, Yasujima M, Chiba S, Sakurai Y, Irokawa N, Miyazaki S, Saito K, Ito T, Otsuka Y, Yoshinaga K: Studies on renomedullary prostaglandin and renal kallikrein-kinin system in hypertension. Jpn Circ J 41:873–880, 1977.
79. Margolius HS, Horwitz D, Geller RG, Alexander RW, Gill JR, Pisano JJ, Keiser HR: Urinary kallikrein excretion in normal man: Relationships to sodium intake and sodium-retaining steroids. Circ Res 35:812–819, 1974.
80. Geller RG, Margolius HS, Pisano JJ, Keiser HR: Effects of mineralocorticoids, altered sodium intake, and adrenalectomy on urinary kallikrein in rats. Circ Res 31:857–861, 1972.
81. Scriabine A, Watson LS, Russo HF, Ludden CT, Sweet CS, Fanelli GM Jr, Bohidar NR, Stone CA: Diuretic and antihypertensive effects of 2-Aminoethyl-4-(1, 1-Dimethylethyl)-6-Iodopheonol hydrochloride (MK-447)[1]. J Pharmacol Exp Ther 208:148–154, 1979.
82. Duarte DG, Chomety F, Geibisch G: Effect of amiloride, ouabain and furosemide on distal tubular function in the rat. Am J Physiol 221:632–639, 1971.
83. Burg M, Stoner LC, Cardinal J, Green N: Furosemide effect on isolated perfused tubules. Am J Physiol 225:119–124, 1973.
84. Burg M, Green N: Effect of ethacrynic acid on the thick ascending limb of Henle's loop. Kidney Int 4:301–308, 1973.
85. Kaplan NM: Personal communication. Arch Intern Med. (In press.)
86. Manner RJ, Brechbill SO et al.: Prevalence of hypokalemia in diuretic therapy. Clin Med 79:15, 1972.
87. Kochlar MS, Itskov HD: Effects of hydrochlorothiazide in hypertensive patients and the need for potassium supplementation. Curr Ther Res 15:298, 1973.

88. Louis WJ, Doyle AE, Dawborn JK, Johnston CI: Comparison of chlorothiazide, chlorthalidone and cyclopenthiazide in the treatment of hypertension. Med J Aust 2:23-25, 1973.
89. Pederson OL: Comparison of metoprolol and hydrochlorothiazide as antihypertensive agent. Eur J Clin Pharmacol 10:381, 1976.
90. Bartels CC, Evans JA et al.: Chlorothiazide – survey of its effects in hypertensive patients. JAMA 170:1796, 1959.
91. O'Haug T: Time course of changes in concentration of some plasma components after frusemide. Br Med J ii:622, 1976.
92. Read AE, Laidlaw J, Haslem RM, Sherlock S: Neuropsychiatric complications following chlorothiazide therapy in patients with hepatic cirrhosis: possible relation to hypokalemia. Clin Sci 18:409-423, 1959.
93. Morgan DB, Davidson C: Occasional review: Hypokalemia and diuretics: an analysis of publications. Br Med J 280:905-908, 1980.
94. Anderson J, Godfrey BE, Hill DM, Munro-Faure AD, Sheldon J: A comparison of the effects of hydrochlorothiazide and of frusemide in the treatment of hypertensive patients. Q J Med 160:541-560, 1971.
95. Leemhuis MP, Van Damme KJ, Struyvenberg A: Effects of chlorthalidone on serum and total body potassium in hypertensive patients. Acta Med Scand 200:37-45, 1976.
96. Wilkinson PR, Issler H, Hesp R, Raftery EB: Total body and serum potassium during prolonged thiazide therapy for essential hypertension. Lancet 1:759-765, 1975.
97. Davidson S, Susawicz B: Ectopic beats and atrioventricular conduction disturbances. Arch Int Med 120:280-285, 1967.
98. Steiness E, Olesen KH: Cardiac arrhythmias induced by hypokalemia and potassium loss during maintenance digoxin therapy. Br Heart J 38:167-172, 1976.
99. Cremer W, Bock KD: Symptoms and cause of chronic hypokalemic nephropathy in man. Clin Nephrol 7:112-119, 1977.
100. Lindeman RD: Hypokalemia: causes, consequences and correction. Am J Clin Sci 272:5-17, 1976.
101. Knochel JP, Schlein EM: On the mechanisms of rhabdomyolysis in potassium depletion. J Clin Invest 51:1750-1758, 1972.
102. Messerli FH, Frohlich ED: High blood pressure. A side effect of drugs, poisons, and food. Arch Intern Med 139:682-687, 1979.
103. Blachley JD, Knochel JP: Tobacco chewer's hypokalemia: licorice revisited. N Engl J Med 302:784-785, 1980.
104. Schwartz WB, Van Ypersele de Strihou C, Kassirer JP: Role of anions in metabolic alkalosis and potassium deficiency. N Engl J Med 2:630-639, 1968.
105. Sopko JA, Freeman RM: Salt substitutes as a source of potassium. JAMA 238:608-610, 1977.
106. Messerli FH, Pappas ND: Potassium chloride and thromboembolic complications: a hypothesis. Lancet 2:919-920, 1980.
107. Schwartz AB, Swartz CD: Dosage of potassium chloride elixir to correct thiazide-induced hypokalemia JAMA 230:702-704, 1974.
108. Earley LE, Orloff J: The mechanism of antidiuresis associated with the administration of hydrochlorothiazide to patients with vasopressin-resistant diabetes insipidus. J Clin Invest 41:1988-1997, 1962.
109. Schrier RW, Berl T, Anderson RJ: Osmotic and nonosmostic control of vasopressin release. Am J Physiol 236:F321-332, 1979.
110. Abramow M: Effects of ethacrynic acid on the isolated collecting tubule. J Clin Invest 53:796-804, 1974.
111. Hantman D, Rossier B, Zohlman R, Schrier R: Rapid correction of hyponatremia in the

738

syndrome of inappropriate secretion of antidiuretic hormone; an alternative treatment to hypertonic saline. Ann Intern Med 78:870–875, 1973.

112. Decaux G, Waterlot Y, Genett F, Mockel J: Treatment of the syndrome of inappropriate secretion of antidiuretic hormone with furosemide. N Engl J Med 304:329–330, 1981.

113. Rocha AS, Magaldi JB, Kokko JP: Calcium and phosphate transport in isolated segments of rabbit Henle's loop. J Clin Invest 59:975–983, 1977.

114. Sutton RA, Dirks JH: Renal handling of calcium. Fed Proc 37:2112–2119, 1978.

115. Edwards BR, Baer PG, Sutton RAL, Dirks JH: Micropuncture study of diuretic effects on sodium and calcium reabsorption in the dog nephron. J Clin Invest 52:2418–2427, 1973.

116. Middler S, Pak CYC, Murad F, Bartter F: Thiazide diuretics and calcium metabolism. Metabolism 22:139–146, 1973.

117. Duarte CG, Winnacker JL, Becker KL, Pace A: Thiazide-induced hypercalcemia. N Engl J Med 284:828–830, 1971.

118. Brickman AS, Massry SG, Coburn JW: Changes in serum and urinary calcium during treatment with hydrochlorothiazide: studies on mechanisms. J Clin Invest 51:945–954, 1972.

119. Pickleman JR, Straus FH, Forland M, Paloyan E: Thiazide-induced parathyroid stimulation. Metabolism 18:867–873, 1969.

120. Balizet L: Recurrent parathyroid adenoma. Association with prolonged thiazide administration. JAMA 225:1238–1239, 1973.

121. Pak CY, Ruskin B, Diller E: Enhancement of renal excretion of zinc by hydrochlorothiazide. Clin Chim Acta 39:511–517, 1972.

122. Wester PO: Trace elements in serum and urine from hypertensive patients before and during treatment with chlorthalidone. Acta Med Scand 194:505–512, 1973.

123. Wester PO: Urinary zinc excretion during treatment with different diuretics. Acta Med Scand 208:209–212, 1980.

124. Lim P, Jacob E: Magnesium deficiency in patients on long-term diuretic therapy for heart failure. Br Med J 620:622, 1972.

125. Seelig MS, Heggtvelt HA: Magnesium interrelationships in ischemic heart disease: a review. Am J Clin Nutr 27:59–79, 1974.

126. Whang R, Aikawa JK: Magnesium deficiency and refractoriness to potassium repletion. J Chron Dis 30:65–68, 1977.

127. Burch GE, Giles TD: The importance of magnesium deficiency in cardiovascular disease. Am Heart J 94:649–657, 1977.

128. Petersen V, Hvidt S, Thomsen K: Effect of prolonged thiazide treatment on renal lithium clearance. Br Med J 3:143–145, 1974.

129. Macfie AC: Letter: Lithium poisoning precipitated by diuretics. Br Med J 1:516, 1975.

130. Wilkins RW: New drugs for the treatment of hypertension. Ann Intern Med 50:1–10, 1959.

131. Schwab RH, Perloff JK, Porus RL: Chlorothiazide-induced gout and diabetes. Their sequential occurrence in the same patient. Arch Intern Med 111:465–470, 1963.

132. Toivonen S, Mustala O: Diabetogenic action of frusemide. Br Med J 1:920–921, 1966.

133. Kohner EM, Dollery CT, Lowy C, Schumer B: Effect of diuretic therapy on glucose tolerance in hypertension patients. Lancet 1:986–990, 1971.

134. Lewis PJ, Kohner EM, Petrie A, Dollery CT: Deterioration of glucose tolerance in hypertensive patients on prolonged diuretic treatment. Lancet 1:564–566.

135. Conn JW: Hypertension, the potassium ion and impaired carbohydrate tolerance. N Engl J Med 273:1135–1143, 1965.

136. Curtis J, Horrigan F, Ahearn D: Chlorthalidone-induced hyperosmolar hyperglycemic nonketotic coma. JAMA 220:1592–1593, 1972.

137. Cannon PJ, Stason WB, Demartini FE, Sommers SC, Laragh JH: Hyperuricemia in primary and renal hypertension. N Engl J Med 275:457–464, 1966.
138. Breckenridge A: Hypertension and hyperuricemia. Lancet 1:15–19, 1966.
139. Messerli FH, Frohlich ED, Dreslinski GR, Suarez DH, Aristimuño GG: Serum uric acid in essential hypertension – an indicator of renal vascular involvement. Ann Intern Med 93:817–821, 1980.
140. Weinman EJ, Eknoyan G, Suki WN: The influence of the extracellular fluid volume on the tubular reabsorption of uric acid. J Clin Invest 55:283–291, 1975.
141. Hall AP: Correlations among hyperuricemia, hypercholesterolemia, coronary disease and hypertension. Arthritis Rheum 8:846–852, 1965.
142. Beevers DG, Hamilton M, Harper JE: The long-term treatment of hypertension with thiazide diuretics. Postgrad Med J 47:639–643, 1971.
143. Fessel WJ: Renal outcomes of gout and hyperuricemia. Am J Med 67:74–82, 1979.
144. Berger L, Yu T-F: Renal function in gout. IV. An analysis of 524 gouty subjects including long-term follow-up studies. Am J Med 59:605–613, 1975.
145. Ames RP, Hill P: Increase in serum-lipids during treatment of hypertension with chlorthalidone. Lancet 1:721–723, 1976.
146. Goldman AI, Steele BW, Schnaper HS, Fitz AE, Frohlich ED, Perry HM Jr: Serum lipoproteins during chlorthalidone therapy. Results from a Vererans Administration/National Heart, Lung, and Blood Institute cooperative study on antihypertensive therapy: mild hypertension. JAMA 244:1691–1695, 1980.
147. Helgeland A, Leren P, Enger SC, Hjermann I, Holme I: HDL-chlolesterol in antihypertensive treatment: the Oslo study. Acta Med Scand (Suppl 625), 131–133, 1978.
148. Kannel WB, Gordon T, McGee D: Diuretics and serum-cholesterol. Lancet 1:1362–1363, 1977.
149. Grimm RH, Leon AS, Hunninghake DB, Lenz K, Hannan P, Blackburn H: Effects of thiazide diuretics on plasma lipids and lipoproteins in mildly hypertensive patients. Ann Intern Med 94:7–11, 1981.
150. Begilow RS, Pollack H et al.: The therapy of hypertension by accelerated sodium depletion. J Mount Sinai Hosp 15:223, 1948.
151. Kempner W: Treatment of kidney disease and hypertensive vascular disease with rice diet. North Carolina Med J 5:125, 1944.
152. Freis Ed, Wilson IM: Potentiating effect of chlorothiazide in combination with antihypertension agents, Preliminary report. Med Ann DC 26:468, 1957.
153. Finnerty FA, Bucholz JH, Truckman J, Hajjar GT, Hassaro GD: Evaluation of chlorothiazide in the treatment of moderately-severe hypertension. Circulation 20:1037–1942, 1959.
154. Goodman LS, Gilman A: The Pharmacologic Basis of Therapeutics, p. 817. New York: MacMillan, 1975.
155. Beerman B, Groschinsky-Grind M, Rosen A: Absorption, metabolism, and excretion of hydrochlorothiazide. Clin Pharmacol Ther 19:531–537, 1976.
156. Johnston DH, Cornish AL: Acute pancreatitis in patients receiving chlorothiazide. JAMA 170:2054–2056, 1959.
157. Shanklin DR: Pancreatic atrophy apparently secondary to hydrochlorothiazide. N Engl J Med 266:1097–1099, 1962.
158. Jones MF, Caldwell JR: Acute hemorrhagic pancreatitis associated with administration of chlorthalidone. Report of a case. N Engl J Med 267:1029–1031, 1962.
159. Diamond MT: Hyperglycemic hyperosmolar coma associated with hydrochlorothiazide and pancreatitis. NY State J Med 72:1741, 1972.
160. Drerup AL, Alexander WA: Jaundice occurring in patient treated with chlorothiazide. N Engl J Med 259:534, 1958.

161. Steinberg AD: Pulmonary edema following ingestion of hydrochlorothiazide. Ann Intern Med 78:251, 1973.
162. Beaudry C, Laplante L: Severe allergic pneumonitis from hydrochlorothiazide. Ann Intern Med 78:251, 1973.
163. Fuller TJ, Barcenas CG et al.: Diuretic induced interstitial nephritis. JAMA 235:1998, 1976.
164. Fitzgerald EW: Fatal glomerulonephritis complicating allergic purpura due to chlorothiazides. Arch Intern Med 105:303, 1960.
165. Kjellto H, Stakeberg H et al.: Possibility of thiazide induced renal necrotizing vasculitis. Lancet 1:1034, 1965.
166. Dinon LR, Kim YS et al.: Clinical experience with chlorothiazide (diuril) with particular emphasis on untoward responses: a report of 121 cases studied over 15-month period. Am J Med Sci 236:533, 1958.
167. Srivastava G, Agarival KN: Thiazide-induced bone marrow aplasia–report of a case. Indian J Pediatr 34:407, 1967.
168. Gesink MH, Bradfor HA: Thrombocytopenic purpura associated with hydrochlorothiazide therapy. JAMA 172:556, 1960.
169. Reid JM, Stevenson JG, Orr M: Non-thrombocytopenic purpura due to chlorothiazide. Scott Med J 14:309, 1969.
170. Vila JM et al.: Thiazide induced hemolytic anemia. JAMA 236:1723, 1976.
171. Perchuk E: Spastic craniofacial syndrome precipitated by diuretics. NY State J Med 75:91, 1975.
172. Srivastave RN, Travis LB et al.: Prolonged coma and visual loss: unusual reactions to chlorothiazide. J Pediatr 74:126, 1969.
173. Kaplan NM: Clinical Hypertension, 2nd edn. Baltimore: Williams & Wilkins, 1978.
174. Parijs J, Joossens JV, der Linden LV, Verstreken G, Amery AKPC: Moderate sodium restriction and diuretics in the treatment of hypertension. Am Heart J 85:22–34, 1973.
175. Carney S, Morgan T, Wilson M, Matthews G, Roberts R: Sodium restriction and thiazide diuretics in the treatment of hypertension. Med J Aust 1:803–807, 1975.
176. Magnani B, Ambrosioni E, Agosta R, Racco F: Comparison of the effects of pharmacological and a low-sodium diet on mild hypertension. Clin Sci Mol Med 51:625s–626s, 1976.
177. Safar ME, Weiss YA, Corvol PL, Menard JE, London GM, Milliez PL: Antihypertensive adrenergic-blocking agents: effects on sodium balance, the renin-angiotensin system in haemodynamics. Clin Sci Mol Med (Suppl 2) 48:93s–95s, 1975.
178. Guazzi M, Magrini F, Fiorentini C, Polese A: Role of the sympathetic nervous system in supporting cardiac function in essential arterial hypertension. Br Heart J 35:55–64, 1973.
179. Tarazi RC, Dustan HP: Beta adrenergic blockade in hypertension. Practical and theoretical implications of long-term hemodynamic variations. Am J Cardiol 29:633–640, 1972.
180. Wilburn RL, Blaufuss A, Bennett CM: Long-term treatment of severe hypertension with minoxidil, propranolol and furosemide. Circulation 52:706–713, 1975.
181. Huang Cm, Atkinson AJ et al.: Pharmacokinetics of orally administered furosemide. Clin Pharmacol Ther 16:659, 1974.
182. Greenblatt DJ, Duhme DW et al.: Clinical toxicity of furosemide in hospitalized patients. Am Heart J 94:6, 1977.
183. Sherlock S, Walder JG: The complications of diuretic therapy in patients with cirrhosis. Ann NY Acad Sci 139:497, 1958.
184. Kelley MR, Cutler RE et al.: Pharmacokinetics of orally administered furosemide. Clin Pharmacol Ther 15:178, 1974.
185. Macherty I: Sudden death after intramuscular furosemide. Lancet 2:1301, 1968.

186. Sharefkin JB, Silen W: Diuretic agents: inciting factors in non-occulsive mesenteric infarction. JAMA 229:1451, 1974.
187. Jones PE, Oelbaum MH: Furosemide induced pancreatitis. Br Med J 1:133, 1975.
188. Burke GJ: Non-ketotic, hyponatremic, normosmolar, diabetic coma and moderate furosemide therapy. South African Med J 50:2118, 1976.
189. Furey JN, Lawrence JR: Phototoxic blisters from high furosemide dose. Br J Dermatol 94:495, 1976.
190. Hendricks WM, Ader RS: Furosemide induced cutaneous necrotizing vasculitis. Arch Dermatol 113:375, 1977.
191. Greenblatt DJ, Duhme DW et al.: Clinical toxicity of furosemide in hospitalized patients. Am Heart J 94:6, 1977.
192. Lyons H, Pinn VW et al.: Allergic interstitial nephritis causing reversible renal failure in four patients with idiopathic nephrotic syndrome. N Engl J Med 288:124, 1973.
193. Fuller TJ, Barcenas CG et al.: Diuretic induced interstitial nephritis. JAMA 235:1998, 1976.
194. Willets GS: Ocular side effects of drugs. Br J Ophthalmol 53:252, 1969.
195. Schwartz GH, David DS et al.: Ototoxicity induced by furosemide. N Engl J Med 282:1413, 1970.
196. Venkateswaran PS: Transient deafness from high dose furosemide Br Med J 4:113, 1971.
197. Cooperman LB, Rubin IL: Toxicity of ethacrynic acid and furosemide. Am Heart J 85:831–834, 1973.
198. MacGregor GA, Tasker PR et al.: Diuretic induced edema. Lancet 1:489, 1975.
199. Norbiato G, Sommariva D et al.: Diuretic induced edema. Lancet 2:1304, 1975.
200. Churcher A: Diuretic induced edema. Lancet 1:90, 1976.
201. Liddle GW: Specific and non-specific inhibition of mineralocorticoid activity. Metabolism 10:1021–1030, 1961.
202. McMahon FG: Management of Essential Hypertension, p. 138. New York: Futura, 1978.
203. Cranston WI et al.: Effect of triamterene on elevated arterial pressure. Am Heart J 68:455, 1965.
204. Greenblatt DJ, Koch-Weser J: Adverse reactions to spironolactone. JAMA 225:40–43, 1973.
205. Spark RF, Melby JC: Aldosteronism in hypertension: the spironolactone response test. Ann Intern Med 69:685, 1968.
206. Levitt JI: Spironolactone therapy and amenorrhea. JAMA 211:2014, 1970.
207. Rose LI, Underwood RH, Newmark SR, Kisch ES, Williams GH: Pathophysiology of spironolactone-induced gynecomastia. Ann Intern Med 87:398–403, 1977.
208. Cranston WI, Juel-Jensen BE: The effects of spironolactone and chlorthalidone on arterial pressure. Lancet 1:1161, 1962.
209. Hansen KB, Bender AD: Changes in serum potassium levels occurring in patients treated with triamterene and a triamterene-hydrochlorothiazide combination. Clin Pharmacol Ther 8:392, 1966.
210. Ettinger B, Norman OO, Sörgel F: Triamterene nephrolithiasis. JAMA 244:2443–2445, 1980.
211. Lieberman FL,Bateman JR: Megaloblastic anemia possibly induced by triamterene in patients with alcoholic cirrhosis. Ann Intern Med 68:168, 1968.
212. Corcino J et al.: Mechanism of triamterene-induced megablastosis. Ann Intern Med 73:419, 1970.
213. Hansen KB, Bender AD: Changes in serum potassium levels occurring in patients treated with triamterene and a triamterene-hydrochlorothiazide combination. Clin Pharmacol Ther 8:392–399, 1967.

742

214. Crane MG, Harris JJ: Effect of spironolactone in hypertensive patients. Am J Med Sci 260:311, 1970.
215. Flanagan MJ et al.: Primary aldosteronism. J Urology 88:111, 1962.
216. Spark RF, Melby JC: Aldosteronism in hypertension: the spironolactone response test. Ann Intern Med 69:685, 1968.

46. BETA-ADRENOCEPTOR BLOCKING DRUGS AS ANTIHYPERTENSIVE AGENTS

LENNART HANSSON

Following Ahlquist's definition, in 1948, of alpha- and beta-adrenoceptors [1], it took ten years until the first beta-adrenoceptor blocking agent, di-chloroisoprenaline was shown to exert a pharmacological effect [2]. Clinically useful beta-adrenoceptor blocking drugs such as pronethalol and propanolol were introduced in the early 1960s and the first report of the antihypertensive effect caused by beta-adrenoceptor blockade was published by Prichard in 1964 [3].

Since then numerous studies have demonstrated that elevated arterial pressure can be reduced by treatment with 'non-selective' beta-adrenoceptor blockers (i.e. compounds having the same affinity to $beta_1$- and $beta_2$-adrenoceptors) such as propranolol [4-7], alprenolol [8, 9], pindolol [10], oxprenolol [11], and timolol [12] as well as with $beta_1$-selective blockers (i.e. agents with a greater afinity to $beta_1$- than to $beta_2$-adrenoceptors) such as practolol [13], atenolol [14, 15], metoprolol [16] and acebutolol [17]. The antihypertensive potency appears to be quite similar with all these agents and such factors as $beta_1$-selectivity, intrinsic sympathomimetic activity (ISA) or membrane stabilizing activity appear to have no influence on the efficacy in this respect. Several studies in which patients with mild to moderate hypertension have been treated show a reduction in systolic blood pressure of about 20 mm Hg and of diastolic blood pressure of about 15 mm Hg [18-22]. In patients with mild to moderate hypertension the blood pressure lowering effect caused by beta-adrenoceptor blockade is usually of the same order as that obtained during treatment with thiazide diuretics [23, 24]. However, in a few open studies comprising large numbers of patients a more conspicuous antihypertensive effect has been reported from the use of propranolol [25-27]. In these trials patients with severe hypertension were included and the dosage of propranolol was considerably higher than what is commonly recommended today.

SIDE EFFECTS

The antihypertensive efficacy of beta-adrenoceptor blocking agents has already been dealt with above. For practical purposes it can be regarded as

Amery, A. (ed.) Hypertensive Cardiovascular Disease: Pathophysiology and Treatment
© 1982, Martinus Nijhoff Publishers. The Hague / Boston / London
ISBN-13: 978-94-009-7478-4

Table 1. Side effects leading to withdrawal of antihypertensive treatment with diuretics or beta-adrenoceptor blocking drugs during the first year of therapy in 666 male patients

Beta-adrenoceptor blocker group (n = 325)		Diuretic group (n = 341)	
Side effect	Number of withdrawals	Side effect	Number of withdrawals
Gastrointestinal	7	S-potassium <3.4 nmol/l	22
Sleep disturbance	6	S-urate >8.5 mg/100 ml	7
Airways obstruction	2	Gout	3
Bradycardia	1	Diabetes mellitus	4
Miscellaneous	10	Miscellaneous	10
Total	26 (8%)	Total	46 (14%)

almost identical to that of diuretics. The fact that beta-adrenoceptor blocking drugs are frequently taking the place of diuretics as the drug of first choice in the treatment of hypertension thus must be attributed to some other fact. Since efficacy and side effects are the two most important factors for selecting any therapy above another, the side effects of beta-adrenoceptor blocking drugs will be put in relation to those observed during thiazide

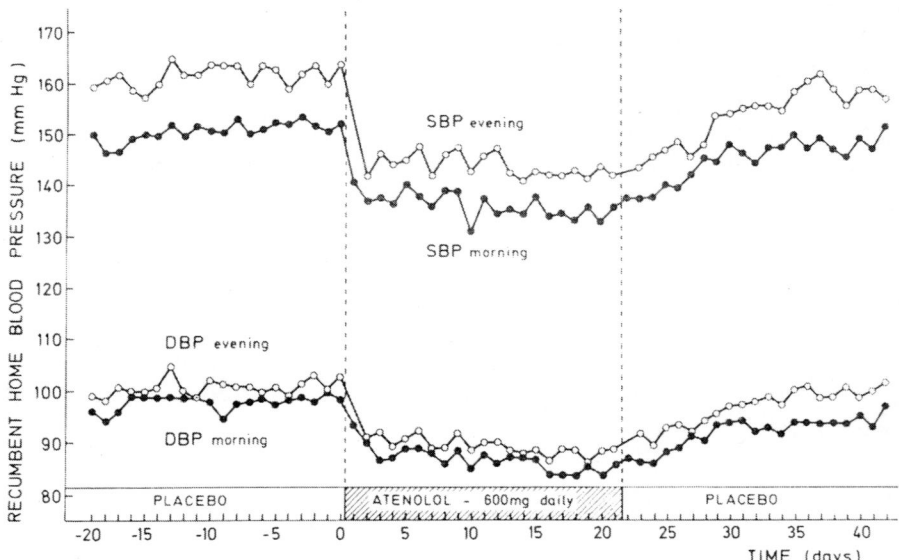

Figure 1. Timing of the fall in blood pressure produced by β-blockade produced ICI 66,082 (Tenormin). From Amery et al.[30], with permission of *Clinical Pharmacology and Therapeutics,* Published by The C.V. Mosby Co.

therapy. Side effects that caused withdrawal of either diuretics or beta-adrenoceptor blockers during the first year of therapy in 666 middle-aged male hypertensive patients are shown in Table 1 [28]. Obviously withdrawal of therapy due to side effects was less common in the beta-adrenoceptor blocker group than in the thiazide group. This is perhaps less important than the fact that electrolyte and metabolic disturbances were more common in the thiazide group, whereas the dominating side effects in the beta-adrenoceptor group were subjectively noticeable. They were also encountered early during therapy and both these facts make it possible to change dosage or to withdraw therapy early after the occurrence of side effects, which is in some contrast to thiazide induced side effects.

The immunological side effects caused by practolol and which in some cases caused blindness and other serious complications appear to have been unique to this particular compound and have not been seen with other beta-adrenoceptor blocking drugs [29].

Side effects related to the blockade of beta-adrenoceptors, e.g. precipitation of cardiac failure or worsening of bronchial asthma were expected to become major problems during the early days of beta-adrenoceptor blocking therapy. However, by and large, it has been possible to avoid these problems by adequate selection of patients.

TIME COURSE OF ACTION

Unlike the beta-adrenoceptor blockade which can be seen within minutes of having administered therapy i.v., e.g. as a reduction in heart rate, the onset of the antihypertensive effect is gradual (Figure 1) [30]. Usually several days will be needed in order to achieve the full antihypertensive effect [31–33]. The antihypertensive effect also disappears gradually following cessation of therapy, whereas heart rate increases more rapidly, perhaps within 24 h of stopping therapy [31]. Some studies have shown that it may take several weeks for the antihypertensive effect to disappear completely [30, 34]. In other words, it is obvious that the time course of the antihypertensive effect of beta-adrenoceptor blocking drugs is different from that of the cardiac beta-adrenoceptor blockade and this is supported by several hemodynamic studies [12, 35–38].

PREDICTABILITY OF RESPONSE

Unless any given therapy is uniformly effective, which is rare indeed and certainly not true of the antihypertensive effect caused by beta-adrenoceptor blocking agents, it is often of interest to find factors or means by which the therapeutic effect can be predicted. As regards the antihypertensive effect of

746

Table 2. Factors that do not predict the antihypertensive response to beta-adrenoceptor blockade

1. Age
2. Weight
3. Heart rate
4. Cardiac output
5. Total peripheral resistance
6. Plasma renin activity
7. Heart rate response to isoprenaline infusion
8. Urinary noradrenelaine excretion
9. Urinary adrenaline excretion
10. Urinary aldosterone excretion

beta-adrenoceptor blockers studies have been performed aiming at identifying such predictive factors [39, 40]. The variables used in one such study [40] are given in Table 2. Unfortunately, all attempts at predicting the therapeutic response have so far been negative. This means that the use of beta-adrenoceptor blocking drugs in hypertension still remains a trial-and-error affair, as it is in most other kinds of antihypertensive therapy.

MODE OF ACTION

Numerous papers have been written about the mechanisms by which beta-adrenoceptor blocking drugs reduce blood pressure. The difference in time course of the antihypertensive effect and the beta-adrenoceptor blocking effect discussed above is easily detected in hemodynamic investigations. After acute administration of a beta-adrenoceptor blocking drug heart rate and cardiac output fall within minutes, whereas a corresponding rise in total peripheral resistance takes place. However, the net effect of these marked hemodynamic changes is that arterial pressure remains unchanged (Figure 2). Not until a few hours or days later does the arterial pressure drop due to a readjustment of total peripheral resistance down towards the initial level. It is by no means clear why this late change of total vascular resistance takes place in patients who respond to therapy. In hypertensive patients not responding to beta-adrenoceptor blocking therapy total peripheral resistance remains elevated, whereas the reduction in cardiac output is the same as in responding patients [41].

In other words two components of the antihypertensive response can be identified: (a) a reduction in cardiac output due to cardiac beta-adrenoceptor blockade, and (b) a 'delayed vasodilator effect'. The mechanism underlying (b) remains to be elucidated and also the fact why (b) fails to take place in non-responding patients. It should be pointed out, though, that the response pattern can show great individual variations. Thus, both during treatment with propranolol and metoprolol, patients have been identified in

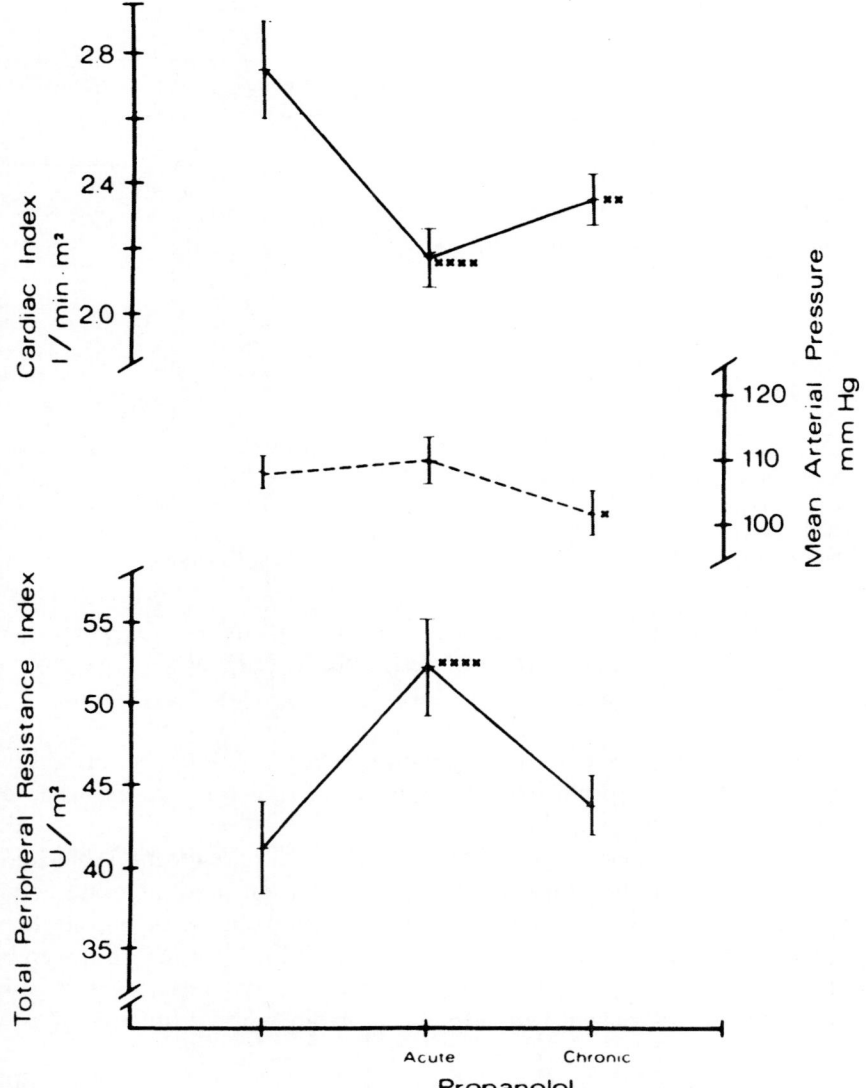

Figure 2. Effects of acute I.V. (0.22 mg/kg) and 4 weeks of oral propanolol (160-320 mg daily) on cardiac index, mean arterial pressure (dashed lines) and total peripheral resistance index [37].

whom the reduction in blood pressure could be ascribed solely to a reduction in total peripheral resistance without any fall in cardiac output [42, 36].

It seems likely that the 'delayed vasodilator effect' is related to beta$_1$-adrenoceptor blockade which causes the reduction in heart rate and cardiac

748

Table 3. Relation between various actions of beta-adrenoceptor blocking drugs and their anti-hypertensive action

Compound	Blocks Beta$_1$-adrenoceptor	Blocks beta$_2$-adrenoceptor	ISA [1]	Membrane stabilizing effect	Antihypertensive effect
Division I [2]					
Group I	+	+	+	+	+
Group II	+	+	−	+	+
Group III	+	+	+	−	+
Group IV	+	+	−	−	+
Division II [3]					
Group I	+	−	+	+	+
Group III	+	−	+	−	+
Group IV	+	−	−	−	+

[1] ISA: Intrinsic sympathomimetic activity.
[2] Group I: Oxprenolol, alprenolol. Group II: Propranolol. Group III: Pindolol. Group IV: Sotalol.
[3] Group I: Acebutolol. Group III: Practolol. Group IV: Atenolol, metoprolol.

output. Many suggestions have been made in an attempt to explain the gradual reduction of total peripheral resistance [43]. However, two principally different explanations emerge [44].

1. Autoregulation. Due to the reduction in cardiac output a certain degree of long standing underperfusion leads to an autoregulatory process whereby total vascular resistance is reduced.

2. Reduced vasoconstrictor nerve activity. Beta-adrenoceptor blockade acting within the central nervous system, possibly on pre-junctional beta$_1$-adrenoceptors [45], would cause a reduced sympathetic nerve activity and in turn a reduction of vascular resistance. Support for this theory is given by the findings that a gradual reduction in transmitter synthesis takes place in sympathetic ganglia during beta-adrenoceptor blocking treatment [46].

Other theories, e.g. that the local anesthetic effect of beta-adrenoceptor blockers would be of importance can be discarded since the dextro-isomer of e.g. propranolol does not possess the antihypertensive effect of the racemic form in spite of possessing the same membrane stabilizing effect [47–49]. The theories involving plasma renin activity as an indicator and mediator of the antihypertensive effect have also been refuted. In some early studies, the observation was made that hypertensive patients with high plasma renin activity in relation to their 24-h urinary sodium excretion, responded particularly well to beta-adrenoceptor blockade, and the claim was made that patients should be selected based upon their renin status and also that the antihypertensive effect was directly related to the renin lowering effect of beta-adrenoceptor blockade [50, 51]. These findings have not been confirmed in several later studies [41, 52–54] and, as pointed out above, plasma renin activity can not be used as a clinical tool in predicting the therapeutic response.

Since many of the beta-adrenoceptor blocking compounds have actions in addition to their ability to block beta-adrenoceptors, it may be worthwhile to point out that, from a pharmacological point of view, the blockade of $beta_1$-adrenoceptor is the conditio sine qua non for the antihypertensive action (Table 3).

COMBINED THERAPY

Beta-adrenoceptor blocking drugs can be combined with most other antihypertensive compounds in order to enhance the blood pressure lowering effect. Although beta-adrenoceptor blockers, in contrast to many other antihypertensive drugs, do not cause an expansion of the plasma volume [55–57] a combination with diuretics is frequently used in order to augment the effect [25, 26]. Of potentially greater interest is the combined use with a vasodilator substance. Since most forms of established hypertension are characterized by a normal cardiac output and an elevated total peripheral resistance [58], a vasodilator would appear to be the ideal drug for correction of the hemodynamic abnormality. However, due to the baroreceptor mediated reflex increase in sympathetic tone a vasodilator alone would not be effective. Obviously, a combination with a beta-adrenoceptor blocking drug would prevent the effects of increased sympathetic discharge, e.g. to the heart or the kidneys. In clinical practice such a combination has been shown to be quite effective [59–62]. Other combinations between antihypertensive agents and a beta-adrenoceptor blocking drug can be used, although the combined use with a diuretic or a vasodilator such as hydralazine (or both) is probably most effective. One combination should be avoided, viz. that between clonidine and a beta-adrenoceptor blocking drug. Since abrupt cessation of clonidine can cause a dramatic rise in blood pressure associated with a marked elevation of plasma catecholamine levels [63], it is obvious that blockade of particularly $beta_2$-adrenoceptors would increase the hazard in this situation, since $beta_2$-adrenoceptor mediated vasodilatation would be prevented.

CARDIOPROTECTIVE EFFECT

Much interest has been devoted to the so called cardioprotective effects of beta-adrenoceptor blocking drugs. The first positive controlled trial was published in 1974 [64]. In this trial a significant reduction in the incidence of sudden death was seen in post-infarction patients treated with alprenolol for two years. Support for this view has been obtained in studies with practolol [65] as well as in further studies with alprenolol [66]. A beneficial, secondary preventive effect with beta-adrenoceptor blocking therapy in post-infarction patients has been shown also with timolol, metoprolol and propranolol. Even if a 'cardioprotective effect' has been established when beta-adrenoceptor blocking therapy was administered to post-infarction patients, it does not immediately follow that such a beneficial effect should be expected also in other kinds of patients, e.g. hypertensives. The claim has been made, however, that hypertensives treated with beta-adrenoceptor blockers have a lower risk of developing a myocardial infarction than patients treated with other forms of antihypertensive agents [67]. This impression gained some support from observations in a large number of middle-aged men with mild hypertension in whom treatment with beta-adrenoceptor blocking drugs, mainly propranolol and alprenolol, reduced the incidence of myocardial infarctions by about 50% in comparison to untreated patients [68]. However, until controlled comparisons between beta-adrenoceptor blockers and other kinds of antihypertensive drugs are available to support the existence of a cardioprotective effect, the matter must be regarded as unresolved.

CONCLUSIONS

All beta-adrenoceptor blocking drugs can be used in antihypertensive treatment. Differences in antihypertensive efficacy between various compounds are negligible, although such a factor as $beta_1$-adrenoceptor selectivity can offer other advantages. Moreover, a compound with marked ISA appears to reduce blood pressure more physiologically by reducing vascular resistance [69]. These drugs can be used as monotherapy in mild cases of hypertension and their efficacy is similar to that of diuretics. Their spectrum of side effects compares favorably with that of diuretics and for this reason beta-adrenoceptor blocking drugs are frequently used as alternatives to diuretics as the drug of first choice in hypertension. Combined therapy with diuretics or vasodilators or both can be useful.

The mode of action is not yet fully elucidated although the hemodynamic effects are well known. Finally, additional positive effects, in particular the so called 'cardioprotective effect' remain to be established. At present, this effect can be regarded as a factor which offers some hope for the future. If the cardioprotective effect were to be confirmed in future studies, it would certainly constitute a valuable positive effect not offered by other presently available anithypertensive compounds.

REFERENCES

1. Ahlquist RP: A study of the adrenotropic receptors. Am J Physiol 153:586–600, 1948.
2. Powell CE, Slater IH: Blocking of inhibitory adrenergic receptors by a dichoroanalogue of isoproterenol. J Pharmacol 122:480–488, 1958.
3. Prichard BNC: Hypotensive action of pronethalol. Br Med J I:1227–1227, 1964.
4. Prichard BNC, Gillam PMS: Use of propranolol ('Inderal') in treatment of hypertension. Br Med J II:725–727, 1964.
5. Prichard BNC, Gillam PMS: Propranolol in hypertension. Am J Cardiol 18:387–391, 1966.
6. Lydtin H, Kusus T, Daniel W, Schierl W, Achenheil M, Kempter H, Lohmöller G, Niklas M, Walter L: Propranolol therapy in essential hypertension. Am Heart J 83:589–595, 1972.
7. Zacharias FJ, Cowen KJ: Controlled trial of propranolol in hypertension. Br Med J I:471–474, 1970.
8. Tibblin G, Åblad B: Antihypertensive therapy with alprenolol, a beta-adrenergic receptor antagonist. Acta Med Scand 186:451–457, 1969.
9. Bengtsson C: Comparison between alpenolol and propranolol as antihypertensive agents. Acta Med Scand 192:415–418, 1972.
10. Morgan TO, Louis WJ, Dawborn JK, Doyle AE: The use of pindolol (Visken) in the treatment of hypertension. Med J Aust 2:309–312, 1972.
11. Eisalo A, Loumanmäki K, Heikkilä J: Hemodynamic effects of Trasicor, a new beta-adrenergic blocking agent, in hypertensive patients. Acta Med Scand 186:105–109, 1969.
12. Franciosa JA, Freis ED, Conway FJ: Antihypertensive and hemodynamic properties of the new beta-adrenergic blocking agent timolol. Circulation 48:118–124, 1973.
13. Esler MD, Nestle PJ: Evaluation of practolol in hypertension. Br Heart J 35:469–474, 1973.
14. Hansson L, Åberg H, Karlberg BE, Westerlund A: Controlled study of atenolol in treatment of hypertension. Br Med J I:367–370, 1975.
15. Amery A, Billiet L, Boel A, Fagard R, Reybrouck T, Willems J: Mechanism of hypertensive effect during beta-adrenergic blockade in hypertensive patients. Hemodynamic and renin response to a new cardioselective agent; tenormin or ICI 66082. Am Heart J 91:634–642, 1976.
16. Bengtsson C: The effect of metoprolol – a new selective $beta_1$-receptor blocking agent – in mild hypertension. Acta Med Scand 199:65–70, 1976.
17. Hansson L, Berglund G, Andersson O, Holm M: Controlled trial of acebutolol in hypertension. Eur J Clin Pharmacol 12:89–92, 1977.
18. Frohlich ED, Tarazi RC, Dustan HP, Page IH: The paradox of beta-adrenergic blockade in hypertension. Circulation 37:417–423, 1968.
19. Richardson DW, Freund J, Gear AS, Mauch HP Jr, Preston LW: Effect of propranolol on elevated arterial blood pressure. Circulation 37:534–542, 1968.
20. Dorph S, Binder C: Evaluation of the hypotensive effect of beta-adrenergic blockade in hypertension. Acta Med Scand 185:443–448, 1969.
21. Hansson L, Åberg H, Jameson S, Karlberg BE, Malmcrona R: Initial clinical experience with ICI 66082, a new beta-adrenergic blocking agent, in hypertension. Acta Med Scand 194:549–550, 1973.
22. Bengtsson C: Comparison between metoprolol and propranolol as antihypertensive agents. A double-blind crossover study. Acta Med Scand 199:71–74, 1976.
23. Paterson JW, Dollery CT: Effect of propranolol in mild hypertension. Lancet II:1148–1150, 1966.
24. Bengtsson C: Comparison between alprenolol and chlorthalidone as antihypertensive agents. Acta Med Scand 191:422–439, 1972.

25. Prichard BNC, Gillam PMS: Treatment of hypertension with propranolol. Br Med J I:7-16, 1969.
26. Zacharias FJ, Cowen KJ, Prestt J, Vickers J, Wall BG: Propranolol in hypertension: a study of long-term therapy, 1964-1970. Am Heart J 83:755-761, 1972.
27. Hansson L, Malmcrona R, Olander R, Rosenhall L, Westerlund A, Åberg H, Hood B: Propranolol in hypertension. Report on 158 patients treated up to one year. Klin Wochenschr 50:364-369, 1972.
28. Werkö L: The place of beta-adrenergic blocking drugs in the treatment of mild to moderate arterial hypertension. In: Pathophysiology and Management of Arterial Hypertension, pp. 228-233. Berglund G, Hansson L, Werkö L, eds. Mölndal: Lindgren & Söner, 1975.
29. Wright P: Ocular reactions to beta-blocking drugs. Br Med J IV:577-580, 1976.
30. Amery A, De Plaen JF, Lijnen P, McKinsh J, Reybrouck F: Relationship between blood level of atendol and pharmacologic effect. Clin Pharmacol Ther 21:691-699, 1977.
31. Simpson FO, Waal-Manning HJ: Hypertension and beta-adrenergic blockade, In: New Horizons in Medicine, p. 59. Sydney: Sandoz, 1970.
32. Bühler FR, Burkart F, Lütold BE, Bertel O, Pristerer M: Plasma-Katecholamine und Hämodynamik im Verlauf der antihypertensiven Betablockade: verschiedene Muster bei 'Propranolol-Responders' und 'Non-Responders'. Schw Med Wochenschr 107:1590-1591, 1977.
33. Zacharias FJ: Propranolol in hypertension: a 5-year study. Postgrad Med J 47 (Suppl):75-80, 1971.
34. Vedin AJ, Wilhelmsson CE, Werkö L: Comparative study of alprenolol and methyldopa in previously untreated essential hypertension. Br Heart J 35:1285-1292, 1973.
35. Tarazi RC, Dustan HP: Beta-adrenergic blockade in hypertension. Practical and theoretical implications of long-term hemodynamic variations. Am J Cardiol 29:633-640, 1972.
36. Sannerstedt R: Hemodynamic effects of adrenergic beta-receptor blocking agents in arterial hypertension. In: Pathophysiology and Management of Arterial Hypertension, pp. 194-200. Berglund G, Hansson L, Werkö L, eds. Mölndal: Lindgren & Söner, 1975.
37. Hansson L, Zweifler AJ, Julius S, Hunyor SN: Hemodynamic effects of acute and prolonged beta-adrenergic blockade in essential hypertension. Acta Med Scand 196:27-34, 1974.
38. Ulrych M, Frohlich ED, Dustan HP, Page IH: Immediate hemodynamic effects of beta-adrenergic blockade with propranolol in normotensive and hypertensive man. Circulation 37:411-416, 1968.
39. Birkenhäger WH, Krauss XH, Schalekamp MADH, Kolsters G, Kroon BJM: Antihypertensive effects of propranolol. Observations on predictability. Folia Med Neerl 14:67-72, 1971.
40. Hansson L, Zweifler AJ, Julius S, Ellis CN: Propranolol therapy in essential hypertension. Observations on predictability of therapeutic response. Int J Clin Pharmacol 10:79-85, 1974.
41. Hansson L: Beta-adrenergic blockade in essential hypertension. Acta Med Scand 550 (Suppl):1-40, 1973.
42. Guazzi M, Polese A, Fiorentini C, Olivari MT, Magrini F: Functional changes of the hypertensive heart following treatment with beta-blocking agents. In: The Arterial Hypertensive Disease, pp. 358-364. Rorive G, Van Cauwenberge H, eds. Liege: Masson, 1975.
43. Lewis PJ: The essential action of propranolol in hypertension. Am J Med 60:837-852, 1976.
44. Åblad B, Almgren O, Ljung B, Sannerstedt R: Mechanism of action of beta-adrenoceptor antagonists in hypertension. In: The Pathophysiology of Human Hypertension pp. 155-167. Lund-Johansen P, ed. Trosa: Trosa Tryckeri, 1979.
45. Dahlöf C, Åblad B, Borg KO, Ek L, Waldeck B: Prejunctional inhibition of adrenergic nervous vasomotor control due to beta-receptor blockade, In: Chemical Tools in Catecholamine Research - II, pp. 201-210. Almgren O, Carlson A, Engel J, eds. Amsterdam: North-Holland, 1975.

46. Raine AEG, Chubb IW: Long term beta-adrenergic blockade reduces tyrosine hydroxylas and dopamine-beta-hydroxylase activities in sympathetic ganglia. Nature 267:265–267, 1977.
47. Waal-Manning HJ: Lack of effect of d-propranolol on blood pressure and pulse rate in hypertensive patients. Proc Univ Otago Med School 48:80–81, 1970.
48. Prichard BNC, Boakes AJ: The use of drugs with beta and alpha inbibitory action to treat hypertension, p. 185. (Abstracts) Fifth Int Congr Pharmacol. San Francisco, 1972.
49. Rahn KH, Hawlina A, Kersting F, Plantz G: Studies on the antihypertensive action of optical isomers of propranolol in man. Naunyn Schmiedebergs Arch Pharmacol 286:319–323, 1974.
50. Bühler FR, Laragh JH, Baer L, Vaughan ED Jr, Brunner HR: Propranolol inhibition of renin secretion. N Engl J Med 287:1209–1216, 1972.
51. Laragh JH, Bühler FR: Propranolol, renin and hypertension: a review. Postgrad Med J 52 (Suppl 4):109–115, 1976.
52. Bravo EL, Tarazi RC, Dustan HP, Lewis JW: Dissociation between renin and arterial pressure responses to beta-adrenergic blockade in human essential hypertension. Circ Res 36 (Suppl 1):1241–1247, 1975.
53. Julius S, Esler M, Hansson L, Zweifler AJ: Dissociation of the renin lowering and antihypertensive actions of propranolol. In: Advances in clinical pharmacology, Hitzenberger G, ed. München-Wien-Baltimore: Urban & Schwartzenberg, 1976, pp. 33–41.
54. Amery A, Billiet L, Fagard R: Beta receptors and renin release. N Engl J Med 290:284, 1974.
55. Tarazi RC, Frohlich ED, Dustan HP: Plasma volume changes with long-term beta-adrenergic blockade. Am Heart J 82:770–776, 1971.
56. Sederberg-Olsen P, Ibsen H: Plasma volume and extracellular fluid volume during long term treatment with propranolol in essential hypertension. Clin Sci 43:165–170, 1972.
57. Parving HH, Gyntelberg F: Albumin transcapillary escape rate and plasma volume during long-term beta-adrenergic blockade in essential hypertension. Scand J Clin Lab Invest 32:105–110, 1973.
58. Lund-Johansen P: Central hemodynamics in essential hypertension. Acta Med Scand, 606 (Suppl):35–42, 1977.
59. Hansson L, Olander R, Åberg H, Malmcrona R, Westerlund A: treatment of hypertension with propranolol and hydralazine. Acta Med Scand 190:531–534, 1971.
60. Gilmore E, Weil J, Chidsey C: Treatment of essential hypertension with a new vasodilator in combination with beta-adrenergic blockade. N Engl J Med 282:521–527, 1970.
61. Katila M, Frick MH: Combined dihydralazine and propranolol in the treatment of hypertension. Int J Clin Pharmacol Ther Toxicol 4:111–115, 1970.
62. Lund-Johansen P: Hemodynamic long-term effects of prazosin plus tolamolol in essential hypertension. Br J Clin Pharmacol 4:141–146, 1977.
63. Hansson L, Hunyor SN, Julius S, Hoobler SW: Blood pressure crisis following withdrawal of clonidine, with special reference to arterial and urinary catecholamine levels, and suggestions for acute management. Am Heart J 85:605610, 1973.
64. Wilhelmsson C, Vedin JA, Wilhelmsen L, Tibblin G, Werkö L: Reduction of sudden deaths after myocardial infarction by treatment with alprenolol. Lancet II:1157–1160, 1974.
65. Multicentre Trial: Improvement in prognosis of myocardial infarction by long-term beta-adrenoceptor blockade using practolol. Br Med J III:735–740, 1975.
66. Andersen MP, Bechsgaard P, Fredriksen J, Hansen DA, Jürgensen HJ, Nielsen B, Pedersen F, Pedersen-Bjergaard O, Rasmussen SL: Effect of alprenolol on mortality among patients with definite or suspected acute myocardial infarction. Lancet II:865–868, 1979.
67. Lambert DMD: Hypertension and myocardial infarction. Br Med J III:685, 1974.
68. Berglund G, Wilhelmsen L, Sannerstedt R, Hansson L, Andersson O, Sivertsson R, Wedel

H, Wikstrand J: Coronary heart disease after treatment of hypertension. Lancet I:1-5, 1978.
69. Svensson A, Gudbrandsson T, Sivertsson R, Hansson L: Metoprolol and pindolol in hypertension: different effects on peripheral haemodynamics. Clin Sci 61:425s–427s, 1981.

47. ALPHA-ADRENOCEPTOR ANTAGONISTS IN HYPERTENSION

S. H. TAYLOR

The therapeutic potential of alpha-adrenoceptor antagonists in patients with sustained elevation of the blood pressure can be fully realised only if based on an understanding of their pharmacodynamic activity when superimposed upon the circulatory pathophysiology of the hypertensive state. This chapter will therefore concentrate on the haemodynamic abnormality in essential hypertension and the way in which this may be modulated by drugs which interfere with the alpha-adrenoceptor neuroeffector mechanisms in the cardiovascular system.

THE HAEMODYNAMIC BASIS OF ESSENTIAL HYPERTENSION

During the past two decades the haemodynamic profile of essential hypertension has gradually emerged [1–3]. Controversies that have arisen have been due to the failure to recognise that each of the many and superficially separate circulatory patterns that have been described have done nothing more than illuminate cross-sectional facets of the longitudinal course of the disease. It is important therefore to review the evolution of the haemodynamic abnormality in hypertension before considering the place of therapeutic intervention with alpha-adrenoceptor antagonists.

Evolution of haemodynamic abnormality

Consideration of the simplistic relationship between the various dynamic components contributing to the blood pressure facilitates understanding of the haemodynamic events that occur during the long drawn out course of the disease.

$$\text{Blood pressure (mean)} \propto CO \times SVR \times V/C$$

At constant arterial volume and capacity the blood pressure is determined by a hyperbolic relationship between cardiac output and systemic vascular resistance (Figure 1). Hypertensive patients are selectively congregated to-

Amery, A. (ed.) Hypertensive Cardiovascular Disease: Pathophysiology and Treatment
© 1982, Martinus Nijhoff Publishers. The Hague / Boston / London
ISBN-13: 978-94-009-7478-4

756

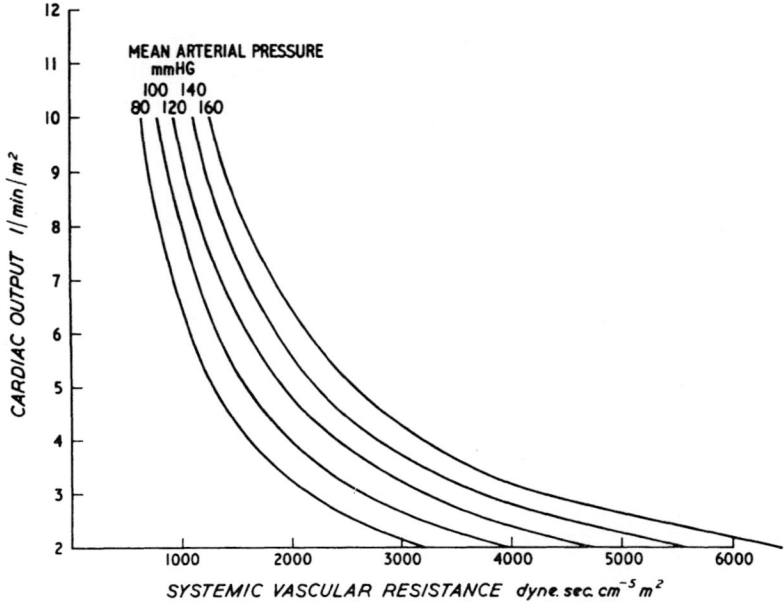

Figure 1. Relationship of minute cardiac output, integrated (mean) arterial blood pressure and calculated systemic vascular resistance at constant arterial volume.

wards the resistance axis so that at any given level of cardiac output the peripheral resistance is greater in the hypertensive than in the normal subject. However, this oft-quoted generalisation obscures the steady haemodynamic progression of the disease. In early, borderline, or labile hypertension the circulatory abnormality is characterised by an elevated cardiac output and an inappropriately normal peripheral vascular resistance, i.e. the resistance is similar in absolute terms to that in normal subjects but greater than would be expected at that level of output. It has been suggested that this increase in cardiac output is in response to an expanded circulating blood volume [4]. However, it is by no means assured that this ingenious explanation is the driving force to the increased cardiac output observed in some patients and it is by no means certain that all patients who eventually develop sustained hypertension pass through this hyperkinetic early stage. Even when it exists, this early cardiac output dominated increase in blood pressure rapidly gives way to a circulatory pattern in which the raised blood pressure is entirely attributable to the raised vascular resistance, i.e. the cardiac output is normal. This is the haemodynamic profile usually described in patients with established essential hypertension, as it is at this stage of the disease that it is usually most frequently detected. Although this pattern apparently persists unchanged for years longitudinal studies have disclosed the insidious haemodynamic progression of the disease with gradually increasing vascular resistance and gradually reducing cardiac output. Eventually the limit of left ventricular myocardial reserve of the ageing heart is reached, which despite hypertrophy can no longer pump efficiently at a normal filling volume. This end stage of essential hypertension is characterised haemodynamically by a subnormal cardiac output and rapid rise in peripheral vascular resistance. Left ventricular failure is the final haemodynamic consequence of untreated elevation of the blood pressure, but this must not be allowed to obscure the intrinsic arterial hazard of hypertension. Although effective antihypertensive treatment, so readily available in so many communities, has vastly reduced the risk of heart failure, high pressure damage to the coronary, cerebral and renal arteries continues to remain a real terminal threat to the hypertensive patient.

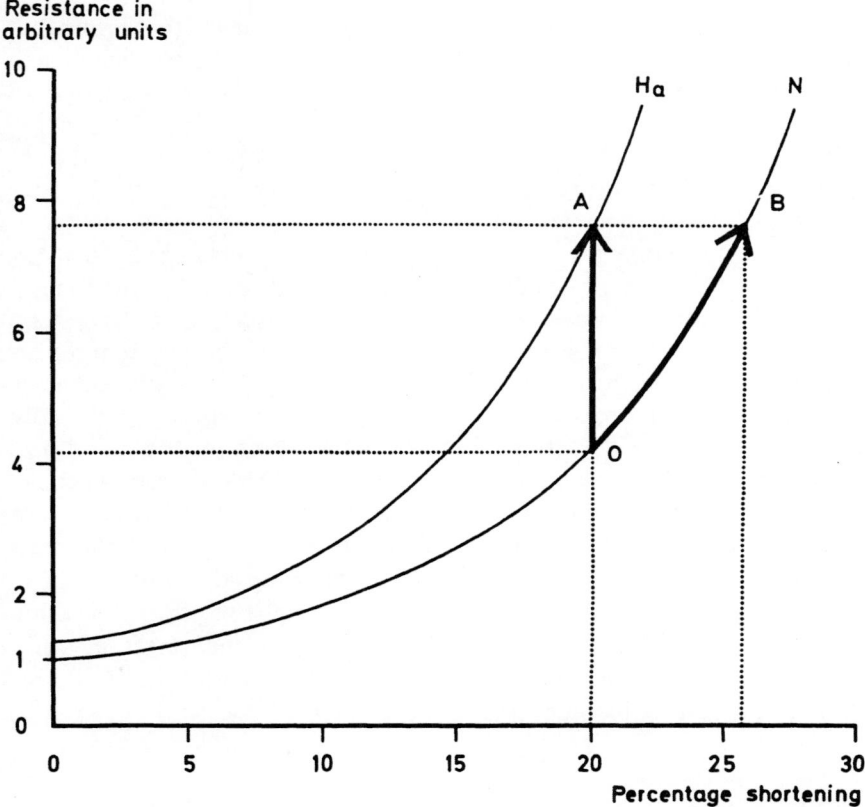

Figure 2. Relationship between the degree of vascular smooth muscle shortening and change in vascular resistance in a normal (N) and hypertensive (H) resistance vessel. In the hypertensive vessel the thickened wall of the arteriole encroaches on the lumen so that a lesser percentage shortening produces the same increase in resistance as a greater shortening in the normal vessel [5].

The pathophysiological implications of this concept are real. The initiating mechanisms in essential hypertension are obscure, but first and foremost the basic haemodynamic abnormality characterising the disease is one of increased resistance to blood flow through the arterial bed in combination with normal cardiovascular reflexes. The increase in vascular resistance is generalised without predeliction for any specific regional circulation until left ventricular failure ensues. Neither is there any convincing evidence that in the absence of heart failure the concentrically narrowed arterioles in any regional circulation are either hypersensitive to neurogenic or humeral stimuli, nor is there evidence that these stimuli are more abundant than in the normal. Although the geometric relationship between the bore of the resistance vessels and the intralumen pressure has potentially sinister haemodynamic implications for the hypertensive patient in that normal contactile stimuli may be expected to produce proportionately similar but greater absolute changes in pressure (Figure 2), there is no evidence that sympathetic control of peripheral vessels is any way abnormal in patients with established uncomplicated essential hypertension or that the baro-receptor reflexes are disturbed.

From the therapeutic viewpoint, the predominantly cardiac output dominated increase in blood pressure in early labile hypertension is exquisitely sensitive to beta-adrenoceptor antagonists; alpha-adrenoceptor antagonists have little or no role to play in the reduction of blood pressure at this stage of the disease. However, once the disease is established, the prime focus of therapeutic attention is most sensibly directed to reduction of the generalised peripheral vascular resistance; this can only be effectively achieved by dilatation of arteriolar resistance vessels. At this stage of the disease, drugs with general vasodilator properties vie for efficacy with specific alpha-adrenoceptor antagonists, at least as far as the reduction in resting blood pressure is concerned. However, in the final stages of the disease, when left ventricular insufficiency ensues, sympathetically mediated functional vasoconstriction is superimposed on the anatomic increase in arteriolar resistance. In this terminal stage of the disease, the pharmacodynamic attractiveness of alpha-adrenoceptor antagonists predominates over drugs with nonspecific vasodilator activity. This outline pinpoints the stages at which alpha-adrenoceptor antagonists may be most usefully employed in the regulation of the resting blood pressure.

Diurnal blood pressure rhythm

Therapeutic interest in the control of high blood pressure has been nearly entirely devoted to that most easily observed by the practicing physician, namely the resting value. Such a confined approach ignores the prognostic

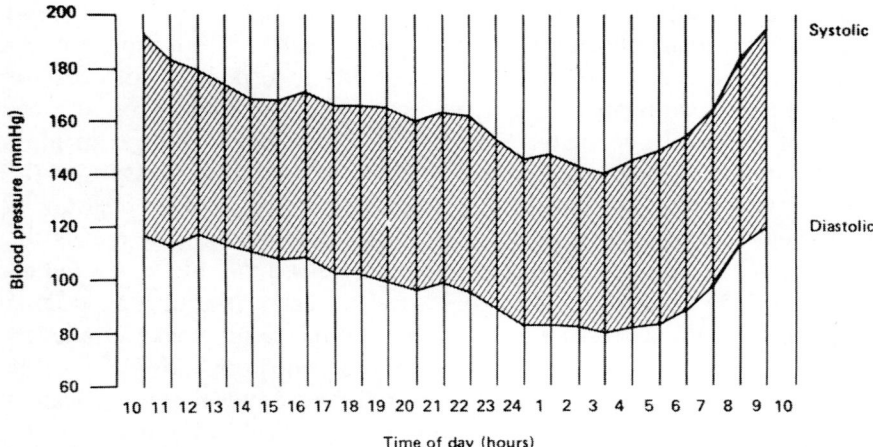

Figure 3. Blood pressure changes constructed from continuous intra-arterial records in ambulant hypertensive patients; measurements averaged in ten patients [37].

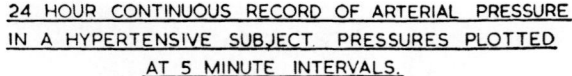

24 HOUR CONTINUOUS RECORD OF ARTERIAL PRESSURE
IN A HYPERTENSIVE SUBJECT. PRESSURES PLOTTED
AT 5 MINUTE INTERVALS.

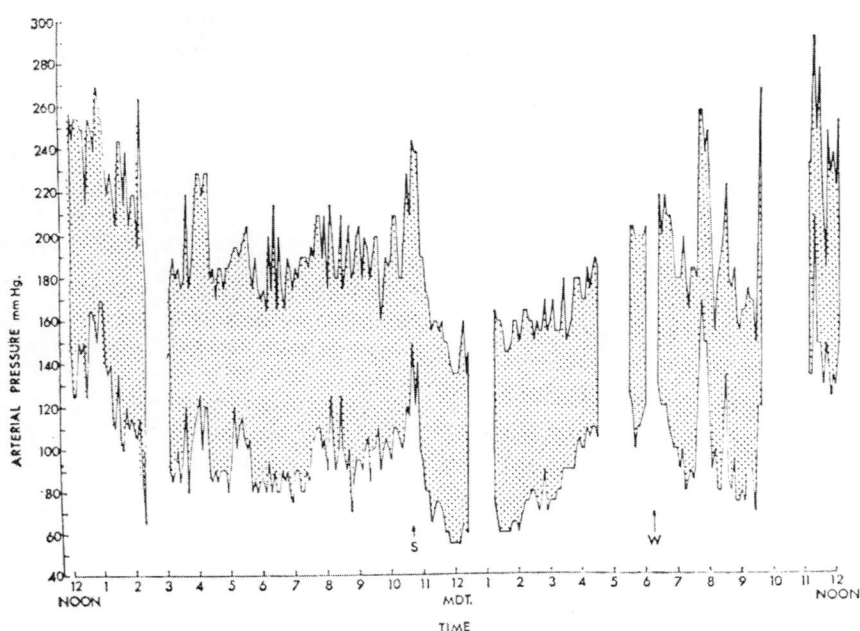

Figure 4. Twenty-four hour intra-arterial blood pressure record in an ambulant 63-year-old female with untreated essential hypertension measured in hospital. S: sleep; W: waking [38].

760

importance of control of hypertension throughout the waking day. Blood pressure varies widely during normal daily life both in the normal subject and in the hypertensive patient. This variability incorporates both pressor and depressor components superimposed upon an underlying diurnal rhythm of the resting pressure. Although the *proportional* changes in pressure are similar to the normal, *absolute* changes in diurnal pressure in the hypertensive subject are particularly marked (Figure 3). The pressure is usually highest soon after waking, subsequently falling gradually during the day. Sleep is associated with an accentuation of this trend, the lowest values being recorded when sleep is deepest. In the early morning as waking approaches, the blood pressure starts to rise and reaches its maximum levels soon after mobilisation. Integrated with this basic diurnal rhythm of the *resting* blood pressure are the pressor and depressor responses associated with the conscious events of normal daily life (Figure 4). In addition to the fall during sleep, blood pressure also falls *after* strenuous dynamic exercise and in conditions of high ambient temperature. In fact, the fall during sleep almost certainly incorporates an ingredient of skin vasodilatation due to retained body heat. Thus in the waking state the chief depressor influence on the blood pressure is heat, whether internally generated in muscles by exercise, or due to external sources. One of the chief mechnamisms by which reflex control of body temperature is achieved is through regulation of blood flow through the skin. The major sympathetic innervation of the skin vessels is dominated by alpha-adrenoceptors, thus illustrating the powerful influence of blockade of such vessels on the blood pressure.

Pressor responses

The major physiological causes of increase in blood pressure are physical exertion, either dynamic or isometric, cold and mental stress singly or in

Table 1. Haemodynamic character and sympathoadrenal mechanisms involved in pressor responses

Dynamic exercise	Isometric exertion
Mental stress	Skin cold
Character	
Systolic > Diastolic	Diastolic > Systolic
Tachycardia + + +	Tachycardia ($\pm$)
Mechanism	
Beta$_1$-adrenoceptors in the heart	Alpha$_1$-adrenoceptors in the arteries

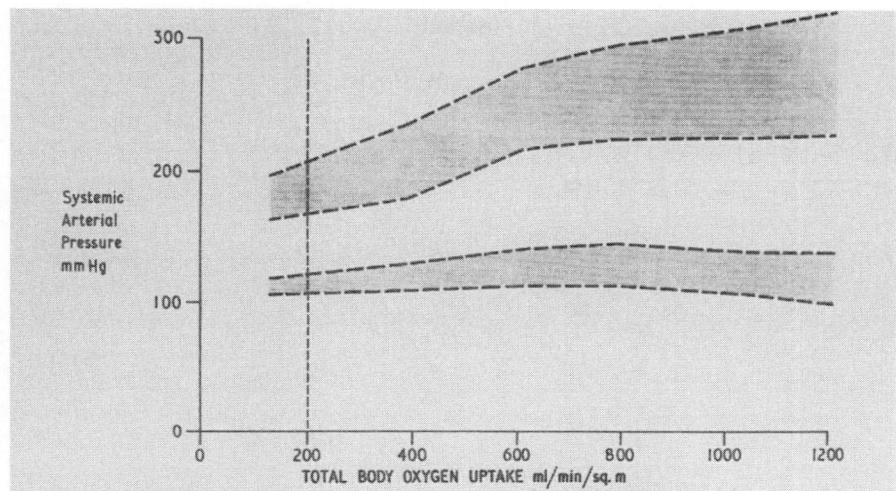

Figure 5. Effects on blood pressure of increasing levels of dynamic exercise (treadmill walking) in patients with uncomplicated essential hypertension. Shaded area includes Mean ±2SD [39].

combination. Although difficult to demonstrate in the case of mental stress, there is a clear relationship between intensity of the stimulus and the resulting pressor responses associated with dynamic exercise, isometric exertion and cold stimuli in both normal and hypertensive patients. Consideration of the physiological mechanisms involved allows the major autonomic components of each to be defined (Table 1).

Dynamic exercise results in a pressor response characterised by a progressive increase in systolic pressure and a biphasic response (initial increase, subsequent reduction) of the diastolic pressure which is directly related both to the intensity of the effort and the muscle mass involved (Figure 5). The major component in this response is sympathetic beta-adrenoceptor stimulation of the heart. Alpha-adrenoceptor stimulation of peripheral vessels in non-exercising regions (e.g. kidney, splanchnic) occurs at the start of such exercise, particularly if it is strenuous, but the heat generated by the working muscles rapidly overrides vasoconstriction of the alpha-adrenoceptor innervated skin vessels.

The pressor response to mental stress frequently follows a similar, if somewhat less clearly defined pattern of blood pressure response. Precise stimulus–response relations are precluded by rapid habituation to repetative stimuli, and the large between-patient variability to any given stress situation. However, in the majority of situations the qualitative circulatory response is a predominant increase in systolic pressure (Figure 6). Sympathoadrenal stimulation of alpha-adrenoceptors occurs to a variable extent, although simultaneous activation of vasodilator beta$_2$-adrenoceptors in

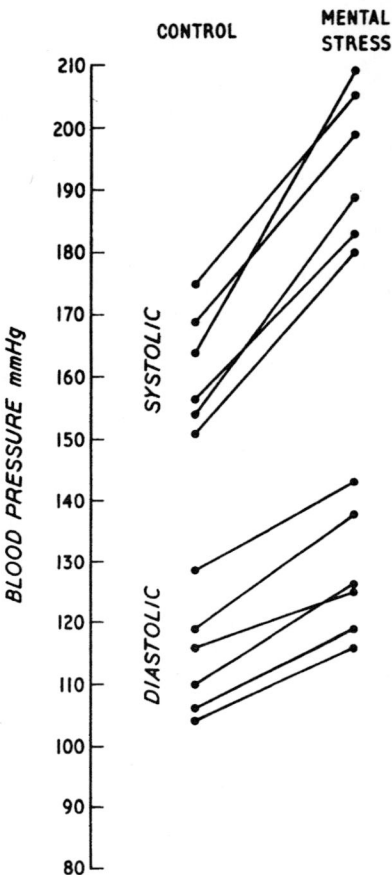

Figure 6. Pressor effects of mental stress (forced arithmetic) in six patients with untreated essential hypertension [2].

striated muscle and skin vessels of the 'blush' area of the face and neck tends to reduce the resulting increase in diastolic pressure. In both these pressor responses, the dominant role of the cardiac beta-adrenoceptor component indicates that they are particularly sensitive to beta- but not alpha-adrenoceptor blockade.

The increase in pressure during isometric exertion is characterised by an increase in diastolic pressure with little or no increase in pulse pressure (Figure 7). This pressor-response is stimulus-related (Figure 8), but independent of the muscle mass involved.

Cold has long been known to be a potent pressor stimulus. The original predictive claim of Hines and Brown [6] has not been upheld, but there is no doubt that cooling of the skin induces marked increases in blood pres-

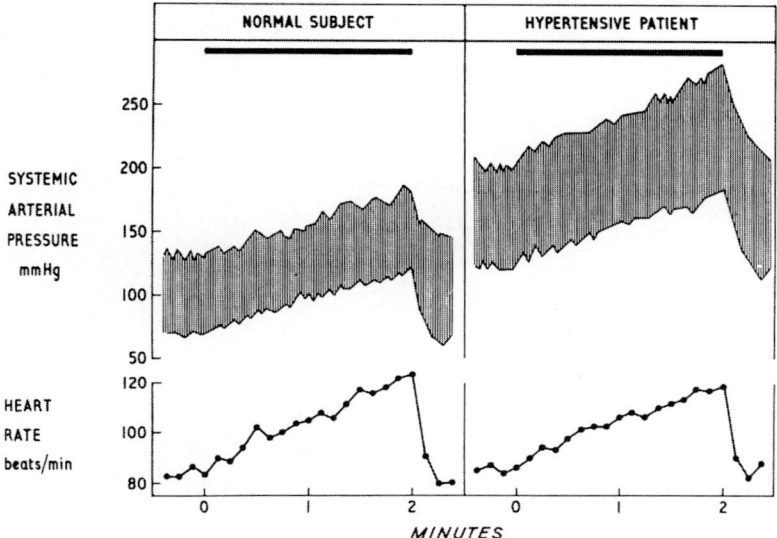

Figure 7. Circulatory effects of sustained handgrip vontraction (30% maximum) in a normal subject (male aged 42 years) and a hypertensive male patient (aged 47 years). Period of contraction indicated by solid bar [39].

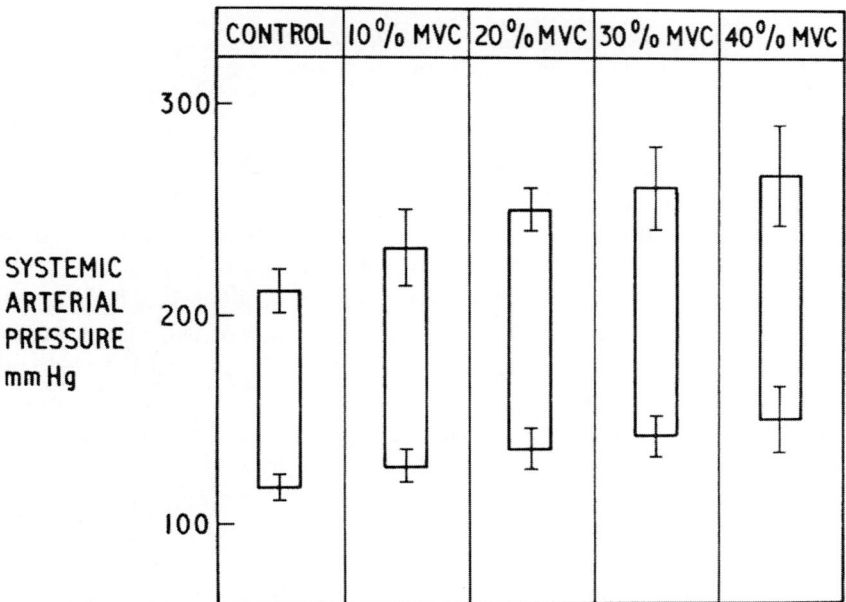

Figure 8. Relationship between intensity of sustained handgrip and increase in systemic arterial pressure inpatients with essential hypertension [39].

764

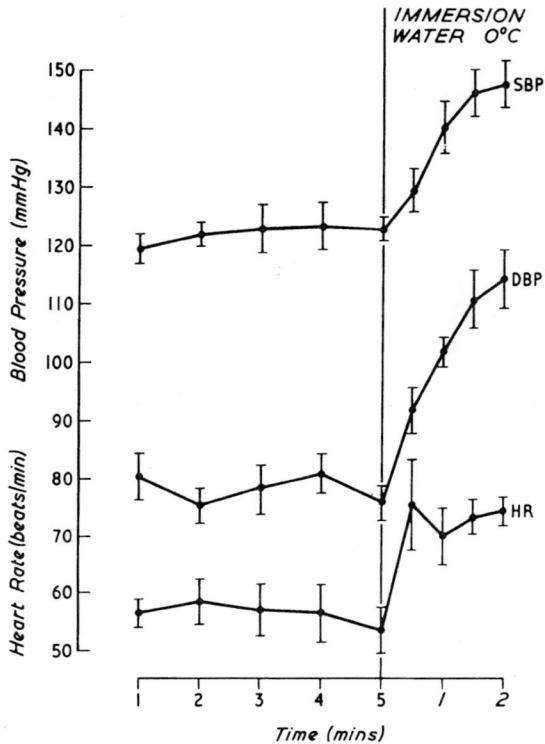

Figure 9. The variability of the circulatory response to
hand cold in twelve normal subjects. Data expressed as
Mean ±2SE [40].

sure. The increase in blood pressure in response to skin cold is specifically
characterised by an increase in diastolic pressure without significant change
in pulse pressure and relatively small increase in heart rate. The pressor
response is rapid, sustained, repeatable (Figure 9), unrelated to the area of
skin involved or the location of the skin cooled, and linearly related to the
intensity of the cold below 20 °C (Figure 10). The mechanism of the pressor
responses to isometric exercise and cold are predominantly mediated
through constriction of arteriolar resistance vessels involving all regional
vascular territories except the coronary circulation. Cardiac beta-adrenoceptor stimulation contributes little to the increase in pressure. Thus in contrast
to the cardiac output dominated pressor responses accompanying dynamic
exercise and mental stress, the major autonomic accompaniment of isometric exertion and cold is sympathetic activation of the peripheral resistance
vessels. These latter pressor increases could, therefore, be expected to be
quantitatively attenuated by drugs which block the peripheral sympathetic
alpha-adrenoceptor pathways. This is the physiological background, on

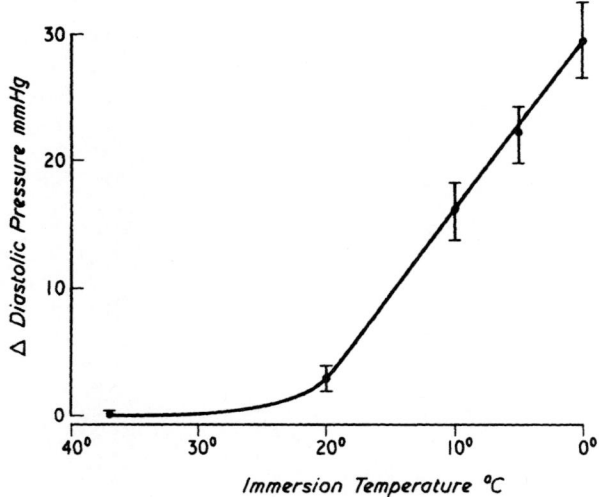

Figure 10. The stimulus-response relationship to hand cold. Data expressed as Mean ±SE [40].

which the pharmacodynamic and therapeutic effects of the alpha-adrenoceptor antagonists will be examined.

PHYSIOLOGY OF ALPHA ADRENOCEPTORS

Understanding of the effects of drugs which block alpha-adrenoceptors on the blood pressure in hypertensive patients, dictates that their distribution and function must be considered in detail. As far as is known, all alpha-adrenoceptors in the vascular system are innervated by the sympathetic nervous system. Receptors are present not only in peripheral blood vessels but also in the central nervous system where their activity may have opposing effects to that in the periphery. This complex situation is clearly demonstrated by the fact that blood pressure may be lowered by stimulation of alpha-adrenoceptors in the central nervous system [7, 8]. Conversely, alpha-adrenoceptor blocking drugs may increase blood pressure [9]. This apparent paradox that diametrically opposed effects, at least on blood pressure, may result from stimulation or blockade of similar alpha-adrenoceptors in different locations is important to an understanding of the mode of action of alpha-blocking drugs. It is also essential to examine the geography of the alpha-adrenoceptors in the pre- and post-synaptic areas before detailed examination of the therapeutic usefulness of drugs which block these receptors is undertaken (see review by Vanhoutte [10]).

766

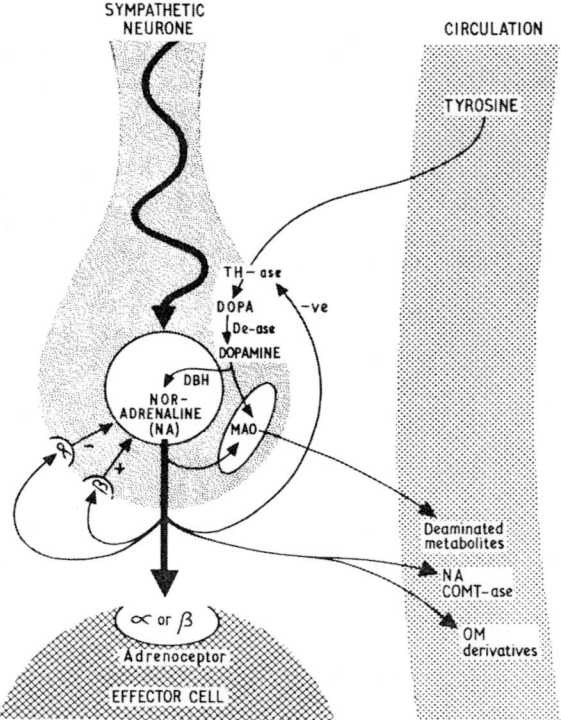

Figure 11. Schematic representation of the synthesis, storage, release and metabolism of noradrenaline at sympathetic neurone terminals. Abbreviations. Th-ase, Tyrosine hydroxylase; Dc-ase, dopa decarboxylase; DBH, dopamine-β-hydroxylase; MAO, Monoamine oxidase; COMT-ase, catechol-O-methyl transferase [43].

Adrenergic innervation of blood vessels

Sympathetic control of blood vessels is accomplished through the functional link between the adrenergic nerve endings and the smooth muscle cells of the pre-capillary resistance vessels and postcapillary venous capacitance vessels. All blood vessels in the body are innervated by sympathetic nerve endings although the geography of their distribution differs widely. The density of innervation is also inconstant, a fact reflected in the different contribution of each regional vascular bed to the overall peripheral vascular resistance. The cerebral, coronary and pulmonary vessels are sparsely supplied with sympathetic nerves and alpha-adrenoceptors. In contrast, the remainder of the circulation is amply innervated, particularly the vessels of the skin and kidney. Postganglionic sympathetic nerves terminate as varicosities near to the effector receptor on vascular smooth muscle.

Neurotransmitter synthesis

The functional characteristics of the sympathetic neurotransmitter endorgan are now clear (Figure 11). The adrenergic neurone takes up tyrosine from the extra cellular fluid which is converted in the neuroplasm to L-DOPA by the enzyme tyrosine hydroxylase. This is the major rate-limiting step in the synthesis of noradrenaline; it is inhibited if the concentration of noradrenaline in the neuroplasm increases but, conversely, is facilitated if the release of noradrenaline is enhanced or if increased levels of angiotensin-II are present. L-DOPA is then transformed to dopamine which is actively taken into the granular storage vesicles where the final step of noradrenaline synthesis is executed by the enzyme dopamine-beta-hydroxylase. The terminal sympathetic neurone also actively takes up noradrenaline from the extracellular fluid, whether this catecholamine has been liberated from the nerve terminal itself or has reached it from the circulating catecholamines in the plasma. The activity of the neuronal amine pump responsible for this active process is inversely related to the volume of sympathetic nerve traffic. It is also linked to the sodium-potassium-ATPase enzyme and thus is influenced by drugs which interfere with this system (e.g. tricyclic antidepressants). Not all of the noradrenaline taken up from the tissue fluids reaches the storage vesicle; a portion is destroyed by the enzyme monoamine-oxidase present in the terminal neurone.

Neurotransmitter Storage

Noradrenaline is stored in the vesicles of the terminal sympathetic neurone as a protein complex, chromogranin A. All terminal sympathetic neurones appear to contain approximately the same number of these noradrenaline containing vesicles; functional sympathetic activity is, therefore, directly related to the number, not character, of terminal sympathetic neurones in any tissue.

Neurotransmitter Release

Noradrenaline is released from the storage vesicle by three processes.
   1. By slow passive diffusion; this does not result in stimulation of post-synaptic receptors as it is largely inactivated by the neuronal monoamine oxidase before it reaches the synaptic cleft.
   2. By displacement from the vesicle by sympathomimetic amines (e.g. amphetamine, tyramine). Part of the displaced noradrenaline is inactivated by neuroplasm monoamine oxidase but a sufficient amount may reach the synaptic cleft to stimulate the post-synaptic receptors.

3) By the action potential generated in the proximal ganglionic cell body (exocytotic release); this is the major release mechanism. The action potential induces an increased concentration of calcium ions in the neuroplasm which results in migration of the storage vesicles towards the synaptic cleft and their contact with the neuronal cell membrane at that pont. The vesicle ruptures at the site of contact so that noradrenaline together with dopamine beta-hydroxylase are released in high concentration into the synaptic cleft thus avoiding destruction by cytoplasmic monoamine oxidase.

Pre-synaptic influences on neurotransmitter release

This simple schema of release of noradrenaline from the terminal sympathetic neurone is complicated by presynaptic modulation of its exocytotic release by a number of physiological variables and neuro-humeral substances. Noradrenaline released into the synaptic cleft stimulates both postsynaptic alpha$_1$- and presynaptic alpha$_2$-adrenoceptors, the latter resulting in negative feedback inhibition of the exocytotic release process. The overall effects of alpha-adrenoceptor antagonists therefore depends upon their selectivity for these two alpha-adrenoceptor sites. In terms of therapeutic relevance, alpha$_2$-receptor autoinhibition of neurotransmitter release is probably the most important of the presynaptic adrenoceptors influencing the release of noradrenaline from the sympathetic neurone. The presynaptic beta$_2$-adrenoceptor enhances the exocytotic release of noradrenaline by a positive feedback system but as the receptor is relatively insensitive to noradrenaline it is probably precluded from a major physiological role. However, the presynaptic beta$_2$-receptors are also activated by circulating adrenaline which may possibly explain the blood pressure lowering effects of some beta$_2$-antagonists.

Angiotensin-II also plays a role in pre-synaptic facilitation. In addition to its many indirect effects on the sympathetic nervous system, which include stimulation of central vasomotor centres, facilitation of ganglionic transmission, and enhancement of noradrenaline synthesis, angiotensin-II also appears to facilitate the release of noradrenaline. Thus the interrelationship between the sympathetic nervous system and renin release constitutes a positive feedback system; sympathetic stimulation affords release of renin, which in turn activates angiotensin and closes the facilitatory feedback loop in the sympathetic chain.

Postsynaptic adrenoceptors

The activation of post-synaptic adrenoceptors is equally complex. Noradrenaline reaches the postsynaptic smooth muscle cell membrane where it binds to the lipoprotein adrenoceptors. The majority of the adrenoceptors in blood vessels are alpha-adrenergic in type; they initiate the biochemical processes that result in contraction of the smooth muscle cell. Postsynaptic alpha-adrenoceptors also comprise both $alpha_1$ and $alpha_2$ sub-types, and although each are pharmacologically distinct, both appear to serve the same contactile-stimulating function. In some blood vessels, particularly those in striated muscle and those in the skin of the face and upper chest, noradrenaline also activates vasodilator $beta_2$-adrenoceptors.

Neurotransmitter Destruction

Noradrenaline released into the synaptic cleft is rapidly removed by:
1. uptake into sympathetic neurones through binding to presynaptic $alpha_2$- and $beta_2$-adrenoceptors
2. extra neuronal uptake by the smooth muscle cell membrane and other tissues, particularly collagen
3. overflow into the tissue space and plasma.

In the sympathetic neurone noradrenaline is inactivated by monoamine oxidase. In smooth muscle cells enzymatic degradation is also achieved by the enzyme catechol-O-methyltransferase.

Distribution of alpha-adrenoceptors

In terms of the functional effects of sympathetic stimulation of alpha-adrenoceptors, the picture is complicated by their geographical distribution. Although $alpha_1$-adrenoceptors are classically regarded as the postsynaptic alpha-adrenoceptor of smooth muscle cells, they also occur in the brain and liver outside the vascular system. $Alpha_2$-adrenoceptors also occur at sites other than the presynaptic; postsynaptic receptors on vascular smooth muscle cell membranes with similar pharmacological characterisation and pharmacodynamic activity have been described [11]. Moreover, in sympathetic cholinergic neurones, $alpha_2$-adrenoceptors mediate inhibition of acetyl choline release. Different alpha-adrenoceptors may respond to the same pharmacological agent with different circulatory results (e.g. phentolamine) or to different agents with similar circulatory results.

Clinical implications

The regional vascular geography and microscopic disposition of these different receptors has important implications for the treatment of hyperten-

770

sion. For instance, clonidine and alpha-methylnoradrenaline, the antihypertensive metabolite of alphamethyldopa [12] are potent agonists at presynaptic alpha$_2$-adrenoceptor sites in the blood vessels. By enhancing autoinhibition of neurotransmitter release they attenuate sympathetically mediated vasoconstriction. Concurrently, however, by facilitation of alpha$_2$-adrenoceptor activity in vasomotor centres in the brain they reduce sympathetic nerve traffic. The end result on blood pressure depends on the relative dominance of each function. This illustrates the complexity of using what are superficially simple sympatholytic agents.

HAEMODYNAMIC EFFECTS OF ALPHA-ADRENOCEPTOR BLOCKADE IN HYPERTENSION

In view of the complexity, distribution and different functions of the vascular and extravascular alpha-adrenoceptors, the circulatory effects of drugs which are used to block this particular sympathetic effector pathway in the hypertensive patient can only be examined from the pragmatic viewpoint. Prazosin and indoramin are relatively selective alpha$_1$-adrenoceptor antagonists; analysis of their haemodynamic effects thus provides basic information of the role of these receptors in blood pressure control in the hypertensive patient.

Selective versus unselective blockade

In the resting state, blockade of alpha$_1$-adrenoceptors is associated with a reduction in systemic arterial diastolic and mean pressure without substantial change in heart rate or cardiac output. The reduction in calculated peripheral vascular resistance implies relaxation of smooth muscle in the arteriolar resistance vessels, confirmed by the direct measurement of vascular resistance in the upper limb [13]. The relatively selective alpha$_1$-adrenoceptor antagonist, indoramin, also appears to result in similar overall haemodynamic changes in hypertensive patients at rest [14]. With both drugs, however, an integrated pattern of the geographical distribution of changes in the regional vascular territories remains to be described. These circulatory changes are in marked contrast to those that occur with unselective alpha-adrenoceptor blockade. Phentolamine competes with noradrenaline at postsynaptic alpha$_1$- and alpha$_2$-adrenoceptor sites, but also blocks neuronal autoinhibition of neurotransmitter release. In hypertensive patients phentolamine results in relaxation of arteriolar resistance vessels accompanied by an increase in circulating catecholamines. This has two effects: it augments the drop in systemic arterial pressure by stimulation of noninnvervated vasodilator beta$_2$-adrenoceptors in striated muscle, but offsets this hypotensive activity by simultaneous stimulation of chronotropic and inotropic beta$_1$-adrenoceptors in the heart (Figure 12).

Thus, nonselective alpha-adrenoceptor antagonists can only be used in combination with drugs which block cardiac beta-adrenoceptors. In the treatment of uncomplicated nonlabile hypertension, selective alpha$_1$-adrenoceptor antagonists are, therefore, the drugs of both physiological and clinical choice. However, the converse is true if hypertension progress to left ventricular failure. In this situation the augmented release of noradrenaline by non-selective blockade of both alpha$_1$- and alpha$_2$-adrenoceptors could be expected to increase myocardial contractility, and activate vasodilator beta$_2$-adrenoceptors as well as block the additional reflex constriction of arteriolar resistance and venous capacitance vessels associated with the reduced cardiac output. Intravenous phentolamine has proved its worth in this situation [15] but as yet no clinically acceptable oral nonselective alpha-adrenoceptor blocking drug is available for the sustained treatment of hypertensive heart failure.

Venous effects

Physiological attention has naturally been primarily directed to the relaxation of systemic arteriolar smooth muscle afforded by the selective alpha$_1$-adrenoceptor antagonists. Clinically, however, it rapidly became apparent that, when first given, the hypotensive potency of these selective agents was

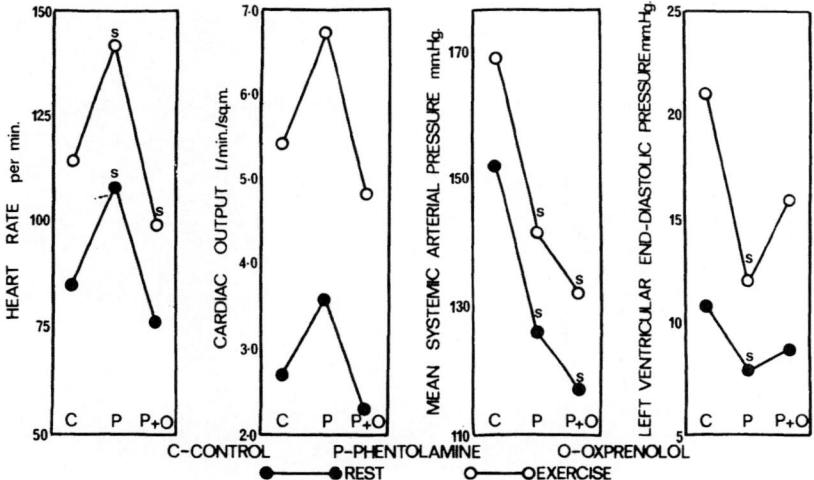

Figure 12. Haemodynamic effects of alpha- and beta-adrenoceptor blockade single and together at rest and during supine leg supine leg exercise in hypertensive patients [41].

772

greatly, if transiently, augmented by their ability to relax smooth muscle in the veins. The increase in venous capacitance can often be so large that when these drugs are first given hypotension, aggravated by posture, is a common clinical event. Salt restriction, or pretreatment with diuretics naturally augments such hypotensive reactions [16]. This highlights the important, if ancillary, role of alpha$_1$-adrenoceptors in the smooth muscle of veins.

Once such venodilatation has occurred, reflex renal retention of fluid leads to an increase in blood volume which offsets the increased capacity of the venous system. The hypotensive response to these drugs is therefore relatively short-lived ('first-dose' effect) so that clinical avoiding action may be taken.

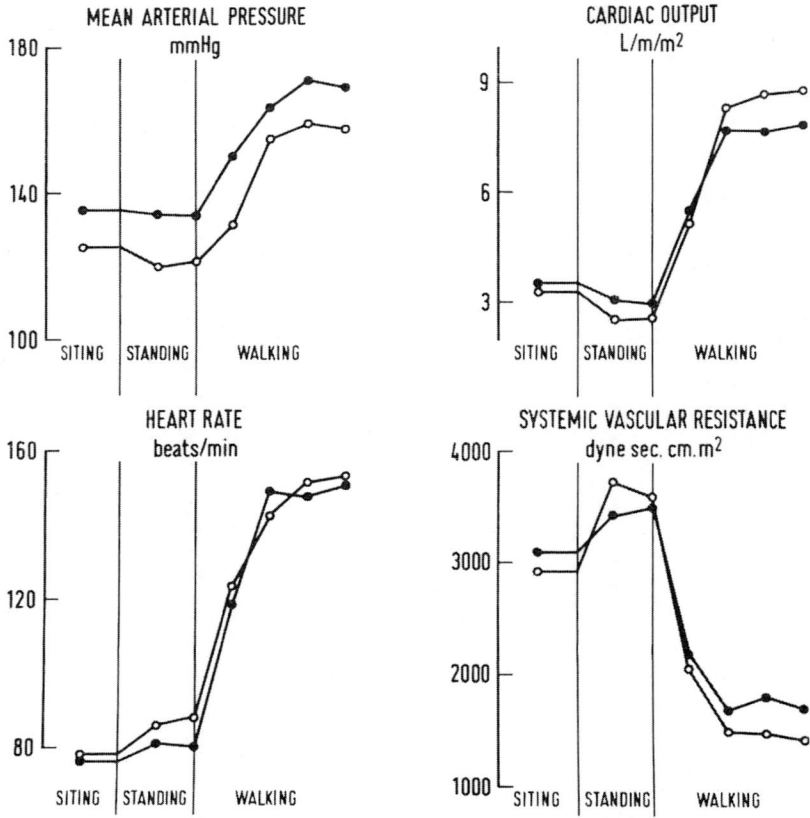

HAEMODYNAMIC CHANGES BEFORE (•)
and AFTER (○) PRAZOSIN IN HYPERTENSION

Figure 13. Effect of chronic treatment with prazosin on the haemodynamic changes during walking in hypertensive patients.

Effects of alpha-adrenoceptor blockade on pressor responses

The foregoing description of the haemodynamic effects of alpha-adrenoceptor blockade in hypertensive patients relates only to those that occur at rest. However, it is of equal therapeutic importance to examine their influence on the pressor responses induced by dynamic exercise, isometric exertion, cold and mental stress.

Dynamic exercise

During chronic treatment, alpha$_1$-adrenoceptor blockade with prazosin is associated with a reduction in systemic arterial diastolic and mean pressure at rest which is maintained during bicycle exercise although the increment in pressure from rest to exercise is uninfluenced by the drug (Figure 13). The heart rate increment from rest to exercise is also unchanged although the cardiac output increment is increased, due to an increase in stroke volume. Thus, the decrement in the calculated systemic vascular resistance during exercise is significantly greater than normal. These results are explicable in the following terms. At rest, the drug induces vasodilatation of peripheral arteriolar resistance vessels by blockade of tonic sympathetic discharges. During dynamic exercise the normal vasoconstrictive influences on the regional circulations not involved in the exercise (e.g. renal, splanchnic, other limbs, etc.) are partially inhibited, resulting in an augmented fall in systemic vascular resistance. The failure to reduce the cardiac output at rest and the greater than normal increase in output during exertion in chronically treated patients may be interpreted as implying that the initial increase in venous compliance and reduction in venous return has been compensated for by an increase in circulating blood volume. Information on the distribution of the drug-induced changes in resistance in the various regional vascular territories during dynamic exercise is lacking. However, the pharmacodynamic spectrum of activity of prazosin and other selective alpha$_1$-adrenoceptor antagonists would suggest that attenuation of vascular resistance in the regional vascular beds would tend to be concentrated in those with high alpha-receptor representation, namely the kidney and skin.

Isometric exercise

The increase in blood pressure during isometric exercise is predominantly due to vasoconstriction induced by stimulation of alpha$_1$-adrenoceptors. It is to be expected, therefore, that blockade of these receptors would attenuate this response. The evidence from studies in man is conflicting. The relatively selective alpha$_1$-adrenoceptor antagonist prazosin does not appear to blunt the pressor response [17]. In contrast, in hypertensive patients pretreated by a beta-blocking drug the nonselective adrenoceptor antagonist, phentolamine, abolished the response [18]. It is possible therefore that this primitive circulatory reflex utilises both alpha$_1$- and alpha$_2$ postsynaptic adrenoceptors. These observations also emphasise the synergistic advantages of combined denervation of the sympathoadrenal system in the treatment of high blood pressure.

Skin cold

The reflex pressor response to cooling of the skin is exercised through a sympathetic neuroeffector pathway similar to that utilised in the response to isometric exercise, namely by stimulation of alpha$_1$-adrenoceptors in systemic arteriolar resistance vessels. Similarly selective alpha$_1$-adrenoceptor blockade with prazosin alone does not appear to influence this pressor response [17]. The influence of nonselective alpha-adrenoceptor blockade or the combination of alpha- and beta-adrenoceptor blockade on this response does not appear to have been tested in hypertension patients.

Mental stress

The influence of selective or nonselective alpha-adrenoceptor blockade on the pressor response to mental stress appears not to have been examined. However, the predominant cardiac beta-adrenoceptor stimulation underlying this haemodynamic response indicates that alpha-adrenoceptor blockade would probably have little modulating effect on the pressure increase.

Effects of alpha-adrenoceptor blockade on baroreceptor control

Baroreceptor sensitivity may be tested by:
1. measuring the effects of changes in systemic arterial blood pressure on the reciprocal changes in heart rate.
2. increasing or reducing tissue pressure around the carotid sinus by a neck cuff.
   Hypertensive patients chronically treated with the alpha$_1$-adrenoceptor blocking drug prazosin, demonstrate no substantial change in these indirect indicators of baro-receptor sensitivity [17].

CLINICAL STUDIES WITH ALPHA-ADRENOCEPTOR ANTAGONISTS
IN HYPERTENSION

At present only two alpha-adrenoceptor antagonists have achieved acceptance for the clinical treatment of hypertension, namely the selective alpha-adrenoceptor antagonists prazosin and indoramin. Nonselective alpha-blocking drugs, e.g. phentolamine and phenoxybenzamine, and those with vascular activity other than that induced by alpha-blockade, e.g. the ergot alkaloids benzodioxans, amidazolines, etc., have no therapeutic standing in this respect and therefore will not be considered further. Drugs which possess both alpha- and beta-adrenoceptor blocking activity, such as tolamolol and labetalol, are also outside the scope of this chapter.

Prazosin

Numerous clinical reports have defined the usefulness of prazosin as an antihypertensive drug and its relative safety during long-term administration [19]. The dose range used has been relatively wide, varying from 2 to 20 mg daily. In terms of comparable blood pressure lowering activity at rst, 1 mg of prazosin is approximately equivalent to 20 mg hydralazine. Due to their different mechanisms of action, it is inappropriate to compare antihypertensive doses of prazosin with other hypotensive agents with different antipressor characteristics. However, a number of direct comparative studies have established that prazosin has similar antihypertensive efficacy to methyldopa, clonidine, and propranolol in patients with mild and moderate essential hypertension.

As would be expected from its mechanism of action, the antihypertensive effects of prazosin are augmented by diuretics and supplemented by combination with a beta-adrenoceptor antagonist. There appear to be no discernible contra-indications to its combination with drugs with a totally different mode of action, such as methyldopa and clonidine.

The only major side effect relates to the 'first dose' phenomenon. In many patients the first dose of the drug induces a greater fall in pressure than can be expected during chronic treatment and this initial fall in pressure is aggravated by posture. It is probably due to the effect of the drug in blocking alpha-adrenoceptors in veins particularly those in the splanchnic region, the resulting increase in venous compliance reducing venous return to the heart. The reflex vasoconstriction in response to the drop in cardiac output is impaired by the primary effect of the drug on arteriolar resistance vessels hypotension ensues. Continued treatment with the drug however leads to an increase in plasma volume which offsets this increase in venous capacity, which is a once-and-for-all phenomenon. Initial doses of the drug

776

are, therefore, recommended to be kept low and the very first dose administered on retirement at night.

Indoramin

Indoramin is a drug with alpha-adrenoceptor blocking activity with a chemical configuration quite different to that of prazosin or any other antihypertensive agent in clinical use [14]. It was developed more than a decade ago but has only recently attracted interest for the treatment of hypertension. Numerous studies are available which confirm its hypotensive properties in patients with mild or moderate essential hypertension. It is pharmacodynamically intriguing that the 'first-dose phenomenon' observed with prazosin does not appear to be a problem with indoramin. However, this finding and scrutiny of the dose-related blood pressure lowering effects leads to the conclusion that it is probably a less potent alpha-adrenoceptor blocking drug than prazosin. The major side effect experienced with the drug appears to be that of sedation.

ALPHA-ADRENOCEPTOR ANTAGONISTS IN HYPERTENSIVE HEART FAILURE

The effectiveness of detection of raised blood pressure in Western communities and the efficacy of antihypertensive treatment has greatly reduced the frequency of hypertensive heart failure. By whatever method it is achieved, reduction of aortic impedance by reduction of the systemic vascular resistance can be expected to reverse the progression of this terminal event. The infrequency of hypertensive heart failure explains the rarity of comparative studies of the efficacy of different antihypertensive compounds on its reversal. However, there is no doubt that vasodilator drugs in general, and alpha-adrenoceptor antagonists in particular, rapidly reverse the deteriorating haemodynamic situation created by failure of left ventricular pumping activity whatever its cause [2, 15, 20, 21]. Drugs with non-specific vasodilator activities (e.g. hydralazine) can be expected to exert their major pharmacodynamic activity by selectively reducing arteriolar resistance with little change in venous compliance. In contrast, alpha-adrenoceptor blocking drugs can be expected to result in a more balanced reduction of both preload (due to increase in venous compliance and reduction in venous return) and aortic impedance (due to reduction in reflex sympathetic increase of systemic vascular resistance) and thus achieve a more complete reduction of left ventricular afterload (Figures 14 and 15). This expectation has also been fulfilled in a number of comparative studies [22, 23].

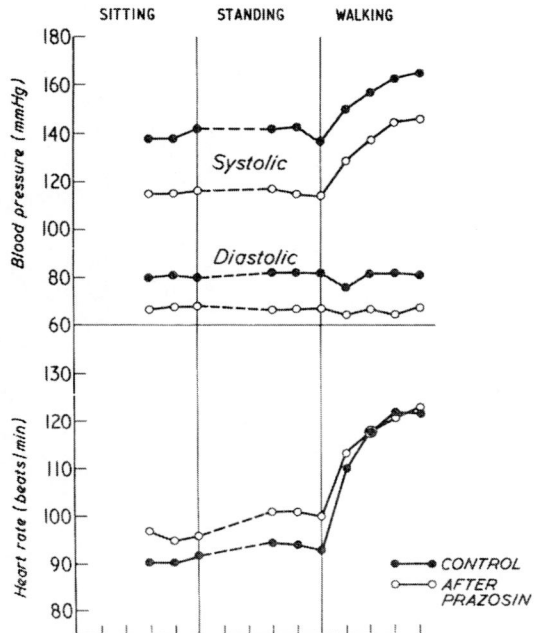

Figure 14. Haemodynamic effects of prazosin in patients with severe heartfailure sitting, standing and during treadmill walking [36].

In heart failure the ability of the terminal sympathetic neurone in the heart to synthesize noradrenaline is quickly depressed with the result that myocardial catecholamine stores are rapidly depleted [24]. This lack of neurotransmitter, forming as it does a vital emergency mechanism to increase myocardial contractility, compounds the reduction in cardiac pumping activity. In this situation the exhibition of nonselective alpha-adrenoceptor antagonists which block both vascular smooth muscle alpha$_1$-adrenoceptors and also the autoinhibitory pre-synaptic alpha$_2$-adrenoceptors could be expected to have advantages over drugs whose blocking activity is confined to the alpha$_1$-receptors. The nonselective alpha-adrenoceptor antagonist, phentolamine, has been shown to be highly effective in the treatment of severe left ventricular failure [15, 25]. Comparative studies of nonselective and selective alpha-blocking drugs in heart failure have so far been precluded by the incompatible formulations of the compounds available; phentolamine is only available for intravenous use and prazosin only for oral administration at the present time. But whatever the outcome of future comparisons, there is no doubt that alpha-adrenoceptor blocking drugs are physiologically the most sensible and therapeutically the most efficacious

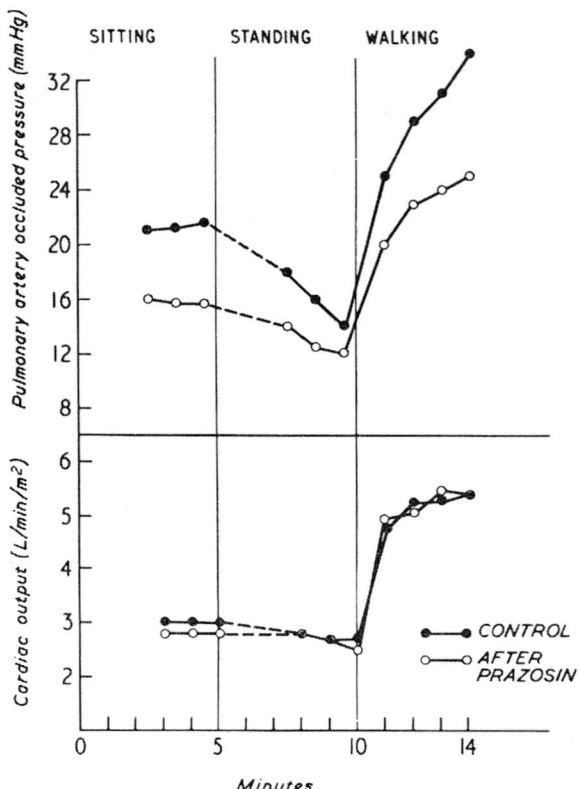

Figure 15. Haemodynamic effects of prazosin in patients with severe heart failure during sitting, standing and tread-mill walking [36].

agents at present available for the treatment of heart failure, including that due to raised blood pressure.

ANCILLARY ACTIVITIES OF ALPHA-ADRENOCEPTOR ANTAGONISTS

There is no doubt that the major haemodynamic and therapeutic forte of alpha-adrenoceptor antagonists is their ability to competitively block sympathetically induced contraction of vascular smooth muscle. However, this should not obscure other avenues of their pharmacodynamic activity of potential clinical importance.

Myocardial metabolism in the failing heart is critically dependent upon the utilisation of carbohydrate, particularly glucose. Assimilation of glucose is dependent upon the insulin transport mechanism. In heart failure, of whatever origin, insulin release is suppressed thus imperilling myocardial survival [26, 27]. Inhibition of secretion of insulin is due to two mechanisms, both the result of stimulation of alpha-adrenoceptors in the splanchnic circulation. Blood flow through the pancreas is reduced in addition to which insulin secretion is further suppressed by the specific inhibitory influence of noradrenaline [28]. This inhibited release mechanism in heart failure is unlocked by alpha-adrenoceptor blockade [29]. This emphasises once more the potential value of alpha-adrenoceptor blocking drugs in this situation.

The major clinical complication and the most frequent terminal event in hypertension is myocardial infarction due to coronary heart disease and the most frequent cause of demise is a ventricular dysrhythmia arising soon after the onset of symptoms. Until recently it was thought that these intrinsic dysrhythmias, often resistent to drug treatment, were facilitated solely by sympathoadrenal stimulation of myocardial beta-adrenoceptors. Recent evidence, however, suggests that myocardial alpha-adrenoceptors may play an important role in the origin of these life threatening disturbances of rhythm [30, 31]. If human studies support these animal experiments then the role for alpha-adrenoceptor antagonists in the treatment of hypertension is further assured.

Renin holds a sinister prognostic implication in essential hypertension [32]. Nonspecific vasodilator drugs are invariably associated with increased secretion of renin and subsequent activation of the vasoconstrictor angiotensin and salt-retaining aldosterone [33]. It is intriguing therefore that despite their hypotensive effects neither prazosin [19] nor indoramin [14] appear to increase plasma renin activity. This once more underlines the potential value of selective alpha$_1$-adrenoceptor antagonists in the treatment of uncomplicated essential hypertension.

Catecholamines appear to be responsible for inducing aggregation of human platelets [34]. Platelets carry both alpha$_1$- and alpha$_2$-adrenoceptors, but it appears that the alpha$_2$-receptor is primarily responsible for mediating the aggregation that occurs in response to adrenaline [35]. In view of the known threat of coronary thrombosis and sudden death in patients with high blood pressure, and the fact that platelet thrombi are probably involved in both events, the effect of alpha-adrenoceptor blocking drugs on platelet aggregation forms an exciting avenue for further research.

CONCLUSIONS

Essential hypertension is outstandingly characterised by the generalised increase in the resistance offered by the systemic arterioles at all stages of the disease. Theoretically, therefore, the ideal antihypertensive drug would relax arteriolar smooth muscle and at the same time attenuate the sympathetically mediated increases in blood pressure that occur in response to the pressor stimuli met in normal daily life. Superficially, alpha-adrenoceptor blocking drugs would appear to go some way towards such a therapeutic ideal. That they do not entirely achieve this purpose is due to our lack of precise knowledge of the sympathetic neuroeffector mechanisms responsible for peripheral vascular control. However, there is no doubt that selective blockade of alpha$_1$-adrenoceptors in the peripheral vasculature more nearly achieves this aim than any other single anti-hypertensive preparation available at the present time. These drugs, by inducing relaxation of vascular smooth muscle, tend to induce a haemodynamic profile approaching the normal. They reduce diastolic blood pressure without significant change in pulse pressure, heart rate, cardiac output or stroke volume. The geographical distribution of this reduction in arteriolar resistance and increase in venous compliance in the various regional vascular territories awaits clarification but it can probably be expected to follow the anatomical distribution of the peripheral sympathetic nerves. Baroreceptor reflex sensitivity appears to be unaltered by these drugs and, although the haemodynamic responses to dynamic exercise, isometric exertion, cold and mental stress are little changed, these pressor reactions occur from a lower absolute level of blood pressure. The relatively small increase in sympathetic stimulation of the heart in response to the fall in blood pressure is intriguing; its cause is obscure but it is an extremely useful clinical characteristic of these drugs and contrasts markedly with the symptomatic impact that accompanies the administration of drugs with nonselective alpha-blocking activity.

The haemodynamic effects of selective alpha$_1$-adrenoceptor blockade in hypertensive patients have favourable prognostic implications. Reduction of the resting blood pressure without substantial increases in circulating catecholamines or increase in plasma renin activity may be highly beneficial to the hypertensive patient. Preservation of the normal pressor responses to such excitatory stimuli as exercise, cold and mental stress implies that circulatory homeostasis is not significantly compromised so that the normal daily life of these patients should be affected. However, the lower resting pressure, and therefore the lower peak pressures that result from such stimuli, may promise significant arterial protection. Drugs with autonomic blocking functions can all be expected to have extravascular and central nervous system pharmacodynamic activity. However, in the case of the selective alpha$_1$-adrenoceptor blocking drugs at present available, these effects to not appear to exert clinically imposing adverse effects.

In the absence of discovery of the initiating and sustaining cause of essential hypertension its treatment must remain based on multi-drug therapy. These deliberations suggest that drugs with alpha$_1$-adrenoceptor blocking activity should probably be an ingredient of all antihypertensive regimes.

REFERENCES

1. Freis ED: Haemodynamics of hypertension. Physiol Rev 40:27–57, 1960.
2. Taylor SH: The circulation in hypertension and cardiovascular reflexes. In: The Hypertensive Patient, pp. 39–112. Marshall AJ, Barritt DW, eds. New York: Pirman Medical, 1980.
3. Lund-Johansen P: Haemodynamics in essential hypertension. Clin Sci, 343–354, 1980.
4. Guyton AC, Coleman TG, Cowley AW, Norman RA, Manning RD, Liard JF: Relationship of fluid and electrolytes to arterial pressure, control and hypertension. Quantitative analysis of an infinite-gain feedback. In: Hypertension: Mechanisms and Management I, pp. 25–36. Onesti G, Kim KE, Moyer JH, eds. New York: Grune & Stratton, 1973.
5. Sivertsson, R: The haemodynamic importance of structural vascular changes in essential hypertension. Acta Physiol Scand (Suppl) 343.
6. Hines EA, Brown GE: A standard test for measuring the variability of blood pressure: its significance as an index of the pre-hypertensive state. Ann Intern Med 7:209–217, 1953.
7. Schmitt H, Schmitt H: Localisation of the hypotensive effect of 2-(2-6-dichlorophenyamino)-2-imidazoline hydrochloride. Eur J Pharmacol 6:8–12, 1969.
8. Henning M, Rubenson A: Evidence that the hypotensive action of methyldopa is mediated by central actions of methylnoradrenaline. J Pharm Pharmacol 23:407–411, 1971.
9. Heise A, Kroneberg G: Control nervous alpha-adrenergic receptors and the mode of action of methyldopa. Naunyn Schmiedebergs Arch Pharmacol 279:285–300, 1973.
10. Vanhoutte PM: The adrenergic neuroreflector interaction in the normotensive and hypertensive blood vessel wall. Cardiovasc Pharmacol 2 (Suppl 3):253–267 S, 1980.
11. Starke K, Docherty JR: Recent developments in alpha-adrenoceptor research. Cardiovasc Pharmacol 2 (Suppl 3):269–286 S, 1980.
12. Kobinger W: Central alpha-adrenergic systems as targets for hypotensive drugs. Rev Physiol Biochem Pharmacol 81:39–100, 1978.
13. Collier JG, Lorge RE, Robinson BF: Comparison of the effects of tolmesoxide, diazoxide, hydralazine, prazosin, glyceryl trinitrate and sodium nitroprusside on forearm arteries and dorsal hand veins of man. Br J Clin Pharmacol 5:35–44, 1978.
14. Archibald JL: Indoramin. In: Pharmacology of Anti-hypertensive Drugs, pp. 161–177. Scriabine A, ed. New York: Raven Press, 1980.
15. Majid PA, Sharma B, Taylor SH: Phentolamine for vasodilator treatment of severe heart failure. Lancet 2:719–724, 1971.
16. Stokes GS, Graham RM, Gain JM, Davis PR: Influence of dosage and dietary sodium on the first-dose effects of prazosin. Br Med J 1:1507–1508, 1971.
17. Mancia G, Ferrari A, Gregorini L, Ferrari MC, Bianchi C, Terzoli L, Leonetti G, Zanchetti A: Regulation of circulation during anti-hypertensive treatment with prazosin. Cardiovasc Pharmacol 2 (Suppl 3):249–361 S, 1980.
18. McAllister RG: Effect of adrenergic receptor blockade on the responses to isometric handgrip: studies in normal and hypertensive subjects. J Cardiovasc Pharmacol 1:253–263, 1979.
19. Scriabine A: Prazosin. In: Pharmacology of Anti-Hypertensive Drugs, pp. 151–160. Scriabine A, ed. New York: Raven Press, 1980.
20. Cohn JN: Vasodilator therapy for heart failure; the influence of impedance on left ventricular performance. Circulation 48:5–8, 1973.
21. Chatterjee K, Parmley WW: The role of vasodilator therapy in heart failure. Prog Cardiovasc Dis 19:301–325, 1977.
22. Mehta J, Iacona M, Pepine CJ, Conti CR: Comparison of haemodynamic effects of oral prazosin, oral hydralazine and intravenous nitroprusside in some patients with chronic heart failure. Br Heart J 42:664–670, 1979.
23. Fitchett DH, Pathe M, Pardy R, Despas P: Effect of vasodilator drugs on exercise perfor-

mance in cardiac failure: comparison of hydralazine and prazosin. Br Heart J 44:215–220, 1980.

24. Chidsey CA, Braunwald E, Morrow AG: Catecholamine excretion and cardiac stores of norepinephrine in congestive heart failure. Am J Med 39:442–451, 1964.

25. Taylor SH, Gould LA: Phentolamine in heart failure and other cardiac disorders. Bern: Hans Huber, 1975.

26. Taylor SH, Majid PA: Insulin and the heart. J Mol Cell Cardiol 2:301–325, 1971.

27. Taylor SH, Majid PA, Saxton C, Sharma B: Insulin secretion in heart failure. Am Heart J 83:281–283, 1972.

28. Porte D, Williams RG: Inhibition of insulin release by norepinephrine in man. Science 152:1248–1251, 1966.

29. Majid PA, Saxton C, Dykes JRW, Galvin MC, Taylor SH: Autonomic control of sinsulin secretion and the treatment of heart failure. Br Med J 4:328–331, 1970.

30. Corr PB, Gillis RS: Autonomic neural influences on the dysrhythmias resulting from myocardial infarction. Circ Res 43:1–9, 1978.

31. Sheridan DJ, Penkoske PA, Sobel BE, Corr PB: Alpha-adrenergic contributions to dysrhythmias during myocardial ischaemia and reperfusion in cats. J Clin Invest 65:161–171, 1980.

32. Laragh JH, Baer L, Brunner HR, Buhler F, Sealy JE, Vaughan ED: Renin, Angiotensin and aldosterone system in pathogenesis and management of hypertensive vascular disease. Am J Med 52:633–652, 1972.

33. Correa-Suarez: The effect of vasodilators on the renin-angiotensin-aldosterone system. In: Arterial Hypertension, pp. 96–103. Velasco M, ed. Amsterdam: Elsevier, 1977.

34. Mills DCB, Roberts GCK: Effect of adrenaline on human blood platelets. J Physiol (London) 193:443–453, 1967.

35. Grant JA, Scruten MC: Novel alpha-2 adrenoceptors primarily responsible for inducing human platelet aggregation. Nature 277:659–661, 1979.

36. Silke B, Hendry WG, Taylor DH: Immediate and sustained haemodynamic effects of prazosin during upright exercise. Br Heart J 46:663–670, 1981.

37. Millar-Craig MW, Raftery EB: The effect of conventional and slow-release oxprenolol on the 24-hour arterial blood pressure in essential hypertension. Br J Clin Prac 32 (Suppl 1):33–41, 1978.

38. Pickering G: High Blood Pressure. London: J and A. Churchill, 1968.

39. Taylor SH: The Circulation in Hypertension. In: Hypertension – Its Nature and Treatment, pp. 29–53. Burley DM, ed. Ciba: Publications Ltd., Horsham, England, 1975.

40. Taylor JA, Watt SJ, Belfield P, Taylor SH: Circulatory response to skin cooling. Clinical Science, 58:10 P, 1979.

41. Majid PA, Meeran MK, Benaim ME, Sharm B, Taylor SH: Alpha- and beta-adrenergic blockade in the treatment of hypertension. Br Heart J 36:588, 1974.

42. Taylor SH: Theory and practice in the treatment of heart failure. In: European Prazosin symposium. Rawlins MD, Geyer G, Bleifeld W, eds. Amsterdam: Elsevier, 1979.

43. Taylor SH: Pharmacology and Clinical Applications of β-adrenoceptor Antagonists. In: Theories and Use of β-blockade in Hypertension and Angina. pp 71–88. Roberts, RH, ed. Chicago: Year Book Medical Publications, 1979.

48. VASODILATORS AS ANTIHYPERTENSIVE AGENTS

M. WORCEL and J. C. GAIGNAULT

In this chapter, we will analyse the mode of action and therapeutic use of the 'direct-acting smooth muscle relaxant antihypertensor drugs'. We will include in this class of drugs those antihypertensive compounds which are supposed to relax vascular smooth muscle without interfering with identified cell receptors (adrenergic, dopaminergic, angiotensin II receptors, etc.). For historical reasons, hydralazine and its analogues will be presented in this chapter, but some recent experimental results suggest that these compounds may act at the neurovascular junction [1].

The smooth muscle relaxant antihypertensor drugs share some pharmacological properties:

1. Their antihypertensive action is independent from the sympathetic tone, as demonstrated in either denervated preparations or spinal animals.
2. They antagonize the vasoconstriction induced by exogenous or endogenous spasmogens (noradrenaline, 5.HT*, KCl, angiotensin II, vasopressin and others).
3. They have similar side effects induced by the reflex stimulation of the sympathetic nervous system: tachycardia and salt and water retention.

HYDRALAZINE

Hydralazine was one of the first effective vasodilating drugs introduced in the early fifties with the purpose of the treatment of arterial hypertension. Since the initial publication by Gross et al. [2] the pharmacology of hydrazinophtalazines has been analyzed in numerous papers. Hydralazine lowers the blood pressure of animals and man in a very similar manner. The hypotension appears slowly, even following intravenous injection, the plateau effect being attained half an hour after administration. There is a simultaneous vasodilation associated with local increases in the femoral, renal, mesenteric and carotid flows. Furthermore, this action was confirmed in man, who develops an enhancement of renal and mesenteric blood flows

* 5.HT: SEROTONIN.

Amery, A. (ed.) Hypertensive Cardiovascular Disease: Pathophysiology and Treatment
© *1982, Martinus Nijhoff Publishers. The Hague / Boston / London*
ISBN-13: 978-94-009-7478-4

NH2-NH2

R

Brands:
Apresoline®, Ciba
Ipolina®, Lafare: Italy
etc.

R = H (hydralazine)
R = NH-NH$_2$ (dihydralazine)*

under the action of hydralazine. The drug induces a decrease in the peripheral resistance which appears to be consecutive to the vasodilation of the precapillary vessels. In vivo studies have further shown that hydralazine has a poor effect on capacitance vessels [3, 4].

It appears that hydralazine's hypotensive action results from a rather specific arterial and arteriolar relaxant effect. In vitro experiments further confirm the selectivity of hydralazine for some vascular smooth muscles. Visceral smooth muscles, as well as large vessels, are not affected by low concentrations of the drug. Rat myometrium and vas deferens are relaxed by concentrations of hydralazine higher than 0.1 mM. Rabbit aorta is even less sensitive, 1.5 mM being necessary to inhibit the contractions induced by different spasmogens. Smaller arteries, like the rabbit ear artery and the rat tail artery are, in contrast, very sensitive to the relaxant effect of the antihypertensor drug. In fact, it has been observed that under certain conditions the in vitro response to hydralazine, of the rat tail artery [5] and rabbit ear artery (N. Brown, personal communication), is modulated by the sympathetic nerve terminals remaining in the tissue. Actually, it has been observed that the rabbit ear artery as well as some portions of the rat tail arteries from normotensive rats are practically unsensitive to hydralazine, unless previously denervated. Under these conditions, the drug reduces the maximal contractile response to different spasmogens, without lateral displacement of their dose-response curves. This non-competitive antagonism is non-specific, since hydralazine relaxes in the same way the contractions induced by phenylephrine, 5.HT and vasopressin.

Hydralazine has a very marked dose-dependent action on sensitive segments. Cumulative concentration effect curves may be constructed, characterized by a very steep slope [5]. These effects are obtained at micromolar concentrations of the drug, which appear to be relevant for its in vivo hypotensive action [3].

Further experiments have shown that the vascular smooth muscle response to hydralazine and hydralazine-like drugs might be affected by the

* The generic drug used in some European countries is dihydralazine. Dihydralazine appears to have the same pharmacological properties of the parent compound. Brands of dihydralazine: Nepresol®, Ciba-Geigy; Depressan, Apogetha: D.D.R.; Ileton, Pliva: Jugoslavia; Nonpressin, Farmosgroup: Finland.

release of natural purines from sympathetic nerve terminals [6], or the addition of exogenous purines. It has been proposed [7] that hydralazine and hydralazine-like drugs relax arterial smooth muscle by activating a smooth muscle receptor, sensitive to ATP or adenosine released from sympathetic nerves, simultaneously with the putative transmittor noradrenaline. Although it is generally admitted that hydralazine exerts its main effect by acting on the arteriolar smooth muscle, some data suggest that the antihypertensive agent may also have a central site of action: a centrally mediated hypotensive action of hydralazine was observed by Craver et al. [8] and by Tangri and Bhargava [9]. We are tempted to analyse these last results on the basis of the prejunctional action of hydralazine observed on peripheral vessels [10]. The possibility of hydralazine having a central inhibitory effect is further suggested by the results of Baum et al. [11] who showed that the antihypertensor drug reduces the spontaneous spike discharge of peripheral sympathetic nerves.

In summary, in vitro studies indicate that hydralazine may have a presynaptic inhibitory effect. This action may explain the fact that under some in vivo conditions, the drug appears to have some clear-cut effects on the central and peripheral nervous system. Nevertheless, its main overall effect in human and animals is an arterial and arteriolar vasodilatation. Hydralazine has strong chelating effects and this property of the drug was actually used to develop a dosage method. Subsequently, it was proposed that hydralazine's hypotensive effects might be related to its copper binding properties [12]. It is still not possible to ascertain whether the interactions between Cu^{2+} and hydralazine are relevant to the arterial effects of the drug, the results not being conclusive.

Pharmacokinetics
It has been recognized that hydralazine metabolism is phenotype dependent. Fast acetylator patients need higher doses of the drug than slow acetylators to attain a given hypotensive effect. Specific more sensitive methods for the dosage of hydralazine have been developed recently [13]. After single or repeated administration it is possible to detect the presence in the blood of hydralazine and different metabolites, the more important being the inactive compound hydralazine pyruvic acid hydrazone (HPH). The bio-avaibility is 6.6–9.5% in fast acetylator subjects and 31.3–39.3% in low acetylators. Peak plasma levels are of 0.32 μM for the single dose and 0.14 μM for repeated doses in the fast acetylator group and 1.03 μM for the single dose and 0.06 μM for repeated doses for the slow acetylator group.

Clinical use
The use of hydralazine alone is not recommended for the treatment of arterial hypertension, because of the incidence of side effects, particularly

with high doses of the drug. Hydralazine is specially indicated in association with β-blockers, with or without diuretics. Under these conditions, the unwanted reflex sympathetic stimulation and sodium and water retention is controlled, and a full benefit from the vasodilating action of hydralazine can be obtained.

The most suitable patient for the use of hydralazine is the one needing and additional drug because of an inappropriate control of blood pressure under the treatment with a β-blocker alone or in association with a diuretic.

Hydralazine treatment is initiated with low doses of 25 mg given two to four times a day, increasing the dosage every two to three days, until control is attained with 200 mg/day. It has been proposed earlier to administer the total dose in four times/day, but it appears that a schedule of two doses/day gives the same results. In any case, the patients should not receive more than 300 mg/day, in order to avoid the risks of hydralazine induced lupus [14].

Side effects
The drug may induce headache and flushing, as well as dyspnea, nausea and vomiting. The reflex stimulation of the sympathetic nervous system may produce an hyperkinetic heart response which in patients suffering from cardiac ischemia may precipitate anginal attacks. Otherwise, the incidence of this type of complication is reduced in patients receiving β-blocking drugs.

An increased incidence of joint pains has been observed, particularly in subjects having a past history of rhumatoid disease. Furthermore, a reversible kind of 'lupus syndrome' has sometimes been observed mainly in females treated with doses of hydralazine higher than 300 mg/day [14]. Otherwise, this complication has been observed with other drugs like procainamide, isoniazide and diphenylhydantoin.

In conclusion, hydralazine should still be considered as a usefull adjuvant for the treatment of hypertension, when added to β-blockers, with or without diuretics.

MINOXIDIL

The work on the chemical series of minoxidil began when it was discovered that the compound 2,4-diamino-6-(diallylaminotriazine) (U-7720) possessed potent and prolonged hypotensive activity when administered orally to trained, unanesthetized dogs [15]. The onset of the hypotensive activity was delayed by 1–3 h. Furthermore U-7720 was found to be very poorly active in man. Pharmacokinetic studies have later shown that the compound undergoes an extensive metabolic transformation in the dog. An essential step which leads to the active hypotensive metabolites is the N-oxidation on the ring nitrogen para to the tertiary amino group. This metabolic step is practically absent in man. The identification of the metabolic products, guided the synthesis of a second generation of compounds of which minoxidil 2,4-diamino-6-piperidinopyrimidine-3-oxide, is an example.

Brand:
Loniten®, Upjohn

Minoxidil lowers the blood pressure when administered to experimental animals [16] given orally to normotensive rats it has an hypotensive action which may last after a single dose more than 24 h. There is a dose-dependent effect which extends over a long range: from 0.15 to 150 mg/kg without attaining a plateau. A similar blood lowering action was obtained in normotensive rhesus monkeys and renal hypertensive dogs. The hemodynamic effects of single oral doses of minoxidil was studied on unanesthetized dogs. The compound increases cardiac output and heart rate coincidently with the decrease in blood pressure and in calculated peripheral resistance. It is interesting to note that minoxidil increases the heart rate at low doses which do not modify yet the blood pressure. On chronic administration to dogs the decrease in blood pressure remains constant without the development of tolerance. Furthermore, the increase of heart rate and cardiac output tends to return to pretreatment values under these conditions. The hypotensive effect of minoxidil cannot be blocked by adrenergic, cholinergic or histamine receptors antagonists, thus suggesting that the drug exerts a direct relaxant effet. Indeed minoxidil has a vasodilating effect in the perfused hind limb of anesthetized dogs which seems to be independent of sympathetic innervation. It has been also shown that the hypotensive effect of the drug is associated with an increase of the blood flow to the skin, skeletal muscles, gastrointestinal tract and myocardium, without alteration of the flows to the central nervous system, adrenal glands, kidney, liver and spleen [17]. On the other hand, the drug has little or no effect on capacitance vessels [18]. Despite the multiple in vivo evidences for an arterial smooth muscle effect of minoxidil, it has not been possible to demonstrate any in vitro myorelaxant effect of the drug on different vascular smooth muscle preparations. Hence it is possible to suggest that the vasodilation induced by the antihypertensor agent is due to a metabolite.

788

As expected, consequent to its hemodynamic action, the antihypertensor drug induces an increase in plasma renin activity, as well as sodium and fluid retention, which can be controlled by β-blockers and diuretics which potentiate its hypotensive effects.

Pharmacokinetics
Minoxidil is rapidly and completely absorbed following oral administration in man, rat, dog and rhesus monkey. Peak plasma levels are achieved within 1 h and the drug rapidly disappears from the plasma (half-life, 2–3 h, and is extensively metabolized. Its antihypertensive effect does not appear to bear any relationship to its plasma concentrations. Over 90% of an oral dose is eliminated in the urine within 48 h, mainly in the form of metabolites. The excretion of the drug is not related to glomerular filtration; therefore, excessive accumulation does not occur in the presence of azotemia [19]. The major excretory product in primates is minoxidil-O-glucuronide [20].

Clinical use
Because of its side effects, the use of minoxidil is reserved to severe hypertension, unmanageable by the combined use of two or more drugs at maximal doses. This potent vasodilator is remarkably effective in the management of high blood pressure in patients with renal failure and has practically eliminated the need for bilateral nephrectomy for the hypertension in these patients [21]. The usual maintenance dose is 10–40 mg orally in a single daily dose. Under these conditions it lowers effectively blood pressure, especially when combined with β-adrenergic blockade with propranolol. This combination appears to have a synergistic effect [22] and inhibits the sympathetic reflex increase in blood pressure. Furthermore, an oral diuretic may be added to the minoxidil plus β-blocker treatment in order to minimize fluid retention [13].

Side effects
The major adverse reaction to the treatment with this compound besides tachycardia and fluid retention, is hypertrichosis. Other more infrequent side effects are angina pectoris, congestive heart failure and pericardial effusion, particularly in patients under hemodyalisis. Hypertrichosis is characterized by elongation, increased pigmentation and thickening of fine body hair. This phenomenon develops within the first month of treatment, and ceases with its interruption. Normal appearance returns after two or six months of the last administration of the drug [23].

In conclusion, considering the untoward effects of minoxidil, the benefit to risk ratio appears to be acceptable only for patients with life threatening hypertension, resistant to other drugs.

DIAZOXIDE

Diazoxide (7-chloro-3-methyl-2H-1,2,4-benzothiadiazine-1,1-dioxide) is a benzothiadiazine derivative, devoid of diuretic properties. It was synthetized by J. G. Topliss, M. M. Sherlock and N. S. Perber from the Schering Corporation in 1961, with the purpose of dissociating the antihypertensive and diuretic properties of this type of molecules.

Brands:
Eudemine®, Allen & Hanbury's
Hyperstat®, Shering Corp.
etc.

Mode of action
The cardiovascular effects of diazoxide were first explored by Rubin et al. [24] in animals. The intravenous injection of diazoxide to anesthetized dogs and cats produces a rapid hypotention, with a maximal effect at 30 s, and lasting for 30–120 min. The blood lowering effect of the drug is not affected by phentolamine, atropine, the ganglion blocker hexamethonium, reserpine, the surgical transection of the spinal cord or antihistaminics. Diazoxide administration increases cardiac output in animals [24] and man [25]. This hemodynamic effect is associated with tachycardia, enhanced dP/dt max, and a marked decrease in the calculated peripheral resistance. As with other vasodilator drugs, the cardiac effects of diazoxide are due to the simultaneous decrease of the afterload, and to an increase of the sympathetic discharge, as a result of the baroreceptor reflex [26].

Diazoxide reduces non-specifically the hypertensive response to noradrenaline, angiotensin and serotonin and reduces the resistance in the femoral, renal and coronary artery territories in the dog [24]. This direct vasodilating effects of the drug are due to an arteriolar myorelaxant effect. Indeed, diazoxide lowers arterial pressure without modifying venous pressure [27].

The cellular mechanism responsible for the myorelaxant effects of diazoxide is not well understood yet. Wohl et al. [28] reported that diazoxide blocks the contractions induced by Ca^{2+} in the presence of KCl depolarizing solutions. The blocking action of the drug on Ca^{2+} contraction appears to have a competitive kinetics, with a pA_2 of 4.3. Furthermore, it has been shown that diazoxide is able to block spike triggering in the isolated rat portal vein.

These results suggest that diazoxide blocks the membrane potential dependent transmembrane Ca^{2+} fluxes, thus interfering with the excitation-contraction coupling of the vascular smooth muscle as a calcium antagonist [29]. It is worthwhile mentioning that the rat aorta is relaxed by concentrations of diazoxide of the order of 0.02 mM. This response appears to be relevant to the in vivo action of the drug. Indeed, the antihypertensor effect of diazoxide coincides with plasmatic concentrations of 0.05 to 1 mM [30]. Besides its hemodynamic effects, diazoxide appears to have an hyperglycemic action, particularly marked in patients with a diabetic predisposition. Hyperglycemia results in part from the simultaneous reduction of insulin secretion and the stimulation of catecholamine release [31].

Pharmacokinetics
Diazoxide is well absorbed by the oral route [30]. Following intravenous administration, peak plasma levels are reached in a few seconds, but it is rapidly bound to serum albumin. This protein bound form of the drug represents 90 % of the diazoxide present in the plasma. So protected from glomerular filtration, the half life of the drug is extremely long (10–57 h) [32], and does not bear any relation with the duration of the hypotensive effect. In man, diazoxide and its metabolites are mainly eliminated in the urine. They are devoid of hypotensive activity, the most important compounds being the 3-hydroxymethyl or 3-carboxy and the sulfate conjugates [33].

Clinical use
Because of its undesirable side effects observed during chronic administration, diazoxide is exclusively used nowadays in the treatment of hypertensive emergencies, when rapid reduction of blood pressure is necessary [34]. Diazoxide is extremely usefull to prevent organ damage from hypertensive encephalopathy, hypertensive crisis and accelerated hypertension. In preeclamptic toxemia and eclampsia, the antihypertensor is particularly effective in arresting convulsions and lowering blood pressure. Following the intravenous injection of the drug in hypertensive patients, there is a rapid pressure fall which starts in one minute, reaching a plateau within two or three minutes. The intensity of the effect of a given dose is higher when diazoxide is injected rapidly, in order to avoid the intense binding of the drug to serum albumin. Interestingly enough the reduction of blood pressure below normotensive levels is uncommon. The magnitude of the effect of diazoxide increases with the pretreatment level of blood pressure, the antihypertensor being effective in 75–85 % of the patients, even when they are resistant to other treatments.

The usual dose of diazoxide is 300 mg or 5 mg/kg given intravenously in less than 30 s. This rapid injection should be made in an established venous line in order to avoid extravasation. Injections may be repeated at intervals of half to three hours, the maximal dose being 1.2 g/day. As opposed to sodium nitroprusside, it has the advantage of having a very rapid effect (1-2 min) after a single injection, blood pressure staying at near normotensive levels at least for 3 h, avoiding the need of continous monitoring.

Blood pressure gradually increases to pretreatment levels following a single administration, within 3–15 h. Diazoxide has been contraindicated in patients with coronary or cerebral vascular insufficiency. However, it has been shown recently that arterial pressure can be controlled with diazoxide even in these patients, by the intermittent injection of smaller doses of diazoxide (50–100 mg) at 15 min intervals, until a satisfactory control of blood pressure is obtained.

Side effects
Salt and water retention, which may precipitate congestive heart failure, appears after repeated injections, especially in uremic patients. It can be controlled by furosemide administration. In some cases, diazoxide may precipitate angina pectoris, cardiac infarction or cerebral ischemia in patients with hypertensive crisis. The incidence of this complication may be diminished by the fractionation of the dose of diazoxide in repeated injections (vide supra). Nausea and vomiting occur sometimes and can be reduced or avoided by the administration of the drug in between meals. As with other vasodilators, the administration of diazoxide may sometimes induce flushing and headache. Used for the treatment of preeclampsia and eclampsia, diazoxide may relax the uterus and interrupt labor. Uterine contractions may be restored by the administration of oxytocic agents [34]. Otherwise, the use of intravenous diazoxide in those cases in which the induced increase in cardiac output may be an endangering event is contraindicated: dissecting aneurism, pheochromocytoma and compensatory hypertensions like those due to coarctation of aorta or arteriovenous shunts. It should be avoided in patients with known coronary and cerebral vascular insufficiency. Of practical importance is the local burning sensation which results from the extravasation of the very alkaline solutions of diazoxide used for intravenous administration. No serious consequences originate from this complication. This inconvenient can be avoided by the administration of the drug on an established venous line.

Some complications have been more frequently or exclusively observed after chronic oral administration of diazoxide, no longer recommended: extrapyramidal symptoms, hyperglycemia, hypertrichosis and hirsutism [35].

In conclusion, we can say that diazoxide may be life saving when administered intravenously for the management of hypertensive crisis. Its use should be restricted to this indication.

SODIUM NITROPRUSSIDE

The medical interest on nitroprusside arose in 1955 after Page et al. [36] described its cardiovascular actions in animals and hypertensive patients. Comprehensive reviews of the pharmacology of nitroprusside have been published [37].

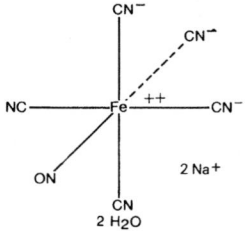

Brands:
Nipride®, Roche
Nipruton®, Berlin Chemie, D.D.R.

Mode of action

Sodium nitroprusside is a strong and fast-acting hypotensive agent when administered intravenously the active component in sodium nitroprusside is the free nitroprusside radical rather than its decomposition products. The short duration of the hypotensive effects are due to the destruction of the active radical which is converted in the body to cyanogen [36].

In the conscious dog, the infusion of nitroprusside determines a precipitous fall in blood pressure, accompanied by an increase in cardiac output which tended to return to control values even during a sustained infusion. On the other hand, tachycardia was maintained during all the infusion time. Simultaneously there is a big increase in the coronary flow, with intermediate vasodilation in the mesenteric and iliac vascular beds, with the least increase in blood flow in the renal circulation. The administration of Na nitroprusside to the conscious dog determines very intense reflex adjustements [38]. Otherwise, the hypotension induced by nitroprusside in anesthetized dogs is associated with a marked decrease in total peripheral resistance and central venous pressure, as well as a reduction of pulmonary arterial pressure [37]. The antihypertensor agent thus appears to have a vasodilator effect in the arterial bed and capacitance vessels. The simultaneous decrease of preload and afterload improves cardiac performance. As a consequence, sodium nitroprusside is especially indicated in hypertensive emergencies in patients suffering from heart failure.

It has been shown in in vitro experiments performed by Kreye et al. [39] that the drug is very active on smooth muscles with a predominantly tonic response, otherwise characterized by an absence of spontaneous contractions, e.g. rat aorta or guinea pig tracheal muscle. These preparations are highly sensitive to nitroprusside, being relaxed with and IC50* in the nanomolar range.

* IC50: Concentration of a substance which produces an inhibitory response corresponding to 50% of the maximal response.

Nitroprusside appears to have an unusual action at the cellular level. The drug reduces the membrane permeability to chloride in rabbit aorta smooth muscle [40]. Indeed, since the equilibrium potential for chloride is lower than the membrane potential in smooth muscle cells, this action could induce an increase in the membrane potential. Indeed, it has been shown by intracellular recording, that nitroprusside hyperpolarizes the rabbit pulmonary artery smooth muscle coincidently with relaxation [41]. Furthermore, it has been shown that the pretreatment with a relatively specific inhibitor of the cGMP phosphodiesterase enhances the relaxation as well as the increase in cellular cGMP levels induced by nitroprusside [42].

In summary, sodium nitroprusside has a direct relaxant effect on vascular smooth muscle. Its cellular mode of action is not completely clear yet. The relaxant effect may be partly due to membrane hyperpolarisation, associated with a decrease in the membrane permeability to chloride. The role of cGMP in the mediation of the nitroprusside relaxation remains to be established.

Pharmacokinetics
Nitroprusside is quickly metabolized in vivo, loosing the cyanide groups. Cyanide is rapidly converted to thiocyanate which appears to be excreted mainly by the kidneys. Some of the thiocyanate can be oxidized back to cyanide [43], nevertheless, even after prolonged administration, cyanide blood concentrations stays well below the lethal level (0.05–0.10 mg/100 ml of blood).

Clinical use
Sodium nitroprusside must be administered by continuous venous infusion, since its hypotensive action is very short-lasting. Blood pressure drops within seconds of starting an infusion, and rapidly rises in less than 10 min, following the interruption of the drug [43]. One of the disadvantages of the sodium nitroprusside therapy is that it requires a continuous nursing care. It is normally given as a 100 mg/l solution, infused through a venous line, with a microdrop dosage device, or even better with an infusion pump. The required doses vary considerably, anywhere from 15–800 μg/min. The main indication for nitroprusside therapy is the hypertensive emergency associated with hypertensive encephalopathy, pheochromocytoma, severe burns, drug-induced hypertension and intracerebral or subarachnoid hemorrage. Nitroprusside is the drug of choice when hypertension is associated with heart failure and/or cardiac infarction. In this case, it is safer than diazoxide. Nitroprusside is effective even in cases in which the patients have been resistant to other types of antihypertensive treatment. The drug allows a satisfactory and rapid control of blood pressure, with a carefull manipulation of the infusion and continuous supervision. Usually, the sensitivity to

other medications is restored after a variable time, and oral antihypertensive treatment can be substituted gradually after a period of hours or several days. In any case, patients already under treatment with hypotensive drugs appear to require lower doses of nitroprusside.

Side effects
They are usually related to the rapid decrease in blood pressure and include the signs of circulatory collapse. Furthermore, the patients may complain of nausea, restlessness and muscular twitching. It has been proposed that the maximal dose of nitroprusside should not exceed 0.5 mg/kg for brief infusions in order to avoid the danger of cyanide poisoning. Hypothyroidism and retention of thiocyanate have been observed after the administration of the drug for periods longer than a week [44]. The prolonged use of nitroprusside is not justified any longer.

In conclusion, nitroprusside infusion should be reserved to the treatment of hypertensive emergencies, under continuous nursing care.

CALCIUM ANTAGONISTS

Since the discovery of verapamil [45], a series of molecules have been synthetized, which act qualitatively in a similar way on cardiac and smooth muscles. At the cellular level, these compounds inhibit the membrane conductance through the slow sodium-calcium channel, and/or the release of Ca^{2+} from external or internal cell stores. In any case as an end result, calcium antagonists by reducing the influx of Ca^{2+} through the cell membrane, have negative inotropic and chronotropic actions on heart muscle, as well as a relaxant effect on smooth muscles. Despite this common mechanism, the members of this class of drugs have rather dissimilar effects, when administered to whole animals. Indeed, verapamil or gallopamil act preferentially on the heart and coronary arteries. In fact, the main clinical indication for verapamil is the treatment of arrythmia associated or not with cardiac ischemia. In the middle of the spectrum we find diltiazem whose main action appears to be exerted on the coronary arteries. These drugs have been indicated in the treatment of angor pectoris and Prinzmetal angina. Diltiazem appears to have a preferential effect on coronary smooth muscle, where it inhibits calcium release from intracellular stores. Additionally, this compound has a weak hypotensive effect and a rather small negative chronotropic action [46, 47].
Other compounds of this pharmacological series have a coronary vasodilator effect, associated with a relaxant action on the peripheral arterial system, responsible of an hypotensive effect. Nifidipine [48], whose main indication is the treatment of cardiac ischemia, has been used in the treatment

of arterial hypertension. More recently, it has been suggested that some compounds like Nitrendipine (Bay e 5009) [49] may have a preferential antihypertensive effect. It is possible that new calcium antagonists will be obtained in the near future, characterized by a higher selectivity for arterial smooth muscle.

DRUGS ACTUALLY USED IN THE TREATMENT OF ARTERIAL HYPERTENSION

Brands:
Adalat®, Bayer
Corinfar, Arzneimittelwerk, Dresden, DDR
Nigelat®, Sidus, Argentina
Oxcord®, Biosintetica, Brazil

Nifedipine

This molecule was described in 1971 by Bossert and Vater [50], and first studied in pharmacology by Vater et al. [51]. Like Verapamil, its main therapeutic indication is as a coronary vasodilator [52]. Nifedipine has a strong relaxant effect on the coronary arteries. Administered to the dog intraveneously or through the perlingual route, it increases rapidly the coronary flow by more than 50%. Furthermore, it has been observed that in vivo this compound produces a strong arterial vasodilation [51], being devoid under these conditions of a negative inotropic effect. On these grounds it was suggested that its main target may be the arterial smooth muscle [52]. Nifedipine has been used for the acute and chronic treatment of arterial hypertension. After oral or sublingual administration of a 10 mg dose, Guazzi et al. [48] observed a large pressure reduction in patients with severe primary hypertension. The hypotensive effect was associated with a marked decrease of peripheral resistance and increase in pulse and cardiac output. Olivary et al. [53] administered 10 mg doses of Nifedipine to 27 patients with primary essential hypertension. Under these conditions, they observed that there is an hypotensive response which lasts during 8-12 h. Administered orally, 10 mg every 6 h during the waking hours (3/day), Nifedipine reduces significantly blood pressure through the 24 h apparently without postural hypotension. Some short-lasting side effects were observed in a reduced number of patients: headache, sporadic extrasystoles, palpitations without arrythmias, symptoms which tended to disappear with continued treatment. Nifedipine did not modify renal function, nor produce edema or any obvious change in sodium handling. It is interesting to note that plasma renin activity was not altered by the treatment with the calcium antagonists. It has been observed that the administration of verapamil to the rat results in a complete inhibition of the tubuloglomerular feedback operation responsible of the control of renin secretion [54, 55]. These results may suggest that as a common feature, calcium antagonists may have vasodilating and hypotensive actions, without a concomitant activation of renin secretion.

Pharmacokinetics

Nifedipine is well absorbed following oral administration. There is not a good correlation between the blood levels of the drug and the hypotensive effects [56]. Nevertheless, the plasma concentration of the drug appears to be correlated to the decrease in peripheral resistance.

Indications

Nifedipine is just in experimental use for the treatment of hypertension. Further clinical evaluation is necessary to determine its long term action and side effects as well as the persistence of its antihypertensive action.

Indapamide

Indapamide has been recently introduced for the treatment of hypertension. This molecule is a sulfamyde diuretic presenting an antihypertensive action which has been attributed to a direct vasodilating effect. This interesting substance is a 3-sulfamoyl-4-chlorobenzamide indolin derivative.

Brands:
Fludex®, Servier, France
Natrilex®, Servier, France

Kyncl et al. [57] have shown that indapamide lowers blood pressure after oral administration to spontaneous hypertensive, DOCA + salt, or renal hypertensive rats. The drug is effective beyond 3 mg/kg p.o., doses 30–300 times higher being necessary to achieve a similar acute hypotensive action with other diuretics. Finch et al. [58] were able to show that indapamide lowers the vascular reactivity in hypertensive rats treated chronically, hydrochlorothiazide being devoid of action under the same conditions. On the basis of experiments performed in vitro, using different isolated vessels, it has been claimed that indapamide has a direct myorelaxant effect on vascular smooth muscle, due to a calcium antagonist effect [59]. Unfortunately, the preparations used are rather insensitive to the drug, indapamide being active at concentrations beyond 10^{-4} M, it is hardly relevant to explain the in vivo effect of the drug. There are no current publications reporting in detail the diuretic effects of indapamide in experimental animals. According to some information the drug appears to have a saline diuretic effect in rat and dog at doses beyond 0.1–0.3 mg/kg p.o., lower than those necessary to induce an hypotensive effect [60]. Otherwise, the drug seems to be well tolerated and endowed with a low toxicity range.

Indapamide has been introduced in the European market for the purpose of the treatment of arterial hypertension in some countries (France) and as a diuretic agent in others (Belgium). It has been used in the treatment of mild to moderate hypertension, administered to patients at a single oral dosage of 2.5 mg/day. Under these conditions it appears to control satisfactorily the blood pressure levels, its antihypertensive effect being installed gradually. The long-term treatment with the drug is sometimes associated with the usual complications of diuretic therapy: hyperuricemia and hypokalemia.

In conclusion, indapamide appears to be a usefull drug for the treatment of mild to moderate hypertension. Nevertheless, it is not clear as yet if the mode of action of this agent is really different from the basic mechanism common to other diuretics. In particular, its singularity as a smooth muscle relaxant needs to be confirmed.

REFERENCES

1. Chevillard C, Saiag B, Worcel M: Hydralazine. In: Vasodilation. pp. 477–489. Vanhoutte P, Leusen I, eds. New York: Raven Press, 1981.
2. Gross F, Druey J, Meier R: Eine Gruppe blutdrucksenkender Substanzen von besonderem Wirkungscharakter. Experientia 6:11–12, 1950.
3. Worcel M, Saiag B, Chevillard C: An unexpected mode of action for hydralazine. Trends Pharmacol Sci 1:136–138, 1980.
4. Gross F: Drugs acting on arteriolar smooth muscle (vasodilator drugs). In: Antihypertensive Agents, pp. 397–476. Gross F, ed. Berlin: Springer-Verlag, 1977.
5. Worcel M: Relationship between the direct inhibitory effects of hydralazine and propildazine on arterial smooth muscle contractility and sympathetic innervation. J Pharmacol Exp Ther 207:320–330, 1978.
6. Chevillard C, Saiag B, Worcel M: Interactions between hydralazine, propildazine and purines on arterial smooth muscle. Br J Pharmacol 73:811–817, 1981.
7. Worcel M, Chevillard C: Mechanism of action of antihypertensive drugs acting on arterial smooth muscle. In: Trends in Arterial Hypertension. Eds., Worcel M, Bonvalet JP, Langer SZ, Menard J, Sassard J, Inserm, Amsterdam: Elsevier/North-Holland. (In press.)
8. Craver BN, Barrett W, Cameron A, Jonkman FF: The activities of 1. hydrazinophtalazine (Ba 5968) a hypotensive agent. J Am Pharm Ass Sci, 40:559–564, 1951.
9. Tangri KK, Barghava KP: The central hypotensive action of 1-hydrazinophtalazine (C 5968). Arch Int Pharmacodyn Ther 125:331–342, 1960.
10. Chevillard C, Mathieu MN, Saiag B, Worcel M: Hydralazine: effect on the outflow of noradrenaline and mechanical responses evoked by sympathetic nerve stimulation of the rat tail artery. Br J Pharmacol 69:415–420, 1980.

11. Baum T, Shropshire AT, vasner LL: Contribution of the central nervous system to the action of several antihypertensive agents (Methyldopa, Hydralazine and Guanethidine). J Pharmacol Exp Ther 182:135-144, 1972.

12. Schroeder HA: The pharmacology of hydralazine. In: Hypertension. The first Hanhemann symposium on hypertension disease, pp.332-344. Meyer H, ed. Philadelphia: Saunders, 1959.

13. Haegele KD, McNay JL, Skadlant HB, Clementi WA, Shepherd AM: Pharmacokinetics and cardiovascular effects in rabbits of a major hydralazine metabolite, the hydralazine-pyruvic-acid hydrazone. J Pharmacol Exp Ther 211:509-513, 1979.

14. Alarcon-Segovia D, Worthington JW, Ward LE, Wakim KG: Clinical and experimental studies on the hydralazine syndrome and its relationship to systemic lupus erythematosus. Medicine 46:1-33, 1967.

15. Freyburger WA, Weeks JR, Ducharme DW: Cardiovascular actions of the hypotensive agent, n, N-diallylmelamine (U-7720). Naunyn-Schmiedeberg's Arch. Pharmacol, 251:39-47, 1965.

16. Ducharme DW, Freyburger WA, Graham BE, Carlson RG: Pharmacologic properties of minoxidil: a new hypotensive agent. J Pharmacol Exp Ther 184:662-670, 1973.

17. Humphrey SJ, Wilson E, Zins GR: Whole body tissue blood flow in conscious dogs treated with minoxidil. Fed Proc, 33:583, 1974.

18. O'Malley K, Velasco M, Wells J, McNay J: Mechanism of the interaction of propranolol and a potent vasodilator antihypertensive agent: Minoxidil. Eur J Clin Pharmacol 9:355-366, 1976.

19. Gottlieb TB, Thomas RC, Chidsey CA: Pharmacokinetic studies of minoxidil. Clin Pharmacol Ther 13:436-441, 1971.

20. Thomas RC, Hsi RSP, Harpootlian H, Judy RW: Metabolism of minoxidil, a new hypotensive agent — I. Absorption, distribution and excretion following administration to rats, dogs and monkeys. J Pharm Sci 64:1360-1366, 1975.

21. Pettinger WA, Mitchell HC: Minoxidil. An alternative for nephrectomy for refractory hypertension. N Engl J Med, 289:167-171, 1973.

22. Gilmore E, Weil J, Chidsey CA: Treatment of essential hypertension with a new vasodilator in combination with beta-adrenergic blockade. N Engl J Med 282:521-527, 1970.

23. Ducharme DW, Zins GR: Minoxidil. In: Pharmacology of antihypertensor drugs, pp 415-421, Scriabine A, ed. New York: Raven Press, 1980.

24. Rubin AA, Roth FE, Taylor RM, Rosenkilde H: Pharmacology of diazoxide, an antihypertensive, nondiuretic benzothiadiazine. J Pharmacol Exp Ther 136:344-352, 1962.

25. Wilson WR, Okun R: The acute hemodynamic effects of diazoxide in man. Circulation 28:89-93, 1963.

26. Schmitt H, Fenard S: Modifications par le diazoxide de la réponse électrique des nerfs sympathiques à des hypertensions aiguës. Therapie 24:523-530, 1969.

27. Rubin AA, Zitowitz L, Hausler L: Acute circulatory effects of diazoxide and sodium nitrite. J. Pharmacol Exp Ther 140:46-51, 1963.

28. Wohl AJ, Hausler LM, Roth FE: The role of calcium in the mechanism of the antihypertensive action of diazoxide. Life Sci, 7:381-387, 1968.

29. Rohdes HJ, Sutter MC: The action of diazoxide on isolated vascular smooth muscle, electrophysiology and contraction. Can J Physiol Pharmacol49:276-287, 1971.

30. Calesnick B, Katchen B, Black J: Importance of dissolution rates in producing effective diazoxide blood levels in man. J Pharm Sci 54:1277-1280.

31. Loubatieres A, Mariani MM, Alric R: The action of diazoxide on insulin secretion, medullo-adrenal secretion and the liberation of catecholamines. Ann NY acad Sci 150:226-241, 1968.

32. Sellers EM, Koch-Weser J: Displacement of warfarin from human albumin by diazoxide

and ethacrynic, mefenamic and nalidixic acids. Clin. Pharmacol Exp Ther 11:524–529, 1970.
33. Pruitt AW, Faraj BA, Dayton PG: Metabolism of diazoxide in man and experimental animals. J Pharmacol Exp. Ther 188:248–256.
34. Paulissian R: Diazoxide. Int Anesthesiol Clin 16:201–237, 1978.
35. Opie LH: Drugs and the heart. VI: Vasodilating drugs. Lancet, 966–972, 1980.
36. Page IH, Corcoran AC, Dustan HP, Koppanyi T: Cardiovascular actions of sodium nitroprusside in animals and hypertensive patients. Circulation 11:188–198, 1955.
37. Kreye VAW: Sodium nitroprusside: approaches towards the elucidation of its mode of action. Trends Pharmacol Sci 1:384–388, 1980.
38. Pagani M, Vatner SF, Braunwald E: Hemodynamic effects of intravenous sodium nitroprusside in the conscious dog. Circulation 57:144–151, 1978.
39. Kreye VAW, Baron GD, Lüth JB, Schmidt-Gayk H: Mode of action of sodium nitroprusside on vascular smooth muscle. Naunyn-Schmiedebergs Arch Pharmacol 288:381–402, 1975.
40. Kreye VAW, Kern R, Schleich I: ^{36}Chloride efflux from noradrenaline-stimulated rabbit aorta inhibited by sodium nitroprusside and nitroglycerine. In: Excitation-contraction coupling in Smooth Muscle, pp. 145–150. Casteels R, Godfraind T, Rüegg JC, eds. Amsterdam: Elsevier/North-Holland, 1977.
41. Hausler G, Thorens G: The pharmacology of vasoactive antihypertensives. In: Vascular Neuroeffector Mechanisms, pp. 232–241. Bevan JA, Burnstock G, Johansson B, Maxwell-RA, Nedegaard OE, eds. Basel: S. Karger, 1976.
42. Kukovetz WR, Holzmann S, Worm A, Poch G: Evidence for cyclic GMP-mediated relaxant effects of nitro-compounds in coronary muscle. Naunyn Schmiedebergs Arch Pharmacol 310:129–138, 1979.
43. Tuzel IH: Sodium nitroprusside: a review of its clinical effectiveness as a hypotensive agent. J Clin Pharmacol 14:494–503, 1974.
44. Kreye VAW: Sodium nitroprusside. In: Pharmacology of Antihypertensive Drugs, pp. 373–396. Scriabine A, ed. New York: Raven Press, 1980.
45. Fleckenstein A: Specific pharmacology of calcium in myocardium, cardiac pacemakers and vascular smooth muscle. Ann Rev Pharmacol Toxicol, 17:149–166, 1977.
46. Opie LH: Drugs and the heart – III: calcium antagonists. Lancet 806–811, 1980.
47. Ito Y, Kuriyama H, Suzuki H: The effects of diltiazem (CRD-401) on the membrane and mechanical properties of vascular smooth muscles of the rabbit. Br. J. Pharmacol, 64:503–510, 1978.
48. Guazzi M, Olivari MT, Polese A, Fiorentini C, Magrini F, Moruzzi P: Nifedipine, a new antihypertensive with rapid action. Clin Pharmacol Exp Ther 22:528–532, 1977.
49. Towart R, Stoepec K: The vascular mechanism of action of Bay e 5009, a new calcium antagonist with a potent antihypertensive action. Arch Pharmacol 308:70, 1979.
50. Bossert F, Vater W: Dihydropyridine, eine neue Gruppe stark wirksamer Coronartherapeutika. Naturwissenschaften 58:578,1971.
51. Vater W, Kronenberg G, Hoffmeister F, Kaller H, Meng K, Oberdorf A, Puls W, Schlossmann K, Stoepel K: Zur Pharmakologie von 4-(2'-Nitrophenyl)-2,6-dimethyl-1,4-dihydropyridin-3,5-dicarbon, Sauredimethylester, (Nifedipine) Bay a 1040, Arzneim Forsch 22:14, 1972.
52. Editorial: Nifedipine. Lancet 352–354, 1980.
53. Olivari MT, Bartorelli C, Polese A, Fiorentini C, Moruzzi P, Guazzi MD: Treatment of hypertension with nifedipine, a calcium antagonistic agent. Circulation 59:1056–1062, 1979.
54. Watanabe AM, Besch HR: Subcellular myocardial effects of verapamil and D600: comparison with propranolol. J Pharmacol Exp Ther 191:241–250, 1974.

55. Lederballe-Pedersen O, Mikkelsen E, Christensen NJ, Kornerup MJ, Pedersen EB: Effect of nifedipine on plasma renin, aldosterone and catecholamines in arterial hypertension. Eur J Clin Pharmacol 15:235–240, 1979.
56. Lederballe-Pedersen O, Christensen CK, Mikkelsen E, Rämsch KD: Relation between the antihypertensive effect and steady-state plasma concentration of nifedipine given alone or in combination with a beta-adrenoceptor blocking agent. Eur J Clin Pharmacol 18:287–293, 1980.
57. Kyncl J, Oheim K, Seki Y, Solles A: Antihypertensive action of indapamide. Comparative studies on several experimental models. Arzneim Forsch 25:1491–1495, 1975.
58. Finch L, Hicks PE, Moore RA: The effects of indapamide on vascular reactivity in experimental hypertension. Curr Med Res Opin 5:S1:44–54, 1977.
59. Mironneau J, Gargouil YM: Action of indapamide on excitation-contraction coupling in vascular smooth muscle. Eur J Pharmacol 57:57–67, 1979.
60. Moore RA, Seki T, Ohsumi S, Omeim K, Kyncl J, Desnoyers P: Action antihypertensive de l'indapamide et revue des travaux de pharmacologie et de toxicologie. Symposium International sur l'Indapamide. L.B.F. Biopharmaceutherapie, Neuilly-sur-Seine, France, 1977.

49. METHYLDOPA AS AN ANTIHYPERTENSIVE AGENT

B. N. C. PRICHARD

ALPHA METHYLDOPA

Mode of action

How α-methyldopa exerts its antihypertensive action has been a matter of debate, but the evidence suggests a central mode of action [1–4].

Methyldopa is an inhibitor of dopa-decarboxylase reducing the rate of catecholamine synthesis. However, as other inhibitors of the enzyme are not antihypertensive this is unlikely to be responsible for the hypotensive effect [5]. It was shown that α-methyldopa is metabolised to α-methyldopamine and then to α-methylnoradrenaline. The α-methylnoradrenaline is formed in sympathetic nerves after methyldopa administration [6] and it is liberated on nerve stimulation [7]. Experiments in man showed that there was a reciprocal relationship between noradrenaline and α-methylnoradrenaline excretion, a finding that is consistent with α-methylnoradrenaline replacing noradrenaline in the neurosecretory pool [8]. Day and Rand [9, 10] proposed that α-methyldopa exerted its anti-hypertensive effect by being converted to α-methylnoradrenaline which then acted as a false transmitter when liberated at sympathetic nerve endings. However, it was found that α-methylnoradrenaline is about equipotent to noradrenaline in the cat and dog both species in whom a-methyldopa exerts a hypotensive effect [11]. It has similarly been shown in man that α-methylnoradrenaline is only slightly less potent that noradrenaline on human smooth muscle [12]. On the other hand in the rat renal artery, in vitro, α-methylnodradrenaline has only one-eighth the vasoconstrictor potency of noradrenaline and the responses to nerve stimulation are reduced by the acute administration of methyldopa [13]. Although the acute administration of α-methyldopa depresses the function of sympathetic nerves, as also shown by the reduction of the response of the cat nictitating membrane to nerve stimulation [10], no effect was seen on the responses after chronic treatment [14]. Lastly, it was also found that hypotensive doses of α-methyldopa failed to reduce the pressor response that is seen when the entire sympathetic outflow is stimulated [13].

Amery, A. (ed.) Hypertensive Cardiovascular Disease: Pathophysiology and Treatment
© *1982, Martinus Nijhoff Publishers. The Hague / Boston / London*
ISBN-13: 978-94-009-7478-4

Another previous hypothesis unlikely for the reasons just discussed, was the proposal that α-methyldopamine, a weak alpha stimulant, was synthetised in the liver and then acted as a competitive inhibitor with noradrenaline at alpha-receptors [15].

A number of observations suggest that the central nervous system is probably the site of the anti-hypertensive action of methyldopa, besides being the site of a number of important side effects. Henning and van Zwieten [16] noted that a dose of 20 mg/kg of α-methyldopa injected into the vertebral artery in the cat under chlorolose anaesthesia produced a fall of blood pressure while intravenous administration of a similar amount produced no effect. However, experiments in the dog found no difference in the hypotensive response to methyldopa between intravenous, intravertebral infusion, or infusion into the internal carotid [17]. Then Ingenito et al. [18] found that the administration of α-methyldopa into the vascularly isolated perfused cat brain caused a fall in blood pressure in the rest of the animal. Moreover, Baum et al. [19] have shown that there is a reduction of sympathetic nerve traffic following the administration of methyldopa to renal hypertensive rats, but Finch and Haeusler [13] failed to show any reduced spontaneous sympathetic nerve activity.

Alpha-methyldopa is converted into α-methylnoradrenaline in the brain [20, 21], which then appears to stimulate central α-adrenergic receptors. The resultant hypotensive effect is blocked by α-adrenoceptor blocking drugs [13, 22] and the prevention of the metabolism of methyldopa and thus the formation of α-methylnoradrenaline by the administration of a centrally active dopa-decarboxylase inhibitor abolishes the anti-hypertensive effect of α-methyldopa [13, 23]. This does not occur when a dopa-decarboxylase inhibitor which does not penetrate the brain is given [21, 23]. The same is true in man, where peripheral decarboxylose inhibition with alpha methyl hydrazine failed to alter the hypotensive response to methyldopa [24]. The prevention of α-methylnoradrenaline synthesis by the destruction of central adrenergic neurones by intraventricular 6-hydroxydopamine also prevented the hypotensive effect of α-methyldopa [25], whereas intravenous 6-hydroxydopamine reduced the fall in blood pressure, but did not prevent it. The exact site of action may be the anterior hypothalamic pre-optic region as injection of α-methylnoradrenaline here lowers the blood pressure [26, 27]. Finch and Haeusler [13] found that the rise in blood pressure after stimulation of the posterior hypothalamus in the anaesthetised cat was reduced by methyldopa.

The anti-hypertensive action of methyldopa does not appear to be due to its renin suppressing action [28].

In conclusion, the evidence points to a central site of action of methyldopa most probably involving the formation of α-methylnoradrenaline.

Cardiovascular effects of α-methyldopa

The intravenous administration of α-methyldopa reduces blood pressure principally by reducing peripheral resistance. There was no significant change in cardiac output for both supine and erect positions [29, 30]. After short-term administration there was no change in the supine cardiac output accompanying the fall in blood pressure [31–33]. Chamberlain and Howard [34] did not observe any fall in cardiac output from short-term doses of 0.75-3G of α-methyldopa daily; the decline in blood pressure in the supine position was associated with a reduction in peripheral resistance. There was an increased fall in blood pressure on standing and on exercise that was associated with a failure of the peripheral resistance to increase, as it did prior to the administration of α-methyldopa. There was no evidence to indicate any increased venous pooling on standing as the normal fall of cardiac output on adopting the erect position was not enhanced after α-methyldopa. However, the blood pressures in many of these patients were relatively high even after treatment with α-methyldopa and thus these results may not be fully applicable to patients when blood pressure is adequately controlled, although all except one patient showed at least some postural hypotension. When there is more adequate control of the blood pressure, venous pooling may play some part as a venodepressor effect has been demonstrated after oral administration of α-methyldopa (2.0–5.0 g daily) over periods of between 21 and 49 days [35]. In contrast to other work, when Lund-Johansen [36] studied a series of 13 mild hypertensives before and after treatment with α-methyldopa for one year (500–1500 mg/day, average 896 mg/day) he found that the fall in blood pressure at rest, standing and on exercise was associated with a fall in cardiac output, no change in peripheral resistance being observed. There was no postural drop in blood pressure; the supine and blood pressures after α-methyldopa were 139/84 mm Hg, standing 150/93 mm Hg. There is little effect on heart rate following intravenous administration [29], whereas after oral administration there is a modest reduction, supine, standing and after exercise [34, 36]. Alpha-methyldopa causes less of a reduction in heart rate than bethanidine or guanethidine for a similar anti-hypertensive effect [37].

It is apparent that larger doses of α-methyldopa used in the treatment of hypertension are associated with postural and exercise hypotension, although less than that seen with sympathetic inhibiting drugs, bethanidine or guanethidine [37, 38]. There is an alteration of the cardiovascular response to Valsalva's Manoeuvre in a way characteristic of inhibition of vasoconstriction; overshoot is abolished [32, 39] and the rise in blood pressure during the effort phase is inhibited [40]. Intravenous α-methyldopa has been found to reduce vascular resistance in the skin [41] and in the coronary circulation [30].

Onesti et al [29] found an insignificant fall in renal blood flow following intravenous α-methyldopa in the supine position (8%) but a significant fall in glomerular filtration rate of 13% (p<0.05). As there was a relatively greater fall in arterial blood pressure, calculated renal vascular resistance was decreased. The short-term oral administration of methyldopa produced a fall in renal vascular resistance and no reduction in renal blood flow or glomerular filtration [31, 42]. This was confirmed by Mohammed et al. [43] in patients with diminished renal function.

Meyer et al. [44] found a slight increase in cerebral flow in spite of a reduced blood pressure after two weeks administration of methyldopa to hypertensive patients with cerebrovascular disease.

Pharmacokinetics

The absorption of methyldopa is rapid but incomplete, about 30–70% according to radio-labelled recovery from the urine [24, 45–47]. There is no information on biliary excretion in man but it is minimal in the rat [48]. Absorption occurs probably at least partly by a stero-specific system, as only 8–13% of carbon-14 appeared in the urine after the administration of radio-labelled D-α-methyldopa [47]. There are differences in the metabolites formed after oral and intravenous administration that suggests first-pass metabolism [49].

Methyldopa is widely distributed in the body. Animal studies reveal that it is taken up and stored in peripheral adrenergic neurones [7] and it penetrates the central nervous system [20]. Peak levels of methyldopa occur between 2–6 h after oral administration [24, 45, 49]. The plasma half-life is about two hours [50]. The short plasma half life contrasts with the time course of the antihypertensive effect, maximum at 3 to 8 hours and lasting up to 24 hours, findings that are consistent with the formation of an active metabolite.

About 10% of a single dose of methyldopa is metabolised to α-methyldopa and then to α-methylnoradrenaline; this is excreted or further metabolised to the 3-methoxyderivative [8, 51, 52]. There are several other metabolites [45, 46, 53], that are formed to a variable extent. The major urinary metabolite is the sulphate conjugate between 20–80% of the urinary excretion products being handled in this way. An approximately similar amount is excreted unchanged. Other excretion products include free and conjugated 3-0-methyl methyldopa (0–15%), α-methyldopamine and 3-0-methoxy-α-methyldopamine, up to 20% of total, and finally, small amounts of 3-4-dihydoxyphenylacetone.

The half-life of unchanged methyldopa after intravenous administration was found to be 1.4–1.8 h [24], whereas the peak hypotensive effect occurred 6-8 h after administration, consistent with the formation of an active metabolite as with oral administration [54]. Metabolism is different after parenteral administration; 86-94% is excreted unchanged, while only 2% of the recovered drug is excreted as α-methyldopamine. The absence of the sulphate conjugation product indicates that this is formed after oral administration during the absorption from the intestinal tract and passage to the systemic circulation.

Clinical use

The effectiveness of α-methyldopa as an antihypertensive agent was first observed by Oates et al. [55]. If a level of standing diastolic pressure of 100 mm Hg is taken as a reasonable control α-methyldopa has been found to control about half of the hypertensive patients to this degree; for instance, 42% of 33 patients [56], 54% of 59 patients [57], 67% of 69 patients [58], 49% of 100 patients [59]. Johnson et al. [59] observed a fall in blood pressure in 37 patients on α-methyldopa, which was similar to that found in 66 patients of similar severity on guanethidine. This confirmed a previous within-patient study in 19 patients by Oates et al. [38], who found α-methyldopa, guanethidine and pargyline had a similar antihypertensive action. Likewise Prichard et al. [37] in a within patient study in 30 patients found α-methyldopa produced similar control to bethanidine and guanethidine, although 6 of these patients could not tolerate α-methyldopa. In a further study (n = 17) it has been confirmed that α-methyldopa produces similar control of the standing blood pressure to bethanidine, and also to propranolol [60].

The usual starting dose of methyldopa is 250 mg two to three times daily, but some would start with an even smaller dose to minimise initial side-effects, unless blood pressure was unduly high. Side-effects tend to become less as a lower blood pressure is maintained [37]. A smaller starting dose would be normally used if the patient is already on other antihypertensive drugs. Increments of 250 mg per dose may be made. Some physicians only use up to 2 grams a day, others have used higher doses, e.g. 6 grams a day [58]. A diuretic should be used in addition if any side-effects occur such as sedation and most usually would be added in any case if a daily dosage of 2 grams is reached. The development of tolerance is not uncommon, but it can usually be overcome by increasing the dose [61].

Side effects

One of the most frequent side-effects from α-methyldopa is tiredness and it is the most common factor limiting dosage. It may occur in about half of the patients treated, occurring in 41% of the patients [59] and more frequently than with other drugs [38]. Prichard et al. [37] found tiredness to occur in 75% of their patients on methyldopa compared with 10% on bethanidine and 17% on guanethidine. Bulpitt and Dollery (1973) also found sleepiness to be associated with methyldopa administration. There may be a general impairment of mental activity of particular trouble to professional people [62]. Patients on methyldopa may be susceptible to dementia when haloperidol is given in addition [63]. Other central nervous system side-effects occur such as dreams [37, 59] and depression in 2 out of 59 patients [57], 3 out of 69 patients [58], 4 out of 100 patients [59], 5 out of 47 patients [61], and 2 severe and 3 mild cases out of 30 patients [37]. There were lower central nervous system side-effects reported in hospital in-patients, perhaps as sedation would then be less noticeable [64]. The estimates of impotence from methyldopa varies; it has been denied [65], found to have a 2% incidence [59] or to occur in 25% of male patients [66]. There are two rare central nervous system side-effects from methyldopa. The administration of methyldopa in single doses of 750–1000 mg and long-term administration has been found to elevate prolactin [67] and this may be responsible for the galactorrhoea that has been reported from methyldopa in women [68, 69]. Methyldopa may increase prolactin concentration by reducing hypothalmic dopamine concentration which may be the prolactin inhibitory factor [67]. This reduction in dopamine may also be responsible for Parkinsonian side-effects that have been reported with methyldopa [69–71].

Weight gain is another common side-effect and has even been reported in 64% of cases [59]. Diarrhoea may occur with α-methyldopa in about 4% [59] to 8% of patients [37], but is much less frequent than with guanethidine. There has been a report of diarrhoea associated with dilation of the small intestine and malabsorption [72], and one case with colitis and hepatitis has been reported (see below).

Symptoms of postural or exertional hypotension are relatively unusual on α-methyldopa [37, 59], a number of trials not reporting these symptoms [61]. Excessive hypotension from methyldopa, however, has been reported particularly in younger patients under 55 years with elevated blood ureas [64]. This series was unusual in that hypotension, often postural, had rate of occurrence of over 10% with drowsiness, and with depression only occurring in less than 3%. Hypotension was more common in patients taking over 1 g a day, and most cases occurred within the first week of treatment. This suggests that the initial dosage was too high.

There have been reports of various skin rashes, urticaria, seborrhoeic dermatitis, eczema [73, 74], particularly in patients with previous skin disorders [74]. Lichenoid reactions have occurred [75–77] which may ulcerate [78]. It may be responsible for ulceration of the oral mucous membrane, oral lichen planus and other reactions [79].

An incidence of 20% of positive Coombs' test in a series of 202 patients receiving α-methyldopa in periods exceeding six months has been found [80]. The incidence was dose-dependent, 9% at less than 1 g, 19% between 1 and 2 g, and 36% when patients were receiving over 2 g a day of methyldopa [80]. However, an autoimmune haemolytic anaemia of the warm antibody type (IgG) only develops in about 0.02% of patients receiving α-methyldopa; most were on 1 g or less a day [81]. Haemolysis may be more likely to occur in women [82]. The prognosis of the anaemia is usually good, haemoglobin normally responding rapidly when methyldopa is stopped and/or steroids are given. In a series of 30 patients, two died while still anaemic, one with multiple pulmonary emboli possibly attributable to the haemolytic process, and one from duodenal ulceration perhaps exacerbated by prednisone [80]. The nature of the warm active IgG antibody is of interest as, unlike previous examples of drug haemolysis (e.g. penicillin), the alpha-methyldopa antibody was not enhanced or inhibited by the drug or its metabolites in vitro [83]. The receptor for the antibody appears to be part of the Rh antigen complex [84]. In vitro incubation of methyldopa with gamma globulin results in a dose dependent covalent binding of methyldopa or one of its metabolites to gamma globulin. Gamma globulin is structurally modified and presumably this is responsible for its adherence to the red cell [85]. Rarely, reversible leucopenia [86] or thrombocytopenia may occur [87, 88]. A positive reaction for antinuclear factor has been reported in just under 15% of patients on α-methyldopa [89].

Methyldopa administration may be associated with a febrile reaction, occasionally to levels 105°F, in 1-2% of patients usually within 1-3 weeks of starting treatment. The mechanism is unclear but it appears to be associated with a depressed metabolism of methyldopa [90]. While fever occurs without hepatic dysfunction it also occurs in association with hepatocellular damage in about a third of such patients [91].

Minor abnormalities of liver chemistry have been assessed to occur in about 6% of patients treated with methyldopa [92], serious reactions in about 0.19% of cases [93]. However rarely, methyldopa may cause an illness clinically and histologically similar to viral hepatitis, the onset being from 1 week to 1 year after starting the drug [92, 94, 95], or possibly up to, say, 5 years [96]. However, the histological picture may be that of chronic agressive hepatitis [94, 95, 96]. Methyldopa has been found to be the cause of almost a quarter of cases of active chronic hepatitis [98]. Most cases make a clinical recovery when methyldopa is stopped. The cases occurring soon after methyldopa is started, have been found to resolve more rapidly than those which occur after a long period of drug administration [96]. Acute submassive hepatic necrosis has been reported [99]. Rarely, there may be fatal progression of liver injury [91, 100, 101]. In one of two patients with subacute hepatic necrosis, in a total series of 7 with liver injury, there was progressive hepatic failure, despite corticosteroids. Post mortem diagnosis showed continuing necrosis with changes of postnecrotic cirrhosis [95].

Inadvertent re-administration of methyldopa has led to a dramatic recurrence of symptoms supporting suggestions that a hypersensitivity mechanism is involved [97, 95], although apparent desensitisation has been reported with less reaction on re-exposure [92]. The basis for methyldopa liver damge is obscure; possibly a drug metabolite protein complex may act as a hapten and, because of a familial incidence, a genetic predisposition has been suggested [96]. The reaction appears more common amongst women [82].

Rarely methyldopa may produce a cholestatic jaundice without any evidence of hepatocellular damage [94, 102]. There has also been a report of acute severe colitis in association with hepatitis after methyldopa, subsiding when the drug was stopped, recurring with re-administration. The patient had fever, skin rash and eosinophilia, suggesting drug allergy [103].

Methyldopa was blamed for the formation of renal stones in two patients on the grounds that the urine darkened on standing and a brown precipitate containing methyldopa then formed [104]. However, a retrospective survey of hypertensive patients with renal calculi failed to reveal any association with methyldopa [105].

A pressor response to intravenous methyldopa has been reported in a patient who apparently did not have a phaeochromocytoma judged by normal vanylmandelic acid excretion [106]. There have been two isolated reports of rebound hypertension following abrupt withdrawal of methyldopa [107, 108].

SUMMARY AND CONCLUSIONS

Methyldopa is a centrally acting antihypertensive drug. It is converted by the metabolic pathway for noradrenaline to α-methyl noradrenaline, which acts to produce stimulation of central alpha receptors to lower the blood pressure. Most studies have indicated that methyldopa produces a reduction in peripheral resistance without significantly dropping cardiac output. There has however been some work to indicate that a fall in cardiac output may be important. The use of methyldopa in the treatment of hypertension is not usually associated with significant postural or exercise hypotension but this may be seen when large doses are used.

As might be expected from a centrally acting drug, central nervous system-side effects, particularly tiredness, are not uncommon. Methyldopa also may occasionally cause a number of important side-effects, an autoimmune haemolytic anaemia, liver damage, pyrexia.

Notwithstanding these side-effects methyldopa has for many years been the most frequently used drug and although its preeminance has been challenged by beta-adrenoceptor blocking drugs, it remains in wide use.

The important differences that exist between α-methyldopa and other anti-hypertensive drugs reside in the effect on cardiovascular responses and the nature of side-effects. The control of the blood pressure with methyldopa is associated with less postural and exercise fall in blood pressure than that seen with adrenergic neurone inhibitory drugs.

ACKNOWLEDGEMENTS

I am most grateful for the help of Miss J. Cashin, S. R. N., Miss I. Clements and Miss F. Bothwick in the preparation of this paper.

REFERENCES

1. Laverty R: The mechanisms of action of some antihypertensive drugs. Br Med Bull 29:152–157, 1973.
2. Day MD, Roach AG, Whiting RL: The mechanism of the antihypertensive action of alpha-methydlopa in hypertensive rats. Eur J Pharmocol 21:271–280, 1973.
3. Haeusler G: Cardiovascular regulation by central adrenergic mechanisms and its alteration of hypotensive drugs. Circ Res 36 (Suppl I):223–232, 1975.
4. Kroneberg G, Heise A: Evidence for an activation of central alpha-adrenoceptors as the cause of the central hypotensive effect of alpha-methyldopa and its metabolites. In: Recent Advances in Hypertension, Milliez P, Safar M, eds. Vol 1, pp. 57–61. Reims: Societe Alina, 1975.
5. Levine RJ, Sjoerdsma A: Dissociation of thedecarboxylase-inhibiting and norepinephrine depleting effects of α-methyldopa, α-ethyldopa, 4-bromo, 3-hydroxy-benzloxymine and related substance. J Pharmacol Exp Ther 146:42–47, 1964.
6. Schumann HJ, Gorbecker U, Schmidt K: Über die Wirkung von α-methyldopa auf den Brenzcatechinamingehalt von Meerschweinchenorganen. Naunyn-Schmiedebergs Arch Pharmacol 251:48–61, 1965.
7. Muscholl E, Maitre L: Release by sympathetic stimulation of α-methylnoradrenaline stored in the heart after administration of α-methyldopa. Experientia, 19:658–659, 1963.
8. Muscholl E, Rahn KH: Über den Nachweis und die Bedeutung von α-Methylnoradrenalin im Harn von Hypertonikern bei Verabreichung von α-Methyldopa. Pharmacol Clin I:19–29, 1968.
9. Day MD, Rand MJ: A hypothesis for the mode of action of α-methyldopa in relieving hypertension. J Pharm Pharmacol 15:221–224, 1963.
10. Day MD, Rand MJ: Some observations on the pharmacology of α-methyldopa. Br J Pharmacol Chemother 22:72–86, 1964.
11. Trinker FR: The significance of the relative potencies of noradrenaline and α-methylnoradrenaline for the mode of action of α-methyldopa. J Pharm Pharmacol 23:306–308, 1971.
12. Coupar IM, Turner P: Relative potencies of some false transmitters on isolated human smooth muscle. Br J Pharmacol 38:463p–464P, 1970.

810

13. Finch L, Haeusler G: Further evidence for a central hypotensive action of α-methyldopa in both the rat and cat. Br J Pharmacol 47:217–228, 1973.
14. Haefely W, Hürlimann A, Thoenen H: Adrenergic transmitter changes and response to sympathetic nerve stimulation after differing pretreatment with α-methyldopa. Br J Pharmacol Chemother 31:105–109, 1967.
15. Holtz P, Palm D: On the pharmacology of α-methylated catecholamines and the mechanism of the antihypertensive action of α-methyldopa. Life Sci 6:1847–1857, 1967.
16. Henning M, Van Zwieten PA: Central hypotensive effect of α-methyldopa. J Pharm Pharmacol 20:409–417, 1968.
17. Blower PR, Poyser RH, Robertson MI: Effects of α-methyldopa on blood pressure in the anaesthetised dog. J Phar Pharmacol 28:437–440, 1976.
18. Ingenito AJ, Barrett JP, Procita L: A centrally mediated peripheral hypotensive effect of α-methyldopa. J Pharmacol Exp Ther 175:593–599, 1970.
19. Baum T, Shropshire AT, Varner LL: Contribution of the central nervous system to the action of several antihypertensive agents (methyldopa, hydrallazine and guanethidine). J Pharmacol Exp Ther 182:135–144, 1972.
20. Carlsson a, Lindqvist M: In-vivo decarboxylation of α-methyldopa and α-methyl metatyrosine. Acta Physiol Scand 54:87–94, 1962.
21. Henning M, Rubenson A: Evidence that the hypotensive action of methyldopa is mediated by the central actions of methylnoradrenaline. J Pharm Pharmacol 23:407–411, 1971.
22. Heise A, Kroneberg G: α-sympathetic receptor stimulation in the brain and hypotensive activity of α-methyldopa. Eur J Pharmacol 17:315–317, 1972.
23. Henning M: Studies on the mode of action of α-methyldopa. Acta Physiol Scand 75 (Suppl 322):1–37, 1969.
24. Sjoerdsma A, Vendsalu A, Engelman K: Studies on the metabolism and mechanism of action of methyldopa. Circulation 28:492–502, 1963.
25. Uretsky NJ, Iversen LL: Effects of 6-hydroxydopamine on catecholamine containing neurones in the rat brain. Journal of Neurochemistry, 17:269–278, 1970.
26. De Jong W, Nijkamp FP, Bohus B: Role of noradrenaline and serotonin in the central control of blood pressure in normotensive and spontaneously hypertensive rats. Arch Int Pharmacodyn Ther 213:272–284, 1975.
27. Struyker-Boudier H, Smeets G, Brouwer G, Van Rosum JM: Central nervous system α-adrenergic mechanisms and cardiovascular regulation in rats. Arch Int Pharmacodyn Ther 213:285–293, 1975.
28. Leonetti G, Terzoli L, Morganti A, Manfrin M, Bianchini C, Sala C, Zanchetti A: Relation between the hypotensive and renin-Suppressing activites of alpha-methyldopa in hypertension patients. Am J Cardiol 40:762–767, 1977.
29. Onesti G, Brest AN, Novack P, Kasparin H, Moyer JH: Pharmacodynamic effects of α-methyldopa in hypertensive subjects. Am Heart J 67:32–38, 1964.
30. Cohen A, Maxmen JS, Ragheb M, Baleiron H, Zaleski EJ, Bing RJ: Effects of alpha-methyldopa on the myocardial blood flow, utilizing the coincidence counting method. J Clin Pharmacol 7:77–83, 1967.
31. Sannerstedt R, Varnauskas E, Werko L: Haemodynamic effects of methyldopa (Aldomet®) at rest and during exercise in patients with arterial hypertension. Acta Med Scand 171:75–82, 1962.
32. Dollery CT, Harington M, Hodge JV: Haemodynamic studies with methyldopa: effect on cardiac output and response to pressor amines. Br Heart J 25:670–676, 1963.
33. Safar ME, London GM, Levenson JA, Khedar MA, Aboras NE, Simon AC: Effect of alpha-methyldopa on cardiac output in hypertension. Clin Pharmacol Ther 25:266–272, 1979.
34. Chamberlain DA, Howard J: Guanethidine and methyldopa: a haemodynamic study. Br Heart J 26:528–536, 1964.

35. Mason DT, Braunwald :: Effects of guanethidine, reserpine, and methyldopa on reflex venous and arterial construction in man. J Clin Invest 43:1449–1463, 1964.
36. Lund-Johansen P: Haemodynamic changes in long term α-methyldopa therapy of essential hypertension. Acta Med Scand 192:221–226, 1972.
37. Prichard BNC, Johnston AW, Hill ID, Rosenheim ML: Bethanidine, guanethidine, and methyldopa in the treatment of hypertension; a within-patient comparison. Br Med J 1:135–144, 1968.
38. Oates JA, Seligmann AW, Clark MA, Rousseau P, Lee RE: The relative efficacy of guanethidine, methyldopa, and pargyline as antihypertensive agents. N Eng J Med 273:729–734, 1965.
39. Wilson WR, Fisher FD, Kirkendall WM: The acute hemodynamic effects of α-methyldopa in man. J Chronic Dis 15:907–913, 1961.
40. Prichard BNC, Gillam PMS, Graham BR: Beta receptor antagonism in hypertension; comparison with the effect of adrenergic neurone inhibition on cardiovascular responses. Int J Clin Pharmacol 4:131–140, 1970b.
41. Mendlowitz M, Naftchi NE, Wolf RL, Gitlow SE: The effects of guanethidine and of alpha methyldopa on the digital circulation in hypertension. Am Heart J 69:731–739, 1965.
42. Morin Y, Turmel L, Fortier J: Methyldopa. Clinical studies in arterial hypertension. Am J Med Sci 248:633, 1964.
43. Mohammed S, Hanenson IB, Magenheim HG, Gaffney TE: The effects of alpha-methyldopa on renal function in hypertensive patients. Am Heart J 76:21–27, 1968.
44. Meyer JS, Sawada T, Kitamura A, Toyoda M: Cerebral blood flow after control of hypertension in stroke. Neurology 18:772–781, 1968.
45. Prescott LF, Buhs RP, Beattie JO, Speth OC, Trenner NR, Lasagna L: Combined clinical and metabolic study of the effects of alpha-methyldopa on hypertensive patients. Circulation 34:308–321, 1966.
46. Au WYM, Dring LG, Grahame-Smith DG, Isaac P, Williams RT: The metabolism of ^{14}C-labelled α-methyldopa in normal and hypertensive human subjects. Biochem J 129:1–10, 1972.
47. Kwan KC, Foltz EL, Breault GO, Baer JE, Totaro JA: Pharmacokinetics of methyldopa in man. J Pharmacol Exp Ther 198:264–277, 1976.
48. Porter CC, Titus DC: Distribution and metabolism of methyldopa in the rat. J Pharmacol Exp Ther 139:77–87, 1963.
49. Saavedra JA, Reid JL, Jordan W, Rawlins MD, Dollery CT: Plasma concentration of alpha methyldopa and sulphate conjugate after oral administration of methyldopa hydrochloride ethyl ester. Eur J Clin Pharmacol 8:381–386, 1975.
50. Barnett AJ, Bobok A, Carson V, Korman JS, McLean AJ: Pharmacokinetics of methyldopa. Plasma levels following single intravenous, oral and multiple oral dosage in normotensive and hypertensive subjects. Clin Exp Pharmacol Physiol4:331–339, 1977.
51. Stott A, Robinson R, Smith P: Total metadrenaline excretion in patients treated with α-methyldopa. Lancet 1:266–267, 1963.
52. Murscholl E, Rahn KH: Nachweis von αMethylnoradrenalin in Harn von Hypertonikern während einer Behandlung mit αMethyldopa. Klin Wochenschr 44:1412–1413, 1966.
53. Buhs RP, Beck JL, Speth OC, Smith JL, Trenner NR, Cannon PJ, Laragh JH: The metabolism of methyldopa in hypertensive human subjects. J Pharmacol Ther 143:205–214, 1964.
54. Gillespie L, Oates JA, Crout JR, Sjoerdsma A: Clinical and chemical studies with α-methyldopa in patients with hypertension. Circulation 25:281–291, 1962.
55. Oates JA, Gillespie L, Udenfriend S, Sjoerdsma A: Decarboxylase inhibition and blood pressure reduction by α-methyl-3, 4-dihydroxy-DL phenylalamine. Science 131:1890–1891, 1960.

56. Cannon PJ, Whitlock RT, Morris RC, Angers M, Laragh JH: Effect of alpha-methyldopa in severe and malignant hypertension. J Am Med Assoc 179:673-681, 1962.
57. Dollery CT, Harington M: Methyldopa in hypertension. Clin Pharmacol Stud Lancet 1:759-763, 1962.
58. Hamilton M, Kopelman H: The treatment of severe hypertension with methyldopa. Br Med J 1:151-155, 1963.
59. Johnson P, Kitchin ah, Lowther CP Turner RWD: Treatment of hypertension with methyldopa. Br Med J 1:133-137, 1966.
60. Prichard BNC, Boakes AJ, Graham BR: A within patient comparison of bethanidine, methyldopa and propranolol in the treatment of hypertension. Clin Sci Mol Med 51 (Suppl 3):567s-570s, 1976.
61. Smirk H: Hypotensive action of methyldopa. Br Med J 1:146-151, 1963.
62. Adler S: Methyldopa-induced decrese in mentalactivity. J Am Med Assec 230:1428-1429, 1974.
63. Thornton WE: Dementia induced by methyldopa with haloperidol. N Eng J Med 294, 1222.
64. Lawson DH, Gloss D, Jick H: Adverse reactions to methyldopa with particular reference to hypotension. Am Heart J 96:572-579, 1978.
65. Bulpitt CJ, Dollery CT: Side effects of hypotensive agents evaluated by a self administered questionnaire. Br Med J 3:485-490, 1973.
66. Newman RJ, Salerno HR: Letter: Sexual dysfunction due to Methyldopa. Br Med J 4:106, 1974.
67. Steiner J, Cassar J, Mashiter K, Dawes I, Russel Frazer T, Breckenridge A: Effects of methyldopa on prolactin and growth hormone. Br Med J 1:1186-1188, 1976.
68. Pettinger WA, Horwitz D, Sjoerdsma A: Lactation due to methyldopa. Br Med J 1:1460, 1963.
69. Vaidya RA, Vaidya AB, Van Woert MH, Kase NG: Galactorrhea and Parkinson-like syndrome: an adverse effect of α-methyldopa. Metabolism 19:1068-1070, 1970.
70. Groden BM: Parkinsonism occuring with methyldopa treatment. Br Med J 1:1001, 1963.
71. Peaston MJT: Parkinsonism associated with alpha-methyldopa therapy. Br Med J 2:168, 1964.
72. Shneerson JM, Gazzard BG: Reversible malabsorption caused by methyldopa. Br Med J 2:1456-1456, 1977.
73. Peterkin GAG, Khan SA: Iatrogenic skin disease. Practitioner 202:117-126, 1969.
74. Church R: Eczema provoked by methyldopa. Br J Dermatol 91:373-378, 1974.
75. Stevenson CJ: Lichenoid drug eruption from methyldopa. Br J Dermatol 85:600, 1971.
76. Burry JN, Kirk J: Lichenoid drug reaction from methyldopa. Br J Dermatol 91:475-476, 1974.
77. Holt PJA, Navaratnam A: Lichenoid eruption due to methyldopa. Br Med J 3:234, 1974.
78. Burry JN: Ulcerative lichenoid eruption from methyldopa Arch Dermatol 112:880, 1976.
79. Hay KD, Reade PC: Methyldopa as a cause of oral mucous membrane reactions. Br Dent J 145:195-203, 1978.
80. Carstairs KC, Breckenridge A, Dollery CT, Worlledge SM: Incidence of a positive direct Coombs Test in patients on α-methyldopa. Lancet 2:133-135, 1966.
81. Worlledge SM, Carstairs KC, Dacie JV: Autoimmune haemolytic anaemia associated with α-methyldopa therapy. Lancet, 2:135-139, 1966.
82. Furhoff AK: Adverse reactions with methyldopa – a decade's reports. Acta Med Scand 203:425-428, 1978.
83. Lobuglio AF, Jandl JH: The nature of alpha-methyldopa red-cell antidoby. N Eng J Med 276:658-665, 1967.

84. Masouredis sp, Sudora E: Ultra-structural mapping of methyldopa and anti-D IgG ery-throcyte antigen receptors. J Clin Invest 55:771–782, 1975.
85. Gottlieb AJ, Wurzel HA: Protein-quinone interaction: in vitro induction of indirect anti-globulin reaction with methyldopa. Blood 43:85–97, 1974.
86. Clark KG: Case history: haemolysis and agranulocytosis complicating treatment with methyldopa. Br Med J 4:94, 1967.
87. Benraad AH, Schoenaker AH: Thrombopenia after use of methyldopa. Lancet, 2:292, 1965.
88. Marcus GJ, Stencon M, Brown T: Alpha-methyldopa indiced immune thrombocytopenia. Am J Clin Pathol 64:113–115, 1975.
89. Breckenridge A, Dollery CT, Worlledge SM, Holborn EJ, Johnson GD: Positive direct Cooms' Tests and antinuclear factor in patients treated with methyldopa. Lancet 2:1265–1268, 1967.
90. Valnes K, Hillestad L, Hansen T, Arnold E: Alpha-methyldopa and drug fever: study of the metabolism of alpha-methyldopa in patients and normal subjects. Acta Med Scand 204:21–25, 1978.
91. Rodman JS, Deutsch DJ, Gutman SL: Methyldopa hepatitis. A report of six cases and review of the literature. Am J Med 60:941–948, 1976.
92. Elkington SG, Schreiber WM, Conn HO: Hepatic injury caused by 1-alpha-methyldopa. Circulation 40:589–595, 1969.
93. Cacace LG, Cohen M: Alpha-methyldopa (Aldomet) hepatitis. Report of a case and review of the literature. Drug Intell 10:144–152, 1976.
94. Toghill Pj, Smith PG, Benton P, Brown RC, Matthews HL: Methyldopa liver damage. Br Med J 3:545–548, 1974.
95. Thomas E, Rosenthal WS, Zapiach L, Micci D: Spectrum of methyldopa liver injury. Am J Gastroenterol 68:125–133, 1977.
96. Sotaniemi EA, Hokkanen OT, Ahokas JT, Pelkonen RO, Ahlqvist J: Hepatic injury and drug metabolism in patients with alpha-methyldopa-induced liver damage. Eur J Clin Pharmacol 12:429–435, 1977.
97. Maddrey WC, Boitnott JK: Severe hepatitis from methyldopa Gastroenterology 68:351–360, 1975.
98. Goldstein GB, Lam KC, Mistilis SP: Drug-induced active chronic hepatitis. Digest Dis 18:177–184, 1973.
99. Schweitzer IL, Peters RL: Acute submassive hepativ necrosis due to methyldopa. Gastroenterology 66:1203–1211, 1974.
100. Hoyumpa AM, Connell AM: Methyldopa hepatitis. Digest Dis 18:213–222, 1973.
101. Rehman OU, Keith TA, Gall EA: Methyldopa-induced submassive hepatic necrosis. J Am Med Assoc 224:1390–1392, 1973.
102. Hoffbrand BI, Fry W, Bunton GL: Cholestatic jaundice due to methyldopa. Br Med J 3:559, 1974.
103. Bonkowsky HL, Brisbane J: Colitis and hepatitis caused by methyldopa. J Am Med Assoc 236:1602–1603, 1976.
104. Murphy KJ: Bilateral renal calculi in patients receiving methyldopa. Med J Aust 2:20–21, 1976.
105. Ramsay LE: Methyldopa and renal stones: a retrospective study. Med J Aust 2:495–497, 1977.
106. Levine RJ, Strauch BS: Hypertensive responses to methyldopa. N Eng J Med 275:946–948, 1966.
107. Burden AC, Alexander CPT: Rebound hypertension after acute methyldopa withdrawal. Br Med J 1:1056–1057, 1976.
108. Frewin DB, Penhall RK: Rebound hypertension after sudden discontinuation of methyl-dopa therapy. Med J Aust 1:659, 1977.

50. CLONIDINE AND IMIDAZOLINES AS ANTIHYPERTENSIVE AGENTS

JOHN L. REID

1. INTRODUCTION

Clonidine is an imidazoline derivative developed from a series of compounds with nasal decongestant activity. Its hypotensive efficacy was recognised early in clinical studies in the 1960s [1]. Clonidine has several novel features and studies on the mechanism of action of this drug have substantially advanced our understanding not only of autonomic pharmacology but also of cardiovascular physiology and circulatory regulation. The concept of central nervous control of autonomic outflow, and thus blood pressure and heart rate via central alpha adrenoceptors, developed largely as a result of studies with clonidine [2]. Furthermore the hypothesis of presynaptic regulatory receptors controlling transmitter release was an extension of investigations with clonidine and the paradoxes apparent from earlier studies [3].

The central site of action of clonidine was demonstrated in animal studies using local injection into the cisterna magna, vertebral artery, or more recently local brain stem areas [2]. This central mechanism and the accompanying fall in sympathetic activity results from an activation of central alpha receptors very similar to presynaptic alpha receptors in the periphery. Presynaptic alpha receptors differ from classical postsynaptic alpha receptors in the specificity and selectivity of agonist and antagonist drugs in a manner similar to β_1 and β_2 receptors [3, 4]. Indeed, a preferable classification is probably α_1 (for classical postsynaptic) and α_2 (for presynaptic or central) alpha receptors [4]. Clonidine is thus a relatively selective α_2 agonist.

2. PHARMACODYNAMIC ACTIONS OF CLONIDINE IN MAN

2.1. Haemodynamic effects of clonidine

Clonidine lowers blood pressure in man after oral or intravenous administration [5–8]. Although the fall in blood pressure is quantitatively greater in

Amery, A. (ed.) Hypertensive Cardiovascular Disease: Pathophysiology and Treatment
© *1982, Martinus Nijhoff Publishers. The Hague / Boston / London*
ISBN-13: 978-94-009-7478-4

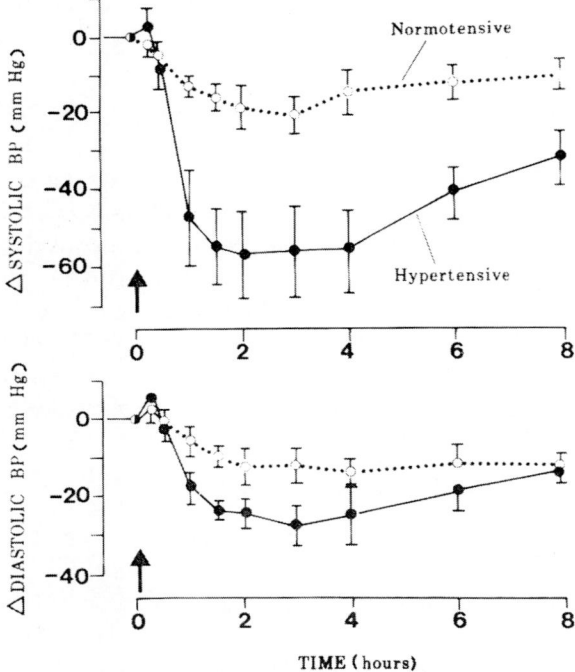

Figure 1. Changes in systolic and diastolic blood pressure
(mean ±S.E.M.) in 5 normotensive subjects (o---o) and 5
essential hypertensives (•—•) after 300 μg of oral clonidine
hydrochloride. (Reprinted from Eur J Clin Pharmacol
12:463–469, 1977.)

patients with essential hypertension compared to normotension, even in the
latter, a significant hypotensive effect can be demonstrated [9] (Figure 1). If
clonidine is given intravenously by rapid injection a brief (1–5 min) hypertensive effect may be observed [6, 7], similar to that seen in animal studies [2] and resulting from an action on postsynaptic alpha receptors on
peripheral vascular smooth muscle.

Clonidine lowers blood pressure to a similar extent in the supine and erect
posture and, at least in the supine posture, hypotension is often associated
with a slowing of heart rate. Reflex responses to exercise and Valsalva's
manoeuvre are little influenced [5, 7, 8]. More detailed haemodynamic studies reveal a modest reduction in peripheral resistance associated with small
but variable falls in cardiac output [5–7]. These haemodynamic changes are
consistent with a central nervous site of action. The observation that clonidine does not lower blood pressure in subjects with a tetraplegia resulting
from a high cervical spinal cord transection and thus interruption of path-

ways from the brain stem to spinal sympathetic efferent outflow further supports a central site of action in man [10].

2.2. Clonidine and indices of sympathetic activity

If clonidine acts centrally in man to reduce efferent sympathetic activity, it might be anticipated that the drug would lower plasma catecholamines and urinary catecholamines and metabolites, as these are considered indices of sympathetic tone. In essential hypertension [11] and in normotensive subjects [12] clonidine lowers plasma noradrenaline and reduces urinary catecholamine excretion. These changes are in contrast to the changes in sympathetic activity observed after treatment with beta-blockers [11], diuretics, alpha-blockers or vasodilators, when plasma catecholamines are unchanged or elevated.

2.3. Other effects of clonidine

The principal subjective side effects of clonidine, sedation or drowsiness and dry mouth have been reported in most studies [13–18]. These effects are dose related and most prominent early in the course of treatment. There is considerable clinical experience and some objective evidence to suggest that some degree of 'tolerance' develops to these effects without loss of antihypertensive efficacy [9]. However, sedation and dry mouth remain frequent subjective complaints with long-term clonidine treatment and are commonly dose-limiting [18]. In Table 1 the most frequent side effects of clonidine are shown.

Table 1. Actions and principal side effects of clonidine

Effect	Mechanism
Hypotension	Central a_2 receptors in brain stem reduce sympathetic tone ? Peripheral presynaptic a_2 effect
Sedation, drowsiness	Central a_2 receptor in arousal/sleep mechanism
Dry mouth	Central a_2 receptor reducing sympathetic and increasing parasympathetic tone ? Peripheral local effect
Bradycardia	Central a_2 receptors in brain stem reducing sympathetic and increasing parasympathetic tone
Constipation	Peripheral a_2 receptor on cholinergic neurons of the myenteric plexus of the gut

2.3.1. Sedation

The sedative effect which appears 2–3 h after drug ingestion and lasts for 6–10 h [8] results from an action on α_2 receptors involved in sleep/arousal regulation [19]. At present this effect cannot be separated from the central hypotensive effect either of clonidine or of the analogues discussed later. Clonidine may cause drowsiness during the day and an ability to fall 'asleep' when not engaged actively in conversation or cerebration. While total nocturnal sleep may be increased clonidine markedly reduces or abolishes rapid eye movement (R.E.M.) sleep [20–22].

2.3.2. Dry mouth

Dry mouth also appears within 2–3 h of drug administration. Zerostomia can be severe and may interfere with mastication and articulation [18]. When dry mouth is assessed objectively by measuring basal parotid and submandibular saliva production [8, 9], or stimulated parotid secretion, clonidine 100–300 µg orally reduced saliva production to 10–15% of pre-drug levels. The reduction in saliva flow lasted for 6–10 h and corresponded closely to subjective complaints of dry mouth. Animal experiments suggest that the principal reduction in saliva flow is a further central effect mediated by α_2 receptors and manifested by changes in parasympathetic tone [23], but peripheral effects could also contribute [24].

2.3.3. Bradycardia and constipation

Bradycardia and constipation have been consistently reported, although they have less frequently resulted in cessation of therapy. Both effects can be attributed to the α_2 agonist action of clonidine. Bradycardia results not only from centrally mediated withdrawal of sympathetic tone but also a central increase in vagal outflow [2, 25]. Constipation, which for some patients may contrast favourably with increased stool frequency, or diarrhoea, experienced with methyldopa, guanethidine or bethanidine, appears to result from an action on an α_2 receptor on cholinergic neurons of the myoenteric plexus [26].

3. PHARMACOKINETICS OF CLONIDINE IN MAN AND CONCENTRATION EFFECT RELATIONSHIPS

3.1. Pharmacokinetics

Early studies on the disposition of clonidine in man were undertaken with radioactive ^{14}C-labelled drug [27]. The conclusions from these studies were limited. The very low (microgram) doses of drug used and thus plasma levels achieved, contributed to difficulties in establishing a drug assay in

Table 2. Pharmacokinetic parameters of clonidine in man

	Mean	Range
Elimination half-life (hours)	8.5	6.9–11.1
Volume of distribution at steady state (L/kg)	2.09	1.70–2.79
Clearance (ml/min/kg)	3.05	1.87–4.74
Bioavailability (%)	75.2	70.6–81.5

Five subjects received clonidine 300 μg orally and intravenously and results were analysed using a 2-compartment open model [29].

plasma. The development of a stable isotope dilution gas chromatographic mass spectrometric (G.C.M.S.) assay [28] permitted a systemic evaluation of plasma clonidine concentration in man after oral and intravenous administration [8, 9, 29]. Clonidine is rapidly and extensively absorbed after oral administration with peak plasma levels of 1–2 ng/ml at 60–90 min after a 300 μg dose. Elimination half life ranges from 6–12 h.

In Table 2 the pharmacokinetic parameters are summarised. There were no differences between essential hypertensives and subjects with normal blood pressure [9, 29]. There was no evidence that, over a wide range of daily doses (0.3–5.4 mg), the kinetics were dose dependent.

3.2. Metabolism

Clonidine is extensively metabolised in man by the liver. About half the dose is excreted unchanges in urine. The remainder is eliminated as metabolites after biotransformation [29]. In animals several pathways of metabolism have been described [30], but there is no evidence that pharmacological activity of any of these metabolites is of relevance to the actions of clonidine in man. In view of the substantial contribution of hepatic metabolism to the overall clearance of clonidine, it is not surprising that the drug can be given to patients with hypertension and renal impairment without serious risk of toxicity in doses similar to those used in other patients.

3.3. Concentration effect relationships

Measurements of plasma levels of clonidine have helped to improve the drug's use in clinical practice by demonstrating the profile of the concentration–effect relationship both for hypertension and for the common side effects of sedation and dry mouth.

For both these latter effects there is a linear relationship between intensity of sedation and/or dry mouth and plasma level. This is illustrated for seda-

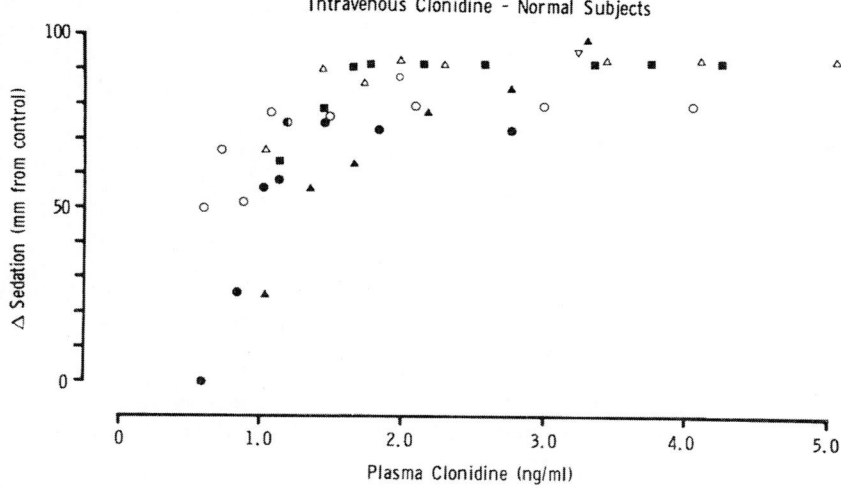

Figure 2. The relationship between the sedative effect of clonidine (measured by self assessment visual analogue rating) and the plasma level of clonidine. (Reprinted from Clin Pharmacol Ther 21:11-17, 1976.

tion in Figure 2. Sedation as assessed by a self-scoring visual analogue scale [8] was prominent at plasma clonidine concentration between 1.0 and 2 ng/ml. The concentration–effect relationship for dry mouth is similar [9, 29]. However, the relationship between plasma level and hypotensive effect is different and appears to be bell-shaped or have a parabolic function. At low plasma levels there is a positive linear relationship but at higher levels (>2 ng/ml) this is lost and at the highest levels the hypotensive effect is less or even absent [9, 29] (Figure 3). There appears to be an optimal range or 'therapeutic window' of plasma concentration of clonidine between 1 and 2 ng/ml. The close relationship of plasma level to effect, together with a plasma half life of 8–12 h, supports the use of a twice or three times a day treatment regimen. It is likely that the hypotensive effect of clonidine is the result of at least two opposite mechanisms [31]: firstly, the central hypotensive effect and, secondly, a direct peripheral pressor effect, apparently at high concentration, particularly after intravenous injection [6, 7]. Other studies in animals [32] and man [33] support the conclusion that clonidine has a narrow optimal therapeutic range and that higher concentrations lead, not only to more severe side effects, but may actually reduce the hypotensive effect. A direct consequence of these observations would be that daily doses of clonidine in excess of 1.2–1.5 mg, which would lead to plasma levels >2 ng/ml, would be unlikely to be of use clinically. In two patients on large doses of clonidine (4–5 mg/day) plasma levels were 14–20 ng/ml and blood pressure was poorly controlled. The same subjects later showed a substantial

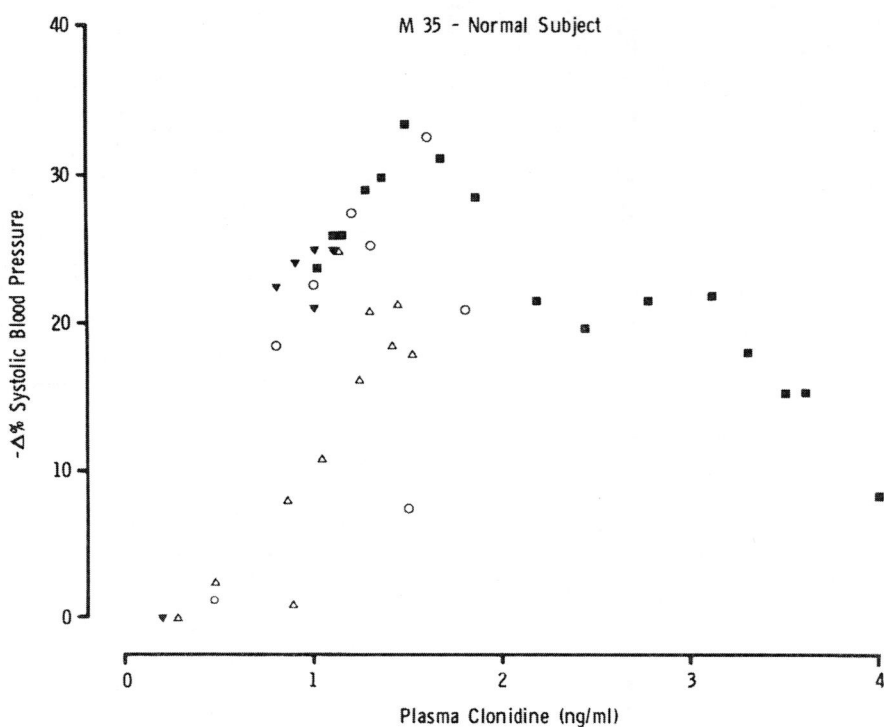

Figure 3. The relationship between hypotensive effect and plasma clonidine concentration in a normotensive subject studied on several occasions after oral and intravenous clonidine. (Reprinted from Clin Pharmacol Ther 21:11–17, 1976.

fall in blood pressure after 0.3 mg clonidine, when plasma levels were tenfold lower [34], further supporting the desirability of maintaining the daily dose at 1.2 mg or less for optimal therapeutic effect.

4. THERAPEUTIC EFFICACY AND THE PRESENT ROLE OF CLONIDINE

When clonidine was first introduced it offered potential advantages over existing agents. It was relatively free of postural and exercise-induced hypotension, did not cause diarrhoea, and at least in some male patients, was less likely to interfere with normal sexual activity. Furthermore, it did not appear to result in significant toxicity with damage to tissues such as liver or bone marrow. As discussed earlier, the disadvantages of clonidine were dry mouth and sedation. These, while troublesome in some patients, were accepted by many.

However, the demonstration that beta-blockers alone, or in combination with diuretics, lowered blood pressure without postural effects or sexual effects, has led to a reappraisal of the role, not only of clonidine, but of methyldopa, reserpine and the postganglionic adrenergic neurone blocking drugs, guanethidine, bethanidine and debrisoquine. Although it would be unwise to underestimate the frequency of symptom side effects with beta-blockers and diuretics, side effects which trouble the patient are more common with centrally acting drugs [35]. When diuretics (diabetes, gout) or beta-blockers (asthma, peripheral vascular disease, bradyarrhythmias) are relatively contraindicated, centrally acting drugs may be considered. However, the number of occasions when clonidine would be an unequivocal choice for monotherapy in mild to moderate hypertension are few. Thus in the 1980s trials of the efficacy of clonidine compared to thiazides [15] or its comparable activity to methyldopa [18] are now not sufficient justification for extensive use of the drug. The alternatives available with fewer symptom side effects are particularly attractive for long-term treatment of otherwise asymptomatic young hypertensives in whom patient acceptability of the drug, and thus good 'compliance' with medical instruction, is the key to good management. Undoubtedly, the recognition that rapid reversal of hypotension occurs within 24–36 h of interruption of therapy and association of rebound hypertension and increased sympathetic activity, even after only a few days withdrawal of drug, is another factor which limits clonidine's usefulness, especially in patients who are 'poor compliers'.

4.1. Mild to moderate hypertension

Early experience with clonidine as monotherapy was not uniformly successful [36]. Only a minority of patients were controlled without symptoms on the drug alone. Addition of a diuretic improved control and often permitted a reduction in clonidine dose [37]. In comparison with guanethidine [17], clonidine showed a favourable side effect profile and efficacy, while in comparison with methyldopa [15, 18] clonidine had a similar profile of symptom side effect. However, neither methyldopa nor clonidine are extensively used as first line treatment of new hypertensive drugs, as centrally acting drugs and their inevitable central nervous side effects have been replaced by beta-blockers (much as centrally acting drugs themselves replaced ganglion blockers) with a more acceptable side effect profile.

If clonidine is used as monotherapy, it should be given as twice or thrice daily divided doses. As discussed above daily doses greater than 1.2 mg are unlikely to be successful. Symptom side effects can usually be controlled by dose reduction, although often at loss of antihypertensive efficacy. Patients should be adequately warned of the problems of interrupting treatment, encouraged to comply and to attend their physician if intermittent illness

822

prevents drug taking. In patients with depression tricyclic antidepressants, which have α_2 antagonist properties, may attenuate or reverse the effects of clonidine [38].

4.2. Severe hypertension

Clonidine has been successfully used in combination with other antihypertensive drugs in the management of severe hypertension [39, 40]. Clonidine with a diuretic is a useful regime [37] and combination with guanethidine, debrisoquine and diazoxide helped control blood pressure [40]. Although it has been suggested that non-selective beta-blockers like propranolol might interfere with the hypotensive effects of clonidine [41], this has not been the general practical clinical experience of many, and beta blocker and clonidine regimen have been used successfully [39]. Beta-blockers, however, may exacerbate withdrawal symptoms if clonidine treatment is interrupted [42].

However, although clonidine can be useful in the management of severe hypertension, the side effects of sedation and dry mouth remain troublesome and the risks or consequences of withdrawal rebound hypertension possibly increased [42]. While diuretics and beta-blockers have become established treatment for moderate hypertension, a triple therapy regime of diuretic, beta-blocker and vasodilators like hydrallazine [43] or minoxidol [44], or alpha-blockers (prazosin or labetalol) has been effective and well tolerated. Clonidine like methyldopa remains an alternative to the third line drug, or can even replace the beta-blocker [40] in patients who cannot tolerate these agents, or in whom there are relative clinical contraindications to beta-blockade or vasodilators. Thus clonidine has its principal role as an alternative to second and third stage drugs in the stepped care triple therapy approach to the management of severe hypertension.

4.3. Secondary hypertension

Clodinine can be used in patients with hypertension and renal impairment in similar doses to patients with normal renal function as elimination by the liver is an important pathway [29] and this is supported by clinical experience.

Clonidine should not be used in phaeochromocytoma. Blood pressure does not fall and autonomic tumour production of catecholamines will not be affected [45].

Although clonidine has been used in patients with renovascular hypertension and may lower plasma renin activity [46], there are now available more specific antagonists of renin release and the renin–angiotensin system.

4.4. Emergency reduction of blood pressure

Intravenous clonidine is available and can be used to control severe hypertensive emergencies. However, it should be given by slow intravenous injection to avoid the pressor effect [6, 7] and marked sedation is inevitable. Experience with clonidine in this setting has not been universally favourable [7] and clonidine cannot be considered parenteral treatment of first choice.

5. WITHDRAWAL SYNDROME AND HYPERTENSION

Several factors have contributed to the markedly reduced use of clonidine. Central nervous side effects of sedation are troublesome; the conventional formulation of the drug must be given in two or three divided daily doses. However, an additional and not unimportant factor is the recognition that interruption of drug treatment is associated with a rapid reversal of hypotensive effect which may be accompanied by symptoms and biochemical evidence of sympathetic overactivity and an overshoot of blood pressure above pre-treatment levels [11–49]. The hypertensive reaction, which resembles a hypertensive crisis in phaeochromocytoma, may last for several days and could in hypertensive patients be a contributory factor to short term cardiovascular morbidity. The frequency of the full reaction is disputed but may occur over 10 % of patients. Symptoms of anxiety, insomnia, nausea, headache, palpitations and raised plasma and urinary catecholamines probably occur in a higher percentage of patients withdrawn [47, 48]. The frequency and severity of the withdrawal syndrome is increased in more severe hypertensives, on higher doses of clonidine for prolonged periods [48]. Co-administration of beta-blockers [41] and, possibly, of diuretics also contribute. The syndrome may appear after only one or two doses of clonidine have been missed and hypotension is reversed within 12 h. Rebound hypertension has occurred even during gradual stepwise reduction in dose [50]. Treatment should be preventative with patient, family and doctor aware of the risks of drug withdrawal. If a patient does present, symptoms can be controlled either by reintroduction of clonidine orally or intravenously, or by administration of an alpha-blocker (phentolamine, phenoxybenzamine or prazosin), or a vasodilator (hydrallazine, diazoxide or sodium nitroprusside). Beta-blockers are rarely necessary and should never be given before the alpha-blocker/vasodilator. Intravenous labetalol, an alpha- and beta-blocker, has been used [51] but has not always controlled hypertension [52].

824

6. OTHER IMIDAZOLIDINES AND RELATED DRUGS

Many analogues have been developed which share with clonidine a relative specificity as α receptor agonists. Several of these drugs have been evaluated in man, including guanfacine [53], guanabenz [54] and tiamenidine [55]. If any of these agents are to be useful in practice, they must exhibit at least comparable efficacy to clonidine with less side effects. In particular such a drug would have to show less sedation and drowsiness and be less likely to cause rebound hypertension. Both these points are difficult to establish objectively. Central α-receptors controlling blood pressure and arousal appear to be very similar and there is no evidence that any newer agent has a substantially more attractive profile of side effects. Withdrawal symptoms and hypertension have been reported after tiamenidine [56, 57] with a similar frequency as after clonidine.

Guanfacine has been extensively studied and, while it also causes withdrawal reactions, these may be less frequent [58]. Guanfacine has a longer plasma half life (15–20 h) and duration of hypotensive action (>20 h) compared to clonidine [59] and these observations suggest that pharmacokinetic and pharmaceutical developments may minimise the problems of withdrawal.

7. CONCLUSIONS

Clonidine is a novel antihypertensive agent which has greatly helped extend knowledge of the role of the central nervous system in blood pressure regulation and alpha adrenoceptors both in the brain and the periphery.

Its use in man is accompanied by symptom side effects of sedation related to its central action. These side effects and the development of simpler regimes with less side effects make clonidine a second choice drug in monotherapy, as does the risk of rebound hypertension when treatment is interrupted deliberately or accidentally.

In more severe hypertension clonidine has a role as second line treatment in patients who cannot take either diuretic, beta-blocker or vasodilator.

REFERENCES

1. Graubner W, Wolf M: Kritische Betrachtungen zum Wirkungsmechanismus des 2(2,6 dichlorophenylamino)-2-imidazolin-hydrochloride. Arzneim Forsch 16:1055–1058, 1966.
2. Van Zwieten PA: Antihypertensive drugs with a central action. Prog Pharmacol 1:1–63, 1975.
3. Langer SZ: Presynaptic receptors and their role in the regulation of transmitter release. Br J Pharmacol 60:481–498, 1977.

4. Berthelsen S, Pettinger WA: A functional basis for classification of α adrenergic receptors. Life Sci 21:595–606, 1977.
5. Barnett AJ, Cantor S: Observation on the hypotensive action of Catapres (ST155) in man. Med J Aust 1:87–)1, 1968.
6. Muir AL, Burton JL, Lawrie DM: Circulatory effects at rest and exercise of clonidine, an imidazoline derivative with hypotensive properties. Lancet ii:181–185, 1969.
7. Mroczek WJ, Davidov M, Finnerty FA: Intravenous clonidine in hypertensive patients. Clin Pharmacol Ther 14:847–851, 1973.
8. Dollery CT, Davies DS, Draffan GH, Dargie HJ, Dean C, Reid JL, Clare RA, Murray S: Clinical pharmacology and pharmacokinetics of clonidine. Clin Pharmacol Ther 19:11–18, 1976.
9. Wing LMH, Reid JL, Davies DS, Neill EM, Tippett P, Dollery CT: Pharmacokinetic and concentration effect relationships of clonidine in essential hypertension. Eur J Clin Pharmacol 12:463–469, 1977.
10. Reid JL, Wing LMH, Mathias CJ, Frankel HL, Neill E: The central hypotensive effect of clonidine: studies in tetraplegic subjects. Clin Pharmacol Ther 21:375–381, 1977.
11. Hokfelt B, Hedeland H, Hansson B-G: The effect of clonidine and penbutolol respectively on catecholamines in blood and urine, plasma renin activity and urinary aldosterone in hypertensive patients. Arch Int Pharmacodyn Ther 213:307–321, 1975.
12. Wing LMH, Reid JL, Hamilton CA, Sever PS, Davies DS, Dollery CT: Effects of clonidine on biochemical indices of symathetic function and plasma renin activity in normotensive man. Clin Sci Mol Med 53:45–53, 1977.
13. Bock KD, Hermsoth V, Merguet P, Schoenermark J: Clinical and Clinical experimental studies with a new hypotensive agent. Dtsch Med Wochenschr 91:1761–1772, 1966.
14. Ng J, Phelan EL, McGregor DD, Laverty RR, Taylor KM, Smirk H: Properties of Catapres: a new hypotensive drug – a preliminary report. NZ Med J 66:864–870, 1967.
15. Amery A, Verstraete M, Bossaert H: Hypotensive action and side effects of clonidine-chlorthalidone and methyldopa-chlorthalidone in treatment of hypertension. Br Med J 4:392–395, 1970.
16. MacDougall AI, Addis GJ, Mackay N: Treatment of hypertension with clonidine. Br Med J 3:440–442, 1970.
17. Hoobler SW, Sagastame E: Clonidine hydrochloride in the treatment of hypertension. Am J Cardiol 28:67–73, 1971.
18. Conolly ME, Brant RH, George CF, Dollery CT: A crossover Comparison of clonidine and methyldopa in hypertension. Eur J Clin Pharmacol 4:222–227, 1972.
19. Delbarre B, Schmitt H: Sedative effects of α-sympathomimetic drugs and their antagonism by adrenergic and cholinergic blocking drugs. Eur J Pharmacol 13:356–363, 1971.
20. Kleinlogel H, Scholtysik G, Sayers AC: Effects of clonidine and BS100141 on the EEG sleep patterns in rats. Eur J Pharmacol 33:159–163, 1975.
21. Autret A, Minz M, Beillevaire T, Cathala H-P, Schmitt H: Effect of clonidine on sleep patterns in man. Eur J clin Pharmacol 12:319–322, 1977.
22. Maling TJB, Dollery CT, Hamilton CA: Clonidine and sympathetic activity during sleep. Clin Sci 57:509–514, 1979.
23. Rand MJ, Rush M, Wilson S: Some observations on the inhibition of salivation by ST155. Eur J Pharmacol 5:168–172, 1969.
24. Green GJ, Wilson M, Yates MS: The effect of clonidine on centrally and peripherally evoked submaxillary salivation. Eur J Pharmacol 53:297–300, 1979.
25. Kobinger W, Walland A: investigations into the mechanism of the hypotensive effect of 2,(2,6 dichlorophenylamono 2-imidazoline HCl. Eur J Pharmacol 2:155–162, 1967.
26. Starke K, Docherty JR: Recent developments in alpha-adrenoceptor research. J Cardiovasc Pharmacol 2 (Suppl 3):269–286, 1980.

27. Rehbinder D, Deckers W: Untersuchungen zur Pharmacokinetik und zum Metabolismus des 2-(2-6 dichlorophenylamino)-2-imidazolin-hydrochloride. Arzneim Forsch (Drug Res) 19:169–176, 1969.
28. Draffan GH, Clare RA, Murray S, Bellward GD, Davies DS, Dollery CT: The determination of clonidine in human plasma. Proc 3rd Int Symp. Mass Spectr Biochem Med, Sardinia, 1975.
29. Davies DS, Wing LMH, Reid JL, Neill E, Tippett P, Dollery CT: Pharmacokinetic and concentration effect relationships of intravenous and oral clonidine. Clin Pharmacol Ther 21:593–601, 1977.
30. Baillie TA, Neill E, Hughes H, Davies DL, Davies DS: Application of stable isotope labelling in studies of the metabolism of clonidine in rat liver. In: Stable Isotopes, pp. 415–425. Proc 3rd Int Conf. Klein ER, Klein PD, eds. London: Academic Press, 1979.
31. Reid JL, Barber ND, Davies DS: The Clinical Pharmacology of clonidine: relationship between plasma concentration and pharmacological effect in animals and man. Arch Int Pharmacodyn Ther (Suppl) pp. 11–16, 1980.
32. Frisk Holmberg M, Paalzow L: Relationship between clonidine kinetics and its blood pressure effects. Acta Med Scand [Suppl] 625:68–73, 1979.
33. Frisk Holmberg M, Edlund OP, Paalzow L: Relationship between clonidine kinetics and its therapeutic effect. Br J Clin Pharmacol 6:227–232, 1978.
34. Wing LMH, Reid JL, Davies DS, Dargie HJ, Dollery CT: Apparent resistance to the hypotensive effect of clonidine. Br Med J 1:136–138, 1977.
35. Bulpitt CJ, Hoffbrand BI, Dollery CT: In: Mild Hypertension: Natural History and Management PP.291–301. Gross F, Strasser T, eds. Tunbridge Wells: Pitman Medical, 1979.
36. Gifford RW: Catapres in the management of hypertension. In: Catapres in Hypertension, pp. 183–196. Conolly ME, ed. London: Butterworths, 1969.
37. Mroczek WJ, Davidov M, Finerty FA: Prolonged treatment with clonidine: comparative antihypertensive effects alone and with a diuretic. Am J Cardiol 30:536–541, 1972.
38. Briant RH, Reid JL, Dollery CT: Interaction between clonidine and desipramine in man. Br Med J 1:522–523, 1973.
39. Raftos J, Bauer GE, Lewis RG, Stokes GS, Mitchell AS, Young AA: Clonidine in the treatment of severe hypertension. Med J Aust 1:786–793, 1973.
40. Pettinger W, Mitchell HC, Gullner HG: Clonidine and the vasodilating beta-blocker antihypertensive drug interaction. Clin Pharmacol Ther 22:164–171.
41. Saarimaa H: Combination of clonidine and sotalol in Hypertension. Br Med J 1:810, 1976.
42. Bailey RR, Neale TJ: Rapid withdrawal with blood pressure overshoot exaggerated by beta blockade. Br Med J 1:942–943, 1976.
43. Zacest R, Gilmore E, Koch Weser J: Treatment of essential hypertension with combined vasodilatation and beta adrenergic blockade. N Engl J Med 286:617–622, 1972.
44. Dargie HJ, Dollery CT, Daniel J: Minoxidol in resistant hypertension. Lancet II:515–518, 1977.
45. Reid JL, Mathias cj, Jones DH, Wing LMH: The contribution of central and peripheral adrenoceptors to the actions of clonidine and alpha methyldopa in man. In: Central Adrenaline Neurons, pp. 317–325. Fuxe K, Goldstein M, Hokfelt B, Hokfelt T, eds. Oxford: Pergamon, 1980.
46. Weber MA, Drayer JIM, Laragh JH: The effects of clonidine and propranolol separately and in combination on blood pressure and plasma renin activity in essential hypertension. J Clin Pharmacol 18:233–240, 1978.
47. Hunyor JN, Hansson L, Hansson TS, Hoobler SW: Effects of clonidine withdrawal: Possible mechanisms and suggestions for management. Br Med J 2:209–211, 1973.
48. Reid JL, Dargie HJ, Davies DS, Wing LMH, Hamilton CA, Dollery CT: Clonidine withdrawal in hypertension. Lancet i:1171–1174, 1977.

49. Feyskes GG, Boer P, Dorhout–Mees EJ: Clonidine withdrawal, Mechanism and frequency of rebound hypertension. Br J Clin Pharmacol 7:55–62, 1979.
50. Cairns SA, Marshall AJ: Clonidine withdrawal. Lancet i:368, 1976.
51. Rosei EA, Brown JJ, Lever AF, Robertson AS, Robertson JIS, Trust PM: Treatment of phaeochromocytoma and of clonidine withdrawal with labetalol. Br J Clin Pharmacol 3 (Suppl):809–815, 1976.
52. Hurley DM, Vandongen R, Beilin LJ: Failure of labetalol to prevent hypertension due to clonidine withdrawal. Br Med J 1:1122, 1979.
53. Dubach UC, Huwyler R, Radielovic P, Singeisen M: A new centrally acting antihypertension agent guanfacine (BS100-141). Arzneim Forsch 27:674–676, 1977.
54. Leary WP, Asmal AC, Williams PC: Evaluation of the efficacy and safety of guanabenz versus clonidine. S Afr Med J 55:83–85, 1979.
55. Lindner E, Kaiser J: Tiamenidine (Hoe440) a new antihypertensive substance. Arch Int Pharmacodyn Ther 211–212:305–325, 1974.
56. Campbell BC, Elliott HL, Hamilton CA, Reid JL: Changes in blood pressure, heart rate and sympathetic activity on abrupt withdrawal of tiamenidine (Hoe440) in essential hypertension. Eur J Clin Pharmacol 18:449–454, 1980.
57. Hansson BG, Hokfelt B: Changes in blood pressure, plasma catecholamines and plasma renin activity during and after treatment with tiamenidine and clonidine. Br J Clin Pharmacol 11:73–78, 1981.
58. Zamboulis C, Reid JL: Withdrawal of guanfacine after longterm treatment in essential hypertension. Eur J Clin Pharmacol 19:19–24, 1981.
59. Reid JL, Zamboulis C, Hamilton CA: Guanfacine: effects of long-term treatment and withdrawal. Br J Clin Pharmacol 10:183–188S, 1980.

51. BLOCKERS OF THE NEUROMUSCULAR JUNCTION AS ANTIHYPERTENSIVE AGENTS

GORDON S. STOKES and HELEN F. OATES

There are three groups of drugs in clinical use for the treatment of hypertension which may produce therapeutic effects by competitive blockade at the neuromuscular junctions of vascular smooth muscle. These are the rauwolfia alkaloids, the guanidinium group of adrenergic neurone blocking drugs and the alpha-adrenoreceptor antagonists. The latter are of sufficient current importance to warrant discussion in a separate chapter. Controversy exists as to whether reserpine, the main active principle of rauwolfia, exerts its antihypertensive effect peripherally, in the central nervous system or at multiple sites. Certainly, consideration of the clinical side effects of reserpine suggest that this drug should be categorized with centrally active antihypertensive agents. Hence, this chapter will focus on adrenergic neurone blocking agents, including guanethidine, bethanidine, debrisoquine and guanadrel.

MECHANISM OF ANTIHYPERTENSIVE ACTION

In Figure 1 the action of adrenergic neurone blockers is contrasted with that of prazosin, an alpha-blocker with predominantly post-junctional activity. The antihypertensive action of the guanidinium group is pre-junctional, involving intereference with the release of neurotransmitter. The blood pressure lowering effects of guanethidine, and of the related guanidinium compounds, bethanidine and debrisoquine, can be attenuated by tricyclic antidepressant drugs [1] and by phenethylamines, phenothiazines and other agents which compete for an amine pump receptor on the sympathetic neurone membrane. This receptor activates a carrier-mediated transport process which also functions as the mechanism for the neuronal re-uptake of neurotransmitter noradrenaline, known as 'uptake$_1$'. The therapeutic effects of the guanidinium compounds depend upon their transport into the neurone by 'uptake$_1$'. Once inside the nerve terminals they may accumulate, being bound to the same particulate fraction as the neurotransmitter, whence they can be released following adrenergic neural stimulation [2]. It is unlikely that they function as 'false' transmitters [3]. Rather, they seem to

Amery, A. (ed.) Hypertensive Cardiovascular Disease: Pathophysiology and Treatment
© 1982, Martinus Nijhoff Publishers. The Hague / Boston / London
ISBN-13: 978-94-009-7478-4

NEUROTRANSMITTER RELEASE AT SYNAPSE

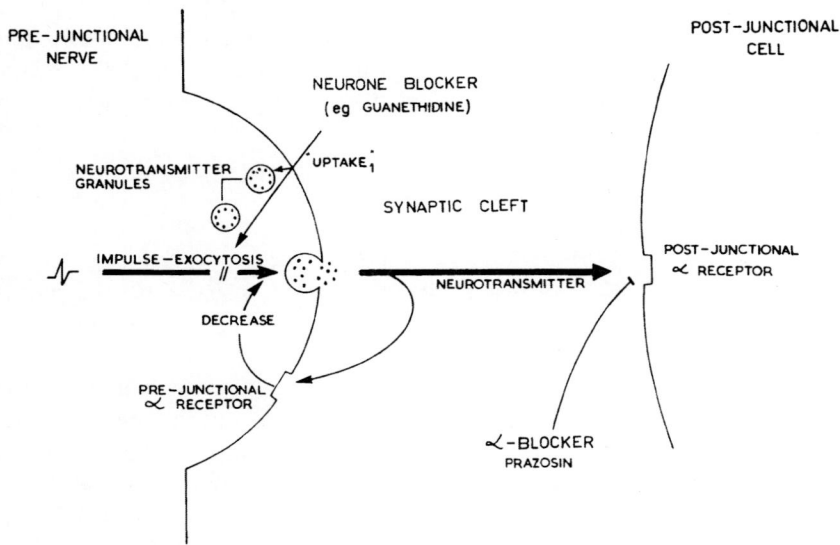

Figure 1. This diagram shows the sites of action at the sympathetic neuromuscular junction of neurone blockers of the guanidium group and of prazosin, the most widely used of the alpha-adrenoreceptor blockers. Whereas the action of prazosin is post-junctional, the guanidium group act after transport into the sympathetic nerve terminal.

interfere with the coupling of nerve impulses to the process of exocytotic release of neurotransmitter storage granules, perhaps by a local anaesthetic action which stabilises the neuronal membrane [4].

The guanidinium compounds show little penetration across the blood-brain barrier and do not appear to exert any important part of their action centrally. As they compete for the re-uptake of catecholamines and interfere with the intra-neuronal storage of neurotransmitter, they can produce a sudden release of catecholamines into the circulation if they are given intravenously, and, following chronic administration, cause marked depletion of catecholamines. Important clinical consequences of catecholamine depletion are hypersensitivity to injected pressor amines (analogous to 'denervation hypersensitivity'), pronounced orthostatic hypotension, and failure of seminal ejaculation. These effects may persist for some weeks after suspension of guanethidine therapy, though no irreversible functional or structural disorders of sympathetic neurones have been documented following guanethidine therapy in man. However, guanacline, a congener now withdrawn from clinical use, has reportedly induced protracted sympathetic disturbances in some patients, and, in experimental animals, severe changes in sympathetic ganglion cells which were still visible 12 weeks after cessation of treatment [5].

Whilst the principal antihypertensive action of the guanidinium adrenergic neurone blocking agents operates through the interruption of sympathetic vasomotor tone, these compounds also have a direct negative inotropic effect, and cause a relative predominance of parasympathetic drive, with consequent bradycardia.

CLINICAL USE OF NEURONE BLOCKERS IN HYPERTENSION

Adrenergic neurone blockers in current use and the usual doses employed are listed in Table 1. Guanethidine has a long duration of action, and a once-daily dosage is sufficient for maintenance therapy or for instituting non-urgent treatment. It is usual to start with 10 mg given as a single morning dose and to increase by increments of 10 mg/day each week until the desired blood pressure reduction is achieved. The target diastolic blood pressure reading is generally the lowest which is compatible with the patient's comfort and safety during normal activity (including exercise) in the upright posture. Orthostatic symptoms often intervene to prevent increase in dosage to a level which adequately controls blood pressure in the recumbent posture. In order to reduce blood pressure rapidly in severely hypertensive patients, a loading regimen may be used for guanethidine [6]. The patient should be admitted to hospital and given an initial oral dose of 75 mg followed by doses at 6 a.m., 12 noon and 6 p.m., each calculated to increase the total amount administered by about 25%. Once the desired response is obtained, the single daily maintenance dose is calculated as one-seventh of the cumulated loading dose.

Side effects with guanethidine include syncope or faintness associated with postural hypotension, failure of ejaculation, diarrhoea and muscular weakness of the lower limbs. The latter may be confused with intermittent claudication. Fluid retention commonly occurs requiring the concomitant use of a diuretic to control oedema and to sustain the antihypertensive effect.

Table 1. Adrenergic neurone blocking agents

Generic Name	Registered name	Usual dose range (mg)
Guanethidine	Ismelin	10–100 mg once daily
Bethanidine	Esbatal	5–100 mg twice daily
Debrisoquine	Declinax	5–100 mg twice daily
Guanadrel	Hylorel	30–100 mg three times daily

Bethanidine, debrisoquine and guanadrel differ from guanethidine mainly by having a shorter duration of action. They are also said to produce a lower incidence of diarrhoea. They allow more rapid dosage titration, whereas guanethidine has the advantage of maintaining blood pressure control with once-daily administration.

For all the guanidinium compounds, dosage requirements vary widely between individuals. In the case of debrisoquine the major determinant of response has been shown to be the systemic availability of the drug [7]. Significant correlations were found between the fall in standing blood pressure induced by oral debrisoquine and the urinary excretion or plasma concentration of the drug. A poor response appears to be associated with extensive metabolism rather than with poor absorption, and can be countered by the use of larger doses.

CONTRAINDICATIONS TO THE USE OF ADRENERGIC NEURONE BLOCKERS

1. Cerebrovascular insufficiency

Patients with a history of transient ischaemic attacks, or of completed stroke accompanied by hypotension, are particularly at risk from the orthostatic hypotension associated with adrenergic neurone blockers. Likewise, a history of recurrent syncope or an occupation in which even transient loss of consciousness would be dangerous are absolute contraindications.

2. Phaechromocytoma

Increased sensitivity to circulating pressor amines during adrenergic neurone blockade renders the use of antihypertensive agents of the guanidinium group hazardous in patients with phaeochromocytoma.

3. Pre-operative management of hypertension

Guanidinium adrenergic neurone blockers, particularly guanethidine, with its long effective half-life, can precipitate vascular collapse and hypotension during anaesthesia or haemorrhage. They may, on the other hand, induce hypersensitivity to pressor agents given for the control of intra-operative falls in blood pressure.

4. With tricyclic antidepressant, phenothiazine or monoamine oxidase inhibitor therapy

Psychotropic drugs commonly used in states of depression and agitation tend to counteract the antihypertensive action of the guanidinium adrenergic neurone blocking agents. Thus, it has clearly been shown that patients undergoing chronic therapy with guanethidine, bethanidine or debrisoquine respond, within one or two days, to the introduction of desipramine by significant rises in blood pressure [1]. This type of response, which is provoked by a wide range of tricyclic compounds, amphetamines and phenothiazines, results from potent antagonism of the uptake of the guanidinium compounds at the amine pump receptor. The high affinity of desipramine for the receptor is illustrated by the long period (5–7 days) required for the antihypertensive effects of the guanidinium compounds to reappear after cessation of the antagonist [1]. In patients receiving chronic tricyclic antidepressant therapy, very large doses of a guanidinium-type agent may be given without much effect on blood pressure control. Should, however, the antidepressant be withdrawn and the adrenergic neurone blocker be continued, severe hypotension may ensue. Monoamine oxidase inhibitors appear to have a somewhat weaker antagonistic effect than amphetamines [8].

5. With sympathomimetic therapy

The use of ephedrine and related amines in 'cold cures' and preparations for bronchitis or asthma can counteract the effect of guanidinium compounds, again by competition for the amine pump.

6. In patients with severe fluid retention due to renal or cardiac failure

The use of guanethidine or its congeners in renal failure or congestive cardiac failure is best avoided. However, if these situations are associated with fluid retention, it may be critically exacerbated by guanethidine. The guanidinium group of antihypertensive agents should never be used in states of fluid retention without adjunctive use of a diuretic.

INDICATIONS FOR THE USE OF ADRENERGIC NEURONE BLOCKERS

It is the authors' belief that the day of the guanidinium adrenergic neruone blocking drugs as drugs of first choice in treating hypertension has now passed. This is mainly a reflection of the orthostatic hypotension and other side effects commonly associated with their use, particularly interference with ejaculation in the male. Their role is now restricted largely to use as second or third line agents in patients who cannot tolerate the newer adrenoreceptor blocking drugs or centrally acting antihypertensive compounds. Their use, even in combination therapy is, however, becoming debatable because of alternative, less toxic, antihypertensive drugs which are available to reduce alpha-adrenoreceptor-mediated sympathetic tone.

REFERENCES

1. Mitchell JR, Cavanaugh JH, Arias L, Oates JA: Guanethidine and related agents – III. Antagonism by drugs which inhibit the norepinephrine pump in man. J Clin Invest 49:1596–1604, 1970.
2. Boullin DJ, Costa E, Brodie BB: Discharge of tritium-labelled guanethidine by sympathetic nerve stimulation as evidence that guanethidine is a false transmitter. Life Sci 5:803–808, 1966.
3. Shand DG, Morgan DH, Oates JA: The release of guanethidine and bethanidine by splenic nerve stimulation: a quantitative evaluation showing dissocation from adrenergic blockade. J Pharmacol Exp Ther 184:73–80, 1973.
4. Maxwell RA, Wastila WB: Adrenergic neurone blocking drugs. In: Antihypertensive Agents, p. 246. Gross F, ed. Heidelberg: Springer-Verlag, 1977.
5. Burnstock G, Doyle AE, Gannon BJ, Gerkens JF, Iwayama T, Mashford ML: Prolonged hypotension and ultrastructural changes in sympathetic neurons following guanadine treatment. Eur J Pharmacol 13:175–187, 1971.
6. Shand DG, Nies AS, McAllister RG, Oates JA: A loading-maintenance regimen for more rapid initiation of the effect of guanethidine. Clin Pharmacol. Ther 18:139–144, 1975.
7. Silas JH, Lennard MS, Tucker GT, Smith AJ, Malcolm SL, Marten TR: Why hypertensive patients vary in their response to oral debrisoquine. Br Med J 1:422–425, 1977.
8. Day MD, Rand MJ: Antagonism of guanethidine and bretylium by various agents. Lancet 2:1282–1283, 1962.

52. GANGLION BLOCKERS AS ANTIHYPERTENSIVE AGENTS

HELEN F. OATES and GORDON S. STOKES

1. MECHANISM OF ANTIHYPERTENSIVE ACTION

Transmission through autonomic ganglia can be blocked either by drugs that prevent acetylcholine-induced depolarization or by drugs that induce persistent depolarization of the postsynaptic membranes, but the term 'ganglion blocking drugs' is usually reserved for agents with the former mode of action [1]. According to the generally accepted mechanism of autonomic ganglionic transmission, neurotransmitter acetylcholine is released from intraneuronal storage sites by presynaptic nerve impulses and is liberated into the synaptic clefts. The neurotransmitter then excites postsynaptic cholinergic receptors, eliciting a localized depolarization, which, in turn, initiates an action potential in the postsynaptic fibre. Ganglion blocking drugs bind competitively to postsynaptic cholinergic (nicotinic) receptors, thus interfering with the binding of acetylcholine. They do not interfere with the release of acetylcholine from presynaptic storage sites. Since no major differences are known to exist in the mode of transmission in sympathetic and parasympathetic ganglia, ganglion blocking agents that selectively interfere with sympathetic transmission have not been developed, but the hypotensive activity of ganglion blocking drugs in general is predominantly a reflection of net decreases in cardiac output and total peripheral resistance consequent upon a reduction in sympathetic outflow.

2. INDIVIDUAL AGENTS

Ganglion blocking agents are not only among the most powerful blood pressure lowering drugs, but were also the first substances to be found capable of inducing a therapeutically significant antihypertensive effect. They may be grouped as quaternary ammonium compounds or nonquaternary compounds on the basis of differing absorption from the gastrointestinal tract, the latter group compromising secondary and tertiary amines and triethylsulfonium salts [1]. The generic and proprietary names and approximate dose ranges of some of the better known ganglion blocking agents are listed

Amery, A. (ed.) Hypertensive Cardiovascular Disease: Pathophysiology and Treatment
© *1982, Martinus Nijhoff Publishers. The Hague / Boston / London*
ISBN-13: 978-94-009-7478-4

Table 1. Generic ánd registrered names and usual doses* of ganglion blocking agents

Generic name	Proprietary name	Approximate dose range (mg)
Chlorisondamine	Ecolid	Initial dose 10 mg orally, maximum daily oral dose 250 mg, i.v. 1–2 mg, or s.c. 1–15 mg.*
Hexamethonium	Vegolysen	Initial dose 5–15 mg s.c. or i.m., usually repeated every 4–6 hours.*
Mecamylamine	Inversine Versamine	Initially, 2.5 mg orally twice daily, increasing to a maximum of 50 mg daily.*
Pempidine	Perolysen Tenormal	Initially, 2.5 mg orally every 6 hours, gradually increasing to a maximum of 80 mg daily.*
Pentolinium	Ansolysen	Orally, 10–20 mg twice daily, increasing to 100–900 mg;* s.c. initial dose 1–2.5 mg up to 20 mg; or 1–50 mg i.m.
Trimethaphan	Arfonad	Administration of 3–4 mg/min to start, by slow i.v. infusion, and adjusting according to the response.

* This information is of historical interest only, and it is not advisable to prescribe these agents in the routine treatment of hypertension.

in Table 1. Chlorisondamine and hexamethonium, quaternary ganglion blockers, are very poorly and irregularly absorbed from the gastrointestinal tract. Mecamylamine, in contrast, a nonquaternary ganglion blocker, though equipotent to hexamethonium, is almost completely absorbed, so that much smaller doses are effective. Since, however, the drug passes freely across cellular barriers in the body, it can produce central nervous system side effects (such as tremor, confusion, mania or depression) in addition to side effects attributable to autonomic ganglion blockade. Pempidine, like mecamylamine, is well absorbed, but serious side effects that cannot be attributed to autonomic ganglion blockade have not been reported with this drug. Pentolinium tartrate, a quaternary ganglion blocker, is four times as potent as hexamethonium, but if given intravenously, slow and inconstant dissociation of the salt may result in unpredictable effects and a peak response occurring some hours after injection. For this reason, the drug is not suitable for inducing controlled hypotension during surgery. Trimethaphan, on the other hand, is a sulfonium compound with a short duration of action and, when administered by constant intravenous infusion, it may be used to induce controlled hypotension during surgical procedures.

836

3. CONTRAINDICATIONS

A prominent feature of the blood pressure lowering effect of ganglion blocking drugs is the dependence upon posture. In the supine position, the blood pressure may be lowered only slightly or not at all, but in the upright position, the pressure may fall considerably, and postural hypotension and fainting may ensue. This effect is explained by blockade of the sympathetic reflex mechanisms which normally would increase vascular tone in the lower parts of the body. After ganglion blockade, blood is pooled in the lower limbs, and venous return and cardiac output are decreased.

Ganglion blocking agents are seldom used any more because of the effects induced by their parasympathoplegic action, including dryness of mouth, blurring of vision, urinary retention, constipation and impotence. Also, the development of tolerance to the antihypertensive effect over a period of one to two months may make a progressive increase in dosage necessary. Since the advent of drugs that selectively inhibit the sympathetic nervous system at specific sites, and which produce far fewer adverse side effects than do ganglionic blocking drugs, the latter are no longer agents of first choice in the long term management of hypertension, but are largely only of historical interest. The intravenous administration of trimethaphan is still useful in two situations: hypertensive crises (particularly when associated with dissecting aortic aneurysm, encephalopathy, subarachnoid haemorrhage or acute pulmonary edema) and surgical procedures in which hypotension is desirable to reduce bleeding [2]. Even so, trimethaphan is contraindicated in conditions where hypotension may subject the patient to undue risk, e.g. uncorrected anaemia, hypovolaemia, shock, asphyxia, uncorrected respiratory insufficiency and severe arteriosclerosis, coronary, renal or hepatic disease.

REFERENCES

1. Kreye VAW: Ganglion-blocking drugs in antihypertensive therapy. In: Antihypertensive Agents, pp. 61–76. Gross F, ed. Heidelberg: Springer-Verlag, 1977.
2. McMahon FG: Ganglionic-blocking agents. In: Management of essential hypertension, pp. 355–359. Mount Kisco, NY: Futura, 1978.

53. INHIBITORS OF THE RENIN–ANGIOTENSIN SYSTEM AS ANTIHYPERTENSIVE AGENTS

J. Staessen, R. Fagard, P. Lijnen and A. Amery

I. introduction

Renin is a proteolytic enzyme that is synthesized, stored and secreted mainly by the juxtaglomerular apparatus of the kidney. The release of renin is regulated a.o. by renal baroreceptors, by sodium-sensitive mechanisms at the level of the macula densa, by the sympathetic nervous system, prostaglandins and angiotensin II. Renin acts on its substrate, angiotensinogen, an alpha-2-globulin produced in the liver and present in the plasma to form the decapeptide angiotensin I, which is practically devoid of pressor activity. The converting enzyme, a peptidyl-dipeptidase, converts angiotensin I to angiotensin II by splitting off the dipeptide histidyl-leucine at the C-terminal of the decapeptide. The pulmonary circulation is the main site of conversion, but converting enzyme is also present in the plasma, in the splanchnic system, in the kidney and in several other tissues. Angiotensin II is the effector hormone of the system in man. Its most important actions are direct pressor effects on the arteriolar smooth muscle, stimulation of the aldosterone secretion by the adrenal gland, and effects on the central and peripheral nervous system; these actions result in an increase of blood pressure and in salt and water retention. Finally, the heptapeptide angiotensin III appears to have biological significance mainly for aldosterone secretion at least in some animal species.

The renin–angiotensin–aldosterone system may be blocked more or less selectively at several levels. Pharmacological agents which depress sympathetic activity decrease renin release, as is the case with beta-adrenoceptor blocking agents. The action of renin on renin substrate has been antagonized by nonspecific proteases such as pepstatin, and antibodies to renin and to angiotensinogen as well as structural analogues of the latter have been developed. Peptide and nonpeptide converting enzyme inhibitors interfere with the conversion of angiotensin I into angiotensin II, but also with the degradation of bradykinin. Angiotensin II analogues, acting as antagonists by competing with angiotensin II at its receptor sites, have been synthesized, but are not completely devoid of agonist actions. Also analogues of angiotensin

Amery, A. (ed.) Hypertensive Cardiovascular Disease: Pathophysiology and Treatment
© *1982, Martinus Nijhoff Publishers. The Hague / Boston / London*
ISBN-13: 978-94-009-7478-4

III have been produced. Finally the effects of aldosterone are antagonized by spironolactone.

This chapter will deal only with the angiotensin II analogues and with the converting enzyme inhibitors.

II. ANGIOTENSIN II ANALOGUES

1. Development and pharmacology

In the first approach to the development of angiotensin II antagonists a thorough study of structure–activity relationship of angiotensin II was performed [1]. As a result of these studies, it was shown that the side group in position 8 on angiotensin II was responsible for the transmission of the information which caused smooth muscle contraction. The information led to the development of the 8-substituted analogues that are competitive inhibitors of angiotensin II. Moreover, it was found that substitution of sarcosine in position 1 potentiates the biological activities already existing in the molecule.

The derivates of angiotensin II which have been used most in clinical and/or experimental studies are:

1-sarcosine-8-alanine-angiotensin II (saralasin) [2]
1-sarcosine-8-isoleucine-angiotensin II
1-sarcosine-8-threonine-angiotensin II.

These substances have antagonist properties, but also agonist angiotensin II-like activities which is not surprising for agents which arose from modification of angiotensin II. The agonist effects of the three angiotensin analogues on several target organs, relative to the effects of angiotensin II, are summarized in Table 1 [3].

Table 1. Intrinsic activities of angiotensin II analogues relative to angiotensin II*

Octapeptide	Pressor activity in ganglion-blocked vagotomized rats	Myotropic activity in rabbit aortic strips	Secretory activity in isolated cat adrenal medulla	Secretory activity in isolated cat adrenal cortex
Angiotensin II	100.0	100.0	100.0	100.0
1-sar-8-ala		0.5	3.0	0.5
1-sar-8-ile	1.0	1.0	3.0	1.0
1-sar-8-thr	0.6	0.5	0.1	1.0

* From [3].

Agonist effects have also been observed when, e.g., saralasin was administered to man: pressor effects and increases in renal vascular resistance [4], rises of plasma catecholamine levels [5], and of plasma aldosterone concentration [6].

Of the developed angiotensin II analogues, 1-sar-8-ala-angiotensin II (saralasin) has been most widely used. Therefore some of the characteristics of this agent are described below [7].

Saralasin has a molecular weight of 912.07 daltons and is highly soluble in either water or 5% aqueous dextrose and in 90% and 95% aqueous alcohol. Preclinically the drug has been used by most parenteral routes. Clinically it has been administered only by the intravenous route. The drug has been given by bolus of 10 mg over a period of 2 min, as a constant rate infusion of usually 10 µg/kg/min for 30–60 min, and as an increasing titrated dose with each dose continuing for about 10 min, starting as low as 0.1 µg/kg/min.

Saralasin has a short half-life. Reported biologically effective $t\frac{1}{2}$ and pharmacological $t\frac{1}{2}$ are between 3 and 12 min. There appears to be little transport of saralasin across the blood-brain barrier.

Saralasin, which is usually administered over short periods of time, appears to be a drug with a high degree of safety. In clinical studies untoward effects are largely related to the pharmacological action of the drug, namely changes of blood pressure. The transient initial pressor effect may be striking in sodium replete low renin hypertension: severe hypotension has been observed in patients with a volume deficit [8]; rebound hypertension has occurred in severe hypertension and in feochromocytoma. Overall, 39 adverse experiences (21 mild, 17 moderate and 1 severe) were reported among 24 of 342 patients studied in a collaborative study [9].

2. Hemodynamic effects of angiotensin II analogues

2.1. Effects of angiotensin II analogues in normotensive man

Sodium replete. When angiotensin II analogues are infused in normotensive men on their 'regular' diet or on a controlled sodium intake exceeding 100 mmol/24 hours, blood pressure remains unchanged or increases slightly when the subjects are supine or erect [4, 10–12]. However when the renin-angiotensin system is stimulated by physical exercise saralasin lowers blood pressure by approximately 9/4 mm Hg [13].

Sodium depleted. When normal subjects are placed on a daily sodium intake of 10 mmol for 4 or more days, sometimes in conjunction with a diuretic, angiotensin II antagonists usually produce no change or a slight decrease of

840

blood pressure in the supine position, depending on the degree of sodium depletion. The maximum decrease of diastolic pressure appears to be 10 mm Hg. When the renin–angiotensin system is further activated by standing, or by physical exercise, pressure usually decreases in response to angiotensin II antagonists [10–12, 14], related to a fall of systemic vascular resistance [14].

2.2. Effects of angiotensin II analogues in hypertensive man

Sodium replete. In their first study on the use of saralasin in human hypertension, Brunner et al. [15] report that the effectiveness of the inhibitor was often modified by changes in the state of sodium balance and that relatively small increases in cumulative sodium balance could abolish the antihypertensive effect of the drug which was observed during sodium depletion. Similar findings are reported by Streeten and Anderson, even in patients with renal arterial stenosis [16].

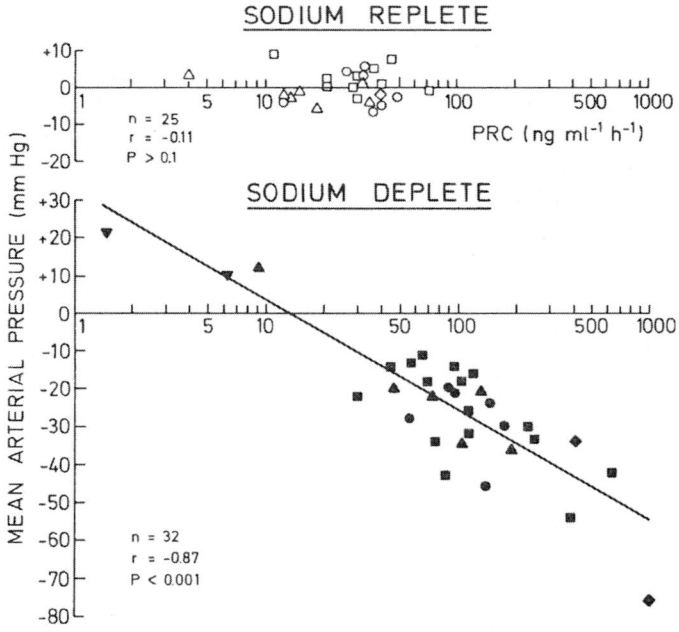

Figure 1. Relationship between changes in mean arterial pressure and log plasma renin concentration (PRC) in sodium replete (open symbols) and in sodium deplete patients (closed symbols) with hypertension of various aetiology (O, essential hypertension; □, renal artery stenosis; ◇, renal artery aneurysm; △, renal parenchymal disease; ▽, primary hyperaldostenosism).

In a few studies [17-20] saralasin has been infused into supine sodium replete hypertensive patients, whose sodium intake was between 95 and 150 mmol/24 h. A vasodepressor response, usually defined as a decrease of diastolic or mean arterial pressure of 7-8 mm Hg, occurred in 0-40% of the patients. Differences between studies may be explained by the etiology of hypertension, prevailing plasma renin levels and possibly by differences in plasma volume which may have been decreased with a consequent rise in plasma renin in severe hypertensives [21]. Furthermore, stimulation of the renin-angiotensin system in the seated position may increase the number of responders [22].

Sodium deplete. In several studies saralasin was administered in both sodium replete and sodium deplete conditions [17-20]. The results of one such study are summarized in Figure 1. Except for low renin hypertension the hypotensive response was greater during sodium depletion, usually achieved with a diuretic, and falls of mean arterial pressure of up to 76 mm Hg occurred. This is ascribed to the higher plasma renin and angiotensin levels, but it is possible that sodium depletion per se has an independent role in the saralasin response. Relationships between the saralasin-induced changes of arterial pressure and prevailing plasma renin levels are highly significant.

Whereas in these studies 0-40% of the patients responded to saralasin with a significant vasodepressor response in sodium replete conditions, the percentage was 30-90% after sodium depletion. Differences between studies are mainly due to patient's selection, but also to the degree of sodium depletion. Indeed, the number of responders and the magnitude of the pressure fall rose with increasing degree of sodium depletion [20] and even low renin patients respond to saralasin after severe sodium depletion [23].

When blood pressure decreases in response to saralasin this is usually related to a reduction of systemic vascular resistance [5].

3. Hormonal effects of angiotensin II analogues

Saralasin may cause a rise in plasma renin activity and consequently in plasma angiotensin I and plasma angiotensin II [24]. The rise of plasma renin is ascribed to the decrease of blood pressure but also to interruption of the negative feedback of angiotensin II on renal renin secretion. There is no effect on plasma-converting enzyme activity [24].

Its effect on plasma aldosterone is more complex and reflects a balance between agonist and antagonist effects of saralasin on the adrenal receptors. In sodium replete conditions saralasin produces a rise of plasma aldosterone, whereas the plasma aldosterone level remains unchanged or decreases in the sodium deplete state [6].

4. Clinical use of angiotensin II analogues

4.1. Screening for angiotensin II dependent hypertension

A potential role for angiotensin II analogues is to seek out and unmask patients with secondary and curable forms of the disease, particularly 'angiotensin II dependent' renovascular hypertension. To determine whether the blood pressure response to saralasin (0.8 mg/min i.v. for 30 min) could be used accurately and safely as a diagnostic screening procedure a collaborative study was set up, involving 342 patients in thirteen centers [9]. Sodium depletion was achieved with 80 mg of oral furosemide the day prior to the saralasin test. A high degree of correlation was found to exist between the blood pressure response to saralasin and levels of plasma renin activity, renin classification and arteriographic findings. Furthermore, of the patients diagnosed as pure renovascular hypertensives, usually on the basis of a successful surgical intervention, 76% exhibited a depressor response to saralasin. Of these diagnosed as pure or mixed forms of essential hypertension only 15% showed a depressor response. From similar data Krakoff et al. [25] concluded that, when the prevalence rate of renovascular hypertension among hypertensive patients is 5%, only 25% of positive saralasin tests will correctly predict its presence for large screening purposes, and merely 10% for a prevalence rate of 2%.

4.2. Treatment of hypertension

The use of angiotensin II antagonists for the treatment of hypertension is up to now limited by the fact that they have to be administered parenterally. Therefore they can only be used for short periods of time. Brunner et al. [15] reported that when given to seven patients with malignant or advanced hypertension, saralasin lowered blood pressure to close to normal levels in three patients, whose peripheral plasma renin activity was elevated, and reduced the blood pressure slightly or not at all in the remaining four with normal or low renin levels. A similar experience was reported by Streeten et al. [26], but they found intravenous infusions of nitroprusside more reliable in those circumstances.

Finally, it is possible that angiotensin II analogues may predict the response to oral drugs which act at least partially through interference with the renin–angiotensin system such as captopril [24] and beta-adrenoceptor blocking agents [27].

III. ANGIOTENSIN CONVERTING ENZYME INHIBITORS

1. Introduction

The angiotensin-converting enzyme is responsible for the conversion of angiotensin I to the potent vasopressor angiotensin II and is identical with kininase II, which is one of the enzymes, degrading the vasodepressor bradykinin into inactive peptide fragments.

A potent and specific competitive inhibitor of converting enzyme has been isolated from the venom of the snake Bothrops Jararaca [28]: the structure of this nonapeptide (Glu-Trp-Pro-Arg-Pro-Gln-Ile-Pro-Pro) has been identified, allowing its synthesis. The clinical use of the nonapeptide inhibitor, commonly known as teprotide (SQ 20881) is limited by the necessity of intravenous or other parenteral routes of administration.

Accumulated knowledge of the chemical and enzymatic properties of the angiotensin-converting enzyme, however has enabled the design and development of powerful orally active inhibitors. D-3-mercapto-2-methyl-L-proline (Figure 2) or captopril (SQ 14.225) was the first orally active inhibitor of the angiotensin-converting enzyme to become available [29, 30] and has been widely used not only in experimental animals, but also clinically for the evaluation and treatment of hypertensive patients [31].

Other converting enzyme inhibitors have been synthesized and are currently investigated for application in human hypertension [32–36]. The present review, however, will be confined to captopril and the nonapeptide teprotide, since up to now most experience with converting enzyme inhibition in human hypertension has resulted from the use of the latter drugs.

2. Pharmakinetics

When captopril is administered to healthy fasting volunteers about 70–75% of the drug is rapidly absorbed. Following oral intake of a single radiolabelled dose of 100 mg, radioactivity can be detected in the blood after 15 min and maximum blood concentrations are reached 15–75 min later [37]. Absorption is reduced by 35% if the drug is ingested in the nonfasting state. Captopril is bound to plasma proteins for about 30% [38].

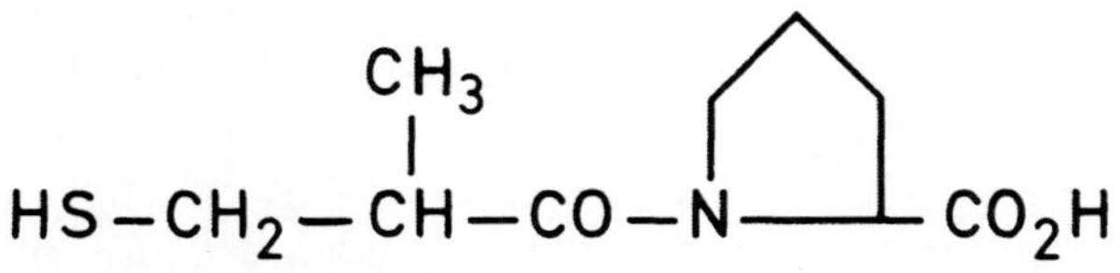

$$HS-CH_2-\underset{\underset{CH_3}{|}}{CH}-CO-N\diagup\diagdown\ CO_2H$$

Figure 2. Structure of captopril (D-3-mercapto-2-methyl-L-proline).

Captopril is rapidly distributed to most tissues, with the exception of the central nervous system. Transfer of the drug to the breast milk of lactating women is minimal [39], but captopril seems to cross the placental barrier in pregnant rats [40].

Captopril is partially oxidised at the mercapto-group to its disulfide [41]. One hour after a single radiolabelled dose (100 mg) unchanged captopril accounts for about 50% of the total radioactivity in the blood: 10% is attributed to its disulfide dimer and the remaining radioactivity to polar metabolites [37]. In blood unchanged captopril, as a percentage of total reactivity, decreases from 73% at 20 min to 6% at 6 h after dosing, while metabolites, consisting of protein-bound and -unbound radioactivity, increase from 26 to 94%. On average, 75% of a radiolabelled dose of captopril is excreted in urine within 1 day. Urinary excretion, as a percentage of the oral dose, consists of unchanged drug (34%), disulfide (4%) and other metabolites (33%) [42]. In patients with renal dysfunction the drugs elimination rate is closely related to the creatinine clearance [43]. In patients with impaired renal function (creatinine clearance less than 70 ml/min) the maximum daily dose should therefore be reduced or dosage intervals increased. In these patients therapy must be carefully individualized, but the following rules may be applied as an approximating guideline: maximum daily dose (mg) = 2.5 × creatinine clearance (ml/min) + 25; or, alternatively, dosage interval (hours) = 600 : creatinine clearance (ml/min).

The disposition profile is similar, when a radiolabelled dose is administered to hypertensives, either acutely or after 10 days of captopril treatment [42].

3. Haemodynamic effects of converting enzyme inhibition

3.1. Effects of converting enzyme inhibition in normotensive subjects at rest and during exercise

In our experience [44] converting enzyme inhibition with 25 mg captopril does not produce a significant effect on intra-arterially measured blood pressure in supine sodium-replete healthy volunteers. Swartz et al. [45] have demonstrated a significant and dose-dependent decrease of diastolic blood pressure in response to increasing doses of captopril (5, 12,5 and 25 mg), when they followed blood pressure in supine subjects during 2 h with an automatic recorder. However, these authors did not include a control group. Our findings [44] confirm other studies [46], which did not show changes in arterial pressure in supine salt-replete normotensives during converting enzyme inhibition.

At rest in the sitting position and during graded exercise on the bicycle ergometer Fagard et al. [47] did demonstrate a significant decrease of intra-arterial pressure in sodium-replete healthy volunteers which was indepen-

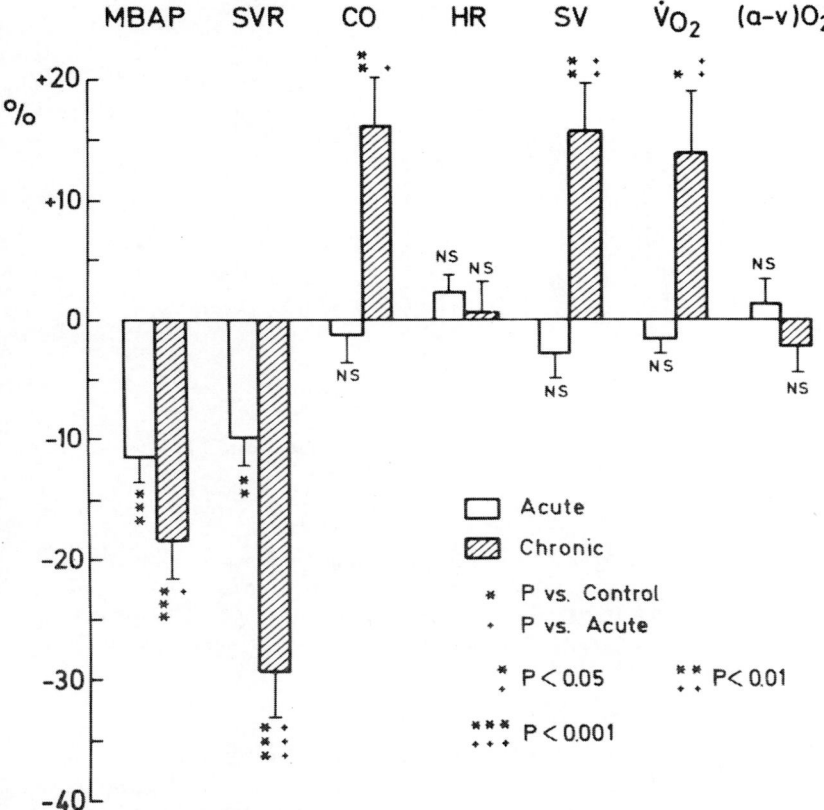

Figure 3. Percent changes from control values in mean brachial arterial pressure (MBAP), systemic vascular resistance (SVR), cardiac output (CO); heart rate (HR), stroke volume (SV), oxygen consumption ($\dot{V}O_2$) and arteriovenous oxygen content difference [(a-v) O_2] during acute (14 patients) and long-term (11 patients) treatment with captopril). Probability (p) values are given for the differences from control values and for the comparisons between acute and long-term changes for 10 pairs. NS = not significant.

dent of the level of physical activity. The hypotensive effect of converting enzyme inhibition in the erect position [47, 48] and during exercise [47] is based on a reduction of systemic vascular resistance. Cardiac output at rest in the erect position and during exercise was not affected in these studies, while heart rate was reported to remain unchanged [47] or to increase slightly [48].

3.2. *Effects of converting enzyme inhibition in hypertensive subjects at rest*

The acute and chronic systemic and pulmonary haemodynamic effects of angiotensin-converting enzyme inhibition in hypertensive subjects during moderate sodium restriction are summarized in Figures 3 and 4.

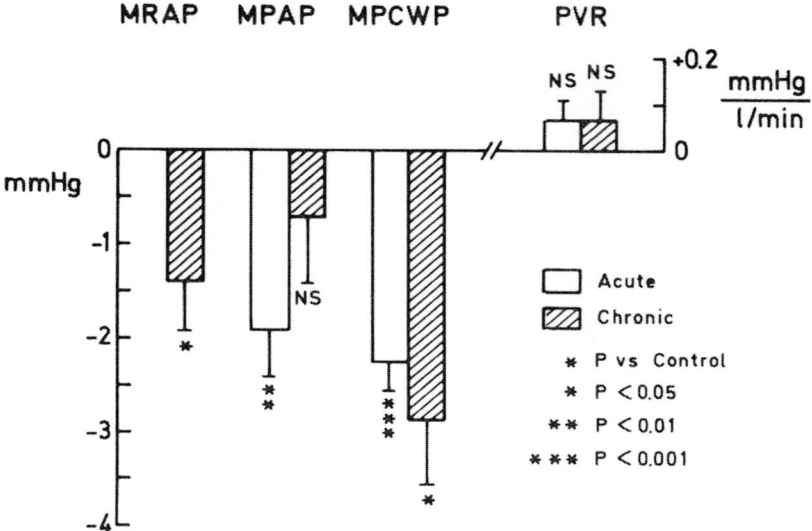

Figure 4. Changes from control values in mean right atrial pressure (MRAP), mean pulmonary artery pressure (MPAP), mean pulmonary capillary wedge pressure (MPCWP) and pulmonary vascular resistance (PVR) during acute and long-term treatment with captopril in 14 hypertensive patients. Probability (p) values are given for the differences from control values.

In acute studies angiotensin converting enzyme inhibition effectively decreases systemic arterial blood pressure, particularly in sodium-volume deplete patients and this acute depressor effect is mediated via a decrease of systemic vascular resistance [49–55]. Converting enzyme inhibitors do not affect cardiac output, when they are administered to hypertensive patients, either acutely [49, 50, 53] or for 3–7 consecutive days [51, 53]. However, cardiac output was reported to increase promptly when teprotide was infused to reduce arterial pressure in patients with acute hypertension after coronary artery bypass surgery [54].

In spite of the marked depressor response observed in most acute and short-term studies, heart rate remains either unchanged or accelerates only slightly. This haemodynamic pattern of reduction in peripheral resistance with constant heart rate and stroke volume is similar to that produced by vasodilators, acting at both arteriolar and venous vascular beds. It has also been shown that angiotensin II causes tachycardia [56], so that inhibition of its generation may counteract the baroreceptor reflex induced tachycardia. Furthermore, as a result of the Bainbridge reflex, a reduction in right atrial pressure may prevent an increase of heart rate. However, captopril does not affect the haemodynamic responses to head-up tilt, regardless of sodium intake [51].

Teprotide [55] and captopril [49, 50] acutely decrease pulmonary capillary wedge pressure: this may be due to unloading of the left ventricle by the reduction of arterial pressure and/or to pooling of the blood by arteriolar or venous vasodilation or both, although the effect of angiotensin on the capacitance vessels remains controversial [57, 58]. Pulmonary vascular resistance remains unchanged, when captopril is administered acutely [49–51, 53].

When captopril treatment is continued for periods ranging from 3 days to 2 months [49–51, 53, 59, 60] both the depressor response and the decrease of total peripheral vascular resistance are maintained. In patients with essential and renovascular hypertension, Fagard et al. [49, 50] have compared the acute haemodynamic effect of captopril observed 75 min after oral intake of 25 mg, with the haemodynamic pattern observed after 2 months of therapy with 150–600 mg/day. Patients were studied in the supine position and cardiac output was measured by the direct Fick method. The acute dose of captopril produced a significant decrease in mean intra-arterial pressure (-12%) and in systemic vascular resistance (-11%) with unchanged cardiac output, heart rate, stroke volume, oxygen consumption, and arteriovenous oxygen content difference. After 2 months of treatment, mean arterial pressure (-18%) and also systemic vascular resistance (-30%) had decreased further, while cardiac output had increased by 15%.

Sullivan et al. [60] found no change in cardiac output in patients with essential and renovascular hypertension, studied by echocardiography, in the supine position, 3–14 days after initiation of captopril therapy. Other investigators [51, 53, 59] using thermodilution and dye dilution techniques reported important variations in cardiac output during long-term therapy, which were related to alterations in blood volume: an inverse relationship between changes in total peripheral resistance and blood volume was also demonstrated by these authors.

The increase in cardiac output, which may occur during long-term captopril therapy [49, 50, 59] is essentially achieved by an augmentation of stroke volume since, like in acute and short-term studies heart rate is not significantly affected.

The decrease in pulmonary wedge pressure is maintained during long-term treatment and also right atrial pressure is decreased, indicating either reduced blood volume, dilation of the venous capacitance vessels or both [49, 50].

3.3. Effects of converting enzyme inhibition in hypertensive subjects during exercise

The response of the systemic and pulmonary circulation to acute converting enzyme inhibition with 25 mg captopril has recently been studied during

848

exercise in hypertensive subjects [47]. Only sodium-replete hypertensives were investigated, since a single dose of captopril may produce adverse hypotension after sodium depletion [48, 61]. Patients were allocated to either a placebo- or to a captopril-treated group; each patient was investigated at rest, recumbent and sitting, and during an uninterrupted graded submaximal exercise up to the anaerobic threshold before treatment and 75 min after treatment (placebo or captopril). The results are summarized in Figures 5 and 6 for the systemic circulation and in Figure 7 for the pulmonary haemodynamics.

Compared to the observations in the placebo group, captopril decreased intra-arterial pressure during exercise via a reduction of systemic vascular resistance, while cardiac output remained unchanged, though heart rate increased slightly during exercise. Captopril decreased pulmonary artery and capillary wedge pressure with unchanged pulmonary vascular resistance. These findings indicated that the depressor effect of converting enzyme inhibition is somewhat more pronounced during exercise than at rest, suggesting that the role of angiotensin II in maintaining arterial pressure

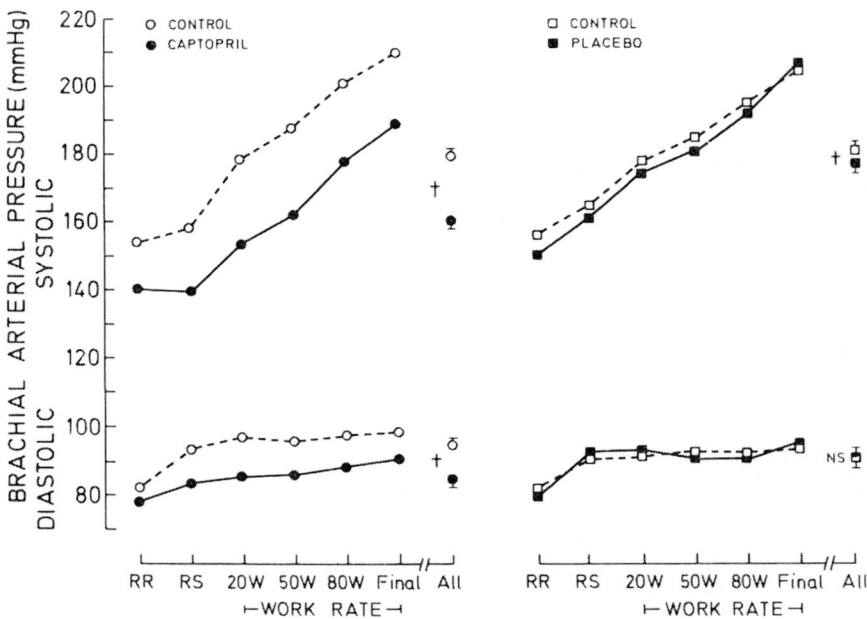

Figure 5. Systolic and diastolic brachial artery pressures at rest recumbent (RR), at rest sitting (RS), during graded exercise, at the final work load and for all data combined before (control) and during captopril or placebo treatment.

Data are means. Statistical analysis was performed by three-way analysis of variance. Statistical significance of the effect of treatment, either captopril or placebo, is indicated. +, p<0.001; n.s., not significant.

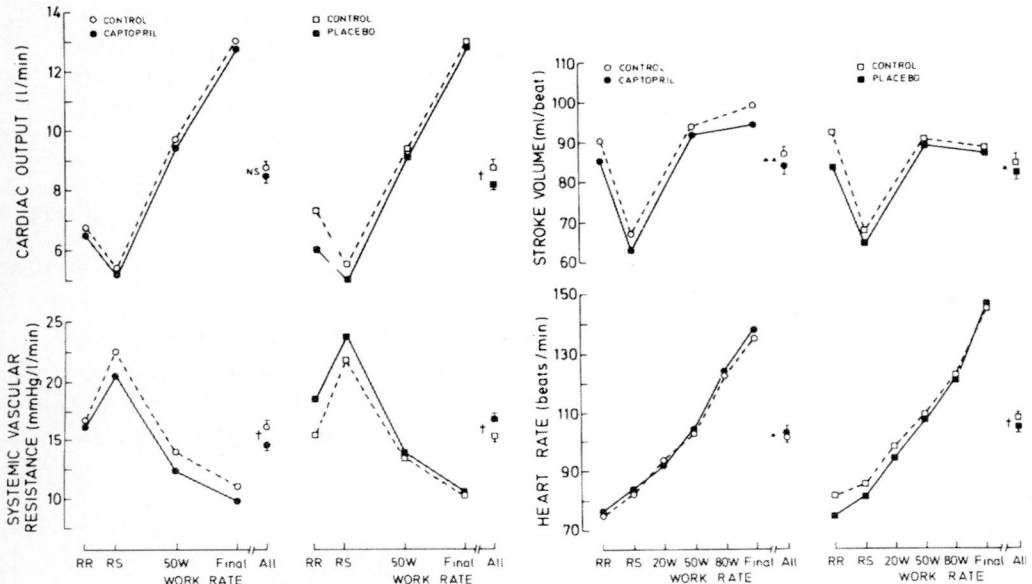

Figure 6. Cardiac output, systemic vascular resistance, stroke volume, and heart rate at rest recumbent (RR), at rest sitting (RS), during graded exercise, at the final work load and for all data combined before (control) and during captopril or placebo treatment.

Data are means. Statistical analysis was performed by three-way analysis of variance. Statistical significance of the effect of treatment, either captopril or placebo, is indicated. $+$, $p<0.001$; **, $p<0.01$; *, $p<0.05$; n.s. not significant.

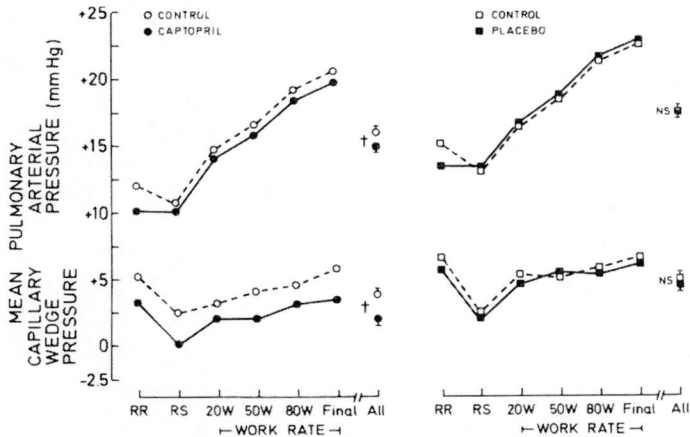

Figure 7. Mean pulmonary arterial pressure and capillary wedge pressure at rest recumbent (RR), at rest sitting (RS), during graded exercise, at the final work load and for all data combined before (control) and during captopril or placebo treatment.

Data are means. Statistical analysis is performed by three-way analysis of variance. Statistical significance of the effect of treatment, either captopril or placebo, is indicated. $+$, $p<0.001$; n.s., not significant.

becomes more important with physical activity or that accumulation of bradykinin or interference with prostaglandin metabolism is greater during exercise. Furthermore, the data demonstrate that also during exercise the depressor effect of captopril is characterized by systemic arteriolar and probably also venous vasodilation, while pulmonary vascular resistance is not affected.

4. Mechanism of hypotensive action

Despite intensive and continuing research, the mechanism of captopril's blood pressure lowering effect remains incompletely understood. The possibilities include: (1) interference with the pressor effect of angiotensin II by blockade of its formation; (2) inhibition of the aldosterone secretion; (3)

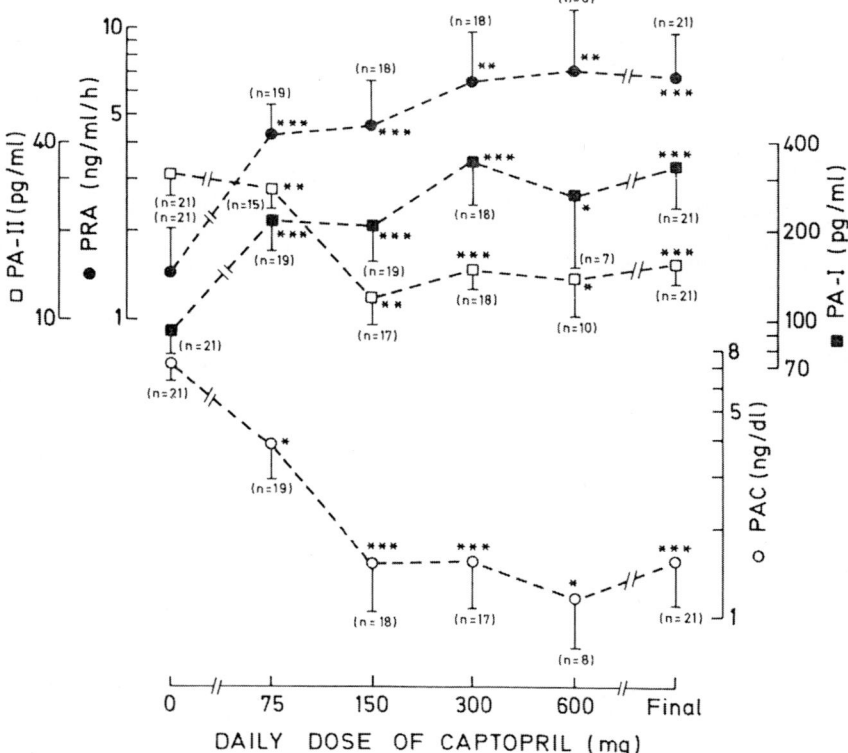

Figure 8. Plasma renin activity (PRA), plasma angiotensin I (PA I), angiotensin II (PA II) and aldosterone (PAC) concentration during placebo (0) and during treatment with increasing doses of captopril for 2 months.

Values given are means ± standard error. Significance of the difference with control (placebo period). *, p<0.05; **, p<0.01; ***, p<0.001.

impairment of the degradation of vasodilatory plasma kinins; (4) interference with the prostaglandin metabolism, leading to an increased production of vasodepressor prostaglandins, and/or a decreased synthesis of vasopressor prostaglandins; (5) direct central nervous effects or a blood pressure lowering effect mediated via the peripheral autonomous nervous system, and (6) a direct vasodilatory effect.

In man, most authors report a suppression of the plasma concentration of angiotensin II [62, 63] during both acute and sustained converting enzyme inhibition, while plasma renin and angiotensin I are increased (Figure 8). However, several lines of evidence suggest that the decreased production of angiotensin II in the circulating blood, cannot be wholly responsible for captopril's effect on blood pressure.

1. The first order correlation coefficient between the acute hypotensive effect of captopril and the suppression of angiotensin II in the blood is rather low (− 0.60) in hypertensive sodium-deplete subjects [49], indicating that in these conditions angiotensin II suppression explains only 30–40% of the observed blood pressure reduction; the low correlation coefficient may result at least partly from the methodology used to measure, either blood pressure or plasma angiotensin II.

2. The hypotensive effect of captopril exceeds that of the angiotensin II antagonist, saralasin, at any prevailing level of plasma renin activity by about 10 mm Hg [49]. Part of the observed difference in hypotensive potency between both drugs may be attributed to the intrinsic pressor activity of saralasin [64].

3. Restoration of control blood pressure during angiotensin converting enzyme inhibition with teprotide (SQ 20881) requires amounts of exogenous angiotensin II, which produce plasma angiotensin II levels, significantly higher than control [65].

4. In sodium-replete normotensive men plasma angiotensin II is not significantly lowered, although captopril in these subjects reduces arterial pressure, either at rest in the supine [45] and sitting [47] position, or during a graded exercise on the bicycle ergometer [47].

5. In anephric animals, captopril conserves its capability to reduce blood pressure [66, 67]: in patients, blood pressure has been reported to be lowered by captopril after bilateral nephrectomy [68, 69], although not by all investigators [70]. It is possible that the hypotensive effect of captopril is dependent on the suppression of angiotensin II formation in tissues, such as the brain [71], the vascular smooth muscle [72] and the kidney [73] or even may be partly unrelated to the renin–angiotensin system. Although captopril does not cross readily the blood-brain barrier [74, 75] there is good evidence that chronic oral treatment may have central effects and that these contribute to the drug's antihypertensive effect by interference with central peptidergic blood pressure regulating systems [76].

In man captopril acutely decreased the plasma aldosterone concentration. It is difficult to conceive how this mechanism might contribute to the acute vasodepressor response to converting enzyme inhibition, since the ensuing changes in the sodium and fluid balance occur only slowly. Nevertheless, inhibition of the adrenal aldosterone secretion may play a role in the long-term hypotensive effect, though a negative sodium balance could not be demonstrated uniformously in all studies [77–80]. Furthermore, Staessen et al. [81, 82] have observed that plasma aldosterone initially decreases during long-term converting enzyme inhibition with captopril, but after three months, in spite of continuously suppressed plasma angiotensin II levels, rises again and may even exceed its pretreatment level after one year (Figure

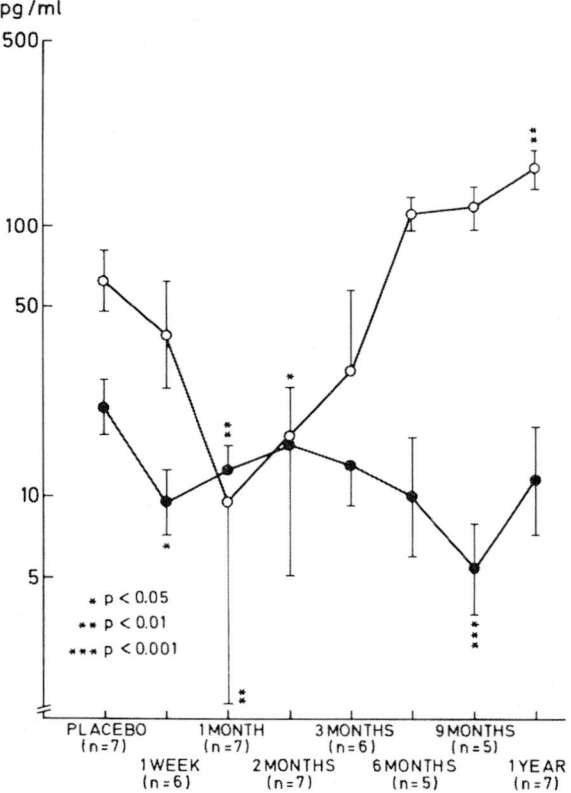

Figure 9. Plasma levels of aldosterone (open circles) and angiotensin II (solid circles) before and during long-term captopril treatment. The number of patients is indicated for each treatment interval. Values are expressed as means ± standard error. P indicates the significance of the difference between values in the placebo period and those in the treatment period.

9). Other investigators [83–85] have even not been able to demonstrate a sustained decrease of plasma aldosterone during short-term studies.

Captopril has no direct effect on vascular smooth muscle or on alfa- and beta-adrenoceptors, and it has no ganglionic or adrenergic neurone blocking activity [86–88]. Converting enzyme inhibition does not interfere with circulating catecholamines [84, 89].

Converting enzyme inhibition not only affects the renin–angiotensin-aldosterone system, but also the kallikrein-kinin and prostaglandin system. Bradykinin acts as a vasodepressor by its direct vasodilator effect and via its renal action, leading to an increase in sodium and water excretion, and is inactivated by converting enzyme (kininase II). Therefore, converting enzyme inhibitors simultaneously antagonize the generation of a powerful vasopressor, angiotensin II, and impair the degradation of a potent vasodepressor, bradykinin. Indeed, in patients with moderate to severe hypertension captopril increases the blood pressure lowering response to exogenous bradykinin [90]. However, the hypothesis that the hypotensive response during chronic converting enzyme inhibition might be enhanced by a decrease of bradykinin's degradation is difficult to ascertain, since the bradykinin assay in the blood is difficult. Moreover, local accumulation of bradykinin in tissues might have important haemodynamic effects through vasodilation and in the kidneys also by natriuresis, but is probably not wholly reflected in circulating bradykinin. Animal studies, which have been reviewed elsewhere [88, 91] have presented divergent conclusions. Also, in humans some investigators [92–94] have reported no significant changes in blood bradykinin, while others did find significantly increased bradykinin levels in the blood after converting enzyme inhibition [65, 95–98]. Aprotin, an inhibitor of kinin generation, decreases the hypotensive response to captopril in patients with renovascular, but not essential hypertension [99]. Correlations between the depressor response to converting enzyme inhibition and the increase in blood bradykinin were found to be significant by some authors [45] but not by others [97]. The hypotensive effect of teprotide has been reported to be related more closely to the changes of urinary kinins than to the decrease of plasma angiotensin II [93].

During converting enzyme inhibition urinary kallikrein excretion decreases [100, 101]. This phenomenon may result from a negative feed-back mechanism activated by the captopril-induced increase in blood kinins [101], or alternatively, may be secondary to the drug's aldosterone inhibiting effect and reflect the positive association, usually observed between mineralocorticoids and urinary kallikrein, the underlying mechanism of which remains unknown [102, 103].

Renal prostaglandins may play an important role in bradykinin-induced hypotension, since the depressor response to bradykinin is attenuated in captopril-treated animals by nephrectomy and in intact animals by pretreatment with indomethacine [104]. Also in hypertensive patients the blood pressure lowering effect of captopril can be attenuated by inhibition of the endogenous prostaglandin synthesis with indomethacine [105]. These observations suggest that both, the kallikrein-kinin and prostaglandin system, may be functionally interrelated and that prostaglandins, per se, may be involved in mediating the hypotension response to converting enzyme inhibition.

However, conflicting observations on the effects of converting enzyme inhibition on prostaglandin metabolism in man have been reported. Urinary excretion of prostaglandin E_2, $F_{2\alpha}$ and 6-keto $F_{1\alpha}$ has been reported to remain unchanged in one study [107], while other invetigators [108] have found increases in urinary prostaglandin E. After acute administration of captopril Lijnen et al. [109] have observed a decrease of the plasma levels of vasopressor prostaglandin $F_{2\alpha}$, but also of vasodepressor prostaglandin E_2: the pressure response in these patients was negatively correlated with the change in plasma prostaglandin E_2. Several investigators [45, 93, 98, 106] have reported significant increases in the plasma concentrations of prostaglandins E_2 or $F_{2\alpha}$ metabolites and in some studies [93, 106] a correlation was demonstrated between the increase in depressor prostaglandins and the hypotensive response to converting enzyme inhibition.

5. Clinical usefulness in the treatment of hypertensive patients

The usefulness of captopril in congestive heart failure will not be discussed here [110].

Captopril reduces arterial blood pressure in many patients with essential hypertension. If the blood pressure lowering effect is mediated via inhibition of angiotensin II formation, the drug would be expected to have a hypotensive action in proportion to the pretreatment renin level. However, studies relating pretreatment plasma renin activity to the blood pressure response have produced divergent results: while some investigators [78, 79] have reported a significant relationship between the initial plasma renin activity and both the early and sustained decrease in blood pressure, others [84, 94, 111] were not able to demonstrate such a relationship, especially for the sustained hypotensive effect during long-term treatment [112–114]. These conflicting findings can be reconciled if one accepts that the plasma renin activity, prevailing before captopril administration, is only a reliable predictor of the drug's hypotensive effect, when measurements of blood pressure and renin are obtained in rigorously standardised conditions, and when the range of the initial plasma renin activity is wide enough. In moderately sodium-deplete hypertensives, Fagard et al. [24] have demonstrated a highly significant correlation between the reduction of mean intra-arterial pressure, produced by a first dose of captopril (25 mg) and the initial plasma renin activity ($r = -0.82$) and angiotensin II levels ($r = -0.72$). In a chronic study Fagard et al. [49] reported a similar but weaker relationship, when intra-arterial pressure was measured 1 h after the morning dose of the converting enzyme inhibitor: the sustained hypotensive effect was also correlated with the pretreatment plasma renin activity ($r = -0.68$) and angiotensin II concentration ($r = -0.46$) in these conditions. However, when in the same patients blood pressure was followed during dose titration at the out-patient clinic such a correlation could not be demonstrated for systolic blood pressure, and for diastolic only inconstantly at some of the doses prescribed [63]. In contrast, Laragh and coworkers [115, 116] have reported a good correlation between plasma renin activity and both the acute and long-term response to captopril. These investigators observed also a close correlation between the initial and sustained blood pressure response and suggested that the response to the first dose of the drug may have predictive value for its long-term influence on blood pressure.

In human renovascular hypertension captopril produces an early fall in blood pressure, which seems to be proportional to the pretreatment plasma renin activity and angiotensin II levels and which parallels the decrease in circulating angiotensin II [62, 79]. Captopril is extremely efficacious in the syndrome of severe hyponatraemia and hypertension, associated with unilateral renal artery occlusion, where it corrects rapidly both high blood pressure and electrolyte abnormalities [117]. Furthermore, captopril has also been reported to lower blood pressure in patients with renal artery stenosis, whose peripheral plasma levels of renin and angiotensin II were within the normal range [62, 111, 118]. In our experience long-term converting enzyme inhibition does not restore normal blood pressure in a substantial proportion of patients with renal artery stenosis: in about 60% of such patients a daily dose of 600 mg captopril did not reduce diastolic blood pressure below 100 mm Hg: however, blood pressure levels during long-term converting enzyme inhibition, both systolic ($r = 0.54$) and diastolic ($r = 0.56$), were correlated with those observed two months after unilateral nephrectomy or reconstructive renal artery surgery, without antihypertensive therapy [119].

In most placebo-controlled studies [63, 78, 79, 85, 94, 120–123] the hypotensive effect of captopril was similar in patients with essential and renovascular hypertension: on average a reduction in both systolic and diastolic blood pressures of 15–25% was reported. In patients with mild to moderate hypertension, captopril (daily dose ⩽450 mg), compared with hydrochlorothiazide (daily dose ⩽100 mg) [124–126] or propranolol (daily dose ⩽360 mg) [124, 127–129] seemed to be equally effective in lowering blood pressure. However, in many of these studies, several patients required, besides captopril, additional drugs to become normotensive.

The addition of a diuretic enhances the effectiveness of captopril and most patients with moderate hypertension can be controlled, if not by captopril alone, by this combination [130, 131]. Also, propranolol produces an additional decrease in blood pressure [132, 133] confirming the hypothesis that the hypotensive action of beta-adrenergic receptor blocking drugs is not wholly due to suppression of the renin release and the angiotensin–aldosterone system at least in these conditions (Figure 10).

In patients with severe treatment resistant hypertension captopril alone may produce about the same blood pressure reduction, as can be achieved with standard triple therapy [134–136]. Nevertheless, additional drugs are needed in the majority of these patients to achieve and maintain a satisfactory blood pressure control. Captopril has also been used successfully in patients with malignant hypertension and encephalopathy [137], in patients with end stage renal failure and dialysis resistant hypertension [138, 139]

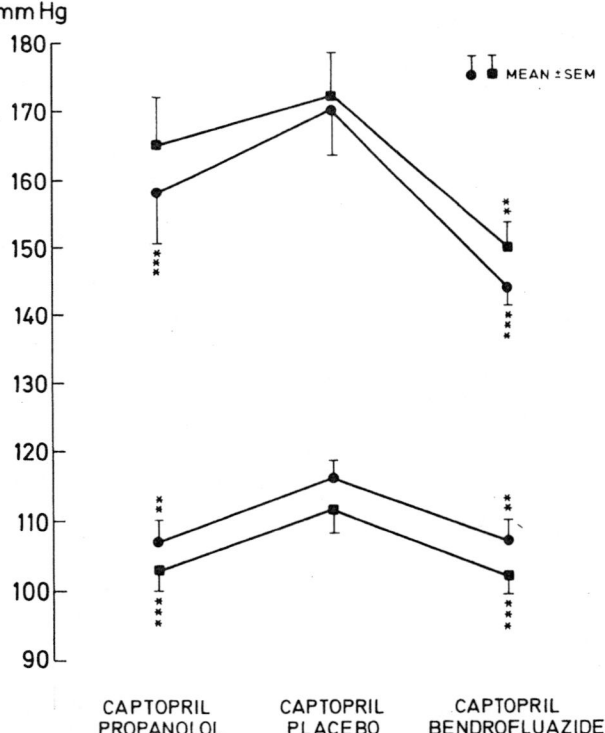

Figure 10. Standing (circles) and recumbent (squares) systolic and diastolic blood pressures when placebo, propranolol (3 × 80 mg) or bendrofluazide (3 × 2,5 mg) were combined with captopril (3 × 200 mg) in 19 patients. P values indicate the significance of the difference with placebo. **, p<0.01; ***, p<0.001.

857

and in hypertensive emergencies, associated with systemic lupus erythematosus [140–142] and scleroderma [143, 144].

While in most studies captopril was administered in three or four divided daily doses, Brunner et al. [145] presented data showing that a twice daily dosage schedule may also provide adequate blood pressure control throughout the day. However, in patients with normal renal function, receiving two or three daily doses of captopril [146, 147] plasma-converting enzyme activity intermittently returns to its pretreatment value, though the hypotensive effect is sustained (Figure 11).

In a chronic out-patient study, inhibition of angiotensin converting enzyme by 75 mg of captopril daily lowered the blood pressure significantly [63]. Except for a slight further reduction of blood pressure at 150 mg of captopril, increasing doses of captopril up to 600 mg daily, did not induce further lowering of systolic or diastolic blood pressure in the supine or

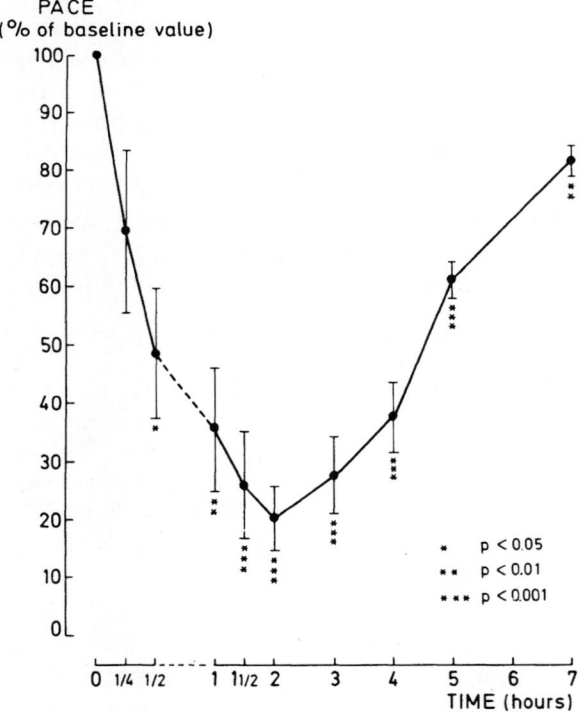

Figure 11. Plasma angiotensin I converting enzyme (PACE) activity before and during 7 hours after intake of the morning dose (200 mg) in 5 patients, treated chronically with 600 mg captopril, in 3 divided daily doses. The results are expressed as percentage (mean ± standard error) of the reference value, determined immediately before the morning dose. Significance of the difference with the reference value is indicated.

858

standing position. Thus, 150 mg appears to be the ceiling hypotensive dose of captopril in most hypertensives, although in some a higher dose may be needed. However, a maximum daily dose of 5–6 mg/kg should not be exceeded (manufacturer's recommendation) to avoid drug-induced toxicity. As mentioned in other sections of this chapter, the daily dose should be reduced in patients with impaired renal function, in patients with immune disorders and in those receiving concomitantly a immunosuppressant drug such as azothioprine.

6. Side-effect of captopril

6.1. First dose effect

A very pronounced depressor effect can be observed, when a first dose of captopril is administered to patients in whom blood pressure is angiotensin II dependent. Thus, serious and sometimes life-threatening hypotension has been reported when captopril therapy was initiated in patients who had previously been sodium-depleted by diet and/or diuretics [61], in patients with unilateral renal artery occlusion [117] and in normotensive subjects with activated renin–angiotensin system [148]. Immediate intravenous infusion of saline may be life-saving in the face of excessive hypotension [61, 79, 117]: the bradycardia, which in some cases accompanies the fall in blood pressure can be counteracted by intravenous injection of atropine [61].

6.2. Skin rash and mucosal irritation

Skin rash is undoubtedly the commonest side-effect observed with captopril: its incidence varies from 8% in one studie [111] to 58% in another one [149]: on average skin eruptions occur in about 14% of patients from combined published and unpublished series [150].

In most cases a morbilliform or maculopapular rash develops, on average nine days after the initiation of captopril treatment and is localized on the head, neck, trunk, arms, the palms of the hand and/or the soles of the foot [149]. However, skin rashes may also appear on the first day of treatment or after several weeks of captopril intake. They usually clear rapidly after dose reduction or drug withdrawal or in some cases may even disappear, while captopril administration is continued at the same daily dose.

Skin rashes are sometimes accompanied by a clinical picture of serum sickness, characterized by fever, adenopathies and arthralgia, but these symptoms resolve upon dose reduction or drug withdrawal.

859

Other cutaneous lesions include: urticaria, angioneurotic oedema of the
face and forearms, maculosquamous, skin eruptions resembling pityriasis
rosea [149], and pemphigus erythematosus [151]. Ulcerations of the tongue [152] and aphtous lesions of the mouth [153] have been reported, while
respiratory symptoms may be caused by irritation of the laryngeal and tracheal mucosa.

6.3. Haematological and immunological side-effects

Several patients developing agranulocytosis or neutropenia during captopril
treatment have been reported [140–142, 150, 154–159] and also one patient
with fatal pancytopenia [160].

Captopril-associated haematological side-effects occur most commonly
3–6 weeks after initiation of treatment [150]. All but one patient [155] had
complex medical problems, such as metastatic malignant disease, polyclonal
gammapathy, scleroderma, lupus erythematosus, membranous glomerulonephritis and tuberculosis or were on multiple drug therapy; most of these
drugs have been associated with bone marrow suppression. Several of these
patients also had an impaired renal function, which may be of particular
relevance, since captopril and its metabolites are excreted by the kidneys.

Table 2. Blood pressure, hemoglobin and blood cell counts in a patient, presenting captopril-
associated agranulocytosis*

Date	Captopril daily dose (mg)	Recumbent blood pressure (mmHg)	Hemoglobin (g/100 ml)	White Cell count (n/mm^3)	Neutrophil count (n/mm^3)	Platelet count (n/mm^3)
Nov. 26	0	216/130	13.2	4.200	2.900	—
Dec. 11	0	230/112	14.4	5.700	2.390	175.000
Jan. 30	600	136/92	12.4	4.100	1.550	—
Febr. 15	600	—	11.2	2.400	—	328.000
Febr. 16	200	108/66	11.0	3.900	—	—
Febr. 17	0	136/96	11.2	3.000	—	—
Febr. 18	0	136/90	12.2	3.500	126	280.000
Febr. 19	0	118/96	10.9	3.200	192	285.000
Febr. 20	0	128/86	9.9	3.200	288	305.000
Febr. 21	0	138/90	10.8	3.100	313	335.000
Febr. 22	0	132/94	9.6	3.400	272	312.000
Febr. 23	0	140/86	9.5	3.500	490	350.000
Febr. 27	0	174/112	11.0	5.900	2.880	390.000
March 5	0	190/114	10.5	7.900	4.800	—
March 19	0	190/118	11	7.900	6.320	360.000
April 23	0	186/114	12.8	8.400	4.530	—

* From [156].

This one patient [155] is thus of particular interest since to our knowledge she was the only case where no other drugs than captopril were administered, and where besides renovascular hypertension no other disease could be identified. The evolution of her blood pressure, haemoglobin values, white blood cell, neutrophil and platelet counts is summarized in Table 2. Co-culturing this patient's bone marrow with increasing captopril concentrations (up to 10^{-4} M) did not influence colony or cluster growth. During the neutropenic period she developed a serum-sickness-like syndrome, while also antinuclear antibodies, together with circulating immune complexes could transiently be demonstrated [156]. This case strongly suggests a direct causal relationship between captopril treatment and bone marrow suppression, though rechallenge in other patients with captopril-associated agranulocytosis, all with complex medical histories and on multiple drug therapy, has produced divergent results [142, 157–159].

The precise mechanism by which captopril or one of its metabolites may induce bone marrow suppression is not clear, but the cytotoxicity seems not to be primarily directed against circulating cells [140, 156], while a direct toxicity of captopril to bone marrow precursor cells could not be demonstrated either [156]. The associated serum-sickness-like syndrome in our patient [155] and the transient development of antinuclear antibodies together with circulating immune complexes strongly support an immunological mechanism. Recent reports on captopril-induced immune complex glomerulonephritis, also associated with positive antinuclear antibodies and a serum-sickness-like syndrome [161, 162]; the inhibition of bone marrow cultures with acute phase serum [140] and the immunosuppressive effect of long-term captopril treatment in hypertensive patients [163], have provided additional evidence for a captopril induced immunodysregulation. Eosinophilia has been reported in about one third of patients treated for one year [164].

The manufacturer now recommends to perform complete blood counts every two weeks for the first three months of captopril treatment and once a month thereafter. If, compared to the pretreatment value, the total leucocyte count decreases by 50% or more or, regardless of the pretreatment value, falls below 3500/mm^3 treatment should be discontinued.

6.4. Renal side-effects

Proteinuria can be demonstrated intermittently or continuously in about 2% of patients treated with captopril for 8 months or longer [40]. However, if patients with pre-existing renal disease are excluded, the incidence of proteinuria is less than 1% [150]. A reversible nephrotic syndrome may develop in some patients [165–167].

During long-term captopril treatment, proteinuria (protein excretion exceeding 200 mg/24 h) has been reported in 6 of 81 patients given captopril for at least 4 months [167]. In all these patients the increased protein excretion occurred by the fourth month of treatment. It subsided partially in 2 and completely in 2 patients despite continued therapy, while in 2 patients a nephrotic syndrome, associated with hypoalbuminaemia and hypercholesterolaemia persisted as long as captopril was given. Renal biopsy specimens in 2 patients showed mild membranous glomerulopathy. Also in another series [161, 162] histological findings indicated an early stage of membranous glomerulopathy in 4 of 13 patients, while in the other patients electron microscopy showed scanty, small subepithelial deposits and immunofluorescence revealed a patchy granular pattern along the glomerular basement membrane. From these observations it has been suggested that prolonged captopril therapy might be associated with the development of immune complex glomerulopathy. However, other investigators [168] could not confirm the occurrence of membranous glomerulonephritis in captopril-treated patients developing proteinuria. Nevertheless, they did find small dens deposits along the glomerular basement membranes, but in their opinion such lesions may also be encountered under a wide variety of conditions.

Reversible renal failure has been described in a few patients with pre-existing renal impairment [169, 170] or renal allografts [171, 172]. A transient rise of serum creatinine seems to occur more frequently [62, 84, 111] and may be caused by a decreased renal blood flow, resulting from the depressor response or by a direct nephrotoxic action.

Several investigators [63, 80, 111] have observed increases in the serum potassium level, serious life-threatening hyperkalaemia being reported once [170]. The increase in the serum potassium level is independently related to the changes of plasma aldosterone and serum creatinine and can therefore be explained by a decreased tubular action of the mineralcorticoid and variations in the kidney function [63].

6.5. Other adverse effects

Next to skin rash reversible loss of taste or taste disturbances are the most commonly observed side-effects occurring in 6–19% of captopril treated patients [40, 173]. Dysgeusia may subside spontaneously, even when treatment is continued. Zinc depletion in humans is commonly associated with decreased taste acuity: captopril binds to the zinc ions, that are present at the active centre of the converting enzyme and might be expected to reduce tissue zinc levels. However, the mechanism underlying the loss of taste remains unclear, since captopril does not decrease the plasma zinc concentration and zinc supplementation does not restore taste acuity [173].

Neurological dysfunction, Guillain Barré syndrome and sensimotor peripheral neuropathy have been reported in patients receiving captopril and cimetidine concurrently, but a causal relationship between these phenomena and either of the drugs or their combination is not established with certainty [174].

Captopril does not affect heart rate consistently, though in some studies slight increases of heart rate were reported and a few patients may even show tachycardia, especially when a diuretic is added [62, 134]. Also cardiac output may increase during converting enzyme inhibition. Both tachycardia and increased cardiac index may precipitate myocardial ischaemia in patients with coronary heart disease. Indeed, chest pain has been observed by ourselves and by others [120, 175] during captopril treatment, and myocardial infarction has occurred in some patients soon after initiation of therapy [175] or during prolonged captopril administration [134]. However, in most of these cases the causal relationship between ischaemic symptoms and converting enzyme inhibition is difficult to ascertain. Nevertheless, it may be advisable to associate a beta-adrenergic blocking agent to captopril given either alone or in combination with a diuretic; beta-adrenergic blocking drugs will moreover potentiate the hypotensive effect [134, 176].

There is no rebound hypertension on abrupt drug withdrawal [84].

IV. CONCLUSIONS

The converting enzyme inhibitors are a new and interesting group of antihypertensive agents. Captopril was the first orally active converting enzyme inhibitor to become available for treatment of hypertensive patients. This first compound has been used on a worldwide scale by many clinical investigators and its therapeutic efficacy in several forms of clinical hypertension is now well appreciated [40, 150, 177, 178]. The toxicity of this first molecule remains a serious problem, however. Side-effects, some of them life-threatening occur frequently. Using captopril routinely for the treatment of mild or moderate essential hypertension can therefore not be recommended. For the present captopril should be reserved for some cases of renovascular hypertension [117], for medical treatment of renin producing tumors [179] and for malignant or otherwise refractory hypertension.

Molecular manipulation has produced new compounds: if new molecules can be found which would have a lower toxicity and possibly an even greater therapeutic efficacy, converting enzyme inhibition may develop in the future to a new and exciting therapeutic approach of essential and some forms of secondary hypertension in man.

863

ACKNOWLEDGMENTS

The authors gratefully acknowledge the secretarial assistance of Ms L. Lommelen, Mrs M. Cober-Stinissen, Mrs K. Van Horenbeek-Byttebier and Mrs Y. Vanhulst-Toremans in the preparation of this manuscript.

Some of the studies referred to in this review were performed in our laboratory with the financial support of the belgian Research Institutes N.F.W.O. and I.W.O.N.L.

REFERENCES

1. Khosla MC, Smeby RR, Bumpus FM: Structure activity relationship in angiotensin II analogs. In: Angiotensin, p. 162. Berlin: Springer-Verlag, 1974.
2. Pals DT, Masucci FD, Denning GS, Sipos F, Fessler DC: Role of the pressor action of angiotensin II in experimental hypertension. Circ Res 29:673–681, 1971.
3. Bumpus FM, Khosla MC: Pathogenetic factors involved in renovascular hypertension. Mayo Clin Proc 52:417–423, 1977.
4. Hollenberg NK, Williams GH, Burger B, Ishikawa I, Adams DF: Blockade and stimulation of renal, adrenal and vascular angiotensin II receptors with 1-sar-8-ala-angiotensin II in normal man. J Clin Invest 57:39–46, 1976.
5. Fagard R, Amery A, Lijnen P, Reybrouck T, Joossens JV, Billiet L, Moerman E, De Schaepdryver A: Effects of 1-sar-8-ala-angiotensin II on systemic and pulmonary haemodynamics in hypertensive patients. Clin Exp Pharmacol Physiol 5:457–464, 1978.
6. Fagard R, Lijnen P, Amery A, Reybrouck T: Effects of 1-sar-8-ala-angiotensin II on arterial pressure, renin and aldosterone in hypertension. Contr Nephrol 11:175–178, 1978.
7. Castellion AW, Fulton RW: Preclinical pharmacology of saralasin. Kidney Int 15:511–519, 1979.
8. Fagard R, Amery A, Timmermans U: Severe hypotension during infusion of saralasin. Lancet i:1136, 1978.
9. Horne ML, Conklin VM, Keenan RE, Varady PD, Dinaro J: Angiotensin II profiling with saralasin: summary of Eaton Collaborative Study. Kidney Int 15:S115–S122, 1979.
10. Posternak L, Brunner HR, Gavras H, Brunner DB: Angiotensin II blockade in normal man: interaction of renin and sodium in maintaining blood pressure. Kidney Int 11: 197–203, 1977.
11. McGregor GA, Dawes PM: Agonist and antagonist effects of Sar[1]-ala[8]-angiotensin II in salt-loaded and salt-depleted normal man. Br J Clin Pharmacol 3:483–487, 1976.
12. Mulrow PJ, Noth R: The role of renin in the control of blood pressure in normotensive man. Progr Biochem Pharmacol 12:163–169, 1976.
13. Fagard R, Amery A, Reybrouck T, Lijnen P, Moerman E, Bogaert M, De Schaepdryver A: Effects of angiotensin antagonism on hemodynamics, renin and catecholamines during exercise. J Appl Physiol 43:440–444, 1977.
14. Fagard R, Amery A, Reybrouck T, Lijnen P, Billiet L, Bogaert M, Moerman E, De Schaepdryver A: Effects of angiotensin antagonism at rest and during exercise in sodium-deplete man. J Appl Physiol 45:403–407, 1978.
15. Brunner HR, Gavras H, Laragh JH, Keenan R: Hypertension in man, exposure of the renin and sodium components using angiotensin II blockade. Circ Res 34 (Suppl 1):35–43, 1974.
16. Streeten DHP, Anderson GH: Outpatient experience with saralasin. Kidney Int 15:S44–S52, 1979.

17. Baer L, Parra-Carillo JZ, Radichevich I: Angiotensin II blockade: evidence for baroreceptor mediated renin release and the role of sodium balance. Kidney Int 15:S60–S67, 1979.

18. Marks LS, Maxwell MH, Kaufman JJ: Renin, Sodium, and vasodepressor response to saralasin in renovascular and essential hypertension. Ann Intern Med 87:176–182, 1977.

19. Fagard R, Amery A, Lijnen P, Reybrouck T: Effects of angiotensin II antagonist 1-sar-8-ala-angiotensin II in hypertension in man. Eur J Clin Invest 7:473–479, 1977.

20. Thananopavarn C, Golub MS, Eggena P, Barrett JD, Sambhi MP: Angiotensin II, Plasma renin and sodium depletion as determinants of blood pressure response to saralasin in essential hypertension. Circulation 61:920–924, 1980.

21. Romero JC, Holmes DR, Strong CG: The effect of high sodium intake and angiotensin antagonist in rabbits with severe and moderate hypertension induced by constriction of one renal artery. Circ Res 40 (Suppl 1):17–23, 1977.

22. Case DB, Wallace JM, Keim HJ, Sealy JE, Laragh JH: Usefulness and limitations of saralasin, a partial competitive agonist of angiotensin II, for evaluating the renin and sodium factors in hypertensive patients. Am J Med 60:825–836, 1976.

23. Gavras H, Ribeiro AB, Gavras I, Brunner HR: Reciprocal relation between renin dependency and sodium dependency in essential hypertension. N Engl J Med 295:1278–1283, 1976.

24. Fagard R, Amery AK, Lijnen PJ, Reybrouck TM: Comparative study of an angiotensin II analog and a converting enzyme inhibitor. Kidney Int 17:647–653, 1980.

25. Krakoff LR, Ribeiro AB, Gorkin JU, Felton KR: Saralasin infusion in screening patients for renovascular hypertension. Am J Cardiol 45:609–613, 1980.

26. Streeten DHP, Anderson GH, Dalakos TG: Angiotensin blockade: its clinical significance. Am J Med 60:817–824, 1976.

27. Kreft C, Menard J, Corvol P: Value of renin measurements, saralasin test and acebutolol treatment in hypertension. Kidney Int 15:176–183, 1979.

28. Ferreira SH: A bradykinin-potentiating factor (BPF) present in the venom of Bothrops Jararaca. Br J Pharmacol 24:163–169, 1965.

29. Ondetti MA, Rubin B, Cushman DW: Design of specific inhibitors of angiotensin converting-enzyme: new class of orally active antihypertensive agents. Science 196:441–444,1977.

30. Rubin B, Laffan RJ, Kotler DG, O'Keefe EH, Demaio DA, Goldberg ME: SQ 14,225 (D-3-mercapto-2-methylpropanoyl-L-proline), a novel orally active inhibitor of angiotensin I converting enzyme. J Pharmacol Exp Ther 204:271–280, 1978.

31. Ferguson RK, Brunner HR, Turini GA, Gavras H: A specific orally active inhibitor of angiotensin-converting enzyme in man. Lancet i:775–778, 1977.

32. Patchett AA, Haris E, Tristram EW, Wyvratt MJ, Wu MT, Taub D, Peterson ER, Ikeler TJ, ten Broeke J, Payne LG, Ondeyka DL, Thorsett ED, Greenlee WJ, Lohr NS, Hoffsommer RD, Joshua H, Ruyle WV, Rothrock JW, Aster SD, Maycock AL, Robinson FM, Hirschmann R, Sweet CS, Ulm EH, Gross DM, Vassil TC, Stone CA: A new class of angiotensin converting enzyme inhibitors. Nature 288:280–283, 1980.

33. Weare JA, Stewart TA, Gafford JT, Erdös EG: Inhibition of human converting-enzyme in vitro by a novel tripeptide analog. Hypertension 3 (Suppl I):I 50–I 53, 1981.

34. Burnier M, Turini GA, Porchet M, Brunner DB, Blasucci D, Vukovich RA, Nics ES, Gavras H, Brunner HR: RHC 3659: a new converting enzyme inhibitor administered orally to healthy volunteers. International symposium on angiotensin-converting enzyme inhibition: a developing therapeutic concept. Milan, 1981.

35. Gavras H, Biollaz J, Waeber B, Brunner HR, Gavras I, Davies RO: Antihypertensive effect of the new oral angiotensin-converting enzyme inhibitor 'MK-421'. Lancet ii:543–547, 1981.

36. Takata Y, DiNicolantonio R, Hutchinson JS, Mendelsohn FAO: An in vivo comparison of the biological activity of three orally active inhibitors of angiotensin converting enzyme. International symposium on angiotensin-converting enzyme inhibition: a developing therapeutic concept. Milan, 1981.

37. Kripalani KJ, McKinstry DN, Singhvi SM, Willard DA, Vukovich RA, Migdalof BM: Disposition of captopril in normal subjects. Clin Pharmacol Ther 27:636–641, 1980.

38. McKinstry DN, Singhvi SM, Kripalani KJ, Dreyfuss J, Willard DA, Vukovich RA: Disposition and cardiovascular-endocrine effects of an orally active angiotensin-converting enzyme inhibitor, SQ 14,225, in normal subjects. Clin Pharmacol Ther 23:121–122, 1978.

39. Devlin RG, Fleiss PM: Selective resistance to the passage of captopril into human milk. Clin Pharmacol Ther 27:250, 1980.

40. Heel RC, Brogden RN, Speight TM, Avery GS: Captopril: a preliminary review of its pharmacological properties and therapeutic efficacy. Drugs 20:409–452, 1980.

41. Dean AV, Kripalani KJ, Migdalof BH: Disposition of captopril (SQ 14,225) in spontaneously hypertensive and normotensive rats. Fed Proc 38:743, 1979.

42. Kripalani KJ, Meeker FS, Dean AV, McKinstry DN, Migdalof BH: Biotransformation of ^{14}C-captopril in hypertensive patients and normal subjects. Fed Proc 39:307, 1980.

43. Rommel AJ, Pierides AM, Heald A: Captopril elimination in chronic renal failure. Clin Pharmacol Ther 27:282, 1980.

44. Fagard R, Lijnen P, Vanhees L, Amery A: Responses of the systemic circulation and of the renin–angiotensin system to converting enzyme inhibition at rest and during exercise in normal man: effects on maximal exercise capacity. (Submitted for publication.)

45. Swartz SL, Williams GH, Hollenberg NK, Crantz FR, Levine L, Moore TJ, Dluhy RG: Increase in prostaglandins during converting-enzyme inhibition. Clin Sci 59:133S–135S, 1980.

46. Sancho J, Re R, Burton J, Barger AC, Haber E: The role of the renin–angiotensin system in cardiovascular homeostasis in normal human subjects. Circulation 53:400–405, 1976.

47. Fagard R, Bulpitt C, Lijnen P, Amery A: Response of the systemic and pulmonary circulation to converting enzyme inhibition (captopril) at rest and during exercise in hypertensive patients. Circulation 65:33–39, 1982.

48. Niarchos AP, Pickering TG, Case DB, Sullivan P, Laragh JH: Role of the renin–angiotensin system in blood pressure regulation: the cardiovascular effects of converting enzyme inhibition in normotensive subjects. Circ Research 45:829–837, 1979.

49. Fagard R, Amery A, Lijnen P, Reybrouck T: Haemodynamic effects of captopril in hypertensive patients: comparison with saralasin. Clin Sci 57:131S–134S, 1979.

50. Fagard R, Amery A, Reybrouck T, Lijnen P, Billiet L: Acute and chronic systemic and pulmonary hemodynamic effects of angiotensin-converting enzyme inhibition with captopril in hypertensive patients. Am J Cardiol 46:295–300, 1980.

51. Cody RJ, Tarazi RC, Bravo EL, Fouad FM: Haemodynamics of orally-active converting enzyme inhibitor (SQ 14,225) in hypertensive patients. Clin Sci Mol Med 55:453–459, 1978.

52. Fouad FM, Ceimo JMK, Tarazi RC, Bravo EL: Contrasts and similarities of acute hemodynamic responses to specific antagonism of angiotensin II (sar[1] thr[8] A II) and to inhibition of converting enzyme (captopril). Circulation 61:163–169, 1980.

53. Tarazi RC, Bravo EL, Fouad FM, Omvit P, Cody RJ: Hemodynamic and volume changes associated with captopril. Hypertension 2:576–585, 1980.

54. Niarchos AP, Roberts AJ, Case DB, Gay WA, Laragh JH: Hemodynamic characteristics of hypertension after coronary bypass surgery and effects of converting enzyme inhibitor. Am J Cardiol. 43:586–593, 1979.

55. Niarchos AP, Roberts JA, Laragh JH: Effects of the converting enzyme inhibitor (SQ 20881, teprotide) on the pulmonary circulation in man. Am J Med 67:785–791, 1979.

866

56. Bunag RD: Circulatory effects of angiotensin. In: Angiotensin. Page IH, Bumpus FM, eds. Berlin: Springer-Verlag, 1974.
57. Borucki LJ, Levenson D, Hollenberg NK: Cardiovascular responses to blockade of angiotensin and alpha-adrenergic receptors. Am J Physiol 235:F199–F202, 1978.
58. Coleman TG, Cowley AW, Guyton AC: Angiotensin and the hemodynamics of chronic salt deprivation. Am J Physiol 229:167–171, 1975.
59. Bravo EL, Tarazi RG, Fouad FN: Hemodynamic effects of long-term captopril therapy in hypertensive man. In: Angiotensin Converting Enzyme Inhibitors: Mechanisms of Action and Clinical Implications, pp. 263–272. Horovitz ZP, ed. Baltimore: Urban & Schwarzenberg, 1981.
60. Sullivan JM, Ginsburg BA, Ratts TE, Johnson JG, Barton BR, Kraus DH, McKinstry DN, Muirhead EE: Hemodynamic and antihypertensive effects of captopril an orally active angiotensin converting enzyme inhibitor. Hypertension 1:397–401, 1979.
61. Fagard R, Amery A, Lijnen P, Staessen J: First dose effect of the oral angiotensin converting enzyme inhibitor captopril. Arch Intern Pharmacodyn Ther (Suppl) Symposium: Clinical Pharmacology of Antihypertensive Agents, pp. 178–187, 1980.
62. Atkinson AB, Brown JJ, Fraser R, Leckie B, Lever AF, Morton JJ, Robertson JIS: Captopril in hypertension with renal artery stenosis and in intractable hypertension; acute and chronic changes in circulating concentrations of renin, angiotensin I and II and aldosterone, and in body composition. Clin Sci 57:139S–143S, 1979.
63. Lijnen P, Fagard R, Staessen J, Verschueren LJ, Amery A: Dose response in captopril therapy of hypertension. Clin Pharmacol Ther 28:310–315, 1980.
64. Fagard R, Amery A, Lijnen P: Angiotensin II and not sodium status in the major determinant of the agonistic/antagonistic balance of saralasine's actions. Clin Sci 59:75S–78S, 1980.
65. Swartz SL, Williams GH, Hollenberg NK, Moore TJ, Dluhy RG: Converting enzyme inhibition in essential hypertension: the hypotensive response does not reflect only reduced angiotensin II formation. Hypertension 1:106–111, 1979.
66. Hutchinson JS, Mendelsohn FAO, Doyle AE: Hypotensive action of captopril and saralasin in intact and anephric spontaneously hypertensive rats. Hypertension 2:119–124, 1980.
67. Vollmer RR, Boccagno JA, Harris DN, Murthy VS: Hypotension induced by inhibition of angiotensin converting enzyme in pentobarbital-anesthetized dogs. Eur J Pharmacol 51:39–45, 1978.
68. Man in 't Veld AJ, Wenting GJ, Schalekamp MADH: Does captopril lower blood pressure in anephric patients. Br Med J 2:1110, 1979.
69. Man in 't Veld AJ, Schicht IM, Derkx FM, de Bruyn JHB, Schalekamp MADH: Effects of an angiotensin-converting enzyme inhibitor (captopril) on blood pressure in anephric subjects. Br Med J 1:288–290, 1980.
70. Leslie BR, Case DB, Sullivan JF, Vaughan ED: Absence of blood pressure lowering effect of captopril in anephric patients. Br Med J 280:1067–1068, 1980.
71. Ganten D, Hutchinson JS, Schelling P: The intrinsic brain iso-renin–angiotensin system in the rat: its possible role in central mechanisms of blood pressure regulation. Clin Sci Mol Med 48:265s–268s, 1975.
72. Thurston H, Swales JD: Blood pressure response of nephrectomized hypertensive rats to converting enzyme inhibition: evidence for persistent vascular renin activity. Clin Sci Mol Med 52:299–304, 1977.
73. Leckie B, Gavras H, McGregor J, McElwee G: The conversion of angiotensin I to angiotensin II by rabbit glomeruli. J Endocrinol 55:229–230, 1972.
74. Vollmer RR, Boccagno JA: Central cardiovascular effects of SQ 14,225, an angiotensin-converting enzyme inhibitor in chloralose-anesthetized cats. Eur J Pharmacol 45:117–125, 1977.

75. Mann JFE, Rascher W, Dietz R, Schömig A, Ganten D: Effects of an orally active converting enzyme inhibitor, SQ 14225 on pressor responses to angiotensin administered into the brain ventricles of spontaneously hypertensive rats. Cli Sci 56:585–589, 1979.
76. Unger T, Rockhold RW, Kaufmann-Bühler I, Hübner D, Schüll B, Speck G, Ganten D: Effects of angiotensin converting enzyme inhibitors on the brain. In: Angiotensin Converting Enzyme Inhibitors: Mechanisms of Action and Clinical Implications. Horovitz ZP, ed. Baltimore: Urban & Schwarzenberg, 1981.
77. Hollenberg NK, Swartz SL, Passan DR, Williams GH: Increased glomerular filtration rate after converting enzyme inhibition in essential hypertension. N Engl J Med 301:9–12, 1979.
78. Brunner HR, Gavras H, Waeber B, Kershaw GR, Turini GA, Vukovich RA, McKinstry DN, Gavras I: Oral angiotensin-converting enzyme inhibitor in long-term treatment of hypertensive patients. Ann Intern Med 90:19–23, 1979.
79. Case DB, Atlas SA, Laragh JH, Sealey JE, Sullivan PA,McKinstry DN: Clinical experience with blockade of the renin–angiotensin–aldosterone system by an oral converting-enzyme inhibitor (SQ 14,225, captopril) in hypertensive patients. Progr Cardiovas Dis 21:195–206, 1978.
80. Atlas SA, Case DB, Sealey JE, Laragh JH, McKinstry DN: Interruption of the renin-angiotensin system in hypertensive patients by captopril induces sustained reduction in aldosterone secretion, potassium retention and natriuresis. Hypertension 1:274–280, 1979.
81. Staessen J, Lijnen P, Fagard R, Verschueren LJ, Amery A: Rise of plasma aldosterone during long-term captopril treatment. N Engl J Med 304:1110, 1981.
82. Staessen J, Lijnen P, Fagard R, Verschueren LJ, Amery A: Rise of plasma aldosterone during long-term angiotensin II suppression. J Endocrinol 91:457–465, 1981.
83. Gavras H, Gavras I, Textor S, Volicer L, Brunner HR, Rucinska EJ: Effect of angiotensin converting enzyme inhibition on blood pressure, plasma renin activity and plasma aldosterone in essential hypertension. J Clin Endocrin Metabol 46:220–226, 1978.
84. Bravo EL, Tarazi RC: Converting enzyme inhibition with an orally active compound in hypertensive man. Hypertension 1:39–46, 1979.
85. Johns DW, Baker KM, Ayers CR, Vaughan ED, Carey RM, Peach MJ, Yancey MR, Ortt EM, Williams SC: Acute and chronic effect of captopril in hypertensive patients. Hypertension 2:567–575, 1980.
86. Rubin B, Laffan RJ, Kotler DG, O'Keefe EH, Demaio DA, Goldberg ME: SQ 14,225 (D-3-mercapto-2-methylpropranoyl-L-proline), a novel orally active inhibitor of angiotensin-I converting enzyme. J Pharmacol Exp Ther 204:271–280, 1978.
87. Harris DN, Heran CL, Goldenberg HJ, High JP, Laffan RJ, Rubin B, Antonaccio MJ, Goldberg ME: Effects of SQ 14,225, an orally active inhibitor of angiotensin-converting enzyme on blood pressure heart rate and plasma renin activity of conscious normotensive dogs. Eur J Pharmacol 51:345–349, 1978.
88. Cushman DW, Ondetti MA, Cheung MJ, Antonaccio MJ, Murthy VS, Rubin B: Inhibitors of angiotensin-converting enzyme. In: The renin-angiotensin system. Johnson JA, Anderson RR, eds. Plenum Publishing Corp, New York, 1980.
89. Lijnen P, Verschueren LJ, Fagard R, Staessen J, Amery A: Acute changes in the renin-angiotensin-aldosterone system, catecholamines and prostaglandines during captopril in man. Methods Find Exp Pharmacol 2:293–301, 1980.
90. Donker JM, Prins EJL, Hoorntje SJ: The responsiveness to exogenous angiotensin I (A I), angiotensin II (A II) and bradykinin (BK) after incremental doses of captopril (SQ 14,225). Kidney Int 16: 904, 1979.
91. Antonaccho MJ, Rubin B, Horovitz ZP: Effects of captopril in animal models of hypertension. Clin Exp Hyp 2:613–637, 1980.

868

92. Millar JA, Johnston CI: Sequential changes in circulating levels of angiotensin I and II, renin and bradykinin after captopril. Med J Austr 2 (Suppl 8):15–17, 1979.
93. Vinci JM, Horwitz D, Zusman RM, Pisano JJ, Catt JJ, Keiser HR: The effect of converting enzyme inhibition with SQ 20881 on plasma and urinary kinins, prostaglandin E_1 and angiotensin II in hypertensive man. Hypertension 1:416–426, 1979.
94. Johnston CI, Millar JA, McGrath BP, Matthews PG: Long-term effects of captopril (SQ 14,225) on blood pressure and hormone levels in essential hypertension. Lancet ii:493–496, 1979.
95. Mersey JH, Williams GH, Hollenberg NK, Dluhy RG: Relationship between aldosterone and bradykinin. Circ Res 40 (Suppl 1):i-84–i-88, 1977.
96. Williams GH, Hollenberg NK: Accentuated vascular and endocrine response to SQ 20881 in hypertension. N Engl J Med 297:184–188, 1977.
97. Anderson GH, Springer J, Tivnan E, Kearney M, Streeten DHP: Hypotensive mechanism of captopril. Clin Research 28:328A, 1980.
98. Moore TJ, Crantz FR, Hollenberg NK, Koletsky RJ, Leboff MS, Swartz SL, Levine L, Podolsky S, Dluhy RG, Williams GH: Contribution of prostaglandins to the antihypertensive action of captopril in essential hypertension. Hypertension 3:168–173, 1981.
99. Mimran A, Targhetta R, Laroche B: The antihypertensive effect of captopril: evidence for an influence of kinins. Hypertension 2:732–737, 1980.
100. McCaa RE, Hall JE, McCaa CS: The effects of angiotensin I converting enzyme inhibitors on arterial blood pressure and urinary sodium excretion. Role of the renal renin–angiotensin and kallikrein–kinin systems. Circ Research 43 (Suppl I):32–39, 1978.
101. Karlberg BE, Ohman KP, Nilsson OR, Wettre S: Captopril lowers urinary kallikrein in hypertensive patients. Lancet i:150–151, 1980.
102. Cunningham RJ, Brouhard BH: Captopril and kallikrein. Lancet I:832, 1980.
103. Marin-Grez M, Bonner G, Gross F: Captopril, kallikrein and hypertension. Lancet i:1033, 1980.
104. Murthy VS, Waldron TL, Goldberg ME: The mechanism of bradykinin potentiation after inhibition of angiotensin converting-enzyme by SQ 14,225 in conscious rabbits. Circ Res 43 (Suppl I):i-40–i-45, 1978.
105. Abe K, Itoh T, Imai Y, Sato M, Haruyama T, Sakurai Y, Goto T, Otsuka Y, Yoshinaga K: Implication of endogenous prostaglandin system in the antihypertensive effect of captopril, SQ 14,225, in low renin hypertension. Jpn Circ J 44:422–425, 1980.
106. Swartz SL, Williams GH, Hollenberg NK, Levine L, Dluhy RG, Moore TJ: Captopril induced changes in prostaglandin production: relationship to vascular responses in normal man. J Clin Invest 65:1257–1264, 1980.
107. Luderer JR, Schneck DW, Demers LM, McKinstry DN, Vary JE, Hayes AH: The humoral effects of captopril and furosemide in hypertensive patients. Clin Pharmacol Ther 27:268, 1980.
108. Abe K, Sato M, Haruyama T, Sato K, Hiwatari M, Tajima J, Miyazaki S, Yoshinaga K: Interaction of prostaglandin (PG) and renin-angiotensin (R-A) in regulation of blood pressure (BP): different pathogenesis of hypertension (HT) in low- and in high-normal renin HT. International symposium on angiotensin converting enzyme inhibition: a developing therapeutic concept. Milan, 1981.
109. Lijnen P, Fagard R, Staessen J, Verschueren LJ, Amery A: Role of various vasodepressor systems in the acute hypotensive effect of captopril in man. Eur J Clin Pharmacol 20:1–8, 1981.
110. Turini GA, Brunner HR, Gribic M, Waeber B, Gavras H: Improvement of chronic congestive heart failure by oral captopril. Lancet i:1213–1216, 1979.
111. Gavras H, Brunner HR, Turini GA, Kershaw GR, Tifft CP, Cuttelod S, Gavras I, Vukovich RA, McKinstry DN: Anti-hypertensive effect of the oral angiotensin converting-enzyme inhibitor SQ 14225 in man. N Engl J Med 298:991–995, 1978.

112. Maruyama A, Ogihara T, Naka T, Mikami H, Hata T, Nakamura M, Iwanaga K, Kumahara Y: Long-term effects of captopril in hypertension. Clin Pharmacol Ther 28:316–323, 1980.
113. Saragoca M, Tarazi RC, Bravo EL, Fouad FM: Contrast between acute and longer term responses to oral converting enzyme inhibitor (CEI). Clin Research 27:317A, 1979.
114. Weinberger MH: Angiotensin converting enzyme inhibition (ACEI) in treatment of resistant hypertension. Clin Pharmacol Ther 27:293, 1980.
115. Case DB, Atlas SA, Laragh JH, Sullivan PA, Sealey JE: Use of first-dose response or plasma renin activity to predict the long-term effect of captopril. Identification of triphasic pattern of blood pressure response. J Cardiovasc Pharmacol 2:339–346, 1980.
116. Laragh JH, Case DB, Atlas SA, Sealey JE: Captopril compared with other antirenin system agents in hypertensive patients: its triphasic effects on blood pressure and its use to identify and treat the renin factor. Hypertension 2:586–593, 1980.
117. Atkinson AB, Brown JJ, Davies DL, Fraser R, Leckie B, Lever AF, Morton JJ, Robertson JIS: Hyponatraemic hypertensive syndrome with renal artery occlusion corrected by captopril. Lancet ii:606–609, 1979.
118. Atkinson AB, Brown JJ, Davies DL, Leckie B, Lever AF, Morton JJ, Robertson JIS: Renal artery stenosis with normal angiotensin II values: relationship between angiotensin II and body sodium and potassium on correction of hypertension by captopril and subsequent surgery. Hypertension 3:53–58, 1981.
119. Staessen J, Fagard R, Lijnen P, Amery A: Comparison of converting enzyme inhibition with surgery in renovascular hypertension. (Submitted for publication.)
120. Larochelle P, Genest J, Kuchel O, Boucher R, Gutkowska Y, McKinstry D: Effect of captopril (SQ 14225) on blood pressure, plasma renin activity and angiotensin I converting enzyme activity. Can Med Assoc J 121:309–316, 1979.
121. Mac Gregor GA, Markandu ND, Roulston JE, Jones JC: Essential hypertension: effect of an oral inhibitor of angiotensin converting enzyme. Br Med J 2:1106–1109, 1979.
122. Alexander JC, Meyer JH: Comparison of captopril with placebo in the treatment of essential hypertension. In: Angiotensin Converting enzyme Inhibitors: Mechanisms of action and Clinical Implications, pp. 379–392. Horovitz ZP, ed. Baltimore: Urban & Schwarzenberg, 1981.
123. Brunner HR, Gavras H, Waeber B, Turini GA, McKinstry DN, Vukovich RA, Gavras I: Orally active angiotensin converting enzyme inhibitor (SQ 14225) as a treatment for essential hypertension. Br J Clin Pharmacol 7 (Suppl 2):2059–2119, 1979.
124. Jenkins AC, McKinstry DN: Review of clinical studies of hypertensive patients treated with captopril. Med J Austr 2 (Suppl 8):32–37, 1979.
125. McNeil JJ, Anderson A, Christophidis N, Mendelsohn FAO, Coghlan J, Louis WJ: Comparison of captopril and hydrochlorothiazide in the treatment of moderate hypertension. Med J Austr 2(Suppl 8):22–24, 1979.
126. Sharpe DN: Comparison of captopril (SQ 14225) with hydrochlorothiazide in the treatment of mild and moderate essential hypertension. Med J Aust 2 (Suppl 8):24–26, 1979.
127. Friedlander DH: Comparison of captopril with propranolol in the treatment of essential hypertension. Med J Austr 2 (Suppl 8):30–32, 1979.
128. Seedat YK: Comparison of captopril with propranolol in the treatment of mild and moderate essential hypertension. S Afr Med J 56:983–986, 1979.
129. Whitworth JA, Walter NMA, Kincaid-Smith P: Clinical trial of an orally administered converting-enzyme inhibitor (captopril). Med J Austr 2 (Suppl 8):27–30, 1979.
130. Atkinson AB, Brown JJ, Lever AF, Robertson JIS: Combined treatment of severe intractable hypertension with captopril and diuretic. Lancet ii:105–108, 1980.
131. White NJ, Rajagopalan B, Yahaya H, Ledingham JGG: Captopril and furesemide in severe drug-resistant hypertension. Lancet ii:108–110, 1980.

870

132. Staessen J, Fagard R, Lijnen P, Verschueren LJ, Amery A: Beta-blockade during captopril treatment for hypertension. N Engl J Med 303:1121-1122, 1980.
133. Staessen J, Fagard R, Lijnen P, Verschueren LJ, Amery A: The hypotensive effect of propranolol in captopril-treated patients does not involve the plasma renin–angiotensin-aldosterone system. Clin Sci 61:441s-445s, 1981.
134. Ferguson RK, Vlasses PH, Koplin JR, Shirinian A, Burke JF, Alexander JC: Captopril in severe treatment-resistant hypertension. Am Heart J 99:579-585, 1980.
135. McCaa CS, Langford HG, Cushman WC, McCaa RE: Response of arterial blood pressure and aldosterone to long-term administration of captopril in patients with severe, treatment-resistant accelerated hypertension. Clin Sci 57 (Suppl 5):371S-373S, 1979.
136. Zweifler AJ, Julius S, Nicholls MG: Efficacy of an oral angiotensin converting enzyme inhibitor (captopril) in severe hypertension. Arch Intern Med 141:907-910, 1981.
137. Case DB, Atlas SA, Sullivan P, Laragh JH: Successful acute and chronic treatment of severe and malignant hypertension with oral converting enzyme inhibitor captopril. Circulation 59-60 (Suppl 2):130, 1979.
138. Vaughan ED, Carey RM, Ayers CR, Peach MJ: Hemodialysisresistant hypertension: control with an orally active inhibitor of angiotensin-converting enzyme. J Clin Endocrin Metabol 48:869-871, 1979.
139. McCredie DA, Powell HR: Use of a converting-enzyme inhibitor in severe hypertension of end-stage renal function. Austr NZ J Med 10:123, 1980.
140. Van Brummelen P, Willemze R, Tan WD, Thompson J: Captopril-associated agranulocytosis. Lancet I:150, 1980.
141. Amann FW, Buhler FR, Conen D, Brunner F, Ritz R, Speck B: Captopril-associated agranulocytosis. Lancet I:150, 1980.
142. Case DB, Whitman HH, Laragh JH, Spiera H: Successful low-dose captopril rechallenge following drug-induced leucopenia. Lancet i:1362-1363, 1981.
143. Lopez-Ovejero JA, Saal SD, D'Angelo WA, Cheigh JS, Stenzel KH, Laragh JH: Reversal of vascular and renal crises of scleroderma by oral angiotensin converting enzyme blockade. N Engl J Med 300:1417-1419, 1979.
144. Zawada ET, Clements PJ, Furst DA, Bloomer HA, Paulus HE, Maxwell MH: Clinical course of patients with scleroderma renal crisis (src) treated with captopril (c) Kidney Int 16:910, 1979.
145. Brunner HR, Gavras H, Waeber B, Textor SC, Turini GA, Wauters JP: Clinical use of an orally acting converting enzyme inhibitor: captopril. Hypertension 2:558-566, 1980.
146. Waeber B, Brunner HR, Brunner DB, Curtet AL, Turini GA, Gavras H: Discrepancy between antihypertensive effect and angiotensin converting enzyme inhibition by captopril. Hypertension 2:236-242, 1980.
147. Staessen J, Fagard R, Lijnen P, Verschueren LJ, Amery A: Fluctuations in the plasma angiotensin I converting enzyme activity during long-term treatment with captopril. Acta Cardiol, 1981. (In press.)
148. Niarchos AP, Pickering TG, Case DB, Sullivan P, Laragh JH: Role of the renin–angiotensin system in blood pressure regulation. The cardiovascular effects of converting enzyme inhibition in normotensive subjects. Circ Res 45:829-837, 1979.
149. Wilkin JK, Hammond JJ, Kirkendall WM: The captopril-induced eruption. Arch Dermatol 116:902-905, 1980.
150. Editorial. Captopril: Benefits and risks in severe hypertension. Lancet ii:129-130, 1980.
151. Parfrey PS, Clement M, Vandenburg MJ, Wright P: Captopril-induced pemphigus. Br Med J 281:194, 1980.
152. Nicholls MG, Maslowski AH, Ikram HI, Espiner EA: Ulceration of the tongue: a complication of captopril therapy. Ann Intern Med 94:659, 1981.
153. Seedat YK: Apthous Ulcers of mouth from captopril. Lancet ii:1297-1298, 1979.

154. Elijovich f, Krakoff LR: Captopril associated granulocytopenia in hypertension after renal transplantation. Lancet I:1927, 1980.
155. Staessen J, Fagard R, Lijnen P, Amery A: Captopril and agranulocytosis. Lancet i:926–927, 1980.
156. Staessen J, Bogaerts M, Fagard R, Amery A: Mechanism of captopril-induced agranulocytosis. Acta Clin Belg 36:87–90, 1981.
157. Forslund T, Borgmästers H, Fyhrquist F: Captopril-associated leucopenia confirmed by rechallenge in patient with renal failure. Lancet i:166, 1981.
158. Edwards CRW, Drury P, Penketh A, Damluji SA: Successful reintroduction of captopril following neutropenia. Lancet i:723, 1981.
159. Kirchertz EJ, Gröne HJ, Rieger J, Hölcher M, Scheler F: Successful low dose captopril rechallenge following drug-induced leucopenia. Lancet i:1363, 1981.
160. Gavras I, Graff LG, Rose BD, McKenna JM, Brunner HR, Gavras H: Fatal pancytopenia associated with the use of captopril. Ann Intern Med 94:58–59, 1981.
161. Hoorntje SJ, Weening JJ, Kallenberg CGM, Prins EJL, Donker AJM: Serum-sickness-like syndrome with membranous glomerulopathy in patient on captopril. Lancet ii:1297, 1979.
162. Hoorntje SJ, Weening JJ, The TH, Kallenberg CGM, Donker AJM, Hoedemacker PJ: Immune-complex glomerulopathy in patients treated with captopril. Lancet i:1212–1215, 1980.
163. Kallenberg CGM, Van Der Laan S, De Zeeuw D: Captopril and the immune system. Lancet ii:92, 1981.
164. Kayanakis JG, Giraud P, Fauvel JM, Bounhoure JP: Eosinophilia during captopril treatment. Lancet ii:923, 1980.
165. Prins EJL, Hoorntje SL, Weening JJ, Donker AJM: Nephrotic syndrome in patient on captopril. Lancet ii:306–307, 1979.
166. Seedat YK: Nephrotic syndrome from captopril. S Afr Med J 57:390, 1980.
167. Case DB, Atlas SA, Mourandian JA, Fishman RA, Sherman RL, Laragh JH: Proteinuria during long-term captopril therapy. JAMA 244:346–349, 1980.
168. Kincaid-Smith P, Whitworth JA, Walter NMA, Dowling JP: Immune complex glomerulopathy and captopril. Lancet ii:37, 1980.
169. Woodhouse K, Farrow PR, Wilkinson R: Reversible renal failure during treatment with captopril. Br Med J 2:1146–1147, 1979.
170. Grossman A, Eckland D, Price P, Edwards CRW: Captopril: reversible renal failure with severe hyperkalaemia. Lancet i:712, 1980.
171. Collste P, Haglund K, Lundgren G, Magnusson G, Ostman J: Reversible renal failure during treatment with captopril. Br Med J 2:612–613, 1979.
172. Farrow PR, Wilkinson R: Reversible renal failure during treatment with captopril. Br Med J 1:1680, 1979.
173. McNeil JJ, Anderson A, Christophidis N, Jarrott B, Louis WJ: Taste loss associated with oral captopril treatment. Br Med J ii:1555–1556, 1979.
174. Atkinson AB, Brownn JJ, Lever AF, McAreavey D, Robertson JIS, Behan PO, Melville ID, Weir AI: Neurological dysfunction in two patients receiving captopril and cimetidine. Lancet ii:36–37, 1980.
175. Baker KM, Johns DW, Ayers CR, Carey RM: Ischemic cardiovascular complications concurrent with administration of captopril. A clinical note. Hypertension 2:73–74, 1980.
176. Staessen J, Fagard R, Lijnen P, Amery A: Double-blind comparison between propranolol and bendrofluazide in captopril-treated resistant hypertensive patients. (Submitted for publication.)
177. Editorial: Inhibitors of angiotensin I converting enzyme for treating hypertension. Br Med J 281:630–631, 1980.

872

178. Atkinson AB, Robertson JIS: Captopril in the treatment of clinical hypertension and cardiac failure. Lancet ii:836–839, 1979.
179. Aurell M, Rudin A, Tisell LE, Kindblom LG, Sandberg G: Captopril effect on hypertension in patient with renin- producing tumour. Lancet ii:149–150, 1979.

54. GENERAL STRATEGY OF ANTIHYPERTENSIVE TREATMENT

F. Olaf Simpson

The general strategy of antihypertensive treatment has to be considered under two headings. Firstly, there is the strategy for dealing with hypertension as a national problem, i.e. on a population basis, and secondly the strategy for dealing with hypertension in the individual patient.

1. STRATEGY FOR THE TREATMENT OF HYPERTENSION ON A NATIONAL SCALE

1.1. Past developments

It cannot be said that the development of antihypertensive treatment has proceeded with any coherent plan. However, this was hardly to be expected, as it has never been possible accurately to predict what drugs will be available in the future. A retrospective view over the last 30 years allows various trends to be recognised:

1. A gradual, though enormous, improvement in antihypertensive drugs.
2. An increase in knowledge of the epidemiology of hypertension and the relationship of coronary artery disease and cerebrovascular disease to hypertension.
3. A lowering of the level of BP at which drug therapy is thought, or known, to be of benefit.
4. A gradual increase in the proportion of medical practitioners who believe in antihypertensive treatment and are capable of applying it reasonably well.
5. An increasing acceptance by the general population that hypertension should be treated.
6. An increase in the time and money spent on lowering BP.
7. An increasing realisation of the desirability of preventing hypertension.

These trends have been the result of a complicated interaction of forces. The primary drive has come from physicians and epidemiologists interested

Amery, A. (ed.) Hypertensive Cardiovascular Disease: Pathophysiology and Treatment
© *1982, Martinus Nijhoff Publishers. The Hague / Boston / London*
ISBN-13: 978-94-009-7478-4

in reducing the toll of hypertensive cerebrovascular, cardiac and renal disease and of coronary disease. They have been propagating for many years, sometimes with a note of despair [1], the message that every person must have BP checks and that high blood pressure must be treated. This message has of course suited the pharmaceutical firms very well and they have put a great deal of effort into spreading the message, fortunately to the benefit also of people with hypertension.

1.2. Possibilities for prevention

One of the results of all this has been the increasing time, effort and money that are expended on the treatment of hypertension. It is a curious fact that success in treating hypertension seems to have stimulated interest in preventing [2] hypertension. One wonders whether this is partly because the cost of hypertension to the community now has to be measured in terms of money rather than in terms of mere mortality and morbidity. A kinder explanation perhaps is that hypertension can no longer be ignored and that many physicians, while basically in favour of lowering blood pressure, are uneasy about the very large numbers of people who seem likely to be going to take antihypertensive drugs. Prevention of hypertension would clearly have many advantages and there are two possibilities: (a) weight reduction, which is theoretically likely to lower the average blood pressure of the population very considerably, but is in practice virtually impossible to achieve on a large scale; (b) reduction of sodium intake and perhaps an increase in potassium intake, both of which could probably be achieved to some extent if people became convinced that they were worth while (see Chapter 16).

1.3. Case-finding and selection for treatment

It is only in the last few years that any semblance of on overall plan has emerged, in the shape of recommendations from WHO [3] and from national committees such as the US Joint National Committee on Detection, Evaluation and Treatment of High Blood Pressure [4, 5]. There is agreement that BP must be checked regularly (e.g. every 3–5 years) in everybody and that high BP must be reduced. In fact, hypertension is one of the few conditions where population screening is acknowledged to be worthwhile.

The level of BP at which it is recommended that treatment be commenced tends to vary however. The author's own views [6] on this are reproduced in Table 1; with the passage of 3 years, the recommendations might be thought by some to be a trifle conservative. However, neither of the recently reported large trials (Hypertension Detection and Follow-up

875

Table 1. A guide to the selection of patients for antihypertensive treatment

	D.B.P. mmHg Age <40	D.B.P. mmHg Age 40–59	D.B.P. mmHg Age 60+	Antihypertensive treatment	Factors militating against drug treatment at these levels
BP values must be based on at least 3 readings (taken sitting on each of 3 different occasions).	130	130	130	Essential	Factors militating against drug treatment at these levels: no symptoms, low systolic BP, normal ECG, normal heart size, reluctance to be treated, mental disease, physical disability, obesity, gout, diabetes, asthma, alcoholism etc.; poor response to simple treatment.
	125	125	125		
The figures are intended to represent phase 5; if phase 4 is used, the limits should in theory be set slightly higher.	120	120	120		
	115	115	115	Advisable	
	110	110	110		
Treatment at these levels is advisable when any of the following are present: definite symptoms, high systolic BP, bad family history, ECG signs of LV hypertrophy, enlarged heart, hyperlipidaemia, ischaemic heart disease, renal disease, migraine.	105	105	105	Optional (but if not given, then observation essential)	
	100	100	100		
	95	95	95	Unnecessary (nearly always)	
	90	90	90		

Male sex is a factor for treatment in borderline cases.
Age >70 years is a factor against treatment in borderline cases.

Reproduced, by permission, from Blood Pressure Screening in New Zealand, a report by a working group of the National Heart Foundation of New Zealand (P.O. Box 17128, Green Lane, Auckland).

Program [7, 8], Australian National Blood Pressure Study [9]) have shown clearly that patients with diastolic pressures of 90–94 mm Hg do better with treatment [10].

The broad outlines of strategy are thus clear enough; the problem is to see that the recommendations are put into effect and also to make sure that the right priorities are maintained. For instance, it seems illogical to treat people with diastolic pressure of 95 mm Hg when others whose diastolics are 120 mm Hg or more are going undetected and untreated. Ideally, the strategy should be to put more effort into case-finding and less into the treatment of the milder cases. If such a policy could have been put into effect over the last 25 years, the benefits of antihypertensive therapy would probably have been even more striking. Unfortunately, the quality of care tends to vary and while, for instance, some general practitioners are assiduous in recording BP on their patients [11, 12] there is evidence [13, 14] that others are not. These data come from the UK and while it is possible that the capitation mode of remuneration gives too little incentive to already busy doctors to embark on screening and long-term treatment of hypertension, surveys in other countries also have brought to light plenty of cases of hypertension that were previously unrecognised. It may be that this unsatisfactory state of affairs is changing fairly rapidly, as reported for Chicago [15] and Finland [16]. There is wide agreement that screening is best done by general practitioners.

1.4. Social effects and costs

The treatment of hypertension on a national scale has, of course, huge ramifications. Though superficially simple, antihypertensive treatment is in fact a sophisticated form of medicine, particularly now that treatment is being given on such a large scale even to symptomless people with 30 or 40 years of life ahead of them. It is clearly vital that the treatment does more good than harm.

This applies not only medically but also socially and psychologically. The loss of work due to attendances for supervision of treatment is, in aggregate, not negligible [17] and there must inevitably be some unease generated in at least some people by the need constantly to take medication. These problems are compounded by some Health Service arrangements. For instance, in the health service of one country, prescriptions can be given for only two weeks at a time; this really makes treatment of mild hypertension, in particular, unacceptable in terms of the disruption of the patient's life. But even if attendances at doctor's consulting rooms or clinic are at 3- or 4-month intervals, it is important to make these attendances as pleasant and efficient as possible. Probably the best solution will be for the practitioner to arrange some form of 'mini-clinic' for his hypertensive patients, on the lines which have been described for diabetes [18].

The costs of large-scale antihypertensive treatment also have to be kept in proportion. There is obviously no point in using health service funds to treat mild hypertension in a country where malnutrition and infectious diseases are the main health problems. The situation is much less easy to assess in countries which are more affluent but whose health budgets are nevertheless strained. The biggest potential costs are in the elderly and there is no doubt that in a society with good access to primary medical care the proportion of the elderly on antihypertensive therapy (including diuretics and β-blockers given for any cause) can become very high [19]. The results of the current trial of the European Working Party on Hypertension in the Elderly [20] are awaited with much interest. However, as mentioned earlier, the question of prevention of hypertension now looms very large. If it really can be proved that a diet containing less sodium and more potassium will lead to a lower prevalence of hypertension (see Chapter 16), then government action will be needed to help to achieve this, at least to the extent that the amounts of sodium present in foodstuffs should be stated on the packing.

2. STRATEGY FOR THE TREATMENT OF HYPERTENSION IN THE INDIVIDUAL

2.1. Work-up

A prerequisite for all antihypertensive therapy is that a proper history must be taken, a full clinical examination (see Chapter 41) done and suitable tests (see Chapters 42 and 43) carried out. The purpose is to determine (a) how hypertensive the individual is, (b) how much organ damage is present, (c) whether any primary causes of hypertension or factors which may be aggravating the hypertension are identifiable, and (d) whether any associated or coincidental conditions are present which could affect prognosis or choice of drugs.

2.2. Treatment of hypertension without drugs

Opportunities for treatment without drugs must not be missed. Coarctation of the aorta (Chapter 32) and the well-known endocrine (Chapters 35 and 36) and renal (Chapters 33 and 34) causes of hypertension are usually not forgotten, but it is equally important to remember that oral contraceptives (Chapter 40), licorice and overuse of nasal vasoconstrictors can cause, or aggravate, hypertension.

Dealing with these factors is usually not too much of a problem. Far more difficult is dealing with aspects of the life-style of people with elevated pressures. There is ample evidence (Chapter 17) that *obesity* and hypertension are related and it should be good strategy to get a person's weight down to normal before antihypertensive drugs are started. But the tactics to achieve this are sadly defective, and the campaign often ends in failure. One essential point is to use an adequately sized cuff before concluding that a person with a large arm is hypertensive; there is, after all, no point in giving antihypertensive drugs to someone whose BP is, in reality, normal. The relationship of *alcohol* to hypertension is rather less certain and evidence does not justify a major effort to reduce alcohol intake on this account, however desirable in other ways. However, a really heavy drinker will often be somewhat careless about therapy, so that long-term treatment of hypertension is undoubtedly made more difficult.

Cigarette smoking has not itself been shown to be associated with hypertension. This is sometimes ascribed to a reduced tendency to obesity in heavy smokers but in a survey in New Zealand [21] the heavy smokers had a higher mean body mass index and yet had a significantly lower BP than the non-smokers. However, there is evidence that once they become hypertensive, smokers are more liable to enter the accelerated phase of hypertension [22–24]. Smokers are also more liable to develop myocardial infarction and peripheral arterial disease [25]. There is, therefore, good justification for trying to get hypertensives to stop smoking.

Finally, there is *salt* or more correctly, *sodium* (see Chapter 16), easily the most important unresolved problem in hypertension at present. In the context of the individual hypertensive patient, the question is whether a moderate degree of salt restriction helps to lower blood pressure. It is generally acknowledged that a very strict low sodium diet is impracticable and current recommendations have been to reduce sodium intake until 24-h sodium output falls below 84 mmol/day [5] or even 70 mmol/day [26]. However, the benefits of this have as yet not been proved [27] and at present it seems reasonable to aim at a compromise: to measure urinary Na^+ output for 24 h and if it is higher than the average for the population, to try to persuade the patient to reduce his or her sodium intake at least to 170 mmol or 140 mmol, respectively. But if patients wish to try to restrict sodium intake more vigorously, they should certainly be allowed to do so. It may be that the important thing is the Na/K ratio rather than the absolute level of sodium intake [28]. Clearly this is a field where more data are badly needed.

Apart from the question of whether sodium restriction lowers blood pressure, there is also the question of how we should look on it in relation to drug therapy. Sodium restriction has been put forward [5] as an adjunct to all forms of antihypertensive treatment, but there would seem to be a fundamental difference between using it as an *adjunct to* diuretic therapy and using it *in place of* diuretic therapy. The latter is the more logical and attractive proposition and indeed it has been suggested by one protagonist [26] of salt restriction that the use of diuretics is particularly appropriate for those who are unable to maintain their daily sodium intake below 150 mmol/day. In a different study [29], patients on antihypertensive therapy (mainly beta-blockers), had a considerable fall in blood pressure when sodium intake was restricted and a greater fall when a diuretic was given without sodium restriction, but a combination of a diuretic and sodium restriction was not significantly better than administration of a diuretic alone. Thus, it seems possible that if a diuretic has to be given, it may be unnecessary to restrict sodium; however, there is evidence [30] that an additional 340–500 mmol of sodium daily will nullify the antihypertensive effects of a diuretic, so that enormous intakes of sodium are clearly best avoided even if a diuretic is being given.

2.3. Treatment of hypertension with drugs

There are a number of different systems of drug treatment, though they tend to shade over into one another:
1. Complete empiricism
2. Stepped care system
3. Individual care system
4. Vasoconstriction–volume analysis system.

2.3.1. Complete empiricism
In the early years of antihypertensive therapy, the patients being treated nearly all had pretty severe hypertension and there was little choice of drugs. Whatever was available was used, though naturally two types of Rauwolfia drug or two types of ganglion blocker would not be used together. The use of combinations of drugs emerged early, for instance in the use of hydrallazine and hexamethonium [31] and in Smirk's advocacy of 'background therapy' [32] with Rauwolfia (and later, diuretics) in order to minimise the dosage required of the more powerful and symptom-causing drugs.

The advent of the thiazide diuretics made the treatment of hypertension enormously easier, but did not initially change any principles of treatment. They were used partly as 'background therapy', (sometimes sufficient by themselves in mild cases), partly to overcome the fluid retention caused by the more specific antihypertensive drugs. It was a matter of trial and error, and, fortunately, it was common experience that results were usually good.

Unexpectedly, the beta-blockers were found to lower BP and they are still used largely empirically. Like the diuretics, they have greatly improved the care of hypertensive subjects. In addition, the difference between their mode of action and that of the diuretics is so great that it raises theoretical possibilities of tailoring therapy to the predominant factors in an individual patient's hypertension.

While empiricism has really served pretty well (and undoubtedly is still present in much antihypertensive therapy), nevertheless it seem reasonable to hope that some rationality could be introduced and a number of guidelines have been put forward.

3.3.2. Stepped care system
This system [4, 5], which developed in the United States, has both strengths and weaknesses.

Step 1. Thiazide-type diuretic; starting dose: hydrochlorothiazide 50 mg, or bendrofluazide 5 mg, or chlorthalidone 25 mg (or equivalent) and increasing to 100 mg, 20 mg or 100 mg, respectively. Spironolactone or triamterene or potassium supplements to be added if serum K falls below 3.3 mmol/l. Asymptomatic hyperuricaemia up to 0.59 mmol/l (10 mg/dl) is to be ignored.

Step 2. Add propranolol 40 mg/day (or other beta-blocker), or methyldopa 500 mg/day or reserpine 0.1 mg/day, and increase the dose if necessary to a maximum of 480 mg/day, 2000 mg/day or 0.25 mg/day, respectively. Clonidine or prazosin may be used instead of abovementioned drugs. If resistance develops and fluid retention occurs, sodium should be restricted, or an additional diuretic given (presumably frusemide, initial dose 80 mg).

Step 3. Add hydrallazine 50 mg/day, increasing if necessary to a maximum dose of 250 mg/day; or clonidine or prazosin can be used at this step. (Note that clonidine is no longer included in step 3 in 1980 recommendations.)

Step 4. Add or substitute guanethidine 25 mg/day, increasing if necessary to 300 mg/day.

The stepped-care system is essentially an off-shoot of empiricism, enunciated in a clear-cut way to help ensure that antihypertensive therapy will not appear too complicated and will be applied with reasonable efficiency. The strengths of this approach are fourfold

1. It gives a definite framework within which to operate,

2. It stresses that drugs should be started singly. Unfortunately, this principle is ignored for patients with average diastolic pressures of 130 mm Hg or more, or with heart failure, encephalopathy, microscopic findings of RBCS or casts when 'treatment may be initiated with several drugs simultaneously' [4]. The wisdom of this is very doubtful; only hypertensive encephalopathy and LV failure are really urgent, and while there is a place for

starting a diuretic and some other drug together in an emergency, it is difficult to see why several drugs need be started simultaneously. In fact, in the latest statement [5] this recommendation no longer appears.

3. It stresses that initial doses should be small in non-urgent cases. However, the actual doses quoted are by no means always small. Hydrochlorothiazide should preferably be started at doses no higher than 25 mg/day, bendrofluazide 2.5 mg/day, methyldopa 250 mg/day, and frusemide 40 mg/day.

4. It makes very *full use of diuretics,* which are cheap.

The weaknesses of the stepped-care approach are also fourfold:

1. It is rather rigid and somewhat slow to change.
2. It does not suit some patients, e.g. those with gout or diabetes.
3. It is doubtful whether it is wise to push daily dosage of thiazide-type diuretics to such limits (e.g. hydrochlorothiazide 100 mg, chlorthalidone 100 mg, bendrofluazide 20 mg) before adding some other drug.
4. The relative simplicity of the system is inevitably getting lost as more and more new drugs come along that do not fit neatly into it. Where will labetalol be placed when it gets accepted in the U.S.A.? Or the Ca^{2+}-antagonists with their individual differences?

2.3.3. Individual care system
This [33, 34] is also an off-shoot of empiricism, is not put forward with any claim to originality, has never previously been given a name, and indeed scarcely deserves the title of 'system'. It probably represents what many physicians do, either consciously or subconsciously. Other authors have also stressed the need for individualisation of treatment [35, 36].

Once the decision is taken to treat a patient, a number of questions have to be answered:

1. *What drugs can I not give to this patient?* Beta-blockers should not be given to people with asthma or chronic obstructive respiratory disease, heart failure, heart block of grade II or III, or peripheral vascular disease, and may cause problems in diabetics. Thiazide diuretics should preferably not be given to people with diabetes (overt or subclinical) or hyperuricaemia; in people with impaired renal function, frusemide is preferable to a thiazide. Patients with a past or present history of depression should not be given Rauwolfia and preferably not methyldopa, clonidine or propranolol either. Posturally acting drugs are less used now but they should in particular not be given to the elderly. The effects of adrenergic neurone blockers on sexual function are usually more marked, and more unwelcome, in young or middle-aged men. Methyldopa should not be used in patients with liver problems. Clonidine should especially not be used in patients who may be erratic in their tablet-taking.

2. *What drugs may have particular benefits for this patient?* If there is fluid retention, or dyspnoea of cardiac origin, or cardiac enlargement, or if the patient is aged 50 years or more, then a diuretic should preferably be included. If the patient has sinus tachycardia (provided this does not represent early cardiac failure), or is particularly nervous, or has angina or ventricular ectopics, then a beta-blocker should be included. If, as is much less common, a phaeochromocytoma is present, or if the hypertension is due to an MAO-cheese reaction or a vasoconstrictor, then an alpha-blocker is needed.

3. *How urgent is it to bring down the blood pressure?* The answer will determine one's procedure but it is *never* necessary, and always unwise, to reduce a very high blood pressure to normal levels in the course of a few minutes or even a few hours. The state of the cerebral blood flow is somewhat precarious in patients with extremely high pressure and must be given time to adjust to lower perfusion pressures. It is far better to lower the blood pressure first to an intermediate level, e.g. from an initial 260/150 mm Hg to, say, 170/110 mm Hg. The urgency should also interfere as little as possible with the general rule that drugs should be started singly; the only major exception is that in some acute cases a diuretic and a specific antihypertensive drug may need to be started more or less together.

4. *How old is the patient?* As already mentioned, patients aged 50 years or more should normally be started first on a diuretic. Younger patients often respond well to a beta-blocker alone, and this can well be tried first. In cases, if response to moderate doses of a single drug is unsatisfactory, then the other type of drug should be added. This simple guide-line evolved from experience and there are probably several reasons for its success. Firstly, older people are more liable to develop heart failure when given drugs with a negative inotropic effect and therefore should, if possible, have a diuretic in their regimen. Secondly, PRA decreases with age [37] and therefore if the response to beta-blockers is related to PRA [38], then young people should on average respond better to these drugs than older people do. Thirdly, sympathetic drive and cardiac output tend to be higher in younger people [39]; beta-blockers could thus be expected to be more effective in this age group.

In general, then, initial treatment will be either with a diuretic or with a beta-blocker starting with low dosage and working up. If response to moderate dosage is unsatisfactory, then the alternative drug is added (again starting with low dosage and working up). If response is still unsatisfactory, then either labetalol can be substituted (by degrees) for the beta-blocker or prazosin or hydrallazine can be added.

The possibility of inadequate diuresis should also be considered at this stage. The addition of spironolactone or amiloride or triamterene can be helpful, and frusemide is usually more effective and better tolerated than a thiazide when renal function is impaired. If control of blood pressure is still not acceptable, one can add methyldopa or an adrenergic neurone blocker, or clonidine, but one or more of the previously started drugs should then be withdrawn. The Ca^{2+}-antagonist nifedipine can be useful and perhaps also verapamil, though their place in therapy is not yet settled. Finally, there is the question of minoxidil or converting enzyme blockade, of which the latter is much the mosre attractive alternative. Captopril (see Chapter 53) can certainly be very effective in difficult cases, but the problems of toxicity have not yet been settled.

2.3.4. Vasoconstriction–volume analysis system

This system, devised and vigorously propounded by Laragh [38, 40], holds that the classification of hypertensive subjects according to their plasma renin activity (PRA) is vitally useful in the selection of the most suitable antihypertensive drug. Patients who have a high PRA are best treated with a beta-blocker, those who have a low PRA with a diuretic. There is a good deal of data supporting this concept, but also some data suggesting that it is not the complete and universal truth (see Chapters 45 and 46).

There are also some anomalies. For low renin hypertension, 'relatively predominant features' [40] are said to be vasodilatation, high cardiac output and high tissue perfusion; for high renin hypertension the features include low cardiac output and low tissue perfusion. The basis for these statements is by no means clear [41–43] and the system seems to ignore the influence of the sympathetic nervous system.

Also, most would disagree with the description [40] of propranolol as a 'renin lowering antivasoconstrictor drug'. It can in fact lead to vasoconstriction, though conceivably not in patients who had high PRA to start with; there seem to be no data on this. It can, and certainly does, lower cardiac output [39] and this can hardly be ignored in the consideration of its mode of action. It is curious also to see methyldopa, clonidine and reserpine described as 'renin-lowering antivasoconstrictor drugs'; their other effects on the sympathetic nervous system presumably deserve some mention.

Like the other systems discussed, the vasoconstriction–volume analysis system has both strengths and weakness. Among its strengths are that (a) it accepts that beta-blockers can be very useful when used alone in some patients and has shown at least partly why; (b) it has helped to emphasize which patients respond best to a diuretic; (c) it has stimulated thinking about what drugs do *not* suit certain patients.

Its weaknesses are that (a) it assumes certain points which are of doubtful validity. (b) It largely ignores the sympathetic nervous system; (c) it would require a massive effort to provide PRA estimations on a large scale, and there would be problems of both accuracy and cost. It is at present scarcely a practical proposition.

2.3.5. *Points relevant to all strategies*

Finally, there are a number of points which are common to all antihypertensive therapy, regardless of the 'system' used:

1. The patient must trust the doctor sufficiently to take the doses as instructed or to tell the doctor why he feels the doses ordered are not suiting him.
2. Initial doses must be small. Increases in dosage must be gradual.
3. Drugs should be started singly, unless there is a special emergency.
4. Drugs should preferably also be stopped gradually and singly.
5. Patients must be provided with a dosage card and must be made to carry it so that it can be a basis for discussion at visits.
6. Poor BP control in spite of one's best efforts may indicate that the patient is not taking his drugs.
7. If BP is persistently normal for many months, a gradual withdrawal of therapy is warranted. Close follow-up is then essential.
8. Failure to keep appointments must be investigated under some form of follow-up system.
9. Attendance at consulting-room or clinic must be made as pleasant and efficient as possible.

SUMMARY

On a national scale, management of hypertension requires an efficient system of detection (preferably based on the general practitioner service), knowledgeable and interested doctors and, for the patients, access to antihypertensive drugs without financial hardship.

At the level of the individual patient, there has to be a good work-up to make sure that hypertension is really present and to detect primary causes, organ damage and conditions which may influence the course of the disease or the choice of drugs. Aggravating factors must be dealt with. The decision to start drug treatment depends on the level of the blood pressure and, in the borderline area, also on other factors. Choice of drugs has to be on an individual basis; drugs should be started singly and at low dosage and cessation should preferably also be gradual. There must be meticulous attention to detail, and a good doctor–patient relationship is vital.

Sodium restriction is currently a burning topic. If moderate restriction is demonstrated definitely to lower blood pressure, or to prevent the development of hypertension, then strategies will have to be devised to reduce sodium intake on a national scale. Meantime, the evidence is still not compelling.

885

ACKNOWLEDGEMENTS

The work on which the author's views are based is supported by the Medical Research Council of New Zealand and the National Feart Foundation of New Zealand.

REFERENCES

1. Page IH: The continuing failure to understand and treat hypertension. JAMA 241:1897-1898, 1979.
2. Editorial. Lowering blood pressure without drugs. Lancet 2:459-461, 1980.
3. Arterial hypertension. Report of a WHO Expert Committee. WHO, Geneva, 1978.
4. Report of the Joint National Committee on Detection, Evaluation, and Treatment of High Blood Pressure. A cooperative study. JAMA 237:255-261, 1977.
5. The 1980 report of the Joint National Committee on Detection, Evaluation, and Treatment of High Blood Pressure. Arch Intern Med 140:1280-1285, 1980.
6. Simpson FO: Hypertension. BR Med J 2:882-883, 1978.
7. Hypertension Detection and Follow-up Program Cooperative Group: Five-Year findings on the hypertension detection and follow-up program - I. Reduction in mortality of persons with high blood pressure, including mild hypertension. JAMA 242:2562-2571, 1979.
8. Hypertension Detection and Follow-up Program Cooperative Group: Five-year findings of the hypertension detection and follow-up program, - II. Mortality by race, sex and age. JAMA 242:2572-2577, 1979.
9. Management Committee Report: The Australian therapeutic trial in mild hypertension. Lancet 1:1261-1267, 1980.
10. Editorial. Mild hypertension. Br Med J 280:1062-1063, 1980.
11. Tudor Hart J: The management of high blood pressure in general practice. JR Coll Gen Pract 25:160-192, 1975.
12. Coope J: A screening clinic for hypertension in general practice. JR Coll Gen Pract 24:161-166, 1974.
13. Heller RF, Rose G: Current management of hypertension in general practice. Br Med J 1:1442-1444, 1977.
14. Barber JH, Beevers DG, Fife R et al.: Blood-pressure screening and supervision in general practice. Br Med J 1:843-846, 1979.
15. Berkson DM, Brown MC, Stanton H et al.: Changing trends in hypertension detection and control: the Chicago experience. Am J Public Health 70:389-393, 1980.
16. Tuomilehto J, Nissinen A, Salonen JT, Kottke TE, Puska P: Community programme for control of hypertension in North Karelia, Finland. Lancet 2:900-903, 1980.
17. Haynes RB, Sackett DL, Taylor DW, Gibson ES, Johnson AL: Increased absenteeism from work after detection and labeling of hypertensive patients. N Engl J Med 299:741-744, 1978.
18. Thorn PA, Russell RG: Diabetic clinics today and tomorrow: mini-clinics in general practice. Br Med J 2:534-536, 1973.
19. Simpson FO: Long-term follow-up of elderly subjects on antihypertensive therapy. In: Hypertension in the Young and Old, pp. 331-334. Onesti G, Kim KE, eds. New York: Grune & Stratton, 1981.
20. Amery A, Berthaux P, Birkenhäger W et al.: Antihypertensive therapy in patients above age 60 years (Fourth Interim Report of the European Working Party on High Blood Pressure in Elderly: EWPHE). Clin Sci Mol Med 55:263s-270s, 1978.

21. Simpson FO, Waal-Manning HJ, Bolli P, Spears GFS. A community study of risk factors for high blood pressure: possibilities for prevention. In: Prophylactic Approach to Hypertensive Diseases, pp. 31-39. Yamori Y et al., eds. New York: Raven Press, 1979.

22. Bloxham CA, Beevers DG, Walker JM: Malignant hypertension and cigarette smoking. Br Med J 1:581-583, 1979.

23. Isles C, Brown JJ, Cumming AMM et al.: Excess smoking in malignant-phase hypertension. Br Med J 1:579-581, 1979.

24. Elliott JM, Simpson FO: Cigarettes and accelerated hypertension. NZ Med J 91:447-449, 1980.

25. Kannel WB, McGee D, Gordon T: A general cardiovascular risk profile: the Framingham study. Am J Cardiol 38:46-51, 1976.

26. Hunt JC. Management and treatment of essential hypertension. In: Hypertension, physiopathology and treatment, pp. 1068-1085. Genest J, Koiw E, Kuchel O, eds. New York: McGraw-Hill, 1977.

27. Simpson FO: Salt and hypertension: a sceptical review of the evidence. Clin Sci 57:463s-480s, 1979.

28. Parfrey PS, Vandenburg MJ, Wright P et al.: Blood pressure and hormonal changes following alteration in dietary sodium and potassium in mild essential hypertension. Lancet 1:59-63, 1981.

29. Carney S, Morgan T, Wilson M, Matthews G, Roberts R: Sodium restriction and thiazide diuretics in the treatment of hypertension. Med J Aust 1:803-807, 1975.

30. Shah S, Khatri I, Freis ED: Mechanism of antihypertensive effect of thiazide diuretics. Am Heart J 95:611-618, 1978.

31. Schroeder HA: Control of hypertension by hexamethonium and 1-hydrazinophthalazine. Arch Intern Med 89:523-540, 1952.

32. Smirk FH: Drug therapy in hypertension. Clin Pharmacol Ther 2:110-120, 1961.

33. Simpson FO: Principles of drug treatment for hypertension: indications for treatment and for selection of drugs. Pharmacol Ther 7:153-172, 1979.

34. Simpson FO: Hypertensive disease. In: Drug Treatment, pp. 639-682. Avery GS, ed. Sydney: ADIS Press, 1980.

35. Koch-Weser J: Individualization of antihypertensive treatment, pp.251-255. Clinical Pharmacology and Therapeutics, Turner P, ed. Proceed 1st World Conf, London: MacMillan, 1980.

36. Zanchetti A. Rational approaches to clinical therapy. pp. 270-274. Clinical Pharmacology and Therapeutics, Turner P, ed. Proceed 1st World Conf, London: MacMillan, 1980.

37. Kaplan NM, Kem DC, Holland OB et al.: The intravenous furosemide test: a simple way to evaluate renin responsiveness. Ann Intern Med 84:639-645, 1976.

38. Laragh JH: Modern system for treating high blood pressure based on renin profiling and vasoconstriction–volume analysis: a primary role for beta blocking drugs such as propranolol. Am J Med 61:797-810, 1976.

39. Lund-Johansen P: Hemodynamic alterations in hypertension — spontaneous changes and effects of drug therapy. A review. Acta Med Scand (Suppl) 603:1-14, 1977.

40. Laragh JH: Vasoconstriction–volume analysis for understanding and treating hypertension: the use of renin and aldosterone profiles. Am J Med 55:261-274, 1973.

41. Schalekamp MA, Lebel M, Beevers DG et al.: Body-fluid volume in low-renin hypertension. Lancet 2:310-311, 1974.

42. Schalekamp MADH, Birkenhäger WH, Zaal GA, Kolsters G: Haemodynamic characteristics of low-renin hypertension. Clin Sci Mol Med 52:405-412, 1977.

43. Dunn MJ, Tannen RL: Low renin essential hypertension. In: Hypertension, Physiopathology and Treatment, pp. 349-364. Genest J, Koiw E, Kuchel O, Eds, New York: McGraw-Hill, 1977.

55. THE BENEFITS OF ANTIHYPERTENSIVE THERAPY

Norman M. Kaplan

Successful reduction of elevated blood pressure will reduce disability and death from various cardiovascular diseases. The risk of untreated hypertension is largely mediated by an acceleration of atherosclerosis, so that heart attack, stroke, and renal damage occur 10–20 years earlier among hypertensives than among people with normal blood pressure. The protection offered by successful reduction of the blood pressure is likely to be mediated by a slowing or reversal of atherosclerosis, though a reduction in the purely mechanical force of the elevated pressure may also be involved.

Proof of the benefits of reduction of the blood pressure has come only from studies using antihypertensive drugs. Though it is probable that if the blood pressure were lowered by non-drug modalities (e.g. weight reduction, sodium restriction), similar – or even greater – benefits would accrue, nothing more can be said in the total absence of data. It is unlikely that trials of non-drug therapy large enough in scale to provide such proof will be forthcoming. It has been hard enough to prove the benefits of more potent drug therapy. Non-drug therapies have been shown to lower the blood pressure [1, 2], but it is quite another task to prove that they will thereby reduce cardiovascular morbidity or mortality. The following problems deserve to be taken into consideration: the antihypertensive effect of these non-drug modalities is usually modest at best; a tremendous amount of effort would be needed to apply and control these effects in thousands of patients over many years; and if, after all, success were achieved, the results might be attributable to coincident changes in independent variables such as plasma cholesterol, body weight, glucose tolerance, or stress.

The proof for the benefits of antihypertensive therapy has come in gradual steps down the heights of hypertension: by 1960 an increased survival of patients with malignant hypertension had been shown [3]; in 1967, protection of patients with diastolics between 115 and 129 mm Hg was demonstrated [4]; in 1970, similar protection was shown for those with diastolics between 104 and 115 mm Hg [5]. Not until 1979 and 1980 was the evidence available for those with diastolics between 90 and 104 mm Hg [6, 7].

Since most are well aware of the older data and since there remain skeptics about the applicability of the newer data to the majority of hypertensive

Amery, A. (ed.) Hypertensive Cardiovascular Disease: Pathophysiology and Treatment
© *1982, Martinus Nijhoff Publishers. The Hague / Boston / London*
ISBN-13: 978-94-009-7478-4

patients [8], the remainder of this chapter will focus on the evidence for the benefits of drugs therapy for those with relatively mild hypertension.

THE RISKS OF MILD HYPERTENSION

Before considering the evidence that antihypertensive drug therapy is beneficial, the risk imposed by relatively mild hypertension should be recognized [9]. By combining the data on the prevalence of various levels of diastolic blood pressure with the eventual mortality associated with these varying levels among the carefully observed population of Framingham [10], more than 40% of the excess mortality related to hypertension can be shown to develop in those patients with relatively small elevations of

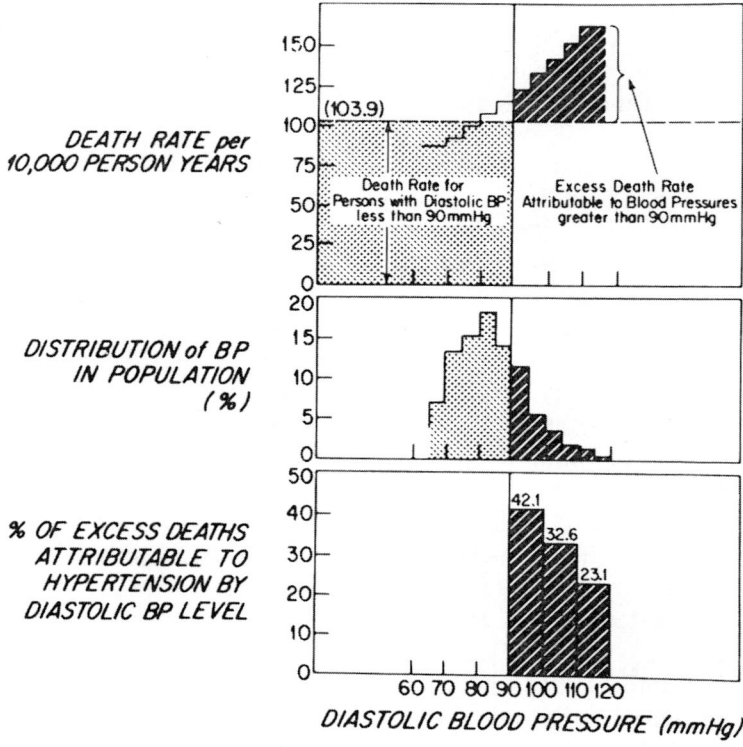

Figure 1. An estimate of the percentage of excess deaths attributable to hypertension by varying levels of diastolic blood pressure is shown in the lower figure. These percentages are derived by multiplying the death rate per 10 000 person years at different levels of diastolic blood pressure in the Framingham study (shown in the top figure) by the distribution of diastolic blood pressures in the population (shown in the middle figure). (Reproduced with permission from [9])

Table 1. Increased mortality for insured men and women with hypertension (20 years of experience with 4 million insured people)

Blood pressure			
Systolic	138–147	148–157	158–167
Men	36%	68%	110%
Women	22%	35%	67%
Diastolic	88–92	93–97	98–102
Men	38%	71%	104%
Women	33%	63%	83%

From: The 1979 Build and Blood Pressure Study, Association of Life Insurance Medical Directors and the Society of Actuaries.

diastolic pressure (Figure 1). Obviously, it takes many years for mild hypertension to cause complications, and individual practitioners seldom observe the long-term consequences. But, with large-scale, long-term observations, the risk becomes apparent.

Affirmation of the risk of even small elevations in blood pressure comes from the recently updated actuarial data from over 4 million insured people in the U.S. [11]. Significant increases in mortality over the next 20 years were observed in those with initial systolic levels above 138 or diastolic levels above 88 mm Hg (Table 1). Men had greater mortality rates at every level of high blood pressure.

A large number of older people (as many as a third of those over 65) have purely or predominately systolic hypertension, presumably from the loss of elasticity in the aorta and major resistance vessels. The risks for cardiovascular disease are increased among such patients [12] (Table 2). In some, it is necessary to ensure that the elevated levels are not artifactual, due to an inability of the sphygmomanometer baloon cuff to collapse rigid arteries and, thereby, giving inappropriately high readings [13].

Table 2. Blood pressure and 3-year risks in patients 65–74

Blood pressure		No.	Coronary deaths	C–V–R deaths	Stroke
Systolic	<180	1973	8.0%	11.1%	5.0%
Diastolic	<95				
Diastolic	>95	493	9.0%	14.9%	8.8%
Systolic	>180	224	13.5%	22.0%	13.4%
Diastolic	<95				
Ratio: 3 vs 1		1.69	1.96	2.53	

From: Chicago stroke study, Shekelde et al.: Stroke 5: 71, 1974.

Table 3. A comparison of the HDFP (stratum I) and Australian therapeutic trial in mild hypertension

	HDFP Stratum I (DBP 90–104)	Australian trial
Source of patients	Community screening	Volunteer screening
Number of patients	7,825	3,427
Blood pressure limits for inclusion	Diastolic >90 (on second screening)	Diastolic >95, <110 (average of two screenings)
Exclusion factors	Bedfast, institution-alized	Current anti-hypertensive therapy; history or evidence of coronary, cerebral, or renal vascular disease; secondary forms of hypertension; ECG evidence of ischemia
Characteristics of patients		
Mean age (years)	50.8	50.5
Percent male	55%	63%
Percent white	61%	100%
Mean screening blood pressure	151.8/96.3	157.4/100.4
Treatment regimen		
Control group	Referred to usual sources: 54% on drugs by year 5	Placebo
Active treatment	Step-wide drugs: (1) Chlorthalidone (2) Reserpine, methyldopa, etc. (3) Hydralazine	Step-wise drugs: (1) Chlorothiazide (2) Methyldopa, propranolol, pindolol (3) Hydralazaine or clonidine
Goal of therapy	Diastolic <90 or 10 mm Hg fall if screening DBP 90–100	Diastolic <90 for first 2 years, then below 80
Duration of therapy	5 years	3 years
Mean diastolic BP at end of trial (mmHg fall)		
Control group	87.6 (−8.6)	93.9 (−6.6)
Active group	83.4 (−12.9)	88.3 (−12.2)
End points	Death: others to be reported	Death Non-fatal: cerebral or coronary vascular disease, CHF, Grade 3 or 4 retinopathy, renal failure (plasma creatinine >2 mg/dl)

891

Table 3 (Cont.). A comparison of the HDFP (stratum I) and Australian therapeutic trial in mild hypertension.

	HDFP Stratum I (DBP 90–104)	Australian trial
Incidence of end-points (control vs active)		
Deaths		
Cardiovascular	165:122	13:4
Non-cardiovascular	126:109	6:5
Non-fatal		127:91

BENEFITS OF THERAPY

Having recognized the risks, we shall now consider the evidence that reduction of elevated blood pressure with antihypertensive drug therapy will reduce the risks. Only recent data relating to the therapy of mild hypertension will be considered. Two large studies provide the best data (although all of their details are not yet available). The first, the Hypertension Detection and Follow-up Program (HDFP), involved 7825 patients with diastolics between 90 and 104 mm Hg [6]. The second, the Australian Therapeutic Trial in Mild Hypertension, included 3427 patients with diastolics between 95 and 109 mm Hg [7]. The two trials differed in numerous ways, but their similarities allow them to be taken together as strong validation of the benefits of antihypertensive therapy for the majority of patients – those with relatively mild hypertension (Table 3 and Figure 2). The HDFP enrolled many patients at greater risk for cardiovascular catastrophes who were excluded from the Australian Trial, including at least 7% who had already had a stroke or a heart attack and 25% who were on antihypertensive therapy at the time of screening and, therefore, likely to have considerably higher underlying blood pressure than recorded at the screening exams. Moreover, 39% of the HDFP population, but none of the Australians were black; they are likely to be at greater risk at any given level of blood pressure than whites are [14].

Nonetheless, the two studies provide a strong affirmation of the benefits of therapy, with a 20% decrease in cardiovascular mortality in the HDFP and a 55% decrease in the Australian trial. The greater protection noted in the Australian trial is not surprising since more than half of the HDFP 'control' group ended up on drug therapy, while the Australian controls were on placebo during the entire study. Thus, though the Australian subjects were at less risk on entry, the presence of a true 'control', placebo-treated group for comparison with active therapy reveals even greater protection by antihypertensive therapy.

CUMULATIVE INCIDENCE OF TRIAL END POINTS

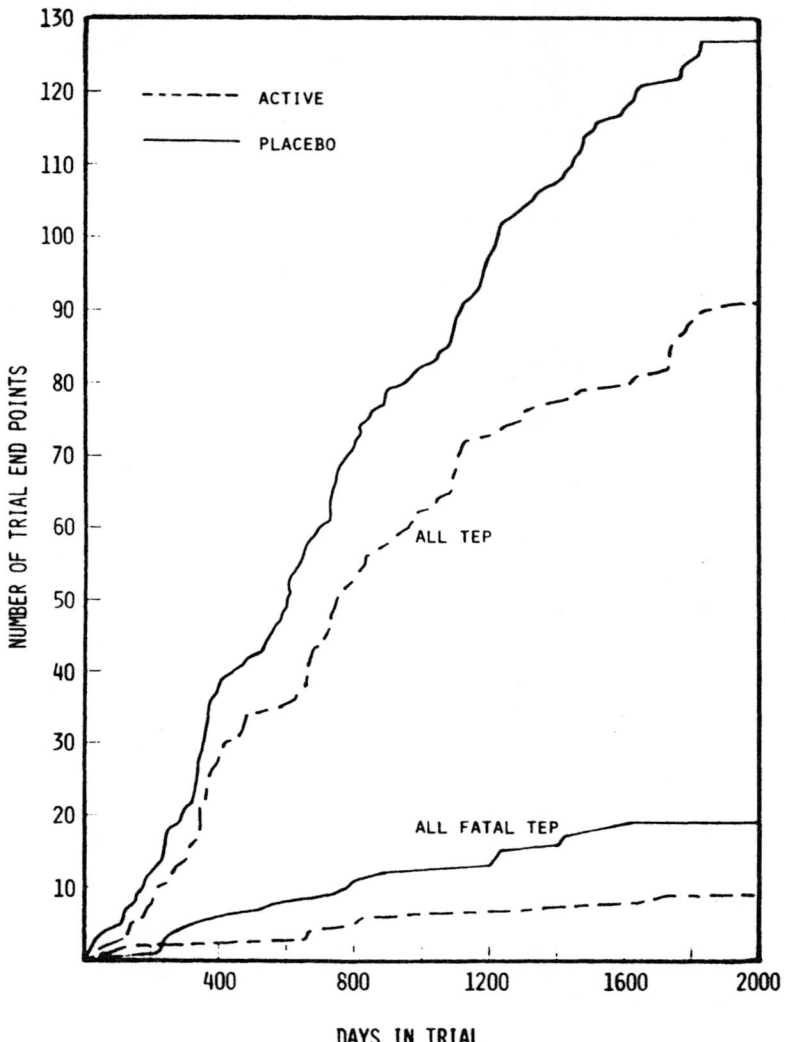

Figure 2. The results of the Australian Therapeutic Trial in Mild Hypertension showing the cumulative occurrence of total end-points (TEP) and of deaths from all causes in 1721 subjects of the active (– – –) and 1706 of the placebo (—) groups. The differences between the two groups are significant for both TEP and deaths. (Reproduced with permission from [7].)

It should be emphasized that these benefits were observed despite relatively small differences in the falls in diastolic pressure between the active and 'control' groups: 4.3 mm Hg in the HDFP and 5.6 mm Hg in the Australian trial. The fall of 8.6 mm Hg in the 'control' group of the HDFP is hardly surprising since 54% of these patients were on antihypertensive drugs by the end of the 5-year study. On the other hand, the 6.6 mm Hg fall of the placebo-treated half of the Australian trial is not unexpected either, since there were only two screening exams performed before start of the trial and similar falls have been observed just with repeated blood pressure measurements over time even without placebo [15]. A greater differential would likely be noted if the screening pressures had been taken while all subjects received a placebo over a longer period so that at least 3 sets of blood pressures could be recorded. But rather than harp on problems with the design of either trial, we should thank the patients and investigators who performed these monumental studies for their perseverance and dedication.

SHORTCOMINGS OF THE HDFP AND THE AUSTRALIAN TRIAL

Despite the statistical proof of the benefit of antihypertensive therapy of mild hypertension provided by these two studies, they leave certain questions unanswered. Firstly, the protection offered patients under the age of 50 was not significant in either trial, probably because of their relatively small number and low mortality rates over such short intervals. Secondly, significant protection was not shown for women in the Australian trial or for white women in the HDFP, though black women were protected [16]. This difference between white and black women is logically explained by the larger number of black women in the trial and their greater decrement in diastolic pressure: 6.3 mm Hg versus 3.5 mm Hg for the white women. Thirdly, the HDFP provided more medical care to the more actively treated stepped-care group, so that the disclaimer has been made that 'This is perhaps as much a trial of medical care as of antihypertensive drugs' [17]. More care could explain the lesser mortality from non-cardiovascular causes observed: 109 in the stepped-care group versus 126 in the referred-care group. This objection was well handled in the Australian trial, where the placebo group averaged 14 visits to the clinic and the active group averaged 16 visits. The non-cardiovascular mortality was identical for the two groups.
   A third large trial that is still in progress, the British Medical Research Council's Mild Hypertension Trial [18], may provide further evidence about the questions left unanswered by the HDFP and Australian trial. The MCR trial involves patients with diastolic pressures within the 90–109 mm Hg range. It involves a larger number of women than were in the Australian trial and compares active drug therapy to placebo, so its differences should be more striking than those seen in the HDFP.

DO THE BENEFITS APPLY TO ALL CARDIOVASCULAR EVENTS?

The VA studies failed to demonstrate clear evidence that antihypertensive therapy protected against coronary artery disease. Another trial involving a relatively small number of patients with mild hypertension, the US Public Health Service Hospitals Cooperative Study, also failed to show a difference in the incidence of coronary disease, though there was a reduction in the development of left ventricular hypertrophy and hypervoltage on ECG [19]. However, such protection was shown in a study on hypertensive men performed in Göteborg, Sweden [20]. Unfortunately, this trial only involved men with diastolic above 115 mm Hg, and it was not randomized or otherwise controlled.

Fortunately, protection from coronary events was noted in the preliminary analysis of the HDFP, with a 45% decrease among the stepped-care group with initial diastolic between 90 and 104 mm Hg [6]. In the Australian trial fewer cases of fatal ischemic heart disease occurred in the active than in the placebo group, but the difference was of borderline statistical significance (p = 0.051) [7].

A detrimental effect of therapy was claimed by an English physician who noted a larger number of myocardial infarctions among his patients whose diastolic pressures were reduced the most [8]. However, the excess number of infarcts occurred in patients who had their pressures lowered to levels considerably lower than advised by any recognized authority [21]. A similar claim of possible harm by antihypertensive therapy, though involving patients with much more severe hypertension who received more aggressive therapy, is also largely invalidated by the inappropriately low levels of blood pressure induced in most of those who suffered ill effects [22].

Protection from cerebrovascular events has been repeatedly shown in every well-controlled trial. In the population at large there are fewer instances of stroke [23] and improved survival among those who suffer a stroke [23, 24]. These improvements in morbidity and mortality from cerebrovascular disease likely reflect, in large part, benefits of antihypertensive therapy.

Table 4. Progression of hypertension in placebo-treated patients with initially mild hypertension.

	VA	USPHS	Australian
Number of patients	194	196	1,706
Initial level of DBP (mmHg)	90–114	90–115	95–109
Threshold level of DBP (mmHg)	125	130	110
Percentage with progression beyond threshold	10	12	12

PROTECTION FROM PROGRESSION OF HYPERTENSION

Beyond the definite protection from stroke and the likely protection from coronary disease afforded by antihypertensive therapy, another benefit has been shown in the three major trials which compared drug therapy to placebo: protection from progression of hypertension (Table 4). Among those who remained on placebo for the three years in Australia, the five years in the VA study, and the seven to ten years in the USPHS trial, the diastolic blood pressure rose to clearly dangerous levels in a significant number. Almost none of those on antihypertensive drugs experienced such progression. A hemodynamic explanation for this protection by therapy has been provided by an intensive study of 13 patients with essential hypertension [25]. These patients were studied before and after twelve months of therapy with diuretics and beta-adrenergic blockers. The second study was done after the diuretic was stopped for four weeks and the beta-blocker for one week. Mean arterial blood pressure was still 15.5 mm Hg lower, but the significant finding was a virtual return to normal of the previously elevated total and non-autonomic component of peripheral resistance. Within four months off therapy, the hypertension had returned to pretreatment levels in 12 of the 13 patients. Thus, the hemodynamic abnormality responsible for hypertension is reversed by successful therapy although the underlying driving mechanisms are still active and capable of reasserting themselves if therapy is stopped.

Hopefully, the return to normal of peripheral resistance by therapy will eventually be reflected in a reversal of the structural thickening of resistance vessels, a process demonstrable in animals but, with available techniques, not yet in humans. We can assume that the lower incidence of vascular complications reflects a decrease in both the tightening and atherosclerotic changes with accompany untreated hypertension.

ARE BENEFITS DETERMINED BY THE TYPE OF THERAPY?

In the small but significant study by Jennings et al., both diuretics and beta-blockers had been used in those who demonstrated a normalization of peripheral resistance [25]. Both of these types of antihypertensive drugs initially cause a *rise* in peripheral resistance, presumably as an autoregulatory response to the decrease in cardiac output they initially invoke. With continuation of diuretic therapy, peripheral resistance clearly does fall [26] but with long-term beta-blocker therapy, peripheral resistance remains high [27].

The protection offered by one or another antihypertensive agent could be affected by its mode of pharmacological action and the responses made by

896

Table 5. The frequency of myocardial infarction and angina among hypertensives on various antihypertensive drugs*

	Diuretic	β-blocker	Diuretic & β-blocker	Other drugs
Men	8.8%	5.2%	2.9%	11.7%
Women	9.0%	9.5%	4.8%	8.6%

* A total of 579 men and 688 women received one of the forms of antihypertensive therapy for one year or longer. Data taken from [28].

the various interacting systems which control the blood pressure, but it is more likely that the protection is largely determined by the degree of blood pressure reduction, regardless of how this is accomplished.

There are really no adequate studies to settle the issue. In one study involving 1247 patients who received various drugs in an uncontrolled manner, the frequency of strokes and myocardial infarction was lowest among those who received a combination of a diuretic and a beta-blocker (Table 5) [28]. In the preliminary report of these data, the severity of the hypertension and the adequacy of blood pressure control was said not to differ significantly between the various therapies.

Beta-blockers may offer additional protection from coronary events, particularly those related to arrhythmias. There is evidence that deaths are significantly reduced in non-hypertensive patients under the age of 65 given beta-blockers after an acute myocardial infarction [29]. However, additional studies are needed to demonstrate primary prevention of coronary disease among hypertensives.

Concern has been expressed about possible ill-effects from diuretics [30], but every trial which has shown protection by antihypertensive therapy has used a diuretic as the initial drug. In a small, uncontrolled study of elderly men with mild hypertension, of the 55 who received a thiazide diuretic, 9 died of a myocardial infarction, whereas only 1 of 40 on a beta-blocker and 1 of 77 on no therapy or diet had a fatal MI [31].

In the absence of definitive evidence that one drug offers better protection than another, I would agree with the Joint National Committee that a diuretic is the best initial drug for almost every hypertensive [32].

THE APPROPRIATE GOAL OF THERAPY

Regardless of the drug chosen, the physician should have a clearly defined goal of therapy. In the past, a diastolic blood pressure of 90 mm Hg was generally accepted. Despite the occasional voice of dissent for a higher pressure as the goal [8], the recently published results of the HDFP and Australian trial will likely lead to a lowering of the goal to below 90 mm Hg.

As shown in Table 3, for those with mild hypertension the goal in both these trials was to bring the diastolic pressure to 90 mm Hg or lower. After two years the pressure was lowered to 80 mm Hg in the Australian trial. In the HDFP, those on stepped-care whose mean diastolic level was reduced to 83.4 had 20% less mortality than those receiving referred-care whose mean DBP was 87.8. Therefore, it seems logical that, in order to achieve the maximal benefits from therapy, the goal should be a pressure of less than 90 mm Hg, probably 85 mm Hg or even lower.

Whether the experts and the medical community will accept these lower levels as the appropriate goal remains to be seen. Epidemiological data can be found both to confirm and to deny the wisdom of a goal lower than 90 mm Hg. Support comes from the Life Insurance actuarial data [11] (Table 6). The least excess mortality among 20 000 hypertensive men receiving antihypertensive therapy at the time of their insurance exam was seen in those with the lowest pressures, less than 127 systolic and less than 83 diastolic.

On the other hand, a careful look at the Framingham data reveals that there was no decrease in cardiovascular morbidity (events) over 18 years of follow-up among those with diastolics below 90 mm Hg [33] (Figure 3). In fact, there is a hint of increased morbidity as the diastolics diminish from 90 down to 70 mm Hg. These low pressures are not the result of antihypertensive therapy, so it may be inappropriate to use them as evidence for possible harm when they are achieved in the treatment of hypertension. Nonetheless, the relationship between diastolic pressure and cardiovascular morbidity may be complicated and there may be a threshold for the greatest benefit to be achieved. At this time I would predict that a goal of 85 mm Hg for the diastolic pressure will be increasingly accepted and recommended.

It should be noted that the Framingham data show lower cardiovascular risk with progressively lower systolic pressures, even below 120 mm Hg. It may be necessary to include the systolic level as part of the goal of therapy, though most trials have disregarded it. The benefit of therapy for those with predominately or purely systolic hypertension has not yet been proved but is based on the clear evidence of increased risk when the pressure is left high

Table 6. Mortality experience among treated hypertensive insured men (1979)*

Systolic	<127	128–137	138–147	148–157	>158
Increased mortality	2%	10%	13%	66%	101%
Diastolic	<83	84–87	88–92	93–97	>98
Increased mortality	4%	24%	24%	67%	102%

* Selected sample of 20,000 on Rx before insurance [11].

898

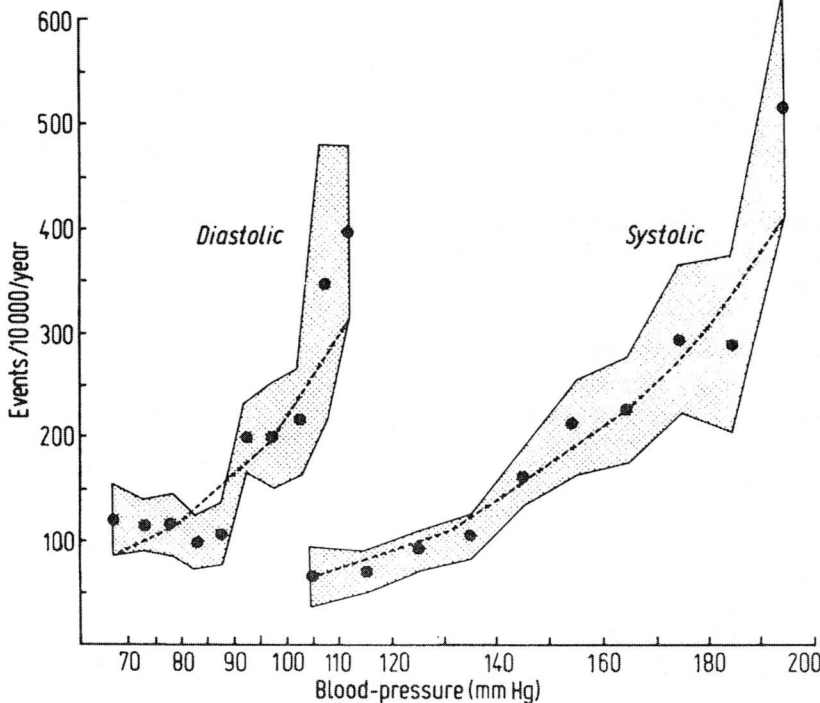

Figure 3. The annual incidence of cardiovascular events per 10 000 subjects in Framingham over 18 years of follow-up, by level of blood pressure for all ages. The individual dots are the means of both male and female rates, the broken lines are the logistic curves, and the shaded area the 95% confidence limits of the individual data points. (Reproduced with permission from reference [33].)

as well as on the epidemiological data that show a lesser risk with lower systolic pressures. The prudent course would now be to lower the systolic pressure to below 160 mm Hg and, if possible without bothersome side effects or large amounts of medications, to below 140 mm Hg. Hopefully, data about the benefits of treating systolic hypertension will soon be available. In the meantime, a gentle, gradual approach to lowering high systolic pressures should be taken.

THE NEED FOR A CHANGE IN ATTITUDE

Though the ideal goal for therapy has not been established, it should certainly be directed at attaining a pressure level that is lower than most practioners now believe. In response to the question: 'At what level of diastolic blood pressure would you begin to treat an asymptomatic 50-year-old man for hypertension?', 17 hospital staff physicians in Birmingham, England, stated they would start treatment in the range of 90–104 mm Hg; another would do so between 105 and 109 mm Hg, and 11 only if the diastolic were 110 mm Hg or higher [34].

The decision to start treatment should not be made lightly. Once started, therapy is likely to cause some side effects, hopefully transient, and it will probably have to be continued for the rest of the patient's life. However, with proper use of currently available drugs, along with appropriate non-drug therapies, almost all hypertensives can have their pressures brought and kept below 140/90. The long-term benefits of such therapy have been proved. What remains to be proved is the willingness of most practitioners to apply this knowledge to the full benefit of their hypertensive patients.

ACKNOWLEDGEMENTS

Supported by an Academic Award in Preventive Cardiology from the National Heart, Lung, and Blood Institute (Award #5-K07-HL00596).

REFERENCES

1. Kaplan NM: Therapy of hypertension. In: Clinical Hypertension, 3rd edn, pp. 105–110. Baltimore: Williams & Wilkins, 1982.
2. Stamler J, Farinaro E, Mojonnier LM, Hall Y, Moss D, Stamler R: Prevention and control of hypertension by nutritional-hygienic means. JAMA 243:1819–1823, 1980.
3. Harrington M, Kincaid-Smith P, McMichael J: Results of treatment in malignant hypertension. Br MedJ 2:969–980, 1959.
4. Veterans Administration Cooperative Study Group on Antihypertensive Agents: Effects of treatment on morbidity in hypertension. JAMA 202:116–122, 1967.
5. Veterans Administration Cooperative Study Group on Antihypertensive Agents: Effects of treatment on morbidity in hypertension – II. Results in patients with diastolic blood pressure averaging 90 through 114 mm Hg. JAMA 213:1143–1152, 1970.
6. Hypertension Detection and Follow-up Program Cooperative Group: Five-year findings of the hypertension detection and follow-up program. I. Reduction in mortality of persons with high blood pressure, including mild hypertension. JAMA 242:2562–2571, 1979.
7. Management Committee: The Australian therapeutic trial in mild hypertension. Lancet i:1261–1267, 1980.
8. Stewart I McD G: Relation of reduction in pressure to first myocardial infarction in patients receiving treatment for severe hypertension. Lancet I:861–865, 1979.
9. Hypertension Detection and Follow-Up Program Cooperative Group: The hypertension detection and follow-up program: a progress report. Circ Res40 (Suppl I):I-106–I-109, 1977.
10. Kannel WB, Dawber TR: Hypertension as an ingredient of a cardiovascular risk profile. Br J Hosp Med 11:508–523, 1974.
11. Society of actuaries: 1979 Build and Blood Pressure Study. Chicago 1980.
12. Shekelle RB, Ostfeld AM, Klawans HL: Hypertension and risk of stroke in an elderly population. Stroke5:71–75, 1974.

900

13. Spence JD, Sibbald WJ, Cape RD: Direct, indirect and mean blood pressures in hypertensive patients: the problem of cuff artefact due to arterial wall stiffness, and a partial solution. Clin Invest Med, 2:165–173, 1980.
14. Gillum RF: Pathophysiology of hypertension in blacks and whites: a review of the basis of racial blood pressure differences. Hypertension 1:468–475, 1979.
15. Laughlin KD, Sherrard DJ, Fisher L: Comparison of clinic and home blood pressure levels in essential hypertension and variables associated with clinic-home differences. J Chronic Dis 33:197–206, 1980.
16. Hypertension Detection and Follow-up Program Cooperative Group: Five-year findings of the hypertension detection and follow-up program — II. Mortality by race, sex and age. JAMA 242:2572–2577, 1979.
17. Peart WS, Miall WE: M.R.C. mild hypertension trial. Lancet, I:104–105, 1980.
18. Report of Medical Research Council Working Party on Mild to Moderate Hypertension: Randomised controlled trial of treatment for mild hypertension: design and pilot trial. Br Med J 1:1437–1440, 1977.
19. U.S. Public Health Service Hospitals Cooperative Study Group: Treatment of Mild hypertension: results of a ten-year intervention trial. Circ Res 40 (Suppl I):I-98–I-105, 1977.
20. Berglund G, Sannerstedt R, Anderson O, Wedel H, Wilhelmsen L, Hansson L, Sivertsson R, Wikstrand J: Coronary heart-disease after treatment of hypertension. Lancet I:1–5, 1978.
21. Kaplan NM: Treatment of severe hypertension. Lancet I:1140, 1979.
22. Ledingham JGG, Rajagopalan B: Cerebral complications in the treatment of accelerated hypertension. Q J Med 48:25–41, 1979.
23. Garraway WM, Whisnant JP, Furlan AJ, Phillips LH, Kurland LT, O'Fallon WM: The declining incidence of stroke. N Engl J Med 300:449–452, 1979.
24. Christie D: Improved survival from stroke: an effet of antihypertensive therapy? Med J Aust, 2:391–393, 1979.
25. Jennings GL, Esler MD, Korner PI: Effect of prolonged treatment on haemodynamics of essential hypertension before and after autonomic block. Lancet II:166–169, 1980.
26. De Carvalho JGR, Dunn FG, Lohmoller G, Frohlich ED: Hemodynamic correlates of prolonged thiazide therapy: comparison of responders and nonresponders. Clin Pharmacol Ther 22:875–880, 1977.
27. Lund-Johansen P: Hemodynamic consequences of long-term beta-blocker therapy: a 5-year follow-up study of atenolol. J Cardiovasc Pharmacol 1:487–495, 1979.
28. Beevers DG, Johnston J, Devine BL, Dunn FG, Larkin H, Titterington DM: Relation between prognosis and the blood pressure before and during treatment of hypertensive patients. Clin Sci Mol Med 55:333s–336s, 1978.
29. Andersen MP, Frederiksen J, Jurgensen HJ, Pedersen F, Bechsgaard P, Hansen DA, Nielsen B, Pedersen-Bjergaard O, Rasmussen SL: Effect of alprenolol on mortality among patients with definite or suspected acute myocardial infarction: preliminary results. Lancet II:865–868, 1979.
30. Laragh JH: Modern system for treating high blood pressure based on renin profiling and vasoconstriction-volume analysis: a primary role for beta blocking drugs such as propranolol. Am J Med 61:797–810, 1976.
31. Morgan T, Adam W, Carney S, Gibbard R, Brown S, Wheeler D: Treatment of mild hypertension in elderly males. Clin Sci 57:355s–357s, 1979.
32. Report of the Joint National Committee on Detection, Evaluation, and Treatment of High Blood Pressure. Arch Intern Med 140:1280–1285, 1980.
33. Anderson TW: Re-examination of some of the Framingham blood-pressure data. Lancet II:1139–1141, 1978.
34. Taylor L, Foster MC, Beevers DG: Divergent views of hospital staff on detecting and managing hypertension. Br Med J 1:715–716, 1979.

56. HYPERTENSIVE EMERGENCIES

RUNE SANNERSTEDT

1. INTRODUCTION

The widespread use of drugs today for active treatment of arterial hypertension has considerably reduced the number of patients with life-threatening blood pressure elevations that require acute measures and often include parenteral administration of blood pressure lowering agents. However, such states of various etiological backgrounds occasionally occur even today and will then need prompt care so as to avoid irreparable organ damages. The advent over the latest three decades of highly effective antihypertensive drugs with different mechanisms of action has made a correct handling of patients with hypertensive crises even more important than before, as their adequate use may safely reduce dangerously high blood pressure levels in the patient.

A number of conditions, underlying the common denominator of dangerously high blood pressure levels, but otherwise different with regard to etiology and pathophysiology, may be identified. As shown in Table 1, they may be subdivided according to symptomatology or according to etiology.

2. HYPERTENSIVE EMERGENCIES, SUBGROUPED ACCORDING TO SYMPTOMATOLOGY

2.1. Malignant hypertension

This condition, defined by the presence of papillary edema in the eyegrounds, hemorrhages and exudates, can be the end stage of severe arterial hypertension of any etiology. Although infrequent today in many countries with the advance of early antihypertensive treatment, it has to be ruled out in patients with diastolic blood pressures in the range of 130 mm Hg and above, especially if there are any visual symptoms present.

Hemodynamically, the salient features are often a hypokinetic circulation with markedly elevated mean arterial blood pressure, a grossly elevated systemic vascular resistance and a subnormal cardiac output.

Amery, A. (ed.) Hypertensive Cardiovascular Disease: Pathophysiology and Treatment
© 1982, Martinus Nijhoff Publishers. The Hague / Boston / London
ISBN-13: 978-94-009-7478-4

902

Table 1. Hypertensive emergencies

Subgrouped according to symptomatology	Subgrouped according to etiology
1. Malignant hypertension	1. Pheochromocytoma
2. Hypertensive encephalopathy	2. Paroxysmal hypertension
3. Left ventricular failure	3. Acute glomerulonephritis
	4. Eclampsia
	5. Dissecting aneurysm of the aorta
	6. Intracranial bleedings

2.2. Hypertensive encephalopathy

Just as malignant hypertension, hypertensive encephalopathy is a non-specific entity characterized by the presence of cerebral symptoms of varying severity up to general fits and unconsciousness, together with severe blood pressure elevation of varying etiology. However, hypertensive encephalopathy may sometimes occur in patients with more moderate blood pressure elevations in the range of 120 mm Hg diastolic.

Little is known about the systemic and local hemodynamics of hypertensive encephalopathy, but it is believed that the cerebral blood flow, through intensive vascular contraction, may cause severe impairments leading to ischemia of vital parts of the cerebrovascular bed. However, there are also indications, that hypertensive encephalopathy may be caused by cerebral hyperperfusion leading to cerebral edema and increased intracranial pressure.

2.3. Left ventricular failure

Left ventricular failure may be the result of any hypertensive disease severe enough to jeopardize the pumping ability of the myocardium. Usually, the high blood pressure has been present for an extended period of time, progressively turning the circulation into an afterload failure with low stroke volume and cardiac output.

3. HYPERTENSIVE EMERGENCIES CONNECTED WITH SPECIFIC ETIOLOGIES

3.1. Pheochromocytoma

In contrast to the abovementioned types, this type represents a hypertensive emergency of defined etiology. One important feature of pheochromocytoma is the disposition to cause hypertensive crises in connection with attack-wise influxes of catecholamines.

Depending on the relation between the incretion of epinephrine and norepinephrine different hemodynamic patterns may be expected, but usually tachycardia and an elevated cardiac output result.

Although rare, the possibility of a pheochromocytoma should always be kept in mind as the cause of a hypertensive crisis, as this will be of significance for the choice of acute treatment. Further, a correct diagnosis will lateron enable radical cure from an otherwise life-threatening condition.

3.2. Paroxysmal hypertension

A clinical picture similar to that of pheochromocytoma and similarly caused by excessive release of catecholamines may be seen in patients on monoamine oxidase (MAO) inhibitors in relation to ingestion of tyramine-rich foods like cheese.

Paroxysmal hypertension, occasionally leading to hypertensive crises can also occur after abrupt withdrawal of treatment with certain antihypertensive drugs, especially clonidine.

3.3. Acute glomerulonephritis

Another etiologically traceable disease that occasionally gives rise to hypertensive emergencies, is acute glomerulonephritis. Depending on the height of the blood pressure and the extent of cardiovascular involvement, the clinical picture may be dominated by cardiac failure or by hypertensive encephalopathy, or by the full-blown picture of malignant hypertension. Hemodynamically, a hyperdynamic circulation may be present with an increased cardiac output and a markedly elevated intravascular fluid volume.

3.4. Eclampsia

Another specific type of hypertensive emergency, although still of unknown etiology, is the severe hypertensive state seen during the latter stage of pregnancy. Typically, it is prone to general convulsions already at relatively low blood pressure levels with diastolic blood pressures not higher than in the range of 110 mm Hg.

Hemodynamically, the eclamptic state is characterized by an intense elevation of the systemic vascular resistance and, in relation to a normal pregnancy, a lowered intravascular fluid volume.

3.5. Dissecting aneurysm of the aorta

Although not regularly connected with alarmingly high blood pressure, dissecting aneurysms of the aorta should be included among hypertensive emergencies calling for immediate blood pressure lowering measures.

3.6. Intracranial bleedings

Subarachnoid and intracerebral hemorrhages are examples of other states that are often connected with dangerously high blood pressure levels indicating the prompt use of antihypertensive agents.

4. GENERAL MEASURES

Today we have at our disposal a wide range of potent pharmacological agents allowing us to acutely lower any increased blood pressure to predetermined levels. This may make us forget to take general, in themselves rather self-evident and simple measures that still play a vital part in the recovery of the patient.

4.1. Environment

A calm and quiet atmosphere will effectively help the patient to relax. Distressing factors like noise, dazzling light, uncomfortable room temperature etc. should actively be avoided.

4.2. Bed rest

Physical activity may increase any severely elevated blood pressure level. Therefore, patients with hypertensive emergencies should be kept at bed rest. Particularly, any type of static exercise should be avoided, as even low levels of isometric stress may lead to dramatic blood pressure increases, especially the diastolic blood pressure. The stress of toilsome bowel movements should be recognized, and tendencies to obstipation be counteracted.

4.3. Supervision

It goes without saying that the blood pressure has to be checked constantly with short intervals, using adequate recording technics and indicating the blood pressure figures on a special chart. Together with the measuring of the blood pressure it is advisable to record the pulse rate.

In addition, the general condition of the patient should be regularly observed, noticing any changes in the cerebral, cardiac and renal functions.

4.4. Sedation

If the patient is anxious and alarmed, a tranquilizing agent, preferably from the benzodiazepine group, should be given. Tricyclic antidepressants and MAO inhibitors are contraindicated, as they interfere with the circulatory regulation and may counteract the effect of antihypertensive agents.

4.5. Convulsion prophylaxis

Hypertensive patients who are judged to be in the risk zone for developing convulsions should be given adequate prophylaxis, including agents like barbiturates and benzodiazepines. In eclamptic patients magnesium sulphate has been widely used.

4.6. Fluid restriction

Patients with known or suspected hypervolemia and those prone to left ventricular failure may benefit from fluid restriction. A strict fluid balance record should be kept in such cases.

4.7. Diagnostics

Obviously, appropriate measures have to be taken to clarify the extent of any target organ engagement evaluating the status of the cerebral, cardiac and renal functions. The possibility of secondary hypertension, like pheochromocytoma, must be ruled out.

5. TREATMENT WITH ANTIHYPERTENSIVE AGENTS

When general measures as outlined above are taken adequately it is possible in many cases of apparent hypertensive emergencies to administer any specific antihypertensive agents via the oral route, thereby following the drug regimens presently suggested for the active pharmacological treatment of arterial hypertension.

However, parenteral administration has to be relied on in order to secure a rapid and effective blood pressure control in cases where general measures turn out to be insufficient, and in patients, who are in immediate danger of serious cerebral, cardiac or renal consequneces due to their blood pressure elevation. As soon as possible the parenteral therapy should then be exchanged for an appropriate oral medication, that may also be started parallel to and overlapping the parenteral treatment.

Below various aspects of the most common antihypertensive drugs for parenteral use are discussed. Some relevant features are summarized in Table 2.

5.1. Sympatholytic agents

5.1.1. Reserpine. This agent, depleting the body stores of catecholamines and serotonin, is probably the sympatholytic agent that has been in clinical use for the longest time and with which a considerable amount of practical experience has been gathered over the years.

Given intramuscularly or intravenously in a dose of 0.5–2.0 mg reserpine causes a slowly developing blood pressure decrease of moderate degree. The maximal effect is reached after 2–3 h. The duration of action is about 6–8 h, after which another injection may be given. Given more frequently, there is a risk for cumulative effects. Drastic blood pressure drops and orthostatic reactions are usually not seen, and the local circulations are not jeopardized.

The mechanism behind the blood pressure fall induced by reserpine is characterized by decreases of both the heart rate, cardiac output and systemic vascular resistance.

The delayed onset of action may in the individual case be of either positive or negative value, but makes the drug of limited value in patients, where rapid blood pressure lowering is indicated.

As side effects sedation and drowsiness may be seen, which in some cases may be of benefit and contribute to the clinical effect, while it is a definite drawback when evaluation of the patient's sensorium is critical, and when the drug is given repeatedly over a long period of time. Nose stuffiness occurs and may be annoying to the patient.

Today reserpine is of limited value for treating hypertensive emergencies, but it may occasionally still be used in patients in whom a moderate, slowly developing blood pressure decrease is wanted that does not require meticulous supervision.

Table 2. Antihypertensive drugs for parenteral treatment of hypertensive emergencies

Drug	Administration	Dose	Time to maximal effect	Duration of action	Note
Sympatholytic agents					
Reserpine	im, iv	0.5–2.0 mg	2–3 h	6–8 h	Causes sedation and drowsiness
Methyldopa	iv	250–500 mg	2–3 h	4–6 h	Causes sedation and drowsiness
Clonidine	sc, im, iv (slow)	150 μg	15–30 min	4–6 h	Causes sedation and drowsiness. Risk for rebound effects after withdrawal
Trimethaphan	iv (infusion)	0.5–10 mg/min	5–10 min	5–10 min	Very potent. Requires constant supervision
Adrenoceptor blockers					
Phentolamine	iv (rapid)	5–15 mg	1–2 min	10–15 min	Limited clinical usefulness
Propranolol and similar	iv	5–15 mg	–	–	No acute antihypertensive effects
Labetalol	iv	50–100 mg	2–4 min	4–10 h	Clinical experiences limited
Peripheral vasodilators					
Hydralazines	im, iv (slow)	5–20 mg	10–20 min	3–6 h	May raise intracranial pressure
Diazoxide	iv (bolus injection)	150 mg (may be repeated with 5–15 min intervals)	3–5 min	4–24 h	Very potent. Causes water retention and hyperglycemia
Sodium nitroprusside	iv (infusion)	25–250 μg/min	<1 min	2–3 min	Extremely potent. Requires meticulous supervision
Diuretic agents					
Furosemide or similar	iv	40–80 mg	2–4 h	12–24 h	No true antihypertensive effect. Contracts intravascular volume

5.1.2. Methyldopa. By and large this agent has a similar clinical profile as reserpine when given parenterally, but has the disadvantage of requiring the intravenous route.

As methyldopa in the acute situation does not offer any definite advantages over reserpine, its parenteral administration is rarely indicated.

5.1.3. Clonidine. This agent acts mainly through stimulation of central α-adrenoceptors. Given subcutaneously, intramuscularly or slowly intravenously in a dose of 150 µg it effects a fairly rapid blood pressure fall of moderate extent. The pressure decrease is maximal after 15–30 min and lasts for 4–6 h. Occasionally, more marked blood pressure drops may be seen to be accompanied by tendencies to orthostatic reactions.

Hemodynamically, decreases in heart rate and cardiac output are the main contributors to the decrease in blood pressure. Immediately after administration a brief period of blood pressure increase may be noticed. Unfavorable influences on local blood flows have been reported.

Although having a quite different mechanism of action, clonidine, just as reserpine, may give rise to sedation and somnolence, and this must be kept in mind when evaluation of the patient's sensorium is needed. It should also be pointed out that sudden withdrawal of clonidine after its repeated administration may result in rapid return of the blood pressure up to and above the initial level.

Clonidine may be regarded as an alternative to reserpine when a moderate blood pressure reduction is aimed at, and the onset of action is usually somewhat more rapid compared to that of reserpine. Like reserpine, clonidine has flexible possibilities for parenteral administration.

5.1.4. Trimethaphan. This is the only ganglionic blocking agent that blocks both sympathetic and parasympathetic ganglia, that still today will find some use in routine clinical practice. Given parenterally as a slow intravenous infusion of 0.5–10 mg/min, trimethaphan offers the possibility of continuous adjustment of the blood pressure to any predetermined level. The effect sets in promptly within a few minutes, and will then disappear within some minutes after stopping the infusion, thus allowing a precise titration of the blood pressure level.

The main hemodynamic effect is on the cardiac output, that is lowered due to decreases in both heart rate and stroke volume. The local blood flows will be reduced, and especially the cerebral, coronary and renal circulations may become negatively affected. The degree of blood pressure drop is highly dependent on body position, and severe orthostatic reactions may occur if the patient's head is raised.

A successful use of trimethaphan requires a meticulous control of the blood pressure. If overdosed, very low pressure levels can be attained endangering the blood supply to vital areas. Given over longer periods trimethaphan may give rise to troublesome symptoms of atonia from the bladder and bowel.

Trimethaphan is an agent to be used by specialists and cannot be recommended for general use. However, trimethaphan is still one of the most powerful antihypertensive agents allowing from-moment-to-moment adjustment of the blood pressure level.

5.2. α-adrenoceptor blocking agents

5.2.1. Phentolamine. This is the only α-adrenoceptor blocking drug, that has an established, albeit limited, clinical use. Thus, the only indication is hypertensive states associated with increased levels of circulating catecholamines.

Accordingly, the main use of phentolamine is to control hypertensive crises in patients with pheochromocytoma. Given rapidly, intravenously to such patients in a dose of 5–15 mg, it has an immediate effect bringing the elevated blood pressure down to normal or near-normal levels. However, the effect of a single injection is short-lived, usually lasting no longer than 10–15 min. To secure a continued blood pressure control using phentolamine, the initial injection must be followed by an intravenous infusion of phentolamine, which is adjusted to keep the blood pressure at an adequate level.

Other situations in which phentolamine may be used are hypertensive crises after sudden withdrawal of clonidine and in the rare patient with increased circulating amounts of catecholamines due to interaction between monoamine-oxidase (MAO) inhibitors and tyramine-rich foods.

Among the side effects that are caused by phentolamine when given parenterally, tachycardia and flushing are the most distressing ones.

5.3. β-adrenoceptor blocking agents

The β-adrenoceptor blocking agents have no immediate hypotensive effects generally; therefore, they are rarely indicated for the acute treatment of hypertensive emergencies. Tentatively, they could be tried in hypertensive states, where an increased heart rate and consequent elevated cardiac output are supposed to be main hemodynamic features behind the blood pressure elevation. Thus, β-adrenoceptor blockade may be expected to have favorable effects on both the heart rate and the blood pressure in the occasional patient with a combination of hyperthyreosis and severe arterial hypertension. Preferably, a β-adrenoceptor blocking agent without intrinsic sympathomimetic effect should then be used such as *propranolol*, given slowly intravenously in a dose of 5–15 mg.

5.4. α- and β-adrenoceptor blocking agents

5.4.1. Labetalol. This agent is a novel antihypertensive drug that is still not available for routine clinical use in many countries. It is characterized by having both α- and β-adrenoceptor blocking properties in a proportion of 1:3.

Labetalol can be given intravenously in doses of 50–100 mg. Maximal effect on the blood pressure has been said to be present already after 2–4 min and the effect will last for 4–10 h.

The experiences from the use of labetalol for treating hypertensive emergencies are still limited. Experimental studies in humans showing a prompt antihypertensive effect through lowering of both the cardiac output and the systemic vascular resistance suggest, however, that labetalol may be of benefit in hypertensive patients with tachycardia and other indications of increased levels of circulating catecholamines.

5.5. Peripheral vasodilators

5.5.1. Hydralazine. This agent and its congener *dihydralazine* have now been used for treatment of hypertension, both acutely and on a chronic basis, for more than 25 years.

Hydralazine acts directly on the smooth muscles of the small vessels on the arterial side producing a general vasodilatation. This results in a decrease of the systemic vascular resistance, which is the main hemodynamic feature behind the hypotensive effect of hydralazines. As a homeostatic reflex to maintain the systemic blood pressure, the heart rate and cardiac output increase.

Given intramuscularly or as a slow intravenous injection in a dose of 5–20 mg, hydralazine and dihydralazine usually achieve a moderate hypotensive effect within 10–20 min, which will then fade away during the next 3–6 h. Marked blood pressure drops may sometimes occur, possibly more often in elderly people. It is advisable, therefore, to use relatively low doses, and repeated rather than single injections, to patients over the age of 60.

As there is a possibility that, in the acute phase, hydralazines may raise the intracranial pressure, it might be recommendable not to use hydralazines for acute treatment of hypertensive disorders in patients with proven or suspected increases of the intracranial pressure.

Side effects are common and include, besides flushing, tachycardia and throbbing headache, as well as nose stuffiness.

Peripheral vasodilators, including hydralazines, presently experience a renaissance, as they are increasingly being used for treating both acute and chronic heart failure as they are supposed to improve the pump action of the heart by reducing afterload. Hydralazines might therefore be especially indicated in hypertensive patients with overt or incipient cardiac failure, where a favorable effect on the cardiac function may be anticipated in addition to the antihypertensive effect as such.

Thus, today hydralazines can still be of great benefit in the care of hypertensive emergencies, but a careful consideration is required to secure an optimal outcome.

5.5.2. Diazoxide. This agent is chemically closely related to the thiazides, but contrary to them has no diuretic properties at all. Instead, just as the hydralazines, it is a powerful peripheral vasodilator acting directly on the vascular wall muscles.

The hemodynamic profile of diazoxide is similar to that of hydralazines, i.e. it causes a decrease in systemic vascular resistance leading to blood pressure fall and compensatory increases of the heart rate and cardiac output.

Diazoxide given intravenously as a rapid bolus injection of 150 mg results in a drastic blood pressure drop in a majority of patients, lowering even extremely high blood pressures to normotensive levels within 3–5 min. Its effect duration is variable lasting from a few hours up to 24 hours or even more.

To obtain an optimal blood pressure lowering effect from diazoxide the drug must be injected very rapidly – within 10–20 sec. Given more slowly most of diazoxide (80–90%) is rapidly bound to serum albumin, which will reversibly render it inactive, and only a small fraction of the unchanged and active drug will reach the target organ, viz. the smooth muscle cells of the vessel wall.

Not only does diazoxide lack diuretic activity, it also has strong sodium and water retaining properties. If the drug has to be administered repeatedly, it is, therefore, recommendable to give a diuretic agent simultaneously. Diazoxide will also rapidly lead to hyperglycemia, and after prolonged administration diabetes eventually develops in a high proportion of the treated patients. Other side effects include nausea and flushing. These serious drawbacks of diazoxide strictly limit its use to the initial therapy of hypertensive emergencies. Its administration in repeated quantities should be done with adequate time intervals and under close observation of the glucose metabolism.

In spite of its disadvantages diazoxide has been shown to be a most valuable drug for the treatment of hypertensive emergencies making it possible to acutely lower almost any severely elevated blood pressure. Its great potency also means, however, that it has to be used with a great deal of caution in patients with deranged cerebral or coronary circulations in whom abrupt blood pressure falls may turn out to be detrimental.

5.5.3. Sodium nitroprusside. This agent is another peripheral vasodilator exerting its action directly on the smooth muscles of the small vessels at both the arterial and the venous side of the circulation. As a result sodium nitroprusside does not cause any compensatory increase in the cardiac output. However, just as hydralazines and diazoxide its hypotensive effect is accomplished through a marked decrease of the systemic vascular resistance.

Administered as an intravenous infusion at a rate of 25–250 µg/min sodium nitroprusside promptly affects the blood pressure within seconds. The blood pressure lowering effect is very short-lived lasting only for a couple of minutes after stopping the infusion. This, together with the prompt onset of action, will allow an exact titration of the blood pressure to any level aimed at. Naturally, the blood pressure must be continuously supervised, if too abrupt swings are to be avoided.

Sodium nitroprusside is metabolised to thiocyanate, that may accumulate and cause psychic symptoms. If treatment with sodium nitroprusside is extended over several days, it is advisable therefore to look for any signs of impending thiocyanate intoxication such as confusion and, if possible, to analyse the blood for its content of thiocyanate.

Similar to other potent blood pressure reducing agents sodium nitroprusside may precipitate cerebral or coronary symptoms in patients with insufficient circulations in these areas, if the blood pressure is allowed to fall too steeply.

Provided that the local pharmacy can supply with fresh solutions of sodium nitroprusside, that is not commercially available in many countries, and further that adequate patient supervision can be arranged, sodium nitroprusside is a highly effective hypotensive agent that will allow precise blood pressure control in all kinds of hypertensive emergencies. It is effective also in cases where other remedies, including diazoxide, have failed.

5.6. Diuretic agents

Among the manifold types and groups of diuretic agents available for routine clinical use, only so called high-ceiling diuretics can be justified as part of the therapeutic arsenal for the acute treatment of hypertensive emergencies. Generally speaking, diuretic agents have no acute hypotensive effects, and their antihypertensive effect in connection with its diuretic action takes several days before it becomes optimal. The diuresis leads to shrinkage of the circulating blood volume and a subsequent decrease in the cardiac output, which will eventually result in a blood pressure fall of moderate extent.

5.6.1. Furosemide. This agent, or one of its derivatives, is the drug of choice when using a high-ceiling diuretic to treat hypertensive emergencies. One reason for this is that furosemide, contrary to ethacrynic acid, another high-ceiling diuretic, does not seem to carry the risk of provoking acute deafness when given parenterally.

Given intravenously in doses of 40–80 mg, furosemide will induce a prompt diuresis to such a degree as to accomplish a substantial fall in the circulating blood volume within hours. It will be especially indicated to patients in whom fluid retention and enlarged intravascular volumes are part of the hemodynamic pattern of their hypertensive disease, and in such cases furosemide may be expected to achieve a blood pressure drop as the blood volume shrinks and the cardiac output declines.

Furosemide administered acutely may also benefit hypertensive patients with established or impending left heart failure, in whom the diuresis induced by furosemide decreases preload and unloads the pumping action of the heart.

Finally, furosemide or one of its congeners may be used to neutralize any sodium and water retaining effect caused by antihypertensive agents that have such properties, e.g. peripheral vasodilators like diazoxide, and sympathetic inhibitors like trimethaphan.

When furosemide is used for treating hypertensive emergencies, the risk for provoking potassium depletion must always be kept in mind, especially in patients already in a state of electrolyte imbalance due to, e.g., aldosteronism, and in patients on digitalis. However, on the whole parenteral administration of furosemide may be considered to be fairly safe and of benefit in all patients with established or impendent volume overload.

6. GENERAL CONCLUSIONS

Many cases of seemingly alarming cases of hypertensive emergencies may be treated simply by relying on general measures. This is particularly true of patients in whom anxiety etc. significantly contributes to rise in blood pressure from the level of an average benign hypertensive disease to the alarmingly high level of accelerated hypertension and true hypertensive crisis.

Nevertheless, patients with truly life-threatening blood pressure increases are a clinical reality. They represent a wide range of different conditions,

914

Table 3. Drug suggestions for treatment of hypertensive emergencies

Clinical background	Suggested drug treatment				Avoid
	Preferred drug	Alternative drug(s)	Supporting therapy	In resistant cases	
Severe hyp. (diast. BP ≧140 mmHg) but no symptoms from target organs	Diazoxide	Hydralazine Labetalol Clonidine	Furosemide	Na-nitropruss. Trimethaphan	
Hypertensive encephalopathy	Diazoxide	Labetalol	Furosemide	Na-nitropruss. Trimethapan	Hydralazines, reserpine, methyldopa, clonidine
Hypertensive stroke	Labetalol	Diazoxide		Na-nitropruss.	Hydralazines, reserpine, methyldopa, clonidine
Eclampsia	Diazoxide	Hydralazines	Mg-sulphate	Na-nitropruss.	Furosemide
Catecholamine excess	Phentolamine	Na-nitropruss.	Propranolol		
Severe hyp. with volume overload/left heart failure	Furosemide	Hydralazines		Na-nitropruss. Trimethaphan	Diazoxide
Severe hyp. with coronary insufficiency	Labetalol	Reserpine Clonidine	Furosemide	Na-nitropruss.	Hydralazines, trimethaphan
Diss. aneurysms of the aorta	Trimethaphan	Labetalol		Na-nitropruss.	
Severe hyp. with renal insufficiency	Hydralazines	Diazoxide Labetalol	Furosemide	Na-nitropruss.	Diazoxide, hydralazines

and Table 3 summarizes the type of pharmacological approach that is most appropriate for the treatment of the individual patient, both from an etiological and pathophysiological point of view.

In this chapter emphasis has been laid on the fact that today the main problem is not how to lower a severely elevated blood pressure, but how to achieve this without exposing the patient to cerebrocardiovascular impairment. Recent reports have stated that patients with malignant hypertension have become permanently blind when their blood pressure levels apparently were reduced too drastically [1]. Therefore, rapid blood pressure lowering and parenteral administration of potent antihypertensive agents should only be resorted to on very strict indications, and in situations when the physician in charge feels convinced that the level of the blood pressure is a serious threat to the patient.

REFERENCE

1. Editorial: Dangerous antihypertensive treatment, Br Med J 2:228–229, 1979.

57. ANESTHESIA AND SURGERY IN THE HYPERTENSIVE PATIENT

LEE GOLDMAN

Because of the prevalence of hypertension in the adult population, a substantial proportion of major surgical procedures will be performed on patients who either are hypertensive or are receiving antihypertensive medications. Such patients represent a challenge to the internist, the surgeon, and the anesthesiologist, not only because of the association of hypertension with more serious cardiovascular disease but also because of the special attention that must be given to such patients during anesthesia and surgery.

GENERAL PREOPERATIVE CONSIDERATIONS

Because of the stress associated with hospital admission, it is common for a patient to be more hypertensive than usual when he or she is first admitted. Later during the hospitalization, however, the blood pressure readings of a hypertensive patient are often better controlled in the hospital than they had been when the patient was ambulatory. Such an observation may be partly related to the forced compliance with antihypertensive medications and the restricted salt diets that often accompany hospitalization, but it is also likely that bed rest alone contributes to better antihypertensive control.

The first decision to be made regarding the hypertensive patient about to undergo surgery is whether or not to continue the medications up to the morning of surgery. Early studies [1–3] suggested that patients receiving reserpine were at higher risk for intraoperative hypotension if the medication were continued up to the day of surgery. Later studies, however, suggested that all hypertensive patients had more labile blood pressures than did nonhypertensive patients, but that the risk of such lability in patients whose blood pressures were treated medically was not greater than the risk among patients whose blood pressures were left untreated [4, 5]. Prys-Roberts and colleagues [6, 7], in a series of elegant hemodynamic studies, also found greater absolute changes in intraoperative blood pressures among patients with higher preoperative blood pressure values. In their early report [6], Prys-Roberts et al. showed markedly lower intraoperative blood

Amery, A. (ed.) Hypertensive Cardiovascular Disease: Pathophysiology and Treatment
© *1982, Martinus Nijhoff Publishers. The Hague / Boston / London*
ISBN-13: 978-94-009-7478-4

pressure values in untreated hypertensive patients, but in a subsequent report they showed no significant difference between the treated and untreated hypertensive patients at any time after the induction of anesthesia [7]. Based on their findings regarding intraoperative hypotension and on the presumption that continuation of the relatively short-acting antihypertensive medications may reduce the probability of postoperative hypertension, Prys-Roberts and his colleagues suggested that antihypertensive medications be continued up to and including the morning of surgery, and that perhaps untreated hypertensive patients should have their blood pressures controlled prior to elective surgery [8].

In a large epidemiologic study, my colleagues and I [9] demonstrated that the mean intraoperative systolic blood pressure nadir was not different among hypertensive patients based on whether the patient had been made normotensive by therapy, had remained hypertensive despite therapy, or was untreated. Similarly, the percentage of patients who required intraoperative fluid challenges or adrenergic agents to maintain blood pressure was not different, based on the degree of preoperative, antihypertensive control (see Table 1). However, because the preoperative systolic blood pressure values were higher among the inadequately treated and untreated hypertensive groups, their absolute blood pressure declines during surgery were larger than those found among the group of patients who had been made nor-

Table 1. Systolic blood pressure changes during elective surgery under general anesthesia in hypertensive patients

	Preoperative systolic blood pressure (mean +/− SEM) [a]	Lowest intra operative systolic blood pressure (mean +/− SEM) [b]	Percent of patients receiving a fluid challenge [c] or adrenergic agents to maintain blood pressure [a]
1. History of hypertension, normotensive on therapy (n = 79)	136±2 mmHg	100±2 mmHg	20
2. Hypertension persists despite anti-hypertensive medications (n = 40)	154±2 mmHg	97±3 mmHg	33
3. Untreated hypertension (n = 77)	161±2 mmHg	98±2 mmHg	27

[a] Each group is significantly (P≤0.05) different from each other group.
[b] No significant differences among the three groups.
[c] Defined as 500 ml in no more than 15 min or 1000 ml in no more than 30 min.
From Goldman et al. [9], with permission of the American Society of Anesthesiologists, Lippincott, Harper & Row, Park Ridge, IL, U.S.A.

motensive by therapy. In our series, the blood pressure changes observed during anesthesia and surgery did not vary according to whether the medications had been continued up to the morning of surgery or had been discontinued 24 or more hours preoperatively.

Based on present data, it appears that elective anesthesia and surgery can be performed without risking severe intraoperative hypotension when antihypertensive medications are continued up to the morning of surgery. Also, provided that the preoperative diastolic blood pressure is stable and is no higher than 115 mm Hg and that the patient is carefully monitored through the intraoperative and recovery room period, elective anesthesia and surgery need not be postponed until adequate hypertensive control is achieved [9, 10].

PREOPERATIVE MEDICATION GUIDELINES

The first major intervention associated with anesthesia and surgery is premedication. Premedication is recommended in the hypertensive patient, especially because apprehension may result in severe hypertension. However, the potential side effects of the drugs used for premedication must be kept in mind. Benzodiazepines, such as diazepam, may cause substantial hypotension when given intravenously, but usually cause less blood pressure changes when given orally. Intramuscular diazepam should be avoided because of its erratic absorption. Premedication with narcotics such as morphine tends to decrease venous return and hence to lower systemic blood pressure. Premedication with phenothiazine derivatives causes peripheral arterial dilatation and can also lower systemic blood pressure.

There are several antihypertensive agents that are associated with specific potential problems during the perioperative period. Clonidine, whose association with severe rebound hypertension is a subject of debate [11–13], should be continued orally up to and including the morning of surgery.

Both guanethidine and reserpine exert their antihypertensive effects partly by causing depletion of norepinephrine at adrenergic sites. If such patients develop hypotension, indirect agents such as ephedrine, which acts largely by causing a secondary release of norepinephrine from nerve endings, may have a markedly blunted effect. Conversely, the use of direct acting agents such as norepinephrine, methoxamine, or phenylephrine may cause exaggerated hypertension based on the denervation–hypersensitivity principle.

Although it was originally feared that propranolol might be dangerous in patients undergoing anesthesia [14], two subsequent studies [15, 16] did not show any increased risk. Similarly, a careful hemodynamic study of patients undergoing coronary artery bypass surgery showed that patients on propranolol had slightly lower heart rates during intubation and surgery, but were

919

able to maintain cardiac outputs, arterial blood pressures, stroke volumes, and peripheral arterial resistances that were similar to those of patients who were not on propranolol [17]. Prys-Roberts and colleagues, in their study of noncardiac surgery in hypertensive patients, also showed that pretreatment with beta-adrenergic agents resulted in less tachycardia, cardiac arrhythmias, hypertension, and ischemia by electrocardiogram during laryngoscopy and intubation without causing any recognized complications [18]. Further data from Prys-Roberts and his group suggest that patients who take less than 7 mg/kg of propranolol per day (480 mg or less in the average size person) have normal responses to atropine and usually do not have excessive bradycardia when given drugs such as neostigmine [19]. Patients on propranolol, however, do have consistently blunted responses to beta-adrenergic agents such as isoproterenol. Prys-Roberts has suggested that in order to increase the heart rate by 20 beats per minute the patient must receive a 10 µg bolus of isoproterenol if the daily propranolol dose was 120 mg, a 30 µg bolus if the daily dose was 240 mg, an 80 µg bolus if the daily dose was 480 mg, and higher doses if the propranolol dose was even higher [19]. It is important to remember that hypotension and bradycardia in the patient on propranolol should first be treated with atropine and/or isoproterenol; treatment with pure alpha-adrenergic agents such as methoxamine or phenylephrine may cause marked hypertension because the patient's usual beta-adrenergic response to alpha-adrenergic agents will be blunted. Similarly, epinephrine may cause a pure alpha-adrenergic response because its alpha-adrenergic effects will be unopposed while its beta-adrenergic effects will be blunted by the propranolol. Because of the small but real risk of propranolol withdrawal rebound [20–22], continuation of the medication up to and including the morning of surgery is recommended, especially if prior use of propranolol has played an important role in controlling angina [23].

Patients who are receiving chronic thiazide diuretics probably have some reduction in blood volume, although such reductions are less dramatic when the patient receives chronic thiazide therapy than when the patient receives acute therapy [24, 25]. The implications of this 5–20% reduction in chronic blood volume and also of the hypokalemia commonly associated with thiazide therapy will be discussed later.

INDUCTION, LARYNGOSCOPY AND INTUBATION

The next major stress that the surgical patient undergoes is the induction of anesthesia. With the exception of ketamine, all agents used for the induction of anesthesia often lower the blood pressure. Such decreases in blood pressure are usually 20–30% in healthy patients but may be substantially greater in hypertensive patients [26].

Laryngoscopy and tracheal intubation commonly cause a modest 20–30 mm Hg increase in arterial pressure in the normal patient, but they may cause dramatic increases in blood pressure in the hypertensive patient [26]. Among the patients studied by Prys-Roberts, such hypertensive episodes during intubation were associated with evidence of myocardial ischemia by electrocardiography in at least 40% of patients [6, 7]. Because the main stimulus for hypertension appears to be laryngoscopy rather than a passage of a tube into the trachea, topical anesthesia of the upper airways, larynx, and trachea may blunt this hypertensive response if it can be performed without prior laryngoscopy. Similarly, blind nasal intubation is associated with substantially less hypertension than is laryngoscopy with direct intubation [27]. Beta-adrenergic blockade is also effective in reducing the degree of hypertension induced by laryngoscopy and intubation [27].

MAINTENANCE OF ANESTHESIA

For the maintenance of anesthesia, the degree of reduction in systolic blood pressure appears to be similar under both general anesthesia and spinal anesthesia [28], whereas epidural anesthesia may be associated with a slightly greater degree of hypotension than is found with spinal anesthesia [29]. As shown in Tables 1 and 2, systolic blood pressure often falls to a nadir in the 95–100 mm Hg range during general anesthesia. Such nadirs are often brief, and the blood pressure may respond to a lightening of the anesthesia. In 20–30% of patients, however, either a brisk fluid challenge or the use of an intravenous adrenergic agent will be needed to maintain the blood pres-

Table 2. Systolic blood pressure changes during elective surgery under general anesthesia in always normotensive patients

	Preoperative systolic blood pressure (mean +/− SEM)	Lowest intra operative systolic blood pressure (mean +/− SEM)	Percent of patients receiving a fluid challenge or adrenergic agents to maintain blood pressure*
1. Always normotensive, not receiving diuretics (n = 431)	126±1 mmHg	94±1 mmHg	19
2. Always normotensive, receiving diuretics for other reasons (n = 49)	129±3 mmHg	95±3 mmHg	18

* P = N.S.

From Goldman et al. [9], with permission of the American Society of Anesthesiologists, Lippincott/Harper & Row, Park Ridge, Illinois, U.S.A.

sure (see Table 2). In our experience, neither the intraoperative systolic blood pressure nadir nor the need for fluid or adrenergic agents to maintain blood pressure was any different in normotensive patients on no diuretics than in always normotensive patients who were on diuretics for reasons other than hypertension [9]. Thus, although chronic diuretics seem to cause a mild decrease in blood volume, patients on chronic diuretics do not appear to be at substantially increased risk for intraoperative hypotension.

Among the various anesthetic agents, nitrous oxide, usually given in a 50–75% concentration, will result in a modest (15%) decrease in cardiac performance [30], but arterial pressure is usually rather well-maintained because of a reflex vasoconstriction. Conversely, halothane results in fairly similar degrees of myocardial depression but seems to inhibit reflex vasoconstriction. In our experience, halothane anesthesia was an independently significant correlate of the intraoperative systolic blood pressure nadir [9]. Similarly, Prys-Roberts [7] found that halothane, when combined with nitrous oxide, resulted in further blood pressure reductions because of decreased cardiac output without a change in peripheral vascular tone. The data from these two sources suggest that the use of halothane in hypertensive patients is associated with a higher risk of intraoperative hypotension.

During artificial ventilation, it is common for the PCO_2 to fall and for systemic vascular resistance to increase as a result of the hypocapnia [7]. Another potential problem associated with artificial ventilation and hypocapnia is related to changes in the distribution of potassium as a result of the associated alkalosis. The patient who has a borderline serum potassium value preoperatively may have a markedly decreased serum potassium value when alkalosis is acutely induced by hyperventilation. Such a risk is especially common now that many hypertensive patients are being maintained without supplemental potassium because of evidence that mild hypokalemia has no important side effects in otherwise healthy ambulatory hypertensive patients who are not receiving digitalis [31]. It is imperative that hypertensive patients receiving diuretics have a serum potassium value checked prior to surgery and that potassium supplements be given if the preoperative potassium level is below 3.5. If the patient is on digitalis, some experts would want the potassium to be at least 4.0.

If fluids must be given in large quantities to treat intraoperative hypotension, it must be remembered that such fluid therapy may result in fluid overload during the postoperative course. This is especially likely because antidiuretic hormone and aldosterone secretion will increase during surgery, therefore reducing free water and sodium clearances. It may be advisable to restrict the salt intake of the severe hypertensive patient to no more than the equivalent of one liter of normal saline per 24 h for the first two postoperative days. Postoperative fluid overload may present with symptoms of congestive heart failure, but it may also present as postoperative hypertension without clear signs of heart failure.

Not surprisingly, more extensive operative procedures are more likely to be associated with intraoperative hypotension. For example, in my own experience [9], anesthesiologists used fluid challenges or adrenergic agents to maintain blood pressure in 39% of patients having abdominal aortic aneurysm resections, in 25% of patients having intraperitoneal or intra-thoracic operations, in 24% of patients having peripheral vascular procedures, but in only 14% of patients having other major noncardiac operations. In that series, the type of operative procedure was the single most important predictor of the probability that a fluid challenge or adrenergic agents would be required. Among patients with a history of hypertension, however, the use of halothane anesthesia was a second independently significant correlate.

PERIOPERATIVE HYPERTENSION

As noted above, systolic blood pressure commonly increases acutely during laryngoscopy and intubation, but such blood pressure responses are short-lived. During the operative procedure, marked hypertension is unusual because of the hypotensive effects of most general anesthetic agents. There are, however, several exceptions to this general rule: intraoperative hypertension may develop because of manipulation of the aorta or the carotid arteries, or it may develop during intracranial procedures. Also, if the anesthesia is too light, painful stimuli may elevate the blood pressure.

Hypertension during anesthesia can be controlled by the use of hydralazine (as described below) or by the use of halothane or enflurane in concentrations high enough to lower the blood pressure. These anesthetic agents lower blood pressure primarily by reducing cardiac output, and therefore they may produce diminished tissue perfusion or central nervous system depression during the early recovery period. In addition, such patients are at risk for the recurrence of hypertension in the recovery room.

The most common time for perioperative hypertension to occur is in the recovery room. As shown in Table 3, patients with a past history of hypertension develop perioperative hypertensive episodes in 20–27% of cases, whereas normotensive patients develop perioperative hypertension only 6–8% of the time. Among patients with a history of hypertension, our data [9] indicated that the risk of perioperative hypertension was not dependent on the degree of preoperative blood pressure control, but patients who had higher prehospital blood pressure values, especially if their diastolic values had been above 110 mm Hg, were at greater risk for perioperative hypertension [9]. Thus, it appears that the risk of perioperative hypertension is more

923

Table 3. Risk of perioperative hypertension in patients having elective surgery under general anesthesia

	Percent of patients with perioperative hypertension*
1. Always normotensive, not receiving diuretics (n = 431)	8
2. Always normotensive, receiving diuretics for other reasons (n = 49)	6
3. History of hypertension, normotensive on therapy (n = 79)	27
4. Hypertension persists despite anti-hypertensive medications (n = 40)	25
5. Untreated hypertension (n = 77)	20

* Defined as a patient who had an intraoperative or recovery room systolic blood pressure above 200 mmHg or more than 50 mmHg above its preoperative value, or as a patient who received intravenous antihypertensive medications for the expressed purpose of lowering blood pressure.
From Goldman et al. [9], with permission of the American Society of Anesthesiologists, Lippincott/Harper & Row, Park Ridge, Illinois, U.S.A.

dependent on the patient's history, and hence on the underlying severity of the hypertensive state, rather than on the immediate preoperative blood pressure.

Another independently significant correlate of perioperative hypertension is the type of operative procedure. In our experience [9], hypertensive events occurred during or after 57% of abdominal aortic aneurysm resections, 29% of peripheral vascular procedures (including carotid endarterectomies), 8% of intraperitoneal or intrathoracic procedures, and only 4% of other noncardiac, nonneurologic procedures. Similarly, Lehv and colleagues [32] have reported the increased risk of postoperative hypertension among patients having carotid endarterectomies.

Postoperative hypertension usually occurs soon after the end of anesthesia: in the series by Gal and Cooperman [33], about 80% of perioperative hypertensive episodes occurred within 30 min after the end of anesthesia and virtually all cases occurred within 60 min after the end of anesthesia. In their series, the mean duration of hypertension was approximately two hours, and complications of the hypertension occurred only in patients whose hypertension lasted for three hours or longer. Although my colleagues and I [9] found no association between the type of anesthesia and the incidence of perioperative hypertension, Gal and Cooperman [33] found significantly more hypertension after procedures performed using fluroxene.

In additional to the factors such as a history of hypertension and the type of operative procedure that are associated with perioperative hypertension, early postoperative problems may often precipitate the hypertension. In the series by Gal and Cooperman [33], conditions such as pain, sudden excitement, a reaction to or discomfort with the endotracheal tube, hypercarbia, hypoxia, hypothermia, and fluid overload were commonly associated with hypertensive events.

Based on these common correlates of hypertensive events, it is not surprising that many such events will be treated most effectively by measures other than the intravenous use of specific antihypertensive medications. The patient must be carefully examined, and then interventions such as small doses of intravenous narcotics for pain, oxygen for hypoxia, improved ventilation for hypercarbia, warming blankets for hypothermia, furosemide for fluid overload, or the appropriate removal of an endotracheal tube may be the best way to abort the hypertensive event.

A subgroup of patients, however, will either not have such precipitating factors or have persistent hypertension despite the appropriate treatment of abnormalities that were present at the time the hypertension began. In such patients, the precise blood pressure values that warrant therapy are uncertain. Some anesthesiologists will not allow diastolic blood pressure in adults to remain over 100 mm Hg for a prolonged period, whereas others will use a diastolic blood pressure above 120 mm Hg or a systolic blood pressure above 200 mm Hg for any prolonged period of time as their thresholds for therapy [34].

The most uniformly safe and effective treatment for severe hypertension in the postoperative period, especially if the hypertension is associated with myocardial ischemia or marked congestive heart failure, is nitroprusside. Nitroprusside, prepared as 50 mg/500 cc of 5% glucose in water, will have an onset of action in less than 1 min, maximum action within 2 min, and a duration of action of only about 5 min. Thus, intravenous nitroprusside is quickly effective but can be tapered rapidly. Such intravenous infusions of nitroprusside require constant monitoring of blood pressure and nitroprusside dose, and the medication is most safely used if the patient has an intra-arterial catheter in place for the monitoring of blood pressure.

A more frequently used antihypertensive agent in the recovery room is hydralazine. Although hydralazine is effective intramuscularly, absorption from intramuscular sites will be erratic in the postoperative patient and therefore intravenous therapy is preferred. For a diastolic blood pressure above 120 mg or for evidence of congestive heart failure, hydralazine can be given usually as a 5 mg intravenous dose, most safely preceded by a 2.0 or 2.5 mg test dose. The dose can be repeated every 10 min, and doses as large as 10 mg can be given once the patient's response to the medication has been assessed. The main complication of hydralazine is a reflex tachycardia that may aggravate myocardial ischemia, especially if such ischemia has already been precipitated by the hypertension itself. If the heart rate is above 100 beats per minute and if there is no evidence of congestive heart failure, propranolol should be given at a rate up to 1 mg intravenously every 5 min to keep the heart rate below 100 in a patient who is also receiving hydralazine. Such treatment with propranolol is also appropriate in the occasional cases where intravenous hydralazine precipitates supraventricular tachycardia or frequent premature ventricular contractions.

Because most postoperative patients will have at least some degree of pain, small doses of morphine, usually given in 2 or 2.5 mg increments intravenously, should usually accompany specific antihypertensive therapy. Similarly, intravenous furosemide, usually given as a 40 mg bolus, will cause an almost immediate peripheral vasodilatation that is later followed by diuresis; such therapy is mandatory in patients with signs of fluid overload, but is often helpful in patients in whom gross fluid overload is not clinically evident, especially if such patients have received substantial intravenous fluids during the operative procedure.

Some anesthesiologists [26] also use chlorpromazine in doses of 5-10 mg when systolic hypertension is not associated with tachycardia. However, such therapy will often cause the patient to sleep deeply for several hours, and the peripheral vasodilation induced by chlorpromazine may result in a marked reflex tachycardia.

Diazoxide, which is commonly used for hypertensive crises in the emergency room, is rarely required in the operating room or in the recovery room. Methyldopa does not have its onset of action for 2-3 h or its peak of action for 3-5 h, even when given intravenously. Although this agent is therefore inappropriate for the acute control of severe hypertension, its delayed onset of action and a duration of 6-12 h will help to control blood pressure after the more acute medications have lost their effects. Similarly, methyldopa is an excellent agent for patients who have mild to moderate degrees of postoperative hypertension but who do not have severe hypertension or hypertension complicated by congestive heart failure or myocardial ischemia.

If a patient on clonidine preoperatively develops perioperative hypertension, clonidine can be given intramuscularly as needed, usually in doses that are about one-half as large as the patient's chronic daily dose [13]. If such treatment is not available or is not successful, treatment with methyldopa, propranolol, or chlorpromazine will often be successful.

In the patient who has been taking propranolol, propranolol withdrawal rebound usually will not occur in the recovery room. This is because propranolol, although it has a plasma half-life of only about 6.5 h, has a tissue half-life of about 24 h. Thus, in a recent study [22], abrupt discontinuation of propranolol did not result in supersensitivity to isoproterenol until 2-6 (median 4) days after propranolol withdrawal; such supersensitivity lasted for 3-13 (median 6) days, with a maximum sensitivity on about day six.

The signs of increased beta-adrenergic activity or of the propranolol withdrawal syndrome are tachycardia, hypertension, and electrocardiographic ischemia. If the clinician can be sure that such postoperative findings are not caused by fluid overload, agitation, hypoxia, or blood loss, the reinstitution of propranolol is mandatory. If the patient can take medications orally or via a nasogastric tube, propranolol should be reinstituted orally. Often, a patient with an otherwise non-functional gastrointestinal tract will absorb sufficient propranolol if the nasogastric tube is clamped for one hour after each dose. Patients will rarely require prophylactic intravenous propranolol if the propranolol was being used for hypertension, but patients may require intravenous medication if they were taking the propranolol for angina. If marked hypertension, which is thought to be related to propranolol withdrawal, develops, the patient can be treated with intravenous nitroprusside followed by intravenous methyldopa or can receive intravenous propranolol. If the propranolol is given intravenously, it should be given as a 0.5–1 mg test dose, with a second or third mg given carefully at 5–10 min intervals to control the syndrome. Subsequently, propranolol can be given as 1 mg intravenously every 20–60 min or, after a total loading dose of about 5–10 mg over 60 min, the patient can be given a constant infusion of 0.01–0.05 mg/minute [35].

BLOOD PRESSURE LABILITY AND MAJOR CARDIOVASCULAR COMPLICATIONS

In our series, after controlling for other cardiac risk factors [28, 36], hypertension, whether treated adequately, treated inadequately, or left untreated, was not correlated with the probability of cardiovascular complications. While other studies have shown a correlation between preoperative hypertension and cardiovascular complications, it is probably because the importance of other preoperative cardiac conditions that may be associated with hypertension, such as the degree of left ventricular dysfunction or the presence of arrhythmias or of a recent myocardial infarction, were not taken into account.

Although prolonged perioperative hypertension may cause acute or more long-lasting electrocardiographic findings, in our series there was no correlation between perioperative hypertensive events and postoperative cardiovascular complications [9]. Similarly, brief hypotensive events are usually well-tolerated, even if the blood pressure falls to rather low levels. However, if the systolic blood pressure is reduced by 33% or more for more than 10 min or by 50% during the operation, the risk of major perioperative cardiovascular complications is increased significantly even after all other factors have been taken into consideration [9, 37].

SUMMARY

The hypertensive patient who has major noncardiac surgery faces a variety of potentially serious problems. Nevertheless, the combination of careful preoperative preparation and close intraoperative and postoperative monitoring has permitted such patients to undergo all types of surgical procedures at an acceptable risk.

REFERENCES

1. Foster MW Jr, Gayle RJ JR: Dangers in combining reserpine (serpasil) with electroconvulsive therapy. JAMA 159:1520-1522, 1955.
2. Coakley CS, Alpert S, Boling JS: Circulatory responses during anesthesia of patients on rauwolfia therapy. JAMA 161:1143-1144, 1956.
3. Ziegler CH, Lovette JB: Operative complications after therapy with reserpine and reserpine compounds. JAMA 176:916-919, 1961.
4. Munson WM, Jenicek JA: Effect of anesthetic agents in patients receiving reserpine therapy. Anesthesiology 23:741-745, 1962.
5. Katz RL, Weintraub HD, Papper EM: Anesthesia, surgery and rauwolfia. Anesthesiology. 25:142-147, 1964.
6. Prys-Roberts C, Meloche R, Foëx P: Studies of anesthesia in relation to hypertension. I: Cardiovascular responses of treated and untreated patients. Br J Anaesth 43:112-137, 1971.
7. Prys-Roberts C, Foëx P, Greene LT, Waterhouse TD. Studies of anesthesia in relation to hypertension – IV. The effects of artificial ventilation on the circulation and pulmonary gas exchanges. Br J Anaesth 44:335-48, 1972.
8. Foëx P, Prys-Roberts C: Anaesthesia and the hypertensive patient. Br J Anaesth 46:575-588, 1974.
9. Goldman L, Caldera DL. Risks of general anesthesia and elective operation in the hypertensive patient. Anesthesiology 50:285-292, 1979.
10. Prys-Roberts C: Hypertension and anesthesia – fifty years on. Anesthesiology 50:281-284, 1979.
11. Hansson L, Hunyor SN, Julius S, Hoobler SW: Blood pressure crisis following withdrawal of clonidine (catapres, catapresan), with special reference to arterial and urinary catecholamine levels, and suggestions for acute management. Am Heart J 85:605-610, 1973.
12. Whitsett TL, Chrysant SG, Dillard BL, Anton AH: Abrupt cessation of clonidine administration: a prospective study. Am J Cardiol 41:1285-1290, 1978.
13. Bruce DL, Croley TF, Lee JS: Properative clonidine withdrawal syndrome. Anesthesiology 51:90, 1979.
14. Viljoen JF, Estafanous FG, Kellner GA: Propranolol and cardiac surgery. J Thorac Cardiovasc Surg. 64:826-830, 1972.
15. Moran JM, Mulet J, Caralps JM, Pifarre R. Coronary revascularization in patients receiving propranolol. Circulation (Suppl II)49, 50:116-121, 1974.
16. Kaplan JA, Dunbar RW, Bland JW Jr, Sumpter R, Jones EL: Propranolol and cardiac surgery: a problem for the anesthesiologist? Anesth Analg (Cleve) 54:571-578, 1975.
17. Kopriva CJ, Brown MB, Pappas G: Hemodynamics during general anesthesia in patients receiving propranolol. Anesthesiology. 48:28-33, 1978.
18. Prys-Roberts C, Foëx P, Roberts JG. Studies of anaesthesia in relation to hypertension. Br J Anaesth. 45:671-680, 1973.

19. Prys-Roberts C: Hemodynamic effects of anesthesia and surgery in renal hypertensive patients receiving large doses of beta-receptor antagonists. Anesthesiology 51 (Suppl): 122, 1979.

20. Alderman EL, Coltart DJ, Wettach GE, Harrison DC: Coronary artery syndromes after sudden propranolol withdrawal. Ann Intern Med 81:625-627, 1974.

21. Miller RR, Olson HG, Amsterdam EA, Mason DT: Propranolol-withdrawal rebound phenomenon. Exacerbation of coronary events after abrupt cessation of antianginal therapy. N Engl J Med 293:416-418, 1975.

22. Nattel S, Rangno RE, Van Loon G: Mechanism of propranolol withdrawal phenomena. Circulation 59:1158-1164, 1979.

23. Goldman L: Noncardiac surgery in patients on propranolol: case reports and a recommended approach. Arch Intern Med 141:193-196, 1981.

24. Leth A: Changes in plasma and extracellular fluid volumes in patients with essential hypertension during long-term treatment with hydrochlorothiazide. Circulation 42:479-485, 1970.

25. Tarazi RC, Dustan HP, Frohlich ED: Long-term thiazide therapy in essential hypertension. Evidence for persistent alteration in plasma volume and renin activity. Circulation. 41:709-717, 1970.

26. Prys-Roberts C, Meloche R: Management of anesthesia in patients with hypertension or ischemic heart disease. Int Anesthesiol Clin 18:181-217, 1980.

27. Prys-Roberts C, Greene LT, Meloche R, Foëx P: Studies of anaesthesia in relation to hypertension - II. Haemodynamic consequences of induction and endotracheal intubation. Br J Anaesth 43:531-546, 1971.

28. Goldman L, Caldera DL, Southwick FS, Nussbaum SR, Murray B, O'Malley TA, Goroll AH, Caplan CH, Nolan J, Burke DS, Krogstad D, Carabello B, Slater EE. Cardiac risk factors and complications in non-cardiac surgery. Medicine. 57:357-70, 1978.

29. Defalque RJ: Compared effects of spinal and extradural anesthesia upon the blood pressure. Anesthesiology 23:627-630, 1962.

30. Eisele JH, Reitan JA, Massumi RA, Zelis RG, Miller RR: Myocardial performance and N_2O analgesia in coronary-artery disease. Anesthesiology 44:16, 1976.

31. Kassirer JP, Harrington JT: Diuretics and potassium metabolism: a reassessment of the need, effectiveness and safety of potassium therapy. Kidney Int 11:505-515, 1977.

32. Lehv MS, Salzman EW, Silen W: Hypertension complicating carotid endarterectomy. Stroke 1:307-312, 1970.

33. Gal TJ, Cooperman LH: Hypertension in the immediate postoperative period. Br J Anaesth 47:70-73, 1975.

34. Albrecht RF, Toyooka ET, Polk SLH, Zahed B: Hydralazine therapy for hypertension during the anesthetic and postanesthetic periods. Int Anesthesiol Clin 16:299-312, 1978.

35. Woolsey RL, Shand DG: Pharmacokinetics of antiarrhythmic drugs. Am J Cardiol 41:986-995, 1978.

36. Goldman L, Caldera DL, Nussbaum SR, Southwick FS, Krogstad D, Murray B, Burke DS, O'Malley TA, Goroll AH, Caplan CH, Nolan J, Carabello B, Slater EE: Multifactorial index of cardiac risk in noncardiac surgical procedures. N Engl J Med. 297:845-850, 1977.

37. Mauney FM, Ebert PA, Sabiston DS Jr: Postoperative myocardial infarction. A study of predisposing factors, diagnosis and mortality in a high risk group of surgical patients. Ann Surg 172:497-503, 1970.

58. QUALITY OF LIFE IN HYPERTENSIVE PATIENTS

C. J. BULPITT

1. WHAT IS THE 'QUALITY OF LIFE'?

The quality or 'degree of excellence' of life embraces many features not usually related to health. Such components would include freedom, security and equality. When examining the quality of life as affected by health, I propose to discuss only certain aspects of this quality and how it may be affected by illness or its treatment.

Table 1 lists certain elements of the quality of life together with the mechanisms whereby this quality can be disrupted by ill health. Personal relationships, work, hobbies, eating, drinking and enjoyment of sex may all be adversely influenced by hypertension or its treatment. Hypertension may lead to headaches or left ventricular failure; be complicated by a stroke or other cardiovascular event or associated with psychiatric problems. These consequences or associations may seriously impair the quality of life. If the presence of hypertension leads to anxiety or depression then the quality of life may be disrupted by an effect on personal relationships: by lessening the patient's ability to work or play, or by the psychological abnormality producing symptoms. The effects of a change in psychological welfare may be subtle and difficult to assess and in this chapter we will pay particular attention to the question whether labelling a patient as hypertensive produces deleterious effects. We shall also briefly consider whether or not depression or anxiety leads to hypertension and which anti-hypertensive drug treatments can produce depression or anxiety.

Table 1 also indicates certain aspects of the quality of life, for example eating, drinking and enjoyment of sex, that may be affected by the side effects of treatment. Table 2 gives the frequency of adverse reactions to drugs as reported by MacMahon [1]. Clonidine, guanethidine, methyldopa, propranolol, hydralazine and thiazide diuretics are considered.

The frequency of adverse reactions is given as follows: ($\times \times$), the effect occurring in more than 5% of treated patients; ($\times$), the effect occurring in 0.1 to 5%; and ($-$), indicating a smaller or zero frequency of a particular side effect. Many associations graded as ($\times$) may, in fact, have little to do with the drug and conversely some associations graded ($-$) may be incor-

Amery, A. (ed.) Hypertensive Cardiovascular Disease: Pathophysiology and Treatment
© *1982, Martinus Nijhoff Publishers. The Hague / Boston / London*
ISBN-13: 978-94-009-7478-4

930

Table 1. Aspects of the quality of life affected by hypertension or its treatment

Aspects of the quality of life	Mechanism whereby these aspects can be disrupted
1. Enjoyable personal relationships and social contacts	a) Depression or anxiety may be associated with hypertension or produced by anti-hypertensive medication. Such psychiatric problems may interfere with personal relationships.
2. Ability to follow usual occupation: wage earning, housework or self-care	b) Mental alertness and abilities can be influenced by a cerebrovascular accident or by sedative drugs. Similarly physical mobility may be affected by a stroke or drugs producing postural hypertension
3. a) Ability to pursue hobbies and other leisure interests b) Enjoyment of organised entertainment: eg. radio, television, theatre, sports programmes	c) These pursuits may be affected by a) and b) above, sporting activities by the disease or its treatment and even sedentary activities may be affected, for example reading may be impaired by retinal vascular accidents.
4. Eating and drinking	d) Side-effects of anti-hypertensive drugs may interfere with the enjoyment of food or alcohol.
5. Enjoyment of sex	e) Anti-hypertensive drugs can interfere with potency and ejaculation in men and orgasm in women
6. General symptomatic well-being	f) Side-effects of drugs may interfere with the patients' well-being in general.

Table 2. Frequency of adverse reaction to drugs*

	Cloni-dine	Guane-thidine	Methyl-dopa	Propra-nolol	Hydral-lazine	Thia-zides
Anxiety	×	—	×	—	×	—
Depression	—	×	×	×	—	×
Sedation	× ×	—	× ×	—	—	×
Fatigue	× ×	× ×	× ×	× ×	× ×	×
Dizziness	× ×	× ×	× ×	× ×	× ×	×
Blurred vision	—	×	—	—	—	×
Dry mouth	× ×	×	× ×	×	—	×
Poor appetite	×	—	—	× ×	—	—
Nausea	×	×	×	× ×	× ×	×
Diarrhoea	—	× ×	×	×	×	—
Male impotence	×	× ×	×	×	—	—
Failure ejaculation	—	× ×	×	—	—	—

* × ×:problem in >5%; × : problem in 0.1–5%; — : no problems. From [1].

rect. For example, hydrallazine may be associated with male impotence [2]. However, the table does indicate the extent to which drug treatment can interfere with the quality of life. Three of the drugs may produce anxiety, depression or sedation, thus interfering with personal relations and the ability to pursue work or hobbies; fatigue and dizziness have been reported with all six drugs and can interfere with work or play; a dry mouth has been reported with five of the drugs, poor appetite with two, nausea with all six and diarrhoea with four. All gastrointestinal symptoms may be expected to interfere with an interest in food and drink. Impotence in men has been reported with four of the drugs and failure of ejaculation with two, thus interfering with a man's enjoyment of sexual intercourse.

2. HOW MAY THE QUALITY OF LIFE BE QUANTIFIED?

Fanshel and Bush [3] have suggested that on any one day a patient may be given a score representing the quality of life. Over a period of time the scores for each day may be summed to give a total score or aggregated Health Status Index (HSI). Using the index, patients can be compared, say over a five-year period, and these summed scores should be useful in quantifying the effects of different treatments.

2.1. The states of well-being/illness that have to be allocated a score

Fanshel and Bush discussed these states in terms of function/dysfunction and defined them as follows.

State 1 (S_1) – *Total well-being*
  The state of a normal young child.

State 2 (S_2) – *Minor dissatisfaction*
  The patient may have caries or other unsatisfactory condition producing a 'very slight, but significant', deviation from wellbeing. S_2 will be the state when an adult feels completely well.

State 3 (S_3) – *Discomfort*
  The patient may have a headache or other symptom, but daily activities are continued 'with no significant reduction in efficiency'.

State 4 (S_4) – *Minor disability*
  Illness or emotional disturbance allows daily activities to be continued but with a 'significant reduction of efficiency'.

State 5 (S_5) – *Major disability*
  The patients will exhibit a 'severe reduction of efficiency in the performance of their expected functions'. Such patients will require continuous help and support at home. They may be able to work at a suitable job.

932

State 6 (S_6) – Disabled
'Ambulatory and can move about the community' but unable to go to work.
State 7 (S_7) – Confined
Not bedridden but institutionalised or the equivalent.
State 8 (S_8) – Bedridden
Bedridden but can communicate with family, friends etc.
State 9 (S_9) – Isolated
For example in an intensive care unit or operating room.
State 10 (S_{10}) – Comatose
May recover.
State 11 (S_{11}) – Dead
Will not recover or, as the authors put it, 'with a zero transitional probability to a higher state'!

2.2. The score to be allocated to a state

Fanshel and Bush allocated S_1 (total well-being) a score of 1 and S_{11} (death) a score of 0. These scores can easily be accepted but what about the scores between these extremes?

The attitude of patients may provide a clue. They often make one of the following statements.

'I prefer a short happy life to a miserable long life. I do not wish to be old anyway.'

'When I have to 'go' I want to die quickly'.

These responses may arise when a patient is asked to stop smoking, drinking alcohol or to diet. It is doubtful whether their unwillingness to be old will persist if they do indeed progress through middle age, but these sentiments do give a clue whereby the states of health can be scored. It may be reasonable to prefer 10 years in state S_6 (disabled) to 20 years of life in state S_7 (confined or institutionalised).

The duration of disability can be measured and the disability scored, thus quantifying the concept that disablement can be traded for years of life lost. The scores will indicate the importance of the quality of life.

2.3. Scores chosen to indicate how many years early a patient would be prepared to die in order to return to state S_1 (total well-being)

Table 3 is freely adapted from Fanshel and Bush's work although the scores are not identical [3]. The scores are arranged to allow the patient to trade a disability for a reduced expectation of life.

Table 3. Disability scores calculated on the theoretical principal that a patient can opt to achieve the age of 80 in his or her present state of health or to resume the state of total well-being and lose a certain number of years of life (3). The last column lists the number of years of life that would be lost to regain health state S_1 at the age of 40

Dysfunction		Score	Number of years of lost life to regain S_1 at 40 years of age
Total well being	(S_1)	1	0
Minor dissatisfaction	(S_2)	0.975	1
Discomfort	(S_3)	0.875	5
Minor disability	(S_4)	0.8	8
Major disability	(S_5)	0.75	10
Disabled	(S_6)	0.625	15
Confined	(S_7)	0.375	25
Bedridden	(S_8)	0.125	35
Isolated	(S_9)	0.025	39
Comatose	(S_{10})	0	40
Dead	(S_{11})	0	40

For the calculation of the reduction in length of life the patient is assumed to be aged 40 years, in a health state S_1 to S_{11}, and be able to live until the age of 80. The patients can opt for a better health state but with a corresponding loss of life. The calculation is as follows:

$$\text{loss of life} = (S_1 - S_n)e,$$

where S_1 is the score for total well-being, S_n the state the patient is in at the age of 40, e the normal expectation of life at age 40 (40 years in this example).

The health scores are calculated to give the acceptable loss of life in the last column of the table. Thus an isolated patient in an intensive care unit is assumed to trade 40 years in the intensive care unit for one year of life in a state of total well-being (39 lost years). Similarly, a disabled person is assumed to trade 15 lost years of life for 25 years of total well-being.

The acceptable years lost can also be calculated for a change between state S_n and an improved state, S_m, not equal to S_1. Then, loss of life $= (S_m - S_n)e$ and a patient may prefer to live 10 years in state S_6 (disabled) to 20 years in state S_7 (confined).

The reader will realise that these scores have been chosen to give a numerical basis for the quality of life. But we must prove that such computations can be helpful.

3. HOW MAY A HEALTH STATUS INDEX BE USEFUL?

The choice may have to be made between treatment which makes the patient feel less well and no treatment and the possibility of early death. A

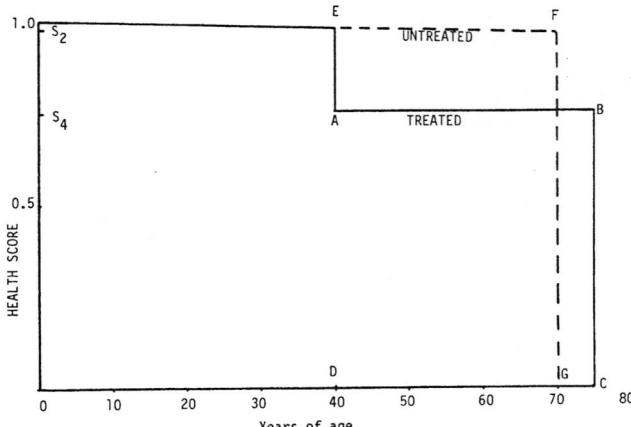

Figure 1. Health score plotted against age for a theoretical group of patients given anti-hypertensive treatment at the age of 40, and a second group who were not treated but died earlier at the age of 70. The quality of life as measured from the aggregated scores (a Health Status Index) is given by the area ABCD for the treated patients and EFGD for the untreated patients.

Health Status Index (HSI), computed over a period of time may aid the decision to treat or not to treat. Figure 1 gives the theoretical results for drug treatment that reduces the average patient from state S_2 (minor dissatisfaction, score 0.975) to S_4 (major disability score 0.75) at the age of 40, yet allows the patient to reach the age of 75. The area under the graph is 35×0.75, an aggregated HSI of 26.3. Without treatment, let us assume that the average patient lives at state S_2 until the age of 70 and then dies suddenly of a cerebral haemorrhage giving, an HSI score of 30×0.975, or 29.3. If we accept that the health scores are reasonable then the computation indicates that if this result was observed in a randomised controlled trial, we should decide not to treat such patients.

The Veterans Administration Trial of Antihypertensive Agents in male patients with an initial diastolic blood pressure of 90–114 mm Hg [4, 5] provides data from which we can compile an aggregated health status index. Of 186 patients given active treatment, 39 had had a previous myocardial infarction, episode of congestive heart failure or cerebral thrombosis. These patients can be given the score S_5 (major disability) = 0.75. At the end of the trial 48 patients were in this category owing to an event prior to the start of the trial or during the trial. Table 4 (row 3) gives these numbers (n), the scores (S) and the aggregated health status indices (n × s). The numbers and aggregated indices are also given for the control group. During the trial 10 actively treated patients and 21 placebo treated patients died to reach state S_{11} and scores of zero (row 4), leaving 147 patients in the actively treated

Table 4. Health status scores in treated and control groups for the Veterans Administration trial of antihypertensive agents in patients with initial diastolic pressures 90–114 mm Hg (4, 5)

Health state	Score (S)	Treated group				Control group			
		Start of trial		End of trial		Start of trial		End of trial	
		n	nxs	n	nxs	n	nxs	n	nxs
S_3	0.875	87	76	17	15	68	60	19	17
S_4	0.8	60	48	111	89	90	72	98	78
S_5	0.75	39	29	48	36	36	27	56	42
S_{11}	0	0	0	10	0	0	0	21	0
Total		186	153	186	140	194	159	194	137

group to be assigned a health state at the beginning of the trial and 128 at the end. The authors estimated that in the actively treated group 59% had no symptomatic complaint. Patients without a complaint could not be allocated a health status higher than S_3 as they were attending hospital as outpatients. However, 59% of 147 patients (87) can be allocated to health state S_3 (discomfort, row 1) and the remaining symptomatic patients to health state S_4 (minor disability) and score 0.80 (row 2). In a similar manner 128 patients at the end of the trial can be allocated at health scores S_3 or S_4. In the placebo group only 43% had no initial complaint and 16% had made no complaint by the end of the trial. The patients in the placebo group can be allocated a health score as were patients in the active group.

The health scores for the patients were aggregated and a total HSI score of 153 for 186 actively treated patients fell to 140 after an average of 3 years in the trial: a reduction of 8%. In the placebo group a HSI of 159 for 194 patients fell to 137 after being in the trial, a reduction of 14%. The calculation of a HSI for the groups in this trial therefore confirms a benefit for actively treated patients. The symptomatic side effects of treatment did not negate the advantages of active therapy in preventing morbid or mortal events. The calculations are more important when the quality of life of patients on similar treatments has to be compared. A trial designed with the above analysis in mind could be structured so that it provides information dividing patients not into four states but into the ten or eleven states given in Table 3.

4. THE HEALTH STATUS OF HYPERTENSIVE PATIENTS

4.1. Psychoneurotic status

Early writers were convinced that hypertensive patients had a particular personality. Features of this personality are given in Table 5. Modern drug

Table 5. Psychological features of hypertensive patients before modern drug treatment was available

Psychological feature	Reference*
1. Worry over trivialities	6, 7
2. Irritable	6–8
3. No hobies — does not play	6
4. Dynamic, hyperactive (sluggish, no exercise)	6-8
5. Unusually shy, less dominant and less self-assertive	7-8
6. Less social activity and fewer friends	8

* 6: Moschcowitz, 1919.
 7: Ayman, 1933.
 8: Hamilton, 1942.

treatment could not have been responsible for these abnormalities, but the earliest observations were subjective, although possibly still correct. In 1919 Moschcowitz stated 'The patients are overweight... The neck is short the muscles are soft, their bodily movements are sluggish... Psychically, these people are tense, they persue their vocation with tremendous seriousness and worry over trivialities. In consequence they are irritable... We cannot help recognize... the "tired business man"... He eats well, drinks alcohol to obtain the stimulation that his mental faculties do not afford, and his most violent daily exercise is his walk to and from the conveyance that takes him to his business. As a rule these people are "successful", and they may be said to die of "success".' Who does not feel uncomfortable, 62 years later, when he reads these words and who does not wonder if the quality of such a

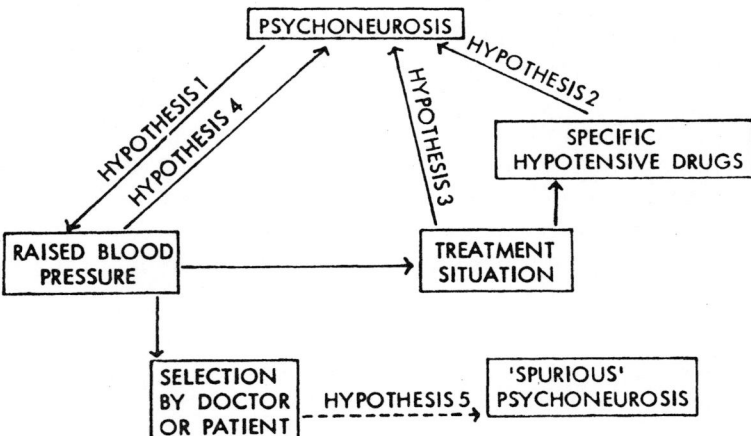

Figure 2. Five possible hypotheses to explain the association between psychoneurosis and hypertension. Reproduced with the kind permission of the Journal of Psychosomatic Research [11].

life really leads to hypertension? We still do not known whether or not 'stress' can lead to sustained elevations of blood pressure. Table 5 shows that Moschcowitz had some support for his views. In 1933 Ayman [7] tried to standardise his interviewing techniques but examined hypertensive out-patients whose personality may have led to this diagnosis and presentation to a hospital clinic, but not all Hamilton's subjects appeared to be aware of their hypertension [8].

More recently several authors have employed validated personality questionnaires and all have agreed that hypertensive patients attending hospital out-patient departments tend to suffer from psychological disabilities [9–11]. We found that treated hypertensive patients had increased scores for free-floating anxiety and depression when compared with the general population [11], but not when compared with patients attending hospital with rheumatoid arthritis [12]. However, phobic anxiety scores were greater for hypertensive patients than for either the general population or rheumatoid arthritis patients. The possible hypotheses relating psychoneurosis to hypertension are given in Figure 2.

4.2. Why may hypertensive patients appear to be psychoneurotic?

The hypotheses are as follows:

1. Psychoneurosis or stress leads to hypertension. This is not definitely disproved, but studies or patients prior to diagnosis do not reveal any overt psychological abnormality [10, 13–16].

2. Anti-hypertensive drugs produce psychological disorders. This will be discussed further in section 4.4.

3. The treatment situation produces psychoneurosis. This is now known as the effect of 'labelling' and will be discussed in section 4.3.

4. A raised blood pressure produces psychoneurosis. Psychological changes may accompany cerebral arteriosclerosis and impaired blood flow but it would appear likely that, with a normal cerebral vasculature and moderate elevations of blood pressure, autoregulation will prevent any changes in cerebral blood flow volume. Thus moderate increases in pressure or reductions due to treatment are not expected to produce psychological changes.

5. Biased selection due to patient or doctor. A hypertensive patient who does not have a psychological problem may not visit his doctor, whereas an anxious patient may do so. The latter will stand a greater chance of having his or her blood pressure taken and the condition diagnosed. Similarly the anxious patient may have more symptoms (see below), be more difficult to treat, and be referred to the hospital out-patients. Thus the hospital sees a high proportion of neurotic patients, their neuroses having precipitated either their initial diagnosis or referral to hospital or both.

The psychological state of the patient is crucial to any discussion of his or her quality of life and we shall consider further how anxiety or depression may be produced in hypertensive patients. The two most popular hypotheses are that psychological changes may be due either to labelling the patient with the diagnosis of hypertension, or to the drug treatment employed.

4.3. The effect of labelling a patient with a diagnosis of hypertension

A recent symposium on patient labelling in hypertension examined the effects of labelling on absenteeism from work and psychological features.

Two studies suggest an increase in absenteeism after labelling and treating patients with hypertension [17, 18]. It is possible that patients believe that they are more ill after a diagnosis of hypertension has been made or that when they feel ill they feel more justified in taking time off from work.

Several studies have failed to show that hypertensives who are unaware of their condition differ from normotensive controls [10, 13–16]. However, most studies indicate that aware hypertensives feel significantly less well than normotensive controls and that this situation is not affected by treatment [15, 16]. This would suggest that labelling but not treatment may be detrimental to psychological welfare. On the other hand, in the Medical Research Council trial of the treatment of mild hypertension, psychiatric morbidity was reduced when the patients were labelled. Moreover, psychiatric morbidity was reduced when the patients were treated [19]. A victory for 'tender, loving care'!

4.4. Does anti-hypertensive drug treatment produce anxiety or depression?

Reserpine has been shown to produce depression but there is controversy as to whether other anti-hypertensive agents can have this adverse effect. Methyldopa has been reported to produce depression in a frequency between 0 [20] and 13% [21]. Similarly, propranolol has been claimed not to produce depression [22] or to cause it in up to 22% [23]. We used the Middlesex Hospital Questionnaire to measure an anxiety score (free-floating and phobic anxiety) and a depression score [24]. Patients referred to hospital were followed for 1 year to measure changes in these scores [25].

Table 6 gives some of the results. The changes in anxiety and depression scores in those not initially on treatment and subsequently untreated are given in the first column. The changes in those given a diuretic alone or propranolol in combination with other drugs, were similar and the two groups were combined to give the results in the second column. The results

Table 6. Change in Middlesex Hospital Questionnaire anxiety and depression scores over a one-year period

	Labelled initially but untreated	Starting diuretic alone or propranolol [a]	Starting methyldopa [a]	Continuing methyldopa [a]	Stopping methyldopa
Number	72	112	33	48	21
Initial anxiety score	4.9	5.0	5.5	5.3	4.9
Change in anxiety score	+0.4	+0.1	−1.6 [b]	+1.1	+1.2 [b]
Initial depression score	4.3	4.3	5.1	5.0	5.2
Change in depression score	+0.3	+0.1	−0.2	+1.2 [c]	+0.8

[a] Usually in combination with other treatment.
[b] $P<0.05$
[c] $P<0.01$ for comparison of change with zero change

are also given for 33 patients who started on methyldopa; 48 who were referred to the hospital clinic while taking this drug and were continued on the same medication; and 21 patients who were referred on methyldopa and in whom the treatment was stopped.

The patients who were given methyldopa at some stage were both more hypertensive at the first visit and tended to be more anxious and depressed (Table 6). This fact makes the results difficult to interpret. The analyses of these data are incomplete but some provisional interpretations can be suggested:

1. Patients labelled with a diagnosis of hypertension but not subsequently treated did not exhibit statistically significant changes in anxiety or depression scores over a one-year period.

2. No changes were observed when a diuretic alone was started nor when propranolol was started alone or in combination with other drugs. It is therefore probable that starting treatment in a hospital out-patient department does not influence anxiety or depression scores.

3. When methyldopa was started there was a significant fall in anxiety score. This may have been due to the sedative effect of the drug and this concept is reinforced by the observation that the anxiety score increased significantly when the drug was stopped.

4. There was an increase in depression score in those who continued with methyldopa for a one-year observation period. In patients who continued

on a variety of other medications no such change was observed and methyldopa may have produced this effect. However, we must have reservations about this concludion. The Middlesex Hospital Questionnaire depression score was derived from eight questions and was not intended for use in patients on sedative drugs. Thus one question was on the ability of the patient to think quickly. This question may be useful in discriminating depressed from normal patients in the general community but may be less useful in patients on sedative drugs.

When considering the quality of life of hypertensive patients we can conclude that the more severely hypertensive patients who attend hospital clinics tend to be both depressed and anxious. Moreover, certain drug treatments such as reserpine can produce depression and make matters worse. Any increase in anxiety or depression must have a profound adverse effect on the quality of life. We have little knowledge on how such psychological changes may affect the activities of hypertensive patients but we do know how their symptoms are increased when they have high anxiety and depression scores [26].

5. THE SYMPTOMATIC WELL-BEING OF HYPERTENSIVE PATIENTS

Patients aware of severe hypertension may be more willing to admit readily to symptoms than before they are diagnosed [27, 28]. Symptomatic complaints are probably higher in those referred to hospital out-patients and higher still when they receive drug treatment. The symptomatic complaints to be expected in these different circumstances will be discussed in turn.

5.1. Symptoms of hypertensive patients who are not aware of their diagnosis

There has been much discussion as to whether or not a high blood pressure can produce symptoms. Early papers tended to attribute many symptoms to uncomplicated hypertension, including flushing, cold hands, fainting and dizzy spells, epistaxis, increased menstrual flow, headache, and migraine [29]. However, Ayman and Pratt attributed these symptoms not to hypertension but to psychoneurosis [30]. Robinson failed to demonstrate any symptoms (apart from breathlessness) as more frequent in the unaware hypertensive then in other patients presenting to their general practitioner [31]. Furthermore, one large study [32] and a smaller study [33] were unable to relate headache to the level of blood pressure in the general population. However, the number with 'severe' hypertension in the general population is necessarily small and others have suggested that headache [34, 35] and even dizziness and nocturia may result from severe hypertension [35]. Whether or not symptoms can be associated with hypertension. in the absence of cardiovascular complications, we must agree that the unaware hypertensive patient with symptoms due to hypertension is rare.

When assessing the prevalence of symptoms we require a standardised question asked in a consistent manner. Table 7 gives estimates of symptom prevalence where eight constant self-administered questions were asked for a general population, not consulting a physician and with an average age of 53 years [35]. We can assume that the frequency of these symptoms will approximate the expected frequency for unaware hypertensives. The high prevalence of complaints was due to the exact nature of the questions. For example the question: 'In the last three months, have you often felt sleepy during the day?', elicited a high number of positive responses (31 %). The data provide a baseline against which the characteristics of hospital treated hypertensive patients can be compared.

5.2. Symptoms of hypertensive patients who are not referred to hospital out-patients

Such patients are presumably aware of their diagnosis and are receiving treatment. We are uncertain as to the prevalence of symptoms in these patients and assume the level lies between that of the unaware hypertensive and the aware hypertensive referred to hospital out-patients.

5.3. Symptoms of patients referred to hospital out-patients prior to treatment

The second column of Table 7 gives the prevalence of eight symptoms in untreated patients referred to hospital out-patients [35]. As discussed above these patients selected themselves and had been selected by their general practitioner on account of their symptoms. The prevalence of symptoms was therefore high and the high prevalence was associated with high scores for anxiety and depression [26]. Other factors which influenced the prevalence of symptoms were age, sex and race [28].

5.4. Symptoms of patients treated in hospital out-patients

In Table 7 the results of two cross-sectional surveys in treated out-patients are given. Column 3 gives the results in 477 patients under treatment in 1972 [36] and column 4 gives the results for 859 patients studied in

Table 7. Prevalence of certain symptoms in four surveys where the same questions were asked on self-administered questionnaires

	General population	Hypertensive patients referred to out-patients			Treatment				
		Untreated	Treated		Diuretic alone	Methyldopa	Propranolol	Bethanidine	Guanethidine
n	78	99	477	859	91	456	169	159	46
Waking headache (%)	15	31	16	–	–	–	–	–	–
Depression (%)	34	45	29	44	–	–	–	–	–
Unsteadiness, dizziness, etc. (%)	13	60	39	44	–	+5	+7	+12	+21
Sleepiness (%)	31	43	51	68	–	+6	–	–11	–
Diarrhoea (%)	16	26	30	30	–	+9	–	–	+32
Weak limbs (%)	18	34	26	43	–	–	+12	+14	–
Male impotence (%)	7	17	25	33	–	–	–	+10	–
Failure ejaculation (%)	0	7	26	14	–	–	–	–	+23
Survey	35	35	36	37	37	37	37	37	37

1975 [37]. A comparison of these results with those for the untreated patients shows a tendency to improve with three symptoms, headache, depression and unsteadiness; whereas treatment led to an increase in complaints of sleepiness, diarrhoea and impaired male sexual function. These findings were largely confirmed in a longitudinal study of patients where an improvement in certain symptoms with treatment was almost exactly counteracted by deterioration in certain other symptoms [35]. The new symptoms were side effects of anti-hypertensive drugs.

Columns 5–9 of Table 7 list the effect of various treatments as measured in the 859 patients in column 4 [37]. Treatment effects are only reported when statistical significance was reached. A diuretic given alone did not affect the prevalence of symptoms, but the administration of methyldopa increased the complaint of unsteadiness by 5% (an increase in prevalence from 44 to 49%) and increased the complaint of sleepiness by 6% and diarrhoea 9%. Similarly propranolol increased the complaint of unsteadiness by 7% and weak limbs by 12%. Bethanidine increased unsteadiness by 12%, reduced sleepiness by 11% (an unexplained finding), increased the complaint of weak limbs by 14% and impotence in males by 10%. Guanethidine produced unsteadiness and diarrhoea in a considerable number of patients and failure of ejaculation in males. Clonidine (not reported in the table) also was associated with a high prevalence of certain symptoms, namely sleepiness (+23%) and dry mouth (+43%) [37].

5.5. An overall view of the symptoms of hypertensive patients

When assessing the symptoms of patients we must remember that the symptoms are usually due neither to drug treatment nor to the level of blood pressure. Of the symptoms in Table 7, headache, depression, unsteadiness and sleepiness usually result from or are associated with anxiety and depression. On the other hand, we have been able to show that diarrhoea and impairment of male sexual function are not statistically related either to anxiety nor depression [26]. When assessing the symptoms of a patient we must realise that a complaint of headache is less likely to be drug-related than a complaint of impotence. However these 'rules' are rules of probability and we are aware of exceptions, for example headache due to hydrallazine and impotence due to psychological problems. Table 8 gives six symptoms most often associated with psychological problems and six symptoms least often occuring in association with anxiety and depression.

When assessing the symptom side-effects of anti-hypertensive drugs, clonidine and guanethidine appear to produce the most problems, methyldopa, propranolol and bethanidine occupy an intermediate position, and diuretic treatment is the most free of symptom side-effects. We do not know to what

Table 8. Results of a survey into the relationship between symptoms and depression and anxiety [26]

Six symptoms most often associated with anxiety and depression
  1. Complaint of depression
  2. Vertigo
  3. Vivid dreams
  4. Nausea
  5. Tired and exhausted
  6. Tingling of the limbs

Six symptoms mostly NOT associated with anxiety and depression
  1. Lessened interest in sex
  2. Diarrhoea
  3. Impotence in males
  4. Failure of ejaculation in males
  5. Nocturia
  6. Number of hours slept

---

extent side-effects affect the quality of life but if we consider the health status scores discussed earlier in this chapter, a patient in state S_1 (total well-being) through to state S_6 (disabled) is likely to have his health status reduced at least to the next state when affected by side effects (Table 3 and section 5.4).

6. HOW SHOULD THE HEALTH STATUS OF A PATIENT OR GROUP OF PATIENTS BE DETERMINED?

How can we determine discomfort (S_3) minor disability (S_4), major disability (S_5), and disablement (S_6)?

6.1. Discomfort and minor disability

A self-administered questionnaire can be used to assess symptomatic complaints. Some patients have symptoms with no apparent cause and doctors may chose to recognise their complaints or to ignore problems that are very real to the patient. If we employ a self-administered questionnaire can the patient's concept of his or her well-being be accepted?

When considering complaints it must be agreed that only the patient can decide whether or not he or she is suffering from a particular symptom. If the patient states that he suffers from a headache, this must be accepted, even if the patient has several other complaints and there seems to be no reason for the headache. Only the patients know how they feel and their reports must be the basis of deciding whether they are in a state of minor dissatisfaction (S_2), discomfort (S_3), or minor disability (S_4). The medical practitioner should not make a value judgement on whether or not the patient's complaints are commensurate with the observed pathology.

The occurrence of a positive response to a certain proportion of questions may be useful in categorising the patient as S_2, S_3 or S_4. For example, when considering the symptoms discussed in section 4, under 30% of positive responses could place the patient in state S_2 (minor dissatisfaction), 30–49% in state S_3 (discomfort) and 50% or more in state S_4 (minor disability).

Table 9. Self-administered questionnaire to determine disability and disablement

---

1. Have you been going out to work during the last 3 months?
   (Answer Yes/No)

2. If 'yes', how many days have you been off sick in the last 3 months?
   (Answer in days.)

3. Have you been able to do all your usual jobs about the house in the last 3 months?
   (Answer Yes/No)

4. If 'yes', for how many days in the last 3 months were you unable to do these jobs through illness?
   (Answer in days.)

5. Are you able to go out and about?
   (Answer Yes/No)

6. Do you require assistance with bathing?
   (Answer Yes/No)

7. Do you require assistance with dressing?
   (Answer Yes/No)

8. What hobbies do you have?
   (Open ended question).

9. Has your high blood pressure or treatment interefered with these hobbies in the last 3 months?
   (Answer Yes/No)

10. If 'yes', which hobbies?
    (Open ended question)

11. Has your high blood pressure or treatment interfered with your life in any way in the last 3 months?
    (Answer Yes/No)

    If yes, in what way?
    (Open ended question)

12. How far can you walk without stopping?
    (Answer in units of distance)

13. How many flights of stairs can you climb at one go?
    (Answer in flights)

14. Can you travel by bus on your own?
    (Answer Yes/No)

Thank you for answering this questionnaire.

6.2. Is the patient disabled in any way?

Most studies of disablement have been concerned with severe disability such as arises with arthritis in the elderly or a stroke. For example Katz and colleagues [38] reported various degrees of disability according to the level of difficulty in performing functions. They found that bathing is impaired before dressing, and dressing before going to the toilet. Getting about the house is impaired before incontinence of urine or faeces occurs or before problems with feeding arise. Such degrees of disablement may be relevant to stroke patients, but not applicable to the average patient under treatment for hypertension. But in order to indicate health status scores S_5 (major disability) and S_6 (disabled) we can ask whether the patient is able to move about the community, to do a limited job, to go to work normally and if he works, how many days a year he is off sick.

Table 9 lists the questions we are proposing to use in a survey of hypertensive patients in order to decide who has a major disability (S_5) and who is disabled (S_6).

7. CONCLUSIONS

This chapter has considered the nature of the 'quality of life', how it may be scored or quantified, how such a score may be useful in reaching a decision about treatment. It has also paid attention to the relationship between the quality of life and the symptomatic well-being of hypertensive patients as well as to the question of how the quality of life can be determined in our patients.

The aim in treating a hypertensive patient is shifting from simply prolonging life to a prolongation of active, useful life which the patient will enjoy.

REFERENCES

1. McMahon FGI: Management of Essential Hypertension. New York: Futura, 1978.
2. Ahmad S: Hydralazine and male impotence. Chest 78: 358, 1980.
3. Fanshel S, Bush JW: A health status index and its application to health services outcomes. Operations Res 18:1021–1066, 1970.
4. Veterans Administration Co-operative Study Group on Antihypertensive Agents. Effects of treatment on morbidity in hypertension – II. Results in patients with diastolic blood pressure averaging 90 through 114 mm Hg. JAMA 213:1143–1152, 1970.
5. Veterans Administration Co-operative Study Group an Antihypertensive Agents. Effects of treatment on morbidity in hypertension – II. Influence of age, diastolic pressure and prior cardiovascular disease; further analysis of side effects. Circulation 45:991–1004, 1972.
6. Moschcowitz E: Hypertension its significance, relation to arteriosclerosis and nephritis and etiology. Am J Med Sci 158:668–684, 1919.

7. Ayman D: The personality type of patients with arteriolar essential hypertension. Am J Med Sci 186:213–223, 1933.
8. Hamilton JA: Psychophysiology of Blood pressure 1. Personality and behaviour ratings. Psychosom Med 42:125–133, 1942.
9. Sainsbury P: Neuroticism and hypertension in an out-patient population. J Psychosom Res 8:235–238, 1964.
10. Kidson MA: Personality factors in hypertension. Aust NZ J Psychiatry 5:139–145, 1971.
11. Bulpitt CJ, Hoffbrand BI, Dollery CT: Psychological features of patients with hypertension attending hospital follow-up clinics. J Phsychosom Res 20:403–410, 1976.
12. Crown S, Crown JM: Personality in early rheumatoid disease. J. Psychosom Res 17:189–196, 1973.
13. Robinson JO: A study of neuroticism and casual arterial blood pressure. Br J Soc Clin Psychol 2:56–64, 1963.
14. Cochrane R: Neuroticism and the discovery of high blood pressure. J. Psychosom. Res 13:21–25, 1969.
15. Monk M: Blood Pressure awareness and Psychological well-being in the U.S. Health and Nutrition Examination Survey. Presented at Symposium on patient labelling in hypertension. Hamilton, Ontario, 1979.
16. Soghikian K, Fallick-Hunkeler EM, Ury HK, Fischer AA: The effect of high blood pressure treatment and awareness on emotional well-being. Presented at symposium on patient labelling in hypertension. Hamilton, Ontario, 1979.
17. Taylor DW, Haynes RB, Sackett DL: Longterm follow-up of absenteeism among working men following the detection and treatment of their absenteeism. Presented at symposium on patient labelling in hypertension. Hamilton, Ontario, 1979.
18. Alderman MH, Charlson ME, Melcher LA: Labelling and absenteeism: the Massachusetts Mutual experience. Presented at symposium on patient labelling in hypertension. Hamilton, Ontario, 1979.
19. Mann AH: Factors affecting psychological state during one year on a hypertension trial. Presented at Symposium on patient labelling in hypertension. Hamilton, Ontario, 1979.
20. Snaith RP, McCoubrie M: Antihypertensive drugs and depression. Psychol Med 4:393–398, 1974.
21. Bauer GE, Baker J, Hunyor SN, Marshall P: Side effects of anti-hypertensive treatment: a placebo controlled study. Clin Sci Mol Med 55:341s–344s, 1978.
22. Hansson L, Malmcrona R, Olander R, Rosenhall L, Westerlund A, Aberg H, Hood B: Propranolol in hypertension. Report on 158 patients treated up to one year. Klin Wochenschr 50:364–369, 1972.
23. Waal HJ: Propranolol-induced depression. Br Med J 2:50, 1967.
24. Crown S, Crisp AH: A short clinical diagnostic self-rating scale for psychoneurotic patients. Br J Psychiatry 112:917–923, 1966.
25. Bulpitt CJ, Clifton P, Hoffbrand BI, Dollery CT: Does either methyldopa or propranolol produce depression in hypertensive patients? (In preparation.)
26. Bulpitt CJ, Dollery CT, Hoffbrand BI: The contribution of psychological features to the symptoms of treated hypertensive patients. Psychological Medicine 77:661–665, 1977.
27. Stewart I: Headache and hypertension. Lancet 1:1261–1266, 1953.
28. Bulpitt CJ, Dollery CT, Carne S: A symptom questionnaire for hypertensive patients. J Chron Dis 27:309–323, 1974.
29. Ohler WR: The signs and symptoms of hypertension. Am Heart J 2:609–612, 1927.
30. Ayman D, Pratt JH: Nature of the symptoms associated with essential hypertension. Arch Intern Med 47:675–687, 1931.
31. Robinson JO: Symptoms and the discovery of high blood pressure. J. Psychosom Res 13:157–161, 1969.

948

32. Weiss NS: Relation of high blood pressure to headache, epistaxis and selected other symptoms. N Eng J Med 287:631–633, 1972.
33. Waters WE: Headache and blood pressure in the community. Br Med J 1:142–143, 1971.
34. Badran RHA, Weir RJ, McGuiness JB: Hypertension and headache. Scot Med J 15:48–51, 1970.
35. Bulpitt CJ, Dollery CT, Carne S: Change in symptoms of hypertensive patients after referral to hospital clinic. Br Heart J 38:121–128, 1976.
36. Bulpitt CJ, Dollery CT: Side effects of hypotensive agents evaluated by a self-administered questionnaire. Br Med J 3:485–490, 1973.
37. Bulpitt CJ, Hoffbrand BI, Dollery CT: Contribution of drug treatment to symptoms of hypertensive patients. In: Mild Hypertension: Natural History and Management. Gross F, Strasser T, eds. Tunbridge Wells: Pitman Medical, 1979.
38. Katz S et al.: Studies of illness in the aged. JAMA 185:914–919, 1963.

59. COMPLIANCE TO ANTIHYPERTENSIVE THERAPY

JOEL MENARD, PIERRE-FRANÇOIS PLOUIN, PATRICE DEGOULET and PIERRE CORVOL

It is generally agreed that the results of the Veterans Administration's trial into the benefits of treatment of permanent arterial hypertension in 1970 gave the decisive impulse to a worldwide fight against arterial hypertension. The trial, commencing in 1963, showed that medically based treatment with diuretics, reserpine, and hydralazine greatly reduced the incidence of cardiovascular events: only 25 events occured in 259 actively treated subjects, compared with 89 in 264 untreated [1, 2]. Following these results several new trials were set up to solve other problems. A number of questions still needed to be answered. Is drug treatment beneficial to less seriously afflicted patients, in particular to those with lower arterial pressures (i.e. diastolic pressures of 90–105 mm Hg) [3]? Does the use of other groups of antihypertensive drugs reduce the incidence of coronary complications, which remained unchanged in the first studies [4]? Does treatment benefit hypertensive patients over 60 years of age [5]?

Between 1970 and 1975 several reports were addressed to another fundamental question. To what extent are the proven benefits of treatment reduced in practice, if patients do not follow their prescriptions? Sackett and Haynes, at McMaster University in Hamilton, Canada, began an extensive investigation of the problem of patient adherence to prescribed treatments [6]. After the paper of Blackwell in 1973 [7], they reviewed and critised 371 articles. Another important work is the thesis of Podell [8], which analysed the numerous factors determining adherence by hypertensive patients to their treatments. The problem has captured the attention of the medical world to such an extent that, in 1977, two-thirds of drug advertisements claimed that treatment with a particular drug was more effective because the simplicity of its prescription favored compliance [9]. *Compliance is a concept which defines the concordance that exists between the recommendations of health personnel and the behavior of the patient.*

I. COMPLIANCE: ITS IMPORTANCE IN ARTERIAL HYPERTENSION

The Veterans Administration's trials can be analysed on different aspects. A

Amery, A. (ed.) Hypertensive Cardiovascular Disease: Pathophysiology and Treatment
© *1982, Martinus Nijhoff Publishers. The Hague / Boston / London*
ISBN-13: 978-94-009-7478-4

definite and affirmative answer to the initial question: 'Is a reduction in blood pressure beneficial?', was obtained after comparing two groups of similar patients, randomly selected and subjected to either active treatment or placebo. However, the results obtained over the total hypertensive population attending the Veterans' Hospital at that time is much less encouraging. Indeed, 50% of patients initially meeting the inclusion criteria for the trial had to be excluded after a preliminary period of follow-up. It appeared that they did not attend their consultations regularly, or that they did not take the entire course of prescribed treatment. This was revealed by the absence of fluorescence in their urine (the tablets contained tracer amounts of riboflavin) or by the number of tablets remaining in containers [1]. Lack of compliance was detected in half of the patients.

Such an incidence of poor compliance weighs heavily against any effort in current medical practice to extend the results of the V. A. trials to a complete population initially exposed to the hypertensive risk. Even after eliminating 50% of the subjects, 44 patients out of 380 disappeared from medical surveillance during the four-year course of these trials (on average within 17,6 months of being selected, with extremes ranging from 1 to 49 months).

There are several reasons why it is not surprising that the general medical problem of non-compliance [10] should be particularly relevant in the course of medical treatment of arterial hypertension.

1. Many hypertensives do not suffer from any symptoms at the time when their condition is recognised. They are not automatically inclined to look for a beneficial effect of drug-taking since they exhibit no need for attention. Furthermore, psychologically, long-term risk of poor health always is of less importance than the various immediate problems encountered in everyday life, such as socio-professional, domestic, and financial difficulties [11].

2. Treatment takes a long time. Problems of compliance exist even in courses of short duration, and increase further with time. This was shown, for example, in the treatment of tuberculosis [12]. Any event capable of modifying the hypertensive's perception of his own state of health could interfere with compliance at any time, particularly extramedical events such as occupational or family problems.

3. Prescriptions are often complex. They frequently contain many antihypertensive medications and it is known that increasing the number of drugs and doses per day lowers patient compliance; even a prescription for three doses per day incurs this problem [13]. Early treatment of moderate hypertension would thus favor compliance since its treatment is simpler than that for severe hypertension. On the other hand, it is certain that extending the period of treatment is unfavorable for compliance. Moreover, drug prescription is only a part of many other recommendations which include loss of

body weight, stopping cigarette smoking, etc. The multiplicity of the medical recommandations could make compliance worse.

4. Antihypertensive medications have unpleasant side effects. These are all the more annoying when they occur in people who believe themselves to be in good health. Prescription of a placebo by itself carries a 5% incidence of side effects in moderate hypertension [14], but these become two to three times more frequent with active treatment [15]. This reason for non-compliance, which is well recognised by doctors, is not one of the main reasons given by patients who were asked why they followed their treatment regimens irregularly.

II. COMPLIANCE TO TREATMENT FOR ARTERIAL HYPERTENSION: METHODS OF MEASUREMENT

The methods are numerous, though those that are simplest often give the best information.

1. Regularity of attendance. The patient who does not keep appointments may have sought other advice or treatment, but alternatively, he could have ceased treatment and supervision altogether. After a short time, he dares not return for his consultation and is lost at follow-up.

2. Interview with the patient. In several studies on compliance, evaluation has been done by an outside person, separate from the doctor prescribing the treatment [16]. Although this is helpful in research, the method cannot be applied in everyday medical practice.

3. Response to the doctor's specific question: 'Do you take your medication every day, in the dosage prescribed?' The manner in which this question is posed is important. It should never sound like a police investigation lest the patient's response be influenced by fear. If the patient answers affirmatively, he still may not be taking his medication. *Only when the patient gives a negative answer, can you be sure that he is not complying.* Among the patients who do not take their medications correctly, about 50% recognise it and admit it; it is these patients who respond most effectively to different strategies aimed at improving their compliance [17].

4. Counting the pills left in containers. This is not easy to accomplish when a patient is supplied directly by his pharmacist. The patient may view it as an unfavorable intrusion into his personal affairs. All kinds of simple trickery are contrived to dodge this control [18–20].

5. The drug measurement in the urine or blood. When this technique can be easily applied, it permits detection of those patients not following their treatment, plus, perhaps, those cases in which the drug is not being absorbed [21, 22]. Therapy with several drugs renders this approach impossible, or at least restricts it to very well equipped centers handling selected

Table 1. The parallel between efficacy of treatment (blood pressure control) and the quality of compliance (the amount of diuretic in the urine)

	Diastolic blood pressure (mmHg)	
	>95	<95
Thiazide −	A (39%)	C (5%)
Thiazide +	B (34%)	D (22%)

patients. Drug levels in the urine or plasma show that the patient has taken his medication before coming to the consultation, but do not prove that he takes it as regularly as required.

6. Measuring other clinical and biological characteristics associated with antihypertensives. The presence of a slowed cardiac rhythm may indicate that beta-blocking drugs have been taken correctly. Similarly, the appearance of hyperuricemia suggests that non-uricosuric diuretics have been correctly taken. These findings are evident for groups of patients [4], but require much more careful interpretation for individuals.

7. Blood pressure control. This is an important factor in judging patient compliance but is not without pitfalls. There is generally a good correspondance between the quality of blood pressure control and correct adherence to the medication [22]. Nevertheless, four possible relationships exist (Table 1).

In case D in Table 1, the patient actually takes the prescribed drugs correctly and arterial pressure is well controlled. This is the ideal situation. Arterial pressure may also be well controlled even when the patient takes only part of the medication or does not take it at all: blood pressure has dropped spontaneously (case C). When the pressure is not well controlled, it could mean either that the patient does not take his medication correctly (case A), or that he is actually resistant to the prescribed treatment (case B). These different possibilities are represented in the decision-making matrix shown in Table 1. The most important comparison is between situations A and B. In B a modification of treatment is mandatory, whereas in A the patient must be persuaded to take his treatment.

The decision-making process is illustrated by the results of Lowenthal et al. [22], who measured the excretion of thiazides in the urine at 207 consultations with hypertensives treated by diuretics. The results are of general value, since 28% of patients were well controlled by diuretic treatment alone, a percentage which is generally observed. The test itself has a low sensitivity (45%), but its specificity is rather good (83%).

III. NON-COMPLIANCE TO ANTIHYPERTENSIVE TREATMENT BEFORE THE GENERAL AWARENESS OF THE PROBLEM

The results published from around 1975 are catastrophic. In a small series, Caldwell et al. in Detroit [24], lost sight of 74% of their 76 severely hypertensive patients within the five years after they had been urgently hospitalised. Of these, 50% stopped treatment within eleven months. Over 1971 and 1972 Finnerty et al. in Washington lost track of 67–74% of their patients in eight months. Amongst those left, only 10% had their blood pressure controlled [25, 26]. In other cities in the United States [27] and Great Britain [28, 29], similar disastrous results were observed.

These studies are of particular merit because causes were sought of these poor results. In the series of Caldwell et al., 39% of patients ceased treatment because they felt healthy, 36% because noone had said anything about the necessity of a long-term treatment, 33% for financial reasons, 24% because their doctor advised them to do so, and 14% because their families were not assisting them. Only 7% ceased treatment on account of side effects [24]. For the study of Finnerty et al., weaknesses in the organisation of the outpatient clinic appeared to be the major factor responsible for poor compliance: an average of $2\frac{1}{2}$ h waiting for a visit of $7\frac{1}{2}$ minutes! Many of the patients knew perfectly well that their hypertension was a serious illness which should have been treated. Many were able to pay the treatment charge, but the poor quality of the doctor–patient relationship, essentially reflected in the short time spent at consultation after a long and usefulness wait, appeared to be the major factor against continuation of the treatment [25].

IV. METHODS OF IMPROVING COMPLIANCE

Since 1975, two complementary approaches, one scientific, the other pragmatic, have been used to study the methods of improving patient compliance. Retrospective analyses have permitted the compilation of a catalogue of close to 200 parameters capable of influencing compliance [6, 10]. Unfortunately, there are multiple interactions between these parameters. The reactions of any one individual facing a given situation are often unpredictable and contradictory. The attitude of medics, in connection with the kind of system of health care which conditions it, varies from one country to the next.

The scientific approach isolates one parameter and, according to the rigorous methodology of a controlled therapeutic trial, studies its influence on patient compliance. The pragmatic approach does not isolate a single factor, but regroups a number of influences which, when applied simultaneously, are able to improve compliance. The scientific approach has precision, because it employs comparable groups, seeks precise definitions of trial strategy and proposes precise criteria for success and failure. However, it is limited by artificiality for it constitutes a unifactorial approach for a multifactorial problem. The pragmatic approach corresponds more with reality, but the results are always difficult to interpret. Is there a dominant factor affecting success or failure? What bias is introduced by the method of selection? Is it valid to compare results obtained at different times and from different systems of health care?

RESULTS OF CONTROLLED CLINICAL TRIALS

These were all performed on groups of randomly selected, comparable patients.

1. The best organisation of health care delivery

Ease of access to care. A group of hypertensive patients were treated at their worksite (87 patients) and compared with a control group treated according to the usual methods by the family doctor (57 patients). Compliance was not better in the first group [30]. This result contradicts that reported by Alderman and Schoenbaum in a pragmatic approach to the problem [31, 32], but the divergence of these results is not surprising considering the fact that the studies were done in different countries and on different populations. Furthermore, in many countries, doctors at the worksite have no official qualification to supervise such courses of treatment.

Organisation of appointments. A secretary was installed in the casualty section of an American hospital to arrange appointments for hypertensive who had consulted the Casualty Service [27]. Seventy-four patients were randomly sampled to benefit from the services of the secretary; meanwhile, 70 others were subjected to the usual hospital routine. After 5 months, 78% of the assisted group were still under medical observation, against only 37% of the control group (p<0.05). Unfortunately, the percentage of patients whose high blood pressure was controlled was exactly the same in both groups. The better organisation of follow-up care had been effective with regards to appointments but ineffective with regards to quality of treatment.

This result is surprising when compared with information from Finnerty et al. [26]. From 98 patients who were randomly selected for follow-up in a specialised clinic having perfect administration of its appointments and a well-structured therapeutical strategy, 82 remained under supervision until 8 months later and 70% of these had normal blood pressure. Of the patients that underwent the usual hospital procedures, many more dropped out and only 10% had normal blood pressures. This study was based on a random selection of two appointment strategies, in which the group attending the special clinic had many more advantages.

2. Patient instruction

When the benefits of instruction given to patients have been evaluated, the results have been surprising, especially to doctors who believe in 'patient participation'.

If patients are told about hypertension, its deleterious effects on certain organs, their life-expectancy, the benefits of anti-hypertensive treatment, the problems of taking daily medication and the principal ways of remembering to do so, their level of awareness is greatly increased. Thus, in one study, 95% of 80 individuals so educated acquired a good knowledge of their illness and its treatment, while only 20% of non-instructed individuals had similar knowledge [19]. But, apparently, such efforts are worthless in the long run, because after 6 months of treatment non-compliance was observed in 44% of instructed subjects and in 41% of non-instructed subjects. This astonishing result, obtained from Canadian industrial workers [19], has been confirmed in a different manner by results collected after interrogation of hypertensive patients in a Swedish clinic [33]. Of the patients who were under observation in the clinic 82% said that they had not received information about their illness, and, moreover, 43% of these did not want to know anything more about it.

From this the conclusion may be drawn that, in order to render the teaching programs more effective, they must be improved by making them more attractive and presenting them on a more personal level.

3. Training the doctors

Many doctors underestimate the difficulties involved in long-term surveillance of patients. For example, in anti-acid treatment of gastroduodenal ulcer, 22 doctors out of 27 overestimated compliance of their patients to the treatment [34].

Underestimation of the problem is due to the fact that the usual doctor–patient dialogues do not show this difficulty, whether it is because the doctor himself does not think of compliance, or because the patient, out of kindness or fear, replies to the questions in the way expected by his doctor. Furthermore, it is difficult to tell at the beginning of the treatment, which patients will not follow the advice of their doctor. In a study involving one month of digitalis and diuretic treatment, doctors were able to predict only 35% of the cases that ceased their treatment, while half of their predictions of compliance were false [35].

It is possible, however, to improve such results through training doctors about the problems of non-compliance, as shown in a study by Inui et al. [36]. Of 62 doctors, 29 were given information on the problems of non-adherence, while the other 33 received none at all. After 6 months of treatment by the trained doctors, a group of 49 patients knew more about their illnes and the difficulties of treating it than did the 53 patients who were treated by the other doctors. Thirty out of the 49 patients took more than 75% of their medications, against 17 out of the 53 patients in the control group. Blood pressure control was satisfactory in 69% of cases in the group treated by the trained doctors, against only 36% of cases in the control group.

Advising a patient takes longer than a simple interview or examination. Instruction given by *one* doctor to *one* patient has the advantage of adapting general rules to the notion that the individual has of his own state of health at a particular time. It is reassuring to observe therefore, that the well-informed doctor can succeed in improving patient compliance irrespective of the patient's age, sex, and level of education. Such a trained doctor will find the most effective form of encouragement for each of his patients, because he realizes that awareness of the social consequences of a badly treated illness is an important disincentive against non-compliance [9].

4. The intervention of the pharmacist

The work of McKenny et al., performed on 49 hypertensives, shows the benefit of active participation of the pharmacist [18]. After initial medical supervision of 6 months, 24 hypertensives received a half-hour consultation with their pharmacist every month for the next 5 months, as well as their usual doctor's visit. The pharmacist tried to identify weaknesses in the patients' knowledge of their illness and in the manner in which they were taking their medications. The pharmacist discussed side effects with patients and indicated difficulties to the doctor. He gave the patients instructive information. Adherence to treatment increased from 25% to 79%, and arterial pressure was well regulated in 79% of the patients compared with 20% in the control group.

Unfortunately, this study also showed that the beneficial effect of pharmacist intervention was only transitory. Six months later, satisfactory adherence was observed in no more than 25% of test patients (16% in the control group), and only 42% had well-regulated blood-pressure.

5. Adapting surveillance and treatment to the behaviour of the patient

A novel, multifactorial strategy was performed by Haynes et al. [30]. Hypertensives on whom study was performed had to take their own blood pressures and to record daily that they had taken their medication. This way the process of medication became part of everyday life. Twice-weekly home visits put more pressure on the patients to comply with the routine. Furthermore, the patients were rewarded by the offer of a sphymmomanometer if they were found to be taking the medication correctly and if blood pressure was decreasing. Such a strategy is multifactorial and complex; it is understandable that under these conditions compliance should have been improved. It must be borne in mind that measurement of blood pressure by the patient himself could be a means of improving compliance. The method showed its effectiveness for those patients who, at the outset, were recognised to have a problem in taking their medication [38].

An analysis of patients' attitudes towards arterial hypertension and its treatment was attempted according to the concepts of the Health Belief Model developed in the application of vaccination programs and in the fight against tubeculosis [6, 10]. This approach attempts to identify personality traits and behavior which facilitate adhesion to a care program. The studies were done on a small number of patients selected during hospital consultations who were already part of a care program [23], or correspondingly represented a very restricted socioprofessional group, viz. Canadian industrial workers [39]. In the first of these two studies, it apears that awareness in the patients of the severity of their illnes and the advantages of the treatment may improve compliance. In the second study, the proposed psychological model contributed little to the analysis of compliance. The use of this general concept in a prospective manner to improve compliance (i.e. by modifying perception of illness and its risk and by developing faith in the treatment and its benefits) has not yet been scientifically studied in a sufficient number of hypertensives.

6. Detection of psychopathological reactions to medical prescription

Refusal to recognise the health problem or opposition to possible treatment may be manifestated by two types of patient reactions which are important to recognise and, if possible, to correct. In certain hypertensives, a side effect systematically follows each medical prescription with or without any relationship with the pharmacological properties of the drug. It is then necessary to analyze in detail with the patient the side effects he has described, and to convince him of their psychological orign, i.e. his refusal to accept the illness and its consequences.

958

In other patients, some of whom are very seriously afflicted, the medication is never taken. Not only does such a patient not state this, but he also ferociously denies the very possibility when the doctor attempts to make such a suggestion, no matter how tactfully. It may be a question of suicidal tendency, or sometimes a threat directed at a particular person in the patients' every day surroundings. The important point is to maintain contact with such patients, and when the opportunity arises, to make them understand their own attitude.

V. PERSONNAL EXPERIENCE: COMPLIANCE IN A SPECIALIZED ARTERIAL HYPERTENSION CLINIC

The general state of opinion on the information available on compliance during the treatment of arterial hypertension has influenced the methods of care distribution used in the Hypertension Clinic at Saint Joseph's Hospital, Paris. Ever since it was put into use in October 1975, the clinic had three objectives requiring special efforts: an organisational, a teaching and a therapeutic objective. The organisational objective has five basic aspects.

1. Creation of a clinical environment, pleasant and functional, with the aim of improving the quality of patient reception. This was facilitated by a health care professional worker who was aware of the importance of these problems.
2. Creation of a special secretarial position for efficient organisation of appointments, and passing on of administrative information to patients.
3. Reduction of waiting time so that it will not exceed the duration of the consultation.
4. Compilation of a minimal work-up as soon as the first visit to the outpatient clinic is due (involving blood creatinine, potassium, uric acid, glucose and cholesterol; urinary protein and sugar; and electrocardiogram).
5. Computerised administration of appointments. At six-monthly intervals, two months prior to the consultation, the computer prints a recall letter which includes information on the treatment, its aim and results ever since the patient was admitted to the service. The recall letter is sent simultaneously to the patient and his family doctor, whom the patient is expected consult every two or three months [40].

The educational objective has three aspects:

1. Training is given to doctors, nurses and dieticians, mainly in the methods of informing the patients about the difficulties which might be encountered during the long course of treatment.

2. Three teaching brochures for hypertensive patients have been produced. One is designed to prepare the patient for his first visit in the hospital. Another aims to inform him during his stay within the hypertensive clinic. The third offers advice and precautions about problems of long-term treatment ('Advice to Treated Hypertensives'). It is given to the patient after several consultations when arterial pressure is well controlled.

3. The computer prints, which are make for each patient's visit and contain a summary of the situation (the change in blood pressure, body weight, cigarette consumption, blood cholesterol, glucose, uric acid and the Sokolow index since the first consultation). This summary is given to the patient so that he will be well informed on the progress of treatment and so that he himself can pass on the information to the doctor that treats him.

The therapeutic objective includes.

1. A stepped-care therapeutic program so as to minimize the initial side effects of treatment.
2. Prescription of medications preferably in one or two dosages per day.
3. Periodic computer recall of previous side effects and past history, so as to avoid contraindicated or poorly tolerated drugs.

The importance of the role played by the computer in improving compliance cannot be overemphasized. It affects all levels of daily practice, such as the facilitation of making appointments, the periodical editing of medical profiles and a contribution to the therapy itself by giving medical contraindications. In addition, the standardised collection and permanent storage of information permits detailed analysis of all aspects of the clinic's activities [40].

RESULTS OF THE FIRST CONSULTATION

From 1976 through 1978, 1616 patients with systolic blood pressures greater than 160 mm Hg and/or diastolic pressures greater than 95 mm Hg were examined for the first time in the clinic. At this first consultation, 156 patients (9.6%) were sent back to their local doctor with a medical advice and were not placed under supervision in the clinic. The remainder were taken in charge at the clinic. Ninety patients (6.1%) no longer turned up after the first visit. Such patients were considered to have dropped out if they did not reappear after one reminder had been sent. A comparison was then made between the three groups of patients from the first consultation, i.e. those who were taken into Artemis System (Group I), those who dropped out (Group II), and those who were sent back to the doctor that treats them (Group III). The latter group was different from the first two in that the mean age of its members was higher (56 ± 13 years, against 50.5 ± 12.7 and 48.9 ± 12.5 in groups I and II, respectively), and by its socioprofessional distribution (it contained the greatest proportion of retired workers, consistent with the mean age of its members).

Two important points emerged from the analysis: 1. There was no significant difference in drop-out incidence for the six doctors who conducted the initial sixty-minute consultation in a very regular manner. (The drop-out rate ranged rom 4.6% to 7.9% between the various doctors.) 2. Socioprofessional categories (giving an indication of the patient's economic situation and degree of education) did not differ between the attending group and the drop-outs.

It is important to consider these points since it has been observed that the representation of socioprofessional categories in the clinic did not correspond to the general distribution of these categories in Paris and its environs [41]. The liberal professions, company directors, industrial managers, businessmen, administrators, craftsmen and small traders were overrepresented, while factory workers, service personnel, office staff and salesmen were underrepresented. This observation suggests a poorer assimilation of less wealthy and less well-educated individuals to the system of health care provisions for hypertensives. This is reinforced by the fact that hypertension is equally distributed throughout the socioprofessional categories and is perhaps more frequent in less fortunate groups [42]. It was important, therefore, to establish whether this deviation from the normal socioprofessional distribution was retained with time in our specialised clinic.

RESULTS AFTER ONE YEAR

The figures drawn from different studies published since 1976 suggest that an 80% compliance rate can be expected after one year, if particular attention is paid to the problem of non-compliance (Table 2). Comparisons between different studies are impossible, however, because the systems of health care vary so much from one country to the next.

In 90% of the cases, the Hypertension Clinic of Saint Joseph's Hospital admitted patients who had been recommended by a doctor. This selection favored compliance to some extent, since patients rejecting these kinds of advice would never have attended the clinic. On the other hand, the supervision maintained by the clinic was, by its nature, partial and intermittent, each patient being sent back to a family doctor after the medical profile was obtained, the patient educated and the treatment commenced. This is different from the Swedish [15] and Finnish procedures [48]. Clearly, our arrangements made it easy for the patient not to return to the Hypertension Clniic, but this did not necessarily mean that treatment had been termi-

Table 2. Compliance to anti-hypertensive treatment: principal results after recognition of the problem (1975-1980)

Study location	Number of patients	Health care system	Study duration (months)	Drop-outs (%)
New york	94	Work-site	12	3
Hamilton	158	Work-site	6	7
Chicago	116	Work-site	12	20
Hamilton	224	GP	12	12
New york	206	Specialist	12	51
Sakyla	78	Clinic	12	4
Goteborg	646	Clinic	12	6
USA	5314	Clinics	12	18.1
Australia	3427	Clinics	36	20.4
Paris	1060	Clinic	12	19.1

nated. Furthermore, regular attendance at appointments is not always synonomous with compliance. Amongst the 25.9% of patients whose diastolic pressure was greater than 95 mm Hg after one year of treatment, it is reasonable to assume, according to the answers registered in the Artemis Data Bank, that several were not taking their complete medication, despite the fact that 94.5% told their doctor otherwise.

Our results were analysed for 1460 patients; 24 of the patients died during the first year of follow-up. In 376 cases we decided to cease observation at the Hypertension Clinic. The characteristics of this group were compared with those who continued to be kept under observation and with those who had dropped out, in order to find out whether the decisions made by the clinic's doctors had introduced any bias into the results. The decision to stop treatment was made on the same grounds by the four doctors that are among the clinic's permanent staff. The mean age of the group was higher $(53.9 \pm 14.4$ years), and, as a consequence, had a greater proportion of inactive subjects (37.7%) than did the patients under observation and the drop-outs. The group had a lower mean diastolic pressure $(102.4 \pm 15.1$ mm Hg), a higher average cholesterol level $(6.46 \pm 1.69$ mmol/l) and contained a smaller percentage of smokers (20.4%).

After one year, 858 patients were still under observation, 727 of whom were examined between the eight and sixteenth month, and 131 had an appointment after the sixteenth month. Thus, 19.1% of the patients dropped out of the treatment program.

These results are comparable with recent observations in other countries such as the United States [31, 43-45], Canada [19, 46], Sweden [15], Australia [47] and Finland [48]; in spite of the different systems of health care, i.e. state of medical affairs at the worksite [19, 31, 43], national health provisions [46] and specialised consultations [15, 44, 45, 47, 48].

CAN IT BE PREDICTED WHICH PATIENTS WILL NOT FOLLOW
MEDICAL ADVICE?

The use of a standardised medical dossier and computer recording system
now enables comparisons to be made between the characteristics of those
patients accepting continued supervision and those who dropped out.

The particular doctor responsible for the patient was not an associated
factor, since the percentage of patients disappearing was identical for each of
the four permanent doctors of the service. The seriousness of the illness may
have had an influence: systolic pressure averaged 175.8 ± 24 mm Hg in
drop-outs, against 179.9 ± 24.9 in the patients followed (p<0.05), and the
diastolic pressure was 102.8 ± 12.9 mm Hg in drop-outs against 106.6 ± 13.9
in the others (p<0.001). In addition, there were several parameters besides
blood pressure readings which differed between the groups. These are summarised in Table 3 and discussed in greater detail below.

1. Referral from the work-site doctor. It could have an effect on group
characteristics before or after registration at the Hypertension Clinic. Patients detected by the worksite doctor were probably not in the health care
system. In effect, the worksite doctor made a diagnosis of arterial hypertension which could already have been made by an efficient family doctor. The
absence of a family doctor may be due to difficulties in adapting to the
medical system. An effect could also take place after treatment in the clinic,
since patients referred by a worksite doctor are not registered with a family
doctor. As a result, neither can the treatment started at the specialized
Hypertension Clinic be continued, nor its advice be put into practice. The
Clinic should therefore be responsible for finding a family doctor for such
patients.

2. Absence of prior treatment and current treatment at the time of consultation was more common in drop-out patients. This shows that prior
intervention by other doctors, recent or otherwise, prepares the patient in a

Table 3. Main differences between hypertensive patients present at appointments and patients
lost for follow-up

Characteristics	Followed patients	Drop-outs	P
1. Referred by work-site doctor	10.4%	29.5%	0.001
2. No previous treatment	32.7%	47.5%	0.001
No current treatment	57.0%	68.8%	0.01
3. Smoker (cigarettes per day)	12.5 ± 10.8	17.3 ± 14.2	0.01
4. Current weight excess (kg)	69.6 ± 13.9	72.9 ± 15.2	0.01
Previous weight excess (kg)	74.8 ± 14.7	77.7 ± 15.5	0.05
5. Lower social classes	36.6%	46.3%	0.05

better way to follow the directions of the Specialised Hypertension Clinic. The opposite effect had actually been expected: previously treated patients having already undergone the initial stages of medical treatment might have been less inclined to follow our directives.

3. Association of arterial hypertension with tobacco use. Smokers accept supervision for arterial hypertension less readily than non-smokers. Here again the effects may occur before or after the specialised consultation. Attitudes of smokers towards various health problems are less compatible with standards expected by the medical profession than one those of non-smokers. Alternatively, the psychological pressure exercised by doctors on the hypertensive smoker after admittance to the Clinic may become unbearable for some who eventually prefer to avoid all medical contact [49].

4. A current or previous tendency to gain overweight is a factor affecting compliance and can be explained in the same way as tobacco usage. The conduct of such patients has long been characterised as one of negligence towards their own health problems as a result of their excessive eating habits. Great pressure is exerted by medical authorities to alter these habits. Indoing so, they impose many restraints that may finally become unbearable for many whose only alternative is to refuse to be medically supervised [50].

5. Social-professional conditions. It must be emphasised that the differences between the various socio-professional categories in the group under observation were significant. In the group of drop-outs, 46.3% of subjects were industrial workers and service personnel, compared with 36.6% in the patients under observation. In the Hypertension Clinic, lower socio-professional categories did perform differently from the other groups. Moreover, they do consult less often, which may be due to the fact that either they express no demand to their local doctor to do otherwise, or their doctor does not refer them to the specialist as frequently as he would patients of higher social positions [41].

VI. CONCLUSIONS

Since the efforts of an Hypertension Clinic have been oriented towards improving patient compliance, it has been observed that approximately 80% of patients are still under observation after one year of supervision, and that 75% of these have a diastolic pressure below 95 mm Hg. This result compares favorably with the most recent information on the subject and is clearly superior to that found around 1975. This satisfactory result is due to efforts made in the organisation of the clinic (i.e. reduction of waiting-time), the education of patients (through informative booklets, summaries of the treatment and its results), and the education of medical staff (in brief, the orientation of all aspects of the work of medical personnel towards improvement of patient compliance).

At all stages the computer has been an active participant and has made possible the analysis of different characteristics of both the patients under observation and those who were lost at follow-up. The information thus obtained enables us to compile a list of patients most likely to drop out during the course of treatment.

In order to increase the efficacy of the treatment of arterial hypertension, a supplementary effort should be made with respect to those patients who have the highest risk for non-complinace. Such an effort is worth the while in that it reduces the consequences that otherwise follow poor compliance affecting both the individual and the community.

All efforts made in the framework of screening and work-up are totally wasted if they do not lead to a permanent decrease in blood pressure. The individual not complying with treatment is still exposed to the consequences of hypertension [51], despite the waste of time and money in diagnosis tests. With non-compliance the community bears the cost of screening work-up, and of the complications, without profiting from this investment. It is useless developing the first two stages of the battle against hypertension, viz. screening and work-up, if the practical performance of the third stage, the actual treatment, is not as near perfect as possible. Fundamental to this is the patient's compliance. It must always be remembered however, that in the area of human endeavour it is not possible – fortunately so – to include 100% of the people in a single system to the satisfaction of each.

ACKNOWLEDGEMENTS

We thank Drs. Marie-Blanche Ducrocq, Alain Tugayé, Patrick Bautier and Daniele Blairvacq who greatly contributed to these results, as well as all the nursing staff and secretaries of the Arterial Hypertension Service at the Saint Joseph's Hospital, Paris.

Andrea Skinner, Melbourne (Australia) translated the text into English.

This work has been supported by a grant from the Ministery of Health in France.

REFERENCES

1. Veterans Administration Cooperative Study Group on Antihypertensive Agents: Effects of treatment on morbidity in hypertension. Results in patients with diastolic blood pressure averaging 115 through 129 mmHg. JAMA 202:116, 1967.
2. Veterans Administration Cooperative Study Group on Antihypertensive Agents: Effects of treatment on morbidity in hypertension. Results in patients with diastolic blood pressure averaging 90 through 114 mmHg. JAMA 213:1143, 1970.

3. Smith McFate W: Treatment of mild hypertension. Results of a ten-year intervention trial. Circ Res 40 (Suppl 1):98, 1977.
4. Report of Medical Research Council Working Party on Mild to Moderate Hypertension: Randomised controlled trial of treatment for mild hypertension: design and pilot trial. Br Med J 1:1437, 1977.
5. Pilot trial of the European Working Party on High Blood Pressure in the Elderly. Gerontology, 23, 426, 1977.
6. Sackett DL, Haynes RB eds: Compliance with therapeutic regimens. Baltimore: Johns Hopkins University Press, 1976.
7. Blackwell B: Patient compliance. N Engl J Med 289:249, 1973.
8. Podell RN: Management of patients with hypertension. N Engl J Med 290:747, 1974.
9. Sackett DL: Patients and therapies: getting the two together. N Engl J Med 298:278, 1978.
10. Haynes RB, Taylor DW, Sackett DL: Compliance in health care. Baltimore: Johns Hopkins University Press, 1979.
11. Rosenstock IM: Why people use health services. Milbank Mem Fund Q 44 (Suppl 94):127, 1966.
12. Luntz GRWNN, Austin R: New Stick test for PAS in urine. Br Med J 1:1679, 1960.
13. Porter AMW: Drug defaulting in a general practice. Br Med J 1:218, 1969.
14. Perry JR HM: Treatment of Mild Hypertension. Preliminary results of a two-year feasibility trial. Circ Res 40 (Suppl 1):180, 1977.
15. Andersson O, Berglund G, Hansson L, Sannerstedt R, Silvertsson R, Wilkstrand J, Wilhelmsen L: Organization and efficacity of an Outpatient Hypertension Clinic. Acta Med Scand 203:391, 1978.
16. Rickels K, Briscoe E: Assessment of dosage deviation in outpatient drug research. J Clin Pharmacol 10:153, 1970.
17. Sackett DL, Haynes RB, Gibson ES, Taylor DW, Roberts RS, Johnson AL: Patient compliance with antihypertensive regimens. Patient counselling and health education 1:18, 1978.
18. McKenney JM, Slining JM, Henderson HR, Devins D, Barr M: The effect of clinical pharmacy services on patients with essential hypertension. Circulation 48:1104, 1973.
19. Sackett DL, Haynes RB, Gibson ES, Hackett BC, Taylor DN, Roberts RS Johnson AL: Randomized clinical trial of strategies for improving medication compliance in primary hypertension. Lancet 1, 1205, 1975.
20. Blackwell B: Treatment adherence in hypertension. Am J Pharm 148:75, 1976.
21. Briggs WA, Lowenthal DT, Cirksena WJ, Price WE, Gibson TP, Flamenbaum W: Propranolol in hypertensive dialysis patients: efficacy and compliance. Clin Pharmacol Ther 18:606, 1975.
22. Lowenthal DT, Briggs WA, Mutterperl R, Aldelman B, Creditor MA: Patient compliance for antihypertensive medication: the usefulness of urine assays. Curr Ther Res 19:405, 1976.
23. Nelson EC, Stason WB, Neutra RR, Solomon HS, McArdle PJ: Impact of patient perceptions on compliance with treatment for hypertension. Med Care 16:893, 1978.
24. Caldwell JR, Cobb S, Dowling MD, De Jongh D: The drop-out problem in antihypertensive treatment. J Chronic Dis 22:579, 1970.
25. Finnerty FA Jr, Mattie EC, Finnerty FA: Hypertension in the inner city – I. Analysis of clinic dropouts. Circulation 47:23, 1973.
26. Finnerty FA Jr, Shaw LN, Himmelsbach CF: Hypertension in the inner city — II. Detection and follow-up. Circulation 47:76, 1973.
27. Flechter SA, Appel FA, Bourgeois MA: Management of hypertension. Effect of improving patient compliance for follow-up care. JAMA 233:242, 1975.

28. Heller RF, Rose G: Current management of hypertension in general practice. Br Med J 1:1442, 1977.
29. Heller RF, Rose G: Current management of hypertension in hospital. Br Med J 1:1441, 1977.
30. Haynes RB, Sackett DL, Gibson ES, Taylor DW, Roberts RS, Johnson AL: Improvement of medication compliance in uncontrolled hypertension. Lancet 1:1265, 1976.
31. Alderman MH, Schoenbaum EE: Detection and treatment of hypertension at the work site. N Engl J Med 293:65, 1975.
32. Alderman MH, Seligman AW, Davis TK: Hypertension control: an alternate view from Gimbels. Am Heart J 96:421, 1978.
33. Aberg H: Patient Compliance. Acta Med Scand 606 (Suppl I):25, 1977.
34. Caron HS, Roth HP: Patients' cooperation with a medical regimen. JAMA 203:922, 1968.
35. Mushlin AI, Appel FA: Diagnosing potential non compliance: physicians' ability in a behavioral dimension of medical care. Arch Intern Med 137:318, 1977.
36. Inui TS, Yourtee EL, Williamson JW: Improved outcomes in Hypertension after physicians tutorials. A controlled trial Ann Intern Med 646, 1976.
37. Blackwell B: Treatment adherence in hypertension. Am J Pharm 148:75, 1976.
38. Johnson AL, Taylor DW, Shimizu A, Dunnett CW, Sackett DL:: Communication to the Hypertension Task Force, 1977, pp. 7–9. Ontario Council of Health.
39. Taylor DW: A test of the health belief model in hypertension. In: Compliance in Health Care, Haynes RB, Taylor DW, Sackett DL, eds. Baltimore: Johns Hopkins University Press, 1979.
40. Degoulet P, Menard J, Berger C, Plouin PF, Devries C, Hirel JC: Hypertension management: the computer as a participant. Am J Med 68:559, 1980.
41. Degoulet P, Devries C, Wolf JPh, Plouin PF, Menard J: L'accès de l'hypertendu aux soins: influence des catégories socio-professionnelles. Nouv Presse Med 9:15, 1980.
42. Action lyonnaise de prevention de l'hypertension et de l'athérosclerose: Hypertension artérielle et catégorie socio-professionnelle. Rôle de la surcharge pondérale. Rev Prat (Paris) 29:99, 1979.
43. Stamler R, Stamler J, Civinelli J, Pritchard D, Gosch FC, Ticho S, Restivo B, Fine D: Adherence and blood pressure response to Hypertension Treatment. Lancet 2:1927, 1975.
44. Hypertension Detection and Follow-up Programme Cooperative Groupe: Patient Participation in a Hypertension Control Program. JAMA 239:1507, 1978.
45. Engelland AL, Aldeman MH, Powell HB: Blood pressure control in private practice: a case report. Am J Public Health 69:25, 1979.
46. Rudnick KV, Sachett DL, Hirst S, Holmes C: Hypertension in family practice. Can Med Assoc J 117:492, 1977.
47. The Australian Therapeutic trial in mild hypertension: Report by the Management Committee. Lancet 1:1261, 1980.
48. Takala J, Niemela N, Rosti J, Sievers K: Improving compliance with therapeutic regimen in hypertensive patients in a Community Health Center. Circulation 59:540, 1979.
49. Gordon T, Kannel WB, Dawber TR: Changes associated with quitting cigarette smoking. The Framingham study. Am Heart J 90:322, 1975.
50. National diet-heart study Research group: The national diet–heart study final report. Circulation 37 (Suppl 1) 241, 1968.
51. Haynes RB, Sackett DL, Taylor W, Gibson ES, Johnson AL: Increased absenteism from work after detection and labeling of hypertensive patients. N Engl J Med 299:741, 1978.

INDEX OF AUTHORS

DRUG INDEX

A. Diuretics

Aldactazine	Searle	spironolactone + altizide
Aldactone A	Searle	spironolactone
Aprinox	Boots	bendroflumethiazide
Aquamox	Lederle	quinethazone
Baycaron	Bayer	mefruside
Brinaldix	Sandoz	clopamide
Burinan	Leo	bumetamide
Chlotride	M.S.D.	chlorothiazide
Dichlotride	M.S.D.	hydrochlorothiazide
Dichlotride K	M.S.D.	hydrochlorothiazide-KCl
Dichlotride K reserpine	M.S.D.	hydrochlorothiazide reserpine-KCl
Dichlotride reserpine	M.S.D.	hydrochlorothiazide reserpine
Disamide	Glaxo	acetazolamide
Diuril	M.S.D.	chlorothiazide
Dytac	R.I.T.	triamterene
Dyta-urese	R.I.T.	triamterene epitizide
Dytenzide	R.I.T.	triamterene + hydrochlorothiazide
Edecrin	M.S.D.	ethacrynezuur
Enduron	Abbott	methylchlorothiazide
Enduronyl	Abbott	methylchlorothiazide deserpidine
Esidrex	Ciba	hydrochlorothiazide
Esidrex K	Ciba	hydrochlorothiazide-KCl
Fluden	Servier	indapamide
Fluitran	Schering	trichloromethiazide
Fluitran KR	Schering	trichloromethiazide reserpine-KCl
Flurese	R.I.T.	epitizide
Fovane	Pfizer	benzithiazide
Haflutan	Curta	clofenamide
Hygroton	Geigy	chlorthalidone
Hygroton-reserpine	Geigy	chlorthalidone reserpine
Infratan	Mead Johnson	ethiazide reserpine meprobamate

Lasix	Hoechst	furosemide 2 ml amp.
Lasix reserpine	Hoechst	furosemide reserpine
Midamor	M.S.D.	amiloride
Moduretic	M.S.D.	amiloride + hydrochlorothiazide
Natrilin		indapamide
Navidrex	Ciba	cyclopenthiazide
Niagar	Simes	hydrochlorothiazide
Pluryl	Leo	bendroflumethiazide 5 ml vial
Pluryl Forte	Leo	bendroflumethiazide
Pluryl K	Leo	bendroflumethiazide-KCl
Pluryl R+K	Leo	bendroflumethiazide reserpine-KCl
Renese	Pfizer	polythiazide amp. 2
Renese R	Pfizer	polythiazide reserpine
Rontyl	Leo	hydroflumethiazide
Rontyl K	Leo	hydroflumethiazide-KCl
Serpasil Esidrex	Ciba	hydrochlorothiazide reserpine
Serpasil Esidrex K	Ciba	hydrochlorothiazide reserpine-KCl
Soldactone	Searle	kalium-canrenoate
Tensionorme	Leo	bendroflumethiazide reserpine
Zaroxolyn		metolazone

B. RAUWOLFIA-DERIVATIVES

Adelphan	Ciba	reserpine + dihydralazine
Anaprel	Servier	trimethoxycinnamoyl methylreserpate
Anaprel 500	Servier	rescinnamine
Brinerdine	Sandoz	dihydro-ergocristine reserpine
Decaserpyl	Roussel	methoserpidine
Gendon	Organon	Rauwolfia-alkaloids
Harmonyl	Abbott	deserpidine
Iso-Triraupine	Boehringer	rescinnamine raubasine reserpine KCl thiabutazide
Lentoserpine	Italseber	reserpine
Paratensol	Latema	dimethylamino ethyl- — reserpilinate diHCl
Preserpine	Ibsa	Rauwolfia-alkaloids vit P factors

Raudosal	Codipha	Rauwolfia vomitoria rescinnamine raubasine
Raupina	Boehringer	Rauwolfia-alkaloids reserpine
Rausedine	Janssen	Rauwolfia-alkaloids
Rauwolfia	Delagrange	Rauwolfia-alkaloids
Rauwopuur	Pharma-chemie	reserpine HCl rescinnamine raupine ajmaline yohimbine
Redouline	Roter	reserpiline
Rescinnamine	Nogepha	rescinnamine
Reserpine	Janssen	reserpine
Reserpinum comp.	Daltafarm	reserpine dihydralazine
Serpasil	Ciba	reserpine
Supressan	S.M.B.	reserpiline rescinnamine
Tensimic	Roussel	
Triraupin	Boehringer	rescinnamine raubasine theofylline
Wolfaserpol		Rauwolfia-alkaloids

C. M.A.O. — INHIBITORS

Eudatine	Abbott	pargyline HCl
Eutron	Abbott	pargyline HCl methylclothiazide

D. ALPHAMETHYLDOPA

Aldomet	M.S.D.	L. alphamethyldopa
Hydromet	M.S.D.	L. alphamethyldopa hydrochlorothiazide
Hyperpax	Organon	L. alphamethyldopa
Mulfasin	Ercopharm	L. alphamethyldopa
Presinol	Bayer	L. alphamethyldopa + ester
Sali presinol	Bayer	L. alphamethyldopa benzthiazide
Sembrina	Boehringer	L. alphamethyldopa

E. CLONIDINE

Catapress	Boehringer Ingelheim USA Ltd.	clonidine
Catapressan	Boehringer Ingelheim	clonidine

F. Ganglion blockers

Ansolysen	May-Baker	pentolinium
		pentapyrrolidinium
Arfonad	Roche	trimetaphan
Ecolid	Ciba	chlorisondamine
Lytensene	Wyeth	pentapyrrolidinium
Mevasine	M.S.D.	mecamylamine
Pendine	Inpharma	pentoloniumbitartraat
Penthonium	Delagrange	penthonium
Pentilium		pentolinium
Bitartras	Nogepha	
Tensilest	Pharma-chemie	pentoloniumder
Tenormae	I.C.I.	pempidinetartraat
Inversine	M.S.D.	mecamylamine
		dydiochloride
Vegolysen	May-Baker	hexanethonium
Wyamine	Wyeth	methylfenylbuthylamine

G. Guanidine-derivatives

Darenthin	Burroughs-Wellcome	bretyliumtosylate
Declinax	Roche	debrisoquine
Envacar	Pfizer	guanoxansulphate
Envarese	Pfizer	guanoxan + polythiazide
Esbatal	Wellcome	betanidinesulphate
Ismeline	Ciba	guanethidinesulphate
Ismeline	Ciba	guanethidine
Navidrex		cyclopenthiazide
Leron	Bayer	guanaclinesulphate
Vatensol	Pfizer	guanoclor
Visutensil	Italsaber	guanethidine

H. Beta-adrenoceptor blockers

Aptin	Astra	alprenolol
Aptin duretter	Astra	alprenolol
Beloc		metoprolol
Betadrenol	Byk	bupranolol
Betaloc		metoprolol
Blacadren	M.S.D.	timolol
Doberol		toliprolol
Gubernal	Geigy	alprenolol
Nideral	I.C.I.	propranolol
Nideral Retard	I.C.I.	propranolol
Seloken	Astra	metoprolol
Seloken duretter	Astra	metoprolol
Lopresar	Geigy	metoprolol
Slow Lopresor	Geigy	metoprolol
Sotalex		sotalol
Stresson		bunitrolol
Temserin		timolol
Tenormin	I.C.I.	atenolol

Trasicor	Ciba	oxprenolol
Slow Trasicor	Ciba	
Visken	Sandoz	pindolol

I. ALPHA-ADRENOCEPTOR BLOCKERS

Dibenzyline	S.K.F.	phenoxybenzamine
Regitine	Ciba	phentolamine
Priscol	Ciba	tolazoline
Minipres	Pfizer	prazosin

J. ALPHA- AND BETA-ADRENOCEPTOR BLOCKERS

| Trandate | Glaxo | labetalol |

K. VASODILATORS

Adelphan	Ciba	dihydralazine reserpine
Adelphan Esidrex	Ciba	dihydralazine reserpine hydrochlorothiazide
Adelphan Esidrex	Ciba	dihydralazine reserpine hydrodichlorothiazide KCl
Apresoline	Ciba	hydralazinechloride
Ipharon	Curta	dihydrazineftalazine--theofillinaat Rauwolfia-alkaloids
Ipharon compr.	Curta	ipharon chlorbenzoldisulfonamide
Nepresol	Ciba	dihydralazine
Hyperstat	Schering/Essen	diazoxide
Nipide		sodium nitroprusside
Loniten	Upjohn	minoxidil

L. ANGIOTENSIN CONVERTING ENZYME INHIBITOR

| Capoten | Squibb | Captopril |

M. ANGIOTENSIN ANALOGUES

| Saressin | Norwich-Eaton | saralasine |

N. CALCIUM ANTAGONISTS

| Isoptin | Knoll | verapamil |
| Adalat | Bayer | nifedipine |

SUBJECT INDEX

A I, *see* Angiotensin I
A II, *see* Angiotensin II
Absenteism, 938
ACTH, *see* Adrenocorticotrophic hormone
Acetylcholine, 23
Acute glomerulonephritis, 903
Acute hypertensive encephalopathy, 400, 902
Adrenal
  adenomas, 547
  arteriography, 680
  computed axial tomography, 683
  hyperplasia
    congenital, 563
    Cushing's syndrome, 555
    diffuse cortical, 547
  medulla, 60
  phlebography, 682
  scintigraphy, 685
  venography, 687
Adrenaline, *see also* Catecholamines, 23, 57, 168
  plasma, 65
  secretion, 62
  urinary, 62
Adrenergic neuronal blocking drugs, 828
α-Adrenergic receptors
  distribution of, 769
  effects of antihypertensive agents on, 775
  hemodynamic effect of, 770
  physiology of, 765
  selectivity, 296
α-Adrenergic receptor blocking agents, *see also*
  Specific α-adrenergic blocking agents, 755
α- and β-Adrenergic receptor blocking agents, 474, 909
β-Adrenergic receptors, 743
  effect of antihypertensive agents on, 744
  role in renin release, 749
  sensitivity, 298, 369

β-Adrenergic receptor blocking drugs, *see also*
  Specific β-adrenergic blocking drugs, 743
  cardioprotective effect of, 749
  in elderly, 360
  in pregnancy, 604
  predictability of response, 745
  time course of action, 645, 746
α-Adrenoceptor antagonists
  ancilliary activities, 778
  effect of baro-receptor control, 774
Adrenocorticotrophic hormone (ACTH), 20
Adrenoceptors, 26, 164
Afterload, 421
Age factor
  and renin, 172, 189
  in arterial pressure rise, 347
  in increased systolic pressure, 347
  in plasma renin activity, 355
Alarm reaction, 22
Alcalosis, 549
  metabolic, diuretics, 719
Alcohol, 878
Aldomet, *see* Methyldopa,
Aldosterone, *see also* Primary Aldosteronism
  effects of prostaglandins, 149
  levels with diuretics, 714
  levels with estrogen intake, 618
Aldosteronism
  primary, *see* Primary Aldosteronism
  secondary, 498
Alpha-methyldopa, *see* Methyldopa
Amygdaloid nucleus, 20
Anemia
  microangiopathic hemolytic
    in malignant hypertension, 469
Anephric state, *see also* Nephrectomy
Anesthesia, 916
  induction of, 919
  maintenance of, 920

Amery, A. (ed.) Hypertensive Cardiovascular Disease: Pathophysiology and Treatment
© *1982, Martinus Nijhoff Publishers. The Hague / Boston / London*
ISBN-13: 978-94-009-7478-4

977

984